The new edition of *Ophthalmic Disease in Veterinary Medicine* is the ideal textbook for trainee and practicing veterinarians needing a quick reference in their daily work. Expert veterinary ophthalmologists will also appreciate this updated completely revised edition, the achievement of a teamwork involving three authors and five contributors, outstanding members of the international veterinary ophthalmology community. Hundreds of beautiful pictures and drawings facilitate a quick, easy, practical consultation and allow direct comparison to clinical cases. For each ophthalmic disease and disorder, the authors provide a detailed description of diagnosis, etiology, clinical signs, prognosis, and therapy. Although the main focus is on small animal species, the readers will appreciate the interesting comparative notes on the horse and the cow, and a section dedicated to presumed inherited eye disorders. *Ophthalmic Disease in Veterinary Medicine* deserves a special space in the library of everyone interested in veterinary ophthalmology. Actually, it is a book to leave on your desk for daily use, so that you can read the notes and show the pictures to owners to help explain what is happening in their pet's eyes.

Prof. Claudio Peruccio, DVM, SCMPA, Dipl ECVO, Hon Dipl ACVO, MRCVS, EBVS®
European & RCVS Specialist in Veterinary Ophthalmology

The most recent edition of *Ophthalmic Disease in Veterinary Medicine* is a welcome addition to the body of literature in veterinary ophthalmology. This text is certainly straightforward and pragmatic enough to be valuable in the library of the general practitioner. But such a statement belies the 700 pages of depth, detail, and scholarship that the specialist in veterinary ophthalmology will find extremely useful and informative; indeed, this text will become required reading for my ophthalmology residents. It is obvious that this work has fallen under the watchful eye of Dr. Charles Martin, whose attention to detail and ability to piece together not-so-obvious connections are legendary in our specialty. Drs. Martin, Pickett, and Spiess have over 100 years of combined experience in veterinary ophthalmology as clinicians, teachers, and researchers. This text provides abundant evidence that they have maintained a cutting edge in vision science and clinical ophthalmology, and their wealth of experience brings context and perspective to new developments in the specialty. The other contributing authors have followed that lead. Photographs, illustrations, schematics, and flowcharts are particularly useful in enriching the reader's understanding in the specialty of ophthalmology, and this book is loaded with extremely well-done examples of these visual aids. The text is very carefully and thoroughly indexed and cross-indexed, which makes it very user friendly. Without question this work will be referenced daily in my clinical work, classroom teaching, and residency training.

Daniel A. Ward, DVM, PhD, Dipl. ACVO
Professor of Ophthalmology
University of Tennessee College of Veterinary Medicine

Ophthalmic Disease in Veterinary Medicine

Ophthalmic Disease in Veterinary Medicine

Second Edition

Charles L. Martin

J. Phillip Pickett

Bernhard M. Spiess

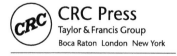

CRC Press
Taylor & Francis Group
Boca Raton London New York

CRC Press is an imprint of the
Taylor & Francis Group, an **informa** business

CRC Press
Taylor & Francis Group
6000 Broken Sound Parkway NW, Suite 300
Boca Raton, FL 33487-2742

First issued in paperback 2020

ISBN 13: 978-0-367-57033-0 (pbk)
ISBN 13: 978-1-4822-5864-6 (hbk)

This book contains information obtained from authentic and highly regarded sources. While all reasonable efforts have been made to publish reliable data and information, neither the author[s] nor the publisher can accept any legal responsibility or liability for any errors or omissions that may be made. The publishers wish to make clear that any views or opinions expressed in this book by individual editors, authors or contributors are personal to them and do not necessarily reflect the views/opinions of the publishers. The information or guidance contained in this book is intended for use by medical, scientific or health-care professionals and is provided strictly as a supplement to the medical or other professional's own judgement, their knowledge of the patient's medical history, relevant manufacturer's instructions and the appropriate best practice guidelines. Because of the rapid advances in medical science, any information or advice on dosages, procedures or diagnoses should be independently verified. The reader is strongly urged to consult the relevant national drug formulary and the drug companies' and device or material manufacturers' printed instructions, and their websites, before administering or utilizing any of the drugs, devices or materials mentioned in this book. This book does not indicate whether a particular treatment is appropriate or suitable for a particular individual. Ultimately it is the sole responsibility of the medical professional to make his or her own professional judgements, so as to advise and treat patients appropriately. The authors and publishers have also attempted to trace the copyright holders of all material reproduced in this publication and apologize to copyright holders if permission to publish in this form has not been obtained. If any copyright material has not been acknowledged please write and let us know so we may rectify in any future reprint.

Visit the Taylor & Francis Web site at
http://www.taylorandfrancis.com

and the CRC Press Web site at
http://www.crcpress.com

CONTENTS

PREFACE

Writing a text has often been compared to marriage as it engenders an obligation to keep the covenant intact short of death. When contemplating another edition of the text *Ophthalmic Disease in Veterinary Medicine*, my considerations were how to improve the book as well as updating the text. Updating the information is quite straightforward, while changing the format is more challenging and risky. Previous editions were essentially single authored, which has the advantage of more consistency between chapters in writing style and philosophy, but it also has the disadvantage of limiting the expression of clinical experience to a single author. For this edition, we have chosen to increase the breadth of clinical expertise with a diverse group of authors from many geographic regions of training and practice and who have actively participated in student training and research in veterinary ophthalmology. They have also demonstrated not only great professional skills but a great deal of patience as the timeline for fruition of publication has been greatly extended from the original target date. I would like to thank all the authors for their participation and thoroughness, and we hope that the readers will appreciate the expertise that this diversity has brought to the text.

I would be remiss if I did not recognize Ms. Alice Oven and Pam Tagg and their staff at CRC Press/Taylor & Francis for keeping faith in the project and the contributors. I am sure it has probably been one of their most challenging projects.

Last but not least I thank my daughter Christena Hughes for her help and patience in the copy editing process and my wife Marilyn for her encouragement and advice.

Charles L. Martin

Charles L. Martin, BS, DVM, MS, Charter Diplomate, American College of Veterinary Ophthalmologist, (ACVO), Emeritus Diplomate ACVO, Professor Emeritus, the University of Georgia, past president of the ACVO and American Society of Veterinary Ophthalmology. Dr. Martin trained at Washington State University, the University of Pennsylvania, and The Ohio State University and taught at the Western College of Veterinary Medicine, Kansas State University, the University of Georgia, and Auburn University.

J. Phillip Pickett, DVM, DACVO, Emeritus Professor, Virginia–Maryland College of Veterinary Medicine is a graduate of Louisiana State University College of Veterinary Medicine. Following three years in a mixed practice, he did a residency in Comparative Ophthalmology at the University of Wisconsin, College of Veterinary Medicine. He is a Diplomate of the ACVO.

He taught at the University of Wisconsin, and was a faculty member at the Virginia–Maryland College of Veterinary Medicine at Virginia Tech where he reached the rank of Professor.

Bernhard M. Spiess, DVM, Dr. med. vet., Diplomate, American and European College of Veterinary Ophthalmologists (ACVO/ECVO), Professor Emeritus is Charter Diplomate and past president of the ECVO. He began his career in Switzerland, at the Veterinary School in Lausanne/Zurich, then moved to the Veterinary Teaching Hospital at the University of Bern. He completed a residency in veterinary ophthalmology at the University of Guelph, Canada, where he stayed on as Assistant Professor after becoming a Diplomate of ACVO. In 1987, he returned to University of Zurich as Assistant Professor of Veterinary Ophthalmology, becoming full Professor in 1994 and Professor Emeritus in 2015.

Eva Abarca obtained her DVM degree from the Veterinary College at the University of Zaragoza, Spain followed by two years in the School of Veterinary Medicine in Alfort, Paris, France. After practicing general medicine for several years, she completed an ACVO residency program and a master's degree at the Biomedical Research Institute of the National Autonomous University of Mexico, becoming a Diplomate of ACVO in 2012. She worked as an ophthalmology research scholar in the Laboratory of Ocular Immunology, Toxicology, and Drug Delivery at North Carolina State University. Dr. Abarca has taught at Auburn University and is currently in the Ophthalmology Service at Vetsuisse-Fakultat, Bern University, Switzerland, where she works as a senior clinician in ophthalmology.

Shannon D. Boveland received her DVM from Tuskegee University, College of Veterinary Medicine. She completed an internship in small animal medicine and surgery at Tuskegee and an ophthalmology residency at the University of Georgia, College of Veterinary Medicine. Following her residency, Dr. Boveland taught at the University of Georgia, Tuskegee University and is currently teaching at Auburn University. Dr. Boveland is a member of the ACVO.

Ursula Dietrich, Dr. med. vet. MRCVS, is senior lecturer in veterinary ophthalmology at the Royal Veterinary College, University of London. She received both her veterinary medical degree and doctorate from the Ludwig Maximilian University in Munich. She is a boarded Diplomate of both ACVO and ECVO and a recognized RCVS specialist in veterinary ophthalmology. Her special interests include corneal disease and corneal surgery, feline ophthalmology, and in particular, glaucoma.

Phillip A. Moore received his DVM from Auburn University, College of Veterinary Medicine. He completed an internship in small animal medicine and surgery and an ophthalmology residency at the University of Georgia, College of Veterinary Medicine. Dr. Moore has taught at Tufts University, School of Veterinary Medicine the University of Georgia, College of Veterinary Medicine, and is currently a Professor in the Department of Clinical Sciences at Auburn University, College of Veterinary Medicine. Dr. Moore is a member of ACVO.

Kate Myrna has a BA from Vassar College and received her DVM from the Virginia–Maryland Regional College of Veterinary Medicine. She completed a one-year internship at the Western College of Veterinary Medicine at the University of Saskatchewan and a one-year specialty internship in small animal ophthalmology at Angell Animal Medical Center—Western New England. Dr. Myrna then completed a residency in comparative ophthalmology and obtained a master of science in comparative biomedical sciences at the University of Wisconsin–Madison. Dr. Myrna is a diplomate of the ACVO.

ANAMNESIS AND THE OPHTHALMIC EXAMINATION

URSULA DIETRICH

ANAMNESIS

Prior to any ophthalmic examination, a thorough history should be obtained including information about the environment of the animal, other pets in the household, diet, previous treatments and medications, but also a complete medical history. Although many ophthalmic diagnoses are anatomic diagnoses, based on direct visual inspection and augmented by known breed-, age-, and species-related syndromes, many systemic diseases may be manifest in the eye and its adnexa as the first and sometimes only clinical symptom (e.g., hypertensive retinopathy, diabetes mellitus, lymphoma).

Breed, age, and occasionally the sex are important data, as many ocular syndromes are inherited or at least have a breed predisposition (see Chapter 15).

The owner's complaints are usually among the following: decreased vision or blindness, ocular discharge, ocular color changes, pain, an opacity or film over the eye, pupillary changes/anisocoria, and exophthalmos/enlarged eye(s). These complaints form the basis for the problem-oriented approach to ophthalmology and are discussed in more detail in subsequent chapters.

Problems observed by the owner

Decreased vision or blindness

Depending on the function of the dog, the environment the animal is kept in, the amount of vision lost, unilateral versus bilateral loss, and the rapidity of development, the historical data may be accurate or misleading. Insidious loss of vision such as progressive retinal atrophy is often diagnosed in an advanced stage when the animal is presented. Most dogs adapt well to vision loss in a familiar environment, and the decrease of vision becomes only noticeable if furniture, and so on, is moved.

Dogs that work by sight are more critically evaluated as to type (moving versus stationary objects) and degree of deficiency. Nonleading questions should be asked regarding night vision, day vision, ability to see moving objects as opposed to stationary objects, and the circumstances under which the visual loss was noted. This information must then be interpreted considering the animal's

function and environment and the owner's ability to discriminate. Most animals are not presented with a complaint of decreased vision unless the condition is bilateral and relatively severe.

Ocular discharge

The type of discharge should be noted and historical data regarding chronicity, progression and modification by therapy, season, and environment should be obtained. While ocular discharge is typical of ocular surface and adnexal disease, intraocular disease and the systemic history should not be overlooked.

Ocular color changes

Color changes may be due to conjunctival and episcleral hyperemia associated with conjunctivitis, scleritis, uveitis, or glaucoma. Bulbar conjunctival hyperemia may be diffuse, involving capillaries and large vessels as with conjunctivitis, or selective, involving mainly the larger conjunctival vessels and deeper episcleral vessels with uveitis, glaucoma, and scleritis. Subconjunctival hemorrhage also produces a red bulbar conjunctiva, either in a sector or, occasionally, involving the entire circumference of the conjunctiva. The normal variation of a unilateral or bilateral nonpigmented third eyelid margin may make the eye look redder and, indeed, a nonpigmented third eyelid is probably more susceptible to irritation than the pigmented conjunctival surface.

Corneal opacities may produce red (granulation, intense neovascularization, hemorrhage), white (lipids, calcium, scar, edema, fungal plaques), or black (melanin pigment, corneal sequestrum in cats, dematiaceous fungi) color changes.

Intraocular color changes may arise from the aqueous humor, iris, or lens. Aqueous humor color changes may be red with hyphema, white to gray with hypopyon, fibrin, or lipids, and brown to black when filled with free-floating iris cysts. Iris color changes are usually most dramatic with unilateral involvement and with lightly pigmented irides. The brown iris becomes darker, and the blue iris becomes yellow with uveitis or brown when infiltrated with pigmented tumors. Iridal redness may be observed with intense neovascularization and engorgement and with pete-chial/ecchymotic hemorrhage in the blue irides. The latter changes are not often obvious in the darker compact irides. Occasionally, a blue iris may turn green in an icteric animal.

Lens color changes are typically in shades of gray-white with aging and white with cataract formation. Rarely, hemorrhage may occur into the lens associated with con-genital vascular anomalies such as persistent hyperplastic primary vitreous (PHPV).

Ocular pain

Blepharospasm and rubbing the eye(s) are obvious signs of pain noted by owners, but ocular pain often manifests in a subtle manner with general malaise, depression, exces-sive sleeping, and a worsening of the temperament. These signs are often not noted by the owners until improve-ment occurs and retrospective comparisons are made. In humans, conjunctival pain is described as a foreign body sensation, corneal pain as a sharp ocular pain, and intra-ocular pain is often a headache pain radiating over the trigeminal nerve distribution. Paradoxically, superficial corneal ulceration is often more painful than deep ulcer-ation due to the concentration of nerve fibers under the corneal epithelium.[1,2] Species variations also exist, as cats and horses are typically more symptomatic with conjunc-tivitis and corneal disease than dogs.

Opacities

Opacities or film over or in the eye may result from pro-lapse of the third eyelid, tenacious ocular discharges, corneal opacities, fibrin, blood, inflammatory cells or masses in the anterior chamber, and cataracts. Historical data regarding chronicity, laterality, constant or intermit-tent occurrence, progression, and precipitating factors should be obtained. Protrusion of the third eyelid is often described by owners as "the eye rolling up into the head."

Pupillary changes

Alterations in pupil size are usually noted when unilateral or when accompanied by another ocular complaint such as blindness, which draws the owner's attention to the eye. Alterations in pupil size are most easily observed in eyes with lightly pigmented irides or against the background of a white cataract. Ocular disease should always be ruled out as the cause for altered pupil size, shape, and mobility before proceeding to neurologic causes.

Exophthalmos/buphthalmos

Enlarged or prominent eyes are most dramatic when uni-lateral. The condition may be acute or chronic in nature and is often accompanied by another complaint such as red eye, pain, ocular discharge, or a film over the eyes.

While buphthalmia is a true enlargement of the globe (most often caused by chronic glaucoma), exophthalmia is forward placement of an otherwise normal-sized globe. Differentiation between exophthalmos and buphthalmos is usually not difficult, but in brachycephalic breeds and ani-mals with only one eye, mild degrees of the problem may be difficult to detect for even the experienced examiner.

General comments

The initial clinical appearance of the problem and its modification with time, therapy, and environmental change should be documented. Measurement of corneal diameters or ultrasonography for measuring globe dimen-sions may be used to determine subtle differences between eyes. Information on the administration of prior "home" or professional remedies should be obtained, particu-larly for chronic cases. With new clients, it is necessary to obtain historical data on previous ocular problems and their course and response to therapy. The disease process may have been modified, and the interpretation of the ocular examination, such as pupillary light reflexes and intraocular pressures, may be complicated by prior ther-apy (such as atropine). Failure of response to previously prescribed therapy should provoke questions to determine the owner's compliance with instructions. Asking to see the remaining medication may allow an assessment of whether the medication has been given as frequently or for as long as was claimed.

Many ocular problems are breed related, and it is often desirable to establish possible inheritance, although the necessary information is often not available. In most instances, genetic syndromes are inferred by the occur-rence of a known syndrome in a particular age and breed of animal (see Chapter 15).

As the eye often manifests systemic illness, it is impera-tive that possible systemic ramifications be considered. In addition, topical medications may have systemic side effects, and, conversely, systemic drugs may have ocular side effects. Candidates for ocular surgery need to be eval-uated preoperatively for systemic disease.

Historical data pertaining to environmental factors such as animal exposure, type of housing, bedding, fenced yard, dusts, irritants such as fumes and fiberglass, and function of the animal may help to establish an etiologic diagnosis for a previously unresolved problem.

> With experience, the clinician will note that many ocular syndromes have predictable histories, but he/she should always be on the lookout for "red her-rings," which are common with historical data.

OPHTHALMIC EXAMINATION

Restraint

The best restraint for ophthalmic examination is usually the least amount possible. The inexperienced examiner usually mistakenly assumes that chemical sedation will facilitate the examination and make up for deficiencies in technique. While sedation is routine in large animal ophthalmic examinations, it is rarely necessary in small animals.

One of the most formidable obstacles to a good ophthalmic examination is protrusion of the third eyelid. Protruding third eyelids can usually be circumvented by keeping the animal alert, off balance, or anxious. Movement of the head, positioning over the edge of the table, or making noises to attract the patient's attention will change the mental status sufficiently so that the eye is exposed for short periods. These maneuvers, combined with exposing the eye to short bursts of light that is no brighter than necessary, allows the experienced clinician enough of a "window of opportunity" to complete most examinations.

In the dog, the muzzle is often held with one hand, and this serves to manipulate the head as well as afford protection to the examiner. Most dogs do not require additional restraint for routine examination, but if there is any doubt as to the examiner's safety, muzzling or, in extreme cases, chemical sedation, is indicated. In the dog, most sedatives or general anesthesia only make the ophthalmic examination more difficult due to protrusion of the third eyelid and infraversion (rolling down) of the eyes.

A gentle and efficient way to restrain a cat during the examination is the "wrap up" method, by gently wrapping the cat into a large, soft towel or small blanket, which is then held by an assistant. The legs and body are securely held, and only the head is exposed with this method. Sedation of a cat is rarely required, but the use of ketamine sedation (10 mg/kg) provides ideal conditions for examination, producing a dilated pupil, eyes straight ahead, and immobilization. The effect of ketamine on the intraocular pressure in cats has been shown to increase by 10%, which needs to be taken into consideration when performing tonometry.[3]

> In small animals, speed and utilization of short bursts of light enables an ophthalmic examination to be performed without chemical sedation in most uncooperative patients.

Regional anesthesia/analgesia in the horse

In the horse, whether presented with or without ocular pain, sedation and palpebral nerve akinesia is routinely performed for a thorough examination. Xylazine (0.5–1.1 mg/kg) intravenously (IV) quiets the animal and drops the head for examination. This not only facilitates the examination but is also safer for the examiner. If ocular pain is present, palpebral nerve blocks are routine, easily performed, and facilitate examination even if sedation is used. Blockage of the palpebral branch of the auriculopalpebral nerve (branch of VII cranial nerve) may be performed at several locations, but the most complete akinesis with the least amount of local anesthetic can be produced by injection at the dorsal margin of the highest point of the zygomatic arch (**Figure 1.1**).[4] Firm palpation of the dorsal rim of the arch usually causes the nerve to snap under the examiner's finger. An alternative site is at the base of the ear between the ear and the zygomatic process (**Figure 1.2**). A 25-gauge needle is placed at the site, a syringe is then attached, and 1–3 mL of a local anesthetic is injected. The resultant block gives sufficient akinesis of the orbicularis oculi muscle such that the lids can be opened with minimal force, but the animal can still blink. The dorsal branches of the palpebral nerve can also be blocked at the supraorbital foramen where it mingles with the supraorbital nerve (sensory, V cranial nerve). The supraorbital foramen can be identified by grasping the margins of the dorsal orbital rim and moving medially until it widens (**Figure 1.3**). At this point, the foramen can be palpated in the middle of the rim.[5] Palpebral nerve blocks do not affect the intraocular pressure (IOP), but attempting to measure the IOP in a blepharospastic horse without a nerve block may result in an artificially elevated IOP. Xylazine sedation may lower the intraocular pressure (IOP) by up to 27% in horses.[6]

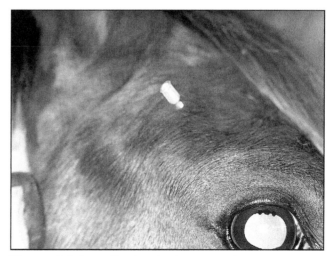

Figure 1.1 A needle placed subcutaneously above the zygomatic arch for a palpebral nerve block in a horse.

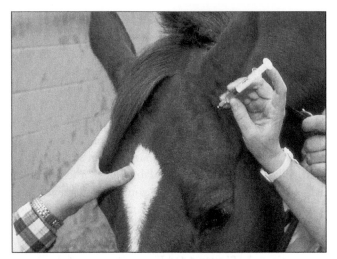

Figure 1.2 Injection at the base of the ear to block the palpebral branch of the facial nerve in a horse.

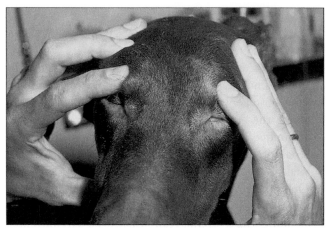

Figure 1.4 Bilateral retropulsion of the globe into the orbit to compare compressibility between orbits. This is different from digital tonometry.

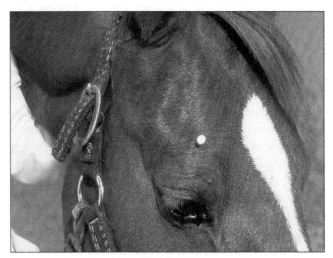

Figure 1.3 A needle in the supraorbital foramen to block the palpebral (motor) and supraorbital (sensory) nerves in a horse.

Diffuse illumination with head unrestrained

Examination with diffuse illumination without head restraint is the initial step in ophthalmic examination and is often ignored in the rush to get a close look at the eye. This is the time to evaluate conformation and symmetry of the eyes and adnexa. It is important to keep the head unrestrained, as simply touching the side of the head will modify lid conformation. In addition, manipulation of the head often precipitates blepharospasm in a dog that is "eye shy" by nature, in pain, or has received prior ocular medication. If some restraint of the head is necessary, the head should be supported under the mandible.

Comparison of ocular and adnexal symmetry is important and should be performed from various angles of observation, that is frontal and dorsal. Palpebral fissures,

third eyelid position, globe size and position, iris color, and pupil size should be evaluated for symmetry. This is the time when the orbit should be evaluated, retropulsion of the globes into the orbit compared (**Figure 1.4**), and the patient examined for exophthalmos by comparing the corneal vertices from a dorsal vantage point. Ocular discharges and lid dermatologic lesions such as swellings, alopecia, and erythema should be noted. The cornea should be inspected for its luster, surface irregularities, and opacities. The specular light reflection off the cornea ("*Purkinje images*") superimposed on the pupils allows accurate assessment of ocular alignment, and gross opacities in the anterior chamber and lens may be noted.

Evaluation for anisocoria (unequal pupils) and the pupillary light reflex (PLR)

The presence of static anisocoria (consistently unequal pupils under varying light conditions) is determined by directing a light at the stop or base of the nose from a distance of 60–90 cm (2–3 feet) in a darkened room. This outlines both pupils simultaneously against the retroillumination of the tapetal reflection. Heterochromia results in a mild anisocoria with the larger pupil in the eye with the blue iris and is considered physiologic. Other forms of anisocoria should be evaluated further.

The PLR is frequently described by authors as either clearly present or absent, but in reality, it is a subjective evaluation that has a great deal of interpretive variation between clinicians of different levels of experience. Pupillary light reflexes should be performed in a darkened room with a bright light, such as a Finoff transilluminator, to produce maximum excursions (**Figure 1.5**). The *swinging light test* employs a bright light shown alternately in each eye for 3–4 seconds at a time. Initial stimulation of the eye elicits the direct response, and the light

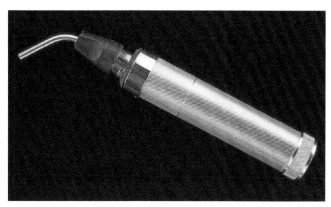

Figure 1.5 Finoff transilluminator used for gross ocular examinations, PLR testing, and mononuclear indirect ophthalmoscopy.

is quickly shifted to the contralateral eye, and the pupil size observed. The initial observation is evaluation of the indirect or consensual reaction, but as it is maintained, it becomes the direct reflex. This is repeated back and forth at 3–4+ second intervals.

Normally, with a relaxed animal in a darkened room, the PLR responses are brisk, and the degree of contraction is significant on direct stimulation. Due to the presence of the relatively cone-rich area centralis, a focal light directed temporally on the retina stimulates a more complete constriction than a light directed on the nasal retina. When the light is moved to the opposite eye, it may be noted that the initial size of the pupil is slightly larger in this eye and then constricts further. This is due to the unequal pupillomotor input to the consensually responding eye in the dog and cat and is a normal dynamic anisocoria.[7] Sustaining the light in the eye may produce a small amount of redilation due to adaptation of the retina to a weak light. If the sustained illumination results in an obvious dilation, the test is positive (Marcus Gunn pupil) and is the result of a retinal or optic nerve lesion. It is relatively common for patients with retinal/optic nerve blindness to have some degree of pupil reaction to a bright light, as vision is a more complex function than the PLR. It is more common to have vision with dilated nonreactive pupils due to efferent arc lesions of the PLR.

If anisocoria and PLR abnormalities are detected, then special attention in the ocular examination should be devoted to vision testing, fundus examination, and diseases of the iris. The detailed examination should rule out synechiae, iris atrophy, iris hypoplasia, lens displacement, elevated IOP, anterior uveitis, and anterior uveal neoplasia, all of which commonly interfere with pupil mobility and/or shape.

If the iris appears normal, evaluation of the anisocoria in darkness and ambient light should be performed.

Anisocoria associated with an afferent arm (usually retina or optic nerve) lesion of the PLR will dilate to equality in a dark room due to an intact sympathetic chain. The anisocoria of Horner's syndrome remains or is more pronounced due to a lack of sympathetic input to the dilator muscle (see section Horner's syndrome, Chapter 4).

Chromatic pupillary light reflex (cPLR)

The physiologic basis of the pupillary light reflex in mammals is a response of the retinal photoreceptor cells (rods and cones) to stimulation with a bright white light source (Finoff transilluminator, slit lamp, or other focused light source). The PLR helps in the assessment of the visual pathway integrity, including the retina, optic nerve, optic chiasm, and anterior visual pathways (optic tracts, midbrain pathways). The phenomenon of a retained pupillary function in rod/cone-less blind mice (by American geneticist Clyde Keeler in 1923) was supported by the more recent discovery of a photosensitive pigment (melanopsin) in the retinal ganglion cells of mammals, which, other than rods and cones, is capable of stimulating nonimage-forming functions, such as a pupillary light reflex.[8-10] This so called intrinsically photosensitive retinal ganglion cell (ipRGC)-mediated PLR activity can be elicited by selective stimulation of the melanopsin pigment with blue light of a narrow wavelength spectrum (480 nm). The commercially available Melan-100 unit is equipped with a powerful diode-based light source and emits blue and red light, which fits the spectral sensitivity of melanopsin (480 nm) and rod–cone opsin (630 nm) (**Figure 1.6**).

The chromatic pupillary light reflex is particularly useful in the diagnosis of retinal disease and optic nerve

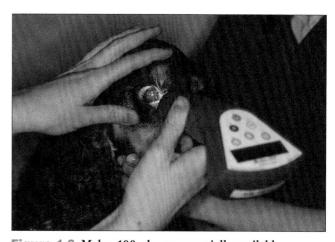

Figure 1.6 Melan-100: the commercially available instrument emits red and blue light which fits the spectral sensitivity of melanopsin (480 nm) and rod–cone opsin (630 nm) which elicits the chromatic pupillary light reflex (cPLR) assisting in the diagnosis of retinal and optic nerve disease.

disease, as clinical studies in healthy dogs and in dogs with retinal or optic nerve disorders showed.[11,12] Assessment of cPLR is especially helpful in eyes with cataracts, prior to cataract surgery to rule out underlying retinal disease, particularly if an electroretinogram is not available. It could be shown that both blue and red light elicited a strong pupillary light constriction in normal eyes and in cataractous eyes without underlying retinal disease.[11]

Retinal degeneration, retinal detachment

Both the blue and red light cPLR responses are significantly decreased in eyes with cataracts and concurrent underlying retinal disease (degeneration or retinal detachment), with the blue light response showing a higher sensitivity and specificity in the detection of retinal degeneration or retinal detachment.[11]

Sudden acquired retinal degeneration (SARDS)

In dogs with SARDS, the red light cPLR response cannot be elicited, but the blue light response is retained in those eyes. This is explained by the complete loss of photoreceptor function but retained intrinsic melanopsin–retinal ganglion cell mediated chromatic PLR.

Optic neuritis

Blue and red light stimulation both show complete absence of cPLR function in dogs with optic neuritis.

Vision evaluation

Vision evaluation in small animals

Vision testing in animals is based on a combination of behavioral abnormalities and visual reflex testing. In many instances, the owner is not aware of an ongoing vision problem if only one eye is affected, as most dogs can adjust very well to decreased vision or blindness in one eye. In the dog with partial decrease in vision, multiple forms of visual testing are performed to satisfy the examiner that there is a deficit and to characterize it. With complete loss of vision, the result of maze or obstacle course testing is usually dramatic. Cats present a special problem in testing their functional vision because they are often reluctant to explore an area, making it difficult to differentiate a normal shy behavior pattern from a visual deficit. Testing cats in their playing behavior (e.g., pulling a string in front of them) or visual cliff testing can be very useful vision testing procedures in this species.

Menace response

The menace response is a threatening, sudden movement presented near the eye, which elicits a blink. Before testing for a menace response, the examiner must make sure the facial nerve is intact by eliciting a blink reflex through the palpebral or corneal reflex. In dogs with facial nerve paralysis but normal vision, the menace response is subtler, and retraction of the globe may be observed due to contraction of all extraocular muscles and the retractor bulbi muscle.

While menacing can still be performed without an intact facial nerve, the response is subtler. The afferent arm of this response is the visual fibers up to the visual cortex and the efferent arm is the facial nerve. Additional centers involved with the menace response are the cerebellum, the rostral colliculus, and the motor cortex. Cerebellar disease produces an ipsilateral deficit in the menace response with retention of vision (**Figure 1.7**) (see Chapter 4).[13–15] The menace response can be altered by nonvisual influences such as mental status and cerebellar disease.

When trying to elicit a menace response, avoid air currents that may stimulate the blink reflex. Presentation of fingers rather than a broad hand are used to avoid air currents. Complacent or trusting animals should have the eyelids occasionally tapped to make them more alert. The contralateral eye should be closed to determine that it was not a binocular response to the stimulus. Due to

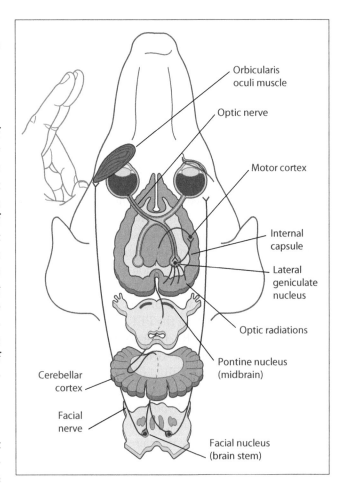

Figure 1.7 Menace response pathways.

Table 1.1 **Comparative visual reflexes with unilateral complete lesions within the visual system.**

LESION LOCATION	PLR	ANISOCORIA	MENACE RESPONSE	ERG
Retina	Direct absent, +MG	Mild static	Absent	Extinguished in most cases
Optic nerve	Direct absent, +MG	Mild static	Absent	Normal
Complete chiasm	Absent OU	Dilated OU	Absent	Normal
Optic tract	Present, −MG	Mild static	Homonymous field defect	Normal
Optic radiations/visual cortex	Present	None	Homonymous field defect	Normal

Source: Modified from Goldbaum et al., 1980. *Principles and Practice of Ophthalmology*, vol II. Peyman, G., Sanders, D., and Goldberg, M. (eds). WB Saunders: Philadelphia, PA, pp. 988–1097.
PLR: pupillary light reflex; **ERG**: electroretinogram; **MG**: Marcus Gunn (pupil); Homonymous: right nasal + left temporal field, or left nasal + right temporal field; **OU**: both eyes.

the mixture of ipsilateral and contralateral visual fibers, unilateral lesions above the chiasm do not produce complete blindness in an eye, and a variable menace response may be obtained depending on the visual field stimulated. The predominance of crossed fibers (65%–75%) in higher lesions results in a larger temporal field (nasal retina) defect in the eye contralateral to the defect. Nasal field defects (lateral retina) are more difficult to detect as they are smaller (25%–35%), and it is easier to stimulate the opposite eye inadvertently with movement if it is not closed. **Table 1.1** summarizes the PLR and menace responses with lesions at different anatomic locations.

Dazzle reflex

The dazzle reflex is a subcortical reflex that involves stimulating the retina with a very bright light, resulting in a bilateral narrowing of the palpebral fissure. The reflex requires the retina, optic nerve, chiasm, optic tract, and, probably, the supraoptic nuclei and the rostral colliculi.[13–15] The dazzle reflex persists with cortical blindness. A positive dazzle response helps to establish the intactness of the lower visual system when vision cannot be evaluated (such as with cataracts), and the PLR is altered due to efferent problems (such as iris atrophy, synechia).

Visual placing

Visual placing is a good test for animals with normal motor function and mental status. The animal is held in space and supported under the chest and head while approaching a flat surface such as a table. The normal response is to extend and raise the legs in anticipation of standing on the surface. If the expected response is not forthcoming, then tactile stimulation should be used to establish the normalcy of proprioception and the efferent arm of the reflex. Testing the response with both eyes open and then alternately holding the lids closed evaluates individual eyes. Approaching the surface from the lateral or medial aspect may give an indication of intactness of the visual fields.

Visual cliff

A visual cliff test evaluates not only vision but depth perception. Some cats that are functionally blind will be able to jump off a table.

Maze or obstacle course

An obstacle course in a nonfamiliar environment for the animal is one of the more common methods of evaluating functional vision. The maze test is usually useful with active animals but is often difficult to evaluate with cats that cower or do not move. The examiner usually scatters objects of varying size through the main pathway of the examination room. Most dogs move toward the exit door or the owner's voice. Repeated trials through the maze under ambient room light and with minimal light are performed. Dramatic differences in scotopic (night) and photopic (light-adapted) vision may be observed with maze testing. Patching of individual eyes can be performed; with monocular blindness, most patients become preoccupied with the bandage and remove it when the good eye is patched.

Cotton ball test

Cotton balls dropped into the visual fields of the patient are a common means to evaluate vision. Animals often get easily bored with this, so initial impressions are the most important.

Basic ophthalmic examination techniques
Schirmer tear test

Schirmer tear testing should be performed before any topical medications are placed in the eye and should be considered part of the basic data collection with every ophthalmic examination and certainly with any ocular surface disease. The test used most often in veterinary ophthalmology is the Schirmer tear test I, which measures basal and reflex secretion rate. The test is performed by bending the strip at the notch and hooking the short end

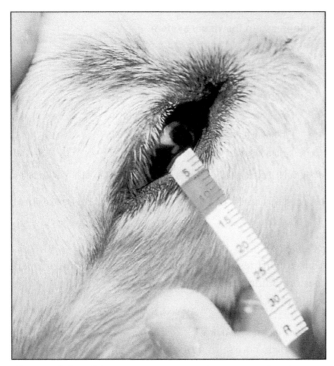

Figure 1.8 Schirmer tear strips with an integral ruler on the strip and dye in the paper.

over the medial lower lid into the conjunctival cul-de-sac (**Figure 1.8**). Once the strip is in place, the retention can be improved by closing the lids. The strip is removed after 1 minute, and the amount of wetting, measured in millimeters, is immediately recorded. The normal values of wetting for the dog are 20 ± 5 mm/min and for the cat are 15–17 mm/min.[16,17] The horse has been variably reported to have Schirmer values of 20–30 mm/min and 13 mm/min.[18,19] Schirmer values in the cat may be quite variable, and often a reading of 0 will be found in a perfectly normal eye. Unless there are clinical signs to reinforce the finding of a low Schirmer value, it is prudent to repeat the test later before prescribing medication for a tear deficiency.

Berger and King[20] found a statistical difference over time and between breeds in the Schirmer values of dogs, but while statistically significant, the variation would rarely be significant in making clinical decisions. Large breeds of dogs have higher Schirmer values than small breeds of dogs.[20] Hamor et al.[21] evaluated the Schirmer values in five breeds of dogs and found a difference only in the Shetland sheepdog, where values were 4–5 mm/min lower. In the dog, ocular signs are usually not associated with decreased tear production until values are between 5 and 10 mm. In the past, variations in the readings were attributable to the type of paper used in manufacture of the strips.[22] Newer strips have the measuring rule on the strip and a dye in the paper that is taken up with the tears to delineate the amount of wetting. No clinically significant differences were noted between brands of Schirmer tear test in two studies.[23,24]

The Schirmer tear test II measures the basal tear secretion by eliminating the reflex irritative component with a topical anesthetic. After application of the topical anesthetic, the lower conjunctival cul-de-sac is dried by swabbing with a cotton-tip applicator, and the tear production is measured. The basal secretion in the dog is approximately 12 mm/min.[25]

Mydriasis

PLRs are evaluated before instilling the mydriatic of choice. Most mydriatics take 10–15 minutes to act, so to conserve time, they should be given early in the examination. Mydriasis is necessary for complete ophthalmoscopy and for a thorough examination of the lens.

The mydriatic of choice for diagnostic use should be effective and short in action. Atropine in the normal dog eye lasts for 3 days and in the horse eye for 5–11 days. Tropicamide 1% (0.5% may be preferred in cats) is the preferred mydriatic for diagnostics (**Figure 1.9**).[26,27] The alkaloid drops traverse the nasolacrimal duct and, when licked from the nose, may stimulate profuse salivation in some animals due to the bitter taste. A transient, dramatic enlargement of the submandibular salivary glands has been occasionally

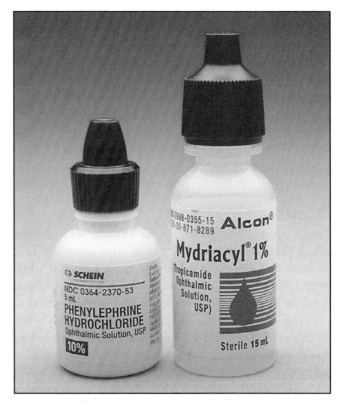

Figure 1.9 The two common mydriatics used in diagnostic work. Note the red caps, which are typical for any mydriatic solution.

noted in cats.[28] In young puppies, maximal mydriasis may not be achieved or may be very fleeting. Combining a parasympatholytic drug with a sympathomimetic drug such as 10% phenylephrine may be necessary for good mydriasis. Phenylephrine alone is a poor mydriatic in several species, having minimal effect in the horse and cat.[27,29] A potential systemic side effect of concentrated phenylephrine solution is systemic hypertension.[30] Mydriatics may produce elevations of the intraocular pressure that may be significant in dogs and cats.[31,32] This should be considered when readings are marginally elevated, and tonometry repeated at a later time without mydriatics.[31]

Detailed examination of the anterior segment

Magnification in the form of a loupe or slit lamp is a critical aid in ophthalmic lesion recognition due to the frequently minute nature of lesions and the structures involved. This technique is mainly limited to the anterior ocular segment and adnexa, unless the eye is aphakic. Various head loupes (**Figure 1.10**) or a magnifying lens can be utilized, but the slit lamp or biomicroscope is the most sophisticated means of accomplishing a magnified examination (**Figure 1.11**).[33–37] A simplified slit lamp consisting of a lens and a battery-operated focused light is marketed for about $500 (**Figure 1.12**) (see section Biomicroscopy, for technical details).

A bright light source such as a transilluminator is directed at various angles and may be utilized in conjunction with magnification to examine the lid margin, conjunctiva, third eyelid, cornea, anterior chamber, iris, and lens. In addition to direct illumination, proximal illumination (lighting the region adjacent to the object of regard) and retroillumination (examination against background lighting) are also helpful (**Figure 1.13**).

> Retroillumination is a rapid and sensitive method of detecting opacities in the clear media, that is, lens, cornea, vitreous, aqueous.

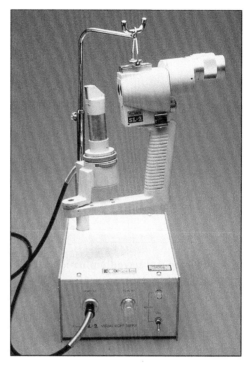

Figure 1.11 Kowa-2 portable slit lamp. It consists of a microscope, focused light, and light source connected to the microscope with a fiber-optic cable.

The lids, lid margins, and canthal regions are examined for abnormalities of the cilia and meibomian glands. The former may be difficult to detect without magnification. Retroillumination of the eyelids may be performed with a transilluminator when searching for imbedded foreign bodies. The conjunctival surfaces are examined for aberrant cilia (palpebral surface), foreign bodies, and presence of follicles, hyperemia, chemosis, symblepharon, and discharges. The cornea is examined by retroillumination of the iris and the fundus (dilated pupil) to detect small opacities and then studied in more detail in direct illumination. Irregularities of the surface, opacities, and

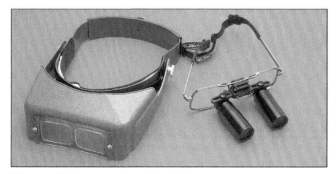

Figure 1.10 Examples of head loupes used for magnification.

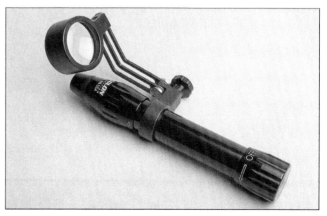

Figure 1.12 Relatively inexpensive portable slit lamp that consists of a 20 D lens and a focused light.

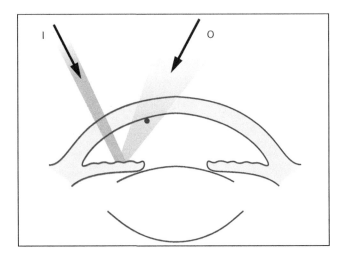

Figure 1.13 Principle of retroillumination of an object against an illuminated background.

neovascularization are searched for and characterized based on extent and depth.

The anterior chamber is examined for changes in depth and abnormal contents. The depth is increased with the loss of lens support (aphakia, microphakia, posterior lux-ated lens, hypermature cataract) and decreased with iris bombe, peripheral anterior synechiae, intumescent lens, or a mass in or behind the iris. Abnormal contents in the anterior chamber such as leukocytes, erythrocytes, fibrin, cysts, the lens, and tumors are noted. Changes in the blood–aqueous barrier can be detected by using a focused light source or thin beam of light to demonstrate the Tyndall effect or "flare" produced by an increased protein content (plasmoid aqueous) and cells in the anterior cham-ber (**Figure 1.14**).

The iris is examined for texture, masses, color, vascu-larity, pupillary membrane strands, and stability. With

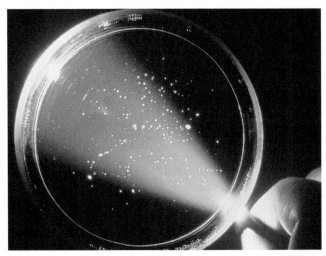

Figure 1.14 Flare or Tyndall effect present in a petri dish that has a colloidal solution. (Courtesy of Dr. M. Wyman.)

loss of the lens support from a displaced lens or periph-eral iris adhesions, the iris trembles on ocular movement (iridodonesis). If the PLRs have not already been exam-ined, they are recorded. The iris, particularly the pupil-lary region, can be examined in the retroillumination of the tapetum to detect areas of atrophy or hypoplasia. If the PLRs are incomplete or anisocoria is present, sphinc-ter atrophy, hypoplasia, or synechiae may be responsible. The pupil is examined for irregularities in shape that may indicate atrophy or adhesions.

The lens is first examined in retroillumination from the fundus to detect opacities rapidly and then in direct and focal illumination to determine the depth of the lesion. Observed opacities are characterized by their shape, number, color, texture, and location. Irregularities on the lens surface (wrinkled capsule in hypermature cat-aracts), shape (coloboma, lenticonus), and size (micropha-kia, intumescent lens) may be observed.

The anterior vitreous can be examined for hyaloid artery remnants, veils, haze (usually protein or cells) and blood clots, and retinal detachment.

A magnification source is critical in ophthalmic examination and manipulations, and it is worth the investment to buy a quality instrument that is comfortable, has good optics and a reasonable focal length, and is easily adjusted.

Lacrimal evaluation tests

Schirmer tear test: See previous discussion

Phenol red thread tear test

A test utilizing a 75-mm thread impregnated with phenol red has been developed in Japan and tested in dogs and cats. The end of the thread is hooked and placed in the lower con-junctival cul-de-sac, similar to a Schirmer tear strip. Tears turn the indicator red as they progress down the thread. The small size of the thread does not create as much irritation on insertion as the Schirmer tear strip, and the reading may be more indicative of the basal tear secretion. The wetting is measured after 15 seconds; the mean wetting for normal dogs is 34 ± 4 mm and 23 ± 2 mm in cats.[38,39]

Tear break-up time (BUT)

While previously discussed tear evaluation tests evaluate quantity, the tear BUT test is an attempt to evaluate the quality of the tears. The test is performed by instilling fluo-rescein on the cornea and not allowing the patient to blink while observing the intactness of the fluorescein in the tear film. The time from instillation of fluorescein to the break-ing up of the fluorescein sheet is the BUT. It can be difficult to perform in animals because while the lids can be held open, the third eyelid cannot be controlled. This test is not performed routinely but may be indicated in various superficial keratopathies. The normal BUT in the dog is reported as 19–20 ± 5 seconds.[40] A recent study in cats showed a significant reduction of the BUT in cats with conjunctivitis and the authors suspect that deficient tear film quality in those cats may predispose to the development of conjunctivitis.[41]

Ocular staining

Fluorescein

Topical sodium fluorescein is an invaluable tool in detecting corneal epithelial defects as well as in monitoring the healing process. Fluorescein is utilized mainly as single-use strips, since it was discovered that the solution was a good culture medium for *Pseudomonas* spp.,[42] although this has recently been brought into question.[43] If used as a 1%–2% solution in multiple-use bottles, care must be taken to avoid contamination. Some clinicians make a fresh solution daily by placing a strip in a 3- to 6-mL syringe and filling it with sterile saline. This may be easier to apply in the horse, but false-negative staining may be encountered with this method because the fluorescein is too dilute.

Hydrophilic fluorescein cannot penetrate the normal lipophilic epithelium, and thus is not normally retained. If intercellular junctions are widened or loss of epithelium occurs, fluorescein is retained by the epithelium or stroma, respectively, and is visible as a bright green stain (**Figure 1.15**).[44] Staining of extensive ulcerations may result in the fluorescein being visible in the aqueous. The corneal staining is transient (about 15–30 min), although in devitalized corneas it may persist for several hours.

If fluorescein strips are used and the ocular surface is not very moist, adding one to two drops of eyewash to the strip ensures an adequate quantity of solution on the eye.

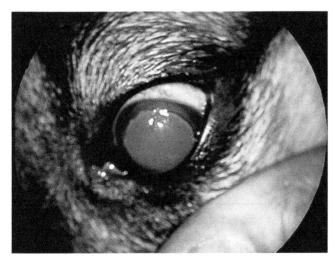

Figure 1.15 Fluorescein staining of a superficial ulcer.

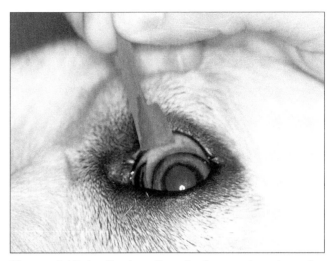

Figure 1.16 Application of a moist fluorescein strip to the conjunctiva.

If a dry strip is touched to the eye for moisture, it should be placed on the conjunctiva rather than the cornea (**Figure 1.16**). Touching the cornea with the strip may give a slight positive staining at the point of contact. The eye is rinsed thoroughly with eyewash to remove excess fluorescein and mucus, and the retention of stain is evaluated. With small defects such as herpes epithelial ulcers in cats, the use of an ultraviolet light (Wood's light) or cobalt-blue filter in a dark room causes fluorescence of the fluorescein, making minute stain retention visible.

Other uses for topical fluorescein stain in ophthalmology are to detect aqueous leaks in perforating corneal wounds (Seidel test) and to determine patency of the lacrimal outflow system. The Seidel test is performed by applying a high concentration of fluorescein at the site in question without rinsing. The concentrated fluorescein is orange; if aqueous is leaking from the site, a dark rivulet forms in the orange background. Evaluation of nasolacrimal duct patency with fluorescein is performed by applying fluorescein to the eye and observing its appearance at the nostril (**Figure 1.17**). Fluorescein can normally be observed at the nostrils within a few minutes. A normal test does not ensure the entire lacrimal ductal system is patent, as only one patent lacrimal canaliculus and punctum is necessary for a positive test. The absence of fluorescein may be due to ductal obstruction or an anomalous orifice into the nasal cavity.

Fluorescein may be given IV as a 10% solution to visualize the fundus vasculature or the iris vessels (see section Fluorescein angiography) and to measure limb-to-retina circulation time.

Rose bengal

Rose bengal is a fluorescein derivative of the xanthene group, and it has been used in ophthalmology as a 1%

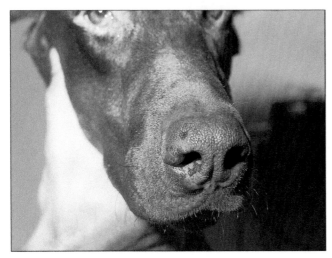

Figure 1.17 Fluorescein staining visible in the nose after application to the eye of a dog.

solution. Rose bengal was originally characterized as a supravital stain that only stained degenerate epithelial cells and mucus. Its main use has been in staining devitalized cells in keratoconjunctivitis sicca (KCS), and it is thought to be more sensitive than the Schirmer tear test (**Figure 1.18**).[45] Rose bengal has also been used to stain herpes epithelial ulcers and dysplastic epithelial cells with squamous neoplasia. Recently, the mechanism of action of rose bengal has been questioned. Cell culture evidence indicates that rose bengal stains cells that do not have a mucus layer or the cornea with a deficiency of the pre-ocular tear film.[46] Rose bengal, therefore, stains healthy cells if they are not protected by mucin, and it is intrinsically toxic to cells in concentrations >0.01%. Exposure to light releases oxygen radicals, which are toxic to cells.[46] Rose bengal is also virucidal and bactericidal, and cultures should be obtained before application of the stain. In a mouse herpesvirus model, no virus could be isolated after a single topical application of 1% rose bengal.[47]

Special ophthalmic examination procedures
Microbiologic cultures of conjunctiva/cornea
If the type of discharge, history of chronicity, lack of response to therapy, or severity of the problem indicates serious or resistant infectious agents are involved, cultures should be obtained early in the examination before the use of topical anesthetics. Topical anesthetics may be bactericidal. Ideally, even if the problem is unilateral, cultures of both eyes are preferred for comparative purposes, but due to the additional expense, this practice is usually not followed. *Staphylococcus* spp. and *Streptococcus* spp. are the most consistent flora of the normal and diseased conjunctiva.[48–53] The swab may be moistened with sterile nutrient broth or saline before use to make the procedure more comfortable and increase the growth rate.[54] Calcium alginate swabs have been reported to yield a higher growth rate.[50] Swabs should be placed in a transport medium or immediately plated to prevent drying of the small samples. Commercial culturettes with transport media and fine tipped swabs are convenient and easy to place on small lesions and avoid contamination from adjacent structures (**Figure 1.19**).

Conjunctival and corneal cytology
Scraping the conjunctiva and/or the corneal surface after topical anesthesia and examining the cells may enable a rapid etiologic diagnosis to be made or may guide initial therapy. The scraping may be performed with various instruments. A metal instrument is used if the surface must be debrided to get to the level of the pathology. A malleable platinum spatula (Kimura) is commercially available but expensive. The author simply uses the noncutting end of a sterile scalpel blade as a convenient disposable sterile scraper (**Figure 1.20**). For surface cytology, a small

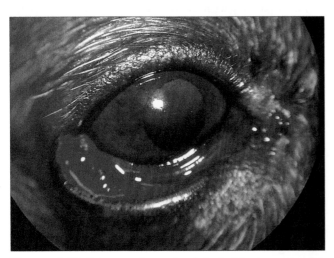

Figure 1.18 Faint rose bengal staining of the cornea and conjunctiva of a dog with KCS.

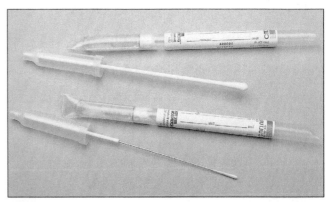

Figure 1.19 Fine- and course-tipped culture swabs with transport media.

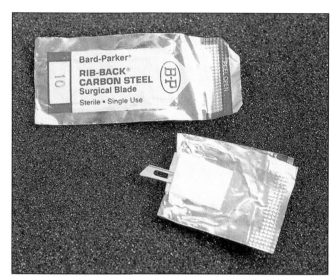

Figure 1.20 Preparation of #10 Bard Parker blade for use as a scraping instrument to obtain cytology and culture specimen.

disposable nylon bristle brush has given superior preparations and is easier to insert into the conjunctival cul-de-sac of cats (**Figure 1.21**).[55,56] Slide preparations made with the brush have fewer cells, but the cells are scattered and not clumped as with a spatula. The material is transferred to glass slides, air dried and fixed, and can be stained with a variety of stains such as Giemsa and Gram stains. The slides are evaluated for cell type, bacteria, viral and chlamydial inclusion bodies, fungi, and foreign material (see Chapter 8).[57]

Cannulation of the lacrimal outflow system

Cannulation and establishing patency of the lacrimal outflow system is indicated with a problem of epiphora or a resistant or relapsing conjunctival infection. This is readily performed in most dogs with topical anesthesia and using restraint in lateral recumbency. A blunt 22-gauge needle, or a commercial malleable lacrimal needle on a 6-mL syringe, is passed into either the upper or lower punctum. The upper punctum is usually more accessible. Ensuring the lid is kept taut, threading the catheter down the canaliculus, and keeping it parallel to the canaliculus all help to prevent kinking and obstruction by the wall of the canaliculus, thus avoiding a false impression of a pathologic obstruction (**Figure 1.22**).

Resting the hand with the syringe against the animal's head minimizes traumatizing the duct if minor head movement occurs. A fountain of fluid should emerge from the opposite punctum and the nostril. If fluid is not observed at the nostril, the opposite punctum is occluded while flushing to force more fluid down the nasolacrimal duct. Imperfect nasolacrimal ducts result in some dogs in fluid running posteriorly into the pharynx, and the patient often starts to choke, sneeze, and swallow. If an obstruction is present, heavy sedation or general anesthesia may be required, as the force necessary to unblock the obstruction is painful.

Cats are more difficult to cannulate because of the small canaliculus and the animal's temperament. A 25- to 27-gauge blunt needle, ketamine sedation, and a loupe should be used to obtain best results.

The horse's nasolacrimal system is most easily evaluated by retrograde flushing from the nasal end of the nasolacrimal duct. A #8 French urinary catheter or infant feeding tube may be passed in a retrograde direction and

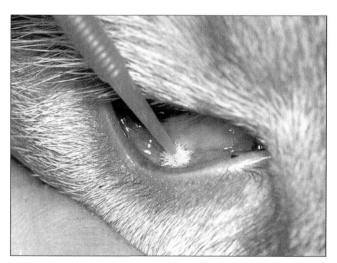

Figure 1.21 Cytobrush used for collecting conjunctival cells. (Courtesy of Dr. M. Willis, The Ohio State University.)

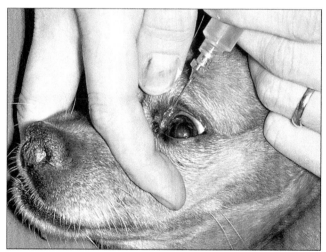

Figure 1.22 Flushing the nasolacrimal duct of a dog through the upper canaliculus, which is usually the easiest to expose and make taut. Note the lateral recumbency of the patient and resting of the examiner's hand on the patient's head.

attached to a syringe for flushing. If the nasolacrimal duct is blocked, the puncta are easily cannulated after sedation.

Double eversion of the eyelids and membrana nictitans

The palpebral conjunctiva and bulbar surface of the third eyelid can be examined by a process of double eversion. Double eversion is performed under topical anesthesia by gently grasping the lid margin with forceps and lifting it up and caudally from the eye, while using an instrument such as a strabismus hook near the base of the lid to push toward the eye. This causes the lid to roll back over the hook, exposing the palpebral conjunctiva (**Figure 1.23**). This maneuver also can be performed on the third eyelid to expose the lymphoid follicles and gland. It is invaluable in searching for hidden foreign bodies and evaluating the tissue pathology.

Tonometry

The measurement of intraocular *pressure* may be made with a variety of instruments, all of which were designed for use on humans. **Indentation tonometry** is exemplified by the Schiotz tonometer, which is of relatively low cost but more difficult to handle and not suitable for all animals. This instrument measures the amount of corneal indention produced by a given weight, and the scale reading is converted to millimeters of mercury with conversion tables (**Figure 1.24**). Conversion tables for dogs and cats have been calculated, and they result in higher IOPs than comparable scale readings on the human conversion table.[58,59] The normal IOP for most species is considered to be <25–30 mmHg (3.3–4.0 kPa) on the human scale.[60–64] The difference in IOP between the two eyes should be ≤8 mmHg (1.07 kPa).[61]

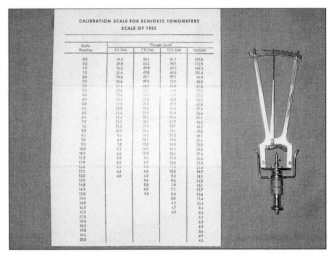

Figure 1.24 Schiotz tonometer with conversion scale.

After topical anesthesia is administered, the animal is placed in dorsal to dorsolateral recumbency so that the eye being measured is directed vertically. The tonometer is allowed to rest with its full weight on the central cornea for 1–2 seconds (**Figure 1.25**). The scale reading is noted, and this is repeated three to four times to determine consistency. Although most animals object to being placed on their sides or backs, the sitting patient usually presents with poor eye position because of the vestibular-ocular reflex that often results in the tonometer being placed near or over the limbus. The body position alters the IOP in man and animals. In the dog, dorsal recumbency increased the mean IOP over sternal and sitting positions

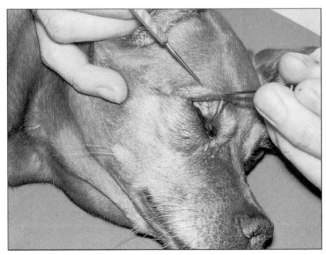

Figure 1.23 Double eversion of the upper eyelid of a dog to examine the palpebral conjunctiva.

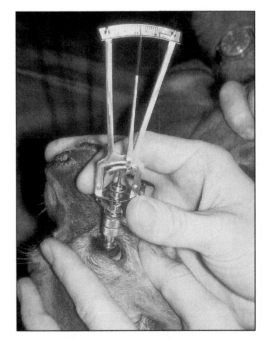

Figure 1.25 Application of the Schiotz tonometer to the axial cornea with the dog in dorsal recumbency.

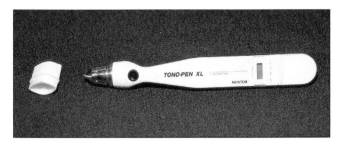

Figure 1.26 **Tono-Pen with cover. The average IOP reading is displayed.**

by 1.5–2 mmHg utilizing the Tono-Pen, but this difference decreased over 3–5 minutes.[65]

Inaccurate or spurious values with the Schiotz tonometer can be produced by dried mucus and tears that have wicked up the plunger, a small corneal curvature (microphthalmos overestimates IOP), a large corneal curvature (such as in buphthalmos, which underestimates IOP), corneal scars, corneal edema, an anterior luxated lens, and transference of pressure to the globe while holding the lids open.

Applanation tonometry measures the force necessary to flatten a given corneal area and may be measured with a variety of instruments. A small handheld electronic applanation tonometer, the Tono-Pen, appears almost ideal for veterinary medicine (**Figures 1.26 and 1.27**). It is portable, consistent, apparently accurate, and easily used on most species including exotics; however, it is expensive. The plunger is 1.5 mm in diameter and is covered with a latex membrane to avoid disease transmission and, more importantly, to avoid tears wicking up the plunger. Light tapping anywhere on the central two-thirds of the cornea perpendicular to the point produces accurate readings.[66] Acceptable readings are indicated by a clicking sound. Three to six acceptable readings are averaged, a tone sounds, and the mean value is displayed in a window with a bar over the coefficient of variance of the readings from 5% to >20%. The Tono-Pen appears to overestimate IOP in the low range, is very accurate in the normal range, and underestimates IOP in the high range in the human, dog, and cat.[67–70] Using the

Tono-Pen, mean IOP in the dog was 19 ± 6 mmHg[71] and 17 ± 4 mmHg,[69,70] and in the cat was 20 ± 6 mmHg.[69,70] In the horse, the instrument underestimated the IOP at all pressures, although by a predictable amount. In the horse, wide fluctuations in IOP can be measured that are not eliminated by auriculopalpebral nerve block. In the horse, when the head was above the heart, the IOP was decreased (mean 17.5 mmHg), and when lowered below the level of the heart, the IOP was increased (mean 25.7 mmHg) in 87% of the subjects. The difference was as much as 28 mmHg, with a mean of 8 mmHg.[72] As unsedated horses frequently raise their head when their eyes are being examined and the head is dropped with xylazine sedation, the difference in IOP measurements may be significant.[72] The mean IOP in the normal horse was 23 mmHg with the Tono-Pen.[73]

Rebound tonometry. A new tonometer, marketed as the TonoVet, is based on measuring the deceleration of the impact of a probe when it strikes the cornea, the soft eye producing less or slower rebound than the firmer eye. This principle is termed impact or rebound tonometry. The advantages of rebound tonometry are no topical anesthetic is required, it is slightly more accurate at all IOP levels, the status of the cornea may not be as critical due to the small contact surface, and the instrument is not as subject to operator error. The instrument must be used on the horizontal plane, it is heavier than the Tono-Pen, and the probes or tips are replaced between patients to minimize contamination (**Figures 1.28 and 1.29**).

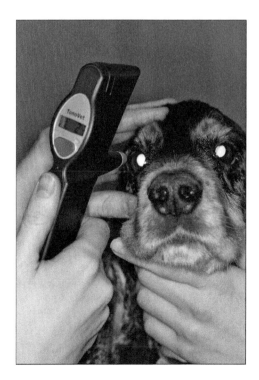

Figure 1.28 **Rebound tonometry using the TonoVet in a dog.**

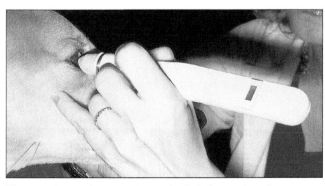

Figure 1.27 **Tono-Pen in use by lightly tapping the cornea.**

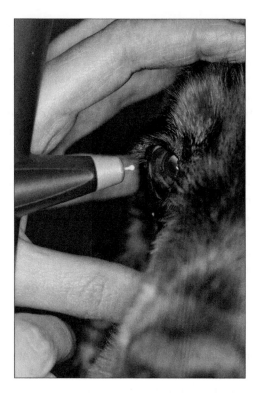

Figure 1.29 The small steel wire covered with a round plastic tip is expelled from the instrument with high speed onto the cornea.

Normal intraocular pressure values using a rebound tonometer have been established for dogs and horses and were 10.8 ± 3.1 mmHg (range, 5–17 mmHg) and 22.1 ± 5.9 mmHg (range, 10–34 mmHg) for dogs and horses, respectively. Comparing the mean measurements of IOP of normal dogs and horses using the Tono-Pen and TonoVet, the TonoVet recorded IOP 2 mmHg lower in the dog and 1 mmHg higher in the horse.[74]

In another study comparing the measurements obtained from a rebound tonometer (Icare) and applanation tonometer (Tono-Pen XL) in dogs, the measurements were comparable, although the values obtained with the rebound tonometer were significantly lower.[75]

Rusanen et al.[76] evaluated and compared the values of the rebound and applanation tonometer readings in normal cats and found that the mean IOP readings obtained with the rebound tonometer were 2–3 mmHg higher than measured with the applanation tonometer. The mean IOP with the rebound tonometer and applanation tonometer were 20.74 and 18.4 mmHg, respectively.[76]

Gonioscopy

Gonioscopy is the act of viewing the iridocorneal angle. This region contains the aqueous outflow pathways and thus is important in the pathogenesis of many glaucomas. To view the iridocorneal angle adequately, a contact lens is

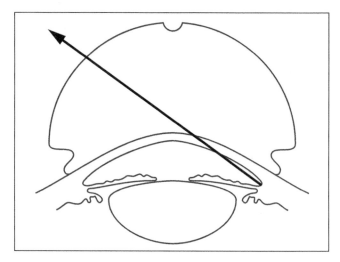

Figure 1.30 Demonstration of light exiting from the angle when a contact lens is applied for gonioscopy. The light can now exit the cornea because the refractive index has changed from the cornea to plastic (or glass), and the curvature of the lens is different from the cornea, allowing light to exit. Note where the examiner must be positioned to view the opposite angle region.

necessary to allow light to exit the cornea (**Figure 1.30**). Gonioscopy is performed after ophthalmoscopy because the coupling fluid utilized under the lens interferes with ophthalmoscopy. The procedure can be accomplished with topical anesthesia and manual restraint in lateral recumbency or in a sitting position (**Figure 1.31**). A variety of gonioscopic lenses designed for use in human medicine are available, and most are applicable to the dog and the cat (**Figure 1.32**). A strong light and a source of magnification are necessary. This can be provided by an otoscope head, a loupe and transilluminator, or by a slit lamp. In addition to investigating the pathogenesis of glaucoma, gonioscopy is useful in evaluating lesions of the peripheral

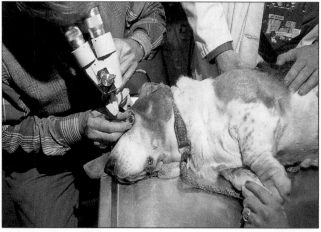

Figure 1.31 Performing gonioscopy in a nonsedated dog utilizing a slit lamp and a Franklin goniolens.

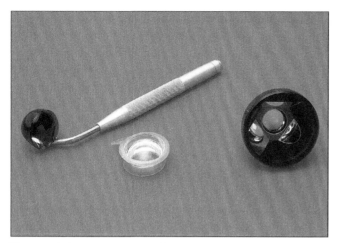

Figure 1.32 Various goniolenses. Left to right are: Cardona-type lens that attaches to a fiberoptic light cable, Franklin lens with sialastic flange, and a three-mirror prism.

anterior chamber such as iris cysts, foreign bodies, tumors of the region, and traumatic lesions.[61,62,77–79]

The normal iridocorneal region in carnivores is dominated by a well-developed pectinate ligament with a bluish-white trabecular region in the background (**Figure 1.33**). (For further discussion on gonioscopic findings see Chapter 12, Glaucoma.)

Ophthalmoscopy

Ophthalmoscopy is one of the most difficult routine procedures that the veterinarian is asked to master. The

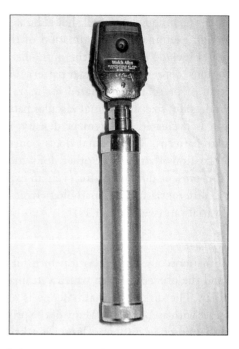

Figure 1.34 Direct ophthalmoscope. Power sources may be battery, rechargeable battery, or wall transformer.

traditional direct ophthalmoscope (**Figure 1.34**) is not the instrument of choice in small animal practice because of the inherent magnification and lack of stereopsis. The technique of direct ophthalmoscopy is most applicable in large animals because the larger eye has less inherent magnification (see **Table 1.1**).[80] Binocular or monocular indirect ophthalmoscopy is preferred in the dog and the cat (**Figure 1.35**). The main disadvantage of the binocular indirect ophthalmoscope is the cost, but essentially, all that is necessary for indirect ophthalmoscopy is a condensing lens and a good light source.

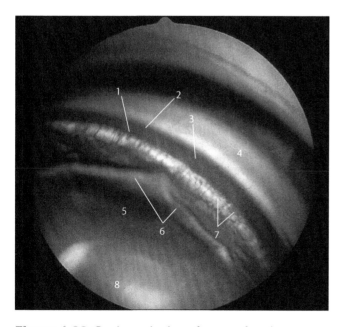

Figure 1.33 Gonioscopic view of a normal canine iridocorneal angle with various anatomic landmarks. (1: Deep pigmented zone; 2: Superficial pigmented zone; 3: Uveal trabeculae in ciliary cleft; 4: Sclera; 5: Iris; 6: Major arterial circle; 7: Pectinate ligament; 8: Pupil.)

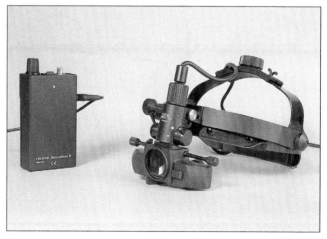

Figure 1.35 Binocular indirect ophthalmoscope. This unit has a rechargeable battery transformer that allows portability.

With either technique, the pupil should be well dilated for a thorough examination. Examination of the ocular fundus should include evaluating the optic disc for size, color, elevations, depressions, vascular pattern, and shape. The tapetum, if present, is evaluated for its reflectivity, mosaic detail, color, size, and retinal vascular pattern. The nontapetum is evaluated for pigment density, mottling, and vascular patterns. The normal dog's ocular fundus has more variations than that of other domestic animals and thus can present difficulties for even an experienced examiner in differentiating mild pathology from extremes in normal variations (see Chapter 14).

Direct ophthalmoscopy

Direct ophthalmoscopy is the classical form of ophthalmoscopy and the procedure with which veterinarians are most familiar. The direct ophthalmoscope is often purchased as a set with an otoscope. Many of the principles of direct ophthalmoscopy involving lesion localization and alignment also apply to the indirect ophthalmoscopy.

The direct ophthalmoscope consists of a power source whose light is reflected through a prism into the patient's eye (**Figure 1.36**). The light is then reflected back through the pupil through a movable lens in the ophthalmoscope to the observer. When examining an animal with frontal eyes and a long nose, it is usually mechanically advantageous for the examiner to avoid the patient's nose by using his/her left eye to examine the patient's left eye and his/her right eye to examine the patient's right eye. This is not as important in the horse and cow, which have laterally placed eyes. Alternating eyes in the examination takes practice as most people have a dominant eye that they prefer to use. Some of the principles that Dr. William Havener espoused when teaching ophthalmoscopy are described in the following section.[81]

There are two dials for adjustment in the basic direct ophthalmoscope. The examiner looks through an aperture of the large dial that contains a series of small lenses that can be rotated into viewing position (**Figure 1.34**). The numbers visible on rotating the large dial indicate the strength of the lens that is in place, expressed in diopters. A diopter is the reciprocal of the focal length of the lens in meters, that is $D = 1/\text{focal length in meters}$. The black or green numbers represent plus (+) lenses that are convex or converging lenses. The red numbers represent minus (−) lenses that are concave or diverging lenses.

The second adjustment possible is one that selects the light beam size, shape, and color. Most of the examinations are performed with white light using the large circular aperture. Additional apertures usually available are a smaller circular aperture, a grid aperture, a streak or slit aperture, and often various filters such as blue and red-free filters. The small circular aperture is usually used for proximal illumination, the grid to measure relative sizes of lesions, and the streak to detect irregular contours such as elevations and depressions. The blue filters are used to examine the nerve fiber layer and the red-free filter to examine blood vessels.

Initially the emmetropic (no refractive error) examiner sets the diopter setting on zero with the large circular aperture and places himself about 46–61 cm (18–24 in) from the patient. The examiner must align with two apertures, the aperture of the ophthalmoscope and the aperture of the pupil of the patient. By placing the ophthalmoscope snugly into the brow, the aperture of the ophthalmoscope is steady and constant, and the peripheral view through the aperture is maximized (**Figure 1.37**). The examiner then aligns the ophthalmoscope light with

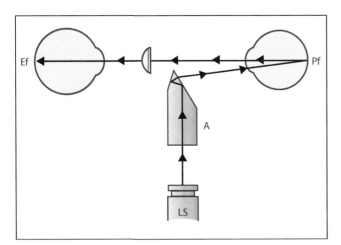

Figure 1.36 Direct ophthalmoscope light pathways. (Pf: patient's fundus; Ef: Examiner's fundus; LS: Light source; A: Prism or mirror.)

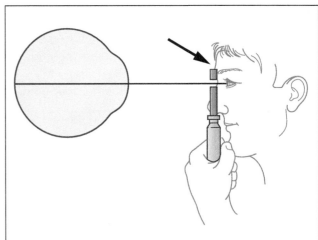

Figure 1.37 Placement of the ophthalmoscope into the brow to eliminate movement in relationship to the ophthalmoscope and to maximize the observer's field of view.

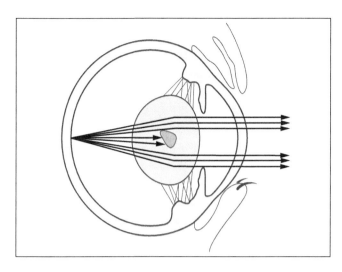

Figure 1.38 Retroillumination of a lenticular lesion from the fundus reflection.

the patient's pupil by finding the fundus or tapetal reflection. This usually is a bright, green-yellow tapetal colored reflection through the dog or cat's pupil. This serves to align the light correctly and quickly, and it is a very sensitive means of picking up central opacities in the clear ocular media in front of the retina, that is vitreous, lens, anterior chamber, and cornea by retroillumination. Even small opacities can be detected as darker regions against the fundus reflection due to the blockage of returned light to the observer (**Figure 1.38**). The examiner often cannot localize the opacity in depth with this method but is alerted to the pathology. This technique is a quick screening technique, and with a trained eye, it is a very sensitive test for detecting axial opacities.

One of the difficulties in veterinary ophthalmoscopy is a lack of patient cooperation, with constant head and eye movement causing the examiner to lose the fundic image. The quickest method of regaining alignment with the patient's pupil is to back up 30 cm (12 in) or more, find the tapetal reflection, and then move close again. It is much easier to regain the alignment at a distance, since small variations in the angle of incident light are magnified at the patient level.

Ophthalmoscopy should be performed close to the eye and through a dilated pupil. The closer to the eye and the more dilated the pupil, the greater the peripheral area that can be examined (**Figure 1.39**). Ophthalmoscopy should also be performed in a dark environment to maximize the contrast to the observer's eye.

A bright specular reflection is present from the corneal surface and is often quite annoying. Specular reflections are the light rays being reflected directly back from the cornea to the observer, and they can drown out fundus detail. If the pupil is dilated, this reflection can be displaced by shifting the light slightly off center on the cornea. If the pupil is miotic, this cannot be done as the light will strike the iris (**Figure 1.40**).

> In summary, find the fundus reflection, and check for opacities of the clear ocular media (anterior chamber, cornea, lens, vitreous), then move in close to the patient and perform ophthalmoscopy through a dilated pupil and in a dark room.

The optic disc in a dog is about 1.5-mm diameter (1,500 μm). With the 17× magnification of the direct ophthalmoscope, structures approximating 30–90 μm in diameter can be visualized (**Table 1.2**; **Figure 1.41**). Because

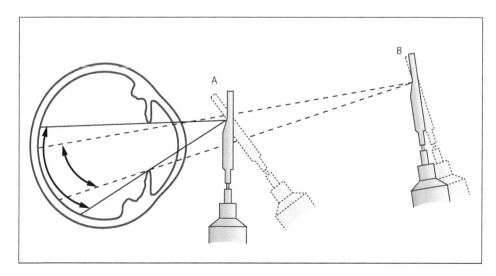

Figure 1.39 Illustration of how dilating the patient's pupil and moving close to the eye (A) increase the field of observation (compare with B).

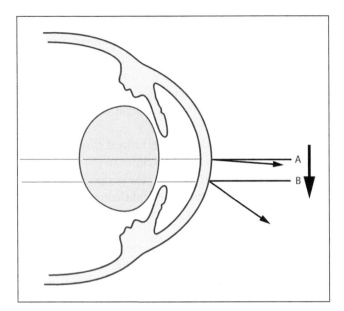

Figure 1.40 Illustration of how to avoid specular corneal reflections by movement of the light slightly off the axis to point B.

lesions are often microscopic, it is important to appreciate the histology of the fundus. The normal sensory retina is transparent, and what are visualized are columns of blood (healthy vessels are transparent), pigment, and the optic nerve. In most domestic animals, the tapetum that is in the superficial choroid and in the dorsal half of the fundus is also observed. The retina consists of the pigment epithelium and the neurosensory layers. A potential space exists between the pigment epithelium and the photoreceptors (**Figure 1.42**), which was the cavity of the embryonic optic vesicle before invagination occurred to form a cup and bring the two layers of the neuroectoderm in apposition. It is at this potential space that retinal detachments occur, which technically are retinal separations.

SPECIES	LATERAL MAGNIFICATION	AXIAL MAGNIFICATION
Horse	7.9	84
Cow	10.59	150
Sheep	13.89	258
Human	14.66	287
Pig	15.15	307
Dog	17.24	397
Cat	19.50	508
Rabbit	25.25	853
Rat	77.18	7,965

Table 1.2 **Magnification factors for direct ophthalmoscopy.**

Source: Modified from Murphy and Howland, 1987. *Vision Research* 27: 599–607.

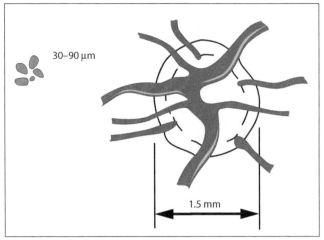

Figure 1.41 Illustration depicting lesions that are <0.1 of a disc diameter (DD) or in the micron range.

The holangiotic (retinal blood vessels over the entire retinal surface) fundus has two sources of blood vessels. The superficial vessels are the retinal blood vessels, which supply the inner half of the retina. In the cow, the retinal blood vessels lie on rather than within the retina, where they protrude into the vitreous. The outer half of the retina receives nutrition by diffusion from the choriocapillaris. In pigmented eyes (the norm), the choroidal vessels are obscured by the pigment epithelium and the tapetum

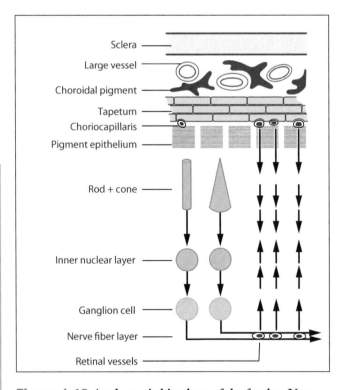

Figure 1.42 A schematic histology of the fundus. Note the location of pigment, blood vessels, and tapetum. Arrows denote source of nutrition for the retina.

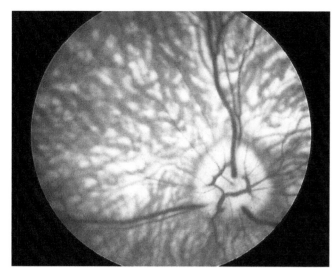

Figure 1.43 A normal canine albinoid, atapetal fundus. Note the two sources of visible blood vessels.

(**Figure 1.42**). In albinoid eyes that lack a tapetum and pigment, both vascular systems can be visualized (**Figure 1.43**). Similarly, there are two sources of pigment, retinal and choroidal. In most domestic animals, the tapetal pigmentation is also in the dorsal choroid (**Figure 1.44**).

When performing ophthalmoscopy, as in all examinations, it is desirable to establish a routine to ensure thoroughness. The usual starting point is to find the optic disc (papilla, nerve head) and then to examine each quadrant peripherally from the disc. The optic nerve in the dog is unique in routinely having myelination extending to the level of the retina. In most species, myelination of the optic nerve stops at the level of the sclera (lamina cribrosa). In the dog, varying degrees of myelination of the nerve produce great variation in the shape, size, elevation, and color

of the disc (**Figure 1.44**). Of particular importance is the vasculature pattern on the disc, its density, origin, vessel size, and color. The retinal arteries in domestic animals are cilioretinal in origin. Domestic animals lack a central retinal artery (as found in humans), and thus the arteries are found at the disc periphery. The surface of the cat's optic disc is not myelinated, resulting in a small, round, dark optic disc, and the vessels all originate from the periphery of the disc (**Figure 1.45**). (See Chapter 14 for further species variations.)

In the dog, the smaller vessels originating near the periphery are the arterioles. The larger, darker primary and smaller secondary veins go further onto the disc surface, usually to an anastomotic arc (**Figures 1.43 and 1.44**).

The vascular pattern on the disc and how the vessels disappear or originate varies with the species, but variations may be a clue to pathology involving the disc. Fish-hooking of vessels over the edge of the disc and being out of focus are often clues that a depression on the disc, such as a coloboma or glaucomatous cupping, may exist (**Figures 1.46 and 1.47**). Due to the lack of stereopsis or depth perception with direct ophthalmoscopy, the depression may not be appreciated without these visual clues.

The color of the disc is quite variable between individuals and between species, but extremes in pallor or hyperemia are usually significant. The dog, for instance, normally has a pinkish-white disc due to a mixture of myelin and capillaries. With atrophy of the nerve head, it becomes whiter to gray in color (**Figures 1.48 and 1.49**). In addition, the myelination is destroyed, so the fullness, shape, and color are affected in the dog. However, in other species without myelination of the nerve head, color change is the main finding of atrophy.

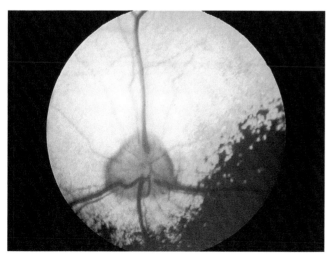

Figure 1.44 A normal canine pigmented fundus with a tapetum. Note the absence of visible choroidal vessels and a triangular pinkish-white optic disc.

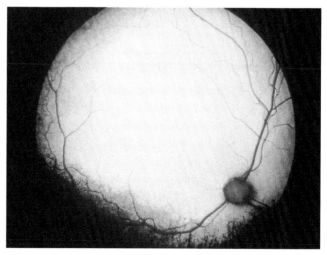

Figure 1.45 A wide-angle photograph of a feline fundus. Note the small, round, darker disc with vessels only at the periphery.

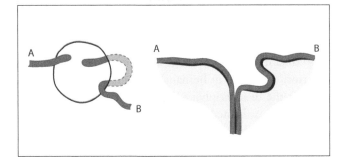

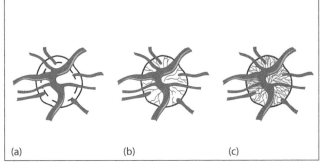

Figure 1.46 Illustration of two views of retinal vessels on the disc: A vessel that can be followed onto the disc until penetrating the nerve head (A); a vessel that disappears at the edge of a shelf and then reappears without obvious continuity (B); (Left panel: Ophthalmoscopic view; right panel: Sagittal section.)

Figure 1.48 Illustration of pathology of optic disc vasculature: Optic atrophy with no capillaries (a); normal (b); hyperemic disc with inflammation or congestion (papilledema) (c).

An increased redness of the disc is usually from capillary engorgement and may be active as in inflammation (papillitis) or passive as in venous stasis that results in edema (papilledema). With both papilledema and papillitis, the disc is swollen and elevated, causing the vessels to bend to get onto the disc (**Figures 1.48 and 1.50**). The vessels are usually dilated, and mild peripapillary edema may be present. Papillitis usually has a more profound effect on the retinal vessels and optic nerve function than papilledema and is accompanied by blindness.

In summary, changes in disc color, shape, and elevation or depression may be important ophthalmoscopic signs. In the dog, the great breadth of normal variation may make it difficult to diagnose early pathologic changes for even the experienced examiner.

As mentioned previously, the clinician can use the grid aperture to measure the size of lesions, but the size of the grid varies with the working distance. A more consistent and convenient means of describing and locating lesions is to relate the lesions to the disc size and location. This method utilizes the disc diameter (DD) size to describe a lesion's size and distance from the disc, and the hands of a clock to locate the lesion in relation to the disc (**Figure 1.51**). This method allows accurate description of a lesion's size and location to compare with at a later date.

There are various clues available for localizing the depth of a lesion with the ophthalmoscope. One useful clue for localization of fluid lesions such as hemorrhages is the morphology of the lesion. Fluid lesions must conform to the anatomy involved and, as a result, have a variety of shapes and sizes. Due to the loose attachment of the vitreous to the retina, the neurosensory retina to the pigment

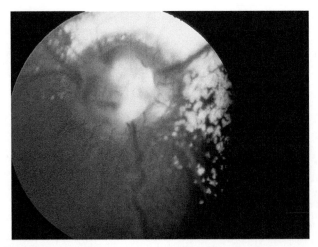

Figure 1.47 *Clinical correlate of 1.46.* The dog has a coloboma of the disc (white area) with vessels falling into this recess. Retinal vessels on one side do not proceed onto the disc as they do on the opposite side.

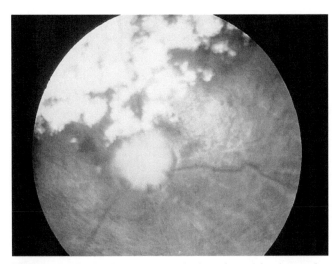

Figure 1.49 Optic nerve atrophy in a dog with advanced progressive retinal atrophy. Note the gray flat disc with scalloped edges.

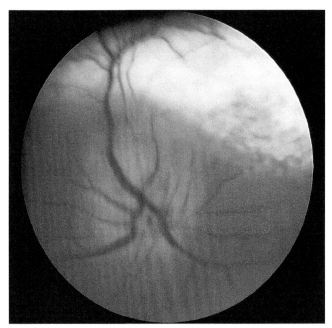

Figure 1.50 Papilledema in a dog with an engorged, elevated disc. Mild peripapillary edema is present.

epithelium, and the loose structure of the choroid, hemorrhages of large size may occur in these three spaces. Intraretinal hemorrhages are confined by the axons, dendrites, and Müller cell processes, which run mainly in a vertical manner, so these tend to be small, round hemorrhages. A hemorrhage in the nerve fiber layer has to insinuate between the fibers so it is typically flat and striated with feathered borders and is often called a flame-shaped hemorrhage (**Figure 1.52**). Preretinal hemorrhages with a formed vitreous are typically large and red, and the

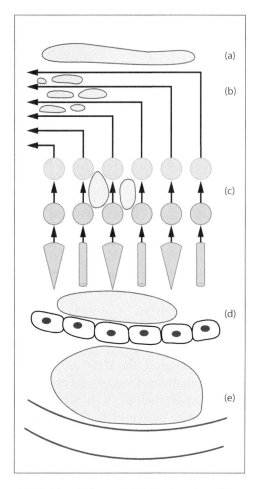

Figure 1.52 Morphology of fluid lesions based on area of fundus: preretinal/subhyaloid area (a); nerve fiber layer (b); intraretinal (c); sub-neuroretina (d); choroidal (e).

erythrocytes may settle out, producing a flat top or keel-boat-shaped hemorrhage (**Figures 1.53 and 1.54**). If the vitreous is liquefied, the preretinal hemorrhage becomes diffuse within the vitreous.

- The first principle of lesion location is that the morphology of fluid lesions is determined by the adjacent anatomy. Familiarity with the tissue architecture can help in localizing the lesion.
- A second principle in lesion localization is to find a structure of known depth and relate it to the lesion.
- The usual structures sought for lesion localization are a retinal or choroidal blood vessel. Other structures such as pigment and the tapetum may also be related to the lesion (**Figure 1.55**).
- A third method of lesion localization is utilizing the phenomenon of parallax. This is a very sensitive method of determining if two points are in apposition or separated. This works well in determining low retinal detachments (**Figure 1.56**).

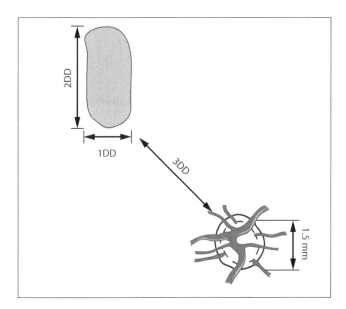

Figure 1.51 Illustration of locating and describing lesions in relationship to the disc and disc diameter (DD).

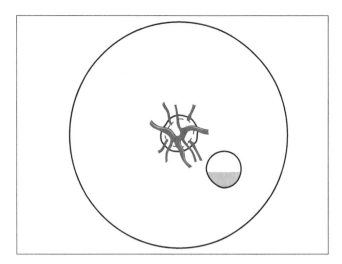

Figure 1.53 Illustration of preretinal hemorrhage that has settled, giving a flat top. The clear top portion may be overlooked by the examiner.

Parallax is looking at the structure in question against the background from two different observation points and determining if the structure moves in relation to the background. This will establish whether the two points are separated.

- The fourth method of lesion localization, unique to the direct ophthalmoscope, is the use of various lenses to focus on the object. Most animal's fundi will be in focus at 0 to –2 diopters (D). A lesion that is blurred can be assumed to lie either in front of

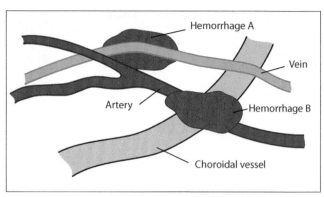

Figure 1.55 Illustration relating the depth of lesions to the two vascular systems.

or at the back of the plane of the fundus. The plus (black or green numbers) lenses converge light, allowing lesions elevated from the surface to come into focus. The negative lenses (red numbers) bring into focus lesions that are below or beyond the level of the normal fundus (**Figure 1.57**). Approximately 4 D is equivalent to 1 mm in the canine eye. This varies by species due to the inherent magnification of the eye.

Summary

The four methods of lesion localization with the direct ophthalmoscope are:

1. Lesion morphology
2. Relating to structures of known depth
3. Utilizing the parallax phenomenon
4. Diopter settings

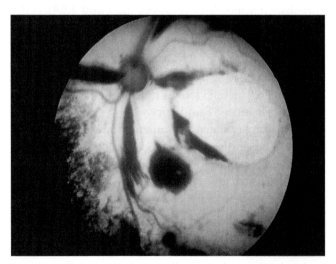

Figure 1.54 Cat fundus with multiple hemorrhages at different levels of the fundus. Preretinal hemorrhages with flat tops (is the packed cell volume normal?) and striated nerve fiber hemorrhages are present.

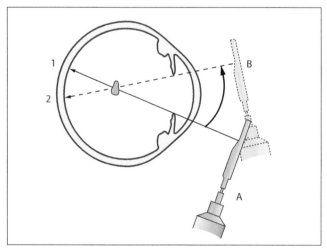

Figure 1.56 Illustration of the principle of parallax by observing the lesion from two perspectives and noting whether the lesion moves against the background. If the lesion moves, it is located in front of the retina and not on it.

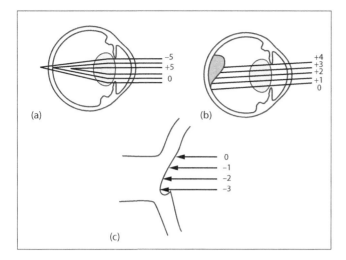

Figure 1.57 Illustration of using the ophthalmoscope lenses to focus on raised or depressed lesions: emmetropic eye focused on 0 (a); + lenses used to focus on a raised lesion (b); − lenses focusing on a depressed lesion (c).

Proximal illumination is a technique whereby the area in question is illuminated by shining the light adjacent to the area being examined. The small circular aperture is used in this instance. This may yield information regarding the structural nature of the lesion. If the lesion is cystic, fluid, or of a low density, the lesion transmits light which is reflected back to the observer's eyes. A dense or heavily pigmented lesion absorbs the light (**Figure 1.58**).

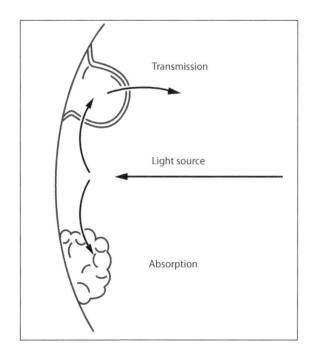

Figure 1.58 Illustration of the technique utilizing proximal illumination.

As with most techniques, competence comes only with practice, practice, and more practice!

Indirect ophthalmoscopy

Although the image may be confusing with the indirect ophthalmoscope because it is upside down and reversed, the technique is easily learned.[82,83] The necessary components of indirect ophthalmoscopy are an adequate light source and a converging lens. The light source with the binocular indirect ophthalmoscope (BIO) is on a headband or fits on spectacle frames, thus freeing the examiner's hands to hold the lens and the patient (**Figure 1.59**). The function of the headset is not only to provide light but to narrow optically the examiner's interpupillary distance (PD) of 60–15 mm (**Figure 1.60**). Narrowing the PD allows both eyes plus the light to be projected through the patient's pupil; this allows the observer binocular vision and stereopsis (**Table 1.3**). Many scopes now have a small pupil feature that narrows the PD to as small as 6 mm. **Table 1.4** gives the minimum pupil size of the patient that is necessary with three different strengths of condensing lenses for binocular observation. The lens strength selected alters the magnification and size of field of the image, the size of pupil that the fundus can be visualized through stereoscopically, and the inherent stereopsis (**Table 1.5**). The higher the diopter strength of the lens, the smaller the image but the larger the field of view, the smaller the pupil that can be examined, and the less the stereopsis.[84,85]

Most of the time when utilizing the BIO, the examiner can handle the animal without having an assistant to restrain the head (**Figure 1.59**). A teaching mirror is also

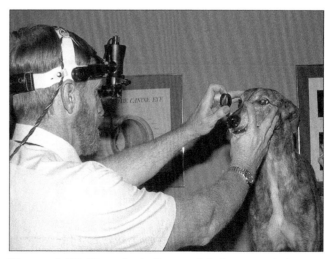

Figure 1.59 Binocular indirect ophthalmoscopy being performed. Note the working distance and lack of an assistant to hold the animal.

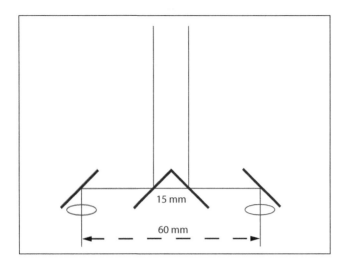

Figure 1.60 Optics of the binocular indirect ophthalmoscope and narrowing the interpupillary distance of the examiner.

available for most models, and video indirect scopes are available.

Before using the BIO, a few adjustments are necessary. The headset band tension is adjusted so that it is firm enough to keep from slipping and allow subtle movement of the light by contraction of the brow, but loose enough to avoid a headache. If the headset is not in front of the examiner's eyes, the headset is moved up or down. The PD is adjusted for each eye by sliding the optics of each eyepiece horizontally. The light should fall in the center of the observation field for that eye, and the two fields should be fused. The adjustment of the light on a vertical basis is performed using the hand as a target. With the hand at the usual, comfortable, bent-arms working distance, the light is adjusted to fall in the upper half of the examiner's field.

The usual binocular indirect ophthalmoscope has three main adjustments to be made before use. They are:

1. Adjustment of the tension of the headband
2. Adjustment of the interpupillary distance of the eyepieces
3. Vertical adjustment of the light in the eyepieces

The light source can be made very bright with a BIO, as it is usually powered by 110 volts from a transformer with a rheostat. In addition, the indirect image is inherently brighter due to all light returning to the observer's eye. The bright light may allow observation through hazy media with the BIO that was previously unsuccessful with the direct form.[83] The light should be no stronger than necessary, as this washes out detail and creates patient discomfort with a resultant lack of cooperation. Anesthetized patients that cannot move may develop retinal burns due to the strong light. The strength of the light must often be decreased for the tapetum and increased for the nontapetal region.

The image formed with a BIO is an aerial image which is upside down, reversed, and formed between the patient and the examiner (**Figure 1.61**).[82]

The lenses used in indirect ophthalmoscopy are biconvex or converging lenses, usually ranging from +14 D lenses to +30 D in strength. When used with the binocular headset, additional magnification is built into the headset, and magnification increases fourfold with the +14 D to twofold with the +28 D lens, although this varies with the species (see **Tables 1.3 and 1.5**). The magnification of the retina is equal to the diopter strength of the eye divided by the diopter strength of the lens used.[84,85] The strength of the lens affects not only the magnification but the amount of stereopsis or depth perception of the

Table 1.3 Magnification factors for indirect ophthalmoscopy.

SPECIES	LATERAL MAGNIFICATION				AXIAL MAGNIFICATION			
	14 D	20 D	30 D	40 D	14 D	20 D	30 D	40 D
Horse	1.18	0.79	0.51	0.38	1.86	0.84	0.35	0.19
Cow	1.58	1.06	0.68	0.50	3.34	1.50	0.62	0.34
Sheep	2.07	1.39	0.90	0.66	5.74	2.58	1.07	0.58
Human	2.19	1.47	0.95	0.70	6.39	2.87	1.19	0.65
Pig	2.26	1.52	0.98	0.72	6.83	3.07	1.28	0.70
Dog	2.57	1.72	1.11	0.82	8.85	3.97	1.65	0.90
Cat	2.91	1.95	1.26	0.93	11.31	5.08	2.11	1.15
Rabbit	3.77	2.53	1.63	1.20	18.99	8.53	3.55	1.93
Rat	11.52	7.72	4.98	3.68	177.44	79.65	33.15	18.06

Source: Modified from Murphy and Howland, 1987. *Vision Research* 27:599–607.

Table 1.4 **Minimum patient pupil size for stereopsis with varying power of condensing lenses using binocular indirect ophthalmoscopy.**

INTERPUPILLARY DISTANCE (MM)	STRENGTH OF CONDENSING LENS (D)	INTERPUPILLARY DISTANCE OF VIEWER'S EYES AS PROJECTED ON THE PATIENT'S EYE (MM)
15	30	1.5
15	20	2.25
IS	15	3.0

Source: Modified from Goldbaum et al., 1980. *Principles and Practice of Ophthalmology*, vol II. Peyman, G., Sanders, D., and Goldberg, M. (eds). WB Saunders: Philadelphia, PA, pp. 988–1097.

Table 1.5 **Ocular characteristics of lenses.**

LENS POWER (D)	APPROXIMATE MAGNIFICATION	FIELD OF VIEW	APPROXIMATE STEREOPSIS
28–35	× 2	60°	× 0.5 normal
20	× 3	51°	× 0.75 normal
14	× 4	30°	× 1 normal

Source: Modified from Goldbaum et al., 1980. *Principles and Practice of Ophthalmology*, vol II. Peyman, G., Sanders, D., and Goldberg, M. (eds). WB Saunders: Philadelphia, PA, pp. 988–1097.

examiner. The higher the diopter strength of the lens, the less the depth perception (**Table 1.5**).

An additional factor in selecting a lens is the size of the patient's pupil. The higher diopter lens can project the examiner's pupil onto a smaller patient pupil (**Figure 1.62, Tables 1.1 and 1.4**[84]). When examining the peripheral fundus, the patient's pupil becomes optically

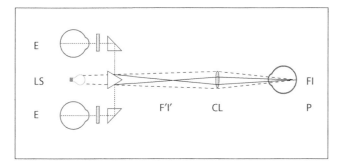

Figure 1.61 Optics of binocular indirect ophthalmoscopy. Note how the examiner's pupil distance is narrowed by the prisms and that a real aerial image is formed between the examiner and the patient. (E = examiner's eyes; LS = light source; P = patient; Ff = patient's fundus; Cl = corrective lens; F′I′ = image patient's fundus in space.) (With permission from Rubin, 1960. *Journal of the American Veterinary Medical Association* 137:648–651.)

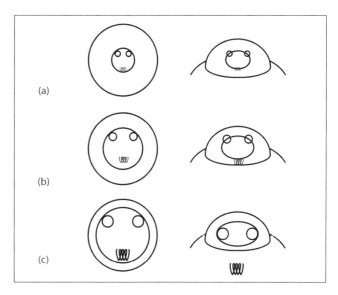

Figure 1.62 Optics comparing pupil size needed for various strengths of condensing lens and the difficulty in projecting the light and viewer's eyes obliquely through the pupil to view the peripheral fundus: 30 D lens image of examiner's eyes and light projecting into a small pupil and when viewing the peripheral fundus (a); 20 D lens image; note the larger pupil size required and that the peripheral fundus can still be examined if the pupil is large (b); 14 D lens; the pupil must be very large and oblique viewing effectively cuts the light out so the peripheral fundus cannot be visualized (c). (With permission from Goldbaum et al., 1980. *Principles and Practice of Ophthalmology*, vol II. Peyman, G., Sanders, D., and Goldberg, M. (eds). WB Saunders: Philadelphia, PA, pp. 988–1097.)

compressed or narrow, so to maintain binocular function, the examiner may have to use a higher diopter lens but lose some depth perception in the process (**Figure 1.62**). A good compromise if only one lens is available is a +20 D lens. The size of the field of view is dependent on the diopter power of the lens and the diameter of the lens. The higher diopter lens produces a more panoramic view, and, for a given lens strength, increasing the diameter of the lens increases the field of view.[84,85] The more recently developed Keeler 2.2 panretinal lens uniquely combines magnification of nearly a +20 D lens with the wider field of view of a +30 D lens and is suitable for the fundic examination through wider and smaller pupils.

Selection of the strength of the lens depends on the patient's pupil size and the amount of stereopsis (depth perception) and magnification desired.

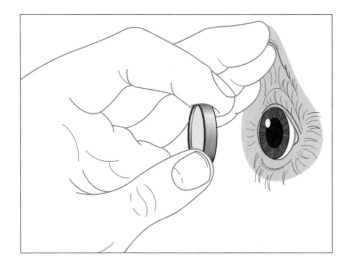

Figure 1.63 Technique of holding the lens so that the upper lid is held open, the lens is aligned, and the hand and the lens move with the head.

The lens is held with the thumb and the forefinger, and the remaining fingers are used to retract the upper lid and steady the lens in space (**Figure 1.63**). The strongest convex surface of the lens should be facing the observer for the best image. Many lenses have an identifying dot or a white ring that identifies the side towards the patient. When using the lens, it will be noted that a bright specular reflection is present from the anterior and posterior lens surface and is located in the center of the lens when the lens is held perpendicular to the light beam. These bright specular reflections are often annoying, as they obscure the area of interest that is usually centered. These specular reflections can be decentered by tilting the lens slightly, which pushes the reflections to the side (**Figure 1.64**).[86] Excessive tilting of the lens creates a prismatic effect, bending the light so that it is not directed through the pupil.

One of the difficulties in learning indirect ophthalmoscopy is created by the reversed image. This confuses the beginner as to the direction to move to bring the object of regard into better view.

> Note: To bring an object into the central view, the observer's head and the hand lens move in the same direction as the area to be viewed in the aerial image.

Movement of the head to bring objects in the image to the center is a simple concept, but it is counterintuitive and requires practice (**Figure 1.65**).

Parallax can be demonstrated with indirect ophthalmoscopy by tilting or shifting the hand lens or the head to observe the object from a slightly different angle. If the

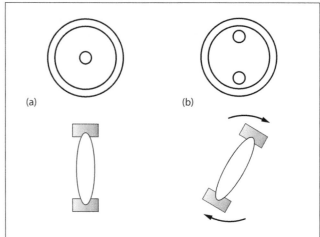

Figure 1.64 Illustration of specular reflections off the handheld lens: specular reflex from each surface is centered in the lens that distracts from viewing (a); slight tilting of the lens pushes the specular reflections to the side leaving the central area clear (b).

object is separated from the background, it then moves in relationship to the background (**Figure 1.66**).

Due to the expense of a BIO, many other light sources can be used instead. Any light source that does not diffuse out excessively can be utilized. If the light source is battery operated, it allows easy portability. The light sources can be as varied as a good penlight, a strong otoscope or direct ophthalmoscope, or any fiber-optic bundle. If the direct ophthalmoscope is used as the light source, more magnification can be produced by adding $1-2+D$ of lenses than if it is set at 0 D. Beyond 2 D, the image becomes blurred. Because there is no optical narrowing of the examiner's PD without a headset, the 60 mm (average PD) must

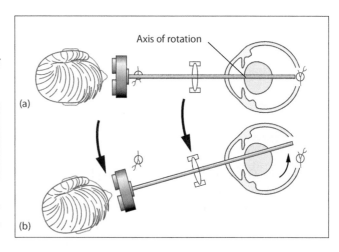

Figure 1.65 The area to the side of the branching vessels in the fundus can be observed by the examiner moving in the direction the vessels are seen in the image.

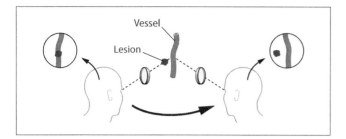

Figure 1.66 Demonstration of parallax of a lesion with a BIO. The lesion when viewed from one perspective is observed against a background vessel; if the lesion is separated from the background vessel, the lesion will move in relation to the vessel by slight rotation of axis of observation.

be projected onto the patient's pupil, and the technique requires a much larger pupil to acquire binocular examination (**Table 1.5**). Consequently, it is termed monocular indirect ophthalmoscopy (**Figure 1.67**). Another form of monocular indirect ophthalmoscopy is available in which the instrument optically rights the reversed and inverted image, thus avoiding this source of confusion. The image is smaller, but there is a wider field than with direct ophthalmoscopy (**Figure 1.68**). The instrument is expensive but extremely easy to use.

Indirect ophthalmoscopy gives a lower magnification but a larger field than direct ophthalmoscopy, and it gives the examiner a better overall picture. With less magnification, the patient's ocular movements are less troublesome. Most forms of indirect ophthalmoscopy utilize both of the examiner's eyes, and thus, stereopsis with depth perception is an important advantage. With good mydriasis, the extreme peripheral retina can be examined. The ora ciliaris retina is routinely visualized temporally and ventrally, less commonly nasally, and rarely dorsally without scleral indention. Peripheral examination requires practice in

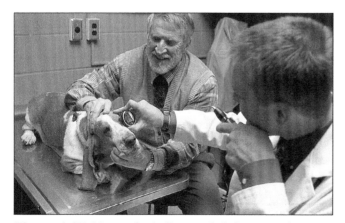

Figure 1.67 Monocular indirect ophthalmoscopy being performed with a Finoff illuminator. Note an assistant is necessary to hold the dog's head.

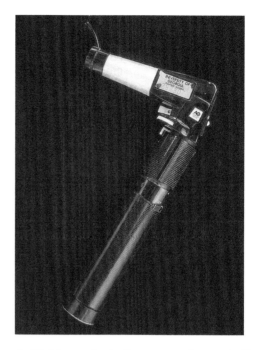

Figure 1.68 Monocular indirect scope that optically corrects the image for the observer.

positioning and manipulating the hand lens to get a prismatic bending of light.

In veterinary medicine, an important advantage of the BIO is that the examiner's head is a distance from the patient. This is important from the standpoint of physical trauma and, occasionally, contagious diseases in laboratory animals. It is always important to compare eyes in the examination, and the BIO allows this to be done quickly and thus to be more valid. Most BIOs have a teaching mirror available, so colleagues or students can gain firsthand observations with an experienced examiner.

> Most texts emphasize the difficulty of using a BIO, but in practice, it is routinely more gratifying to the novice to finally see the overall picture, so that it encourages ophthalmoscopy rather than discourages it.

The most important disadvantage of the usual BIO is the cost. This is not prohibitive for the practitioner, but it is for the student. The monocular version of indirect ophthalmoscopy only requires a lens that may cost from $20 to $300. The magnification with this form of indirect ophthalmoscopy is usually not as much as the BIO, and depending on the source of light, both of the examiner's hands are used, so an assistant is necessary. The patient's pupil must be larger to have binocular vision and stereopsis (**Table 1.6**).

Table 1.6 **Ocular characteristics of lenses.**

AVERAGE INTERPUPILLARY DISTANCE OF HUMANS (MM)	POWER OF CONDENSING LENS (D)	SIZE OF PATIENT'S PUPIL (MM)
0	30	6
0	20	9
0	15	12

Source: Modified from Goldbaum et al., 1980. *Principles and Practice of Ophthalmology*, vol II. Peyman, G., Sanders, D., and Goldberg, M. (eds). WB Saunders: Philadelphia, PA, pp. 988–1097.

Electrophysiologic tests

Electroretinography, visually evoked responses, and electro-oculography are electrophysiologic responses that may be utilized in clinical investigations. While initially limited to institutions, computerization has made the electroretinography equipment less expensive, and it is usually available in specialist practices.

The electroretinogram (ERG) is an action potential that occurs when a sudden change of illumination falls on the retina. The potential is divided into three major components: A-, B-, and C-waves. The A-wave is the first negative deflection and arises from the photoreceptors; the B-wave follows and is the first positive deflection and arises from nonneuronal glia in the inner nuclear layer; and the C-wave is a slow positive potential arising from the pigment epithelium of the retina (**Figure 1.69**).[87–89] **Figure 1.69** is typical of a flash-induced ERG with white light under dark adaptation (rod-dominated response). Fundus photography or indirect ophthalmoscopy reduces the dark adapted ERG amplitudes, and up to 60 minutes of dark adaption may be necessary to return to comparable ERG amplitudes of 20 minutes of dark adaption without previous light stimulation.[90] The usual flash ERG is generated by the outer half of the retina, and diseases that preferentially affect the ganglion cells or optic nerve, such as glaucoma, may result in a normal ERG in a blind animal.

A retinal electrical potential evoked with an alternating patterned grating (patterned ERG, PERG) evokes responses that may have optic nerve and ganglion cell origins.[91] The PERG has also been utilized to estimate the visual acuity of animals.[92]

Oscillatory potentials (OPs) are small oscillations that are superimposed on the B-wave, and there may be up to four to five wavelets. They are observed best during dark adaptation; their origin is the inner retina, and they are thought to be from the amacrine cells. Wavelets O3 and O4 are most easily observed (**Figure 1.69**).[93,94] In humans, alterations in the OPs are observed with alterations in retinal circulation, most notably in diabetes mellitus.

Visual evoked potentials (VEPs) are measured over the occipital cortex after stimulating the retina with light. The potentials are small and require computer averaging and general anesthesia. VEPs measure the integrity of the optic nerve, optic tracts, and occipital cortex.

Fluorescein angiography

Fluorescein angiography is used to study the retinal, choroidal, and iris vasculature. After injection of 10–25 mg/kg of fluorescein IV, the circulation is observed through a camera equipped with an exciter filter (500 nm) to stimulate the fluorescence of fluorescein, a barrier filter that selects light at the peak emission for fluorescein (550 nm), a motorized film advancer, and a rapid strobe recharging unit. The flow of dye through the vessels is sequentially observed as the choroidal, retinal arteriolar, capillary, and venous phases (**Figure 1.70**).[95,96] The tapetum fluoresces at similar wavelengths as fluorescein, thus reducing the contrast, but this can be minimized by a barrier filter that transmits wavelengths over 530 nm.[97]

Ultrasound

Ultrasonography in A and B modes has become routine in most centers for studying ocular lesions when the medium is opaque. It is particularly helpful in detecting neoplasia, phacoclastic uveitis, lens abnormalities and posterior lens rupture, foreign bodies, vitreous pathology, and retinal detachment with opaque media.[98–100]

Ultrasonography detects acoustic interfaces or differences in the density of tissue. The more dramatic the acoustic interface, the more the ultrasound waves are reflected back to the probe. A-mode ultrasonography gives an image of the amplitude of reflections in one spatial dimension (anterior–posterior), whereas B-mode ultrasonography consists of two spatial dimensions. A-mode is best suited for biometric measuring of ocular dimensions, whereas B-mode is usually used for diagnostic imaging,

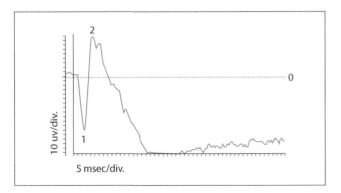

Figure 1.69 ERG from a normal dog: A-wave (1); B-wave (2); no C-wave is recorded. Performed with blue light in a dark room. Note two oscillatory potential wavelets on the B-wave.

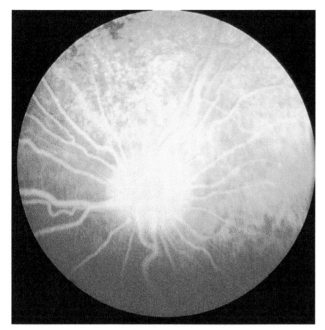

Figure 1.70 Fluorescein angiogram in a dog in the late venous phase. Note the arteries and veins are both filled. (Courtesy of Dr. K. Gelatt.)

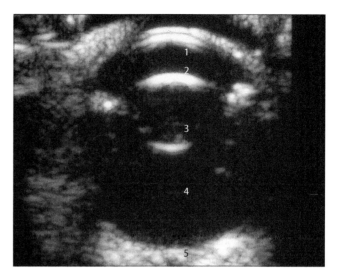

Figure 1.71 B-mode ultrasound image of a normal 11-year-old dog with a 10-MHz probe and direct contact with the cornea. (1: Cornea; 2: Anterior chamber; 3: Lens; 4: Vitreous; 5: Optic nerve.)

although B-mode has been reported to be as accurate as A-mode for biometric measurements.[100,101] The method of probe placement may be through a water bath (surgical glove filled with water) offset on the closed lids, or, more commonly, directly on the cornea utilizing an ultrasound coupling gel. Typical probe frequencies used in ophthalmic ultrasound are 7–10 MHz.

New instruments with probes that can focus at different focal lengths have improved visualizing the anterior segment without an offset (**Figure 1.71**).

The development of high-frequency ultrasound in recent years (with probe frequencies ranging from 20–50 MHz) allows a detailed examination of the anterior ocular segment, including sclera, cornea, anterior chamber, iris, and iridocorneal angle. Although the tissue penetration depth is limited to about 4–5 millimeters, the resolution of the imaged ocular structures is very high and comparable to a low-power sagittal histologic section through the tissue[102] (**Figure 1.72**). Ultrasound biomicroscopy, which uses even higher frequencies of 50–100 MHz, is particularly useful in the examination of the iridocorneal angle and ciliary cleft.[103]

B-mode ultrasonography has greatly expanded our diagnostic capabilities in eyes with opaque media.

Ultrasound biometry is particularly useful for the measurements of intraocular dimensions and determination of the axial length of the eye.[100,101] The reported axial lengths of the dog eye vary with the head type. Mesocephalic dogs have a mean axial length of 19.9 mm and dolichocephalics have a mean of 21.2 mm.[101] Sedated Samoyeds have a mean of 22 mm,[104] and an overall mean of 20.4 mm was found when a variety of breeds was examined.[105] Ultrasound biometry has also been used for accurate measurement of the axial length to calculate

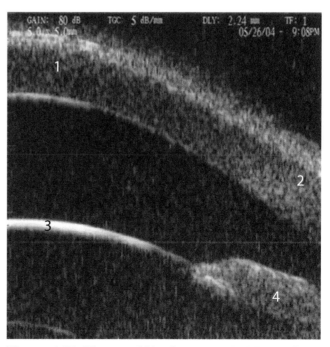

Figure 1.72 Ultrasound biomicroscopy (50-MHz probe). (1: Cornea with epithelium, stroma, and Descemet's membrane; 2: Sclera; 3: Anterior lens capsule; 4: Iris.)

the refractive power for intraocular lens implants in dogs,[105] cats,[106] and horses.[107]

An extension of the use of ultrasound has been color flow Doppler studies of the eye and orbit to study blood flow[108] and ultrasonic pachymetry to measure corneal thickness.[109]

Ocular centesis

Aqueous and vitreous centesis is performed frequently for cultures and cytology of intraocular disease.[110,111] Aqueous centesis can be performed under topical anesthesia in a cooperative patient, but most clinicians feel more comfortable using sedation. Aqueous humor centesis is performed with a 25- to 30-gauge needle entering the anterior chamber at the limbus, with the needle passing parallel with the iris (**Figure 1.73**). The "seal" on the syringe should be broken prior to passing the needle into the eye to avoid awkward movement when aspirating fluid. Unless the anterior chamber is collapsed, about 0.3 mL of aqueous humor can usually be aspirated. Centesis is used not only to obtain aqueous humor but may be used to vacuum cells off lesions on the iris and aspirate cystic lesions. Centesis of the anterior chamber is usually safe, but with opaque corneas or marked iris bombe, trauma to the iris, endothelium, or lens is more likely. (See **Table 1.7** for aqueous humor laboratory values.[110])

Cultures obtained from the aqueous may be negative with septic conditions because of the dilution and turnover of fluid. Vitreous is a more reliable culture media for septic endophthalmitis, but vitreous centesis has more inherent complications (hemorrhage and creation of retinal holes)

Table 1.7 **Baseline values for aqueous humor for the dog and cat.**

FACTOR	DOG	CAT
Refractive index	1.335	1.335
Protein content (mg/100 mL)	24–54	15–55
	11–55	–
Anterior chamber volume (mL)	0.4–0.6	0.6–0.9
	–	0.72
Cytology	Occasional mononuclear cell or melanocyte	

Source: Modified from Olin, 1977. *Journal of the American Veterinary Medical Association* 171:557.

and so is reserved for seriously diseased eyes. A 22-gauge needle is used due to the difficulty in aspirating formed vitreous. The needle is passed 6–8 mm posterior to the limbus in the lateral to dorsolateral quadrant where the pars plana is widest. The needle is pointed to the center of the eye (**Figure 1.74**) utilizing extreme care to avoid hitting the lens. The needle frequently needs repositioning to find pools of liquified vitreous.

Biomicroscopy

The advent of portable slit lamps has made biomicroscopy the standard for examination of the anterior segment. Otto Ueberreiter, an Austrian veterinarian, pioneered the use of the slit lamp in veterinary ophthalmology.[33,34,112]

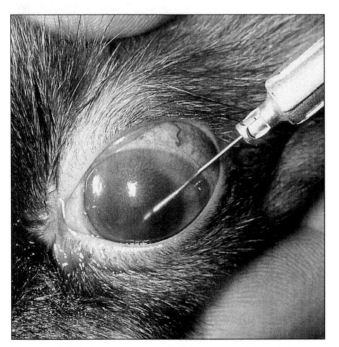

Figure 1.73 Aqueous centesis from a cat with uveitis.

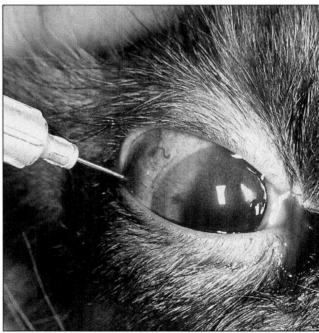

Figure 1.74 Vitreous centesis of a cat eye. Special care should be taken to avoid the lens.

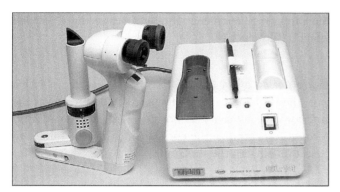

Figure 1.75 Kowa SL-14 slit lamp with recharging stations.

A variety of portable slit lamps are in use today; they range in price from $500 to $3500 (**Figure 1.75**). In veterinary medicine, where patient movement is inherent, a disadvantage of the newer slit lamp models is that the lowest magnification is often 10×, which is too high.

Biomicroscopic techniques

Slit lamps come in many variations, but all consist essentially of an illuminating system with a focused light that usually has various apertures to modify the color and the shape of the light beam and a microscope. The light can be rotated at various angles around the point of observation with the microscope. The slit lamp is unique in that the microscope and the light source have the same focal length (about 7–10 cm [2.8–4 in]). Before using, the oculars of the microscope should be adjusted for the PD of the examiner and the focus of the oculars adjusted by observing the light on a target rod. Some instruments have lines within the oculars to focus on. Because the light is focused, it is important to adjust the oculars for each individual so that the microscope and the light focus coincide. The target rod is located at the focal point of the light source, and the oculars are adjusted so that the margins of the light image are sharp in each ocular. In general, the clinician should utilize the least magnification possible and wider beam widths for preliminary examinations and should selectively utilize higher magnifications for minute lesions. The light beam is placed 20–30° from the axis of the microscope, and in most dogs, it is oriented from the temporal side of the eye because the nose interferes with placement of the light. The light can be utilized from either side in brachycephalic dogs, cats, and horses.

Most common illumination techniques
Direct focal illumination This is the most common form of slit lamp examination with the microscope and light beam focused on the same point. The advantage of the focused light beam is that the sharp demarcation of

illuminated and nonilluminated surfaces reduces scattered light that drowns out detail. When observing the cornea and lens, this produces a parallelepiped or a three-dimensional block of light as it traverses the tissue (**Figure 1.76**). Examination of solid structures such as the iris simply gives a magnified view with minimal glare. The parallelepiped of the cornea and lens allows visualization of the two surfaces of the tissue as well as the intervening tissue. As the surfaces of the cornea and lens are curved, specular reflections are produced. Specular reflections appear as bright reflections near the center of the vertical axis of the light beam. Examination with a broad light beam producing a parallelepiped gives a preliminary or overall impression. This is followed with the optic section, which is produced by narrowing the width of the light so that the block of light becomes two dimensional, namely length and depth (**Figure 1.76**). Coincidentally, the strength of the light usually must be increased. Examination of the tissue with the optic section allows exact localization in depth of lesions. When examining with an optic section, various zones of optical discontinuity can be observed in the cornea and lens.[35–37] The optic section is an *in vivo* histologic section at low magnification.

Retroillumination Retroillumination can be categorized as direct and indirect. Direct retroillumination examines structures or lesions against the background of the retroilluminated light (**Figure 1.13**); indirect retroillumination examines the retroilluminated structure against the adjacent dark background (**Figure 1.77**). The technique of retroillumination uses light that is reflected from deeper intraocular structures such as the iris or the fundus, while focusing the microscope on the nearer structures studied such as the cornea or the lens (**Figure 1.13**).[35–37] Retroillumination is an extremely sensitive and rapid method of detecting opacities

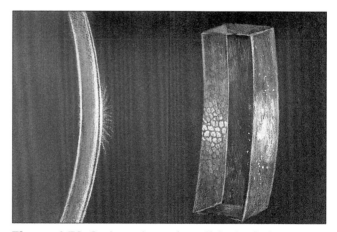

Figure 1.76 Optic section and parallelepiped of cornea. Note the specular reflections. The endothelium can be visualized with a quiet patient utilizing specular reflections.

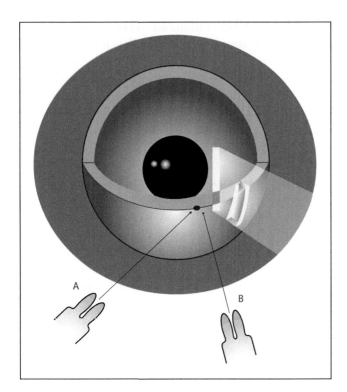

Figure 1.77 Direct and indirect retroillumination of a corneal lesion. At position A, direct retroillumination views the object in the cornea against the retroilluminated iris; at position B, the object is illuminated by the light but is examined against the dark nonilluminated iris. (Modified from Berliner, 1966. *Biomicroscopy of the Eye: Slit Lamp Microscopy of the Living Eye*, vol 1. Hafner Publishing: New York.)

of the clear media. Objects are observed because they obstruct, refract, or reflect light. Structures studied that obstruct light appear darker in direct retroillumination.

Oscillatory illumination Oscillatory illumination is a minor variation of direct focal illumination and retroillumination that utilizes the movement of the light source to study the dynamics of changing illumination on the structure or lesions.

Proximal or indirect illumination Proximal illumination utilizes a focused beam directed adjacent to the object being studied. Proximal illumination may determine the density of the lesion, that is solid versus cystic.

Focal pinpoint illumination The newer generations of slit lamps allow the examination of the anterior chamber with a pointed, focal light, which is a highly specific feature on the slit lamp dial settings. This pinpoint light source allows the detection of aqueous flare within the anterior chamber as a pathognomonic sign of intraocular inflammation. Aqueous flare is an accumulation of cells, causing

the physical phenomenon of light scattering ("Tyndall effect") (**Figure 1.14**).

Examination of the posterior segment In an eye with a lens, the slit lamp can only focus as far posteriorly as the anterior vitreous cavity. Contact or noncontact lenses may be used to neutralize the cornea and allow the fundus to be examined with the slit lamp.[113]

REFERENCES

1. Marfurt, C., Murphy, C., and Florczak, J. 2001. Morphology and neurochemistry of canine corneal innervation. *Investigative Ophthalmology and Visual Science* 42:2242–2251.
2. Reichard, M., Hovakimyan, M., Wree, A., Meyer-Lindenberg, A., Nolte, I., Junghans, C., Guthoff, R., and Stachs, O. 2010. Comparative *in vivo* confocal microscopical study of the cornea anatomy of different laboratory animals. *Current Eye Research* 53(12):1072–1080.
3. Hahnenberger, R.W. 1976. Influence of various anaesthetic drugs on the intraocular pressure of cats. *Albrecht von Graefes Arch Klin Exp Ophthalmol* 199:179–186.
4. Rubin, L. 1964. Auriculopalpebral nerve block as an adjunct to the diagnosis and treatment of ocular inflammation in the horse. *Journal of the American Veterinary Medical Association* 144:1387–1388.
5. Manning, J., St Clair, L. 1976. Palpebral, frontal, and zygomatic nerve blocks for examination of the equine eye. *Veterinary Medicine/Small Animal Clinician* 71:187–189.
6. Trim, C., Colbern, G., and Martin, C. 1985. Effects of xylazine and ketamine on intraocular pressure in horses. *Veterinary Record* 117:442–443.
7. Lowenstein, O., Murphy, S., and Loewenfeld, I. 1953. Functional evaluation of the pupillary light reflex pathways: Experimental pupillographic studies in cats. *Archives of Ophthalmology* 49:656–670.
8. Lucas, R.J., Douglas, R.H., and Foster, R.G. 2001. Characterization of an ocular photopigment capable of driving pupillary constriction in mice. *Nature Neuroscience* 4:621–626.
9. Hattar, S., Liao, H.W., Takao, M., Berson, D.M., and Yau, K.W. 2002. Melanopsin-containing retinal ganglion cells: Architecture, projections, and intrinsic photosensitivity. *Science* 295:1065–1070.
10. Panda, S., Nayak, S.K., Campo, B., Walker, J.R., Hogenesch, J.B., Jegla, T. 2005. Illumination of the melanopsin signaling pathway. *Science* 307:600–604.
11. Grozdanic, S.D., Kecova, H., and Lazic, T. 2013. Rapid diagnosis of retina and optic nerve abnormalities in canine patients with and without cataracts using chromatic pupil light reflex testing. *Vet Ophthalmol* 5:329–340.
12. Grozdanic, S.D., Matic, M., Sakaguchi, D.S., and Kardon, R.H. 2007. Evaluation of retinal status using chromatic pupil light reflex activity in healthy and diseased canine eyes. *Invest Ophthalmol Vis Sci* 48(11):5178–5183.
13. Petersen-Jones, S.M. 1989. Neuro-ophthalmology. *British Veterinary Journal* 145:99–120.
14. Hart, W.M. 1992. The eyelids. In: Hart, W, editor. *Adler's Physiology of the Eye* 9th Edition: Mosby Year Book: St. Louis, MO, pp. 1–17.

15. Scaglliotti, R.H. 1999. Comparative neuro-ophthalmology. In: Gelatt, K, editor. *Veterinary Ophthalmology.* Lippincott, Williams and Wilkins: Philadelphia, PA, pp. 1307–1400.

16. Rubin, L., Lynch, R.K., and Stockman, W.S. 1965. Clinical estimation of lacrimal function in dogs. *Journal of the American Veterinary Medical Association* 147:946–947.

17. Veith, L.A., Cure, T.H., and Gelatt, K.N. 1970. A simple and helpful diagnostic tool: The Schirmer tear test in cats. *Modern Veterinary Practice* 57:48–49.

18. Marts, B.S., Bryan, G.M., and Prieur, J. 1977. Schirmer tear test measurement and lysozyme concentration of equine tears. *Journal of Equine Medicine and Surgery* 1:427–430.

19. Williams, R.R., Manning, J.P., and Peiffer, R.L. 1979. The Schirmer tear test in the equine: Normal values and the contribution of the gland of the nictitating membrane. *Journal of Equine Medicine and Surgery* 3:117–119.

20. Berger, S.L., and King, V.L. 1998. The fluctuation of tear production in the dog. *Journal of the American Animal Hospital Association* 34:79–83.

21. Hamor, R.E., Roberts, S.M., Severin, G.A., and Chavkin, M.J. 2000. Evaluation of results for Schirmer tear tests conducted with and without application of a topical anesthetic in clinically normal dogs of five breeds. *American Journal of Veterinary Research* 61:1422–1425.

22. Hawkins, E.C., and Murphy, C.J. 1986. Inconsistencies in the absorptive capacities of Schirmer tear test strips. *Journal of the American Veterinary Medical Association* 188:511–513.

23. Hirsh, S., and Kaswan, R. 1995. A comparative study of Schirmer tear test strips in dogs. *Veterinary Comparative Ophthalmology* 5:215–217.

24. Woman, M., Gilger, B., Mueller, P., and Norris, K. 1995. Clinical evaluation of a new Schirmer tear test in the dog. *Veterinary Comparative Ophthalmology* 5:211–214.

25. Gelatt, K.N., Peiffer, R.L., Jr., Erickson, J.L., and Gum, G.G. 1975. Evaluation of tear formation in the dog, using a modification of the Schirmer tear test. *Journal of the American Veterinary Medical Association* 166:368–370.

26. Rubin, L.F., and Wolfes, R.L. 1962. Mydriatic for canine ophthalmoscopy. *Journal of the American Veterinary Medical Association* 140:137–141.

27. Gelatt, K.N., Boggess III, T.S., and Cure, T.H. 1973. Evaluation of mydriatics in the cat. *Journal of the American Animal Hospital Association* 9:283–287.

28. Willis, M., Martin, C.L., Stiles, J., and Chaffin, K. 1997. Acute, transient sialoadenomegaly in two cats following topical administration of tropicamide. *Veterinary Comparative Ophthalmology* 7:206–208.

29. Gelatt, K., Gum, G., and MacKay, E. 1995. Evaluation of mydriatics in horses. *Veterinary and Comparative Ophthalmology* 5(2):104–108.

30. Pascoe, P.J., Elkiw, J.E., Stiles, J., and Smith, E. 1994. Arterial hypertension associated with topical ocular use of phenylephrine in dogs. *Journal of the American Veterinary Medical Association* 205:1562–1564.

31. Taylor, N.R., Stanley, R.G., Vingrys, A.J., and Zele, A.J. 2007. Variation in intraocular pressure following application of tropicamide in three different dog breeds. *Veterinary Ophthalmology* 10:8–11.

32. Stadtbaumer, K., Frommlet, F., and Nell, B. 2006. Effects of mydriatics on intraocular pressure and pupil size in the normal feline eye. *Veterinary Ophthalmology* 9:233–237.

33. Ueberreiter, O. 1956. Augenuntersuchungsmethoden mit besonderer Berucksichtigung der Mikroskopie am lebenden Tierauge. *Wiener Tierarztliche Monatsschrift* 43:1–13.

34. Ueberreiter, O. 1956. Die Mikroskopie am lebenden Tierauge. *Wiener Tierarztliche Monatsschrift* 43:77–82.

35. Martin, C. 1969. Slit lamp examination of the normal canine anterior ocular segment. Part I. Introduction and technique. *Journal of Small Animal Practice* 10:143–149.

36. Martin, C. 1969. Slit lamp examination of the normal canine anterior ocular segment. Part II. Description. *Journal of Small Animal Practice* 10:151–162.

37. Martin, C. 1969. Slit lamp examination of the normal canine anterior ocular segment. Part III. Discussion and summary. *Journal of Small Animal Practice* 10:163–169.

38. Brown, M., Galland, J., Davidson, H., and Brightman, A. 1996. The phenol red thread tear test in dogs. *Veterinary Comparative Ophthalmology* 6:274–277.

39. Brown, M., Brightman, A., Butine, M., and Moore, T. 1997. The phenol red thread tear test in healthy cats. *Veterinary and Comparative Ophthalmology* 7(4):249–252.

40. Moore, C., and Collier, L. 1990. Ocular surface disease associated with loss of conjunctival goblet cells in dogs. *Journal of the American Animal Hospital Association* 26:458–465.

41. Lim, C.C., and Cullen, C.L. 2005. Schirmer tear test values and tear film break-up times in cats with conjunctivitis. *Veterinary Ophthalmology* 8(5):305–310.

42. Vaughan, D.G. 1955. Contamination of fluorescein solutions. *American Journal of Ophthalmology* 39:55–61.

43. Claoue, C. 1986. Experimental contamination of minims of fluorescein by *Pseudomonas aeruginosa*. *British Journal of Ophthalmology* 70:507–509.

44. Romanchuk, K.G. 1982. Fluorescein: Physicochemical factors affecting its fluorescence. *Survey of Ophthalmology* 26:269–283.

45. Gelatt, K.N. 1972. Vital staining of the canine cornea and conjunctiva with rose bengal. *Journal of the American Animal Hospital Association* 8:17–22.

46. Feenstra, R., and Tseng, S. 1992. Comparison of fluorescein and rose bengal staining. *Ophthalmology* 99:605–617.

47. Roat, M., Romanowski, E., Araullo-Cruz, T., and Gordon, J. 1987. The antiviral effects of rose bengal and fluorescein. *Archives of Ophthalmology* 105:1415–1417.

48. Jones, W.G. 1955. A preliminary report of the flora in health and disease of the external ear and conjunctival sac of the dog. *Journal of the American Veterinary Medical Association* 127:442–444.

49. Bistner, S.I., Roberts, S.R., and Anderson, R.P. 1969. Conjunctival bacteria: Clinical appearances can be deceiving. *Modern Veterinary Practice* 50:45–47.

50. Urban, M., Wyman, M., Reins, M., and Marraro, V. 1972. Conjunctival flora in clinically normal dogs. *Journal of the American Veterinary Medical Association* 161:201–206.

51. McDonald, P.J., and Watson, A.D.J. 1976. Microbial flora of normal canine conjunctivae. *Journal of Small Animal Practice* 17:809–812.

52. Murphy, J.M., Lavach, J.D., and Severin, G.A. 1978. Survey of conjunctival flora in dogs with clinical signs of external eye disease. *Journal of the American Veterinary Medical Association* 172:66–68.

53. Shewen, P.E., Povey, R.C., and Wilson, M.R. 1980. A survey of the conjunctival flora of clinically normal cats and cats with conjunctivitis. *Canadian Veterinary Journal* 21:231–233.

54. Hackner, D.V., Jensen, H.E., and Selby, L.A. 1979. A comparison of conjunctival culture techniques in the

dog. *Journal of the American Animal Hospital Association* 15:223–225.

55. Bauer, G., Speiss, B., and Lutz, H. 1966. Exfoliative cytology of conjunctiva and cornea in domestic animals: A comparison of four collecting techniques. *Veterinary Comparative Ophthalmology* 6:181–186.

56. Willis, M., Bounous, D., Kaswan, R. et al. 1997. Conjunctival brush cytology: Evaluation of a new cytological collection technique in dogs and cats with a comparison to conjunctival scraping. *Veterinary Comparative Ophthalmology* 7:74–81.

57. Lavach, J.D., Thrall, M.A., Benjamin, M.M., and Severin, G.A. 1977. Cytology of normal and inflamed conjunctivas in dogs and cats. *Journal of the American Veterinary Medical Association* 170:722–726.

58. Peiffer, R.L., Gelatt, K.N., Jessen, C.R., Gum, G.G., Swin, R.M., and Davis, J. 1977. Calibration of the Schiotz tonometer for the normal canine eye. *American Journal of Veterinary Research* 38:1881–1889.

59. Picket, J., Miller, P., and Majors, L. 1988. Calibration of the Schiotz tonometer for the canine and feline eye. *Proceedings of the American College of Veterinary Ophthalmology* 19:45–51.

60. Magrane, W.G. 1957. Canine glaucoma. I. Methods of diagnosis. *Journal of the American Veterinary Medical Association* 131:311–314.

61. Lovekin, L.G. 1964. Primary glaucoma in dogs. *Journal of the American Veterinary Medical Association* 145:1081–1091.

62. Vainisi, S.J. 1970. Tonometry and gonioscopy in the dog. *Journal of Small Animal Practice* 11:231–240.

63. Heywood, R. 1971. Intraocular pressures in the Beagle dog. *Journal of Small Animal Practice* 12:119–121.

64. Walde, V.I. 1982. Glaukom beim hunde. *Kleintier Praxis* 27:343–354.

65. Broadwater, J., Schorling, J.J., Herring, I.P., and Elvinger, F. 2008. Effect of body position on intraocular pressure in dogs without glaucoma. *American Journal of Veterinary Research* 69:527–530.

66. Khan, J.A., Davis, M., Graham, C.E., Trank, J., and Whitacre, M.M. 1991. Comparison of Oculab Tono-Pen readings obtained from various corneal and scleral locations. *Archives of Ophthalmology* 109:1444–1446.

67. Boothe, W., Lee, D., Panek, W., and Pettit, T. 1988. The Tono-Pen: A manometric and clinical study. *Archives of Ophthalmology* 106:1214–1217.

68. Priehs, D., Gum, G., Whitley, D., and Moore, L. 1990. Evaluation of three applanation tonometers in dogs. *American Journal of Veterinary Research* 51:1547–1550.

69. Miller, P., Pickett, P., Majors, L., and Kurzman, I. 1991. Evaluation of two applanation tonometers in cats. *American Journal of Veterinary Research* 52:1917–1921.

70. Miller, P.E., Pickett, J.P., Majors, L.J., and Kurzman, I.D. 1991. Clinical comparison of the Mackay-Marg and Tono-Pen applanation tonometer in the dog. *Progress in Veterinary and Comparative Ophthalmology* 1:171–176.

71. Gelatt, K.N., and MacKay, E.O. 1998. Distribution of intraocular pressure in dogs. *Veterinary Ophthalmology* 1:109–114.

72. Komaromy, A.M., Garg, C.D., Ying, G.S., and Liu, C. 2006. Effect of head position on intraocular pressure in horses. *American Journal of Veterinary Research* 67:1233–1235.

73. Millers, P., Pickett, P., and Majors, L. 1990. Evaluation of two applanation tonometers in horses. *American Journal of Veterinary Research* 51:935–937.

74. Knollinger, A.M., La Croix, N.C., Barrett, P.M., and Miller, P.E. 2005. Evaluation of a rebound tonometer for measuring intraocular pressure in dogs and horses. *Journal of the American Veterinary Medical Association* 227:244–248.

75. Leiva, M., Naranjo, C., and Pena, M.T. 2006. Comparison of the rebound tonometer (ICare[R]) to the applanation tonometer (Tono-Pen XL) in normotensive dogs. *Veterinary Ophthalmology* 9(1):17–21.

76. Rusanen, E. 2010. Evaluation of a rebound tonometer (Tonovet) in clinically normal cat eyes. *Veterinary Ophthalmology* 13:31–36.

77. Martin, C.L. 1969. Gonioscopy and anatomical correlations of drainage angle of the dog. *Journal of Small Animal Practice* 10:171–184.

78. Gelatt, K.N., and Ladds, P.W. 1971. Gonioscopy in dogs and cats with glaucoma and ocular tumors. *Journal of Small Animal Practice* 12:105.

79. Bedford, P.G.C. 1977. Gonioscopy in the dog. *Journal of Small Animal Practice* 18:615–629.

80. Murphy, C., and Howland, H. 1987. The optics of comparative ophthalmoscopy. *Vision Research* 27:599–607.

81. Havener, W.H. 1966. Ophthalmoscopic interpretation: A semi-programmed instruction sequence. *Notes* pp. 1–30.

82. Rubin, L.F. 1960. Indirect ophthalmology. *Journal of the American Veterinary Medical Association* 137:648–651.

83. Havener, W.H., and O'Dair, R.B. 1963. The indirect ophthalmoscope. *Eye, Ear, Nose & Throat Monthly* 42:41–52.

84. Goldbaum, M., Joondeph, H., Huamonte, F., and Peyman, G. 1980. Retinal examination and surgery. In: Peyman, G., Sanders, D., and Goldberg, M., editors. *Principles and Practice of Ophthalmology*, vol II. WB Saunders: Philadelphia, PA, pp. 988–1097.

85. Snead, M., Rubinstein, M., and Jacobs, P. 1992. The optics of fundus examination. *Survey of Ophthalmology* 36(6):439–445.

86. Havener, W.H., and Gloeckner, S. 1967. *Atlas of Diagnostic Techniques and Treatment of Retinal Detachment*. Mosby: St. Louis, MO, pp. 1–200.

87. Parry, H.B., Tansley, K., and Thomson, L.C. 1953. The electroretinogram of the dog. *Journal of Physiology* 120:28–40.

88. Rubin, L.F. 1967. Clinical electroretinography in dogs. *Journal of the American Veterinary Medical Association* 151:1456–1469.

89. Brown, K.T. 1968. The electroretinogram: Its components and their origins. *Vision Research* 8:633–677.

90. Tuntivanich, N., Mentzer, A.L., Eifler, D.M., Montiani-Ferreira, F., Forcier, J.Q., Johnson, C.A., and Petersen-Jones, S.M. 2005. Assessment of the dark-adaptation time required for recovery of electroretinographic responses in dogs after fundus photography and indirect ophthalmoscopy. *American Journal of Veterinary Research* 66:1798–1804.

91. Dawson, W.W., Maida, T.M., and Rubin, M.L. 1982. Human pattern-evoked retinal responses are altered by optic atrophy. *Investigative Ophthalmology and Visual Science* 22:796–803.

92. Sims, M., and Ward, D. 1992. Response of pattern-electroretinograms (PERGs) in dogs to alterations in the spatial frequency of the stimulus. *Progress in Veterinary and Comparative Ophthalmology* 2:106–112.

93. Sims, M., and Brooks, D. 1991. Changes in oscillatory potentials in the canine electroretinogram during

dark adaptation. *American Journal of Veterinary Research* 51:1580–1586.

94. Sims, M., Sackman, J., McLean, R., and Slaymaker, C. 1991. Effects of stimulus intensity and conditioning on the electroretinogram and oscillatory potentials in dark-adapted cats. *Progress in Veterinary and Comparative Ophthalmology* 1:177–185.

95. Gelatt, K.N., Henderson, J.D., Jr., and Steffen, G.R. 1976. Fluorescein angiography of the normal and diseased ocular fundi of the laboratory dog. *Journal of the American Veterinary Medical Association* 169:980–984.

96. Peruccio, C., Helper, L.C., Monti, F., and Brightman III, A.H. 1982. Fundus fluoroangiography in the cat. *Journal of the American Animal Hospital Association* 18:939–945.

97. Kommonen, B., and Koskinen, L. 1984. Fluorescein angiography of the canine ocular fundus in ketamine–xylazine anesthesia. *Acta Veterinaria Scandinavica* 25:346–351.

98. Rubin, L.F., and Koch, S.A. 1968. Ocular diagnostic ultrasonography. *Journal of the American Veterinary Medical Association* 153:1706–1716.

99. Hager, D.A., Dziezyc, J., and Millchamp, N.J. 1987. Two-dimensional real-time ocular ultrasonography in the dog. *Veterinary Radiology* 28:60–65.

100. Schiffer, S.P., Rantanen, N.W., Leary, G.A., and Bryan, G.M. 1987. Biometric study of the canine eye using A-mode ultrasonography. *American Journal of Veterinary Research* 43:826–830.

101. Cottrill, N., Banks, W., and Pecham, R. 1987. Ultrasonography and biometric evaluation of the eye and orbit of dogs. *American Journal of Veterinary Research* 50:898–903.

102. Bentley, E., Miller, P.E., and Diehl, K. 2003. Use of high-resolution ultrasound as a diagnostic tool in veterinary ophthalmology. *Journal of the American Veterinary Medical Association* 223(11):1617–1622.

103. Gibson, T., Roberts, S., Severin, G., Steyn, P., and Wrigley, R. 1998. Comparison of gonioscopy and ultrasound biomicroscopy for evaluating the iridocorneal angle in dogs. *Journal of the American Veterinary Medical Association* 213:635–638.

104. Ekesten, B. 1994. Biological variability and measurement error variability in ocular biometry in Samoyed dogs. *Acta Veterinaria Scandinavica* 35:427–433.

105. Gaiddon, J., Rosolen, S., Steru, L., Cook, C., and Peiffer, R. 1991. Use of biometry and keratometry for determining optimal power for intraocular lens implants in dogs. *American Journal of Veterinary Research* 52:781–783.

106. Gilger, B.C., Davidson, M.G., and Howardson, P.B. 1998. Keratometry, ultrasonic biometry and prediction of intraocular lens power in the feline eye. *American Journal of Veterinary Research* 59(2):131–134.

107. McMullen, R.J., and Gilger, B.C. 2006. Keratometry, biometry and prediction of intraocular lens power in the equine eye. *Veterinary Ophthalmology* 9(5):357–360.

108. Schmid, V., and Murisier, N. 1996. Color Doppler imaging of the orbit in the dog. *Veterinary Comparative Ophthalmology* 6:35–43.

109. Schoster, J., Wickman, L., and Stuhr, C. 1995. The use of ultrasonic pachymetry and computer enhancement to illustrate the collective corneal thickness profile of 25 cats. *Veterinary Comparative Ophthalmology* 5:68–77.

110. Olin, D.D. 1977. Examination of the aqueous humor as a diagnostic aid in anterior uveitis. *Journal of the American Veterinary Medical Association* 171:557.

111. Hazel, S.J., Thrall, M.A.H., Severin, G.A., Lauerman, L.H., Jr., and Lavach, J.D. 1985. Laboratory evaluation of aqueous humor in the healthy dog, cat, horse, and cow. *American Journal of Veterinary Research* 46:657–659.

112. Ueberreiter, O. 1959. Examination of the eye and eye operations in animals. In: *Advances in Veterinary Sciences*, vol. 5. Academic Press, New York, pp. 1–80.

113. Berliner, M.L. 1966. *Biomicroscopy of the Eye: Slit Lamp Microscopy of the Living Eye*. Vol 1. Hafner Publishing, New York.

CHAPTER 2

OPHTHALMIC PHARMACOLOGY

BERNHARD M. SPIESS

ROUTES OF ADMINISTRATION

Topical

Topical administration is the usual route associated with ophthalmic drugs. Some of the many factors to consider when selecting a drug for topical therapy are: what is the target tissue and can the drug reach the targeted tissue in therapeutic levels; is the drug available in ophthalmic form; what form of topical drug to use if it is available in more than one form; what is the desired frequency of administration and practicality of it being administered; owner compliance; patient cooperation; comparative cost of medications; and potential side effects and toxicities.

Ability to penetrate the intact cornea

The intact cornea consists of the epithelium, which has a high lipid content; the stroma, which has a high water content; and the endothelium, which also has a high lipid content. Most drugs penetrate the cornea by a process of passive diffusion, which depends on concentration gradients, solubility characteristics, and for ionizable molecules, the dissociation constant.[1] A drug applied topically must have a differential solubility in water and lipid to penetrate the intact cornea.[2,3] Many drugs do not possess this characteristic; for instance, antibiotics are mainly water soluble, with the notable exception of chloramphenicol and the sulfonamides. The solubility of a drug may sometimes be improved by combining it with certain organic salts (glucocorticoids with acetate) or by producing a prodrug, or chemical derivative of the drug, manipulated to improve a certain characteristic such as solubility, which once absorbed is regenerated into the parent compound (dipivalyl epinephrine to epinephrine). Surfactants, such as benzalkonium chloride, which is a frequent preservative in ophthalmic solutions, also enhance absorption through the epithelial barrier by their epithelial toxicity. The main lipid barrier is broken with ulcerations and lacerations so that in these conditions the water-soluble antibiotics may attain therapeutic concentrations. In conditions such as corneal abscesses, the epithelium may be debrided to enhance drug penetration. In rabbits, removal of 25%–50% of the corneal epithelium increases the drug concentration in the cornea and aqueous ninefold. Defects larger than 50% do not further increase the drug concentrations.[4] In general, topical therapy achieves therapeutic drug levels only on the ocular surface and as far posteriorly as the iris–ciliary body. Topical therapy should not be relied on for posterior segment diseases.[5,6] An exception may be the newer nonsteroidal anti-inflammatory drugs such as nepafenac, the pharmacokinetics of which suggest a potential use in the treatment of posterior disease.[7]

Frequency of application

The frequency of therapy varies with the severity of the condition, the vehicle used, and the duration of action of the drug administered. For instance, one instillation of atropine in the normal eye can maintain mydriasis for 3–4 + days, whereas in an eye with iritis, mydriasis may require instillation three to four times per day. Antibiotics used for minor infections or prophylaxis may be given every 8–12 hours, but for an infected corneal ulcer, the concentration may be increased, and it may be used hourly or by constant infusion.

Placement of topical drugs

Most containers are multiple use and may be used on different patients. Care must be taken so that the container nozzle does not touch the hair or the cornea and become contaminated. A solution should be applied so that the drop falls onto the eye rather than have the container held into the eye and squeezed. The amount of fluid that the conjunctival cul-de-sac can accommodate is about 30 μL, and this is often exceeded by one drop from an ordinary bottle. The moral is that one drop, if it hits the eye, is more than enough, and two drops are excessive, wasteful, and increase the potential for systemic side effects from nasolacrimal absorption.[1] To minimize washout by subsequent drops, if more than one preparation is being given to a patient, a 5- to 10-minute interval should be observed between drops.

Ointments are harder to quantitate but a 1-cm (0.25- to 0.5-in) ribbon of ointment is adequate. After application, it is almost a reflex action to rub the ointment over the cornea, but this should be avoided as it is traumatic, particularly if an ulcer is present.

Vehicle

The vehicle chosen for topical therapy may be a solution, a suspension, an ointment, or a solid ocular insert. The advantages and disadvantages of solutions and ointments are outlined in **Tables 2.1 and 2.2**. Comparable preparations in different vehicles are usually quite acceptable, and it is often a matter of personal preference.

Excipients of topical drugs

Excipients are the therapeutically inactive ingredients in drugs, but they are often critical to the success of the preparation. Excipients in topical medications are used to buffer, maintain sterility, prevent oxidation, and increase absorption. The pH of the preparation may be buffered by products such as acetic, boric, or hydrochloric acid or bicarbonate, borates, citrates, and phosphates to increase the nonionized form of the drug to improve lipid solubility, to increase the drug's stability, and to improve ocular comfort. The viscosity of the solution may be altered by vehicles such as polyvinyl alcohol, polyvinylpyrrolidone, and various forms of methylcellulose; in general, the goal is to increase the corneal contact time with the drug by slowing lacrimal drainage. Surfactants such as benzalkonium chloride are frequently found in ophthalmic solutions, and they act as antibacterial agents or preservatives, increase the solubility of hydrophobic agents, and enhance corneal penetration by their epitheliotoxic

Table 2.1 Advantages and disadvantages of solutions and suspensions.

Advantages

- Less disturbance of vision (questionable importance in veterinary medicine).
- Lower incidence of contact dermatitis.
- Less toxic to interior eye if an unsealed perforating corneal injury is present.
- May be easier to apply for some owners, especially in small animals.

Disadvantages

- Very short contact time (30 seconds), necessitates frequent application.[8,1] Important when considering owner compliance, as the more frequent the application, the less likely it is to be performed.
- Diluted out in irritated eyes with epiphora.
- Often more expensive for short-term therapy when compared with a comparable ointment.
- Suspensions often need excessive shaking to mix and deliver the intended dose.
- Systemic absorption from nasolacrimal duct drainage is greater than ointments.[8]

Table 2.2 Advantages and disadvantages of ointments.

Advantages

- Longer contact time, which means less frequent therapy and higher drug concentrations are usually delivered.
- Not diluted out by epiphora.
- Protects the cornea from exposure and keeps it moist better than solutions.
- Softens crusts and discharges.
- Easier to apply in large animals.
- Often less expensive than the comparable solution.

Disadvantages

- Add to the amount of discharge material from the eye.
- More difficult for some owners to apply.
- Higher incidence of contact dermatitis.
- More toxic to the endothelium if a penetrating injury is present.
- Interfere with epithelial healing more than solutions. However, this is controversial, and some studies have found no significant difference, or, if present, it is not clinically significant.[9]
- Imprecise dosage.
- More difficult to sterilize.
- Drug release from the vehicle is variable so that prolonged contact time may be negated, that is, 0.1% sodium dexamethasone phosphate solution penetrates better than the ointment.[10,9]

action. Other preservatives used are chlorhexidine, chlorobutanol, and thiomersal.

Agents such as dextrans, glycerine, and sodium chloride are added to solutions to bring the tonicity to a physiologic range of approximately 0.9% to minimize ocular discomfort. Antioxidants such as sulfites and EDTA are added to prevent degradation of many drugs to an inactive form by sunlight and oxygen (e.g., epinephrine, proparacaine). In suspensions, the particles that hold the active ingredient are excipients.[11,12]

Packaging of topical medications

To avoid confusion in identifying topical solutions, by convention they are coded by cap colors: mydriatics and cycloplegics are red; miotics are green; carbonic anhydrase inhibitors (CAIs) are orange; β blockers are yellow or blue; glucocorticoids are pink; nonsteroidal anti-inflammatory drugs (NSAIDs) are gray; and anti-infective agents are tan or brown.[6]

Alternative topical delivery systems

Membrane-controlled delivery system

A polymeric membrane containing a reservoir of drug can be placed into the conjunctival cul-de-sac, and this allows the drug to diffuse out at a predictable rate. The rate and duration vary depending on the design. Such delivery systems are commercially available for a few drugs such as pilocarpine and epinephrine, which are used in glaucoma treatment, and these allow placement only once a week into the eye. The drug release is small, but the effect is equal to or better than the pulsed therapy of a drop at intervals. Because of the lower concentration of drug released, the undesirable side effects are not noted.[13] The commercial designs have not been satisfactory in the dog or cat as the third eyelid usually catches on the reservoir and flips it out of the cul-de-sac. It is also a relatively expensive means of therapy, particularly for its main use in treating glaucoma, which is a lifetime therapy.

Pellets

Solid pellet-like particles of methylcellulose that dissolve slowly in the conjunctival cul-de-sac are commercially available. The main purpose is to give a slow continuous release, but in domestic animals, the third eyelid often flips them out of the cul-de-sac.[14]

Collagen inserts

Antibiotics impregnated into collagen inserts designed as rings to be inserted into the conjunctival cul-de-sac have been experimentally utilized in cattle. Mechanical design and physical properties of the collagen produce difficulties that have prevented successful application.[15] Collagen shields, which when hydrated appear as soft contact lenses, are on the market for the cat and the dog. They slowly dissolve over 3–5 days and may act as a drug reservoir when soaked in water-soluble drugs such as antibiotics. The pharmacokinetics vary with each drug and cannot be anticipated but in general are comparable to frequent topical applications. Caution should be exercised as the preservatives in the preparation are often toxic, and they will also be increased in concentration.

Soft contact lens

A soft contact lens can be soaked in water-soluble drugs and used as a drug reservoir. Caution should be taken with preparations containing preservatives as these may reach toxic levels if there is prolonged contact.[16]

Continuous and intermittent irrigation

A tube placed into the conjunctival cul-de-sac and brought out through either lid (subpalpebral lavage, SPL) or placed in the nasolacrimal duct and exiting through the false nostril can be used as a means of applying drops to an uncooperative patient.[17,18] In the past, when the tubes and footplates had to be fashioned individually, there were significant complications with the tube or the footplate rubbing on the cornea when the tube was placed in the upper lid.[19] As a result of the complications, clinicians advocated utilizing the lower medial lid (**Figure 2.1**) where the third eyelid would protect the cornea or the nasolacrimal duct.[18,20] With the advent of a commercial source of SPL sets (Mila International,),

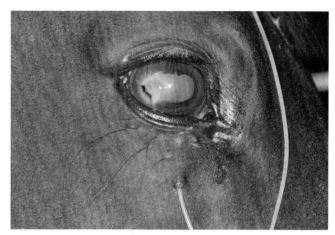

Figure 2.1 Right eye of a horse with a subpalpebral lavage system inserted through the inferior eyelid. The footplate of the tube rests between palpebral conjunctiva and third eyelid to avoid corneal irritation.

corneal ulcerations from rubbing of the footplate on the cornea have become uncommon. The placement of a SPL has become routine in treating horses with painful ocular disease that requires therapy over a prolonged period. Medication is placed in the tube (0.1–0.2 mL) and then pushed through with a bolus of air. Some horses object to the passage of air into the cul-de-sac and may require larger amounts of medication or a flush with saline to push the medication onto the eye. These latter methods increase the volume of drug and the expense or run the risk of diluting the medications.

When administering multiple medications, it is tempting to combine them in one solution. *In vitro* antimicrobial testing of solutions combining gentamicin, tobramycin, miconazole, and atropine for 6 hours did not demonstrate any decrease in effectiveness against *Pseudomonas* spp. or *Aspergillus* spp.[21]

Two basic techniques exist for applying SPL. The first is a two-hole system where the tubing is looped into and back out of the conjunctival cul-de-sac, with one or more holes placed in the portion of the tube exposed to the cul-de-sac. Placing the tube is difficult and requires two punctures by a needle trocar (**Figure 2.2**); this technique was popular before the advent of commercial SPL kits. The second technique is a single-hole SPL system that utilizes a silicone tube with a footplate. Both types of SPL require placement of the holes at the fornix or furthest extreme of the conjunctival cul-de-sac of the upper or preferably the lower eyelid to avoid ulceration. The injection end of the tubing is placed on a braided portion of the mane with a tongue depressor and tape. The tubing is held in place with taped "butterflies" that are sutured to the skin. The placement of the first butterfly close to the eye is the most critical in keeping the tube pulled up away from

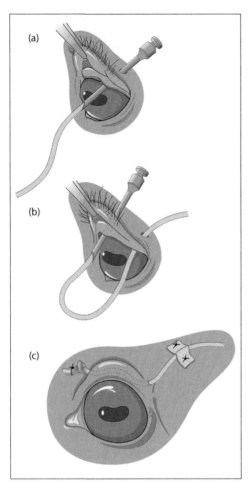

Figure 2.2 Two-hole method of placing a subpalpebral lavage in the horse. The initial hole is created by a 14 gauge needle to thread tubing through (the direction can also be reversed) (a). Placement of a second hole to thread tubing through back onto the lid (b). A knot is tied at the end of the tubing to secure with a suture, and a hole made in the tubing traversing the conjunctival cul-de-sac; taped butterflies are sutured to the skin (c).

the cornea. The tubing is slipped through the barrel of a tuberculin syringe and a blunt 22-gauge catheter threaded onto the tubing. The catheter is seated snugly into the barrel of the tuberculin syringe and a catheter cap placed on the catheter (**Figure 2.3**).

Commercial SPL kits are now available, so they do not have to be custom made. SPL units can be applied for several weeks, but they must be monitored for placement, infection, and function. In a series of 156 SPL placements of a custom-made tube, serious complications requiring premature removal developed in 16% of the placements.[19] One of the most common complications, subconjunctival migration of the footplate, is minimized by using a commercial SPL kit with a larger footplate, which also decreases the rate of corneal ulceration.

Alternatively, in the horse it is easy to place a tube in the nasolacrimal duct and flush retrograde with medications, although the tube is not as well tolerated. Nasolacrimal catheters require larger volumes of medication to reach the eye, and more of the medication is likely to reflux back as the tube does not reach the conjunctival cul-de-sac.

A micropump hooked to the subpalpebral unit delivers medications in a continuous manner. The micropump may be mechanical, for example, the Cormed ambulatory infusion pump (Medina, NY), elastomeric, or osmotic. The osmotic pump may be implanted subcutaneously and connected to a SPL or placed subconjunctivally after priming with medication. Tissue fluids are drawn around the drug reservoir, resulting in pressure that pushes the drug out at a calculated rate for up to 7 days. The amount and duration of medication varies depending on the size of the pump.[22–24] An external elastomeric pump is commercially available that delivers 0.5 mL/h and avoids the need for dissection (Mila International). The pump holds up to 125 mL of medication, but the calculated delivery rate is affected by the temperature and the viscosity of the medication. Pumps are a great work saver when only giving one medication or if several medications are to be given at the same high dosing rate. However, when using multiple medications, drugs are often given on varying dosing schedules. Also, even inexpensive drugs may become expensive when administered in the quantities necessary for continuous infusion.

Subconjunctival

Injection of a drug under the bulbar conjunctiva is also usually under Tenon's capsule, and consequently, the drug is deposited against the sclera, thus bypassing the lipid barrier that the intact cornea presents. Penetration of the drug is mainly by simple diffusion through the sclera, although leakage through the needle hole and topical absorption does occur.[5,6] The use of repositol or long-acting products can produce a prolonged therapeutic effect, but there is nothing inherent in the route that allows the drugs to last for long periods of time. Most animals can have the injection performed under topical anesthesia (**Figure 2.4**). Injection in the usual anterior location achieves therapeutic levels only in the anterior segment, although if injected posteriorly, therapeutic retinal levels may be achieved.[25] Injection of a drug subconjunctivally in the palpebral conjunctiva, as is frequently performed in food animal medicine, loses the advantage of being absorbed through the sclera. Drug uptake is probably topical through leakage from the needle hole and systemic from vascular uptake.

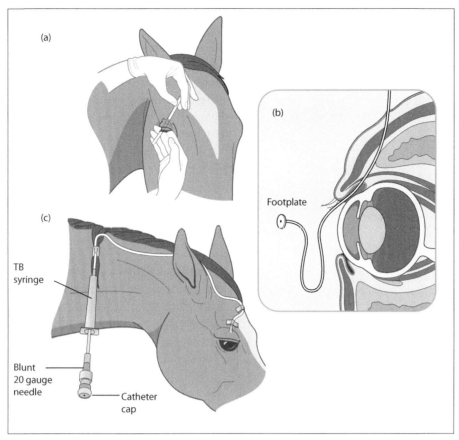

Figure 2.3 Single-hole method of placing subpalpebral lavage system in the horse. A hubless needle trochar is placed in the fornix and through the lid (a). Tubing is threaded into the trochar and pulled through the lid. A cross-section illustration to show placement of tubing in the fornix or as high up in the conjunctival sac as possible (b). The footplate is pulled up to the fornix, taped, and sutured in place and a tuberculin syringe used to stabilize the distal end of the tubing (c). The tubing is threaded into the needle end of a tuberculin syringe barrel, and a blunt 22-g cannula is threaded into the tubing; the hub of the cannula seats or fits snugly into the tuberculin syringe. A catheter cap is added to the cannula; the syringe is then taped to a tongue depressor, and the unit is taped to a piece of braided mane.

Advantages

- Aqueous products can be absorbed into the eye.
- If repositol-type products are used, a prolonged drug level can be obtained without the bother of frequent topical medication.

Disadvantages

- Perforation of the globe with the needle can occur.
- Many drugs are irritating.
- If repositol products are used, it is difficult to discontinue therapy, for instance to stop steroids if they become contraindicated.
- Increased systemic absorption and potential side effects.

Intraocular or intracameral administration

Intraocular injections are given when heroic means are needed to control a problem. The dangers of the trauma of injection plus the toxicity of many drugs to the corneal endothelium, lens, and retina must be balanced against the therapeutic benefit. The concentration of drugs is drastically reduced when intraocular injections are utilized. The injection can be in either the anterior chamber (intracameral) or the vitreous, or both, depending on the condition (see section Ocular centesis, for site). Intravitreal injections are often the only means of achieving significant drug levels in the vitreous.

The most common drugs administered intracamerally are antibiotics for endophthalmitis and tissue plasminogen activator for fibrin formation. Intravitreal implants of polymers surrounding an antiviral drug have been used in humans to treat cytomegalovirus retinitis. Experimentally in horses, cyclosporine intravitreal implants have been used to treat recurrent uveitis (ERU), and implants have been designed to achieve therapeutic cyclosporine levels for up to 10 years.[26,27] Because of serious side effects, a suprachoroidal cyclosporine-releasing device has since been developed and implanted successfully in many horses with ERU.[28]

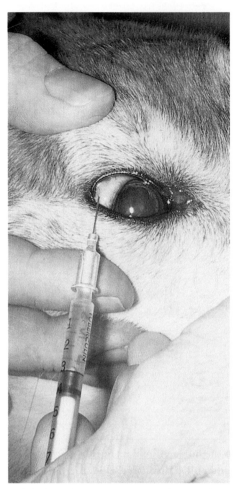

Figure 2.4 Subconjunctival injection being administered in a dog under topical anesthesia with a 25-gauge needle.

Retrobulbar injection

Retrobulbar injection is an infrequent route of drug administration, although this may be a route to obtain good drug levels in the optic nerve, vitreous, and posterior pole.[29] Systemic absorption is significant, with serum drug levels comparable to levels given by systemic routes.[30] Air or positive contrast material may be injected retrobulbarly for radiographic studies of the orbit. With the availability of computed tomography (CT) and magnetic resonance imaging (MRI), these contrast techniques are now rarely utilized. In the horse, retrobulbar local anesthesia is used to position the eye better and decrease ocular movements, thus allowing lighter general anesthesia, or to facilitate surgical procedures in standing horses.[31,32] Retrobulbar injections of anesthetics have also been shown to decrease postoperative pain after enucleation in dogs.[33] However, this is not without possible complications.[34]

Systemic

The systemic route is usually used to achieve therapeutic drug levels in the posterior segment and the optic nerve. Just as in the cornea, the posterior and anterior segments have barriers in the normal eye that limit the penetration of many drugs. A blood–aqueous humor barrier exists in tight cellular junctions of the ciliary body nonpigmented epithelium[35] and iris vascular endothelium, and a blood–retinal barrier exists due to tight junctions in the retinal vascular endothelium and the retinal pigment epithelium.[36,37] These barriers require lipid-soluble drugs to penetrate in the healthy eye, but with inflammation, the barriers become more permeable. Systemic therapy is given when the drug is needed in the posterior segment, severe anterior segment disease is present, or it is the only route available for the desired drug.

ANTIMICROBIAL AGENTS

Considerations in selecting an antimicrobial agent

Spectrum of activity and mode of action of the drug

When the infectious agent is unknown, a broad-spectrum agent or combination product is often used. A preliminary selection of antibiotics is made based on the presence and morphology of bacteria in scrapings or aspirates, combined with previous experience or published studies on sensitivity patterns.[38–40] Devastating intraocular infections require a bactericidal antibiotic to stop the infection as quickly as possible. Antimicrobial antagonisms are theoretically possible, but due to the very specific timing and dose relationships that are required, clinical antimicrobial antagonism is uncommon.[41]

When used prophylactically or for mild surface infections, potent antibiotics should not be used because drug resistance is encouraged.

Where is the agent needed?

The target area for the antimicrobial agent determines the route, the frequency of administration, and often the drug used, based on its known ability to penetrate the various barriers.

Patient comfort

Some preparations such as sulfonamides routinely sting and result in poor owner compliance. Cats are unpredictable in their tolerance to a particular topical antibiotic (gentamicin drops are often not tolerated), and inflammation may increase the irritation for many drugs.

Potential hypersensitivity to an antibiotic

Patients potentially may develop a systemic hypersensitivity to an antibiotic that is used topically and thus preclude future systemic use of that antibiotic. This is a major consideration in humans but less of a concern in animals. Alternatively, certain antibiotics such as neomycin are prone to produce topical hypersensitivity reactions or, rarely, a systemic anaphylactic reaction.

Development of a severe keratitis and/or blepharitis after initiating therapy should prompt the clinician to consider that the reaction is drug induced.

Indications for antimicrobial agents

Topical antibiotics are used for infections or suspected infective processes involving the lids, conjunctiva, cornea, anterior chamber, iris, and ciliary body. The number of antibiotics commercially available as ophthalmic preparations is limited, particularly for resistant Gram-positive organisms. In these cases, it is necessary to formulate topical preparations (often cephalosporins) from systemic antibiotics. The frequency of administration should be at least three to four times a day and may be hourly, depending on the severity and consequences of the infection (blindness with intraocular infection, progressive ulceration). In severe infections, the commercial topical solution may be fortified with the systemic form of the antibiotic to increase the antibiotic concentration. Experimental infections have confirmed the increased efficacy of fortified preparations; for instance, tobramycin and gentamicin have been recommended at a fourfold increase from the commercial topical preparations.[42,43]

The antibiotic selected depends on the sensitivity (known or suspected) of the organism and where the drug is needed. (See **Table 2.3** for intraocular penetration of antibiotics in the nonulcerated, noninflamed eye.) The fluoroquinolone antibiotics have become popular antibiotics when a broad-spectrum and bactericidal antibiotic is needed either systemically or topically. Ofloxacin has become the topical fluoroquinolone of choice because it penetrates the intact cornea better than other fluoroquinolones.[44] The main therapeutic weakness of the fluoroquinolones is their lack of effectiveness against Streptococci. The fourth-generation fluoroquinolones (moxifloxacin and gatifloxacin) have improved their efficacies against Gram-positive organisms while maintaining the similar effectiveness of older fluoroquinolones to Gram-negative organisms. Moxifloxacin penetrates the ocular barriers two to three times better than gatifloxacin and the older generations of fluoroquinolones.[45,46] The fluoroquinolones are also reported to inhibit keratocyte proliferation and produce cytotoxicity in tissue culture preparations.[47] Systemic fluoroquinolones, specifically enrofloxacin, have been associated with acute blindness in cats[48] (see Chapter 14). The toxicity affects the outer half of the retina and appears to be dose dependent. Risk factors are IV dosing, long-term administration, and aged animals.[49]

Table 2.3 **Intraocular penetration of antibacterial agents.**[50-57,59-70]

AGENT	SYSTEMIC	TOPICAL	SUBCONJUNCTIVAL
Penicillin	Fair	Poor	Good
Ampicillin	Poor	Poor	Good
Amoxicillin	Good	Poor	Good
Ciprofloxacin	Good	Poor	–
Ofloxacin	Good	Poor	–
Methicillin	Good	–	Good
Erythromycin	Poor	Good	Good
Cephalosporin	Poor	Poor	Good
Colistin	Poor	Poor	Good
Gentamicin	Poor	Poor	Good
Tobramycin	Poor	Poor	Good
Kanamycin	Poor	Poor	Poor
Amikacin	Good	?	? probably
Lincomycin	Good	–	–
Neomycin	–	Poor	Poor
Chloramphenicol	Poor/fair	Good	Good
Tetracycline	Poor	Good	Good
Minocycline	Good	?	? probably
Bacitracin	–	Poor	Poor
Rosacin	Poor	Good	Good
Polymyxin	–	Poor	Poor
Trimethoprim/ Sulfadiazine	Good	–	–
Sulfonamide	Good	Good	Good

Sources: Compiled from Bloome, M.A. et al. 1976. *Archives of Ophthalmology* 83:78–8350; Rowley, R.A., and Rubin, L.F. 1970. *American Journal of Veterinary Research* 31:43–49; Axelrod, A.J., and Peyman, G.A. 1973. *American Journal of Ophthalmology* 76:584–588; May, D.R. et al. 1974. *Archives of Ophthalmology* 91:487–489; Pohjanpelto, P.E.J. et al. 1974. *British Journal of Ophthalmology* 58:606–608; Purnell, W.D., and McPherson Jr., S.D. 1974. *American Journal of Ophthalmology* 77:578–582; Rieder, J. et al. 1974. *Albrecht von Graefes Archiv fur Klinische und Experimentelle Ophthalmologie* 190:51–61; Faigenbaum, S.J. et al. 1976. *American Journal of Ophthalmology* 82:598–603; Zachary, I.G., and Forster, R.K. 1976. *American Journal of Ophthalmology* 82:604–611; George, F.J., and Hanna, C. 1977. *Archives of Ophthalmology* 95:879–882; Barza, M.B. et al. 1978. *American Journal of Ophthalmology* 85:541–547; Kluge, R.M., and Zimmerman, T. 1978. *Annals of Ophthalmology* 10:1248–1251; Hillman, J.S. et al. 1979. *British Journal of Ophthalmology* 63:794–796; Saunders, J.H., McPherson Jr., S.D. et al. 1980. *American Journal of Ophthalmology* 89:564–566; Sigel, C.W. et al. 1981. *Veterinary Medicine/Small Animal Clinician* 76:991–993; Borden, T.B., and Cunningham, R.D. 1982. *American Journal of Ophthalmology* 93:107–110; Hulem, C.D. et al. 1982. *Archives of Ophthalmology* 100:646–649; Tabbara, K.F. et al. 1983. *Archives of Ophthalmology* 101:1426–1428; Wingfield, D.L. et al. 1983. *Archives of Ophthalmology* 101:117–120; Jay, W.M. et al. *Archives of Ophthalmology* 102:430–432.

In addition to topical antibiotics, systemic and subconjunctival antibiotics may be used in severe anterior segment infections, and the systemic route is indicated for posterior segment infections. **Table 2.4** presents appropriate antibiotic dosages for subconjunctival injections. Fluoroquinolones, specifically enrofloxacin, should be used cautiously in cats and avoided when other antibiotics would be just as effective. When utilized, a dose of 2.5 mg/kg every 12 hours is recommended, and fundus examination should be performed on a weekly basis.

Intraocular antibiotics are given for intraocular infections or to destroy the aqueous humor secreting capacity of the eye. The concentration of antibiotic is critical and must be supported by research data rather than estimates (**Table 2.5**). Gentamicin can be tolerated at a maximum dose of 350–400 µg inside the eye. The larger dose is given for bacterial endophthalmitis and may save the eye if given early. Intravitreal injection is the only route that produces high vitreous drug levels, and therapeutic levels may remain for 48–72 hours.[53,70] Higher doses destroy the retina and produce cataracts. Doses of 25–35 mg of gentamicin injected into the vitreous destroy the ciliary epithelium and result in decreased, or cessation of, aqueous humor production. Intravitreal gentamicin has been used as a chemical means of treating some forms of advanced glaucoma with permanent blindness,[71] but it should not be used in the functioning eye because this concentration will

Table 2.5 Intraocular antibiotic dosages.[52,53,70,74,108,109]

AGENT	DOSAGE
Amikacin	500 µg
Amphotericin B	1–5 µg
Cefazolin	2.25 mg
Cephalothin	2 mg
Cephaloridine	250 µg
Ciprofloxacin	100 µg
Gentamicin	350–400 µg
Methicillin	<10 mg
Moxalactam	1.25 mg

Sources: Compiled from Axelrod, A.J., and Peyman, G.A. 1973. *American Journal of Ophthalmology* 76:584–588; ; May, D.R. et al. 1974. *Archives of Ophthalmology* 91:487–489; Zachary, I.G., and Forster, R.K. 1976. *American Journal of Ophthalmology* 82:604–611; Rutgard, J.J. et al. 1978. *Annals of Ophthalmology* 10:293–298; Fisher, J.P. et al. 1982. *Archives of Ophthalmology* 100:650–652; Fett, D.R. et al. 1984. *Archives of Ophthalmology* 102:435–438; Talamo, J.H. et al. 1986. *Archives of Ophthalmology* 104:1483–1485.

also destroy the retina. In one series,[72] 9% of injected eyes developed phthisis an average of 15 months post injection, and in 65% of the eyes, glaucoma was controlled. In eyes that required a second injection, the success rate was 50%.

Intravitreal aminoglycoside antibiotics vary in toxicity: gentamicin > tobramycin > amikacin = kanamycin.[73] Due to the emergence of Gram-negative organisms resistant to gentamicin and the lower retinal toxicity of amikacin, 400–500 µg of amikacin intravitreally has been recommended over gentamicin for treating endophthalmitis.[74]

Paromomycin, an aminoglycoside antibiotic that is poorly absorbed from the gut and used to treat enteric protozoal infections, produced acute renal failure, cataracts, and deafness in cats after a 5-day course of oral therapy.[75] Three of four cats developed severe cataracts, which were noted by the owners a few weeks after antibiotic therapy.

Due to the limited effectiveness of aminoglycosides against Gram-positive organisms, a cephalosporin is often concurrently injected.

Table 2.4 Subconjunctival antibiotic dosages.

AGENT	DOSAGE
Ampicillin	50–250 mg
Amphotericin B	125 µg
Bacitracin	10,000 U
Carbenicillin	100 mg
Cefazolin	50 mg
Cephaloridine	100 mg
Cephalothin	50–100 mg
Chloramphenicol	50–100 mg
Colistin	15–37.5 mg
Erythromycin	100 mg
Gentamicin	10–20 mg
Tobramycin	10 mg
Lincomycin	150 mg
Methicillin	150–200 mg
Neomycin	250–500 mg
Penicillin G	$0.5–1.0 \times 10^6$
Polymixin B	10 mg
Streptomycin	50–100 mg
Tetracycline	2.5–5.0 mg

The selection of topical antibiotics is not as varied as one might anticipate, resulting in the need to improvise in concentration and compounding of systemic preparations when resistant organisms are encountered. Fortunately, many disease processes break down the barriers to drug absorption, allowing therapeutic levels of antibiotics to be achieved that might otherwise not be effective.

Antibiotic prophylaxis

Topical antibiotics are frequently administered for 1–3 days after lid, conjunctival, and corneal surgery. Also, whenever there is a break in the corneal epithelium (ulcer or laceration), whether or not it is associated with infection, it is routine to use prophylactic topical antibiotics to prevent the native bacterial flora from becoming established in traumatized tissue.[76] Newer antibiotics should not be used indiscriminately for routine prophylaxis to help avoid the development of resistant organisms to the drug. In the horse, which is predisposed to fungal keratitis after corneal ulceration, prophylaxis is often extended to the use of antifungal antibiotics. Subconjunctival and systemic prophylactic antibiotics are also given before and after intraocular surgery by some surgeons.

Antifungal preparations

Topical ophthalmic antifungal preparations are in the "orphan drug" category as fungal ophthalmic conditions are relatively uncommon, and thus it is not economically feasible for companies to develop such products. The only commercially available product marketed in the United States and Europe for ophthalmic use is natamycin 5% suspension. As natamycin (pimaricin) is quite expensive and not widely available, off-label use of topical and systemic antifungal preparations has become almost universally accepted. Systemic antifungal drugs may be formulated for topical therapy, and topical antifungal agents for use on other surfaces may be used for ocular use. Antifungal drugs fall into several categories: polyenes, pyrimidines, imidazoles, and miscellaneous drugs.[77]

The selection of an antifungal drug is difficult because of the lack of choice in commercially available products and often the lack of knowledge regarding the drug sensitivity of the organism. Performing mycotic sensitivity testing is expensive and time consuming, with the results often returning after the patient is cured (which usually takes several weeks)! Knowledge of the local fungal flora and their susceptibility to various antifungal drugs may help in the choice of the initial therapy.[78]

Polyene antifungals

Polyene antifungals increase the cell wall permeability of fungi by binding irreversibly to ergosterol.

- Natamycin 5% (pimaricin): Natamycin is the only commercially available ophthalmic drug marketed for topical therapy. Natamycin is a white suspension that is water insoluble and is effective against filamentous fungi and yeast such as *Candida* spp.[77] An ophthalmic ointment preparation (Infectomyk®) is available but penetrates the intact cornea poorly and leaves a white precipitate on ulcerated surfaces, lids, and inside SPL tubes.

- Amphotericin B: Amphotericin B is best known as an antifungal used in treating systemic mycoses. It has been used in topical ophthalmic therapy as a 0.1%–1.0% solution where it appears to be tolerated but, unless the surface is ulcerated, corneal penetration is poor. Topical 1% amphotericin B solution exhibits the most corneal toxicity and interference with corneal healing of a variety of antifungal agents.[79] Amphotericin B has also been injected subconjunctivally and intravitreally, but these routes have significant problems. Subconjunctival amphotericin B is very irritating, and it is questionable whether there is a safe dose with intravitreal injection. Axelrod and Peyman[52] and Axelrod et al.[80] recommended a very low dose of 5–10 µg in the middle of the vitreous cavity to avoid retinal toxicity. Souri and Green[58] found that even 1 µg of intravitreal amphotericin B was toxic to the retina and the lens in the rabbit.

Imidazoles

Imidazoles alter the fungal cell membrane by inhibiting ergosterol synthesis, resulting in increased permeability of the cell wall. Some may also interfere with mitochondrial oxidation and cause cell death by an accumulation of toxic substances. In one series of fungal sensitivities, *Aspergillus* sp. was the prevalent species, and the imidazoles were the most effective group of antifungals against this organism.[81] The latest *in vitro* sensitivity testing concluded that voriconazole was the most effective antifungal agent for the species of *Aspergillus* isolated from equine mycotic keratitis.[78]

- Miconazole has a broad spectrum of activity against yeast, filamentous fungi, and dermatophytes.[77] It penetrates moderately well, especially if corneal ulceration is present.[82] The IV form of miconazole has been used extensively as a topical 1% solution for equine keratomycosis; 2% vaginal and dermatologic creams have also been used for topical ocular therapy. The IV form has also been administered subconjunctivally.

Intraocular injection of miconazole is of questionable safety due to the toxicity of the vehicle as well as the drug. If injected intraocularly, the dose should not exceed 40 µg in a small eye, such as in a dog;[83] the safe dose for the larger equine eye is unknown. Intravenous miconazole has been taken off the market in the United States, but compounding pharmacies have been formulating a preparation. When compounding, it has been difficult to keep the drug in solution.

- Clotrimazole has been used for topical ophthalmic therapy using 1% vaginal and dermatologic creams.
- Ketoconazole penetrates the cornea well, and dermatologic preparations have been used on the cornea. Ketoconazole has a broad spectrum of activity, and isolates from equine keratomycosis have been susceptible.[40,81] It has been used extensively for treating systemic mycoses in the dog, where cataracts have been a complication of long-term therapy.[84]
- Thiabendazole paste has been used historically for equine keratomycosis but has been supplanted by the newer imidazoles.[85]
- Fluconazole is a newer imidazole that has been used systemically, topically, and intracamerally. It is a triazole and has the advantage of enhanced tissue penetration because it has minimal protein binding. Like miconazole, the IV preparation of fluconazole is used as a topical solution and penetrates very well with corneal debridement.[86] While anecdotal reports are promising, fungal sensitivity testing indicates that most of the isolates are resistant.[40] Systemic therapy has been advocated for deep keratomycosis or corneal abscesses because of the drug's excellent tissue penetration,[87] starting with a loading dose of 2 mg/kg followed by 1 mg/kg every 12 hours by mouth for 2 weeks. With improvement, the dose can be decreased to 1 mg/kg every 24 hours.[88] Latimer et al.[89] studied the pharmacokinetics of fluconazole in the horse and calculated that the loading dose should be 14 mg/kg by mouth, followed by 5 mg/kg every 24 hours. This is a very expensive therapy for a horse. Fluconazole has also been administered intracamerally at 100 µg/0.1 mL.[88]
- Itraconazole is a triazole, and it has improved activity against filamentous fungi.[40] It has poor water solubility; Ball et al.[90] enhanced corneal penetration by dissolving the drug in dimethyl sulfoxide and creating a 1% ointment, with excellent clinical success. Itraconazole (5 mg/kg) is also being used systemically with equine keratomycosis. Systemic itraconazole has been the treatment of choice for systemic mycoses.
- Itraconazole/DMSO 1% ointment was formulated by dissolving 1 g of ultramicronized itraconazole in 33.3 mL 90% DMSO, heated to 80°C (176°F) while agitated, and the heated mixture combined with 66.6 mL of petrolatum that had been heated to 80°C (176°F). The mixture was allowed to cool while agitated until it solidified.[90]

- Voriconazole belongs to the triazoles and inhibits ergosterol synthesis causing cell membrane disruption. A 1% solution is prepared from the commercially available IV solution by reconstituting the lyophilized powder with sterile water for injection.[91] Voriconazole has been shown to have the best efficacy against equine fungal isolates.[78]

Miscellaneous antifungals

- Betadine solution has been used in topical therapy of keratomycosis.
- Silver sulfadiazine has been used as a topical cream for equine and human mycotic keratitis. It generally is well tolerated, is inexpensive, and moderately effective.[92]
- Chlorhexidine gluconate 0.2% has been used as an effective and inexpensive antifungal preparation in humans.[93]

Initiation of antifungal therapy in the horse is often accompanied by a clinical worsening of the condition. This worsening is probably due to the sudden death of fungi. Therapy is monitored by frequent corneal cytology if the condition is superficial. If healthy fungal hyphae continue to be observed on cytology despite therapy, the antifungal drug should be changed.

ANTIVIRAL AGENTS

The topical antiviral agents are mainly directed against the herpesvirus in man, and they are relatively specific for DNA viruses. Their use in veterinary medicine is mainly for ocular herpesvirus in cats and horses. The topical commercial agents are nucleic acid analogs, and they interfere with nucleic acid synthesis. They are virostatic and do not have an effect on viruses that are latent and are not multiplying. There are several commercial topical ophthalmic antiviral preparations available in the United States:

- Idoxuridine (IDU): A first-generation antiviral agent. IDU substitutes for thymidine in the purine building block of the DNA virus and is toxic to other mammalian cells as well. IDU was available as a solution and an ointment. Therapy is frequent: ointment is every 4 hours and solution every hour or every 2 hours. IDU is the least expensive of the antiviral agents. Individuals may experience irritation from the solution, and this is most likely if the product has become oxidized, as evidenced by a brown discolorization.[94] IDU has been discontinued in the United States but can be obtained through compounding pharmacies.

- Adenine arabinoside (Ara-A or vidarabin): Also a structural analog for adenosine. Vidarabin is available as a 3% ointment, given every 4 hours. Vidarabin is less toxic to mammalian cells and more effective than IDU.[94]
- Trifluorothymidine (TFT) (trifluridine): A thymidine analog inhibitor against the DNA virus. It is a 1% solution, administered every 4 hours. It is less toxic and more effective than other antivirals but more expensive. Based on a rabbit herpes keratitis model, it has been suggested that the application of trifluridine might be reduced to as infrequently as every 24 hours.[95]
- Acyclovir (acycloquanosine): An analog for guanosine that becomes a potent inhibitor of viral DNA polymerase. Acyclovir is selectively activated by phosphorylation by viral thymidine kinase but not by cellular thymidine kinase. This concentrates the active form in viral-infected cells and so minimizes toxicity to other mammalian cells.[94] Acyclovir may be given both systemically and topically, although it is not available in the United States as an ophthalmic preparation.
- Ganciclovir has been shown to be effective in a rabbit herpes simplex keratitis model.[96] It is commercially available as an ophthalmic gel preparation (Virgan®).
- Cidofovir (Vistide®) is commercially available as a 7.5% solution for injection. Diluted with 0.9% saline to a 0.5% solution, it can be used topically for the treatment of FHV-1 keratitis in cats.[97] It has the advantage of a twice-daily application only.

The relative efficacies of the antiviral agents are usually quoted for human herpesvirus in man or rabbit. The efficacy with other species of herpesvirus may vary as well as between strains of the same species. A limited *in vitro* study of feline herpesvirus sensitivities indicated that TFT was most effective, followed by IDU, vidarabin, and acyclovir.[98] This has been expanded to: trifluridine > idoxuridine = ganciclovir > cidofovir = penciclovir > vidarabine > acyclovir = foscarnet.[99,100]

Systemic acyclovir has been used in cats but, due to its limited bioavailability and feline herpesvirus resistance, it is of questionable benefit. Attempts at increasing the bioavailability of acyclovir by using valacyclovir, which is converted in the liver to acyclovir, result in systemic toxicity. Cats given valacyclovir exhibited clinical signs of dehydration and lethargy associated with hepatic necrosis and renal tubular necrosis after 12 days of therapy.[101] This toxicity is apparently species specific. Despite the report of systemic toxicity to valacyclovir, ophthalmologists and internists have been using famciclovir orally for several years without apparent toxicity. The dose and

duration has been quite varied, but some caution is in order. Ophthalmologists have been giving between 1/4 of a 125 mg tablet to 1/4 of a 250 mg tablet for an adult cat for 3–6 weeks and 1/4 of a 125 mg tablet for kittens.[102] Some individuals have used famciclovir indefinitely to treat relapsing syndromes. Thomasy et al.[103] evaluated the toxicity and efficacy of famciclovir (90 mg/kg every 8 hours for 21 days) in experimental herpes infection in cats. They detected no adverse affects in the physical or biochemical parameters, and the clinical signs were attenuated with the drug.

The use of topical antiviral therapy with feline herpesvirus infections raises questions of cost/benefit ratio and accuracy of diagnosis. The clearest indication for therapy is with active corneal epithelial ulcers that are characteristic of herpesvirus.

Intravitreal injection of the systemic antiviral cidofovir at a dose of 100–500 μg has been advocated as a treatment for glaucoma. Unlike intraocular gentamicin, cidofovir apparently is not toxic to the retina or the lens.[104] It was originally noted that individuals given systemic cidofovir developed marked hypotony. The safety and efficacy of cidofovir for intraocular injections need further investigation.

Miotics (cholinergic agonists)
Pharmacology
The cholinergic miotics are classified into direct and indirect according to their action. The direct acting miotics, for example, pilocarpine, act directly on the cell to produce an acetylcholine-like action. They maintain their effect upon denervated structures. Pilocarpine has muscarinic action (stimulation of smooth muscle and glands) but not nicotinic action (stimulation of striated muscle). By convention, miotic solutions have a green cap.

The indirect acting miotics are cholinesterase inhibitors, and they act by preserving acetylcholine at the nerve endings. They have no effect on denervated structures where acetylcholine is not released. They are also categorized by their reversible or irreversible binding ability with acetylcholinesterase (**Table 2.6**). The indirect, nonreversible drugs are very potent drugs, and severe side effects from systemic absorption are possible.

Miotic preparations constrict the pupil (miosis), cause contraction of the ciliary muscle that produces accommodation, open the aqueous humor outflow channels, and increase vascular permeability. A transient breakdown of the blood–aqueous humor barrier may occur that resolves after about 48 hours.[109] Miotics are used in man almost exclusively for glaucoma therapy, where the important action is not the outward miotic effect but the contraction of the ciliary muscle, which increases aqueous humor

Table 2.6 Parasympathomimetic miotics used in ophthalmology.

DRUG	CONCENTRATION	FORMS	ACTION
Pilocarpine	0.5%–10%*, 4%**	Solution*, gel**, inserts	Direct cholinergic, muscarinic action
Carbachol	0.75%–3%	Solution	Direct and indirect cholinergic muscarinic and nicotinic actions
Echothiophate iodide	0.03%–0.25%	Solution	Cholinesterase inhibitor; irreversible, muscarinic and nicotinic actions
Isoflurophate (DFP)	Withdrawn	–	Cholinesterase inhibitor; irreversible, muscarinic and nicotinic actions
Demecarium	Withdrawn	–	Cholinesterase inhibitor; reversible, muscarinic and nicotinic actions

Note: *Solution; ** Gel.

outflow.[110] Miotics are usually not very effective for glaucoma therapy in animals because of the typical high intraocular pressure (IOP) when the condition is recognized and the physical obstruction present in the outflow pathway. The miotic and pressure lowering effectiveness also decreases with long-term therapy.[111–113]

Indications for use

Glaucoma

Miotics are used in glaucoma therapy and work most effectively with open-angle glaucoma, which is relatively rare in the dog. Carrier and Gum[111] found a statistically significant decrease in IOP in normal and glaucomatous beagles with 4% pilocarpine gel every 24 hours. However, the animals were only treated for 3 days, and during this time, IOPs drifted back to baseline values. Mean IOP response was 2.0–2.5 mmHg (0.27–0.33 kPa). When testing various concentrations of pilocarpine from 0.5%–8% in the glaucomatous beagle, all concentrations produced statistically significant decreases in IOP; all concentrations were equally effective, although the higher concentrations had more side effects.[114] Carbachol and N-demethylated carbachol both produced similar decreases in IOP as pilocarpine in the glaucomatous beagle and were not concentration-related, indicating that weak solutions were as effective as the higher concentrations.[115,116] The decrease in IOP was associated with an increase in conventional outflow, with the coefficient of outflow increasing from 0.33 μL/min/mmHg to 0.61 μL/min/mmHg in normal beagles, and from 0.15 μL/min/mmHg to 0.38 μL/min/mmHg in glaucomatous beagles.[117]

Demecarium bromide and echothiophate iodide produced similar decreases in IOP as pilocarpine in the glaucomatous beagle, but the effect was for 3–4 days; thus, the drugs decreased the opportunity for pressure fluctuations during the day and would presumably increase owner compliance if frequency of application was reduced.[118] The pressure in acute closed-angle glaucoma (most common in the dog) is usually too high for miotics to be of much benefit, and the angle morphology so disrupted that outflow facility would be unlikely to be improved. When treating acute glaucoma, miosis is not observed until the IOP has been decreased.

Intracameral carbachol (0.5 mL of 0.01%) has been used in humans and dogs after cataract surgery. In the dog, carbachol minimized or eliminated the transient postoperative hypertensive episode that occurs in 50% of operated eyes.[119,120]

Glaucoma prophylaxis

Miotics have been advocated for years for prophylactic treatment of the normotensive eye when a unilateral primary glaucoma is diagnosed (see section Prophylaxis, Chapter 12). Until recently, there were no good clinical trials to support this use,[121] but because of the difficulty in treating this disease, clinicians will use anything that might have theoretical value. Because of their convenience, the long-acting preparations are often selected. Based on the studies to date, the type of glaucoma medication used in prophylaxis does not apparently make a significant difference.[121,122]

Displaced lens

Miotics may be used to try to trap a subluxated lens in the posterior chamber to keep it from luxating forward, or to trap an anterior luxated lens in the anterior chamber before surgery. Long-term miotic therapy results in a decrease in miosis; in the author's experience, cholinergic therapy is usually less successful in producing sustained, marked miosis than the prostaglandin (PG) analog latanoprost.[112,113,123]

Hyphema therapy

Miotics may be recommended for the treatment of hyphema because they increase the outflow of red blood cells (RBCs) from the anterior chamber. Miotics also produce vascular dilation and may induce secondary bleeding. Miotic therapy also aggravates traumatic iritis discomfort by inducing ciliary spasm[110] and may encourage pupillary block.

Keratoconjunctivitis sicca (dry eye)

Patients with some residual tear production may respond to stimulation with a parasympathomimetic drug to increase their tear production.[124] The oral use of ophthalmic pilocarpine had been used successfully for years before the advent of topical cyclosporine. Most clinicians preferred to use pilocarpine in food, but in multiple dog households where food is *ad lib*, the topical route has been recommended. The efficacy of the topical route has been discounted by Smith et al.[125] who found no increase in tear production in normal dogs in treated eyes and, paradoxically, a decrease in tear production in the contralateral untreated eye. Oral application of pilocarpine has been shown to be effective in the treatment of neurogenic keratoconjunctivitis sicca.[126]

The stimulation of lacrimation may take several weeks, and thus, a trial of 4 weeks or more is recommended. The use of topical cyclosporine as a lacrimomimetic has almost completely supplanted the use of pilocarpine (see section Therapy, Chapter 9). On rare occasions, a dog may respond to pilocarpine but not to cyclosporine.

Diagnostics

Miotics may be used to define the cause of a dilated pupil(s). Direct acting miotics should constrict the pupil unless there is a problem with the iris sphincter muscle. Indirect-acting miotics require an intact neuron in the iris to function and thus do not cause miosis with peripheral parasympathetic denervation (**Table 2.7**).

Side effects

- Ciliary muscle contraction or spasm may be stimulated. The discomfort is variable with patients, usually lasts 5–10 minutes, and often a tolerance develops within several days.
- Decreased vision may result if an axial lenticular opacity is present.
- Conjunctival congestion and mild flare (due to increased protein) may occur in the anterior chamber. This is a transient phenomenon.

- Systemic absorption from topical application or overdosing with oral medication produces vomiting, salivation, and diarrhea. Dogs with a heart block may be compromised. Systemic toxicity must be considered when intensive treatment is administered, as is frequently recommended for acute glaucoma.
- Long-term topical use may produce drug hypersensitivity, resulting in a severe follicular conjunctivitis.

Mydriatics
Pharmacology

Mydriatics produce pupillary dilation (mydriasis), and some agents are also cycloplegics (paralyze the ciliary muscles). As with the miotics, there are direct- and indirect-acting mydriatics. The duration of action between drugs and variation between species may be significant. Two groups of drugs are most commonly used for mydriasis, either individually or in combination for maximum effect. By convention, mydriatic solutions have a red cap.

Parasympatholytic agents

Parasympatholytic agents have both mydriatic and cycloplegic actions, and they are direct acting and compete with acetylcholine. The duration and strength of their action varies.[127] The rapidity and degree of mydriasis vary with the age, species, and pigmentation of the iris. Heavily pigmented irises bind many drugs, and the result is a slower onset and a decrease in magnitude of mydriasis, but the duration of action may be prolonged. This may explain why the pupils of some horses remain dilated for weeks after long-term atropinization.[128] Some but not all rabbits produce atropine esterase that inactivates atropine by hydrolysis. Occasionally, a dog may respond, paradoxically, to atropine or tropicamide with miosis. This is usually encountered preoperatively, and subsequent intraocular epinephrine will dilate the pupil. Long-term atropinization in young cats resulted in smaller resting pupils after discontinuation of the drug, and this was thought to be due to a compensatory increase in cholinergic receptors due to deprivation of transmitter.[129] This phenomenon has

DRUG	NORMAL	CENTRAL PARASYMPATHETIC LESION	PERIPHERAL PARASYMPATHETIC LESION (ADIE'S SYNDROME)	IRIS ATROPHY	GLAUCOMA	ATROPINE BLOCKAGE
1% Pilocarpine	+	+	+ (hypersensitive)	0	0	0
0.01% Phospholine iodide	+	+	0	0	0	0

Table 2.7 **Pharmacologic lesion localization with a dilated pupil.**

Note: +: constriction; 0: no response.

been used to explain the previously mentioned paradoxical miosis with mydriatics, but it is lacking in evidence.

While Mughannam et al.[130] were unable to find any change in IOP after atropine instillation in the horse, Herring et al.[131] found an 11% decrease in IOP in 10/11 horses, but one horse had a significant increase in IOP. Stadtbaumer et al. found significant increases in IOP in the cat after 0.5% tropicamide.[132] Unilateral instillation of tropicamide produced bilateral statistically significant increases in IOP of cats, but the mydriatic effect was only unilateral. While the mean increase in IOP was 3 mmHg (0.4 kPa), some individual cats had increases in IOP of 18 mmHg (2.4 kPa), resulting in IOP values of 30–37 mmHg (4.0–4.9 kPa). The phenomenon was age-related, with younger cats responding with higher mean changes in IOP. The mechanism for bilateral response with unilateral treatment is unknown but is thought to be due to a systemic effect. Stadtbaumer et al.[133] repeated the trial later and found a lack of bilateral IOP rise, with the only difference in trials being the lack of a topical anesthetic used for tonometry in the second study. The mydriasis lasted longer than the increase in IOP. The effect of tropicamide on the IOP of dogs is equivocal, with apparently minimal change.[134] Taylor et al.[135] evaluated post-mydriatic IOP in three breeds (Golden retrievers, Siberian huskies, and English Cocker Spaniels) and found that the majority of the dogs had less than a 5 mmHg increase in IOP, but the huskies had the highest IOPs before and after mydriasis.

Examples of parasympatholytics:

- Atropine 0.5%–4% solution: Atropine is the most commonly used mydriatic for therapy. In a normal eye, one administration of atropine may last for 4–5 days, but when used in uveitis therapy, more frequent administration is required (every 6 to 12 hours).
- Homatropine 2%–5% solution: Used in therapy. In a normal dog eye, one administration may last for 2 days.

- Scopolamine 0.25%–0.5% solution: Used in therapy. Duration of action of one administration in a normal eye is 4–5 days.
- Cyclopentolate 1% solution: Potent drug that frequently produces marked chemosis in the dog, so is not routinely used.
- Tropicamide 0.5%–1%: Most common agent used for diagnostic purposes because of its short duration of 6–12 hours.

Adrenergic agents/sympathomimetic agents

Due to the development of new drugs with activity targeted against specific adrenergic receptors, and due to species differences in receptors, not all adrenergic drugs dilate the pupil. For instance, apraclonidine dilates the dog pupil but constricts the cat pupil. Some adrenergic agonists such as nonselective α and β agonists and selective α agonists generally produce mydriasis without cycloplegia. Adrenergic agents may be either indirect (act by stimulating the release of norepinephrine) or direct (act on catecholamine receptors, similar to norepinephrine). Catecholamine receptors are classified as α-1, α-2, β-1, and β-2.

Sympathomimetic agents may be used to augment mydriasis, in glaucoma therapy to increase aqueous humor outflow and decrease aqueous humor production, and in diagnostics to localize sympathetic lesions involving the pupil (**Table 2.8**). Examples are:

- Epinephrine 0.1%–2%: Direct action, used for therapy and diagnostics. It is a nonselective α and β agonist and is used for glaucoma therapy, to dilate the pupil intraoperatively, and for vasoconstriction and hemostatic control in surgery.
- Dipivalyl epinephrine (Propine®): A prodrug of epinephrine. It is the esterified form of epinephrine and penetrates the cornea much better (9–17×) than epinephrine and can thus be used in lower concentrations. Once in the anterior chamber and

Table 2.8 **Pharmacologic lesion localization in Horner's syndrome.**

DRUG	NORMAL	LESION		
		CENTRAL	PREGANGLIONIC	POSTGANGLIONIC
1% Hydroxamphetamine[a]	+	+	+	0
1% Phenylephrine	0	0	0	+
10% Phenylephrine	−	+60 min	+30–45 min	+10–20 min
0.001% Epinephrine	0	0	mild+	+

Note: +: dilates; 0: no response.
[a] No longer available.

in the uvea, it is hydrolyzed to epinephrine, which is direct acting.[136]

- Paradrine® (hydroxyamphetamine) 1%: Indirect action, has been used for diagnostics for localizing the sympathetic lesion in Horner's syndrome.[137,138] It is no longer available as a commercial product.
- Phenylephrine 2%–10% solution: A direct-acting α agonist, used in diagnostics and therapy. Phenylephrine is not effective as a mydriatic in the cat, the cow, and the horse.[139–141] It has been used to localize sympathetic lesions in Horner's syndrome.[142]
- Cocaine: Indirect sympathomimetic, which dilates the pupil, causes vasoconstriction, and is a potent long-acting topical anesthetic. It is rarely used now because it is a Class IV controlled drug. It blocks the uptake of epinephrine by nerve endings, allowing a prolonged action of epinephrine and norepinephrine.[143] It can be used to try to break synechiae or adhesions of the pupil.
- Apraclonidine: α-2 agonist that is used in humans to treat postoperative IOP spikes and augment maximum medical therapy in glaucoma treatment. The selective α-2 agonists have been developed for glaucoma therapy to overcome the side effects that topical epinephrine produces in many patients. Apraclonidine 1% decreases aqueous humor formation by decreasing cyclic AMP, increases uveoscleral outflow in the treated as well as the untreated eye, and produces mydriasis.[143] Tachyphylaxis limits the duration of effectiveness of the drug for many patients.

In normal dogs, 0.5% apraclonidine decreases IOP and produces mydriasis.[144] In normal cats, apraclonidine lowers IOP and produces miosis, bradycardia, and vomiting. The side effects in cats preclude using commercially available 0.5% apraclonidine.[145]

Brimonidine is a selective α-2 agonist that is more selective than apraclonidine. It lowers the IOP by decreasing aqueous humor production as well as increasing uveoscleral outflow. Gelatt et al. tested 0.2% and 0.5% brimonidine in glaucomatous beagles and did not find a statistically significant decrease in IOP, although the pupil dilated.[146] Tachyphylaxis results in a decreased effectiveness over time.

> The adrenergic agonists have not become an important group of drugs for glaucoma therapy because of their minimal effectiveness combined with significant side effects.

Indications for use
Diagnostics
Mydriatics are used for examination of the lens and in ophthalmoscopy. A long-acting agent is undesirable, and tropicamide is the agent of choice.[127,139] Very young animals do not respond as well or as long, and the addition of a sympathomimetic agent may be necessary to achieve good dilation. The use of sympathomimetic drugs for lesion localization in Horner's syndrome (sympathetic denervation to the eye and adnexa) is based on denervation hypersensitivity and the ability, or lack thereof, to stimulate intact sympathetic fibers in the iris. Direct-acting sympathomimetics are used to determine whether the iris is stimulated by dilute concentrations of epinephrine, or similar acting drugs, that are not effective in the normal eye. Hypersensitivity indicates that the lesion is peripheral or in the third neuron and that the nerve endings in the iris have degenerated. Boydell[142] utilized the speed of pupil dilation to topical 10% phenylephrine to distinguish between first-, second-, and third-order neuron involvement in Horner's syndrome in the dog. Dogs with first-order neuron disease responded to 10% phenylephrine in 50–60 minutes, second-order neuron disease in 30–45 minutes, and third-order neuron disease in 10–20 minutes. Similarly, drugs such as Paradrine (hydroxyamphetamine) act by stimulating intact nerve endings to release norepinephrine, and thus a positive response indicates an intact third neuron (**Table 2.8**). The results from these tests are highly variable, and interpretation is based on speed of onset and degree of reaction. Ideally, the opposite eye (if normal) should be used as a control.

Therapy of corneal ulcers
Intraocular pain may be decreased by producing cycloplegia to stop the pain from ciliary muscle spasms. Ciliary muscle spasms may occur with stimulation of the cranial nerve V endings in the cornea. The spasms are thought to arise from antidromic impulses that travel down the sensory nerve to the muscles. Atropine is usually the agent of choice and is administered every 8–12 hours. While some horses appear sensitive to topical atropine-induced colic at moderate doses every 6–12 hours, intensive therapy is more likely to induce colic from systemic absorption. Williams et al. induced colic with topical atropine administered hourly in 4/6 horses.[147] Occasionally, a pupil may remain dilated for weeks after multiple atropine applications, and this is probably due to depletion of atropine esterase or binding of atropine by uveal pigment and subsequent prolonged release.[128]

Therapy of anterior uveitis
Mydriatics, specifically atropine, are used in uveitis therapy to dilate the pupil, minimize adhesions or

complications from complete adhesions, and decrease ciliary muscle pain. Atropine is also used after surgically induced uveitis.

> Unless severe uveitis is present, intensive use of postoperative atropine in cataract surgery has been discontinued by many surgeons in favor of no mydriatics or tropicamide.

Nonsurgical therapy for axial cataracts

Vision can be improved in patients with axial cataracts and a clear periphery by dilating the pupil. Mydriasis allows the patient to see around the central opacity.

Medical therapy of equine glaucoma

The horse has a significant amount of aqueous humor outflow via the uveoscleral route, and it has been hypothesized that atropine may be beneficial in treating glaucoma in this species. Normal horses had an 11% decrease in IOP when treated with atropine compared to the control eye.[148]

Side effects

- Parasympatholytics decrease tear production and may produce transient keratoconjunctivitis sicca (KCS). Atropine administered to one eye decreases the Schirmer tear test (STT) in both eyes and may persist for 5 weeks or more after cessation of therapy. This is commonly observed in postoperative cataract patients.[149]
- Parasympatholytics may produce atony of the gut. While atropine may be used in most horses as often as every 2–4 hours without problems, the gut motility should be monitored.[147,150] Some horses are more sensitive than others to atropine-induced colic.
- Atropine may produce prolonged mydriasis and photophobia.
- Sympathomimetics often sting and may cause self-mutilation or rubbing. This tendency is most critical after intraocular surgery.
- Phenylephrine is toxic to the corneal endothelium and may produce corneal edema when used intensively in 10% concentration or if the absorption is enhanced by breaks in the epithelium.
- Frequent therapy with atropine may result in disorientation and incontinence. This usually occurs in very old or small dogs.
- Topical 10% phenylephrine may induce significant systemic hypertension through systemic absorption.[151]

- Acute, transient enlargement of the salivary glands may occur in cats after administration of tropicamide and atropine. The condition resolves in about 30 minutes.[152]

β-adrenergic blockers

Pharmacology

Topical β-adrenergic blockers decrease the production of aqueous humor by as much as 50% in humans.[153] The mode of action on the inhibition of aqueous humor production is unknown, although β-adrenergic blockers are known to be potent inhibitors of cyclic adenosine monophosphate (AMP) in the ciliary body. The major receptor in the anterior segment is the β-2 receptor; thus, drugs such as βxolol, which are β-1 blockers, are less effective than nonselective blockers, but they have fewer systemic side effects.[154] β-blockers do not affect carbonic anhydrase or the aqueous humor outflow.[153] The effect of β-blockers is variable in different species, due in part to concentration differences necessary to elicit a response.[153,155] In the normal cat and dog, higher concentrations of drug appear to be necessary to produce a reduction in IOP than in humans, and this may explain the early reports that β-blockers were ineffective in the dog.[156] Two studies reported that timolol (Timoptic®), which is a nonselective β-1 and β-2 blocker, was effective in both the dog and the cat and in the normal and glaucomatous beagle.[157–159]

Topical 0.5% timolol applied unilaterally in the normal cat eye reduced IOP by 22% in the treated eye and by 16% in the untreated eye. In addition, the pupil in the treated eye constricted by 38% for over 12 hours but not in the nontreated eye.[158,159] In one study in the normal dog, 0.5% timolol produced a significant mean reduction of 16% (2.5 mmHg [0.33 kPa]) in IOP, a 34% reduction in pupil size in the treated eye, and a 14% decrease in pupil size in the untreated eye, whereas other studies were unable to demonstrate a significant difference in IOP at this concentration.[156,158,159] The beagle with open-angle glaucoma did respond, with a significant drop in IOP using 0.5% timolol, but the decrease was only 4–5 mmHg (0.53–0.7 kPa). In the glaucomatous beagle, concentrations of timolol of 4%, 6%, and 8% did produce a significant drop in IOP of 8–14 mmHg (1.0–1.9 kPa) in the treated eye and a less extensive decrease in the untreated eye. This study did not detect any changes in the pupil size but did note a significant decrease in the heart rate at all concentrations.[157]

Available β-blockers may be either nonselective, blocking both β-1 and β-2 receptors, or selective. Timolol and levobunolol are nonselective β-blockers and are available as 0.25% and 0.5% solutions; as previously indicated, these drugs are minimally effective in the dog and the cat at this concentration. Betaxolol 0.5% is a selective β-1 blocker. While not studied as extensively as nonselective β-blockers, in the dog, it is also questionably effective at this concentration. Therapy is usually administered every 12 hours with both agents.

β-blockers can be additive in their effect when used with carbonic anhydrase inhibitors (61% decrease in IOP), parasympathomimetics, and even with epinephrine (50% decrease in IOP) when treating glaucoma.[160,161] The additive effect with epinephrine is confusing, considering that epinephrine is an adrenergic α and β-1 and β-2 agonist.

Indications for use

β-blockers are used in glaucoma therapy and prophylactic treatment of eyes thought to be susceptible to glaucoma (**Table 2.9**).

Side effects

Systemic absorption of β-2 blockers may produce or exacerbate pulmonary signs of bronchoconstriction and spasms and cardiovascular signs of bradycardia and heart blocks.[162] Decreased exercise tolerance may be noted, and, therefore, these drugs should be avoided in athletic dogs. Corneal erosions may occur and may be related to a decrease in tear production.[163]

DIURETICS

Two specific forms of diuretics are routinely used in ophthalmology, osmotic and carbonic anhydrase inhibitors.

Osmotic diuretics

Osmotic diuretics are used to draw fluid from the eye (aqueous humor and vitreous), and they are of dramatic benefit in the emergency therapy of acute glaucoma.[164] They produce systemic dehydration, so they are limited as to their frequency of use. Since they expand the blood volume, the presence of a weak cardiovascular system should be considered and care taken in the speed of administration.

The preparations usually used are:

- Mannitol: Recommended dose is 1–2 g/kg IV via slow push (over 5 minutes) or 1 mL/kg/min.[165] The author routinely uses 0.5–1.0 g/kg mannitol and obtains the expected results with glaucoma patients. Mannitol may crystallize out of solution if not kept in a fluid warmer. Mannitol tends to remain in the vascular system and exits via the kidneys, thus producing less rebound of fluids into the interstitial spaces. This is not absolute, particularly with inflammation, and with repeated administration, it becomes less effective until a minimal response is achieved after the third or fourth dose. Lowered IOP is evident by 20–30 minutes and may last for 6–72 hours.
- Glycerol or glycerine: Administered orally at 1–2 g/kg. Glycerol is irritating to the stomach and frequently results in vomition unless diluted. Glycerol is less expensive than mannitol and is an alternative in the horse.
- Isosorbide: Administered orally as a 50% solution at a dose of 1.5 g/kg.

Indications for use

- Glaucoma: Mannitol is used in emergency glaucoma therapy until surgery can be performed or until medical therapy becomes effective. Mannitol may also be used to treat transient postcataract surgery ocular hypertensive episodes if the IOP becomes very elevated.
  Topical latanoprost often produces dramatic decreases in IOP in acute glaucoma and may be used instead of mannitol in emergency therapy. If latanoprost does not realize the desired reduction in IOP within 30 minutes, mannitol is then administered.
- Preoperatively, intraoperatively, and postoperatively to reduce the vitreous size and so minimize vitreous prolapse through the pupil.

Carbonic anhydrase inhibitors (CAIs)

CAIs reversibly interfere with the hydration of carbon dioxide to form carbonic acid. CAIs are sulfonamides and are relatively ineffective diuretics, but they decrease aqueous humor production by about 30%–40%.[166,167] CAIs affect only the aqueous humor and not the vitreous. The exact mechanism of CAIs is still unknown, but they are thought to act on the active secretory component of

Table 2.9 **Topical ophthalmic β-blockers and their action.**		
DRUG	**CONCENTRATION/FORMS**	**ACTION**
Timolol	0.25%, 0.5% solutions	Nonselective β-1, β-2 blocker
Levobunolol	0.25%, 0.5% solutions	Nonselective β-1, β-2 blocker
Carteolol	2% solution	Nonselective β-1, β-2 blocker
Metipranolol	0.3% solution	Nonselective β-1, β-2 blocker
Betaxolol	0.25% ointment, 0.5% solution	Selective β-1 blocker
Levoβxolol	0.5% ointment	Selective β-1 blocker

aqueous humor production, and this is independent of the kidney.[167]

Four isoenzymes of carbonic anhydrase have been described. Carbonic anhydrase II is the predominant form present in the eye and is involved with aqueous humor production.[168] It is also present in the corneal endothelium, iris, and retina. In general, CAIs must be given systemically to have an effect as >99% of the enzyme must be inhibited.[169,170] As carbonic anhydrase is ubiquitous in the body, nonselective inhibitors are likely to produce side effects other than the desired decrease in IOP. Systemic CAIs have historically been the backbone of medical maintenance therapy in canine glaucoma therapy.

Enhancing the corneal penetration by increasing the liphophilia of the compounds has allowed topical preparations of CAIs to produce modest decreases in IOP.[171–173] The quest for an effective topical CAI was pursued because of the frequent side effects noted with systemic CAI therapy and consequent poor patient compliance. Dorzolamide was the first commercially available topical CAI. It is not as effective as systemic CAIs but does not have the usual side effects of systemic therapy. It is available as a 2% solution, and every-8-hour therapy is recommended. In humans, dorzolamide decreases the IOP by 17%–20% and is only slightly less effective than timolol.[174,175] Dorzolamide can be given with β-blockers, and the effect is additive. Intraocular penetration of the drug is probably through the limbus and the sclera rather than the cornea. The hypotensive effect is greater in lighter pigmented irises than in the darker irises found more commonly in animals. This is presumably due to drug binding by melanin.

Corneal decompensation or edema might be expected with CAIs as carbonic anhydrase is present in the endothelium and postulated to be responsible for pumping water out of the stroma. To date, corneal decompensation is a rare event.[174] Statistically significant decreases in IOP have been found in the horse, the dog, and the cat after treating with dorzolamide, and the decrease is larger when combined with a β-blocker such as timolol.[176–178] While not as effective as systemic CAIs, the lack of systemic side effects and cost for equine patients has made topical CAIs popular in veterinary ophthalmology.

Brinzolamide 1% is the newest topical CAI. It is equally effective in suppressing aqueous humor secretion as dorzolamide but with less ocular irritation.[179–181]

Systemic preparations
- Acetazolamide: Is available as a tablet, spansule, and IV preparation. It is the most widely available CAI, but at a dose of 10–20 mg/kg every 8–12 hours, many dogs have side effects.
- Dichlorphenamide: Has fewer side effects. It has recently been discontinued by the manufacturer and must be compounded. It was available only as a tablet (50 mg) and administered at 2–5 mg/kg every 8–12 hours.
- Ethoxzolamide: 5 mg/kg every 8–12 hours.
- Methazolamide: 5 mg/kg every 8–12 hours.

Side effects
Side effects are common with systemic CAIs, in particular with acetazolamide at the recommended dose. Systemic acidosis, vomiting, diarrhea, anorexia, panting, poorer temperament, and paresthesia manifesting as lameness are possible. Ataxia is common in cats. In humans, kidney stones and fatal blood dyscrasias have been recorded.[182,183] An individual patient may be sensitive to all or only one of the preparations. Potassium supplementation has been recommended with long-term therapy. Besides ocular irritation, in humans, corneal edema, sterile mucopurulent conjunctivitis, and nephrolithiasis have been rare complications of topical CAIs.[184–186]

Other diuretics
Ethacrynic acid in cell cultures of trabecular cells produced reversible changes in cell shape. In enucleated canine eyes, ethacrynic acid increased the outflow facility and decreased IOP when injected intracamerally in monkeys and humans.[187,188] Pilot studies in dogs with a 2% solution were very disappointing. No changes in IOP were noted, marked ocular irritation was produced, and it was difficult to prepare a stable solution.[189]

ARTIFICIAL TEARS

Artificial tear solutions are used as vehicles for ophthalmic solutions, replace tears if deficient, protect eyes from exposure, and act as a filling substance between the cornea and a diagnostic lens (gonioscopy). They are generally over-the-counter products that do not require a prescription. Their main goal is to lubricate the surface of the eye, and many agents or combinations of agents are capable of this goal to varying degrees. The usual variables between the products are tonicity (isotonic versus hypotonic), presence of preservatives, and type and viscosity of lubricating agent used.

Agents
- Methylcellulose, hydroxypropylmethylcellulose, and carboxymethylcellulose: Preparations with different viscosity are available.
- Polyvinyl alcohol: 1.4%–3%.
- Polyvinylpyrrolidone: Artificial mucus-like agent (mucomimetic).

- Hyaluronic acid: Human studies have indicated no particular advantage, and such viscoelastic agents are expensive. The prolonged contact time, however, imparts better corneal protection and lubrication than other artificial tears. Hyaluronic acid is available commercially in various forms and preparations. Multiuse vials without preservatives, (0.3% i-Drop Vet) are available. Other preparations are Remend 0.4%, Hyasent-S, OptiMend 0.2%, and Opti-Vet.
- Various ointment bases are used as ocular lubricants with tear deficiencies and to protect the cornea from exposure (anesthesia, exophthalmos, cranial nerve VII deficiency). They usually contain some combination of white petrolatum, mineral oil, and lanolin.
- Carbomer (polyacrylic acid) gels have become very popular tear substitutes.[190]

DYES

Most dyes are used for diagnostic purposes. The main dyes used are fluorescein and rose bengal.

Sodium fluorescein

Sodium fluorescein is available as a 1%–2% solution or on sterile strips. The solution is a good culture medium because preservatives are not used as they are inactivated by the dye. Multiple-use vials were found to be a potential culture medium for *Pseudomonas* spp.[191] Single-use strips or small-volume bottles and care in application are recommended to minimize iatrogenic infection.

Indications for use

- To detect corneal epithelial loss and follow the progression of healing. Water-soluble fluorescein does not normally penetrate the intact epithelium, but if breaks in the epithelium exist, it diffuses into the stroma where it is seen as a bright green color. Small breaks can be detected by using a blue light to excite fluorescence.
- To determine the patency of the nasolacrimal duct. Fluorescein applied to the eye usually appears at the nostril within 30–60 seconds. False negatives are possible, so a negative result should be followed by nasolacrimal flushing.
- Fluorescein IV is used to study the fundus vasculature. Fluorescein is a small molecule, and approximately 80% is protein bound. The nonprotein-bound portion is readily diffusible but is retained by tight intercellular junctions. Thus, it is valuable in detecting alterations in vascular permeability and epithelial intercellular barriers.[192]

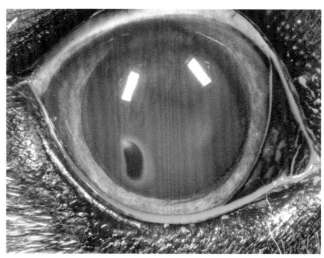

Figure 2.5 Positive Seidel test: Leaking aqueous humor from a small perforation is leaving a dark rivulet in the green tearfilm.

- To detect an aqueous humor leak from a perforating corneal injury (Seidel test).[193] The orange fluorescein applied to the suspicious area develops a dark rivulet in the green tear film where the aqueous humor trickles out of the wound (**Figure 2.5**).

Rose bengal

Rose bengal has been traditionally called a supravital stain that stains devitalized cells. The staining mechanism has been questioned in that it stains healthy cultured cells. Recent evidence suggests that healthy corneal cells are protected from staining by tear components such as albumin and mucin that block the stain uptake.[194] When rose bengal is applied to the cornea and the conjunctiva, it stains unprotected epithelial cells a rose color.

It is used mainly in diagnosing KCS (dry eye), and it is supposed to be more sensitive than the STT tear film deficiencies.[195] Rose bengal is virucidal and should not be used before culturing. It is also photodynamic and intrinsically toxic to cells. Rose bengal is often irritating when applied as a solution; this can be decreased by using a topical anesthetic prior to use or the use of impregnated strips of rose bengal.

Indocyanine green

A 0.5% solution of indocyanine green has been used intracamerally to visualize the capsule while performing curvilinear capsulorrhexis. Visualizing the capsule against a mature white cataract is difficult, and staining aids in identification for grasping with capsular forceps.[196,197] In humans, indocyanine green has also been injected intravenously and used for retinal angiography. Combined with diode laser, it has been used to obliterate retinal neovascularization.

Trypan blue

Trypan blue has been used as a supravital stain to determine the viability of corneal endothelial cells in donor corneas for transplantation. It is also used to stain the capsule to facilitate capsulorrhexis during cataract surgery. Trypan blue is introduced into the anterior chamber under a large air bubble to keep the stain away from the corneal endothelium and against the lens capsule. It is rinsed out after 30 seconds to 2 minutes, leaving a mildly blue-stained lens capsule that is easier to see against the background of a white, mature cataract.

TOPICAL ANESTHETICS

Topical anesthetics are used extensively and exclusively for diagnostic and manipulative procedures of the eye but not for medical therapeutics. They are rapid in their onset, taking effect within 15–30 seconds and lasting about 15 minutes. Herring et al. found that by applying two drops at 1-minute intervals the length of maximal analgesia was extended to 25 minutes.[198] For the most profound analgesia, the author frequently supplements drops with a cotton tip applicator saturated with the anesthetic and placed specifically on the location to be manipulated. As a group, topical anesthetics are readily absorbed from mucosal surfaces but not from the skin. They are very toxic to the epithelium and retard healing of the cornea by inhibiting both mitosis and cellular migration.[199] Repeated usage creates tolerance, which begets increased frequency. It has been demonstrated that a reduced concentration can be used without toxic effects, but the disadvantage of short duration of action still remains.[200] Repeated topical application of anesthetics to diseased epithelium, such as in corneal edema, may result in epithelial erosions.[201] The topical anesthetics are also bactericidal, so conjunctival or corneal cultures should be taken prior to application.

Topical proparacaine has helped to maintain mydriasis or prevent miosis and decrease the breakdown of the blood–aqueous humor barrier as much as topical NSAIDs; therefore, it is being used preoperatively with intraocular surgery.[202]

Do not use topical anesthetics for the treatment of corneal ulcers.

Agents

- Proparacaine 0.5% is the most commonly utilized topical anesthetic.
- Tetracaine 0.5%–2%
- Oxybuprocaine 0.4%
- Piperocaine
- Dibucaine
- Benoxinate 0.4%
- Cocaine 0.5%–4%: The original topical anesthetic, but it is the most toxic to the epithelium. Cocaine is a controlled drug, so is rarely used now for this purpose.

MATRIX METALLOPROTEINASE INHIBITORS

The matrix metalloproteinases (MMPs) are categorized into subgroups according to their structure and matrix specificity, that is collagenases, gelatinases, and stromelysins. The MMPs are a family of zinc-dependent endopeptidases that are present in low levels in normal tissue and upregulated during normal and pathologic remodeling of tissue, such as in embryonic development, inflammation, neoplasia, and angiogenesis. They cleave collagen molecules and are secreted in a latent form. The catalytic domain for proteolytic activity contains a Zn^{2+} binding site that is stabilized by Ca^{2+}[154]. Examples of MMPs are collagenases (MMP-1, MMP-8, MMP-13), gelatinases (MMP-2, MMP-9), stromelysins (MMP-3, MMP-10), elastase, and the serine proteases of plasmin and tissue plasminogen activator.[203–205] These enzymes are present in various cells such as migrating neutrophils, phagocytes, corneal cells, and in infectious agents such as *Pseudomonas* spp.[206,207]

The original ophthalmic interest in MMPs was in their role in corneal ulceration. The regenerating corneal epithelium interacts with the stroma to liberate the enzyme collagenase (MMP-1).[208] Collagenase is liberated in a latent form by corneal cells, is activated by plasmin, and is calcium dependent.[209,210] If present in excessive amounts, collagenase cleaves the stromal collagen and creates a progressive ulcer in both depth and diameter. Once initiated, progression of a superficial ulcer to a perforated ulcer can be a matter of hours.

Strubbe et al.[211] isolated MMP-2, MMP-9, and neutrophil elastase in higher levels from the tear film of horses with corneal ulcerations than from normal aged-matched controls. Levels of MMPs were elevated whether the ulcer was sterile or was associated with bacteria or fungi; MMPs were present in both eyes even with a unilateral ulcer.

Four natural inhibitors of MMPs (tissue inhibitors of MMPs [TIMPs]) have been identified.[212] Various drugs cause collagenase inhibition, and most of these work as chelating agents against calcium and zinc. Clinically, results are often disappointing. A verifiably effective protocol for treating progressive corneal ulcers has yet to be described; however, due to the potential devastating outcome of rapidly progressive corneal ulceration, clinicians utilize empirical treatment with a variety of products.

Glucocorticoid therapy is potentially dangerous with active ulceration because the drugs augment collagenase activity up to $15\times$.[213] Olliviero et al.[214] tested a variety of MMP inhibitors against tears from horses with ulcerative keratitis and found all to have 92%–99% inhibitory activity against MMPs in tears. Drugs tested were: EDTA, acetylcysteine, doxycycline, ilomastat (Galardin), and α-1 proteinase inhibitor.

The interest in MMPs in ophthalmology has expanded from corneal ulceration to aqueous humor outflow regulation, angiogenesis, and cancer.[212]

Agents
- Topical sodium and potassium EDTA reversibly bind calcium and zinc. Calcium binding interferes with the burst of respiratory energy necessary for the neutrophils to degranulate.[215,216]
- Topical acetylcysteine binds calcium, but it also acts by reducing a disulfide bond and consequently is not completely reversible by adding calcium.[215]
- Topical penicillamine binds calcium.[215,216]
- Topical serum globulin: Serum contains α-2 macroglobulins, which are nonspecific, irreversible binders of collagenase[217] and are superior in action on a molar basis than the metal chelators. Brooks et al. found that equine serum had high levels of *in vitro* inhibition of MMP activity that was effective for up to 1 week, whether stored in a refrigerator or at room temperature; no differences were found in activity between fresh or frozen serum.[218]
- Topical sodium citrate inhibits calcium.[216]
- Systemic ascorbate: There is conflicting evidence as to its efficacy.[219–221]
- Tetracycline given intramuscularly at 50 mg/kg/day was effective in treating alkali- and *Pseudomonas aeruginosa*–induced ulcerations in rabbits.[222,223]
- Thiols and hydroxamic acids (MMP inhibitors); for example, Galardin; more effective than previous drugs but experimental and is not yet available.[204,205]

For effective therapy, MMP inhibitors must be administered frequently, probably every hour, to keep the cells bathed in the inhibitor. Acetylcysteine has been used most frequently because it is commercially available as a mucolytic agent for respiratory nebulization therapy. Mucomyst is available as 10% and 20% solutions and should be refrigerated; once opened, it is relatively unstable. Mucomyst at the higher concentrations is toxic to the cornea, so a 5%–10% solution is recommended.[224]

Serum from the patient is another alternative, particularly for horses, but care must be taken to avoid contamination since it is such a good culture medium.

GLUCOCORTICOIDS

Pharmacology
Glucocorticoids found an early use in ophthalmology and were a great therapeutic advance due to the importance of minimizing scarring in the ocular healing process. As with all therapeutic modalities, glucocorticoid therapy was not a panacea, and it has been responsible for many avoidable ocular catastrophes. Their anti-inflammatory and immunosuppressive effects have made the glucocorticoids a powerful tool in preventing scarring, maintaining transparency, and treating the immune-mediated inflammations of some forms of keratitis, uveitis, conjunctivitis, scleritis/episcleritis, and corneal transplants. Glucocorticoids do not eliminate noxious stimuli but appear to only modify the response to the noxious stimuli. Glucocorticoids at therapeutic doses have some action on every facet of the immune response (**Table 2.10**).

A variety of corticosteroid, glucocorticoids, are available commercially in topical preparations. In general, the more potent the steroid the lower the concentration in the solution. Considerations in selecting a glucocorticoid for topical therapy include corneal penetration, anti-inflammatory effect, duration of action, and systemic and topical side-effects.[225] Topical phosphate solutions are water soluble, and acetates and alcohols are suspensions and biphasic. Experimental studies indicate that topical prednisolone acetate 1% produces the best anti-inflammatory effect in the intact cornea, followed by dexamethasone alcohol 0.1% suspension, prednisolone phosphate 0.1% solution, and dexamethasone phosphate 0.05% ointment.[226] Despite the advantage of prednisolone acetate suspension, vigorous shaking of the bottle is necessary to deliver the intended dosage, and marked discrepancies can occur between brands

---

Table 2.10 **Anti-inflammatory effects of therapeutic doses of glucocorticoids.**

- Block permeability of capillary endothelium.
- Prevent intracellular edema.
- Inhibit migration of neutrophils by decreasing vascular permeability and vasoconstriction.
- Reduce neutrophil adherence.
- Inhibit ingestion of bacteria and release of proteolytic enzymes by neutrophils and macrophages.
- Prevent antibody production of B-lymphocytes before humoral recognition.
- Suppression of lymphokines from stimulated T-lymphocytes.
- Interfere with complement subfractions.
- Inhibit histamine synthesis and counteract histamine vascular effects.
- Decrease fibroblastic proliferation and collagen deposition.
- Possibly stabilize lysosomal membranes.
- Possibly affect prostaglandin synthesis.

of the same product. In one study, shaking the bottle 40 times delivered 82% of the maximum concentration of the product with one product and 22% with another product.[227]

All the prednisolone derivatives penetrate the blood–aqueous humor barriers equally when given systemically. Except for methylprednisolone, which is a repositol glucocorticoid, the aqueous humor levels are short lived, that is, 2–3 hours.

Route of therapy

If possible, it is desirable to limit steroid therapy to the topical route to minimize systemic side effects. Even with topical therapy, there is ample evidence to show adrenal suppression and hepatic metabolic changes from systemic absorption (through conjunctiva and oral absorption from licking the nose after exiting from the nasolacrimal duct). Clinical signs of polyuria, polydipsia, and increased appetite may occasionally be noted with topical glucocorticoids.[228–231] Diabetic dogs may be more difficult to control while on topical glucocorticoids.

Subconjunctival repositol steroid products relieve the owner of frequent therapy and produce higher levels in the anterior segment (**Table 2.11**). However, there is potential difficulty in stopping the steroid action if they become contraindicated. There is also an increased systemic effect from the subconjunctival route, and patients routinely develop polyuria and polydypsia.[232] An occasional complication of subconjunctival repositol steroids is a subconjunctival granuloma,[233] which appears as a smooth, circumscribed subconjunctival mass. A white residue from the repositol steroids is often visible for weeks after injection.

The systemic route is utilized for severe intraocular conditions and when topical glucocorticoids may be contraindicated.

Indications for use
- Sterile immune-mediated ocular diseases, for example, pannus, atopic conjunctivitis, VKH.

Two of the most common errors when treating severe inflammatory conditions with topical glucocorticoids are to use a weak product such as hydrocortisone and not to administer the drug frequently enough (every 4–6 hours).
- Post-traumatic ocular inflammation, for example, post-surgical inflammation.
- Ocular infections with significant destructive immune-mediated inflammation, for example, feline infectious peritonitis (FIP) associated uveitis, feline immunodeficiency virus (FIV)-associated uveitis, and *Toxoplasma*-associated uveitis. Therapy with systemic infectious agents is almost always limited to topical glucocorticoid therapy. Glucocorticoids are generally not used with bacterial or mycotic ocular infections.
- Reduction of ocular scarring, neovascularization, and pigmentation.

Contraindications and nonresponsive conditions for topical glucocorticoid therapy
- In the presence of corneal ulcerations and abrasions: Glucocorticoids activate collagenase and may induce a progressive ulceration (**Figure 2.6**).[213,235]
- In general, the presence of bacterial or fungal infections of the eye. The latter applies particularly to the horse.

Glucocorticoids are ineffective against old scars of the cornea or elsewhere in the eye, stromal pigment, primary glaucoma, cataracts, and degenerative corneal diseases

Table 2.11 **Repositol subconjunctival glucocorticoids.**		
DRUG	**DURATION OF ACTION**	**RELATIVE ANTI-INFLAMMATORY POTENCY**
Methylprednisolone acetate	14–30 days	5
Betamethasone sodium phosphate and acetate	7–14 days	25
Dexamethasone sodium phosphate	7–10 days	30
Triamcinolone acetonide	7–30+ days	5

Source: Modified from Krohne, S.D.G., and Vestre, W.A. 1987. *American Journal of Veterinary Research* 48:420–422.

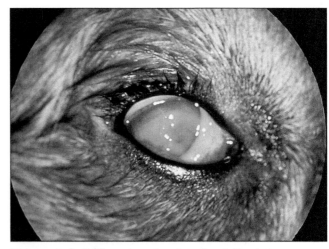

Figure 2.6 Collagenase ulcer in a dog following experimental wounding and administration of repositol methylprednisolone. Five days after wounding, the lesion progressed from a healing superficial lesion to a descemetocele within 6 hours.

such as corneal endothelial degeneration with edema and corneal lipids.

Side effects and complications

- Increase corneal mycotic infections (horse), activate latent herpesvirus infection (cat), and in all species may worsen a bacterial infection if not covered by appropriate antibiotic.
- Progression of corneal ulceration due to augmentation of MMPs.
- Complications of posterior subcapsular cataracts and glaucoma as observed in humans were not thought to develop in domestic animals; however, subcapsular cataracts and ocular hypertension were produced with topical dexamethasone sodium phosphate therapy in cats.[236,237] Anecdotally, dogs on systemic or topical glucocorticoids have been found with rapidly developing cortical cataracts and lipid keratopathy.
- Band keratopathy or superficial calcification of the cornea may occur with topical therapy using phosphate salts of the glucocorticoids.[238]
- Iatrogenic Cushing's syndrome and adrenal suppression.[230]

PROSTAGLANDIN INHIBITORS (NSAIDs) AND PROSTAGLANDIN ANALOGS

Pharmacology

Prostaglandins (PGs) are a group of oxygenated fatty acids that in humans and higher animals are derived mainly from arachidonic acid. The precursors are stored as esterified phospholipids in cell membranes and are released by phospholipase A_2. The precursors are rapidly oxygenated through either cyclooxygenase or lipoxygenase pathways. The cyclooxygenase pathway leads to a variety of PG compounds and thromboxane A_2. In the presence of epinephrine as a cofactor, the main PGs produced are PGD_2, PGE_2, $PGF_{2\alpha}$, PGI_2, and thromboxane. There are two cyclooxygenase isoforms: Cyclooxygenase 1 is present at all times in the tissue and is responsible for the basal prostaglandin synthesis in homeostasis, and cyclooxygenase 2 is inducible and expressed in inflammatory sites by monocytes, macrophages, and fibroblasts. Most NSAIDs are nonselective inhibitors of cyclooxygenase, and this results in many of the undesirable side effects of these drugs.[239]

The lipoxygenase pathway results in the production of various leukotrienes and hydroxyeicosatetraenoic acids (HETEs), which are strong chemotactic agents for polymorphonuclear cells.[240]

PG precursors are abundant in the anterior uvea and conjunctiva and are released whenever the iris is injured. Species variations are present, but in general, the result of PG release is intraocular inflammation, that is, miosis, increased protein content in the aqueous humor, and conjunctival hyperemia. The effect on IOP varies with the species, PG, dose, and time. In general, an initial hypertension is followed by a prolonged hypotension. The signs of inflammation can be reduced by prior treatment with PG inhibitors, and, therefore, they are ideally used before surgery to minimize postsurgical inflammation. Glucocorticoids induce a protein called macrocortin (also called lipomodulin) that interferes with phospholipase A_2 and consequently affects both the cyclooxygenase and lipoxygenase pathways.[241] Glucocorticoids are selective inhibitors of cyclooxygenase 2 (see section Glucocorticoids).

NSAIDs

- Aspirin is a cyclooxygenase pathway inhibitor. Many dogs can tolerate a dose of 10 mg/kg every 12 hours for long periods. Aspirin has been demonstrated to decrease the protein in secondary aqueous humor (newly formed aqueous humor after an ocular insult to the blood–aqueous humor barrier) in the dog.[242,243] The author has been reluctant to use aspirin postoperatively due to an observed higher incidence of postoperative hyphema, nor in equine recurrent uveitis due to perceived ineffectiveness.
- Flunixin meglumine is not approved for use in small animals, but many surgeons use it routinely before eye surgery at a single dose of 0.5 mg/kg IV without problem. Higher doses may produce gastrointestinal ulcerations and renal failure. Flunixin should be used cautiously in patients who are hypotensive or dehydrated.[244] Flunixin indirectly decreases aqueous humor protein after an ocular injury by reducing PG-induced vascular permeability, and it is additive when used in combination with systemic dexamethasone (64% reduction) on postoperative aqueous humor protein values.[234,245] Systemic flunixin and topical flurbiprofen were relatively equal in minimizing miosis after a laser-induced injury, but they also promoted post-injury ocular hypertension.[246] Flunixin is utilized extensively in equine ophthalmology in treating corneal and uveal diseases.
- Flurbiprofen 0.03% was the original topical NSAID preparation and was marketed to prevent intraoperative miosis during cataract surgery. When used as a postoperative anti-inflammatory agent, it does not inhibit corneal stromal healing.[247,248] Intraoperative spontaneous bleeding appears to

be more common with intensive preoperative PG inhibitors, and, therefore, the author has decreased the intensive use of hourly flurbiprofen. It can be used as an alternative anti-inflammatory when corneal ulceration prohibits glucocorticoid therapy or used in conjunction with glucocorticoids. Topical flurbiprofen has been shown to decrease significantly aqueous humor outflow in noninjured and injured eyes.[249] Flurbiprofen was more effective in decreasing aqueous humor protein than systemic or topical steroids in two noninvasive models of inflammation, while in an invasive model, topical 1% prednisolone acetate was more effective than topical NSAIDs.[202,250,251]

- Diclofenac 0.1%, suprofen 1%, 0.5% ketorolac, bromfenac 0.09%, and nepafenac 0.1% are alternative topical NSAIDs, and depending on the model used, they may not be as effective as flurbiprofen in inhibiting miosis and aqueous flare. Diclofenac has some corneal analgesic properties, but like topical anesthetics, the effect is relatively short lived.[252] Bromfenac and nepafenac (and its active metabolite amfenac) are selective cyclooxygenase-2 inhibitors and penetrate the intact cornea well.[253–256]

- Topical NSAIDs are frequently utilized when the cornea is ulcerated and an anti-inflammatory drug is still needed. The author has used flurbiprofen for years in this manner without complications, but melting ulcers have been reported in humans with topical ketorolac and diclofenac.[257,258] NSAIDs, either topical or systemic, are generally not indicated with glaucoma due to the ocular hypertensive effect.

- Indomethacin is rarely used systemically in the dog due to digestive tract complications. Topical preparations are available commercially outside the United States. Indomethacin has been shown to decrease significantly aqueous humor protein content in secondary aqueous humor and prevent miosis.[259,260] Concentrations from 0.1%–1% are equally effective.

- Phenylbutazone at 20 mg/kg intravenously decreased the protein in the secondary aqueous humor after paracentesis to one-third that of controls.[243] Clinically, phenylbutazone is not as effective as flunixin in the horse in treating ocular pain and inflammation. Nevertheless, it is used extensively for mild-to-moderate ocular pain and inflammation because it is much less expensive than flunixin.

- Carprofen is a systemic anti-inflammatory that is a weak cyclooxygenase inhibitor and a free radical scavenger. The effect of carprofen on inhibiting breakdown of the blood–aqueous humor barrier is comparable to aspirin and flunixin.[261]

Carprofen may be associated with gastrointestinal signs and renal and hepatocellular toxicosis.

Most studies have shown that the maximum anti-inflammatory effect is achieved when topical combinations of glucocorticoids and NSAIDs are given, rather than either type of agent alone.[243,248]

Prostaglandin analogs

Latanoprost, which is an esterized prodrug of $PGF_{2\alpha}$, was the first PG analog introduced for topical glaucoma therapy. It is available as a 0.005% solution and, in humans, is normally only given every 24 hours. It has been described as the most potent topical drug to date for treating glaucoma. Additional PG derivatives that have been recently introduced are travoprost 0.004%, bimatoprost 0.03%, and unoprostone 0.15%. In normal dogs and glaucomatous beagles, the IOP lowering effect and side effects of the various prostaglandin analogs appear to be quite similar.[262,263]

The effects of PGs vary with the type, dose, and species, so each species must be explored individually. Latanoprost increases the unconventional outflow (uveoscleral) pathway, which is unique for antiglaucoma medications. Latanoprost is more lipophilic, allowing better corneal penetration than the end product, $PGF_{2\alpha}$.[264] How it affects uveoscleral flow is still under investigation, but one demonstrated effect is to increase matrix metalloproteinases in the ciliary body, which may decrease the resistance to outflow in the extracellular spaces of the ciliary muscle.[265,266]

There is not much information on the use of latanoprost in canine glaucoma, but in the author's experience, it frequently produces a dramatic drop in IOP in dogs within 30–60 minutes of instillation, often when other drugs have not worked. The continued success of treatment has been variable after the initial reduction, as it becomes ineffective in some dogs, while others maintain a low IOP for extended periods. The author routinely uses it every 12 hours. Gelatt and MacKay found that 0.005% latanoprost reduced the IOP in the glaucomatous beagle model by 50%–60%, and every-12-hour therapy resulted in less fluctuation in IOP through the day.[267] The pressure-lowering effect of latanoprost and travoprost in dogs has been well established.[268–270]

Latanoprost can be used with other antiglaucoma medications, including the β-blockers and topical and systemic CAIs. Whether latanoprost should be used in secondary glaucoma associated with breakdown of the blood–aqueous humor barrier is not yet clear. The author has used it where there are postoperative cataract surgery pressure spikes with dramatic but not invariable results and has not noted any increased postoperative inflammation.

Diehl et al. found that latanoprost administered every 24 hours produced a significant lowering of IOP in normal horses, but adverse effects of epiphora, blepharospasm, and blepharedema were common.[271] Clinically, the author has not observed a significant reduction in IOP with latanoprost in glaucomatous horses. Latanoprost is not effective in lowing the IOP in normal cats, although it is a very potent miotic.[272–274] Anecdotally, clinicians have thought it is effective in treating feline glaucoma.

Side effects

Like its action, the side effects of latanoprost are also unique and vary between species. In the cat and the dog, latanoprost produces a dramatic miosis that lasts for several hours.[272] Conjunctival hyperemia is variable but may be marked. In humans, no miosis is noted, but up to 10% of patients may develop iris hyperpigmentation after 3–5 months of therapy. Other side effects reported in humans are hypertrichosis of the cilia, macular edema, choroidal effusion, anterior uveitis, and facial skin rash.[264,275,276] In the rabbit, latanoprost worsened the severity of herpesvirus keratitis and increased the risk of recurrences.[277] If latanoprost proves ineffective in feline glaucoma, concern with aggravating herpesvirus keratitis may not be of significance in veterinary medicine.

> All the effects of latanoprost in dogs are not currently known. The rapid decrease in IOP in responsive dogs would argue against the proposed mechanism of altering MMPs; such a mechanism should have a lag time since MMPs exist in a latent form.

ANTIHISTAMINES AND DECONGESTANTS

Pharmacology

Histamine release from mast cells in the conjunctiva mediates the clinical signs of vasodilatation, edema, and itching through H^1 and H^2 receptors. H^1 and H^2 receptors both dilate small blood vessels. Intraocular effects of histamine are constriction of the pupil and an iris vasodilation, causing an increase in aqueous humor protein.[225] Antihistamines and decongestants are widely used in over-the-counter ophthalmic drugs that are used for "red eyes."

Agents

- Antazoline phosphate is an H^1 blocker that inhibits itching but not conjunctival redness, so it is often combined with a vasoconstrictor.[225] Other H^1 blockers used topically are pheniramine maleate and pyrilamine maleate.
- Sodium cromolyn, a drug that prevents mast cell degranulation, is available as a 4% ophthalmic solution. It inhibits all the signs of histamine release. Unfortunately, to be effective, it must be given before the insult to prevent degranulation.[278]
- Lodoxamide tromethamine 0.1% inhibits mast cell degranulation and is used in allergic conjunctivitis and eosinophilic keratitis in the horse. However, it is expensive, which can prevent its use in routine treatment of atopic or allergic conjunctivitis. Its effectiveness in feline eosinophilic keratitis has not been reported.
- Vasoconstrictive agents utilized in topical preparations include naphazoline, tetrahydrozoline, and phenylephrine.

IMMUNOSUPPRESSIVE DRUGS

Pharmacology

Despite the potential for serious side effects, the immunosuppressive drugs are developing a niche for treating blinding ophthalmic inflammatory conditions that are resistant to conventional glucocorticoid therapy. Most of these drugs function by inhibiting the process of cellular division. While the goal is usually to interfere with lymphocyte proliferation and function, most of them are nonselective in their inhibition, resulting in side effects that are first noted in rapidly dividing cells.

Alkylating agents

Cyclophosphamide and chlorambucil are alkylating agents and are cell cycle-phase nonspecific, affecting cells in either the resting or proliferating phase. The alkylating agents produce cross-linking and breakage of DNA strands and inhibition of DNA synthesis. While these agents affect slow-growing cells, they are most effective on rapidly dividing cells; lymphocytes are very sensitive.[279,280]

The dose of cyclophosphamide depends on the severity of the condition and concurrent drugs that are being used. For immunosuppression, 1.5–2.5 mg/kg every other day has been used.[280]

Purine analogs

Some purine analogs have been used for immunosuppression and others as antiviral agents. The two most important for immunosuppression are 6-mercaptopurine and azathioprine.

Azathioprine is a prodrug that becomes 6-mercaptopurine after reacting with sulfhydryl compounds in the liver. These compounds interfere with the nucleic acid metabolism by inhibiting the incorporation of normal purine compounds. The purine analogs are most effective in inhibiting cell division during the S phase.[281] The immunosuppressive effect is through affecting T-helper lymphocyte function, with little effect on humoral immunity or B-lymphocytes unless large doses are administered within 48 hours of antigenic priming.[282] The purine analogs work best on cell-mediated immune diseases.[282] In the dog, it has been used most frequently in the therapy of Vogt–Koyanagi–Harada (VKH) uveitis and fibrous histiocytomas (nodular episclerokeratitis) of the cornea.[283]

Azathioprine is most commonly used at 50 mg/m² (2 mg/kg) by mouth every 24 hours, reduced after 2 weeks to 1 mg/kg every other day for 2 weeks and then 1 mg/kg once a week if possible.[283] Azathioprine is usually given initially with systemic glucocorticoids because there is a 3- to 5-week lag before clinical effects are evident.[281] Glucocorticoids are tapered once clinical improvement is noted and, hopefully, eventually discontinued. Weekly complete blood cell and platelet counts should be monitored until the minimal maintenance dose of azathioprine is reached, when monitoring can be reduced in frequency, depending on the blood cell counts.

Folic acid analogs

Methotrexate is the major drug in this category. Methotrexate competitively inhibits folic acid reductase, which is involved in folate metabolism. Folic acid is reduced to tetrahydrofolic acid, which is involved with purine metabolism, and thus DNA and RNA synthesis and cellular replication are inhibited. Methotrexate has been recommended for use as a subconjunctival injection at 12.5 mg for treatment of intraocular tumors.[284]

Cyclosporine A

Cyclosporine is the metabolite of two fungi, and unlike other immunosuppressive agents, its action is not mediated via cytotoxicity. Cyclosporine's action is incompletely understood, but it is thought to act by interfering with interleukin-2 and T-cell activation. Cyclosporine is normally administered orally, is expensive, and has potential renal toxicity.[279] A safer, less expensive mode of therapy for ophthalmic use is topical application, and a 0.2% ointment is available commercially for topical use in veterinary medicine. Alternatively, compounding pharmacists are diluting the oral preparation with corn oil to a 1% or 2% solution for topical use.

Cyclosporine is lipophilic and thus is well absorbed through the cornea. A 1%–2% solution and a 0.2% ointment have demonstrated an effect on a variety of experimental immune-mediated ocular inflammations.[285–287] Its main use topically in veterinary ophthalmology is in treating KCS, but it has potential in the treatment of a variety of immune surface diseases such as pannus, pigmentary keratitis, and allergic conjunctivitis.[288–290] Cyclosporine stimulates lacrimal secretion and increases the tear production in normal and deficient dogs. In mice, this action of topical cyclosporine was reversed with capsaicin, which depletes substance P from the lacrimal gland,[291] suggesting cyclosporine causes the release of the neurotransmitter substance P from sensory nerve endings, and that substance P then stimulates parasympathetic nerves in the gland.

Topical cyclosporine either as a 1% or 2% solution is effective in 75%–85% of KCS cases.[292–294] The frequency of therapy varies with the condition treated, but therapy for KCS is usually every 12 hours, and the duration of therapy is indefinite. Inflammatory conditions have been initially treated at 6-hour intervals over a 2- to 3-week period and continued at decreased frequency as long as needed to control the condition.

Cyclosporine has been implanted in the vitreous in an experimental sustained-release device to treat recurrent uveitis in horses. The device was primed with cyclosporine to deliver 4 µg/day for up to 5 years.[295] Complications from the procedure were minimal when the device was implanted in quiet eyes. A newer cyclosporine-releasing device is implanted in the suprachoroidal space of horses with recurrent uveitis and releases cyclosporine for an estimated 36 months.[27]

Tacrolimus and pimecrolimus

Tacrolimus is derived from *Streptomyces tsukabaensis* and is an immunosuppressant that is 10–100 times more potent on a weight basis than cyclosporine. Tacrolimus and pimecrolimus are macrolactam derivatives that bind to macrophilin-12 and inhibit calcineurin, resulting in T-cell activation and some suppression of humoral immunity. Tacrolimus is used systemically to counteract transplant rejections, and both tacrolimus and pimecrolimus are used topically to treat eczema in humans. Tacrolimus is being compounded for topical use as a 0.02%–0.03% solution or ointment and pimecrolimus as a 1% oil solution for treating KCS and chronic superficial keratitis.[296–298,299] Chambers et al.[300] had a 96% success rate, although the severity of cases treated was not stipulated. As tacrolimus utilizes different cell receptors than cyclosporine, it may be effective in cyclosporine-resistant cases of KCS.

ANTIFIBRIN AGENTS

Tissue plasminogen activator

Recombinant tissue plasminogen activator (tPA) is used systemically in humans to break up blood clots in patients with myocardial infarction and stroke. It acts by binding fibrin, and the complex then binds plasminogen and activates it to plasmin. Plasmin then accelerates the breakdown of fibrinogen to fibrin degradation products and fibrin to fibrin-split products. Tissue plasminogen activator injected at 25 µg into the anterior chamber has been successful in lysing fibrin clots and breaking synechiae when used within 24–72 hours of their formation.[301,302] The author has used tPA in acute idiopathic inflammation and postoperatively in cataract and aqueous humor shunt surgery.[303] The use of tPA with hyphema that is not spontaneously resolving is a tempting possibility, but there is a significant danger of recurrent hemorrhage.[304,305]

Tissue plasminogen activator has demonstrated no toxic effects to the corneal endothelium or changes in the IOP when ≤50 µg was injected in the anterior chamber of the normal canine eye.[169] Injection of tPA in the vitreous in doses of ≥50 µg results in photoreceptor cell damage, but at least part of this toxicity is due to the vehicle.[306]

Tissue plasminogen activator is packaged for systemic use and is extremely expensive. Diluting the drug and repackaging into sterile vials that are stored at –70°C (–94°F) until thawed for use has made the cost reasonable ($20 per vial). Anterior chamber doses of 25 µg are safe and effective, but caution should be used with vitreal injections. Most patients can be injected under topical anesthesia using a 30-gauge needle. Topical application of tPA in a 0.1% solution (1 mg/mL) has also experimentally resulted in detectable intraocular concentrations of tPA and dissolution of clots. However, at this concentration, expense is once again a factor.[307]

Tissue plasminogen activator is truly a miracle drug to the surgeon/clinician who has struggled with intraocular adhesions. To watch a large fibrin clot dissolve or synechiae release over 30 minutes is amazing.

Heparin

Heparin impairs the thrombin-mediated formation of fibrin and is utilized intraoperatively during intraocular surgery to minimize fibrin formation during and immediately after surgery. An increased risk of intraoperative and postoperative bleeding may occur. Preservative-free heparin is preferable. The dose is 1 U/mL of irrigating fluids.

Hirudin

Hirudin is a direct-acting antithrombin agent that blocks the formation of fibrin from fibrinogen without an effect on platelets. It was originally isolated from leeches and is now available in a recombinant form. It decreased the amount of fibrin in a rabbit model when used intraoperatively at 100 µg/mL in an infusion, and no intraocular hemorrhage was noted.[308]

VISCOELASTIC AGENTS

Viscoelastic agents are transparent solutions of high viscosity, and they have become important adjuncts to intraocular surgery. These agents are used to maintain spatial relationships, separate tissue to prevent adhesions, contain hemorrhage, act as a lubricant, and protect tissue from mechanical injury.[309] In addition, they have been used on the corneal surface to lubricate and replace tears and maintain optical clarity during surgery (see section Artificial tears). While somewhat slow to be accepted into veterinary ophthalmologic surgery because of their significant cost, they have become almost universally accepted with the advent of phacoemulsification surgery. Their viscous nature helps to maintain the anterior chamber during manipulations through small incisions, and they protect the corneal endothelium from trauma during surgery and introduction of intraocular lenses.

Wilkie and Willis reviewed the properties of viscoelastic agents and compared the various properties available.[310] Viscoelastic agents can be characterized in terms of their rheologic properties of viscosity, pseudoplasticity, viscoelasticity, and surface tension. Viscosity is a measure of the resistance to flow; high-viscosity products have the desirable property of staying in the anterior chamber, but they may be difficult to inject through a small cannula. Pseudoplasticity is the change of viscosity that occurs with increasing shear rate, that is, decreasing viscosity with increasing movement; this property allows the product to be injected through a small cannula. Elasticity of a substance is the ability to return to its original shape after a deforming force has been applied and is related to cohesiveness. Cohesive viscoelastics maintain spaces well and are aspirated more easily from the anterior chamber. A dispersive viscoelastic is lower in molecular weight and viscosity and spreads within available space.[310] Viscoelastics with dispersive properties spread and protect tissues and are not expelled from the eye as rapidly during surgery as cohesive viscoelastics.

Ideally, because of the varying qualities needed from a viscoelastic for different stages of performing extracapsular extraction with phacoemulsification, more than one product would be used during the procedure. In practice, most surgeons utilize only one viscoelastic that happens to be their favorite, often based on cost.

Agents

- Sodium hyaluronate was the first viscoelastic agent. It was initially derived from rooster combs and umbilical cords and most recently from genetic engineering utilizing fermentation with Streptococci. Sodium hyaluronate is the benchmark against which all other viscoelastic agents are compared. There are various hyaluronic acid preparations on the market, and the purity and viscosity may vary. Thus, agents used for treatment of joint disease may not be acceptable for ophthalmology. Ophthalmic sodium hyaluronate is available in a regular viscosity and, more recently, as a supercohesive form.

- Chondroitin sulfate–sodium hyaluronic mixture provides increased coating of tissues and implants due to the dispersive qualities of chondroitin and the cohesiveness of hyaluronate; the mixture thus remains within the eye to maintain spatial relationships.
- Hydroxypropyl methylcellulose 2%, unlike the previous two agents, is not a natural substance in animals. It is readily available and thus less expensive to manufacture, and it is stable and autoclavable. Hydroxypropyl methylcellulose is viscous and dispersive and is less cohesive than the other viscoelastics.

Viscoelastic agents have made all intraocular surgeons better surgeons, allowing manipulations through small incisions that would previously have been difficult to perform.

Side effects

- Postoperative pressure elevations. Postoperative IOP elevations are reported in humans if viscoelastic agents are not completely removed at the termination of surgery but not in the dog. However, transient postoperative pressure elevations are also common without the use of viscoelastic agents.
- Endotoxins from nonophthalmic preparations may produce sterile postoperative inflammations.
- Postoperative corneal edema has been clinically noted with some batches of hydroxypropyl methylcellulose.

REFERENCES

1. Shell, J.W. 1982. Pharmacokinetics of topically applied ophthalmic drugs. *Survey of Ophthalmology* 26:207–218.
2. Ueno, N., Refojo, M.F., and Abelson, M.B. 1994. Pharmacokinetics. In: Ablert, D.A., and Jokobeic, F.A. editor. *Principles and Practice of Ophthalmology: Basic Sciences.* WB Saunders: Philadelphia, PA, p. 916–929.
3. Axelrod, J., Daly, J.S., Glew, R.H., Barza, M., and Baker, A.S. 1995. Antibacterials. In: Ablert, D.A., and Jokobeic, F.A. editors. *Principles and Practice of Ophthalmology: Basic Sciences.* WB Saunders: Philadelphia, PA, pp. 940–961.
4. Johnson, D.A., Johns, K.J., Robinson, R.D., Head, W.S., and O'Day, D. 1995. The relationship of corneal epithelial defect size to drug penetration. *Archives of Ophthalmology* 113:641–644.
5. Mathis, G.A. 1991. Clinical ophthalmic pharmacology and therapeutics. In: Gelatt, K. editor. *Veterinary Ophthalmology*, 3rd Edition: Lippincott, Williams & Wilkins: Philadelphia, PA, pp. 291–336.
6. Bartlett, J.D. 2001. Ophthalmic drug delivery. In: Bartlett, J.D., and Jaanus, S.D. editors. *Clinical Ocular Pharmacology*, 4th Edition: Butterworth Heinemann: Boston, MA pp. 41–62.
7. Koevary, S.B. 2003. Pharmacokinetics of topical ocular drug delivery: Potential uses for the treatment of diseases of the posterior segment and beyond. *Current Drug Metabolism* 4(3):213–222.
8. Robin, J.S., and Ellis, P.P. 1978. Ophthalmic ointments. *Survey of Ophthalmology* 22:335–340.
9. Hanna, C., Fraunfelder, F., Cable, M., and Hardberger, R. 1973. The effects of ophthalmic ointments on corneal wound healing. *American Journal of Ophthalmology* 76:193–200.
10. Cox, W.V., Kupferman, A., and Leibowitz, H.M. 1972. Topically applied steroids in corneal disease. *Archives of Ophthalmology* 88:549–552.
11. Mindel, J.S. 1998. α-adrenergic drugs. In: Tasman, W., and Jaeger, E.A. editors. *Duane's Foundations of Clinical Ophthalmology 3.* Lippincott-Raven: Philadelphia, PA pp. 1–17.
12. Fiscella, R.G., and Burstein, N.L. 2001. Ophthalmic drug formulations. In: Bartlett, J.D., and Jaanus, S.D. editors. *Clinical Ocular Pharmacology*, 4th Edition: Butterworth Heinemann: Boston, MA, pp. 19–40.
13. Richardson, K.T. 1975. Ocular microtherapy. *Archives of Ophthalmology* 93:74–86.
14. Gelatt, K.N., Glenwood, G.G., Williams, L.W., and Peiffer, R.L. 1979. Evaluation of a soluble sustained-release ophthalmic delivery unit in the dog. *American Journal of Veterinary Research* 40:702–704.
15. Punch, P.I., Costa, N.D., Edwards, M.E., and Wilcox, G.E. 1987. The release of insoluble antibiotics from collagen ocular inserts *in vitro* and their insertion into the conjunctival sac of cattle. *Journal of Veterinary Pharmacology and Therapeutics* 10:37–42.
16. Fraunfelder, F.T., and Hanna, C. 1974. Ophthalmic drug delivery systems. *Survey of Ophthalmology* 18:292–298.
17. Gelatt, K.N., Peterson, G.E., Myers, V., and McClure, R. 1972. Continuous subpalpebral medication in the horse. *Journal of the American Animal Hospital Association* 8:35–37.
18. Schoster, J.V. 1992. The assembly and placement of ocular lavage systems in horses. *Veterinary Medicine/Small Animal Clinician* 87:460–471.
19. Sweeney, C.R., and Russell, G.E. 1997. Complications associated with use of a one-hole subpalpebral lavage system in horses: 150 cases. *Journal of the American Veterinary Medical Association* 211:1271–1274.
20. Giuliano, E.A., Maggs, J.D., Moore, C.P., Boland, L.A., Champagne, E.S., and Galle, L.E. 2000. Inferomedial placement of a single-entry subpalpebral lavage tube for treatment of equine eye disease. *Veterinary Ophthalmology* 3:153–156.
21. Hinkle, K.M., Gerding, P.A., Kakoma, I., and Schaeffer, D.J. 1999. Evaluation of activity of selected ophthalmic antimicrobial agents in combination against common ocular microorganisms. *American Journal of Veterinary Research* 60:316–318.

22. Eliason, J.A., and Maurice, D.M. 1980. An ocular perfusion system. *Investigative Ophthalmology and Visual Science* 19:102–105.

23. Glaze, M. 1986. An implantable system for perfusion of the equine eye. *Proceedings of the Scientific Meeting of the American College of Veterinary Ophthalmologists* 17, pp. 52–57.

24. Blair, M.J., Gionfriddo, J.R., Polazzi, L.M., Sojka, J.E., Pfaff, A.M., and Bingaman, D.P. 1999. Subconjunctivally implanted microosmotic pumps for continuous ocular treatment in horses. *American Journal of Veterinary Research* 60:1102–1105.

25. Hyndiuk, R.A. 1969. Radioactive depot-corticosteroid penetration into monkey ocular tissue. II. Subconjunctival administration. *Archives of Ophthalmology* 82:259–262.

26. Gilger, B.C., and Allen, J.B. 1998. Cyclosporine A in veterinary ophthalmology. *Veterinary Ophthalmology* 1:181–187.

27. Velez, G., and Whitcup, S.M. 1999. New developments in sustained release drug delivery for the treatment of intraocular disease. *British Journal of Ophthalmology* 83:1225–1229.

28. Gilger, B.C. et al. 2010. Long-term outcome after implantation of a suprachoroidal cyclosporine drug delivery device in horses with recurrent uveitis. *Veterinary Ophthalmology* 13(5): 294–300.

29. Hyndiuk, R.A., and Reagan, M.G. 1968. Radioactive depot-corticosteroid penetration into monkey ocular tissue. Retrobullar and systemic administration. *Archives of Ophthalmology* 80:499–503.

30. Wiejtens, O., Sluijs, V., and Schoemaker, R. 1997. Peribulbar corticosteroid injection: Vitreal and serum concentrations after dexamethasone disodium phosphate injection. *American Journal of Ophthalmology* 123:358–363.

31. Labelle, A.L., and Clark-Prince, S.C. 2013. Anesthesia for ophthalmic procedures in the standing horse. *Veterinary Clinical Equine* 29:179–191.

32. de Linde Henriksen, M., and Brooks, D.E. 2014. Standing ophthalmic surgeries in horses. *Veterinary Clinical Equine* 30: 91–110.

33. Myrna, K.E. et al. 2010. Effectiveness of injection of local anesthetic into the retrobulbar space for postoperative analgesia following eye enucleation in dogs. *Journal of the American Veterinary Medical Association* 237(2):174–177.

34. Oliver, J.A., and Bradbrook, C.A. 2013. Suspected brainstem anesthesia following retrobulbar block in a cat. *Veterinary Ophthalmology* 16(3):225–228.

35. Smith, R., and Rudt, L. 1973. Ultrastructural studies of the blood-aqueous barrier. 2. The barrier to horseradish peroxidase in primates. *American Journal of Ophthalmology* 76:937–947.

36. Cunha-Vaz, J.G., Shakib, M., and Ashton, N. 1966. Studies on the permeability of the blood–retinal barrier. *British Journal of Ophthalmology* 50:441–453.

37. Hudspeth, A., and Yee, A. 1973. The intercellular junctional complexes of retinal epitheium. *Investigative Ophthalmology and Visual Science* 12:354–365.

38. Moore, C.P., Collins, B.K., and Fales, W.H. 1995. Antibacterial susceptibility patterns for microbial isolates associated with infectious keratitis in horses: 63 cases (1986–1994). *Journal of the American Veterinary Medical Association* 207:928–933.

39. Moore, C.P., Collins, B.K., Fales, W.H., and Halenda, R.M. 1995. Antimicrobial agents for treatment of infectious keratits in horses. *Journal of the American Veterinary Medical Association* 207:855–862.

40. Brooks, D., Andrew, S., Dillavou, C., Ellis, G., and Kubilis, P. 1998. Antimicrobial susceptibility patterns of fungi isolated from horses with ulcerative keratomycosis. *American Journal of Veterinary Research* 59:138–142.

41. Leopold, I.H. 1984. Anti-infective agents. In: Sears, M.L. editor. *Pharmacology of the Eye*. Springer-Verlag: New York, pp. 385–457.

42. Kupferman, A., and Leibowitz, H.M. 1979. Topical antibiotic therapy of *Pseudomonas aeruginosa* keratitis. *Archives of Ophthalmology* 97:1699–1702.

43. Gilbert, M., Wilhelmus, K., and Osato, M. 1987. Comparative bioavailability and efficacy of fortified topical tobramycin. *Investigative Ophthalmology and Visual Science* 28:881–885.

44. Donnenfeld, E.D., Schrier, A., and Perry, H.D. 1994. Penetration of topically applied ciprofloxacin, norfloxacin, and ofloxacin into the aqueous humor. *Ophthalmology* 101:902–905.

45. Schlech, B.A. and Alfonso, E. 2005. Overview of the potency of moxifloxacin ophthalmic solution 0.5% (Vigamox). *Survey of Ophthalmology* 50:7–15.

46. Robertson, S.M. et al. 2005. Ocular pharmacokinetics of moxifloxacin after topical treatment in animals and humans. *Survey of Ophthalmology* 50:32–45.

47. Setz, B., Hayashi, S., Wee, W.R., LaBree, L., and McDonnell, P.J. 1996. *In vitro* effects of aminoglycosides and fluoroquinolones on keratocytes. *Investigative Ophthalmology and Visual Science* 37:656–665.

48. Gelatt, K.N., Van der Woerdt, A., Ketring, K.L. et al. 2001. Enrofloxacin-associated retinal degeneration in cats. *Veterinary Ophthalmology* 4:99–106.

49. Wiebe, V., and Hamilton, P. 2002. Fluoroquinolone-induced retinal degeneration in cats. *Journal of the American Veterinary Medical Association* 221:1568–1571.

50. Bloome, M.A., Golden, B., and McKee, A.P. 1970. Antibiotic concentration in ocular tissues: Penicillin G and dihydrostreptomycin. *Archives of Ophthalmology* 83:78–83.

51. Rowley, R.A., and Rubin, L.F. 1970. Aqueous humor penetration of several antibiotics in the dog. *American Journal of Veterinary Research* 31:43–49.

52. Axelrod, A.J., and Peyman, G.A. 1973. Intravitreal amphotericin B treatment of experimental fungal endophthalmitis. *American Journal of Ophthalmology* 76:584–588.

53. May, D.R., Ericson, E.S., Peyman, G.A., and Axelrod, A.J. 1974. Intraocular injection of gentamicin. *Archives of Ophthalmology* 91:487–489.

54. Pohjanpelto, P.E.J., Sarmela, T.J., and Raines, T. 1974. Penetration of trimethoprim and sulfamethoxazole into the aqueous humor. *British Journal of Ophthalmology* 58:606–608.

55. Purnell, W.D., and McPherson Jr., S.D. 1974. The effect of tobramycin on rabbit eyes. *American Journal of Ophthalmology* 77:578–582.

56. Rieder, J., Ellerhorst, B., and Schwartz, D.E. 1974. Ubergang von sulfamethoxazol und trimethoprim in das augenkammerwasser beim menschen. *Albrecht von Graefes Archiv fur Klinische und Experimentelle Ophthalmologie* 190:51–61.

57. Faigenbaum, S.J., Boyle, G.L., Prywes, A.S., Abel Jr., R., and Leopold, I.H. 1976. Intraocular penetration of amoxicillin. *American Journal of Ophthalmology* 82:598–603.

58. Souri, E.N., and Green, W.R. 1974. Intravitreal amphotericin B toxicity. *American Journal of Ophthalmology* 78:77–81.

59. George, F.J., and Hanna, C. 1977. Ocular penetration of chloramphenicol. *Archives of Ophthalmology* 95:879–882.

60. Barza, M.B., Kane, A.B., and Baum, J. 1978. Intraocular penetration of gentamicin after subconjunctival and retrobulbar injection. *American Journal of Ophthalmology* 85:541–547.

61. Kluge, R.M., and Zimmerman, T. 1978. The penetration of antistaphylococcal antibiotics into the aqueous humor of rabbits. *Annals of Ophthalmology* 10:1248–1251.

62. Hillman, J.S., Jacobs, S.I., Garnett, A.J., and Kheskani, M.B. 1979. Gentamicin penetration and decay in the human aqueous. *British Journal of Ophthalmology* 63:794–796.

63. Saunders, J.H., and McPherson Jr., S.D. 1980. Ocular penetration of cefazolin in humans and rabbits after subconjunctival injection. *American Journal of Ophthalmology* 89:564–566.

64. Sigel, C.W., Macklin, A.W., Grace, M.E., and Tracy, C.H. 1981. Trimethoprim and sulfadiazine concentrations in aqueous and vitreous humors of the dog. *Veterinary Medicine/Small Animal Clinician* 76:991–993.

65. Borden, T.B., and Cunningham, R.D. 1982. Tobramycin levels in aqueous humor after subconjunctival injection in humans. *American Journal of Ophthalmology* 93:107–110.

66. Hulem, C.D., Old, S.E., Zeleznick, L.D., and Leopold, I.H. 1982. Intraocular penetration of rosoxacin in rabbits. *Archives of Ophthalmology* 100:646–649.

67. Tabbara, K.F., Ghosher, R., and O'Conner, R. 1983. Ocular tissue absorption of minocycline in the rabbit. *Archives of Ophthalmology* 101:1426–1428.

68. Wingfield, D.L., McDougal, R.L., Roy, F.H., and Hanna, C. 1983. Ocular penetration of amikacin following intramuscular injection. *Archives of Ophthalmology* 101:117–120.

69. Jay, W.M., Shockley, R.K., Aziz, A.M., Aziz, M.Z., and Rissing, J.P. 1984. Ocular pharmacokinetics of ceftriazone following subconjunctival injection in rabbits. *Archives of Ophthalmology* 102:430–432.

70. Zachary, I.G., and Forster, R.K. 1976. Experimental intravitreal gentamicin. *American Journal of Ophthalmology* 82:604–611.

71. Moller, I., Cook, C.S., Peiffer Jr., R.L., Nasisse, M.P., and Harling, D.E. 1986. Indications for and complications of pharmacological ablation of the ciliary body for the treatment of chronic glaucoma in the dog. *Journal of the American Animal Hospital Association* 22:319–326.

72. Bingaman, D.P., Lindley, D.M., Glickman, N.W., Krohne, S.G., and Bryan, G.M. 1994. Intraocular gentamicin and glaucoma: A retrospective study of 60 dog and cat eyes (1985–1993). *Veterinary and Comparative Ophthalmology* 4(3):113–119.

73. D'Amico, D.J., Caspers-Velu, L., Libert, J. et al. 1985. Comparative toxicity of intravitreal aminoglycoside antibiotics. *American Journal of Ophthalmology* 100:264–275.

74. Talamo, J.H., D'Amico, D.J., and Kenyon, K.R. 1986. Intravitreal amikacin in the treatment of bacterial endophthalmitis. *Archives of Ophthalmology* 104:1483–1485.

75. Gookin, J.L., Riviere, J.E., Gilger, B.C., and Papich, M.G. 1999. Acute renal failure in four cats treated with paromomycin. *Journal of the American Veterinary Medical Association* 215:1821–1823.

76. Starr, M.B. 1983. Prophylactic antibiotics for ophthalmic surgery. *Survey of Ophthalmology* 27(May–June):353–373.

77. Yolton, D.P. 2001. Antiinfective drugs. In: Bartlett, J.D., and Jaanus, S.D., editors. *Clinical Ocular Pharmacology, 4th edition*. Butterworth Heinemann: Boston, MA, pp. 219–264.

78. Voelter-Ratson, K. et al. 2013. Evaluation of the conjunctival fungal flora and its susceptibility to antifungal agents in healthy horses in Switzerland. *Veterinary Ophthalmology* 17 (Suppl 1):31–36.

79. Foster, C.S., Lass, J.H., Moran-Wallace, K., and Giovanoni, R. 1981. Ocular toxicity of topical antifungal agents. *Archives of Ophthalmology* 99:1081–1084.

80. Axelrod, A.J., Peyman, G.A., and Apple, D.J. 1973. Toxicity of intravitreal injection of amphotericin B. *American Journal of Ophthalmology* 76:578–583.

81. Coad, C.T., Robinson, N.M., and Wilhelmus, K.R. 1985. Antifungal sensitivity testing for equine keratomycosis. *American Journal of Veterinary Research* 46:676–678.

82. Foster, C.S., and Stefanyszyn, M. 1979. Intraocular penetration of miconazole in rabbits. *Archives of Ophthalmology* 97:1703–1706.

83. Tolentino, F.I., Foster, C.S., Lahav, M., Liu, L.H., and Rabin, A.R. 1982. Toxicity of intravitreous miconazole. *Archives of Ophthalmology* 100:1504–1509.

84. da Costa, P.D., Meredith, R.E., and Sigler, R.L. 1996. Cataracts in dogs after long-term ketaconazole therapy. *Veterinary and Comparative Ophthalmology* 6:176–180.

85. Upadhyay, M., West, E.P., and Sharma, A.P. 1980. Keratitis due to *Aspergillus flavus* successfully treated with thiabendazole. *British Journal of Ophthalmology* 64:30–32.

86. Yee, R.W., Cheng, C.H., Meenakshi, S., Ludden, T.M., Wallace, J.E., and Rinaldi, M.G. 1997. Ocular penetration and pharmacokinetics of topical fluconazole. *Cornea* 16:64–71.

87. O'Day, D.M., Foulds, G., Williams, T.E., Robinson, R.D., Allen, R.H., and Head, W.S. 1990. Ocular uptake of fluconazole following oral administration. *Archives of Ophthalmology* 108(7):1006–1008.

88. Blair, M.J., Gionfriddo, J.R., and Krohne, S.G. 1996. Fluconazole therapy for mycotic endophthalmitis. *Proceedings of the Scientific Meeting of the American College of Veterinary Ophthalmologists* 27:66.

89. Latimer, F.G., Colitz, C.M.H., Campbell, N.B., and Papich, M.G. 2001. Pharmacokinetics of fluconazole following intravenous and oral administration, and body fluid concentrations of fluconazole following repeated oral dosing in horses. *American Journal of Veterinary Research* 62:1606–1611.

90. Ball, M., Rebhun, W., Trepanier, L., Gaarder, J., and Schwark, W. 1997. Corneal concentrations and preliminary toxicological evaluation of an itraconazole/dimethyl sulphoxide ophthalmic ointment. *Journal of Veterinary Pharmacology and Therapeutics* 20:100–104.

91. Clode, A.B. et al. 2006. Evaluation of concentration of voriconazole in aqueous humor after topical and oral administration in horses. *American Journal of Veterinary Research* 67(2): 296–301.

92. Mohan, M., Gupta, S., Vajpayee, R., Kalra, V., and Sachdev, M. 1988. Management of keratomycosis with 1% silver sulfadiazine: A prospective controlled clinical trial in 110 cases. In: Cavanagh, D., editor. *The Cornea: Transactions of the World Congress*. Raven Press: New York, pp. 495–498.

93. Rahman, M.R., Johnson, G.J., Husain, R., Howlader, S.A., and Minassian, D.C. 1998. Randomised trial of 0.2% chlorhexidine gluconate and 2.5% natamycin for fungal keratitis in Bangladesh. *British Journal of Ophthalmology* 82(8):919–925.

94. Teich, S.A. 1993. Topical and systemic antiviral agents. In: Yanoff, M., Fine, B., Mindel, J.S., and Leonard, N.B., editors. *Duane's Foundations of Clinical Ophthalmology*. Lippincott-Raven: Philadelphia, PA, pp. 1–39.

95. Kaufman, H.E., Varnell, E.D., and Thompson, H.W. 1998. Trifluridine, cidofovir, and penciclovir in the treatment of experimental herpetic keratitis. *Archives of Ophthalmology* 116:777–780.

96. Castela, N. et al. 1994. Ganciclovir ophthalmic gel in herpes simplex virus rabbit keratitis: Intraocular penetration and efficacy. *Journal of Ocular Pharmacology* 10(2): 439–451.

97. Stiles, J. et al. 2010. Stability of 0.5% cidofovir stored under various conditions for up to 6 months. *Veterinary Ophthalmology* 13(4):275–277.

98. Nasisse, M.P., Guy, J.S., Davidson, M.G., Sussman, W., and De Clercq, E. 1989. *In vitro* susceptibility of feline herpesvirus-1 to vidarabine, idoxuridine, trifluridine, acyclovir, or bromovinyldeoxyuridine. *American Journal of Veterinary Research* 50:158–160.

99. Banker, A.S. et al. 1998. Effects of topical and subconjunctival cidofovir (HPMPC) in an animal model. *Curr Eye Res* 17(6):560–566.

100. De Clercq, E. 1996. Therapeutic potential of Cidofovir (HPMPC, Vistide) for the treatment of DNA virus (i.e. herpes-, papova-, pox- and adenovirus) infections. *Verhandelingen - Koninklijke Academie voor Geneeskunde van Belgie* 58(1):19–47.

101. Nasisse, M.P., Dorman, D.C., Jamison, K.C., Weigler, B.J., Hawkins, E.C., and Stevens, J.B. 1997. Effects of valacyclovir in cats infected with feline herpesvirus-1. *American Journal of Veterinary Research* 58:1141–1144.

102. Thomasy, S.M., Lim, C.C., Reilly, C.M., Kass, Lappin, M.R., and Maggs, D.J. 2011. Evaluation of orally administered famciclovir in cats experimentally infected with feline herpesvirus type-1. *American Journal of Veterinary Research*, 72(1):85–95.

103. Thomasy, S.M., Maggs, D.J., Lim, C.C., Lappin, M.R., and Stanley, S.D. 2006. Safety and efficacy of famciclovir in cats infected with feline herpesvirus. *Proceedings of the 37th Annual Conference of the American College of Veterinary Ophthalmologists* 37, San Antonio, p. 43.

104. Peiffer, R., and Harling, D. 1998. Intravitreal cidofovir (Vistide) in the management of glaucoma in the dog and cat. *Proceedings of the Scientific Meeting of the American College of Veterinary Ophthalmologists* 29, Seattle, p. 29.

105. Daily, M.J., Peyman, G.A., and Fishman, G. 1973. Intravitreal injection of methicillin for treatment of endophthalmitis. *American Journal of Ophthalmology* 76:343–350.

106. Rutgard, J.J., Berkowitz, R.A., and Peyman, G.A. 1978. Intravitreal cephalothin in experimental staphylococcal endophthalmitis. *Annals of Ophthalmology* 10:293–298.

107. Fisher, J.P., Civiletto, S.E., and Forster, R.K. 1982. Toxocity, efficacy, and clearance of intravitreal injected cefazolin. *Archives of Ophthalmology* 100:650–652.

108. Fett, D.R., Silverman, C.A., and Yoshizumi, M.O. 1984. Moxalactam retinal toxicity. *Archives of Ophthalmology* 102:435–438.

109. Krohne, S.G. 1994. Effect of topically applied 2% pilocarpine and 0.25% demecarium bromide on blood-aqueous barrier permeability in dogs. *American Journal of Veterinary Research* 55:1729–1733.

110. Zimmerman, T.J. 1981. Pharmacology of ocular drugs. *Ophthalmology* 88:85–88.

111. Carrier, M., and Gum, G. 1989. Effects of 4% pilocarpine gel on normotensive and glaucomatous canine eyes. *American Journal of Veterinary Research* 50:239–244.

112. Pickett, P., Irby, M., and McCain, W. 1991. Short-term and long-term effects of twice daily topical administration of 0.125% demecarium bromide in the normal canine. *Proceedings of the Scientific Meeting of the American College of Veterinary Ophthalmology* 22, p. 42.

113. Pickett, P., Irby, M., and McCain, W. 1991. Short-term and long-term effects of twice daily topical administration of 4% pilocarpine gel in the normal canine. *Proceedings of the Scientific Meeting of the American College of Veterinary Ophthalmology* 22, p. 43.

114. Whitley, R.D., Gelatt, K.N., and Gum, G.G. 1980. Dose response of topical pilocarpine in the normotensive and glaucomatous Beagle. *American Journal of Veterinary Research* 41:417–424.

115. Chiou, C.Y., Trzeciakowski, J., Gelatt, K.N. 1980. Reduction of intraocular pressure in glaucomatous dogs by a new cholinergic drug. *Investigative Ophthalmology and Visual Science* 19:1198–1203.

116. Gelatt, K.N., Gum, G.G., Wolf, D., and White, M.M. 1984. Dose response of topical carbamylcholine (carbachol) in normotensive and early glaucomatous Beagles. *American Journal of Veterinary Research* 45:547–554.

117. Gum, G.G., Metzger, K.J., Gelatt, J.K., Gilley, R.L., and Gelatt, K.N. 1993. Tonographic effects of pilocarpine and pilocarpine-epinephrine in dogs. *Journal of Small Animal Practice* 34:112–116.

118. Gum, G.G., Gelatt, K.N., Gelatt, J.K., and Jones, R. 1993. Effect of topically applied demacarium bromide and echothiophate iodide on intraocular pressure and pupil size in Beagles with normotensive eyes and Beagles with inherited glaucoma. *American Journal of Veterinary Research* 54:287–293.

119. Smith, P.J., Brooks, D.E., Lazarus, J.A., Kubilis, P.S., and Norman, K. 1996. Ocular hypertension following cataract surgery in dogs: 139 cases (1992–1993). *Journal of the American Veterinary Medical Association* 209:105–111.

120. Stuhr, C.M., Miller, P.E., Murphy, C.J., Schoster, J.V., and Thomas, C.B. 1998. Effect of intracameral administration of carbachol on the postoperative increase in intraocular pressure in dogs undergoing cataract extraction. *Journal of the American Veterinary Medical Association* 212:1885–1888.

121. Miller, P.E., Schmidt, G.M., Vainisis, S.J., Swanson, J.F., and Hermann, M.K. 2000. The efficacy of topical prophylactic antiglaucoma therapy in primary closed-angle glaucoma in dogs: A multicenter clinical trial. *Journal of the American Animal Hospital Association* 36:431–438.

122. Slater, M., and Erb, H. 1986. Effects of risk factors and prophylactic treatment on primary glaucoma in the dog. *Journal of the American Veterinary Medical Association* 188:1028–1030.

123. Bito, L.Z., Hyslop, K., and Hyndman, J. 1967. Antiparasympathomimetic effects of cholinesterase inhibitor treatment. *Journal of Pharmacology and Therapeutics* 157:159–169.

124. Rubin, L.F., and Aguirre, G.D. 1967. Clinical use of pilocarpine for keratoconjunctivitis sicca in dogs and cats. *Journal of the American Veterinary Medical Association* 151:313–320.

125. Smith, E., Buyukmihci, N.C., and Farver, T. 1994. Effect of topical pilocarpine treatment on tear production in

dogs. *Journal of the American Veterinary Medical Association* 205:1286–1289.

126. Matheis, F.L. et al. 2012. Canine neurogenic keratoconjunctivitis sicca: 11 cases. (2006–2010). *Veterinary Ophthalmology* 15(4):288–290.

127. Rubin, L.F., and Wolfes, R.L. 1962. Mydriatic for canine ophthalmoscopy. *Journal of the American Veterinary Medical Association* 140:137–141.

128. Salazar, M., and Patil, P.N. 1976. An explanation for the long duration of mydriatic effect of atropine in the eye. *Investigative Ophthalmology* 15:671–673.

129. Smith, E.L., Redburn, D.A., Harwerth, R.S., and Maguire, G.W. 1984. Permanent alterations in muscarinic receptors and pupil size produced by chronic atropinization in kittens. *Investigative Ophthalmology and Visual Science* 25:239–243.

130. Mughannam, A.J., Buyukmihci, N.C., and Kass, P.H. 1999. Effect of topical atropine on intraocular pressure and pupil diameter in the normal horse eye. *Veterinary Ophthalmology* 2:213–215.

131. Herring, I.P., Pickett, J.P., Champagne, E.S., Troy, G.C., and Marini, M. 2000. Effect of topical 1% atropine sulfate on intraocular pressure in normal horses. *Veterinary Ophthalmology* 3:139–143.

132. Stadtbaumer, K., Kostlin, R.G., and Zahn, K.J. 2002. Effects of topical 0.5% tropicamide on intraocular pressure in normal cats. *Veterinary Ophthalmology* 5:107–112.

133. Stadtbaumer, K., Frommelt, F., and Nell, B. 2006. Effects of mydriatics on intraocular pressure and pupil size in the normal feline eye. *Veterinary Ophthalmology* 9(4):233–237.

134. Hacker, D.V., and Farver, T.B. 1988. Effects of tropicamide on intraocular pressure in normal dogs: Preliminary studies. *Journal of the American Animal Hospital Association* 24:411–415.

135. Taylor, N.R. et al. 2007. Variation in intraocular pressure following application of tropicamide in three different dog breeds. *Veterinary Ophthalmology*, 10:8–11.

136. Gwin, R.M. et al. 1978. Effects of topical 1-epinephrine and dipivalyl epinephrine on intraocular pressure and pupil size in the normotensive and glaucomatous Beagle. *American Journal of Veterinary Research* 39(1): 83–86.

137. Thompson, H.S., and Mensher, J.H. 1971. Adrenergic mydriasis in Horner's syndrome: The hydroxyamphetamine test for diagnosis of postganglionic defects. *American Journal of Ophthalmology* 72:472–480.

138. Skarf, B., and Czarnecki, J.S. 1982. Distinguishing postganglionic from preganglionic lesions: Studies in rabbits with surgically-produced Horner's syndrome. *Archives of Ophthalmology* 100:1319–1322.

139. Gelatt, K.N., Boggess III, T.S., and Cure, T.H. 1973. Evaluation of mydriatics in the cat. *Journal of the American Animal Hospital Association* 9:283–287.

140. Hacker, D.V., Buyukmihci, N.C., Franti, C.E., and Bellhorn, R.W. 1987. Effect of topical phenylephrine on the equine pupil. *American Journal of Veterinary Research* 48:320–322.

141. Gelatt, K.N., Gum, G.G., and MacKay, E.O. 1995. Evaluation of mydriatics in cattle. *Veterinary Comparative Ophthalmology* 5:46–49.

142. Boydell, P. 1999. The accuracy of denervation hypersensitivity testing with 10% phenylephrine eyedrops in Horner's syndrome in the dog. *Proceedings of the Scientific Meeting of the American College of Veterinary Ophthalmologists* 30, p. 49.

143. Mindel, J.S. 1995. α-adrenergic drugs. In: Tasman, W., and Jaeger, E.A., editors. *Duane's Foundations of Clinical Ophthalmology*. Lippencott-Raven: Philadelphia, PA, pp. 1–24.

144. Miller, P.E., Nelson, M.J., and Rhaesa, S.L. 1996. Effects of topical administration of 0.5% apraclonidine on intraocular pressure, pupil size, and heart rate in clinically normal dogs. *American Journal of Veterinary Research* 57:79–82.

145. Miller, P.E., and Rhaesa, S.L. 1996. Effects of topical administration of 0.5% apraclonidine on intraocular pressure, pupil size, and heart rate in clinically normal cats. *American Journal of Veterinary Research* 57:83–86.

146. Gelatt, K.N., and MacKay, E.O. 2002. Effect of single and multiple doses of 0.2% brimonidine tartrate in the glaucomatous Beagle. *Veterinary Ophthalmology* 5:253–262.

147. Williams, M.M., Spiess, B.M., Pascoe, P.J., and O'Grady, M. 2000. Systemic effects of topical and subconjunctival ophthalmic atropine in the horse. *Veterinary Ophthalmology* 3:193–199.

148. Herring, I.P., Pickett, J.P., Champagne, E.S., and Troy, G.C. 1997. The effect of topical atropine sulfate on intraocular pressure in the normal horse. *Proceedings of the Scientific Meeting of the American College of Veterinary Ophthalmologists* 28, p. 53.

149. Hollingsworth, S.R., Canton, D.D., Buyukmihci, N.C., and Farver, T.B. 1992. Effect of topically administered atropine on tear production in dogs. *Journal of the American Veterinary Medical Association* 200:1481–1484.

150. McLaughlin, S.A., Whitely, R.D., and Gilger, B.C. 1991. Ophthalmic atropine in horses: Is colic a serious problem? *Equine Veterinary Education* 3:94–96.

151. Pascoe, P.J., Elkiw, J.E., Stiles, J., and Smith, E. 1994. Arterial hypertension associated with topical ocular use of phenylephrine in dogs. *Journal of the American Veterinary Medical Association* 205:1562–1564.

152. Willis, M., Martin, C.L., Stiles, J., and Chaffin, K. 1997. Acute, transient sialoadenomegaly in two cats following topical administration of tropicamide. *Veterinary Comparative Ophthalmology* 7:206–208.

153. Novack, G. 1989. Beta-blockers in ophthalmology. *Clinics of North America* 2:77–96.

154. Allen, R.C., Hertzmark, E., Walker, A.M., and Epstein, D.L. 1986. A double-masked comparison of βxolol vs. timolol in the treatment of open-angle glaucoma. *American Journal of Ophthalmology* 101:535–541.

155. Liu, H., Chiou, G., and Garg, L. 1980. Ocular hypotensive effects of timolol in cat eyes. *Archives of Ophthalmology* 98:1467–1469.

156. Pickett, J., and Majors, L. 1989. Short-term and long-term effects of topical timolol maleate and βxolol on intraocular pressure, heart rate, and blood pressure in normal dogs. *Proceedings of the Scientific Meeting of the American College of Veterinary Ophthalmologists* 20, p. 115.

157. Gum, G., Larocca, R., Gelatt, K., Mead, J., and Gelatt, J. 1991. The effect of topical timolol maleate on intraocular pressure in normal Beagles with inherited glaucoma. *Progress in Veterinary and Comparative Ophthalmology* 1:141–148.

158. Wilkie, D., and Latimer, C. 1991. Effects of topical administration of timolol maleate on intraocular pressure and pupil size in dogs. *American Journal of Veterinary Research* 52:432–435.

159. Wilkie, D., and Latimer, C. 1991. Effects of topical administration of timolol maleate on intraocular pressure and

pupil size in cats. *American Journal of Veterinary Research* 52:436–444.

160. Higgins, R., and Brubaker, R. 1980. Acute effect of epinephrine on aqueous humor formation in the timolol-treated normal eye as measured by fluorophotometry. *Investigative Ophthalmology and Visual Science* 19:420–423.

161. Kass, M., Korey, M., Gordon, M., and Becker, B. 1982. Timolol and acetazolamide: A study of concurrent administration. *Archives of Ophthalmology* 100:941–942.

162. Nelson, W. 1986. Adverse respiratory and cardiovascular events attributed to timolol ophthalmic solution, 1978–1985. *American Journal of Ophthalmology* 102:606–611.

163. Arthur, B., Hay, G., Wasan, S., and Willis, W. 1983. Ultrastructural effects of topical timolol on the rabbit cornea. *Archives of Ophthalmology* 101:1607–1610.

164. Robbins, R., and Galin, M.A. 1969. Effect of osmotic agents on the vitreous body. *Archives of Ophthalmology* 82:694–699.

165. Lorimer, D.W., Hakanson, N.E., Pion, P.D., and Merideth, R.E. 1989. The effect of intravenous mannitol or oral glycerol on intraocular pressure in dogs. *Cornell Veterinarian* 79:249–258.

166. Maren, T.H. 1976. The rates of movement of NA^+, CL^-, and $HCO3$ from plasma to posterior chamber: Effect of acetazolamide and relation to the treatment of glaucoma. *Investigative Ophthalmology and Visual Science* 15:356–364.

167. Friedman, Z., Krupin, T., and Becker, B. 1982. Ocular and systemic effects of acetazolamide in nephrectomized rabbits. *Investigative Ophthalmology and Visual Science* 23:209–213.

168. Wistrand, P.J., Schenholm, M., and Lonnerholm, G. 1986. Carbonic anhydrase isoenzymes CA I and CA II in the human eye. *Investigative Ophthalmology and Visual Science* 27:419–428.

169. Gerding, P., and Essex-Sorlie, D. 1991. Effects of intracameral injection of tissue plaminogen activator on intraocular pressure, corneal endothelium, and fibrin in dogs. *Proceedings of the Scientific Meeting of the American College of Veterinary Ophthalmologists* 22, p. 90.

170. Remis, L.L. 1994. Carbonic anhydrase inhibitors. In: Albert, D.M., and Jakobiec, F.A., editors. *Principles and Practice of Ophthalmology: Basic Sciences*. WB Saunders: Philadelphia, PA, pp. 1070–1075.

171. Stein, A., Pinke, R., Krupin, T. et al. 1983. The effect of topically administered carbonic anhydrase inhibitors on aqueous humor dynamics in rabbits. *American Journal of Ophthalmology* 95:222–228.

172. Bar-Ilan, A., Pessah, N.I., and Maren, T.H. 1984. The effects of carbonic anhydrase inhibitors on aqueous humor chemistry and dynamics. *Investigative Ophthalmology and Visual Science* 25:1198–1204.

173. Flach, A.J., Peterson, J.S., and Seligmann, K.A. 1984. Local ocular hypotensive effect of topically applied acetazolamide. *American Journal of Ophthalmology* 98:66–72.

174. Pfeiffer, N. 1997. Dorzolamide: Development and clinical application of a topical carbonic anhydrase inhibitor. *Survey of Ophthalmology* 42:137–151.

175. Wayman, L., Larsson, L.I., Maus, T., Alm, A., and Brubaker, R.B. 1997. Comparison of dorzolamide and timolol as suppressors of aqueous humor flow in humans. *Archives of Ophthalmology* 115:1368–1371.

176. Cawse, M.A., Ward, D.A., and Hendrix, D. 1999. Effects of topically applied 2% dorzolamide on intraocular pressure and aqueous humor flow in normal dogs. *Proceedings of the Scientific Meeting of the American College of Veterinary Ophthalmologists* 30, p. 48.

177. Willis, A.M., Robbin, T.E., and Wilkie, D.A. 1999. Effect of topical dorzolamide and dorzolamide-timolol on intraocular pressure in normal horse eyes. *Proceedings of the Scientific Meeting of the American College of Veterinary Ophthalmologists* 30, p. 48.

178. Rainbow, M.E., and Dziezyc, J. 2001. Effects of 2% dorzolamide on intraocular pressure in cats. *Proceedings of the Scientific Meeting of the American College of Veterinary Ophthalmologists* 32, p. 5.

179. Ingram, C.J., and Brubaker, R. 1999. Effect of brinzolamide and dorzolamide on aqueous humor flow in human eyes. *American Journal of Ophthalmology* 128:292–296.

180. Willis, A.M. et al. 2002. Advances in topical glaucoma therapy. *Veterinary Ophthalmology* 5(1):9–17.

181. Germann, S.E. et al. 2008. Effects of topical administration of 1% brinzolamide on intraocular pressure in clinically normal horses. *Equine Veterinary Journal* 40(7): 662–665.

182. Kass, M.A., Kolker, A.E., Gordon, M. et al. 1981. Acetazolamide and urolithiasis. *Ophthalmology* 88:261–265.

183. Fraunfelder, F.T., Meyer, S.M., Bagby Jr., G.C., and Dreis, M.W. 1985. Hematologic reactions to carbonic anhydrase inhibitors. *American Journal of Ophthalmology* 100:79–81.

184. Carlsen, J., Durcan, J., Zabriskie, N., and Crandall, A. 1999. Nephrolithiasis with dorzolamide. *Archives of Ophthalmology* 117:1087–1088.

185. Konowal, A., Morrison, J.C., Brown, S.V.L. et al. 1999. Irreversible corneal decompensation in patients treated with topical dorzolamide. *American Journal of Ophthalmology* 127:403–406.

186. Schnyder, C.C., Tran, V.T., Mermoud, A., and Herbort, C.P. 1999. Sterile mucopurulent conjunctivitis associated with the use of dorzolamide eyedrops. *Archives of Ophthalmology* 117:1429–1431.

187. Quinn, R.F., Keller, C.B., and Tingey, D.P. 1994. Evidence of sulfhydryl reactivity in cells cultured from the canine iridocorneal angle. *Veterinary Comparative Ophthalmology* 4:149–154.

188. Quinn, R.F., Keller, C.B., Yamashiro, S., and Tingey, D.P. 1994. The effects of ethacrynic acid on the facility of aqueous outflow in the enucleated canine eye. *Veterinary Comparative Ophthalmology* 4:155–159.

189. Keller, C.H. 1997. The effect of topical ethacrynic acid on the intraocular pressure in normal dogs: A pilot study. *Proceedings of the Scientific Meeting of the American College of Veterinary Ophthalmologists* 28, p. 11.

190. Sullivan, L.J. et al. 1997. Efficacy and safety of 0.3% carbomer gel compared to placebo in patients with moderate-to-severe dry eye syndrome. *Ophthalmology* 104(9):1402–1408.

191. Vaughan, D.G. 1955. Contamination of fluorescein solutions. *American Journal of Ophthalmology* 39:55–61.

192. Kommonen, B., and Koskinen, L. 1984. Fluorescein angiography of the canine ocular fundus in ketamine-xylazine anesthesia. *Acta Veterinaria Scandinavica* 25:346–351.

193. Schnider, C.M. 2001. Dyes. In: Bartlett, J.D., and Jannus, S.D., editors. *Clinical Ocular Pharmacology*, 4th Edition: Butterworth Heinemann: Boston, MA, pp. 349–366.

194. Feenstra, R., and Tseng, S. 1992. Comparison of fluorescein and rose bengal staining. *Ophthalmology* 99:605–617.

195. Gelatt, K.N. 1972. Vital staining of the canine cornea and conjunctiva with rose bengal. *Journal of the American Animal Hospital Association* 8:17–22.

196. Horiguchi, M., Miyake, K., Ohta, I., and Ito, Y. 1998. Staining of the lens capsule for circular continuous capsulorrhexis in eyes with white cataracts. *Archives of Ophthalmology* 116:535–537.

197. Silverman, B.S. 2000. Anterior capsule staining with indocyanine green for continuous curvilinear capsulorrhexis. *Proceedings of the Scientific Meeting of the American College of Veterinary Ophthalmologists* 31, p. 5.

198. Herring, I. et al. 2005. Duration of effect and effect of multiple doses of topical ophthalmic application of 0.5% proparacaine hydrochloride in clinically normal dogs. *American Journal of Veterinary Research* 66:77–80.

199. Gundersen, T., and Liebman, S.D. 1944. Effect of local anesthetic on regeneration of corneal epithelium. *Archives of Ophthalmology* 31:29.

200. Maurice, D.M., and Singh, T. 1985. The absence of corneal toxicity on low-level topical anesthesia. *American Journal of Ophthalmology* 99:691–696.

201. Rubin, L.F., and Gelatt, K.N. 1967. Corneal epithelial sloughing in dogs with glaucoma. *Journal of the American Veterinary Medical Association* 151:1449–1452.

202. Krohne, S., Gionfriddo, J., and Morrison, E. 1998. Inhibition of pilocarpine-induced aqueous humor flare, hypotony, and miosis by topical administration of anti-inflammatory and anesthetic drugs to dogs. *American Journal of Veterinary Research* 59:482–488.

203. Herouy, Y., Trefzer, D., Zimpfer, U., Schopf, E., Vanscheidt, W., and Norgauer, J. 2000. Matrix metalloproteinases and venous leg ulceration. *European Journal of Dermatology* 10:173–180.

204. Schultz, G.S., Strelow, S., Stern, G.A., and Chegini, N. 1992. Treatment of alkali-injured rabbit corneas with a synthetic inhibitor of matrix metalloproteinases. *Investigative Ophthalmology and Visual Science* 33:3325–3331.

205. Barletta, J., Angella, G., Balch, K.C., and Dimova, H.G. 1996. Inhibition of pseudomonal ulceration in rabbit corneas by a synthetic matrix metalloproteinase inhibitor. *Investigative Ophthalmology and Visual Science* 37:20–28.

206. Foster, C.S., Zelt, R.P., Mai-Phan, T., and Kenyon, K.R. 1982. Immunosuppression and selective inflammatory cell depletion. *Archives of Ophthalmology* 100:1820–1824.

207. Seng, W.L., Kenyon, K.R., and Wolf, G. 1982. Studies on the source and release of collagenase in thermally burned corneas of vitamin A-deficient and control rats. *Investigative Ophthalmology and Visual Science* 22:62–72.

208. Brown, S.I., and Weller, C.A. 1970. Cell origin of collagenase in normal and wounded corneas. *Archives of Ophthalmology* 83:74–76.

209. Berman, M., Leary, R., and Gage, J. 1980. Evidence for a role of the plasminogen activator-plasmin system in corneal ulceration. *Investigative Ophthalmology and Visual Science* 19:1204–1221.

210. Wang, H., Berman, M., and Law, M. 1985. Latent and active plasminogen activator in corneal ulceration. *Investigative Ophthalmology and Visual Science* 26:511–524.

211. Strubbe, D.T., Brooks, D.E., Schultz, G.S. et al. 2000. Evaluation of tear film proteinases in horses with ulcerative keratitis. *Veterinary Ophthalmology* 3:111–119.

212. Clark, A.F. 1998. New discoveries on the roles of matrix metalloproteinases in ocular cell biology and pathology. *Investigative Ophthalmology and Visual Science* 39:2514–2516.

213. Brown, S.I., Weller, C.A., and Vidrich, A.M. 1970. Effect of corticosteroids on corneal collagenase of rabbits. *American Journal of Ophthalmology* 70:744–747.

214. Olliviero, F.J., Brooks, D.E., Kallberg, M.E. et al. 1992. In vitro effects of EDTA, doxycycline, N-acetylcysteine, ilomastat, and α-1 proteinase inhibitor on matrix metalloproteinase activity in the tear film of horses with ulcerative keratitis. *Proceedings of the Scientific Meeting of the American College of Veterinary Ophthalmologists* 33, p. 55.

215. Hook, C.W., Brown, S.I., Iwanij, W., and Nakanishi, I. 1971. Characterization and inhibition of corneal collagenase. *Investigative Ophthalmology* 10:496–503.

216. Pfister, R.R., Haddox, J.L., Dodson, R.W., and Deshazo, W.F. 1984. Polymorphonuclear leukocytic inhibition by citrate, other metal chelators, and trifluoperazine. *Investigative Ophthalmology and Visual Science* 25:955–970.

217. Berman, M. 1975. Collagenase inhibitors: Rationale for their use in treating corneal ulceration. In: Pavan, D., editor. Little Brown: Boston, MA, pp. 49–66.

218. Brooks, D.E., Olliviero, F.J., Schultz, G.S. et al. 2002. Duration of *in vitro* inhibitory activity of equine serum against equine tear film matrix metalloproteinases. *Proceedings of the Scientific Meeting of the American College of Veterinary Ophthalmologists* 33, p. 54.

219. Pfister, R.R., and Paterson, C.A. 1977. Additional clinical and morphological observations on the favorable effect of ascorbate in experimental ocular alkali burns. *Investigative Ophthalmology and Visual Science* 16:478–487.

220. Pfister, R.R., Nicolaro, M.L., and Paterson, C.A. 1981. Sodium citrate reduces the incidence of corneal ulcerations and perforations in extreme alkali-burned eyes: Acetylcysteine and ascorbate have no favorable effect. *Investigative Ophthalmology and Visual Science* 21:486–490.

221. Phan, T.M., Zelt, R.P., Kenyon, K.R., Chakrabarti, B., and Foster, C.S. 1985. Ascorbic acid therapy in a thermal burn model of corneal ulceration in rabbits. *American Journal of Ophthalmology* 99:74–82.

222. Seedor, J.A., Perry, H.D., Mcnamara, T.F., Golub, L.M., Buxton, D.F., and Guthrie, D.S. 1987. Systemic tetracycline treatment of alkali-induced corneal ulceration in rabbits. *Archives of Ophthalmology* 105:268–271.

223. Levy, J.H., and Katz, H.R. 1990. Effect of systemic tetracycline on progression of *Pseudomonas aeruginosa* keratitis in the rabbit. *Annals of Ophthalmology* 22:179–183.

224. Sugar, A., and Waltman, S.R. 1973. Corneal toxicity of collagenase inhibitors. *Investigative Ophthalmology and Visual Science* 12:779–782.

225. Abelson, M.B., Allansmith, M.R., and Friedlaender, M.H. 1980. Effects of topically applied decongestant and antihistamine. *American Journal of Ophthalmology* 90:254–257.

226. Leibowitz, H.M., and Kupferman, A. 1974. Anti-inflammatory effectiveness in the cornea of topically administered prednisolone. *Investigative Ophthalmology and Visual Science* 13:757–763.

227. Apt, L., Henrick, A., and Silverman, L.M. 1979. Patient compliance with use of topical ophthalmic corticosteroid suspensions. *American Journal of Ophthalmology* 87:210–214.

228. Roberts, S.M., Lavach, J.D., Macy, D.W., and Severin, G.A. 1984. Effect of ophthalmic prednisolone acetate on the canine adrenal gland and hepatic function. *American Journal of Veterinary Research* 45:1711–1714.

229. Eichenbaum, J.D., Macy, D.W., Severin, G.A., and Paulsen, M.E. 1988. Effect in large dogs of ophthalmic prednisolone acetate on adrenal gland and hepatic function. *Journal of the American Animal Hospital Association* 24:705–709.

230. Murphy, C.J., Feldman, E., and Bellhorn, R. 1990. Iatrogenic Cushing's syndrome in a dog caused by topical ophthalmic medications. *Journal of the American Animal Hospital Association* 26:640–642.

231. Glaze, M.B., Crawford, M.A., Nachreiner, R.F., Casey, H.W., Nafe, L.A., and Kearney, M.T. 1998. Ophthalmic corticosteroid therapy: Systemic effects in the dog. *Journal of the American Veterinary Medical Association* 192:73–75.

232. Regnier, A., Toutain, P.L., Alvinerie, M., Periquet, B., and Ruckebusch, Y. 1982. Adrenocortical function and plasma biochemical values in dogs after subconjunctival treatment with methylprednisolone acetate. *Research in Veterinary Science* 32:306–310.

233. Fischer, C.A. 1979. Granuloma formation associated with subconjunctival injection of a corticosteroid in dogs. *Journal of the American Veterinary Medical Association* 174:1086–1088.

234. Krohne, S.D.G., and Vestre, W.A. 1987. Effects of flunixin meglumine and dexamethasone on aqueous protein values after intraocular surgery in the dog. *American Journal of Veterinary Research* 48:420–422.

235. Martin, C. 1971. The effect of topical vitamin A, antibiotic, mineral oil, and subconjunctival steroid on corneal epithelial wound healing in the dog. *Journal of the American Veterinary Medical Association* 159:1392–1399.

236. Zhan, G.L., Miranda, O.C., and Bito, L.Z. 1992. Steroid glaucoma: Corticosteroid-induced ocular hypertension in cats. *Experimental Eye Research* 54:211–218.

237. Bhattacherjee, P., Paterson, C.A., Spellman, J.M., Graff, G., and Yanni, J.M. 1999. Pharmacological validation of a feline model of steroid-induced ocular hypertension. *Archives of Ophthalmology* 117:361–364.

238. Taravella, M.J., Stulting, D., Mader, T.H., and Weisenthal, R.W. 1994. Calcific band keratopathy associated with the use of topical steroid-phosphate preparations. *Archives of Ophthalmology* 112:608–613.

239. Masferrer, J., and Kulkarni, P. 1997. Cyclooxygenase-2 inhibitors: A new approach to the therapy of ocular inflammation. *Survey of Ophthalmology* 41:35–40.

240. Stjernschantz, J. 1984. Autocoids and neuropeptides. In: Sears, M.L., editor. *Pharmacology of the Eye*. Springer-Verlag: New York, pp. 311–350.

241. Flower, R. 1981. Glucocorticoids, phospholipase A_2, and inflammatory trends. *Pharmacology and Science* 2:186–189.

242. Brightman, A.H., Helper, L.C., and Hoffman, W.E. 1981. Effect of aspirin on aqueous protein values in the dog. *Journal of the American Veterinary Medical Association* 178:572–573.

243. Regnier, A., Bonnefoi, M., and Lescure, F. 1984. Effect of lysine-acetylsalicylate and phenylbutazone premedication on the protein content of secondary aqueous humor in the dog. *Research in Veterinary Science* 37:26–29.

244. Forrester, S.D., and Troy, G.C. 1999. Renal effects of nonsteroidal anti-inflammatory drugs. *Compendium on Continuing Education for the Practicing Veterinarian* 21:910–919.

245. Regnier, A., Whitley, R.D., Benard, P., and Bonnefoi, M. 1986. Effect of flunixin meglumine on the breakdown of the blood-aqueous barrier following paracentesis in the canine eye. *Journal of Ocular Pharmacology* 2:165–170.

246. Millichamp, N.J., and Dziezyc, J. 1991. Comparison of flunixin meglumine and flurbiprofen for control of ocular irritative response in dogs. *American Journal of Veterinary Research* 52:1452–1455.

247. Lee, B.B., Kuperman, A., and Leibowitz, H.M. 1985. Effect of suprofen on corneal wound healing. *Archives of Ophthalmology* 103:95–97.

248. Leibowitz, H.M., Ryan, W.J., Kupferman, A., and Desantis, L. 1986. Effect of concurrent topical corticosteroid and NSAID therapy of experimental keratitis. *Investigative Ophthamology and Visual Science* 27:1226–1229.

249. Millichamp, N.J., Dziezyc, J., and Olsen, J.W. 1991. Effect of flurbiprofen on facility of aqueous outflow in the eyes of dogs. *American Journal of Veterinary Research* 52:1448–1451.

250. Ward, D.A., Ferguson, D.C., Ward, S.L., Green, K., and Kaswan, R.L. 1992. Comparison of the blood–aqueous barrier stabilizing effects of steroidal and nonsteroidal anti-inflammatory agents in the dog. *Progress in Veterinary and Comparative Ophthalmology* 2:117–124.

251. Dziezyc, J., Millichamp, N.J., and Smith, W.B. 1995. Effect of flurbiprofen and corticosteroids on the ocular irritative response in dogs. *Veterinary Comparative Ophthalmology* 5:42–45.

252. Szerenyi, K., Sorken, K., Garbus, J., Lee, M., and McDonnell, P. 1994. Decrease in normal human corneal sensitivity with topical diclofenac sodium. *American Journal of Ophthalmology* 118:312–315.

253. Bucci Jr., F.A., and Waterbury, L.D. 2011. A randomized comparison of to-aqueous penetration of ketorolac 0.45%, bromfenac 0.09% and nepafenac 0.1% in cataract patients undergoing phacoemulsification. *Current Medical Research & Opinion* 27(12): 2235–2239.

254. Henderson, B.A. et al. 2011. Safety and efficacy of bromfenac ophthalmic solution (Bromday) dosed once daily for postoperative ocular inflammation and pain. *Ophthalmology* 118(11):2120–2127.

255. Waterbury, L.D. et al. 2011. Ocular penetration and anti-inflammatory activity of ketorolac 0.45% and bromfenac 0.09% against lipopolysaccharide-induced inflammation. *Journal of Ocular Pharmacology & Therapeutics* 27(2):173–178.

256. Jones, B.M., and Neville, M.W. 2013. Nepafenac: An ophthalmic nonsteroidal antiinflammatory drug for pain after cataract surgery. *Annals of Pharmacotherapy* 47(6):892–896.

257. Guidera, A.C., Luchs, J.I., and Udell, I.J. 2001. Keratitis, ulceration, and perforation associated with topical nonsteroidal anti-inflammatory drugs. *Ophthalmology* 108:936–944.

258. Prasher, P. 2012. Acute corneal melt associated with topical bromfenac use. *Eye & Contact Lens: Science & Clinical Practice* 38(4):260–262.

259. Spiess, B.M., Mathis, G.A., and Leber, A. 1991. Kinetics of uptake and effects of topical indomethacin application on protein concentration in the aqueous humor of dogs. *American Journal of Veterinary Research* 52:1159–1163.

260. Regnier, A.M., Dossin, O., Cutzack, E.E., and Gelatt, K.N. 1995. Comparative effects of two formulations of indomethacin eyedrops on the paracentesis-induced inflammatory

response of the canine eye. *Veterinary and Comparative Ophthalmology* 15:242–246.

261. Krohne, S.G., Blair, M.J., Bingaman, D., and Gionfriddo, J.R. 1998. Carprofen inhibition of flare in the dog measured by laser flare photometry. *Veterinary Ophthalmology* 1:81–84.

262. Gelatt, K.N. and MacKay, E.O. 2004. Effect of different dose schedules of travoprost on intraocular pressure and pupil size in the glaucomatous Beagle. *Veterinary Ophthalmology* 7:53–57.

263. Carvalho, A.B. et al. 2006. Effects of travoprost 0.004% compared with latanoprost 0.005% on the intraocular pressure of normal dogs. *Veterinary Ophthalmology* 9:121–125.

264. Patel, S., and Spencer, C. 1996. Latanoprost: A review of its pharmacological properties, clinical efficacy, and tolerability in the management of primary open-angle glaucoma and ocular hypertension. *Drugs and Aging* 9:363–378.

265. Lindsey, J., Kashiwagi, K., Kashiqagi, F., and Weinreb, R. 1997. Prostaglandins alter extracellular matrix adjacent to human ciliary muscle cells *in vitro*. *Investigative Ophthalmology and Visual Science* 38:2214–2223.

266. Weinreb, R., Kashiwagi, F., Tsukahara, S., and Lindsey, J. 1997. Prostaglandins increase matrix metalloproteinase release from human ciliary smooth muscle cells. *Investigative Ophthalmology and Visual Science* 38:2772–2780.

267. Gelatt, K.N., and MacKay, E.O. 2001. Effect of different dose schedules of latanaprost on intraocular pressure and pupil size in the glaucomatous Beagle. *Veterinary Ophthalmology* 4:283–288.

268. Studer, M.E. et al. 2000. Effects of 0.005% latanoprost solution on intraocular pressure in healthy dogs and cats. *American Journal of Veterinary Research* 61(10):1220–1224.

269. Gelatt, K.N., and MacKay, E.O. 2004. Effect of different dose schedules of travoprost on intraocular pressure and pupil size in the glaucomatous Beagle. *Veterinary Ophthalmology* 7(1): 53–57.

270. Smith, L.N. et al. 2010. Effects of topical administration of latanoprost, timolol, or a combination of latanoprost and timolol on intraocular pressure, pupil size, and heart rate in clinically normal dogs. *American Journal of Veterinary Research* 71(9):1055–1061.

271. Diehl, K.A., Willis, A.M., Hoshaw-Woodard, S., Kobayashi, I., Vittuci, M., and Schmall, M. 2000. Effect of topical 0.005% latanoprost on normal eyes of horses. *Proceedings of the Scientific Meeting of the American College of Veterinary Ophthalmologists* 31, p. 15.

272. Studer, M., Martin, C., and Stiles, J. 2000. The effect of latanoprost 0.005% on intraocular pressure in normal feline and canine eyes. *American Journal of Veterinary Research* 61:1220–1224.

273. Regnier, A. et al. 2006. Ocular effects of topical 0.03% bimatoprost solution in normotensive feline eyes. *Veterinary Ophthalmology* 9:39–43.

274. Bartoe, J.T. et al. 2005. The effects of bimatoprost and unoprostone isopropyl on the intraocular pressure of normal cats. *Veterinary Ophthalmology* 8:247–252.

275. Rowe, J., Hattenhauer, M., and Herman, D. 1997. Adverse side-effects associated with latanoprost. *American Journal of Ophthalmology* 124:683–685.

276. Warwar, R., Bullock, J., and Ballal, D. 1998. Cystoid macular edema and anterior uveitis associated with latanoprost use. *Ophthalmology* 105:263–268.

277. Kaufman, H.E., Varnell, E.D., and Thompson, H.W. 1999. Latanoprost increases the severity and recurrence of herpetic keratitis in the rabbit. *American Journal of Ophthalmology* 127:531–536.

278. Allansmith, M., and Ross, R. 1986. Ocular allergy and mast cell stabilizers. *Survey of Ophthalmology* 30:229–244.

279. Nussenblatt, R., and Palestine, A. 1986. Cyclosporine: Immunology, pharmacology, and therapeutic uses. *Survey of Ophthalmology* 31:159–169.

280. Stanton, M., and Legendre, A. 1986. Effects of cyclophosphamide in dogs and cats. *Journal of the American Veterinary Medical Association* 188:1319–1322.

281. Beale, K.M. 1988. Azathioprine for treatment of immune-mediated diseases of dogs and cats. *Journal of the American Veterinary Medical Association* 192:1316–1318.

282. Foster, S.C. 1994. Pharmacologic treatment of immune disorders. In: Albert, D., and Jakobiec, F., editors. *Principles and Practice of Ophthalmology: Basic Sciences.* WB Saunders: Philadelphia, PA, pp. 1076–1084.

283. Latimer, C., Wyman, M., and Szymanski, C. 1983. Azathioprine in the management of fibrous histiocytoma in two dogs. *Journal of the American Animal Hospital Association* 19:155.

284. Bussanich, M., Rootman, J., Kumi, C., and Gudauskas, G. 1985. Ocular absorption and toxicity of methotrexate in the dog. *Canadian Veterinary Journal* 26:263–266.

285. Wiederholt, M., Kossendrup, D., Schulz, W., and Hoffmann, F. 1986. Pharmacokinetics of topical cyclosporine in the rabbit eye. *Investigative Ophthalmology and Visual Science* 27:519–524.

286. Kaswan, R., Martin, C., and Gardner, S. 1987. Pharmacokinetics of ophthalmic cyclosporin. *Proceedings of the 2nd International Congress on Cyclosporine* 2, p. 59.

287. Kaswan, R., Kaplan, H., and Martin, C. 1988. Topically applied cyclosporin for modulation of induced immunogenic uveitis in rabbits. *American Journal of Veterinary Research* 49:1757–1759.

288. Gratzek, A., Kaswan, R., Martin, C., Champagne, E., and White, S. 1995. Ophthalmic cyclosporine in equine keratitis and keratouveitis: 11 cases. *Equine Veterinary Journal* 27:327–333.

289. Sansom, J., Barnett, K., Neumann, W., Schulte-Neumann, S., Clerc, B. 1995. Treatment of keratoconjunctivitis sicca in dogs with cyclosporine ophthalmic ointment: A European clinical field trial. *Veterinary Record* 137:504–507.

290. Williams, D., Hoey, A., and Smitherman, P. 1995. Comparison of topical cyclosporine and dexamethasone for the treatment of chronic superficial keratitis in dogs. *Veterinary Research* 137:635–639.

291. Yoshida, A., Fujihara, T., and Nakata, K. 1999. Cyclosporin A increases tear fluid secretion via release of sensory neurotransmitters and muscarinic pathway in mice. *Experimental Eye Research* 68:541–546.

292. Salisbury, M., Kaswan, R., Ward, D., and Martin, C. 1990. Topical application of cyclosporine in the management of keratoconjunctivitis sicca in dogs. *Journal of the American Animal Hospital Association* 26:269–274.

293. Morgan, R., and Abrams, K. 1991. Topical administration of cyclosporine for treatment of keratoconjunctivitis sicca in dogs. *Journal of the American Veterinary Medical Association* 199:1043–1046.

294. Olivero, D., Davidson, M., English, R., Nasisse, M., Jamieson, V., and Gerig, T. 1991. Clinical evaluation of 1% cyclosporine for topical treatment of keratoconjunctivitis sicca in dogs. *Journal of the American Veterinary Medical Association* 199:1039–1042.

295. Gilger, B.C., Wilkie, D.A., Davidson, M.G., and Allen, J.B. 2001. Use of an intravitreal sustained-release cyclosporine delivery device for treatment of equine recurrent uveitis. *American Journal of Veterinary Research* 62:1892–1896.

296. Ofri, R. et al. 2009. Clinical evaluation of pimecrolimus eye drops for treatment of canine keratoconjunctivitis sicca: A comparison with yclosporine A. *The Veterinary Journal* 179:70–77.

297. Nell, B. et al. 2005. The effect of topical pimecrolimus on keratoconjunctivitis sicca and chronic supreficial keratitis in dogs: Results from an exploratory study. *Veterinary Ophthalmology* 8:39–46.

298. Berdoulay, A. et al. 2005. Effect of topical 0.02 tacrolimus aqueous suspension on tear production in dogs with keratoconjunctivitis sicca. *Veterinary Ophthalmology* 8:25–232.

299. Ofri, R. et al. 2009. Clinical evaluation of pimecrolimus eye drops for treatment of canine keratoconjunctivitis sicca: A comparison with cyclosporine A. *Veterinary Journal* 179(1):70–77.

300. Chambers, L., Fischer, C., McCalla, T., Parshall, C., Slatter, D., and Yakley, B. 2002. Topical tacrolimus in treatment of canine keratoconjunctivitis sicca: A multicenter preliminary clinical trial. *Poster Presentation at the Scientific Meeting of the American College of Veterinary Opthalmologists.* Denver.

301. Johnson, R., Olsen, K., and Hernandez, E. 1988. Tissue plasminogen activator treatment of postoperative intraocular fibrin. *Ophthalmology* 95:592–596.

302. Jaffe, G. 1989. Treatment of postvitrectomy fibrin pupillary block with tissue plasminogen activator. *American Journal of Ophthalmology* 108:170–175.

303. Martin, C., Kaswan, R., Gratzek, A., Champagne, E., Salisbury, M., and Ward, D. 1993. Ocular use of tissue plasminogen acitvator in companion animals. *Progress in Veterinary and Comparative Ophthalmology* 3:29–36.

304. Sternberg, P.L., Aguilar, H., Drews, C., and Aaberg, T. 1990. The effect of tissue plasminogen activator on retinal bleeding. *Archives of Ophthalmology* 108:720–722.

305. Howard, G. 1991. Intraocular tissue plasminogen activator in a rabbit model of traumatic hyphema. *Archives of Ophthalmology* 109:272–274.

306. Johnson, M. 1990. Retinal toxicity of recombinant tissue plaminogen activator in the rabbit. *Archives of Ophthalmology* 108:259–266.

307. Lim, J. 1991. Intraocular penetration of topical tissue plasminogen activator. *Archives of Ophthalmology* 109:714–717.

308. Mittra, R., Dev, S., Nasir, M., and Toth, C. 1997. Recombinant hirudin prevents postoperative fibrin formation after experimental cataract surgery. *Ophthalmology* 104:558–561.

309. Liesegang, T. 1990. Viscoelastic substances in ophthalmology. *Survey of Ophthalmology* 34:268–293.

310. Wilkie, D.A., and Willis, A.M. 1999. Viscoelastic materials in veterinary ophthalmology. *Veterinary Ophthalmology* 2:147–153.

PROBLEM-BASED MANAGEMENT
OF OCULAR EMERGENCIES

CHARLES L. MARTIN

INTRODUCTION

There are relatively few true emergencies in ophthalmology where delaying treatment for a few minutes or hours will change the outcome of the disease, but there are many that require timely therapy. **Table 3.1** lists the usual ocular emergencies. The veterinarian is often asked to respond to ocular conditions that are either dramatic and/or alarming to the owner but rather benign as far as visual function is concerned. A good philosophy, when in doubt, is to see non-emergencies rather than risk turning away an emergency.

Ocular emergencies can be triaged into acute loss of sight, imminent loss of sight, potential loss of sight, painful conditions but usually not blinding, and dramatic signs with no significant visual sequela (**Table 3.1**). In addition, systemic implications may be superimposed on the ocular scoring, and the general practitioner should decide whether to refer the patient (**Table 3.2**). Most ocular emergencies that have visual implications should probably be seen by a veterinary ophthalmologist, either for definitive therapy or to confirm your diagnosis and advise on therapy. Proptosis (prolapse) of the globe is one of the main exceptions for referral. This condition can usually be readily managed without special instrumentation, and the outcome is mainly dependent on the injury sustained by the eye at the time of proptosis.

Triaging ocular emergencies often begins on the telephone. Knowing what questions to ask comes with the experience of taking countless histories and listening to clients interpret various ocular events (see **Table 3.3** for a list of questions regarding loss of sight). In general, it is difficult to interpret events from an owner's perspective, so when in doubt, timely examination should be encouraged.

Detailed management of all the possible ocular emergencies are not dealt with in this chapter, but the reader will be referred to the appropriate chapter for a detailed discussion. The objective of this chapter is to develop a "mind-set" or mental algorithm for managing ocular emergencies.

Ocular emergencies can be categorized into one or more problems: loss of vision in one or both eyes, unequal pupils, red eye, painful eye, ocular discharge, ocular opacity, and change in position of the eye. It is helpful to have an algorithm to investigate the various problems rationally.

BLINDNESS

History

Historical questions relating to blindness should include the duration of the problem, partial or complete loss of vision, conditions under which it is observed (both environment and light conditions), course, what the animal can and cannot do visually, systemic or neurologic signs, breed, and age of animal (**Table 3.3**).

Many animals that have their environment changed are thought by their owners to become acutely blind, when in reality they have been chronically blind from an insidious problem. True acute blindness is usually associated with disorientation and anxiety, which should be differentiated from signs and symptoms of senile dementia (cognitive dysfunction syndrome), such as pacing, circling, and panting, that are often interpreted by owners as being caused by blindness. When asked, many owners note differences in vision with varying amounts of ambient light. However, this information is not usually spontaneously volunteered.

> The owner should be asked about systemic or topical medications that the patient may have been given in the recent past or is currently taking and any history of systemic problems.

Evaluation of patients with vision deficiency

Clinical testing of vision is usually limited to a maze test, menace response, and the dazzle reflex (**Figure 3.1**). The maze test should be performed in both light and darkened conditions. The pupillary light reflex (PLR) should be evaluated with a bright light and the intraocular pressure (IOP) taken before dilating the pupils if they are not already dilated. Interpretation of the PLR is not as obvious as is often suggested, and incomplete sluggish movement should not be interpreted as a normal response. Conversely,

Table 3.1 Ocular conditions associated with various degrees of clinical urgency.

ACUTE VISUAL LOSS

Acute glaucoma

Luxated lens

Optic neuritis

Proptosis

Acute detachment syndromes

Iris prolapse

Endophthalmitis

Hyphema

Acute cataracts

Ruptured globe

IMMINENT VISUAL LOSS

Descemetocele

Progressive ulcer

Endophthalmitis

Glaucoma

Anterior uveitis

Corneal laceration

POTENTIAL LOSS OF SIGHT

Stromal ulcer

Orbital cellulitis

Myositis of masticatory muscles

Anterior uveitis

Displaced lens

Immune-mediated keratitis

Corneal endothelial decompensation

Cataract

Hyphema

Lipids in aqueous

PAINFUL BUT NOT USUALLY BLINDING

Orbital cellulitis/abscess

Superficial corneal ulcer

Corneal foreign body

Entropion

Distichia

Aberrant cilia

Myositis of masticatory muscles

DRAMATIC SIGNS WITHOUT VISUAL SIGNIFICANCE

Prolapse of the gland of the third eyelid

Protrusion of the third eyelid

Subconjunctival hemorrhage

Chemosis

Blepharoedema

Lacerations involving the third eyelid

Lid lacerations

Lid bruising

Table 3.2 Ocular emergencies that should be referred.

MOST SIGHT-THREATENING CONDITIONS

Glaucoma

Luxated/subluxated lens

Optic neuritis

Progressive ulcers

Descemetoceles

Iris prolapse from various causes

Acute retinal detachments: to determine cause

Endophthalmitis

Acute cataracts

Uveitis workup

Nontraumatic hyphema workup

Table 3.3 History taking questions for patients with vision loss.

QUESTION	VARIABLES
Duration of deficit?	Acute, chronic
Amount of deficit?	Complete, partial, one eye
Type of deficit?	Complete, moving versus stationary, large versus small, near versus far
Changes since first noted?	Static, progressive
Ability to see in various ambient light conditions?	Night blind, day blind, no difference
Environment when first noted?	No change, moved, different
Environment of animal?	Outside, inside, both
Medications past and present?	Preventive, therapeutic, how much, how long, current
Toxin exposure?	House plants, insecticides, pest control
Systemic signs?	PU/PD, weight gain, appetite, seizures, ataxia, weakness
Intact or neutered?	Used for breeding?
Diet?	Commercial, formulated, table food
Other animals in environment?	Related, ages, similar signs, illness
Past medical history?	None, CNS signs, metabolic signs, neoplasia

a lack of response often occurs from something as innocuous as atrophy of the iris sphincter. Examination with a penlight at this time may note other signs such as conjunctival hyperemia, corneal opacification and irregularities, abnormal anterior chamber contents (flare, hypopyon, hyphema), irregularities in the pupil margin and iris, and significant opacities in the axial lens. Once the pupils are dilated, a penlight examination quickly determines whether the vision complaints can be attributable to the clear media by the presence or absence of a clear tapetal reflection.

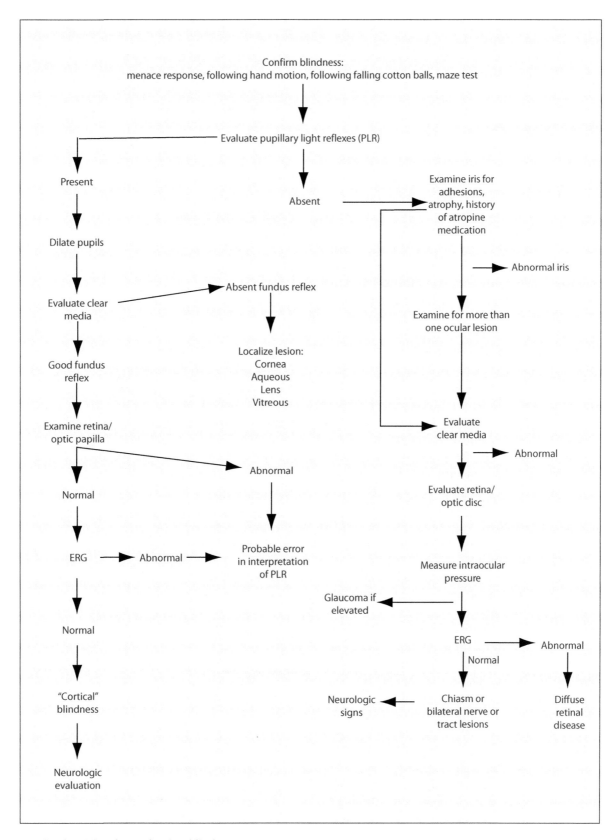

Figure 3.1 Algorithm for evaluating blindness.

Assumptions should not be made until the pupils are dilated; nuclear sclerosis is easily misdiagnosed as blinding cataracts in aged patients.

Causes of blindness

There are usually four broad categories of patients: blind with PLR, with or without clear media, and blind with no PLR, with or without clear media. If possible, a fundus examination should now be performed. If the fundus can be examined, blindness should not be attributed to opacification of the media. If media opacification precludes fundus examination, the challenge is to determine the location of the opacity and whether it is an emergency (needs immediate therapy) or, indeed, needs therapy (**Table 3.4**). Acute corneal edema, large fibrin clots or lipids in the anterior chamber, hyphema, acute cataract formation, hyalitis, and vitreous hemorrhage are examples of opacities in the clear media that may be presented as an emergency.

The two conditions that pose the greatest challenge to recognition are lipids in the anterior chamber and hyalitis (vitreous opacity). True acute cataracts, while not an emergency in themselves, are typically intumescent (swollen) and may have accompanying severe lens-induced uveitis and/or glaucoma. The main rule out for true acute bilateral cataracts is diabetes mellitus and the accompanying systemic implications. Ocular ultrasound is invaluable with opaque ocular media to determine the full extent of the lesions and, sometimes, to diagnose the cause of the opacification, for example foreign bodies, intraocular tumors, or retinal detachment.

If the fundus can be examined, the possibilities include dramatic fundus lesions, optic nerve lesions, minor/focal fundus lesions, or no lesions. Blindness with normal PLRs, clear media, and a normal fundus usually equates to central nervous system (CNS) blindness, either associated with metabolic disease (portocaval shunts) or diffuse or multifocal CNS disease. These cases should have medical and neurologic workup. Hemeralopia (day blindness), a relatively rare disease, can mimic CNS blindness but will date back to a young age and evidence of vision in a darkened environment.

Bilateral blindness with sluggish or dilated pupils and clear media implies an afferent arc lesion in the PLR (bilateral retina, optic nerve, chiasm, or optic tract) (**Table 3.5**). If the lesion is in the retina or anterior optic nerve, dramatic retinal lesions such as detachments, diffuse tapetal hyperreflectivity and vascular attenuation, diffuse inflammatory lesions, diffuse retinal hemorrhages, or disc elevation with hyperemia and edema will be present in most instances (**Table 3.4**). The three main exceptions are sudden acquired

Table 3.4 **Causes of bilateral loss of vision.**

OPACIFICATION OF THE CLEAR MEDIA

Keratitis: Keratoconjunctivitis sicca, immune mediated, multiple ulcerative events, chemical burns

Keratopathy: Lipids, endothelial dystrophy/degeneration/inflammation

Aqueous turbidity: Fibrin, lipids, hemorrhage

Cataracts: Genetic, metabolic, toxic, nutritional, radiation, traumatic, inflammation

Vitreous: Hemorrhage, inflammation, fibrous scars

DISEASES OF THE RETINA

Retinopathies

Genetic: PRA, inborn errors of metabolism, hemeralopia

Nutritional: Taurine deficiency (cats), vitamin E

Glaucoma

Postinflammatory atrophy

SARD

Toxic: Enrofloxacin, ivermectin

RETINAL DETACHMENT SYNDROMES

Genetic: Collie eye anomaly, retinal dysplasia syndromes, Australian shepherd anomaly

Exudative: Systemic mycoses, prototothecosis, ehrlichiosis, toxoplasmosis, FIP, FeLV, immune-mediated choroiditis

Transudative: Hypertension, IV solution overload

Neoplastic: Metastatic, multicentric

CHORIORETINITIS

Distemper, systemic mycoses, brucellosis, FIP, toxoplasmosis, ehrlichiosis, granulomatous meningoencephalitis, bacterial septicemia, VKH syndrome

LESIONS OF THE OPTIC NERVE, CHIASM, OPTIC TRACTS, OR OPTIC RADIATIONS

Hypoplasia of the optic nerves

Granulomatous meningoencephalitis

Distemper encephalitis

FIP

Systemic mycoses

Neoplasia involving the chiasm

Traumatic avulsion

Myositis of masticatory muscles

Vitamin A deficiency

LESIONS OF THE OCCIPITAL CORTEX

Hydrocephalus

Cerebral malformations

Distemper encephalomyelitis

FIP

Systemic mycoses

(Continued)

Table 3.4 (*Continued*) **Causes of bilateral loss of vision.**
Granulomatous encephalomyelitis
Hepatic encephalopathy
Inborn metabolic errors
Ivermectin toxicosis
Hypoxia
Vascular infarcts
Traumatic edema and/or hemorrhage
Postictal

While anisocoria has neurologic connotations to most observers, ocular causes should always be ruled out first as these are much more common.

retinal degeneration (SARD), retrobulbar neuritis, and chiasmal lesions (pituitary tumor). The majority, but not all, of SARD patients may have accompanying cushingoid signs and clinical features. An electroretinogram (ERG) can differentiate SARD (extinguished trace) from retrobulbar neuritis/chiasmal lesions (normal trace).

Focal lesions that may be incidental are the most difficult to interpret. The focal lesions may be clues in piecing the puzzle together or, more likely, be "red herrings." What appears to be a focal "scar" in one eye may be geographic retinal dysplasia and indicates that the retinal detachment in the contralateral eye is part of an inheritable dysplasia/detachment syndrome.

Of the causes of acute blindness, only a small number can be successfully treated. Blindness associated with opacities in the clear media may be reversible (inflammation, lipids, some hemorrhages, glaucoma-induced corneal edema, luxated lens) by treating the ocular disease or by removing the opacity (cataracts). Blindness in eyes with clear media can occasionally be treated. Examples of potentially treatable retinal diseases are bullous detachments from hypertension and sterile (immune-mediated) chorioiditis. Nonseptic optic neuritis may respond to systemic glucocorticoids. Metabolic (liver disease) blindness and some toxicities (ivermectin) that produce CNS blindness may improve with specific therapy or time.

Anisocoria
Evaluation
Cats or dogs with light-colored irides are most likely to be presented for the complaint of unequal pupils. Dark irides are often difficult to evaluate against the black pupil. The first decision is to determine which of the pupils is abnormal; this is not always obvious if the anisocoria is mild and both pupils are mobile.

The pupillomotor pathways are presented in Chapter 4, **Figure 4.6**. Anisocoria is evaluated in a dark room by shining the light at the base of the nose. This results in both pupils being illuminated against the tapetal reflection. Anisocoria should be evaluated under both dark and ambient light conditions. An algorithm for evaluating anisocoria is presented in **Figure 3.2**. The PLRs are evaluated with the swinging flashlight test. Anisocorias can be classified as to whether the PLRs are static (constant) or dynamic (manifest during or after light stimulation).

Causes of anisocoria
Regarding ocular emergencies, static anisocoria is the form most likely to be noted and is often associated with vision complaints (**Table 3.5**). Static anisocoria is associated with disease of the efferent side of the PLR reflex arc from the parasympathetic nuclei to the iris. Evaluation of static anisocoria should start from the eye and work backwards to the brain. Ocular examination should determine if the pupil is constricted, midpoint, or dilated. Constricted pupils are typical of acute uveitis, iris spasm such as from corneal pain, or drug induced. Midpoint irregular pupils are typical of a chronic uveitis. Irregular pupils may be congenital or be due to posterior or anterior synechia, iris atrophy, or a space occupying

Table 3.5 **Pupillary light reflexes with unilateral complete lesions at various levels of the visual system.**

LOCATION OF LESION	PLR	ANISOCORIA	MENACE	ERG
Retina	Absent direct Ipsilaterally, +MG	Mild static	Absent	Extinguished
Optic nerve	Absent direct, Ipsilaterally, +MG	Mild static	Absent	Normal
Chiasm	Absent OU	Mild static	Absent	Normal
Optic tract	Present, −MG	Mild static	Homonymous defect	Normal
Optic radiations/visual cortex	Present	None	Homonymous defect	Normal

PLR: pupillary light reflex; ERG: electroretinogram; MG: Marcus Gunn (pupil); OU: oculus uterque (each eye).

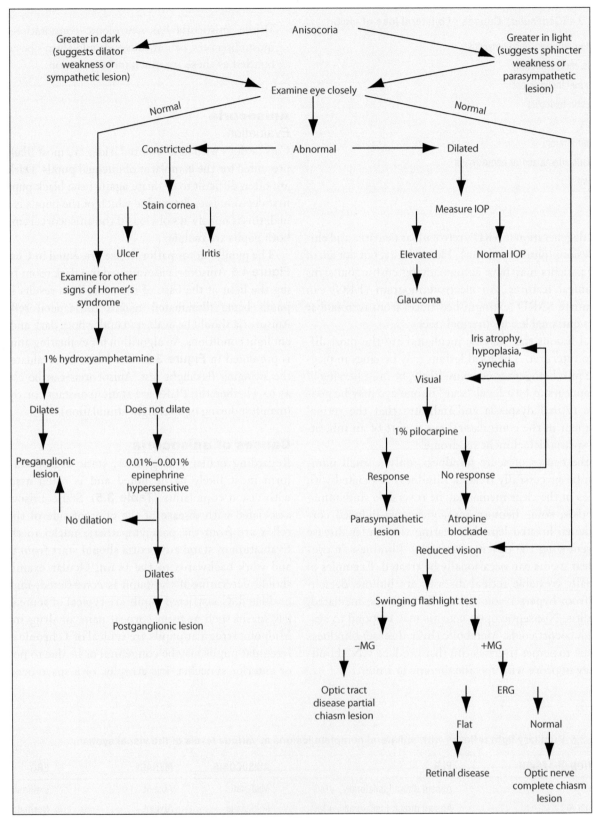

Figure 3.2 Algorithm for evaluating anisocoria. (IOP: intraocular pressure; MG: Marcus Gunn [pupil]; ERG: electroretinogram.)

lesion in the iris. A dilated pupil may be irregular if associated with iris atrophy or synechia and may be regular if associated with oculomotor paralysis, glaucoma, or if drug induced.

If the cause of anisocoria is ocular disease, there are usually other ocular signs such as conjunctival hyperemia, corneal opacity, aqueous humor turbidity, altered anterior chamber depth, and blindness. Oculomotor nerve paralysis may be strictly internal, combined with external ophthalmoplegia (paralysis of extraocular muscles), or present with other neurologic signs that may suggest neighboring lesions.

The main rule outs for static anisocoria associated with blindness and other ocular problems are glaucoma (dilated pupil), uveitis (constricted or midpoint), or a combination of the two. A fixed dilated pupil with blindness but without a red eye may be due to an orbital apex syndrome. The latter is usually due to a space-occupying orbital lesion and may have decreased globe retropulsion. Detailed workups should entail finding the underlying cause for these ocular signs.

Emergency therapy for anisocoria is indicated for the ocular signs of uveitis (see Chapter 11) and glaucoma (see Chapter 12).

Ocular pain
Evaluation
Ocular pain is a frequent cause for presentation of ocular emergencies. The most obvious manifestations of ocular pain are blepharospasm, third eyelid protrusion, and enophthalmos. Since the cornea is one of the most sensitive tissues in the body, it should be evaluated first. **Figure 3.3** is an algorithm for evaluating blepharospasm. The corneal nerve endings are concentrated in the subepithelial region, and thus the degree of pain may be inversely related to the seriousness of the corneal disease; superficial ulcers may cause more pain than deep ulcers. Corneal ulceration is the most common form of corneal disease associated with significant pain. However, nonulcerative disease is also a common cause of pain, especially in horses. All patients with corneal pain should have fluorescein testing of the cornea to detect ulceration. In the cat, evaluation with a blue light and/or rose bengal may be necessary to detect small herpesvirus ulcerations.

Causes of ocular pain
If corneal ulcers are present, the examination should be continued to search for the cause (**Table 3.6**). All ulcers should be evaluated for depth and the likelihood of progression, that is, how serious an emergency is it. Epithelial ulcers, while painful, do not represent a true emergency despite the dramatic signs. Epithelial ulcers have only a thin margin of epithelium visible at the edges without any appreciable depth to the base of the ulcer (see Chapter 10, **Figure 10.76**). These ulcers may present problems with slow healing but rarely become progressive in depth except in some brachycephalic breeds (see Chapter 10).

Stromal ulcers have some depth to the sides of the ulcer, take up fluorescein stain, usually stimulate some neutrophilic infiltration, and have some perilesional edema. If a mucopurulent exudate or a dense yellow perilesional halo accompanies the stromal ulcer, both bacterial sepsis and progression should be anticipated, and intensive therapy should be initiated to arrest further development (see Chapter 10). For the general practitioner, these cases should be referred before they become surgical emergencies. An ulcer with steep edges and a clear bottom that does not take up stain represents a descemetocele and is in

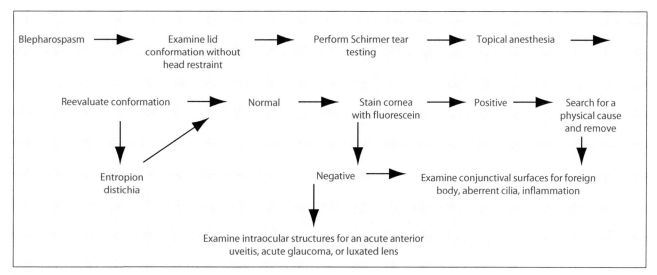

Figure 3.3 Algorithm for evaluating blepharospasm.

Table 3.6 **Rule outs for the cause of corneal ulceration.**

MECHANICAL IRRITATION
Distichia, trichiasis, aberrant cilia, entropion, foreign bodies, dermoid
TRAUMA
KERATOCONJUNCTIVITIS SICCA
Deficiency in serous, mucous, or lipid layers
EPITHELIAL BULLA RUPTURE
Corneal edema from endothelial disease: Degeneration, inflammation, trauma
LAGOPHTHALMOS
Shallow orbits, VII cranial nerve paralysis, exophthalmos
NEUROTROPHIC
V cranial nerve deficit, postsurgical, postlasering of ciliary body
INFECTIOUS
Viral: Herpesvirus in cats
Bacterial: *Moraxella* spp., secondary to trauma
Fungal: Usually secondary to trauma
Immunologic: Peripheral ulcerations and furrows, rarely bullous epithelial diseases
DEGENERATIVE
Calcium and lipid plaques sloughing
THERMAL INJURIES
CHEMICAL INJURIES
Acids, alkalis, soaps
BASAL LAMINA DEFECTS
Indolent ulcers

imminent danger of perforation (see **Figure 10.74**). Care in manipulation of the eye and restraint of the patient are important to avoid applying pressure to a severely weakened globe.

Depending on the surface area of the defect, some descemetoceles may be tolerated for an extended period of time, but it is best to assume they are an urgent problem. Descemetoceles are a surgical problem and should be referred by most general practitioners.

Another source of corneal pain may be from a plant foreign body. The most common appearance is a flat, brownish 1- to 2-mm lesion lying on the corneal surface (see Chapter 10, **Figure 10.10**). This type of foreign body can be easily removed after application of a topical anesthetic. Splinters are much more difficult to remove, requiring general anesthesia and delicate forceps, so they should be referred. Penetrating foreign bodies that are retained should be referred; they pose significant risk to the eye through sterile as well as septic inflammation. Breeching the lens capsules with these injuries may necessitate lens removal to save the eye.

Small, self-sealing, perforating injuries often belie the seriousness of the incident if the lens capsule has been ruptured or vitreous/retinal pathology exists.

Perforations, whether self-sealing or closed by iris entrapment, may be from BB (air gun) shot or pellet injuries, lacerations, perforated ulcers, or ruptured globes following blunt trauma. Recognition of an iris prolapse should prompt immediate referral.

All focal, peracute, perforating lesions, even if sealed, should have ultrasound and/or radiographic examination of the head to diagnose metallic foreign bodies.

Acute anterior uveitis and acute anterior lens luxation, with or without glaucoma, often manifest with acute ocular pain. Concomitant signs of selective conjunctival hyperemia, corneal edema, and pupillary changes may accompany these syndromes. In the dog, if the lens is clear and luxated, it probably represents a primary luxation if in a predisposed breed, such as a terrier (see Chapter 13). If the lens is cataractous, it is probably a secondary luxation, and the prognosis for vision may be guarded. Emergency treatment of a luxated lens consists of controlling the IOP with drugs that do not constrict the pupil. Pupillary constriction with acetylcholine-like drugs or prostaglandin analogs may aggravate a pupillary block. In the cat and the horse, most lens luxations are secondary to uveitis, and the prognosis is more complex.

Acute anterior uveitis is typically treated with anti-inflammatory drugs by topical and systemic routes and with topical atropine. Systemic glucocorticoids should not be used if there is known or suspected systemic bacterial or fungal infection. Antibiotics are indicated with sepsis but are often administered without clear indications.

Ocular discharge
Evaluation
If patients are presented for an ocular emergency because of an ocular discharge, typically the discharge is mucopurulent or purulent and copious. Most patients presented with an ocular emergency will at least have epiphora, although this may not be the presenting symptom.

Virtually all patients with purulent ocular discharge will have conjunctival hyperemia. Additional signs such as pain and corneal lesions are common, as well as intraocular changes. The possible diagnoses with this problem

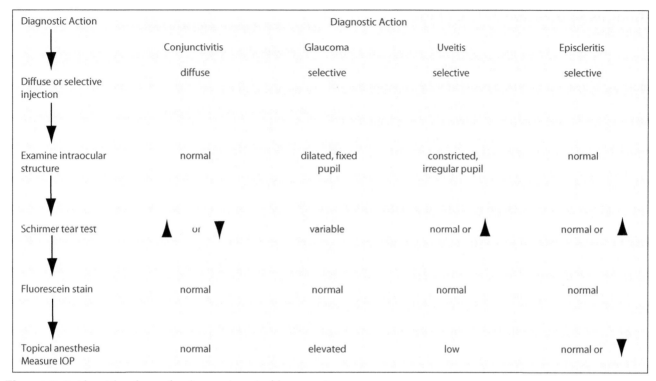

Diagnostic Action	Diagnostic Action			
	Conjunctivitis	Glaucoma	Uveitis	Episcleritis
Diffuse or selective injection	diffuse	selective	selective	selective
Examine intraocular structure	normal	dilated, fixed pupil	constricted, irregular pupil	normal
Schirmer tear test	▲ or ▼	variable	normal or ▲	normal or ▲
Fluorescein stain	normal	normal	normal	normal
Topical anesthesia Measure IOP	normal	elevated	low	normal or ▼

Figure 3.4 Algorithm for evaluating conjunctival hyperemia.

include conjunctivitis, keratitis, and endophthalmitis, and they are differentiated by the associated signs. **Figure 3.4** presents a diagnostic plan. Conjunctival hyperemia with conjunctivitis is typically diffuse and primarily on the palpebral surface (**Figure 3.5**). Selective large conjunctival vessel hyperemia is more typical of intraocular diseases (glaucoma, uveitis) and scleritis (**Figures 3.4 and 3.6**).

Tear production should always be evaluated in patients with ocular discharge. Patients with acute keratoconjunctivitis sicca frequently develop deep corneal ulcers. Patients with acute glaucoma may have decreased tear production with mucopurulent discharge or increased tear production with epiphora.

Conjunctival cultures and cytology are indicated in many patients with acute purulent discharge. Topical antibiotics are indicated for variable periods depending on the underlying cause.

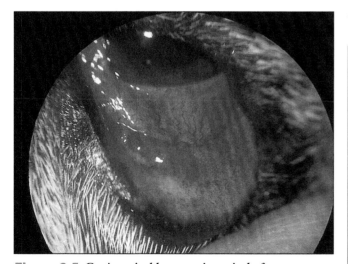

Figure 3.5 Conjunctival hyperemia typical of conjunctivitis in a dog. Note the diffuse hyperemia involving capillaries and the large vessels. This involves both bulbar and palpebral conjunctiva but is usually mainly palpebral.

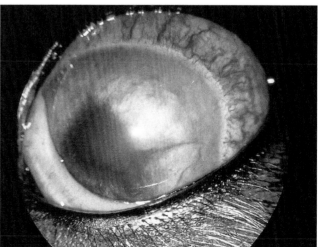

Figure 3.6 Conjunctival hyperemia in a dog, typical of intraocular disease, with selective large-vessel injection of the bulbar surface.

Changes in position of the globe

Evaluation

The ocular emergencies most commonly associated with this complaint are proptosis of the globe and acute orbital cellulitis. Much less common causes for acute exophthalmos are extraocular myositis, as observed in the Golden retriever, and acute masticatory myositis (see Chapter 6). While orbital neoplasia does not produce acute exophthalmos, the owner's observations may be inaccurate. Proptosis of the globe does not represent a diagnostic challenge, and the reader is referred to Chapter 6 for a more detailed discussion on prognosis and therapy. While considered an emergency for humane reasons, the prognosis for vision is altered very little by prompt therapy.

Orbital cellulitis is a questionable emergency from the perspective of affecting vision, but the dramatic pain and periocular swelling prompts the request for emergency examination. Severe forms of orbital cellulitis may affect the optic nerve and vision. Early orbital cellulitis presents with a red eye and a protruding third eyelid. The exophthalmos at this time may not be noted unless specifically evaluated from a dorsal perspective and by testing ocular retropulsion (see Chapter 1, **Figure 1.4**). While not a strict ocular emergency, it is desirable to initiate systemic antibiotics as soon as possible to shorten the course of the disease.

Enophthalmos may be presented with a complaint of "film over the eye" or "the eye is rolling up into the head." These observations are, of course, due to protrusion of the third eyelid. The most common cause of acute enophthalmos that presents as an emergency is ocular pain. (See the previous discussion on ocular pain and Chapter 6.)

Ocular opacity

The emergency patient with an ocular opacity may present with problems as diverse as third eyelid protrusion, pannus, corneal edema, lipids in the aqueous humor, fibrin in the anterior chamber, hyphema, and cataracts. The opacities can be divided into red, white, or black. **Tables 3.7–3.9** present causes of opacities based on color.

Third eyelid protrusion is a frequent cause for emergency presentation and has been discussed with ocular pain. In evaluating protrusion of the third eyelid, it is important for the examiner to keep in mind the factors that control the position of the third eyelid to develop an algorithm for protrusion (see Chapter 8). Emergency conditions that may be presented with this problem would be any condition that produces pain (conjunctivitis, corneal ulcers, glaucoma, acute uveitis, acute lens luxation); acute orbital space-occupying lesion (hemorrhage, inflammation, edema); head, neck, and chest trauma; poisoning (strychnine); tetanus; and systemic states that induce dehydration.

Table 3.7 **Rule outs for a red eye.**

INTRAOCULAR REDNESS
Hyphema
Vitreous hemorrhage
Normal albinotic fundus reflection
Hemorrhage into the lens (rare) associated with congenital vascular anomalies (PHTVL)
OCULAR SURFACE REDNESS
Conjunctivitis
Anterior uveitis
Glaucoma
Episcleritis/scleritis
Subconjunctival hemorrhage
Corneal granulation in healed ulcer, proliferative keratitis
Corneal neovascularization: Ulcerative and nonulcerative keratitis
Corneal hemorrhage: Rare
Corneal neoplasia
Iris prolapse covered by fibrin-laceration, perforated corneal ulcer, ruptured globe, perforating injury

Table 3.8 **Rule outs for white corneal opacities.**

Lipid deposition: Any depth
Calcium deposition: Usually superficial
Stromal scar: Any depth
Edema: Usually full-thickness
Leukocytic infiltration: Any depth
Infectious agents: Mycotic plaques, "Florida spots"
Descemet's membrane scars: PPM, anterior synechia, perforating injuries, inflammatory
Inclusion cyst: Relatively rare, usually superficial
Corneal scleralization: Extends from limbus
Eosinophilic protein: Present with eosinophilic keratitis syndromes in cat and horse
Immune complex formation: Often multifocal or zonular

Opacities of the cornea that are acute and may present as an emergency include corneal edema (white), cellular infiltration (creamy white), stromal hemorrhage (relatively rare), and black lesions produced by uveal prolapse. Profound corneal edema implies endothelial disease or deep corneal involvement and may be caused by trauma, uveitis, glaucoma, or a luxated lens (see Chapter 10, **Figure 10.23**). Therapy should be directed at the underlying cause of the opacity; topical hyperosmotic drugs produce only minimal improvement. Chronic corneal edema may

Table 3.9 **Rule outs for black corneal opacities.**
Chronic keratitis with melanin migration: Superficial, flat
Limbal melanocytoma: Usually raised
Iris prolapse: Superficial, usually raised, pupil distorted, chamber shallowed
Anterior synechia: Deep, distorted pupil, shallow chamber
Persistent pupillary membrane attachments: Deep, may have strands present, pupil usually not distorted
Intraocular melanoma: Extraocular invasion, extension to posterior cornea, mass in globe
Corneal sequestrum: Only in cats, superficial but extends deep
Dematiaceous fungi: Rare, cytology
Plant foreign bodies: Superficial
Drug residues: Rare, silver nitrate, epinephrine

be presented as an emergency due to the formation of sub-epithelial bullae that rupture, producing a painful acute ulcerative syndrome. The causes of chronic edema are similar to the causes of acute edema, with the addition of senile degenerative disease (**Table 3.8**).

Intense leukocytic infiltration, usually accompanied by edema and neovascularization, is a common emergency presentation with septic ulcerative or nonulcerative keratitis (see Chapter 10, **Figure 10.92**). Corneal abscessation is common in the horse but less so in other species. The cause may be bacterial or fungal. Intense topical antibacterial and antifungal therapy is indicated. Systemic antifungal therapy can also be administered but is very expensive. Other causes for white corneal opacities are lipids, calcium, eosinophils, and infectious agents. Lipids and calcium in the cornea are usually incidental findings, although exceptions may occur. Occasionally, lipid degeneration associated with hypothyroidism is diffuse and rapid enough to be presented with a sense of urgency. Calcium is usually deposited superficially in the cornea and denotes a degenerative condition; if rapidly progressing, Cushing's syndrome should be considered. Calcium plaques may slough and produce corneal ulcers.

Eosinophilic keratitis in the horse and the cat may have white plaques or spots in a bed of granulation tissue that, on cytology, reveals numerous eosinophils and mast cells. These patients present with pain or red, granulating opacities (see Chapter 10, **Figures 10.49 and 10.50**). The most common infectious cause for white to yellow plaques on the cornea is fungal infection. The horse is unique in its susceptibility to fungal keratitis, but it may occur occasionally in the dog and the cat (see Chapter 10, **Figures 10.33 and 10.35**). The diagnosis is made from corneal cytology.

Hypopyon (leukocytes in the anterior chamber) is common with septic ulceration and uveitis but is not usually the presenting symptom. It is recognized by the white boat-shaped opacity in the ventral anterior chamber (see Chapter 11, **Figure 11.50**). Hypopyon is not an absolute indicator of intraocular sepsis. Sterile inflammation can also induce hypopyon, but it is safer to assume sepsis and treat with antibiotics until proven otherwise. Rarely, ocular lymphoma syndromes present with marked hypopyon (**Figure 11.49**).

Lipid in the anterior chamber appears as a diffusely white opacity and may be confused with diffuse corneal edema or a cataract with a dilated pupil (see Chapter 11, **Figure 11.65**). The lack of texture may help to differentiate lipid from corneal edema, and the inability to see the iris should differentiate it from a cataract. Lipid in the anterior chamber indicates systemic hyperlipidemia and may occur with systemic metabolic diseases such as diabetes mellitus, pancreatitis, Cushing's disease, liver disease, and essential hyperlipidemia of Schnauzers, or it may result simply from ingestion of a fatty meal (garbage). Lipids gain access to the chamber because of a breakdown of the blood–aqueous humor barrier, and their presence implies underlying uveitis. Consequently, most patients with lipid aqueous humor also have a red eye. Therapy should be directed at any systemic disease, treating the uveitis with anti-inflammatory drugs and atropine, and dietary restriction of fat. Glaucoma may be a complication of lipids in the anterior chamber, so the IOP should be monitored and glaucoma therapy initiated if the IOP is elevated (see Chapter 12).

Fibrin clots may produce acute opacities in the eye and are often intermixed with hemorrhage (see Chapter 11, **Figure 11.54**). Dramatic fibrin clots are most commonly observed in neonatal septicemia in large animals (**Figure 11.60**). The aqueous humor may be sterile, but antibiotics should be administered as well as anti-inflammatories and atropine. Large fibrin clots may undergo dramatic resolution over a 7-day period, but intraocular tissue plasminogen activator (tPA) ensures and hastens the resolution (see Chapter 11).

Subconjunctival hemorrhage is a common finding on ocular examination in trauma patients but is usually not the presenting complaint. Subconjunctival hemorrhage is a benign condition that does not require therapy. The remainder of the eye should always be evaluated to ascertain if other more serious ocular lesions may be present. Subconjunctival hemorrhage is usually due to trauma, but choking injuries and systemic diseases should also be considered if other physical evidence of trauma is not present.

Hyphema is commonly presented as an ocular emergency, but in reality, there is no need for urgent treatment. However, the systemic implications of hyphema may warrant an emergency visit. The outcome of traumatic hyphema is rarely dependent on the therapy but is dependent on the initial damage produced by the trauma and the amount of blood present. While trauma is the most common cause of hyphema, it is not the only cause. Unless there is physical evidence of trauma or trauma was witnessed, an underlying systemic disease should always be considered, such as hypertension, blood dyscrasias, diseases causing vasculitis such as tick-borne infection and clotting and bleeding disorders. It is common for the owner to presume trauma with hyphema and present it as historical fact, when it was not actually observed. Conversely, the patient may have suffered trauma because of hyphema or blindness. The opposite eye and the fundus should also be examined for evidence of hemorrhage. Hyphema may also mask and be caused by other ocular conditions such as neoplasia, glaucoma, retinal detachment (acute or chronic), and chronic uveitis. Ocular ultrasonography is indicated to determine the presence of other lesions and the extent of the ocular hemorrhage (presence in the vitreous).

The prognosis for hyphema depends on the cause and associated ocular lesions. Simple traumatic hyphema involving less than half of the anterior chamber has a good prognosis, whereas complete hyphema has a guarded prognosis. Assessment of the degree of hyphema may vary with the animal's activity level. Hyphema usually settles out in the anterior chamber with rest and becomes dispersed with activity. This apparent worsening of the hyphema is not accompanied by any change in the amount of blood in the anterior chamber.

The main therapy for hyphema is cage rest and tranquilization. While a variety of drugs have been used to treat hyphema, none have shown clear benefit in controlled studies. Patients with traumatic hyphema should be assumed to have traumatic uveitis as well and should be treated accordingly. Surgical removal of the blood is rarely indicated.

Acute onset of cataracts is occasionally presented as an emergency. One of two scenarios is usually present with this complaint: insidious cataracts that have reached a threshold that the owner has noticed, or truly acute onset of bilateral cataracts. Most forms of cataracts are usually asymmetrical in their development with the significant exception of sugar and toxic cataracts. Of these exceptions, diabetic cataracts are by far the most common. Diabetic cataracts may literally appear overnight to the owners, and often the owners do not volunteer information regarding the accompanying systemic signs, such as polyurea and polydipsia. These patients are often poorly regulated and ketotic and can sometimes be diagnosed by smelling their breath. Acute diabetic cataracts are typically symmetrical, intumescent, or swollen and may have complications of uveitis and/or glaucoma. While the systemic state takes precedence, the eyes should be treated for lens-induced uveitis with topical atropine and anti-inflammatory drugs. In some instances, the inflammation and/or IOP is not easily controlled and may require lens removal to control. Sometimes the lens ruptures.

Black opacities on the cornea that are presented as emergencies are most likely to be uveal tissue prolapse from a breech in the surface (**Table 3.9**). The lesion is often raised, and although the uvea is itself pigmented, the exuding of fibrin from the surface often results in a red or gray opacity (see Chapter 10, **Figure 10.108**). Involvement of the iris can usually be confirmed by finding the anterior chamber is partially or completely shallowed or collapsed and the pupil tented or not visible. Concurrent corneal opacification may preclude direct evaluation of intraocular structures. Uveal prolapse may occur from a perforated ulcer, penetrating injury, laceration, or blunt traumatic rupture of the cornea. The prognosis varies according to the cause and the amount of damage to intraocular structures (see Chapter 11). These patients should be referred immediately.

Superficial corneal pigment may also be present because of previous or chronic pathology. Other sources of pigment in the cornea may be the corneal nigrum in the cat and, rarely, dematiaceous fungi that produce pigment.

EMERGENCIES THAT DO NOT THREATEN SIGHT

Injuries and diseases of the lids, conjunctiva, and third eyelid may be presented as emergencies but in general do not threaten sight. As such, they are examined to ensure the process is localized to the adnexa, and they can then be managed at a more convenient time.

Lid emergencies are usually lid lacerations or acute swellings from contusions, infection, angioedema, venomous bites, and burns, either heat or chemical. Of these, only snake bites or chemical burns would indicate urgent therapy. Lid lacerations are easily recognized and are most easily treated within the first 24–48 hours. Accurate apposition of the lid margin is the key to functional and cosmetic success (see Chapter 7). Slips of lid margin that may be hanging loose with lacerations running parallel to the lid margin should not be removed but sutured in place to maintain the normal mucocutaneous junction.

Acute lid swelling from contusions should be further evaluated for globe and orbital injuries, and they may benefit from cold packing in the first 12–24 hours and later from hot packing. Acute cellulitis or abscessation is a common emergency in cats, particularly free-roaming intact males. If treated early, systemic antibiotics should be sufficient, but at the stage of abscessation, drainage plus local and systemic antimicrobial therapy is necessary. Lid abscessation often produces marked chemosis and may drain into the conjunctival cul-de-sac, but the globe is usually spared.

Acute bilateral lid swelling caused by allergic reactions (angioedema) may be accompanied by edema of the nose and urticaria. Angioedema should improve with or without treatment (see Chapter 7) but is usually treated with an injection of antihistamines and/or glucocorticoids.

Acute chemical burns to the lids and globe are, unfortunately, often malicious. The main therapy is immediate and copious flushing with any water or saline solution at hand and removal of any residue from the surface. Alkali burns are the most disastrous to tissue because of their deep penetration. The various self-defense sprays such as mace and pepper spray are often blamed for various ocular lesions without definite proof of exposure. While irritating, no lasting pathology should occur with these chemicals; irrigating the eye and avoiding self-trauma should be sufficient therapy.

Emergency presentation for conjunctival lesions is usually associated with trauma or infection. Laceration, chemosis, and subconjunctival hemorrhage are the usual sequelae to conjunctival trauma. Conjunctival lacerations do not need suturing unless the third eyelid attachments or cartilage are involved. Dramatic chemosis may occur from allergic reactions, trauma, or infection. Differentiation will be based on associated lesions, history, type of ocular discharge, and conjunctival cytology. Traumatic and allergic reactions are treated with topical anti-inflammatory therapy (assuming no corneal abrasions), while antimicrobial therapy is administered for suspected infection.

Emergency presentation due to third eyelid disease is usually due to eversion of the third eyelid gland or protrusion of the third eyelid. Cherry eye or eversion of the gland is a common dramatic but nonemergency event. The diagnosis can usually be made with some confidence over the telephone from the age (up to 2 years) and breed of the dog. Similar signs in older dogs may have more serious implications, such as an orbital lesion, but are not emergencies. Protrusion of the third eyelid has been discussed previously.

CHAPTER 4

NEURO-OPHTHALMIC DISORDERS

BERNHARD M. SPIESS

Neuro-ophthalmology is the science of the interrelationships of the ophthalmic and the central nervous system (CNS). Many CNS diseases cause ophthalmic dysfunction, and, therefore, an understanding of neuro-ophthalmology is often essential for localizing neurologic lesions.

Neuro-ophthalmology encompasses (1) vision, (2) pupillary size and light reflexes, (3) ocular position, (4) ocular motility and movement, (5) eyelid position and movement, (6) lacrimation, and (7) ocular sensation.

Seven of the 12 cranial nerves are of primary importance in clinical neuro-ophthalmologic disease. An astute ophthalmologist can easily evaluate eight of the 12 cranial nerves (CN) on any routine eye examination.

The following gives a description of location and function of the cranial nerves affecting the eye and the adnexa and their functions (**Figure 4.1**).

DIENCEPHALON

The diencephalon is the most rostral part of the brainstem and includes the hypothalamus, thalamus, subthalamus, and metathalamus.

CN II

Optic nerve: This nerve is strictly visual-sensory input to the lateral geniculate nuclei and on to the occipital cortex of the brain, to the rostral colliculi as afferent arch for the dazzle reflex, and to the pretectal nuclei for the afferent arch of the pupillary light reflex. The optic nerve and the chiasm are located on the ventral surface of the hypothalamus near the pituitary gland.

Disease: Optic neuritis and papillitis, primary optic nerve neoplasias, congenital hypoplasia or aplasia, colobomas.

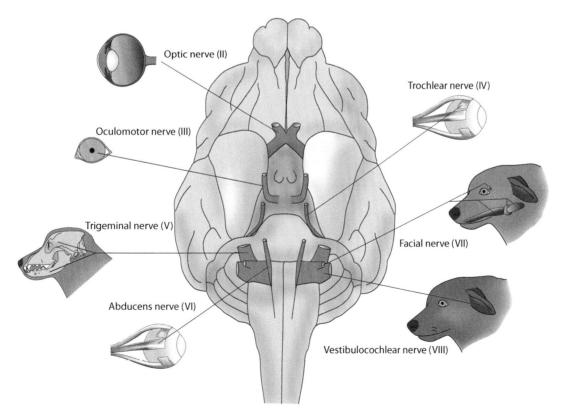

Figure 4.1 Ventral view of the brain and the cranial nerves.

MESENCEPHALON

The mesencephalon or midbrain has many important structures, such as the reticular activating substance for consciousness and sleep, the red nucleus, origin of the rubrospinal tract, and two cranial nerves.

CN III

Oculomotor nerve: Its fibers innervate the ventral, dorsal, and medial rectus muscles; the inferior oblique muscles; and the levator palpebrae muscles. It contains the parasympathetic efferent fibers to the sphincter pupillae muscle and the ciliary muscle.

Disease: Ocular motility abnormalities, strabismus, dilated pupils not associated with iris sphincter muscle deficits, abnormal pupillary light reflex (PLR), ptosis.

CN IV

Trochlear nerve: It is the motor nerve to the superior oblique muscle.

Disease: Ocular motility abnormalities, a torsional strabismus.

METENCEPHALON

The metencephalon contains the pons, the cerebellum, and one cranial nerve.

CN V

Trigeminal nerve: The ophthalmic and maxillary branches transmit pain and pressure sensation from the cornea and lids, is the afferent arch for the blink reflexes, and provides input for reflex lacrimation. Its motor branches control muscle tone in the muscles of mastication. It originates in the pons.

Disease: Abnormal corneal and palpebral reflex, neurotropic keratitis, dropped jaw.

MYELENCEPHALON

The myelencephalon, the medulla oblongata, is composed of many ascending and descending pathways and nuclei. Seven cranial nerves originate in the myelencephalon.

CN VI

Abducens nerve: It is the motor nerve to the lateral rectus muscle and the retractor bulbi muscles. It also carries sympathetic fibers to the third eyelid. It originates in the pons and has the longest course through the cranium of all cranial nerves and is, therefore, most susceptible to compression.

Disease: Ocular motility abnormalities, medial strabismus, Duane's retraction syndrome.

CN VII

Facial nerve: General motor nerve to all muscles of facial expression. It is also the motor nerve to the orbicularis oculi muscle. Parasympathetic fibers innervate the lacrimal gland and third eyelid gland.

Disease: Facial paralysis, abnormal palpebral reflexes, neurogenic KCS, neuroparalytic keratitis, lagophthalmos.

CN VIII

Vestibulocochlear nerve: The cochlear branch is of little neuro-ophthalmic importance. The vestibular branch is intimately involved with ocular motility and position including nystagmus and strabismus.

Disease: Nystagmus, strabismus, head tilt.

CN X

Vagus nerve: Initiates swallowing and is centrally involved in the oculocardiac reflex (efferent arch).

Disease: Dysphagia, bradycardia.

ANATOMY OF THE VISUAL PATHWAYS

Retina

The retinal photoreceptors—rods and cones—convert incoming light energy into electrochemical energy of nerve impulses (see Chapter 14).[1-4]

These impulses are relayed to the retinal bipolar cells, the true first-order neurons. The second-order neurons are the ganglion cells with their axons forming the optic nerve. These axons are nonmyelinated and located in the nerve fiber layer and run towards the optic papilla. The nerve fiber layer thickens towards the papilla.[5] Because the nerve fibers are not myelinated, they are extremely delicate and sensitive to alterations in intraocular pressure.

Optic nerve

At the papilla, the axons turn 90° and leave the globe through the lamina cribrosa to form the optic nerve. In most animals, the nerve fibers can be visualized ophthalmoscopically at the level of the papilla because here they are myelinated. The oligodendroglial cells produce the myelin for the axons of the optic nerve.

The ratio of ganglion cells to nerve fibers is almost 1:1. In the dog, the optic nerve is formed by 145,000–165,000 axons, while the total axon count is 193,000 in cats, 1,080,000 in horses, and 1,100,000 in humans.[6] The optic nerve is surrounded by meninges, including a subarachnoid space. It projects posteriorly through the orbital cone formed by the extraocular muscles and enters the optic canal through the optic foramen in the presphenoid bone.

Optic chiasm

In the dog, 75% of the axons cross over to the contralateral side (decussate) at the level of the optic chiasm just rostral to the hypophysis. The percentage of decussation is 81% for the horse, 83% for cattle, 89% for sheep, 88% for swine, and 65% in cats.[7] In contrast, in man, 50% of the axons remain ipsilateral, while in birds and in most fish, all the axons cross over to the contralateral side. As a rule, the axons arising from the lateral one-third of the retina remain ipsilateral, while the medial two-thirds of the retina project to the contralateral side. The dividing line in the cat is a sagittal section through the area centralis. The visual information is relayed to the visual cortex in the lateral geniculate body.

The degree of decussation is directly related to the forward placement of the eyes and with binocular vision (**Figure 4.2**). Lower vertebrates, such as fish, have no binocular visual field, and 100% of their axons cross over. At the other end of the evolutionary ladder, in man, with parallel visual axes, 50% of the fibers cross.

Optic tract

After the chiasm, the axons run as optic tracts in a caudal-dorsal-lateral direction over the sides of the diencephalon and end in the lateral geniculate body (**Figure 4.3**). While the optic nerve contains only axons from one eye, each optic tract is made up of axons of the medial retina of the contralateral eye and of axons of the lateral retina of the ipsilateral eye. Light from the right side of the visual field thus falls onto the medial retina of the right eye and onto the lateral retina of the left eye. The right visual field projects onto the left visual cortex and vice versa.[8]

Approximately 80% of the axons constituting the optic tracts terminates in the lateral geniculate body, while the remaining 20% subserve pupillomotor function. Some axons terminate in the rostral colliculus and/or supraoptic nuclei and form the afferent arm of the dazzle reflex or photic blink reflex. However, the entire dazzle reflex pathway has not been elucidated in animals.[9]

Lateral geniculate body

The lateral geniculate body is a caudal-dorsal protrusion of the thalamus and the principal relay station between the retina and visual cortex (**Figure 4.4**).

In the lateral geniculate body of the dog and the cat, three layers can be differentiated. In man and primates, there are six different cell layers. The axons of the optic tract terminate primarily in the dorsal parts of the lateral geniculate body. Here, a lamina principalis anterior, a lamina principalis posterior, a lamina parvocellular, and a lamina magnocellular can be distinguished. Uncrossed axons end mostly in the lamina principalis posterior, while crossed fibers terminate in the remaining layers.

The optic tract, however, is not the only influence on the lateral geniculate body. Nonretinal inputs are from the visual cortex as the corticogeniculate pathway from the brainstem and the ventral thalamus. It is thought that these nonretinal inputs are regarded as mechanisms to protect the cortex from unimportant visual information.

Optic radiations, tractus geniculo-occipitalis

After leaving the lateral geniculate body, the axons of the ganglion cells of the lateral geniculate body run as tractus

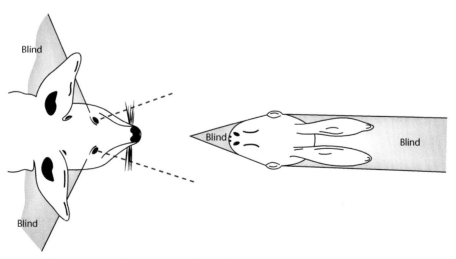

Figure 4.2 The degree of decussation of retinal ganglion cell axons is partly determined by the position of the eyes in the skull and the animal's need for binocular vision.

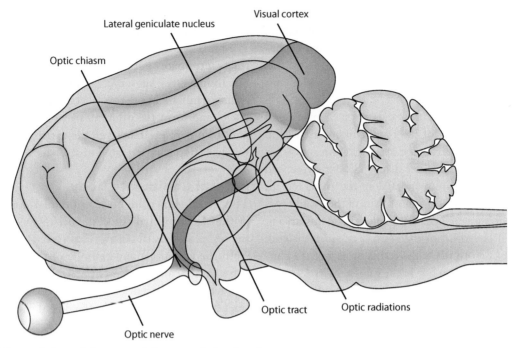

Figure 4.3 Lateral view of the eye and the central visual pathways.

geniculo-occipitalis or optic radiation towards the visual cortex, the area optica or striata of the lobus occipitalis.

Visual cortex

All areas of the gray matter of the occipital lobes participating in visual perception are called visual cortex. It involves primarily the caudal and medial parts and to a lesser amount the lateral aspects of the occipital lobes.

In primates, the gray matter of the brain has been divided into several functional areas. Areas 17 (c), 18 (b), and 19 (a) and part of the suprasylvian gyrus form the visual cortex (**Figure 4.5**). Area 17 is also called area striata. Most of the axons end in area 17, the primary visual cortex. Vision depends on the integrity of area 17. Permanent blindness occurs when this area is destroyed.

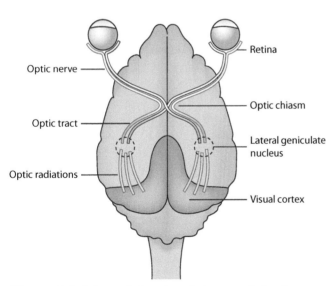

Figure 4.4 Schematic drawing of the central visual pathways with the lateral geniculate body as the primary relay station between the eyes and the visual cortex. Images from the right visual field are received and processed in the opposite (left) cerebral hemisphere.

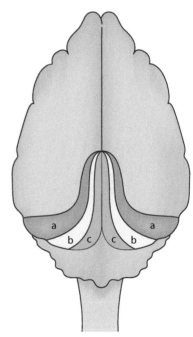

Figure 4.5 Schematic representation of areas a,b,c of the primary visual cortex.

Based on electrophysiologic information, the cells of the visual cortex can be classified into (1) cells responding to direction of movement, (2) cells responding to movement in any direction, (3) cells responding to stationary stimuli, and (4) cells responding to diffuse illumination.

ANATOMY OF THE PUPILLARY REFLEX PATHWAY

About 20% of the axons in the optic nerve do not project to the lateral geniculate body but participate in the pupillary light reflex.[8] They project to the midbrain via the superior brachium of the rostral colliculus and synapse on cells of the third-order neurons, which make up the pretectal nucleus. Thus, lesions to the lateral geniculate body do not affect PLR (**Figure 4.6**).

Pretectal nucleus

As most axons arising from one eye decussate in the chiasm, most axons participating in the reflex pathway end in the contralateral pretectal nucleus. Most of these fibers, however, decussate again in the posterior commissure to the contralateral Edinger-Westphal (E-W) nucleus. Only a minority of fibers arches around the central gray matter to reach the ipsilateral E-W nucleus. This is in sharp contrast to man and the primates and explains some of the differences seen in the PLR in these species.

Edinger-Westphal nucleus: Third nerve nucleus

The E-W nucleus is located rostral and dorsal to the oculomotor nucleus and receives crossed and some uncrossed

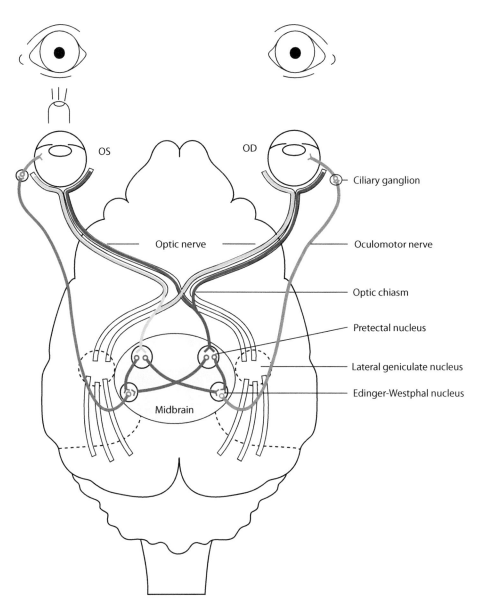

Figure 4.6 Schematic anatomy of the pupillary light reflex pathway.

axons from the pretectal nuclei. From the E-W nucleus, the fibers leave in intimate association with the motor nerve fibers of CN III (oculomotor nerve) and leave this nerve only within the orbital cone to synapse on the ciliary ganglion. The efferent fibers of the reflex pathway remain uncrossed.

Ciliary ganglion

The ciliary ganglion is a collection of postganglionic parasympathetic cells just lateral to the optic nerve. Postganglionic axons form the short ciliary nerves, which terminate in the smooth muscle of the iris sphincter muscle.

Short ciliary nerves

The short ciliary nerves course along the optic nerve and enter the globe at the lamina cribrosa. They then ramify in the uveal tract and innervate the ciliary body and the sphincter muscle. There are important differences in the anatomy of the short ciliary nerves between the dog and the cat.

In the dog, up to eight short ciliary nerves enter the globe. They contain postganglionic (parasympathetic) fibers of the ciliary ganglion, postganglionic (sympathetic) fibers of the superior (cranial) cervical ganglion, and afferent sensory fibers of the ophthalmic branch of the trigeminal (V) nerve.

In the cat, two short ciliary nerves leave the ciliary ganglion containing only postganglionic parasympathetic fibers. Only at the point of entry into the globe are these two nerves joined by sympathetic and sensory fibers (V) via the nasociliary nerve. The lateral short ciliary nerve is also called the malar nerve and innervates the lateral half of the sphincter muscle, while with the medial short ciliary nerve, the nasal nerve is innervating the medial half of the iris. The dilator muscle of the iris is innervated by sympathetic fibers. The central neuron of the tectotegmental spinal tract descends primarily ipsilaterally from the posterior hypothalamus through the brainstem and lateral funiculus of the cervical spinal cord. It synapses with preganglionic cells within the gray matter of the spinal cord at the levels T1 through T3.

The preganglionic fibers leave the spinal cord via the segmental roots to the paravertebral sympathetic chain. These fibers synapse in the cranial cervical ganglion caudomedially to the tympanic bullae. The postganglionic fibers join the tympanic branch of CN IX within the middle ear to form the caroticotympanic nerve. Sympathetic postganglionic fibers eventually join the trigeminal nerve to enter the globe as the long ciliary nerves. Sympathetic fibers run in the suprachoroidal space to innervate the ciliary body and the dilator muscle.

OCULAR PLACEMENT AND MOTILITY

The placement of the globe within the orbit and the situation of the orbit itself is species specific and closely related to the natural behavior and habitat of the animal (**Figure 4.2**).[10] In domestic animals, ocular movements are executed by the four rectus muscles, the inferior and superior oblique muscles, and the retractor bulbi muscles (**Figure 4.7**). The rectus muscles are innervated by CN III with the exception of the lateral rectus muscle, which is innervated by CN VI. The superior oblique muscle is innervated by the trochlear nerve (IV), while the inferior oblique is innervated by CN III. The lateral portion of the retractor bulbi muscle is innervated by CN VI, while the remainder of this muscle is innervated by CN III.[11]

To keep an object in the visual field, the animal relies on the action of the extraocular muscles and the vestibulocochlear reflex arch. So-called saccades are necessary to keep an image in the area centralis and for normal functioning of the retina. Both eyes must execute minute movements in unison. In extraocular muscles, one motor axon innervates five to 10 muscle fibers, whereas one axon innervates thousands of fibers in skeletal muscles. This allows for much finer control of the movement of the eyes.[12]

Rhythmical oscillations of the eyeballs are called nystagmus. Nystagmus is characterized by a slow and a fast component. The direction of a nystagmus refers to the direction of the fast component. Nystagmus can be horizontal or vertical. Nystagmus most commonly accompanies disease of the vestibular system. The vestibular system uses the semicircular canals and the utricular and

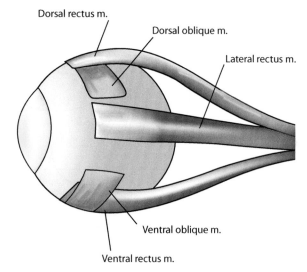

Dorsal rectus m.

Dorsal oblique m.

Lateral rectus m.

Ventral oblique m.

Ventral rectus m.

Figure 4.7 Schematic drawing of the extraocular muscles (the retractor bulbi muscle is not shown).

saccular end organs of the inner ear to transduce angular acceleration, linear acceleration, and gravity into nerve impulses, which activate the vestibular nuclei. The activity produces a continuous tone tending, in the case of the horizontal plane, to deviate the eyes to the opposite side. In normal conditions, the tone of each side remains in balance. Nystagmus usually occurs towards the disordered side.

Listed below are the various types of nystagmus:

1. Congenital nystagmus
   Pendular nystagmus
   Jerk nystagmus
2. Acquired nystagmus
   Vestibular nystagmus
   Nonspecific nystagmus
3. Special types of nystagmus
   Rotary nystagmus (midbrain disease)
   Dissociated nystagmus (unilateral nystagmus in lateral gaze)
   Upbeat nystagmus (thiamine deficiency)
   Downbeat nystagmus (medullary trauma)
   Convergence-retraction nystagmus (head trauma, third ventricle tumor)
4. Induced nystagmus
   Optokinetic nystagmus
   Caloric nystagmus
   Rotatory nystagmus
   Postrotatory nystagmus

A normal induced vestibular nystagmus is the optokinetic nystagmus. In optokinetic nystagmus, the eyelid must be open. The nystagmus is in the opposite direction of the visual stimulus. If, however, the stimulus is stationary, and the head or the body is moved, the nystagmus has the same direction as the movement of the head. Optokinetic nystagmus is best observed in the horizontal plane but can also be induced in the vertical plane by flexion and extension of the head. Optokinetic nystagmus can be used to demonstrate vision in an animal.

A second type of normal nystagmus is rotatory nystagmus. Rotatory nystagmus occurs even when the lids are closed. The rapid phase of this nystagmus is in the same direction as the rotation of the head/body. Postrotatory nystagmus occurs after rotation is stopped and lasts for about 10 seconds. Its fast phase is opposite the previous direction of rotation. Rotatory and postrotatory nystagmus is triggered by acceleration and deceleration, respectively. If rotation of the head/body occurs at a constant speed, there is no nystagmus if the lids are kept closed. If the lids are opened, an optokinetic nystagmus can be observed.

A third normal nystagmus is caloric nystagmus, which can be induced by instillation of warm or cold water into the ear canal.[13] Warm water elicits a nystagmus with the rapid phase towards the stimulated ear, while cold water elicits a nystagmus with the rapid phase towards the opposite side. Both forms of nystagmus are induced by expansion or contraction of the endolymph in the semicircular canals adjacent to the ear canal.

The nystagmus, which can be observed during induction of anesthesia, is thought to be due to decreased inhibition of brain centers that initiate nystagmus.

In congenitally blind animals, a wandering, random, slow nystagmus can be observed (congenital pendular nystagmus). Congenital jerk nystagmus is sometimes seen in animals. It is a nystagmus in the direction of gaze and more obvious with lateral gaze. It is not associated with decreased visual performance.

The absence of ocular movement on any head movement is associated with severe brainstem disease.

Eyelid position and movement

The eyelid receives sensory innervation from branches of the trigeminal nerve.[11] The ophthalmic nerve innervates the middle portion of the upper eyelid and the medial portions of both upper and lower lids via the frontal and infratrochlear nerves, respectively. The maxillary nerve innervates the lateral portions of both lids by the zygomaticotemporal and the zygomaticofacial nerves. Diseases of any of these nerves results in anesthesia of the specific area of innervation and consequently abnormal palpebral reflexes if the lid is touched in this area. If the entire sensory innervation of the lids are damaged but the facial nerve is intact, the lids will close in response to a menacing gesture or a sudden loud noise but not in response to tactile stimuli.

The size of the palpebral fissure is controlled by several muscles. The orbicularis oculi muscle is innervated by the palpebral branch of the facial nerve. Contraction of this muscle closes the palpebral fissure. The levator palpebrae superioris muscle is innervated by the oculomotor nerve. It elevates the superior lid and enlarges the palpebral fissure. Muller's muscle is innervated by postganglionic sympathetic fibers, which enter the orbit together with the ophthalmic nerve. It also elevates the superior eyelid dependent on the state of arousal.

Lacrimation

The lacrimal glands are innervated by parasympathetic fibers in the greater petrosal nerve, a branch of the facial nerve. The preganglionic fibers synapse in the pterygopalatine ganglion. The postganglionic fibers for the main lacrimal gland run via the zygomatic nerve to the lacrimal nerve and with the latter to the gland. The gland of the third eyelid receives its parasympathetic fibers with the infratrochlear nerve.

Postganglionic sympathetic fibers arise from the cranial cervical ganglion and run within the deep petrosal nerve, pass through the pterygopalatine ganglion without synapses, and run with the parasympathetic fibers to the gland.

Within the glands, both parasympathetic and sympathetic fibers are evenly distributed, but there are more cholinergic fibers than adrenergic fibers.

Basal and reflex lacrimation depends on the normal sensory innervation of the cornea and intact parasympathetic innervation of the glands. Mechanical and olfactory stimulation of the nasal mucous membranes also cause an increase in lacrimation, as do paranasal sinus diseases.

Corneal sensitivity

All structures of the eyeball including the cornea receive sensory innervation from the long ciliary nerves, which arise from the ophthalmic branch of the trigeminal nerve.[14] There are approximately 12 corneal stromal nerves entering the cornea at the limbus. A deep layer of corneal nerves penetrates the limbus at approximately midstromal level and extends to the center of the cornea. These nerves branch extensively to form a subepithelial plexus. From this plexus, bundles of nerve fibers extend into the epithelium itself with nerve endings in the wing cell layer. A second layer penetrates the limbus at a subepithelial level. These nerves innervate only a 2- to 4-mm rim of peripheral cornea. Corneal sensitivity in dogs is lower than in other species. It is greatest in the center of the cornea. Brachycephalic dogs and cats have been shown to have lower corneal sensitivity compared to dolichocephalic dogs.[15]

NEURO-OPHTHALMOLOGIC EXAMINATION

Neuro-ophthalmic history

Changes of behavior, seizures, loss of vision, and so on?[16] Other clinical signs relating to systemic disease? Trauma to head/neck?

Examination of pupil size and the pupillary light reflex

Pupil size

At the beginning of the examination, the size of both pupils is evaluated. This is best done with the aid of a direct ophthalmoscope with the diopters set at 0 or +1D. Viewed through the instrument at arm's length, the tapetal reflexes nicely outline the pupils and allow for a rather accurate assessment of their respective size. In the normal animal, both pupils should be of equal size.[10]

Swinging flash light test

This test assesses the integrity of the entire pupillary light reflex. A focal light source is alternately directed into one or the other pupil. This causes constriction of both pupils in the normal animal. The stimulated pupil should be more miotic than the contralateral pupil because most PLR fibers cross to the contralateral side in the chiasm but re-cross to the ipsilateral side at the level of the posterior commissure. This causes a normal dynamic contraction anisocoria. The swinging flashlight test is easier to perform in animals with a large binocular visual field, for example, dogs and cats, than in animals with strongly divergent visual axes, for example, cattle and horse. A slight redilation of the stimulated pupil can sometimes be observed after initial constriction. This is due to light adaptation of the retina and is called pupillary escape. It should not be confused with dilation of the pupil when the light source is moved from the normal to the abnormal eye. A positive swinging flashlight test is present when both pupils constrict when the light is swung from the abnormal to the normal eye and, conversely, when both pupils dilate when the light is moved from the normal to the abnormal eye (this is also referred to as a Marcus Gunn sign). A positive swinging flashlight test is pathognomonic for retinal or prechiasmal optic nerve disease.[17]

Dark adaptation test

The animal is allowed to dark-adapt for 5 minutes, and pupil size is again evaluated with a direct ophthalmoscope. Because of lack of retinal stimulation, both pupils completely dilate in the normal animal and in animals with unilateral or bilateral lesions affecting the afferent arm of the PLR. The dark adaptation test is used to distinguish afferent arm lesions from other forms of pupillary abnormalities, for example, Horner's syndrome.

Chromatic pupillary light reflexes

The PLR is driven by photo pigments (opsins) localized in the outer segments of photoreceptors but also by melanopsin, a photo pigment localized in retinal ganglion cells (RGC). While photoreceptors absorb preferentially wavelengths of 630 nm (red), melanopsin absorbs primarily light of 480 nm (blue). Intensive red and blue stimulation of the retina may aid in differentiating inner and outer retinal function. Outer retinal dysfunction results in poor red PLR with a normal blue PLR.[18,19]

Normal modifications of the PLR

In the conscious and alert animal, the sympathetic nervous system works on the dilator muscle of the pupil, while inhibition of parasympathetic fibers relaxes the sphincter muscle. This can be observed in the excited or startled animal. As the level of consciousness decreases, the inhibitory influence on the Edinger-Westphal nucleus also decreases with resulting miosis.

The time between stimulation of the retina and pupillary constriction is relatively long because of the multisynaptic pathway and the smooth muscles as effector organs. Different areas of the retina have different pupillomotor sensitivities; however, this fact cannot be used in most clinical cases.

Dazzle reflex

The dazzle reflex is a subcortical reflex elicited by a strong light. The exact anatomic pathway of this reflex has not been demonstrated in animals.[9] When strong light is shone into an eye, a slight blinking occurs in both eyes, with the reaction on the contralateral side tending to be weaker. The afferent arm is the optic nerve, while the efferent arm of this reflex requires an intact facial nerve. This reflex can be used to determine whether an animal has an intact retina and optic nerve when there are opacities in the eye (cataract, etc.) or when there is no menace response. Although investigations in decerebrated cats have shown that this reflex remains intact because it is a subcortical reflex, it can still be used to provide valuable information about a patient's potential ability to see.[20] An intact dazzle reflex indicates a functional retina, prechiasmal optic nerve, and a postchiasmal optic nerve to a level just proximal to the lateral geniculate nucleus.

Evaluation of motility and movement of the globe

Observation of eye movements and range of movement

If the animal's head is restrained, the movements of the globes as they view a moving object can be observed. This movement is called version.

Because of the conjugate action of the extraocular muscles, one eye must be covered to accurately evaluate the movement of the other eye. With an attractive object (food), the eye examined is led through the 2° positions of gaze, for example, elevation, depression, adduction, and abduction. This test evaluates the function of CN III and VI. In some animals (cats with a vertically elliptical pupil), the 3° positions of gaze can be evaluated (version); however, this is very difficult to perform in most clinical patients. The 3° positions of gaze involve the action of the two oblique muscles and evaluates also CN IV.

Vestibulo-ocular reflexes

Moving the head left and right causes a normal horizontal nystagmus with the fast phase opposite the direction of head movement. The same is true for head movements in the vertical direction. This nystagmus must be simultaneous and conjugate for both eyes. While the optokinetic nystagmus is a normal nystagmus induced to examine CN III, IV, VI, and VIII, there are several pathologic conditions causing nystagmus even if the head is held still.

Pendular nystagmus: This nystagmus is used to recognize congenitally blind animals, such as collies with severe CEA or an animal with congenital cataracts and other ocular malformations.

Vestibular nystagmus: In acute vestibular disease, nystagmus may be present. Vestibular nystagmus is more obvious when fixation is lost. When the lids are held closed, nystagmus can be palpated through the lids. Alternately, vestibular nystagmus can be observed with the naked eye or by visualizing the optic nerve with the aid of a direct ophthalmoscope. This nystagmus can be vertical, horizontal, rotatory, or a combination of these.[10,16]

Strabismus

Strabismus in vestibular disease is also called skew deviation. With the head held in certain positions, interference with the normal vestibular mechanism that maintains the eyeball in adjustment with the position of the head causes the eye on the affected side to deviate ventrolaterally. Unlike strabismus in CN III palsy, skew deviation is transient and occurs in certain head positions only.

Forced duction test

If a limitation of eye movement is noted in one direction, a forced duction test can differentiate between paralysis of the muscle involved and mechanical restriction of movement.[21] The anesthetized globe is grasped near the limbus with small fixation forceps, and the globe is moved in the direction of the limitation of movement (**Figure 4.8**). Alternately, forced duction can be attempted with a cotton applicator. If the globe can be moved in the direction of limited gaze, this proves a paralysis of the muscle involved. Forced duction is inhibited by mechanical obstructions. This is called a positive passive forced duction test.

In suspected mechanical restriction, the globe is fixated with forceps, and the animal is made to look in the direction of the defective muscle. If the muscle reacts normally, this is felt as a slight pull on the forceps. This is called a positive active forced duction test.

Disease of one or more of the motor nerves innervating the extraocular muscles causes paralysis of the muscles involved with the inability to move the globe in certain directions and a strabismus. True strabismus as encountered in man is rather uncommon in animals.

A bilateral ventrolateral strabismus (down and out) is often seen in animals with severe hydrocephalus. This strabismus is possibly due to the skull formation rather than a true neurologic dysfunction.

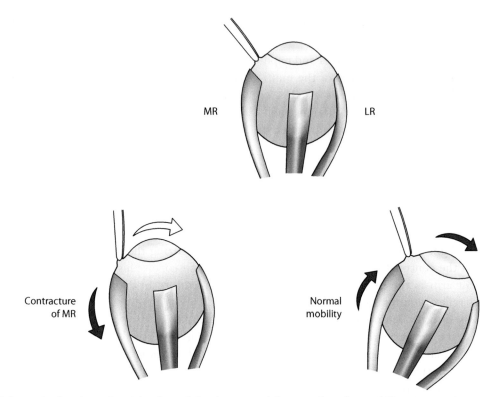

MR   LR

Contracture
of MR

Normal
mobility

Figure 4.8 Schematic drawing of positive forced duction test with normal ocular mobility (top) and contracture of the medial rectus muscle (bottom).

More commonly, strabismus is observed in animals with vestibular disease.

Examination of the blink reflex and lid movement

At rest, normal blinking occurs at a rate of three to five per minute and one to five per minute in the dog and the cat, respectively. It is more frequent in other species and in the dog and the cat during stress/restraint. The closure of the palpebral fissure is controlled by CN VII. The opening of the palpebral fissure is controlled by CN III (m. levator palpebrae) and CN VII (pars palpebralis of the m. colli profundus).

Any stimulation of CN V causes a blink reflex, for example, touching the cornea or the lids. Directing a very strong light source toward an eye causes a rapid blink called the dazzle reflex. This reflex is mediated by CN II and CN VII. It is subcortical and mediated by centers in the rostral colliculus and is, therefore, not a test for vision.

The blink reflex can be evaluated with the palpebral reflex, the corneal reflex, the menace response, and the dazzle reflex.

Facial nerve paralysis

The palpebral reflex is negative. To rule out a CN V deficit, the corneal reflex is performed. With an intact CN V, there is still no blink reflex, but an eyeball retraction may be observed. The menace response and the dazzle reflex are negative. There is a lack of tone of the lids. The palpebral fissure on the affected side is enlarged. Check tear production! The STT is decreased when damage lies proximal to the facial canal. Exposure keratitis (neuroparalytic keratitis) may occur.[22,23]

Hemifacial spasm

Uncommon in dogs. Irritation of CN VII may occur with otitis media. The palpebral fissure may be smaller than normal, mimicking facial paralysis on the normal side. If the underlying cause is not eliminated, this can lead to facial paralysis.[24]

Ptosis

Defined as drooping or a lack of normal elevation of the upper lid; one must distinguish between oculomotor ptosis and ptosis associated with Horner's syndrome. Paralysis of the levator palpebrae muscle is usually associated with internal ophthalmoplegia, while the extraocular muscles are spared.[25–28]

Evaluation of corneal sensitivity

Corneal sensitivity is tested with the corneal reflex. With a cotton-tipped applicator, the cornea is touched gently, and a blink or a retraction of the globe is observed. Semiquantitative assessment of corneal sensitivity can be achieved with a Cochet–Bonnet esthesiometer.[29,30]

Bilateral loss of corneal sensitivity has been observed in neurapraxia of the trigeminal motor neurons and concurrent dysfunction of the ophthalmic branch of CN V. This causes a dropped jaw with the animal's inability to grasp or retain food. Recovery is usually complete after a few weeks, although corneal sensitivity may be slow to return. Severe corneal fibrosis and pigmentation as seen in chronic pigmentary keratitis, chronic superficial keratitis, and keratoconjunctivitis sicca may also significantly reduce corneal sensitivity. Corneal sensitivity is also reduced in diabetes mellitus.[31,32] Neurotrophic keratitis is a rare degenerative corneal disease described in man, where a partial or total loss of trigeminal innervation causes corneal anesthesia.[33] Neurotrophic keratitis in dogs has been reported following orbital trauma and cavernous sinus syndrome.[34]

Evaluation of vision

Subtle alterations of visual function are difficult to assess and to substantiate. The owner is very often helpful in describing minute changes in the visual behavior of his animal. Many visual tests allow for a rather good assessment of the animal's vision.

Pupillary light reflex

The PLR itself is not a test for vision; for example, a normal PLR doesn't mean the animal can see. It is, however, helpful in localizing afferent arm lesions.[8] Animals with cataracts are blind but usually have a normal PLR. Even dogs with advanced retinal degeneration or progressive retinal atrophy (PRA) may still have a near-normal PLR. On the other hand, a negative PLR may be observed in a visual animal with iris atrophy, pharmacological pupillary dilation, or internal ophthalmoplegia.

Menace response

The menace response requires a normal CN II, visual cortex, and CN VII and is a crude method for evaluating an animal's vision. The menace response may be false negative, however, in a visual animal with facial paralysis or false positive when the menacing gesture causes an air drift, which in turn may cause a blind animal to blink.

Obstacle course

A very sensitive method of vision testing is to observe an animal in an obstacle course under photopic and scotopic conditions.[35] An obstacle course is set up, and the animal is allowed to negotiate the course in bright white light. Then the white light is turned off, ideally

leaving only a dim red light source. Animals with photoreceptor disease such as PRA may slow down in dim light or refuse to walk at all. There are several standardized obstacle courses in use that allow the exact measurement of transit or exit times under variable light conditions.[36]

Cotton ball tracking test

With one or the other eye occluded, a cotton ball is thrown from behind the animal through its monocular visual field. Visual and alert animals will follow the passing cotton ball.[16]

However, animals rapidly become indifferent to this ploy, so initial impressions are most accurate.

Visual placing reaction

With both eyes covered, the animal is held high and moved towards a table. If the animal's motor system is intact, it will try to place its feet on the table as soon as it touches the edge of the table. With the eyes uncovered, the visual animal sees the table and tries to place its feet on it. The test can be repeated with one or the other eye covered.

Visual field testing

Visual field testing is very important in human ophthalmology but has serious limitations in veterinary ophthalmology because of lack of patient cooperation. Visual field testing (perimetry) is a routine examination technique in human ophthalmology for the diagnosis of a multitude of diseases associated with loss of visual fields. Automated perimetry devices are usually used.[37]

Electroretinography

ERG can be diagnostic in inflammatory and degenerative retinal diseases. It can also differentiate between bulbar (retinal) and retrobulbar causes of blindness. The ERG itself is not a test for vision but for outer retinal function.[38–41] Since the flash-ERG is generated by outer retinal layers only, retinal ganglion cell loss/damage, for example, optic nerve atrophy or neuritis, is associated with a normal ERG recording.[42] The same phenomenon is seen in early glaucomatous retinal degeneration.

Visual evoked responses

With adequate instrumentation and signal averaging capabilities, visual evoked cortical responses can be recorded from the occipital lobes of the cerebrum in the anesthetized animal. The difficult methodology and the large standard deviations, especially in amplitudes, but also in implicit times, make this diagnostic technique less applicable in veterinary ophthalmology.[43–47]

Pathophysiology of the visual pathways

If abnormalities of the PLR or anisocoria are detected, any structural alteration of the iris and the sphincter muscle (e.g., iris sphincter coloboma or atrophy) must be ruled out.

Afferent arm lesions
Prechiasmal lesions

Lesions of the retina and/or optic nerve cause unilateral blindness, anisocoria with the dilated pupil ipsilateral to the lesion, and a positive swinging flashlight test. As in all afferent arm lesions, the anisocoria disappears after dark adaptation.

Retinal lesions can, of course, be diagnosed ophthalmoscopically or electroretinographically in most cases. Interestingly, even in advanced photoreceptor degeneration, the PLR persists for a long time even if the response is sluggish and incomplete.

In unilateral disease, the pupil on the affected side is mydriatic compared to the normal eye.

Note: Many retinal degenerations are bilateral and symmetrical!

Prechiasmatic optic nerve lesions

Because the prechiasmal optic nerve carries only fibers from one eye, these lesions have the same neurologic signs as retinal lesions, for example, abnormal pupil is larger, positive swinging flashlight test, and so on.

In the absence of obvious ophthalmoscopic signs, a positive swinging flashlight test is pathognomonic for such lesions (**Figure 4.9**).

Lesions of the chiasm

In small animals, neoplastic lesions arising adjacent to the chiasm need to be large to compress the chiasm. Vision loss is noted only late in the disease. Pupillary reflexes show subtle changes according to the exact site of compression. Central chiasmatic lesions affect the uncrossed fibers less than the decussated fibers. The resting pupils are moderately dilated. Light reflexes elicited by stimulation of the lateral retina are better than PLR elicited from the medial retina. This is called a hemianopic pupillary reaction. Affected patients have a heteronymous (binasal or bitemporal) hemianopia (**Figure 4.10**). This can occur normally because of the location of the area centralis laterallly.

Lesion of the optic tract

Postchiasmatic lesions also present with anisocoria, only this time the larger pupil is on the normal, nonaffected side because most of the fibers have decussated. The anisocoria may be less pronounced because of the mixed nature of the optic tracts. The swinging flashlight test is

negative. In dark adaptation, both pupils dilate maximally, again demonstrating that the lesion involves the afferent arm. On the ipsilateral side of the lesion, the pupil always remains relatively miotic compared to the contralateral pupil, whether this eye is stimulated or the other one. Theoretically, there is a homonymous hemianopia, although this may be difficult to substantiate in animals (**Figure 4.11**).

Lesion of the lateral geniculate body

Usually the PLR is normal. There is no anisocoria. Obvious visual disturbance is absent. A congenital lesion of the lateral geniculate body is seen in Siamese cats where their retinotopic cortical projection is aberrant. The laminae of the dorsal nuclei of the lateral geniculate body are disorganized. This leads to convergent strabismus and sometimes nystagmus in these animals.[48]

Lesions of the optic radiation and visual cortex

These are very difficult to localize. PLR and ocular motility are normal if no other areas are involved. There is a homonymous hemianopia or total blindness if bilateral. The dazzle reflex and light perception may persist. This may occur after prolonged anoxia in small animals. The most common causes for unilateral lesions of the visual cortex are neoplasms in small animals and abscesses in large animals. Parasitic cysts of coenurus are seen in sheep.

All the above listed lesions may be readily localized when they are unilateral. Bilateral lesions most often involve the retina (PRA) or the optic nerves (neuritis). Lesions of the chiasm are rare in animals. The occasional neoplasm of adjacent areas of the cerebrum probably causes other neurological signs. In the rare event where a central chiasmatic lesion destroys the decussated fibers leaving the uncrossed fibers intact, the swinging flashlight test should still be negative; however, this time the more miotic pupil is always contralateral to the stimulated eye.

Bilateral and symmetrical lesions of the optic tract have been described in canine distemper but appear to be exceedingly rare and usually accompanied by other neurological signs, as are lesions of the posterior commissure.

Efferent arm lesions

Efferent arm lesions result in so-called *internal ophthalmoplegia*. The lesion can involve the iris sphincter muscle, the ciliary ganglion, and the short ciliary nerves, but it can also be the result of parasympatholytic drug action, for example, atropine.

In general, unilateral lesions of the efferent arm of the PLR cause a (1) dilated pupil on the same side as the lesion, (2) possibly a "D" or "reversed D" pupil in the cat, (3) a pupil that does not react to direct and indirect

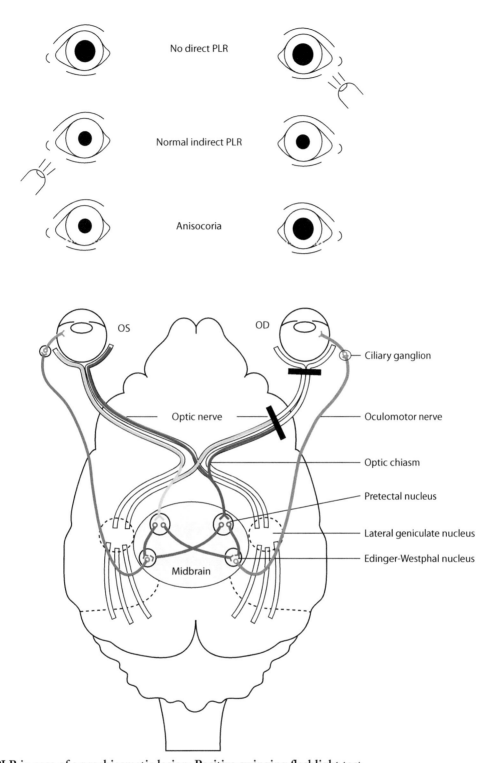

Figure 4.9 **PLR in case of a prechiasmatic lesion: Positive swinging flashlight test.**

stimulation. The dilated pupils will (4) be supersensitive to weak parasympathomimetic drugs, such as 0.2% pilocarpine if the iris sphincter muscle and its receptor sites are functional.

The direct PLR is always reduced or absent on the affected side, while the normal side shows normal direct PLR; this is in contrast to afferent arm lesions.

Because of the close proximity of the efferent parasympathetic fibers of the PLR with the motor fibers of CN III and the close proximity of the E-W-nucleus with the CN III motor nucleus, it is not unusual for central internal ophthalmoplegia to be accompanied by *external ophthalmoplegia*. Damage to the motor fibers of CN III causes (1) ptosis on the side of the lesion (paralysis of the levator

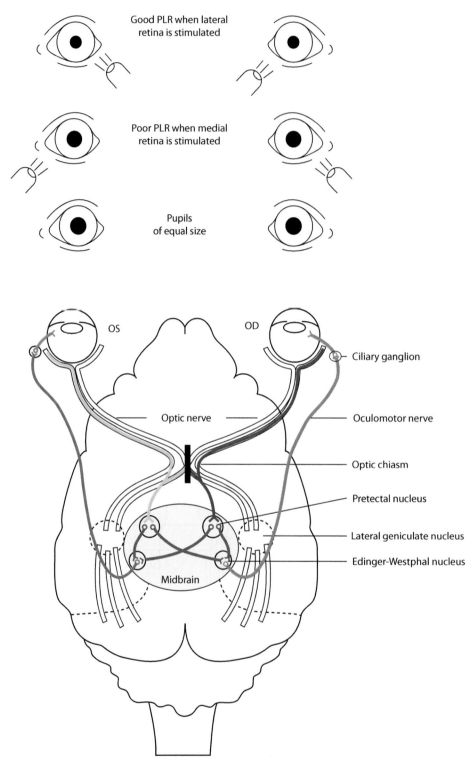

Figure 4.10 **PLR in case of a central chiasmatic lesion: Uncrossed axons from the lateral areas of the retina are spared.**

palpebrae muscle), and (2) exotropia (lateral strabismus) (**Figure 4.12**). The globe cannot be rotated dorsally, ventrally, or medially. A forced duction test demonstrates the absence of a mechanical obstruction. Because external ophthalmoplegia occurs more frequently with central lesions, it can give some localizing information.

Neuro-ophthalmologic conditions
Central blindness
Central blindness is a unilateral or bilateral blindness in the presence of a normal PLR and dazzle reflex. Unilateral lesions of the optic radiation and visual cortex cause a hemianopia, that is, a loss of the contralateral visual field.

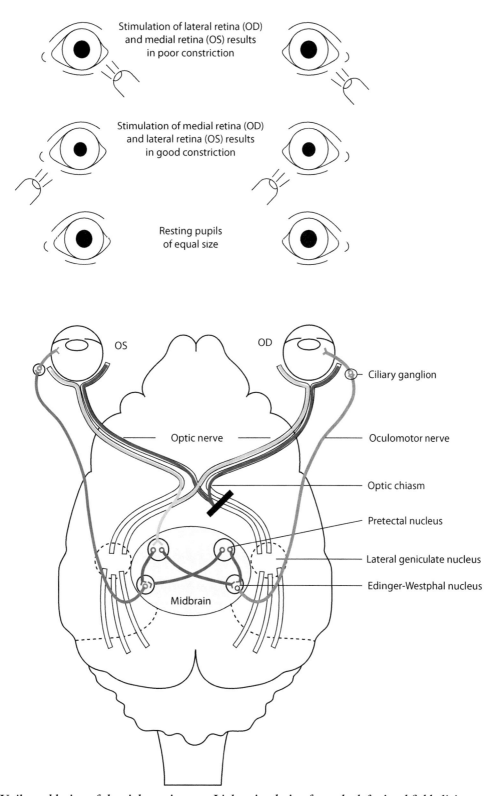

Stimulation of lateral retina (OD) and medial retina (OS) results in poor constriction

Stimulation of medial retina (OD) and lateral retina (OS) results in good constriction

Resting pupils of equal size

OS   OD

Ciliary ganglion

Optic nerve

Oculomotor nerve

Optic chiasm

Pretectal nucleus

Lateral geniculate nucleus

Edinger-Westphal nucleus

Midbrain

Figure 4.11 Unilateral lesion of the right optic tract: Light stimulation from the left visual field elicits a poor PLR.

The cause can be traumatic, inflammatory, vascular, or neoplastic.[49–52] The different storage diseases can also manifest as a central blindness. Hydrocephalus in dogs and cats can cause central blindness as well.[53] Complete blindness with a retained PLR is typical for a bilateral lesion of the visual cortex, as can occur after cerebral herniation or cranial trauma. One of the most common causes of central blindness in animals, however, is an adverse anesthetic event with prolonged hypoxia. Hypoxia for more than 3 minutes can lead to damage in the visual cortex.[54]

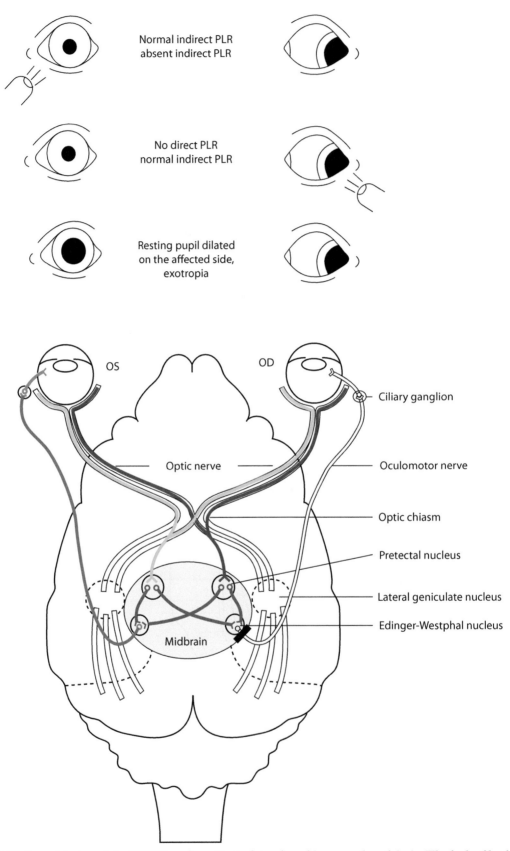

Figure 4.12 Unilateral lesion of the CN III nucleus: Ventrolateral strabismus and mydriasis. The lack of both direct and indirect PLR suggests an efferent arm lesion.

Internal ophthalmoplegia: Adie's tonic pupil

Idiopathic internal ophthalmoplegia or Adie's tonic pupil has been described as a rare event in dogs.

Etiology

The cause of internal ophthalmoplegia remains unknown in most cases.

Clinical signs

The affected pupil is unresponsive to light and is fixed in variable degrees of mydriasis. Dazzle reflex and menace response are normal; the eye is visual. There is a consensual PLR from the stimulated abnormal eye to the normal contralateral eye, but the inverse is not true.

Diagnosis

Affected pupils show denervation supersensitivity to weak parasympathomimetic drugs if the ciliary ganglion or the short ciliary nerves are involved. Instillation of 0.5% physostigmine solution, an indirect-acting parasympathomimetic, in equal quantities to both eyes causes miosis in the affected (dilated) eye about 1 hour before the normal eye if the lesion is preganglionic or central. Instillation of equal quantities of 0.2% pilocarpine solution, a direct-acting parasympathomimetic, causes rapid miosis in the affected (dilated) eye compared to the normal eye.[55,56] If both tests are negative, the internal ophthalmoplegia is not neurologic in origin. In most cases, the cause of mydriasis is due to pharmacologic mydriasis of the pupil, or the animal has come in contact with the plant species *Datura*, which contains the belladonna alkaloids scopolamine, hyoscyamine, and atropine. Iris hypoplasia/atrophy may also mimic internal ophthalmoplegia.

External ophthalmoplegia

External ophthalmoplegia is the complete lack of globe movements due to dysfunction of extraocular muscles, such as extraocular polymyositis, total lack of extraocular muscle nervous innervation by cranial nerves III, IV, and VI, or orbital space-occupying lesions (**Figure 4.13**).[57]

Horner's syndrome

Horner's syndrome is named after the Swiss ophthalmologist Claude Bernard Horner, who in 1869 was the first to describe this syndrome in man.

Etiology

Lesions of the efferent arm of the sympathetic pathway to the pupillary dilator muscles, Mueller's muscle of the upper lid, and adnexa/periocular facial structures. The specific lesion causing Horner's syndrome can be anywhere along

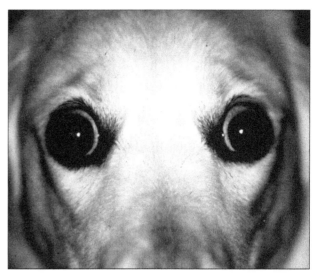

Figure 4.13 **External ophthalmoplegia in a dog with extraocular polymyositis.**

the efferent sympathetic pathway; however, postganglionic lesions are the most common. The causes of Horner's syndrome can be manifold: hypothyroidism, intracranial and intrathoracic tumors, otitis media and interna, and avulsion of the brachial plexus have been reported in dogs and cats. Injuries to the head, the neck, and the thorax in addition to aggressive irrigation of the external ear canal have also been documented to result in Horner's syndrome. No cause can be found in approximately 50% of dogs and 42% of cats with Horner's syndrome. Rare causes for Horner's syndrome are trauma due to bulla osteotomy, surgery of the cervical spine, intrathoracic tube drainage, and infections with *Neospora caninum*.[58–64] An idiopathic Horner's syndrome has been described in Golden retrievers.[65,66]

In horses, trauma to the neck region during jugular injections, guttural pouch infections, and laryngeal hemiplegia are possible causes for Horner's syndrome.

Clinical signs

The lack of sympathetic innervation of the dilator muscle causes miosis on the ipsilateral side as the lesion and anisocoria in dim light. In addition, paralysis of Muller's muscle causes ipsilateral ptosis and narrowing of the palpebral fissure. This gives the impression of an apparent enophthalmos (**Figure 4.14**).

Denervation of the smooth muscles in the periorbita causes true enophthalmos and secondary protrusion of the nictitating membrane (**Figure 4.15**).

In horses, Horner's syndrome is uncommon, and the most common clinical signs are ptosis and sweating on the ipsilateral head and neck, while miosis and enophthalmos are many times lacking.[67]

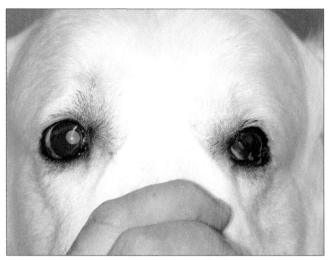

Figure 4.14 Horner's syndrome of the left eye in a Golden retriever. Note the prolapsed nictitans, the apparent enophthalmos, and the miotic pupil.

Diagnosis

The PLR is normal with the miotic pupil always remaining on the same side. The swinging flashlight test is negative. In dark adaptation, the miotic pupil fails to dilate, and the anisocoria is more marked. In very bright light, the anisocoria is not apparent.

Drug testing in localizing Horner's lesion—The best results are obtained with hydroxyamphetamine 1% drops. This is an indirect acting sympathomimetic that causes sympathetic nerve endings to release norepinephrine. One drop instilled into both eyes causes normal mydriasis in both eyes in central and preganglionic lesions, while there will be no or only minimal dilatation in postganglionic lesions. Unfortunately, this drug is no longer available.

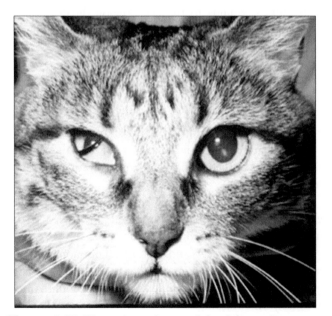

Figure 4.15 Horner's syndrome of the right eye in a cat.

In the presence of postganglionic lesions, denervation hypersensitivity of the dilator muscle causes rapid mydriasis within approximately 10 minutes after instillation of a weak (1%–2.5%) phenylephrine solution. Denervation hypersensitivity may take up to 2 weeks to become apparent. There is no pharmacologic test differentiating first- and second-order neuron lesions.

Therapy

If ptosis and protrusion of the nictitans cause a visual deficit, the clinical signs may be alleviated temporarily with 1% phenylephrine drops.

Prognosis

The prognosis depends on the underlying lesion. Treatment of otitis interna/media may result in relatively quick resolution of clinical signs. Spontaneous resolution of clinical signs can be expected in idiopathic Horner's syndrome within 3–6 months.

Feline and canine dysautonomia

This autonomic syndrome of unknown etiology was first described in cats in the United Kingdom in 1982.[68-78]

It occurs in cats of all ages, breed, and sex. The syndrome has been seen occasionally in continental Europe and the United States but appears to occur mainly in the United Kingdom. The disorder rarely occurs in dogs.[68,69,79]

Etiology

Disturbance of the autonomic nervous system of unknown cause.

Clinical signs

Ocular signs include mydriasis with occasional anisocoria, hyposecretion of lacrimal glands with secondary KCS, blepharospasm, and photophobia.

Diagnosis

The diagnosis is based on the ocular and systemic clinical signs and can only be definitively diagnosed by histology of autonomic ganglia.

Therapy

A specific therapy is not possible, and supportive therapy of affected animals is important. Systemic pilocarpine may enhance aqueous tear production and enhance gut motility to combat megaesophagus and megacolon/constipation.

Prognosis

The prognosis is guarded to poor.

Feline spastic pupil syndrome

Affected cats have anisocoria and abnormal PLR with the affected eye having either a miotic or a mydriatic pupil. Dark adaptation fails to dilate the miotic pupil (therefore not an afferent arm lesion), and light stimulation does not constrict a mydriatic pupil. Anisocoria and abnormal PLR may be unilateral or bilateral or may change sides. Some cats may test positive for either FeLV or FIP and may succumb within 6 months of presentation.[80]

Hemidilation of the feline pupil

In contrast to the dog, the cat has two distinct short ciliary nerves that emerge from the ciliary ganglia, (1) the malaris nerve (ciliaris lateralis) and (2) the nasalis nerve (ciliaris medialis). They innervate the lateral and medial half of the pupillary sphincter muscle, respectively. If lesions affect only one or the other of the two separate nerves, there is only partial dilation/constriction of the pupil resulting in a D-shaped or reverse D-shaped pupil (**Figure 4.16**). As with feline spastic pupil syndrome, some affected cats may test positive for FeLV. The hemidilated pupil must be differentiated from dyscoria due to posterior synechiae.[81]

Facial paralysis

Facial neuropathy is seen in dogs, cats, and horses.[22,23,67]

Etiology

Trauma, neoplasia, hypothyroidism, and otitis media and interna are the most common causes for facial paralysis. In 74% of dogs and 25% of cats, cases are considered idiopathic by ruling out any known cause for facial neuropathy. In horses, halter injuries and prolonged lateral recumbence may cause facial nerve paralysis.

Clinical signs

The clinical signs include a widened palpebral fissure due to lack of orbicularis oculi muscle tone, ipsilateral drooping of lips and nostrils, salivation, and occasionally a slight drooping of the ipsilateral ear (**Figures 4.17 and 4.18**). In small animals, there may be a concomitant reduction in tear production.

Diagnosis

The diagnosis is based on clinical signs. The above-mentioned diseases must be ruled in or out.

Therapy

Until the facial nerve function returns, the ocular surface must be protected from drying by frequent application of tear substitutes. To adequately protect the corneal surface, a temporary temporal tarsorrhaphy is many times necessary. If the facial nerve fails to recover, a permanent partial temporal tarsorrhaphy or even enucleation of an affected globe must be considered, if supportive therapy with tear substitutes is ineffective and secondary corneal ulceration occurs (neuroparalytic keratitis), especially if neurogenic keratoconjunctivitis sicca (KCS) accompanies the inability to blink.

Prognosis

Guarded to poor, depending on the etiology.

Ptosis

Ptosis or drooping of the upper eyelid is a common feature of older dogs of certain breeds, such as the Cocker Spaniel, bloodhound, Saint Bernard, and so on (**Figure 4.19**).

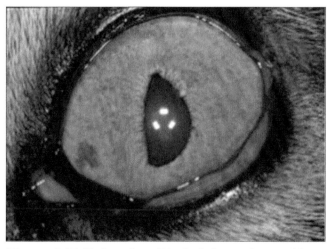

Figure 4.16 D-shaped pupil in the left eye of a cat with a lesion of the malaris nerve (ciliaris lateralis).

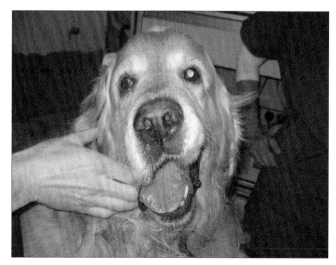

Figure 4.17 Right-sided facial paralysis in a Golden retriever. There is ptosis and drooping of the right lower eyelid.

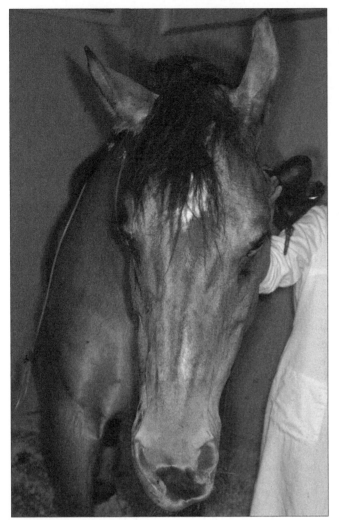

Figure 4.18 Right-sided facial paralysis in a horse.

In the context of neuro-ophthalmology, ptosis is a feature of Horner's syndrome, cavernous sinus syndrome, third nerve palsy, myasthenia, and facial paralysis (**Figure 4.20**).[25–28,82]

Neurogenic keratoconjunctivitis sicca (KCS)

Both basal and reflex tear production are under control of the autonomic nervous system.[8,10,83] The afferent sensory information from the lacrimal gland itself, the periocular structures, and the globe are sent centrally via the ophthalmic (lacrimal nerve, frontal nerve, nasociliary nerve) and maxillary division (zygomatic nerve) of the trigeminal nerve. The efferent arm of lacrimation is under control of the parasympathetic nervous system; the parasympathetic fibers originate from the parasympathetic nucleus of the facial nerve lying in the rostral portion of the medulla oblongata. They run as part of the facial nerve through the facial canal of the petrous temporal bone to the genu, where the geniculate ganglion is located. The facial nerve

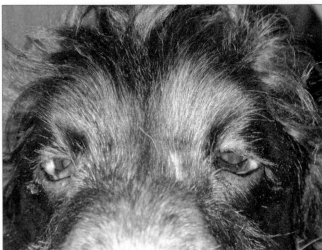

Figure 4.19 Ptosis in a 13-year-old English Cocker Spaniel.

then exits its canal through the stylomastoid foramen and emerges at the surface of the skull, whereas the preganglionic parasympathetic fibers leave the facial nerve as the greater petrosal nerve. It is joined by postganglionic sympathetic fibers from the deep petrosal nerve. It synapses in the pterygopalatine ganglion, and the postganglionic fibers are then distributed to the lacrimal gland via the zygomaticotemporal nerve, the most dorsal branch of the zygomatic nerve.

Etiology

Any lesion along the efferent pathway leads to a decreased tear production and results in neurogenic KCS.[81–84] Depending on the localization of the lesion, other neurological deficits such as Horner's syndrome, facial paralysis, or trigeminal nerve deficits may be present. Any acute-onset unilateral KCS with dry nasal mucous membranes should be considered neurogenic in origin.

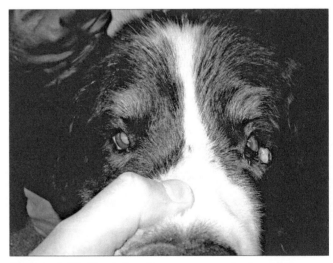

Figure 4.20 Ptosis in a Bernese mountain dog with Horner's syndrome of the left eye.

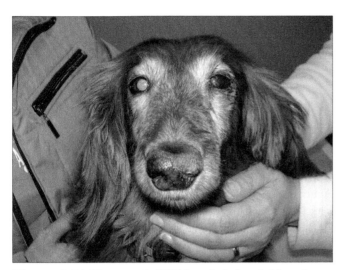

Figure 4.21 **Neurogenic KCS in a dachshund. Note the typical signs of KCS in the left eye and the dry nostril on the same side.**

Clinical signs

Clinical signs of KCS in combination with a dry ipsilateral nose (**Figure 4.21**).

The lack of aqueous tear production is usually quite dramatic (STT = 0 mm/min) with neurogenic KCS.

Diagnosis

The diagnosis of a neurogenic KCS is based on the clinical signs of a unilateral xerophthalmia with ipsilateral dry nose in the absence of signs of systemic disease, drug-induced causes, history of local irradiation, or third eyelid gland removal.

Therapy

Tear stimulation with oral administration of 1% (dogs <10-kg body weight) or 2% (dogs >10-kg body weight) pilocarpine eye drops. Initially, one drop is administered twice daily in food for 2–3 days. If STT values remain low, and if no excessive salivation or vomition occurs, the dosage is increased by one drop every 2–3 days until improved tearing or excessive salivation, vomition, or diarrhea is observed. This is the required maintenance dose. If salivation, vomiting, or diarrhea is excessive, the greatest tolerated dosage is used. Alternatively, topical application of 1/8% to 1/4% ophthalmic pilocarpine diluted with saline-based artificial tears may be tried if oral pilocarpine does not increase tearing when used at the maximum tolerated dose (see Chapter 9). Initially, symptomatic tear substitutes are added to the treatment.

Prognosis

Many dogs respond well to oral pilocarpine (or topical pilocarpine) treatment within 2–4 weeks. With oral pilocarpine treatment, the tear production increases, and the

dry nostril disappears. Topical pilocarpine may improve tearing without resolution of the ipsilateral dry nares. In some cases, where efferent parasympathetic innervation returns, pilocarpine therapy may be reduced and eventually discontinued without a drop in tear production.

Strabismus

Strabismus describes abnormal position and alignment of the globes. Under physiological conditions, both globes are suspended and moved by the extraocular muscles. If one of these muscles is longer or stronger than its counterpart, the globe deviates away from the longer muscle or towards the stronger muscle. Convergent strabismus is called esotropia, while a divergent strabismus is called exotropia. Esotropia is a frequent congenital condition in Siamese cats (**Figure 4.22**).[48,85,86]

Strabismus may be the result of defective innervation of extraocular muscles or be associated with vestibular disease.

Depending on the cranial nerve and extraocular muscles involved, there may be esotropia (lateral rectus muscles, CN VI), exotropia (medial rectus muscles, CN III), hypotropia (dorsal rectus muscle, CN III), hypertropia (ventral rectus muscle, CN III), or cyclotropia (dorsal oblique muscle, CN IV, or ventral oblique, CN III).

Strabismus in vestibular disease is also called skew deviation. With the head held in certain positions, interference with the normal vestibular mechanism that maintains the eyeball in adjustment with the position of the head causes the eye on the affected side to deviate ventrolaterally.

Third nerve palsy causes also a ventrolateral strabismus, which is independent of head position unlike skew deviation, which is transient and occurs in certain head positions only.

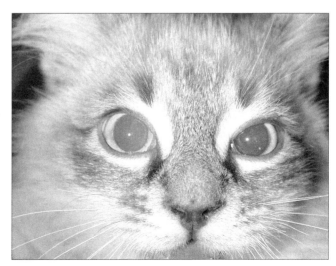

Figure 4.22 **Breed-specific esotropia (convergent strabismus) in a Siamese cat.**

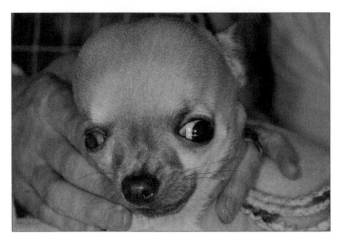

Figure 4.23 Marked hydrocephalus in a Chihuahua pup. There is bilateral ventrolateral strabismus.

Bilateral ventrolateral strabismus is present in dogs and cats with marked hydrocephalus (**Figure 4.23**). This form of strabismus is probably due to the abnormal skull formation rather than a true neurological deficit.

Nictitating membrane protrusion (Haws syndrome)

A poorly understood syndrome of idiopathic bilateral protrusion of the third eyelids in cats has been described.[87] The condition is occasionally associated with diarrhea. The protruded nictitans retracts following instillation of phenylephrine eye drops, suggesting sympathetic denervation, as in Horner's syndrome.[9]

The condition is self-limiting, and spontaneous resolution usually occurs, although this may take several weeks.

Non-neurologic diseases associated with altered PLR or vision

For detailed descriptions, refer to the respective chapters in this book.

Retinal degeneration

Retinal degenerations occur frequently in dogs and cats but are less common in horses.[88–90] They can be a sequel to inflammatory or traumatic diseases of the retina and choroid (chorioretinitis) or may be hereditary degenerations. While postinflammatory retinal degeneration may be unilateral or at least asymmetrical, hereditary retinal degenerations are usually bilateral and symmetrical. If the degeneration is bilateral, the swinging flashlight test is not helpful in localizing the disease; however, the ophthalmoscopic signs are usually obvious and diagnostic.

Acute retinal necrosis (sudden acquired retinal degeneration syndrome: SARDS)

Although seen in any age, sex, or size of dog, SARDS occurs primarily in middle-aged spayed female dogs of small breeds, such as Dachshunds. The etiology of this acute-onset retinal degeneration and blindness is still not fully understood. The diagnosis is confirmed by electroretinography. The chromatic PLR shows a near-normal PLR with blue light stimulation and an absent PLR with red light stimulation. There is no generally accepted therapy, and the prognosis for return of vision is poor.[91–94]

Enrofloxacin-induced retinal degeneration in cats

Acute and irreversible blindness has been reported in cats treated with enrofloxacin at dosages $\geq$5 mg/kg/day. Both the oral and the injectable form of enrofloxacin led to blindness in some feline patients. The reaction appears to be dose-related, and most cases have received dosages of 10–20 mg/kg/day. The pathogenesis of the condition is unknown, but a direct toxic effect on the retinal neurons is suspected.[95]

DISEASES OF THE OPTIC NERVE

Aplasia/hypoplasia of the optic nerve

While aplasia of the optic nerve is extremely rare, hypoplasia has been reported as an inherited problem in several canine breeds, most notably in the miniature and toy poodle.[96–100] It appears to be rare in cats and horses.[79,90]

Clinical signs

Affected eyes are blind from birth. If the condition is bilateral, affected animals have dilated and unresponsive pupils and a pendular nystagmus. Unilateral disease will show slight anisocoria (afflicted eye slightly larger pupil in room light) with a total afferent PLR deficit (Marcus Gunn sign). The optic discs are obviously small and not myelinated (**Figure 4.24**). Only the mesodermal parts

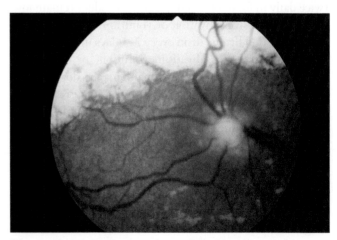

Figure 4.24 Optic nerve hypoplasia in a 12-week-old miniature poodle. Both eyes were affected, and the animal was blind. ERGs were normal.

of the optic nerve (vessels, meninges) are present, but the axons of the RGC are missing. A differential diagnosis is micropapilla in which the optic disc is notably small; however, affected animals are visual.

Diagnosis

The ophthalmoscopic signs are usually diagnostic. Histologically, the retinal ganglion cell layer is lacking completely, while the outer retinal layers are normal. A flash ERG is therefore normal.

Therapy

There is no therapy. Affected animals should not be bred.

Prognosis

Afflicted eyes are irreversibly blind.

Optic nerve coloboma

Coloboma is an apparent defect of ocular tissue due to failure of a part of the fetal fissure to close. It can affect the eyelid, iris, lens, optic nerve, retina, choroid, and/or sclera. Colobomas of the optic disc are a part of collie eye anomaly (see section CEA, Chapter 14).[84–88] Optic nerve colobomas have been reported as an inherited defect in several breeds of cattle (**Figure 4.25**).[101–108]

It is more common than aplasia or hypoplasia of the optic nerve. In collies, the optic nerve coloboma is usually limited to the immediate ocular disc area, and the remainder of the retrobulbar optic nerve is normal in the orbit.

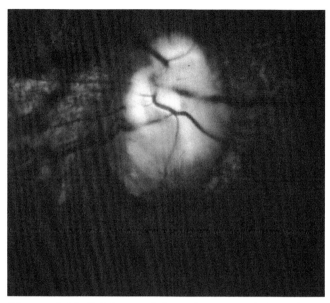

Figure 4.26 Coloboma of the optic nerve and choroidal hypoplasia in a collie pup.

Clinical signs

Depend on the extent of the coloboma. Total optic nerve colobomas may cause a total afferent vision/PLR deficit, but it is usually an incidental finding not associated with noticeable visual disturbance. Ophthalmoscopic signs range from a small "pit" in the optic disc to a large excavation of the disc, with the disc appearing larger in diameter than normal with a depression several millimeters deep (**Figure 4.26**).

Therapy

There is no treatment for this developmental defect.

Prognosis

The prognosis for worsening of vision beyond what is initially noted is usually good. Most optic disc colobomas are static. Peripapillary retinal detachments and hemorrhages may occur with large optic disc colobomas and CEA.

(Retrobulbar) Optic neuritis (see also Chapter 14)

Optic neuritis is rather common in dogs but appears to be uncommon in cats.[89,109–115]

Etiology

Optic neuritis can be traumatic, infectious, neoplastic, toxic, metabolic, and immune-mediated. Traumatic optic neuritis and resultant optic atrophy are often seen associated with proptosis of the globe in dogs and cats and due to trauma to the occipital region in horses. Abrupt displacement of the globe leads to massive traction on the optic nerve with subsequent degeneration. In many cases,

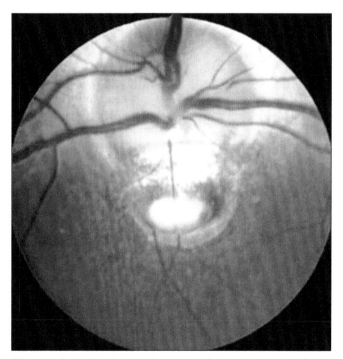

Figure 4.25 Typical optic nerve coloboma in a Charolais bull.

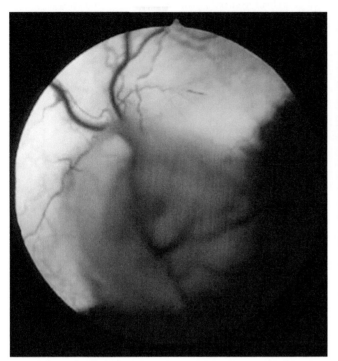

Figure 4.27 Papilledema and peripapillary retinal edema in a dog with optic neuritis.

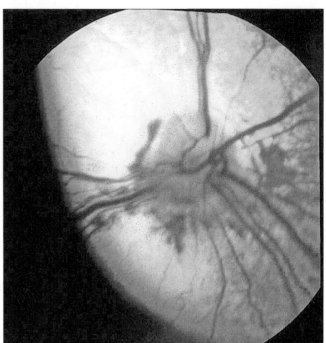

Figure 4.28 Peripapillary hemorrhages in a dog with optic neuritis.

the etiology remains unknown. Granulomatous meningoencephalitis (GME) has been reported as a frequent cause for optic neuritis in dogs. Optic neuritis may also accompany severe, diffuse retinitis, choroiditis, panophthalmitis, and toxicities such as alcohol, arsenic, thallium, trauma, or infectious diseases, especially canine distemper. In MDR1-positive dogs, avermectin may cause optic neuritis.

Clinical signs
Sudden onset of blindness (if bilateral) with fixed, dilated pupils. If unilateral, can have afferent deficit and unilateral blindness. The optic disc may be swollen with hemorrhage on or adjacent to the disc. In retrobulbar optic neuritis, the discs are usually normal in appearance.

Diagnosis
If there is papilledema and hemorrhage, the diagnosis is based on history and clinical signs (**Figures 4.27 and 4.28**).

If the optic discs are normal, and there is vision impairment/blindness with PLR deficit, central nervous system disease or sudden acquired retinal degeneration syndrome (SARDS) must be ruled out. The electroretinogram is very helpful in these cases. If there is a total PLR deficit (afferent PLR defect), and the electroretinogram is normal, this rules out primary retinal disease (SARDS) and supports the diagnosis of optic neuritis.

Therapy
Treatment is in most cases symptomatic and must be initiated as soon as possible to avoid irreversible damage/blindness. High anti-inflammatory concentrations of prednisolone (1–2 mg/kg body weight s.i.d,) are administered and should be continued for several days. Return of vision is often seen within 1–3 days. If there is no resolution within one week, it must be considered permanent.

Prognosis
The short-term prognosis is fair if diagnosed and treated early. If axons have already been damaged, the prognosis is poor. The long-term prognosis is guarded because recurrences are frequent in idiopathic cases, and subsequent optic degeneration is possible.

Optic nerve degeneration/atrophy

Optic nerve degeneration is usually a result of retinal degeneration, optic neuritis, compression from neoplasm, or glaucoma.[88,89,116] In horses, traumatic optic neuritis and subsequent degeneration is relatively common.

Clinical signs
The optic disc appears pale with loss of myelination and vasculature. In glaucomatous optic nerve degeneration, the disc is cupped or excavated and may look sunken in appearance (**Figure 4.29**). Affected eyes are blind with a lack of direct pupillary light response (**Figure 4.30**).

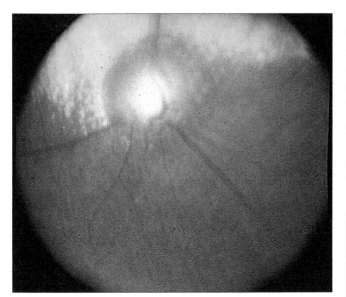

Figure 4.29 Glaucomatous optic nerve atrophy (cupping): The optic disc is demyelinated. The dark halo surrounding the optic disc marks the extent of the previous myelin.

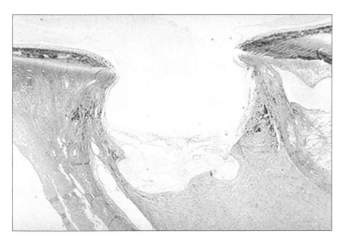

Figure 4.30 Histology of glaucomatous optic nerve cupping. There is severe atrophy of the optic nerve with deformation of the lamina cribrosa.

Diagnosis

The diagnosis is based on history, clinical signs, and ophthalmoscopic appearance. It must be differentiated from optic nerve hypoplasia.

Therapy

There is no treatment possible.

Prognosis

The prognosis for vision is poor.

Neoplasia of the optic nerve

Primary neoplasms of the optic nerve are uncommon. Ganglioglioma, astrocytoma, meningioma, and medulloepithelioma have been described.[117–122]

Clinical signs

Tumors of the optic nerve may present as space-occupying orbital lesions with resultant exophthalmos, possibly external ophthalmoplegia, and strabismus. The affected eye is usually blind. The pupil is unresponsive, but due to contralateral input, there is only minimal mydriasis. Extensive neoplasia with involvement of the chiasm causes bilateral blindness. Occasionally such tumors invade the globe and can be visualized ophthalmoscopically (**Figures 4.31 and 4.32**).

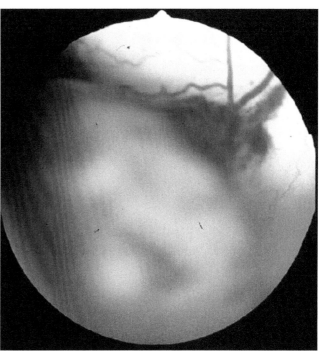

Figure 4.31 Intraocular (vitreous) extension of a myxosarcoma of the optic nerve in a dog.

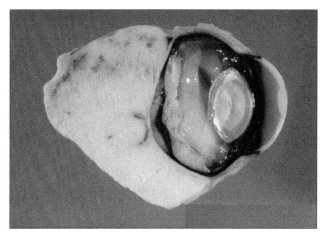

Figure 4.32 Gross pathology of a glioma of the optic nerve with intraocular extension in a dog. The globe has been fixed in Bouin's solution.

Diagnosis

The diagnosis is based on clinical and ophthalmoscopic signs of a retrobulbar mass lesion. Diagnostic imaging techniques (orbital ultrasonography and computerized tomography) determine size, location, and extension of the lesion and allows tissue sampling and planning of possible therapies.

Therapy

In selected cases, such tumors may be removed by orbitotomy with retention of the (blind) globe.[123] In most cases, however, exenteration of the orbit is the only option, provided the animal shows no clinical signs of metastatic disease. Some of these tumors may arise from within the cranial cavity and involve the orbital portion of the optic nerve so that exenteration is of no benefit. Palliative radiation therapy may be an option in selected cases.

Prognosis

The prognosis is often guarded. Many tumors are usually diagnosed at a relatively late stage of the disease.

CLINICAL CASE

A 2-year-old mixed breed dog was presented for what the owner described as "an odd appearance of the left eye." The condition appeared suddenly 10 days ago.

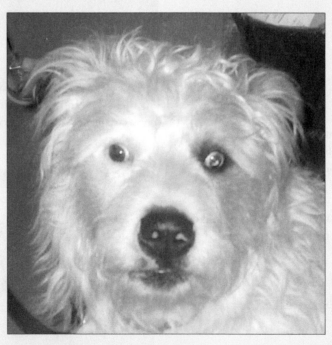

Q1: Describe the two most obvious alterations of the left eye.
Q2: Which cranial nerve is most likely involved?

Answers:
1. Ventrolateral strabismus, mydriasis
2. Oculomotor nerve (III)

REFERENCES

1. Samuelson, D. 1991. Ophthalmic embryology and anatomy. In: Gelatt, K., editor. *Veterinary Ophthalmology*. Lea & Febiger: Philadelphia, PA, pp. 1–123.

2. Gum, G., and MacKay, E.O. 2013. Physiology of the eye. In: Gelatt, K., Gilger, B.C., and Kern, T.J., editors. *Veterinary Ophthalmology*. Wiley-Blackwell: Ames, IA, pp. 171–207.

3. Ofri, R. 2007. Optics and physiology of vision. In: Gelatt, K., editor. *Veterinary Ophthalmology*. Blackwell Publishing: Ames, IA, pp. 183–219.

4. Pearlman, A. 1981. Anatomy and physiology of central visual pathways. In: Moses, E., editor. *Adler's Physiology of the Eye*. CV Mosby Co.: St. Louis, MO, pp. 427–65.

5. Sharma, R.K., and Ehinger, B.E.J. 2003. Development and structure of the retina. In: Kaumtman, P.L., Alm, A., editors. *Adler's Physiology of the Eye; Clinical Application*. Mosby: St. Louis, MO, pp. 319–47.

6. Samuelson, D.A. 2013. Ophthalmic anatomy. In: Gelatt, K.N., Gilger, B.C., and Kern, T.J., editors. *Veterinary Ophthalmology*. Wiley-Blackwell: Ames, IA, pp. 39–170.

7. Herron, M., Martin, J.E., and Joyce, J.R. 1978. Quantitative study of the decussating optic axons in the pony, cow, sheep and pig. *American Journal of Veterinary Research* 37:1137–9.

8. DeLahunta, A. 1977. *Veterinary Neuroanatomy and Clinical Neurology*. WB Saunders: Philadelphia, PA.

9. Webb, A.A., and Cullen, S.L. 2013. Neuro-ophthalmology. In: Gelatt, K.N., Gilger, B.C., and Kern, T.J., editors. *Veterinary Ophthalmology*. Wiley-Blackwell: Ames, IA, pp. 1820–96.

10. Scagliotti, R. 1998. Comparative neuro-ophthalmology. In: Gelatt, K., editor. *Veterinary Ophthalmology*. Lippincott Williams & Wilkins: Philadelphia, PA, p 825–32.

11. Samuelson, D.A. 2007. Ophthalmic anatomy. In: Gelatt, K., editor. *Veterinary Ophthalmology*. Blackwell: Ames, IA, pp. 37–148.

12. Burde, R. 1981. The extraocular muscles. In: Moses, R., editor. *Adler's Physiology of the Eye*. The CV Mosby Company: St. Louis, MO, pp. 84–183.

13. Abrams, R.M. et al. 1998. Vestibular caloric responses and behavioral state in the fetal sheep. *International Journal of Pediatric Otorhinolaryngology* 45(1):59–68.

14. Barrett, P., Scagliotti, R.H., Merideth, R.E., Jackson, P.M., and Lazano Alacron, F. 1991. Absolute corneal sensitivity and corneal trigeminal nerve anatomy in normal dogs. *Veterinary and Comparative Ophthalmology* 1(4):245–54.

15. Blocker, T., and Van Der Woerdt, A. 2001. A comparison of corneal sensitivity between brachycephalic and domestic short-haired cats. *Veterinary Ophthalmology* 4(2):127–30.

16. Spiess, B.M. 2010. Ophthalmological examination. In: Jaggy, A., editor. *Small Animal Neurology*. Schlütersche: Hannover, Germany, pp. 34–37.

17. Enyedi, L.B., Dev, S., and Cox, T.A. 1998. A comparison of the Marcus Gunn and alternating light tests for afferent pupillary defects. *Ophthalmology* 105(5):871–3.

18. Grozdanic, S.D., Kecova, H., and Lazic, T. 2013. Rapid diagnosis of retina and optic nerve abnormalities in canine patients with and without cataracts using chromatic pupil light reflex testing. *Veterinary Ophthalmology* 16(5):329–40.

19. Grozdanic, S.D. et al. 2007. Evaluation of retinal status using chromatic pupil light reflex activity in healthy and diseased canine eyes. *Investigative Ophthalmology & Visual Science* 48(11):5178–83.

20. Gelatt, K.N. 1997. Visual disturbance: Where do I look? *Journal of Small Animal Practice* 38(8):328–35.

21. Rosenberg, S.E., and Shippman, S. 2011. Situational restriction: Using your physical exam to differentiate pulley abnormalities from other vertical deviations secondary to restrictive conditions. *American Orthoptic Journal* 61:13–8.

22. Braund, K.G. et al. 1979. Idiopathic facial paralysis in the dog. *Veterinary Record* 105(13):297–9.

23. Tietje, S., Wisniewski, S., and Feilke, M. 1995. Bilateral facial nerve paralysis in a horse [German]. *Praktische Tierarzt* 76(6):528–9 ff.

24. Roberts, S.R., and Vainisi, S.J. 1967. Hemifacial spasm in dogs. *Journal of the American Veterinary Medical Association* 150(4):381–5.

25. Cho, J. 2008. Surgery of the globe and orbit. *Topics in Companion Animal Medicine* 23(1):23–37.

26. Jones, B.R., and Studdert, V. 1975. Hornerss syndrome in the dog and cat as an aid to diagnosis. *Australian Veterinary Journal* 51(7):329–32.

27. van der Woerdt, A. 2004. Adnexal surgery in dogs and cats. *Veterinary Ophthalmology* 7(5):284–90.

28. Willis, A.M. et al. 1999. Brow suspension for treatment of ptosis and entropion in dogs with redundant facial skin folds. *Journal of the American Veterinary Medical Association* 214(5):660–2.

29. Kaps, S., Richter, M., and Spiess, B.M. 2003. Corneal esthesiometry in the healthy horse. *Veterinary Ophthalmology* 6(2):151–5.

30. Wieser, B., Tichy, A., and Nell, B. 2013. Correlation between corneal sensitivity and quantity of reflex tearing in cows, horses, goats, sheep, dogs, cats, rabbits, and guinea pigs. *Veterinary Ophthalmology* 16(4):251–62.

31. Good, K.L. et al. 2003. Corneal sensitivity in dogs with diabetes mellitus. *American Journal of Veterinary Research* 64(1):7–11.

32. Ledbetter, E.C., Marfurt, C.F., and Dubielzig, R.R. 2013. Metaherpetic corneal disease in a dog associated with partial limbal stem cell deficiency and neurotrophic keratitis. *Veterinary Ophthalmology* 16(4):282–8.

33. Semeraro, F. et al. 2014. Neurotrophic keratitis. *Ophthalmologica* 231(4):191–7.

34. Ledbetter, E.C., and Gilger, B.C. 2013. Diseases and surgery of the canine cornea and sclera. In: Gelatt, K.N., Gilger, B.C., and Kern, T.J., editors. *Veterinary Ophthalmology*. Wiley-Blackwell: Ames, IA, pp. 976–1049.

35. Garcia, M.M. et al. 2010. Evaluation of a behavioral method for objective vision testing and identification of achromatopsia in dogs. *American Journal of Veterinary Research* 71(1):97–102.

36. Annear, M.J. et al. 2013. Reproducibility of an objective four-choice canine vision testing technique that assesses vision at differing light intensities. *Veterinary Ophthalmology* 16(5):324–8.

37. Kedar, S., Ghate, D., and Corbett, J.J. 2011. Visual fields in neuro-ophthalmology. *Indian Journal of Ophthalmology* 59(2):103–9.

38. Leber-Zurcher, A.C. et al. 1991. [Clinical electroretinography in the dog. Part 2]. *Schweiz Arch Tierheilkd* 133(7):301–9.

39. Spiess, B.M., and Leber-Zurcher, A.C. 1991. [Clinical electroretinography in the dog. Part 1]. *Schweiz Arch Tierheilkd* 133(5):217–23.

40. Spiess, B.M., and Leber-Zurcher, A.C. 1991. [Clinical electroretinography in the dog. Part 3]. *Schweiz Arch Tierheilkd* 134(2):61–74.

41. Spiess, B.M., and Leber-Zurcher, A.C. 1992. [Oscillating potentials on the B-wave of the ERG in the dog]. *Schweiz Arch Tierheilkd* 134(9):431–43.

42. Spiess, B., Litschi, B., Leber-Zürcher, A.C., and Stelzer, S. 1991. Bilaterale hypoplasie der nervi optici bei einem pudelwelpen. *Kleintierpraxis* 36:173–8.

43. Boyer, S., and Kirk, G.R. 1973. Maturation of the visual evoked response in the dog. *Experimental Neurology* 38:449–57.

44. Creel, D., Dustman, R.E., and Beck, E.C. 1973. Visual evoked responses in the rat, guinea pig, cat, monkey and man. *Experimental Neurology* 40:351–66.

45. Harding, G. 1974. The visual evoked response. *Advanced Ophthalmology* 28:2–28.

46. Malnati, G., Marshall, A.E., and Coulter, D.B. 1981. Electroretinographic components of the canine visual evoked response. *American Journal of Veterinary Research* 42:159–63.

47. Strain, G.M., Jackson, R.M., and Tedford, B.L. 1990. Visual evoked potentials in the clinically normal dog. *Journal of Veterinary Internal Medicine* 4(4):222–5.

48. von Grunau, M.W., and Rauschecker, J.P. 1983. Natural strabismus in non-Siamese cats: Lack of binocularity in the striate cortex. *Experimental Brain Research* 52(2):307–10.

49. Barrett, P.M., Merideth, R.E., and Alarcon, F.L. 1995. Central amaurosis induced by an intraocular, posttraumatic fibrosarcoma in a cat. *Journal of the American Animal Hospital Association* 31(3):242–5.

50. Hollingsworth, S.R. 2000. Canine prototothecosis. *Veterinary Clinics of North America—Small Animal Practice* 30(5):1091–101.

51. Mayhew, I.G. et al. 1985. Ceroid-lipofuscinosis (Batten's disease): Pathogenesis of blindness in the ovine model. *Neuropathology and Applied Neurobiology* 11(4):273–90.

52. Sreter, T. et al. 2002. Ocular onchocercosis in dogs: A review. *Veterinary Record* 151(6):176–80.

53. Estey, C.M. 2016. Congenital hydrocephalus. *The Veterinary Clinics of North America. Small Animal Practice.* 46(2):217–29.

54. Jurk, I.R. et al. 2001. Acute vision loss after general anesthesia in a cat. *Veterinary Ophthalmology* 4(2):155–8.

55. Spiess, B. 1988. What is your diagnosis? Idiopathic internal ophthalmoplegia (Adie's syndrome) in a dog. *The Canadian Veterinary Journal* 29:73–74.

56. Gerding, P.A., Brightman, A.H., and Brogdon, J.D. 1986. Pupillotonia in a dog. *Journal of the American Veterinary Medical Association* 189(11):1477.

57. Spiess, B.M., and Pot, S.A. 2013. Diseases and surgery of the canine orbit. In: Gelatt, K.N., Gilger, B.C., and Kern, T.J., editors, *Veterinary Ophthalmology.* Wiley-Blackwell: Ames, IA. 793–831.

58. Boydell, P. 1995. Horner's syndrome following cervical spinal surgery in the dog. *Journal of Small Animal Practice* 36(11):510–2.

59. Boydell, P., and Brogan, N. 2000. Horner's syndrome associated with Neospora infection. *Journal of Small Animal Practice* 41(12):571–2.

60. Boydell, P. et al. 1997. Horner's syndrome following intrathoracic tube placement. *Journal of Small Animal Practice* 38(10):466–7.

61. Guard, C.L., Rebhun, W.C., and Perdrizet, J.A. 1984. Cranial tumors in aged cattle causing Horner's syndrome and exophthalmos. *Cornell Veterinary* 74(4):361–5.

62. Kern, T.J., Aromando, M.C., and Erb, H.N. 1989. Horner's syndrome in dogs and cats:100 cases (1975–1985). *Journal of the American Veterinary Medical Association* 195(3):369–73.

63. Morgan, R.V., and Zanotti, S.W. 1989. Horner's syndrome in dogs and cats:49 cases (1980–1986). *Journal of the American Veterinary Medical Association* 194(8):1096–9.

64. Smith, J., and Mayhew, I.G. 1977. Horner's syndrome in large animals. *Cornell Veterinary* 67:529–42.

65. Boydell, P. 1995. Idiopathic Horner's syndrome in the golden retriever. *Journal of Small Animal Practice* 36(9):382–4.

66. Boydell, P. 2000. Idiopathic Horner's syndrome in the golden retriever. *Journal of Neuro-Ophthalmology* 20(4):288–90.

67. Mayhew, I.G. 2010. Neuro-ophthalmology: A review. *Equine Veterinary Journal.* Supplement(37):80–8.

68. Harkin, K.R., Andrews, G.A., and Nietfeld, J.C. 2002. Dysautonomia in dogs:65 cases (1993–2000). *Journal of the American Veterinary Medical Association* 220(5):633–9.

69. Schulze, C., Schanen, H., and Pohlenz, J. 1997. Canine dysautonomia resembling the Key-Gaskell syndrome in Germany. *Veterinary Record* 141:496–7.

70. Wright, J., Bond, A.L., and Humphreys, D.J. 1983. Key-Gaskell syndrome. *The Veterinary Record* 112(5):111.

71. Ruben, J.M. 1983. Key-Gaskell syndrome. *The Veterinary Record* 112(7):159.

72. Alexander, R.W. 1983. Key-Gaskell syndrome. *The Veterinary Record* 112(26):614.

73. Tutt, J.B. 1982. The Key-Gaskell syndrome. *The Veterinary Record* 111(15):353.

74. Nash, A.S., Griffiths, I.S., and Sharp, N.J. 1982. The Key-Gaskell syndrome—An autonomic polyganglionopathy. *The Veterinary Record* 111(13):307–8.

75. Nash, A.S., Griffiths, I.R., and Sharp, N.J. 1982. Key-Gaskell syndrome. *The Veterinary Record* 111(24):564.

76. Kock, R. 1982. The Key-Gaskell syndrome. *The Veterinary Record* 111(20):469.

77. Kidder, A.C. et al. 2008. Feline dysautonomia in the Midwestern United States: A retrospective study of nine cases. *Journal of Feline Medicine and Surgery* 10(2):130–6.

78. Novellas, R. et al. 2010. Imaging findings in 11 cats with feline dysautonomia. *Journal of Feline Medicine & Surgery* 12(8):584–91.

79. Caines, D. et al. 2011. Autonomic dysfunction in a Jack Russell terrier. *Canadian Veterinary Journal* 52(3):297–9.

80. Brightman, A.H., Ogilvie, G.K., and Tompkins, M.T. 1991. Ocular disease in FeLV-positive cats:11 cases 1981–1986. *Journal of the American Veterinary Medical Association* 198:1049–51.

81. Nell, B., and Suchy, A. 1998. "D-shaped" and "reverse-D-shaped" pupil in a cat with lymphosarcoma. *Veterinary Ophthalmology* 1(1):53–56.

82. Shelton, G.D., Schule, A., and Kass, P.H. 1997. Risk factors for acquired myasthenia gravis in dogs: 1,154 cases (1991–1995). *Journal of the American Veterinary Medical Association* 211(11):1428–31.

83. Matheis, F.L., Walser-Reinhardt, L., and Spiess, B.M. 2012. Canine neurogenic keratoconjunctivitis sicca:11 cases (2006–2010). *Veterinary Ophthalmology* 15(4):288–90.

84. Scagliotti, R.H. 1999. Comparative neuro-ophthalmology. In: Gelatt, K.N., editor. *Veterinary Ophthalmology.* Blackwell Publishing: Ames, IA, pp. 1342–5.

85. Rengstorff, R.H. 1976. Strabismus measurements in the Siamese cat. *American Journal of Optometry & Physiological Optics* 53(10):643–6.

86. Johnson, B.W. 1991. Congenital abnormal visual pathways of Siamese cats. *Compendium on Continuing Education for the Practicing Veterinarian* 13(3):374–8.

87. Gruffydd-Jones, T.J., Orr, C.M., and Flecknell, P.A. 1977. A new syndrome in cats. *The Veterinary Record* 101(20):413–4.

88. Nell, B., and Walde, I. 2010. Posterior segment diseases. *Equine Veterinary Journal.* Supplement(37):69–79.

89. Martin, C.L. 2013. Vitreous and ocular fundus. In: Martin, C.L., editor. *Ophthalmic Disease in Veterinary Medicine.* Manson Publishing Ltd: London, pp. 401–70.

90. Wilkie, D.A. 2005. Diseases of the ocular posterior segment. In: Gilger, B.C., editor. *Equine Ophthalmology.* Elsevier Saunders: Maryland Heights, MO, pp. 367–96.

91. Acland, G., Irby, N.L., and Aguirre, G.D. 1984. Sudden acquired retinal degeneration in the dog: Clinical and morphologic characterization of the "silent retina" syndrome. *Transactions of the American College of Veterinary Ophthalmology* 15:86–104.

92. Acland, G., and Aguirre, G.D. 1986. Sudden acquired retinal degeneration: Clinical signs and diagnosis. *Veterinary Ophthalmology* 17:58–63.

93. Venter, I.J., and Petrick, S.W. 1995. [Acute blindness in a dog caused by sudden acquired retinal degeneration]. *Journal of the South African Veterinary Association* 66(1):32–4.

94. van der Woerdt, A., Nasisse, M.P., and Davidson, M.G. 1991. Sudden acquired retinal degeneration in the dog: Clinical and laboratory findings in 36 cases. *Progress in Veterinary & Comparative Ophthalmology* 1(1):11–18.

95. Gelatt, K.N. et al. 2001. Enrofloxacin-associated retinal degeneration in cats. [erratum appears in *Vet Ophthalmology* 2001 Sep;4(3):231]. *Veterinary Ophthalmology* 4(2):99–106.

96. Barnett, K.C., and Grimes, T.D. 1974. Bilateral aplasia of the optic nerve in a cat. *British Journal of Ophthalmology* 58(7):663–7.

97. Negishi, H. et al. 2008. Unilateral optical nerve hypoplasia in a Beagle dog. *Laboratory Animals* 42(3):383–8.

98. da Silva, E.G. et al. 2008. Distinctive histopathologic features of canine optic nerve hypoplasia and aplasia: A retrospective review of 13 cases. *Veterinary Ophthalmology* 11(1):23–9.

99. Kern, T.J., and Riis, R.C. 1981. Optic nerve hypoplasia in three miniature poodles. *Journal of the Veterinary Medical Association* 178(1):49–54.

100. Ernest, J.T. 1976. Bilateral optic nerve hypoplasia in a pup. *Journal of the Veterinary Medical Association* 168(2):125–8.

101. Bedford, P.G. 1998. Collie eye anomaly in the Lancashire heeler. *The Veterinary Record* 143(13):354–6.

102. Bedford, P.G. 1982. Collie eye anomaly in the border collie. *The Veterinary Record* 111(2):34–5.

103. Barnett, K.C., and Stades, F.C. 1979. Collie eye anomaly in the Shetland sheepdog in the Netherlands. *Journal of Small Animal Practice* 20(6):321–9.

104. Roberts, S.R. 1969. The collie eye anomaly. *Journal of the Veterinary Medical Association* 155(6):859–65.

105. Barnett, K.C. 1969. The collie eye anomaly. *The Veterinary Record* 84(17):431–4.

106. Falco, M., and Barnett, K.C. 1978. The inheritance of ocular colobomata in Charolais cattle. *The Veterinary Record* 102(5):102–4.

107. Gelatt, K.N. 1976. Congenital ophthalmic anomalies in cattle. *Modern Veterinary Practice* 57(2):105–9.

108. Barnett, K.C., and Ogien, A.L. 1972. Ocular colobomata in Charolais cattle. *The Veterinary Record* 91(24):592.

109. Stadtbaumer, K., Leschnik, M.W., and Nell, B. 2004. Tick-borne encephalitis virus as a possible cause of optic neuritis in a dog. *Veterinary Ophthalmology* 7(4):271–7.

110. McEntee, K. et al. 1995. Closantel intoxication in a dog. *Veterinary & Human Toxicology* 37(3):234–6.

111. Dakshinkar, N.P., Dhoot, V.M., and Kolte, R.M. 1994. Retrobulbar optic neuritis in dog. *Indian Veterinary Journal* 71(12):1262–3.

112. Paulsen, M.E. et al. 1989. Bilateral chorioretinitis, centripetal optic neuritis, and encephalitis in a llama. *Journal of the American Veterinary Medical Association* 194(9):1305–8.

113. Nuhsbaum, M.T. et al. 2002. Treatment of granulomatous meningoencephalomyelitis in a dog. *Veterinary Ophthalmology* 5(1):29–33.

114. Smith, R.I.E. 1995. A case of ocular granulomatous meningoencephalitis in a German shepherd dog presenting as bilateral uveitis. *Australian Veterinary Practitioner* 25(2):73–8.

115. Nell, B. 2008. Optic neuritis in dogs and cats. *The Veterinary Clinics of North America. Small Animal Practice* 38(2):403–15, viii.

116. Martin, C.L. 2013. Glaucoma. In: Martin, C.L., editor. *Ophthalmic Disease in Veterinary Medicine.* Manson Publishing Ltd.: London, pp. 337–68.

117. Dugan, S., Schwarz, P.D., Roberts, S.M., and Ching, S.V. 1993. Primary optic nerve meningioma and pulmonary metastasis in a dog. *Journal of the American Animal Hospital Association* 29:11–6.

118. Langham, R.F., Bennett, R.R., and Zydeck, F.A. 1971. Primary retrobulbar meningioma of the optic nerve of a dog. *Journal of the American Veterinary Medical Association* 159(2):175–6.

119. Mauldin, E.A. et al. 2000. Canine orbital meningiomas: A review of 22 cases. *Veterinary Ophthalmology* 3(1):11–6.

120. Spiess, B.M., and Wilcock, B.P. 1987. Glioma of the optic nerve with intraocular and intracranial involvement in a dog. *Journal of Comparative Pathology* 97(1):79–84.

121. Martin, E. et al. 2000. Retrobulbar anaplastic astrocytoma in a dog: Clinicopathological and ultrasonographic features. *Journal of Small Animal Practice* 41(8):354–7.

122. Eagle, R.C. Jr., Font, R.L., and Swerczek, T.W. 1978. Malignant medulloepithelioma of the optic nerve in a horse. *Veterinary Pathology* 15(4):488–94.

123. Spiess, B.M., Ruhli, M.B., and Bauer, G.A. 1995. [Therapy of orbital neoplasms in small animals]. *Tierarztl Prax* 23(5):509–14.

CHAPTER 5

PRINCIPLES OF OPHTHALMIC SURGERY

J. PHILLIP PICKETT

INTRODUCTION

The emphasis in this chapter is on the preparation, instrumentation, principles of surgery, and postoperative care of patients for ophthalmic surgery of the adnexa and the cornea. Because of the investment in equipment and the uniqueness of the surgery, intraocular surgery should be delegated to those individuals who perform it on a regular basis. Nevertheless, extraocular surgery is still the most delicate surgery that is performed by the general practitioner. Knowledge of the anatomy involved and the acquisition of a few specialized instruments greatly facilitates performing extraocular surgery. The individual surgical procedures are discussed in detail in the appropriate chapters.

PATIENT PREPARATION FOR SURGERY

Patient selection

Ophthalmic surgery is often indicated for the very young or the very old patient. Patient selection and preparation are, therefore, extremely important to try to avoid unwanted mortalities. Surgery on the very young patient (2–12 weeks) is difficult due to the constraints of size and the increased anesthetic risk. Surgery in the very young puppy or kitten for conformational defects that are not producing significant corneal disease may be postponed until near adult size/conformation is achieved (5–6 months). If the cornea or vision is being affected in the very young patient, either a provisional surgical procedure or medical therapy may extend the time until a definitive procedure can be performed. For example, everting lid sutures for entropion can be placed in the very young puppy, and the cornea in a kitten with eyelid agenesis can be medically protected.

Ophthalmic surgery is often elective and can be performed at a mutually convenient time. The animal's temperament and the owner's expectations are important to assess prior to surgery. Animals that are very nervous or vicious may require at least one additional sedation/anesthetic event for suture removal if absorbable sutures are not used. Complications from wound dehiscence from rubbing the face are more likely in the nervous, compulsive patient. Owners who have unrealistic expectations regarding the correction of complex conformational defects are seldom satisfied and, therefore, require detailed and accurate communication. The owner who is extremely distraught by the inherent risk of surgery should also be thoroughly counseled on the advantages and disadvantages of surgery or perhaps should be encouraged to avoid elective surgery.

The patient presenting for surgery that has a periocular or conjunctival infection should have the infection controlled before proceeding with surgery. A more dramatic dilemma is presented in the patient with a bacterial panophthalmitis that has extended to an orbital cellulitis. The indication for enucleation is clear, but operating in an infected field is contraindicated. Humane considerations must be balanced with good medical principles, and intense medical and supportive care should precede and follow surgery.

> Extraocular surgery is often elective and can be delayed until the animal is older, undergoing an anesthesia episode for another condition, or until the time is mutually convenient.

ANESTHESIA/SEDATION

Some adnexal surgical procedures can be performed with local anesthesia and/or sedation, and this should be considered as an alternative to general anesthesia in the aged or high-risk patient. If the surgery is elective and general anesthesia is indicated, the high-risk patient should be evaluated by performing a thorough physical examination and organ function tests. Age alone is not a contraindication for surgery or anesthesia.

Unless performing a salvage procedure, glaucoma patients should have normalized intraocular pressure (IOP) before surgery. If intensive preoperative systemic diuretic therapy has been administered, electrolyte and acid–base imbalances may be produced and create an increased anesthetic risk. In general, potassium loss and a tendency towards metabolic acidosis can be assumed with the use of carbonic anhydrase inhibitors.[1] Mannitol may be used preoperatively with glaucoma patients or to reduce vitreous volume in intraocular surgery. If possible, mannitol administration should be performed before anesthesia induction as adverse side effects are more common in the hypotensive anesthetized patient.[2]

If surgical intervention is anticipated (particularly intraocular), prolonged preoperative administration of prostaglandin inhibitors (especially aspirin) and topical cholinesterase inhibitors should be avoided. Intraocular hemorrhage is more frequent and severe when these groups of drugs are used. Similarly, the preoperative use of long-acting subconjunctival glucocorticoids is usually contraindicated if a keratectomy is anticipated. Glucocorticoids in high dosages or in a form that cannot be withdrawn may result in corneal perforations in >20% of keratectomy cases.[3] Aminoglycoside antibiotics, systemic cholinesterase inhibitors such as insecticides, and some anthelmintics should be avoided before and during surgery if an anesthetic protocol with neuromuscular blockade (pancuronium, vecuronium, etc.) is to be used. These drugs prolong the respiratory arrest and paralysis of neuroparalytic agents.

> Preoperative topical and/or systemic medications such as mannitol, carbonic anhydrase inhibitors, cholinesterase inhibitors, glucocorticoids, and non-steroidal anti-inflammatory drugs (NSAIDs) may have important ramifications for safe anesthesia.

While some anesthetic protocols are more ideal than others, there is no clear surgical advantage (other than duration) of one anesthetic protocol over another for eyelid surgery. Surgery of the conjunctiva and cornea is facilitated by anesthetics or degree of anesthesia that keep the eye from rolling ventrally or constantly moving. Therefore, barbiturates and some sedatives that negatively affect globe position/movement should not be used when performing corneal surgery.

Neuromuscular blockade with pancuronium, vecuronium, atracurium, or similar agents may be used with intraocular surgery or for the repair of a perforated cornea of the ventral medial region where manipulation is necessary to bring the surgical field into view. If neuromuscular blockade is used, concurrent ventilatory support must be given to avoid respiratory acidosis. Low-dose pancuronium may provide ocular muscle paralysis with apparent intact respirations; however, the respiratory efforts are not sufficient to avoid hypercapnia.[4]

The proper restraint (or lack of it) of an animal with a descemetocele or perforated cornea should be emphasized to personnel who are helping with anesthesia induction. Many of the brachycephalic breeds that develop these kinds of problems are extremely difficult to restrain without putting pressure on the globe. If the patient struggles, restraint of the animal should be reduced to avoid rupture of the eye. Heavy narcotic sedation is indicated for these patients.

> Extreme caution should be used when restraining brachycephalic dogs with weakened globes, such as with corneal lacerations and descemetoceles, to avoid inadvertent perforation of the globe.

The use of atropine to prevent the oculocardiac reflex is not necessary for most procedures, unless pressure on the globe or significant pulling on the optic nerve or extraocular muscles is anticipated, such as with enucleation.[5] The horse seems the most prone to problems with the oculocardiac reflex, and glycopyrrolate is the drug of choice to counteract the bradycardia in this species. Atropine is routinely withheld preoperatively with parotid duct transplantation to facilitate the retrograde passage of a nylon suture up the parotid duct. Appropriate use of a retrobulbar-injected local anesthetic greatly diminishes the oculocardiac reflex in horses needing a central globe position for corneal surgery or in dogs requiring enucleation.

PREPARATION OF THE SURGICAL FIELD

Minor lid surgery

Postoperative eyelid skin infection is uncommon, so relatively minor plastic surgery of the eyelid, such as simple entropion, is managed as a "clean" procedure. The surgical area is prepared by modest shaving with a surgical blade, fine scissors, or clippers (**Figure 5.1**) and scrubbing with a 1:10 dilution of 10% stock povidone–iodine solution in saline for 2–4 minutes.[6] This dilution is nonirritating to the cornea and is as effective a germicide as the concentrated solution. Alcohol is not used in ocular or periocular surface preparation, nor are other antiseptics such as hexachlorophene, which are irritating to the cornea.

The surgery site is covered with a fenestrated drape, and sterile gloves are worn. A surgical gown is not necessary. This protocol may also be used for minor third eyelid surgeries, minor conjunctival surgery, and minor superficial keratectomies. While some practitioners might argue that more stringent asepsis should be adhered to, the cost–benefit ratio does not warrant it; the procedure

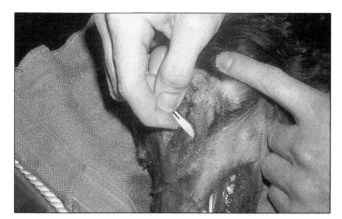

Figure 5.1 Shaving in a dog with a #10 Bard–Parker blade after wetting the hair with a sterile water-soluble jelly. Shaving is with the direction of the hair. Cats and shorthaired dogs do not clip well, but they are also difficult to shave. Fine-bladed scissors coated with sterile water-soluble jelly may also be used for hair removal.

is often only excision of a small piece of skin and suture of the defect similar to a skin biopsy.

Major lid surgery, lid surgery with buried sutures, and corneal surgery

Unlike minor lid surgeries, extensive plastic procedures, such as a large tumor excision or procedures that have buried nonabsorbable sutures, are treated as aseptically as possible. Shaving or clipping the surgical site is more extensive than for minor procedures, although the skin disinfection is similar. Careful shaving with a surgical blade or fine-blade scissors after wetting the hair/scissor blades with a sterile water-soluble lubricant jelly is preferred to clipping (**Figure 5.1**). Clipper blades, when hot, may burn the skin, may be contaminated from previous preparations, and do not cut close on cats or shorthaired dogs. The draping of the surgical site is usually by triangulation with three drapes or covering with a fenestrated drape. For a more impermeable draping of the surgical site, use of a commercially available self-adhesive plastic drape (**Figure 5.2**) is appropriate. Preparation of the surgeon is the same as for all aseptic surgery. The surgeon's gloves should be wiped free of powder with sterile saline moistened gauze to avoid foreign body reaction in tissues or in the eye.

Surgery for deep corneal ulcers and perforated corneas can be managed with little skin preparation to avoid expulsion of intraocular contents and intraocular contamination with surface debris. If the cornea is intact, the skin is prepared for 2–4 cm (0.8–1.5 in) beyond the eyelid margins; pressure should not be exerted on the globe. Water-soluble jelly is placed on the blades of fine scissors that are used to trim the lashes and the periocular hair

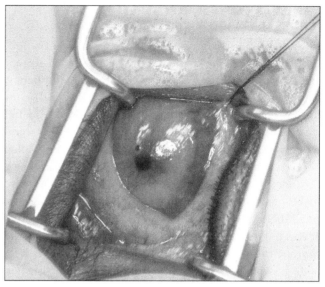

Figure 5.2 Preparation of a dog's eye for sterile surgery with an overlying plastic adhesive drape covering a larger fenestrated drape. Note placement of lid speculum blades and use of a 6-0 silk limbal stay suture to enhance globe positioning.

to prevent the cut cilia from falling onto the globe. If the cornea is perforated, the surgeon may elect no lid shaving or preparation other than cutting the lashes and the long periocular hairs with jelly-coated fine scissors and cautiously cleaning the conjunctival cul-de-sac with saline/diluted povidone-iodine solution moistened cotton tip applicators.

A sterile plastic adhesive drape placed over the eye, covered with a larger fenestrated drape or triangulated with drapes, provides an excellent barrier to facial surface bacteria contaminating the ocular surgical field (**Figure 5.2**). Studies have shown that preoperative rinsing of the conjunctival sac with sterile electrolyte solutions increases the risk of contaminating the conjunctiva and the cornea with skin bacteria from any backwashing that may occur.[7] This may be true in the nonhaired periocular skin in humans, but in veterinary species with nasal folds and hair that may harbor bacteria, yeast, and other infectious agents, attempts to cleanse the ocular/periocular surfaces prior to major surgery are indicated. Because of the incidence of facial skin/nasal folds being contaminated with bacteria (sometimes the same ones that are growing on the ulcerated corneal surfaces), this author recommends trimming hair around the eye, on the face, and in the nasal folds so that these areas can be appropriately cleansed and kept free of mucus, crusts, medication residue, and so on, that may cause increased attempts at postoperative self-trauma and may make the area easier for the owner to keep clean during the postoperative healing period.

PATIENT POSITIONING AND EXPOSURE OF THE GLOBE

Positioning of the patient for ophthalmic surgery can vary from dorsal, sternal, or lateral recumbency, depending on the surgeon's preference, the skull conformation, and the procedure to be performed. Lid and third eyelid procedures are usually performed in lateral or sternal recumbency, and corneal or conjunctival flap surgeries can be better performed in dorsal recumbency (**Figures 5.3 and 5.4**). If bilateral lid procedures are to be performed, the animal may be placed in sternal recumbency with the nose supported. This allows access to both sides without having to move, reprep, and redrape the patient.

Bags containing small plastic beads, which when placed under a vacuum become rigid in the prevacuum conformation, are excellent for immobilization of the head in any position and are a good investment for all types of surgery (**Figures 5.3 and 5.4**). Alternatives are the use of "sand bags" or bags of various size filled with spent soda lime, synthetic cat litter, and so on, and taped to position the nose and the head. All delicate ophthalmic surgery is performed seated, with the hands and arms supported (**Figure 5.5**). Lid surgery may be performed

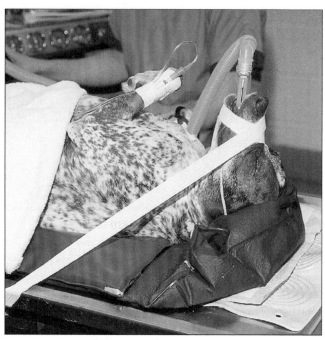

Figure 5.4 Vacuum bag as seen in (Figure 5.3) after molding to the patient/position and applying vacuum. Additional tape is applied to the nose to help better position the head for ophthalmic surgery.

standing, which allows more flexibility in positioning of the patient. Most equine extraocular and surface ocular surgery is performed standing.

After incision of the plastic adhesive drape, a method must be utilized to keep the lids open and expose the area of concern. The usual method of holding the lids open is by using a lid speculum. Because of the diversity of breeds and species, more than one size of speculum is needed.

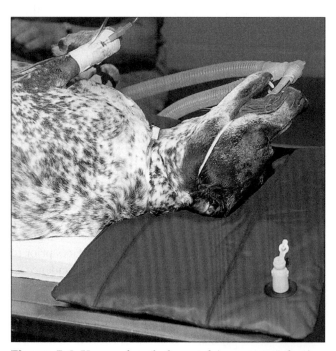

Figure 5.3 Vacuum bag (before applying vacuum) that is utilized to immobilize a dog's head. The bag is filled with plastic beads so that when a vacuum is applied (Figure 5.4), it holds the mold or the shape that was fashioned before applying the vacuum.

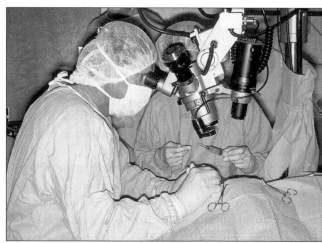

Figure 5.5 Positioning of the practitioner's arms and hands so that they are supported is important for microsurgery to allow smooth precise movement.

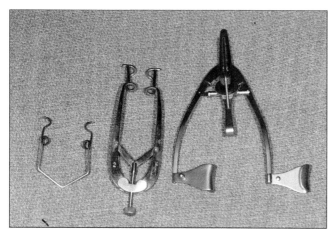

Figure 5.6 Lid speculums appropriate for veterinary use. The wire speculum (left) is appropriate for small dogs and cats, whereas the larger speculum (center) is necessary for large fissures in the dog and may work in the horse. The Guyton-Park speculum (right) is an excellent choice for the horse. The surgeon should be aware that pressure might be inadvertently applied to the globe with the larger speculums.

A pediatric speculum is used for small dogs and cats. Wire lid speculums are preferred because of their simplicity, light weight, and low cost (**Figure 5.6**). Alternatively, sutures can be placed near the lid margins and clamped to the drapes. Larger lid speculums may be used in larger dogs, and special lid speculums are made for horses (**Figure 5.6**). If the globe is weakened or perforated, great caution must be taken with any instrument that is used to hold the lids open to avoid transmitting pressure onto the globe.

Convenient positioning of the globe for surgery is often the most frustrating step for the beginner, and the method used can be critical when dealing with a perforated or weakened globe. One method for increasing the surgical exposure is by doing a lateral canthotomy. This is performed by making a horizontal crimp at the lateral canthus to the depth of the lateral cul-de-sac using a hemostat and then cutting the crimp with scissors. With experience, the need for a canthotomy decreases, except in patients with a very small palpebral fissure. Following completion of surgery on the globe, the lateral canthotomy is closed utilizing a standard two-layer closure as described for closure of a vertical full-thickness lid laceration (see Chapter 7).

Stay sutures of 6-0 silk placed near the limbus in the superficial sclera can be used to manipulate the globe (**Figure 5.2**), but unless meticulously placed with a fine ophthalmic needle, they are often only anchored in the loose conjunctiva and are of minimal benefit. If manipulating an intact globe, such as for a keratectomy, two small mosquito hemostats placed 180° from each other on the perilimbal conjunctiva offer good exposure. This method should not be used for a weakened or ruptured globe, as pressure is transmitted to the globe.

The third eyelid can be retracted with forceps or, less traumatically, with a mattress stay suture that is passed through the medial lower lid and into the third eyelid near its margin and back out of the skin. This pulls the third eyelid into a retracted position, and the friction of the suture through the skin is often enough to hold it in place.

INSTRUMENTATION

Eponyms are common and confusing in ophthalmic instrument nomenclature and many times represent minor changes from one instrument to another very similar instrument. Despite the wide array of names and instruments, most represent variations of a few basic instruments.

Lid and third eyelid surgery instrumentation

Many of the simple ophthalmic lid procedures can be performed without special instrumentation. However, two instruments that facilitate lid procedures are a lid plate and a large chalazion clamp (**Figure 5.7**). The skin of the eyelids is loose, and it is difficult to make a smooth incision on the eyelids unless they are held taut while incising. The lid plate is an inexpensive contoured plate that is placed in the conjunctival sac, elevated by the surgeon/assistant producing a firm, taut, and immobile skin surface

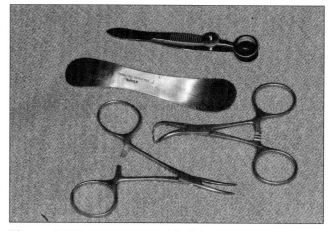

Figure 5.7 Instruments used for lid surgery. A variety of chalazion clamps (top) of different sizes are available. They facilitate excision of tissue and hemostasis. The lid plate (second from top) facilitates clean skin incisions. Baby Bacchus towel clamps and curved mosquito hemostats may be used for retraction/positioning, retaining drapes, and hemostasis.

that facilitates a clean, precise incision. Since it stretches the skin, the surgeon must become accustomed to evaluating the amount of skin to excise under these conditions.

A chalazion clamp facilitates the removal of aberrant cilia and small lid tumors. When clamped over the area to be incised, it provides hemostasis and a firm backing for making an accurate, clean incision.

Forceps that are used for lid and third eyelid surgeries are usually small to medium sized, 1 × 2 rat-toothed forceps with the teeth at right angles, such as Adson or Bishop–Harmon forceps (**Figure 5.8**). These are inexpensive forceps and are preferred to more delicate forceps that are easily damaged. Since the suture material for lid and third eyelid surgery is not usually smaller than 5-0 in size, small nonophthalmic needle holders (**Figure 5.9**) should suffice and are preferable for larger needles. Smaller ophthalmic scissors such as tenotomy scissors (**Figure 5.10**) are an appropriate size for ophthalmic plastic surgery, but misusing them on the skin can easily damage them. Small bladed general surgical scissors (Metzenbaum) should be used for cutting skin.

Although not usually needed for minor lid surgery, a loupe or similar magnification (**Figure 5.11**) is almost mandatory for the presbyopic surgeon and is invaluable for meticulous procedures such as nasolacrimal duct cannulation, fine suture removal, and so on.

A well-stocked extraocular surgery pack for eyelids and third eyelid should include:

- A lid plate
- A chalazion clamp
- Fine Adson 1 × 2 rat-toothed forceps (or multiple-toothed Brown-Adson forceps)
- Medium Bishop–Harmon forceps
- Small needle drivers (nonophthalmic)
- Tenotomy scissors
- Small bladed general surgery scissors
- General scalpel handle (Bard–Parker or equivalent)
- Small curved mosquito forceps (×2)
- Towel clamps (×3)
- Cotton-tipped applicators, gauze sponges

Conjunctival and corneal surgery

Since conjunctival and corneal tissue is inherently more delicate, smaller suture material and cutting instrumentation are utilized, and specialized ocular instruments are preferable. In general, microsurgical instruments are miniaturized and designed to hold like a pencil in each hand. The surgeon's arms should be supported at the wrists on the table or chair arms, and often the hand is steadied by support of at least one finger on the patient's head (**Figure 5.5**). Manipulation of microsurgical instruments involves fine motor movement, rolling the instrument with the fingers instead of gross motor movement rolling of the wrist/forearm. Instruments such as ophthalmic needle holders (**Figure 5.9**) that are designed to roll between the fingers may be round-sided or six-sided for even finer movement involved in delicate corneal surgery (**Figure 5.9**). Instruments that are not rotated, such as scissors

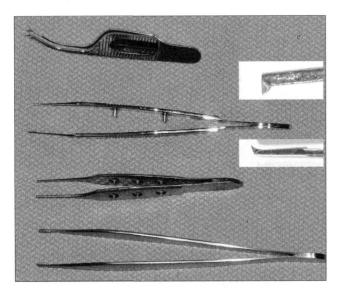

Figure 5.8 Various types/sizes of forceps for adnexal and corneal surgery. Top to bottom: Colibri-type forceps; 45-degree angled teeth forceps (Castroviejo); right-angle toothed 1 × 2 rat-toothed forceps (Bishop-Harmon); and Adson or Brown Adson forceps. Inset images show tips. Castroviejo tips (bottom inset) are at a 45-degree angle with a tying platform behind tips. Bishop-Harmon forceps (top inset) have 90-degree angled teeth.

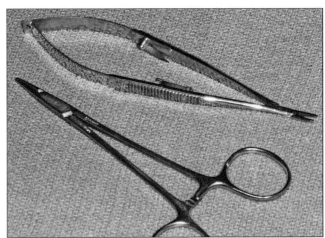

Figure 5.9 Needle holders for ophthalmic surgery. Above, a microsurgical needle holder (medium, curved tipped locking Castroviejo needle driver). Below, a small standard locking needle holder (Derf).

and many forceps, have flattened handles or platforms for the fingers. Locking instruments, such as a needle holder, should be designed to lock and unlock smoothly (**Figure 5.9**) with no change in hand position. Because of the delicate nature of many of these instruments, inappropriate use may damage the instrument (tips and locks).

Lid speculum

See globe exposure, **Figure 5.6**.

Scissors

Small blunt-tipped scissors such as tenotomy scissors should suffice for conjunctival dissection (**Figure 5.10**). They may also be used for cutting fine suture material. Sharp-tipped scissors may create holes in the conjunctiva when bluntly separating tissue.

Forceps

Two or three types of forceps are needed for conjunctival and corneal manipulation. A right-angled rat-toothed forceps of medium to small size (Bishop–Harmon) is used to manipulate the conjunctiva. Grasping with this type of forceps captures only the conjunctiva and Tenon's capsule. They are not used for fixation of, or moving, the globe. If the cornea is to be manipulated or sutured, a pair of curved tissue forceps with very small right-angled teeth, such as the Colibri forceps, or straight forceps with 45-degree angled teeth, such as the Castroviejo forceps, are used to hold the edges of the cornea (**Figure 5.8**). Many corneal forceps also have a tying platform behind the teeth (**Figure 5.8**) to hold fine suture while tying knots ("double instrument tie"). Inappropriate manipulation of

suture with the teeth of a toothed forceps may damage the suture. Unfortunately, corneal forceps are one of the most expensive instruments to purchase because of the delicate teeth. Extreme care should be exercised in the type of tissues grasped with these forceps, as improper use can easily damage the teeth and arms of the instrument.

The third type of forceps is a 45-degree angled rat-toothed or splay-toothed forceps that is used for fixation and manipulation of the globe. When pressed against the globe and closed, they grasp the deeper layers of episclera and sclera rather than the loose conjunctival surface, or when closed over a rectus muscle, they pass under the muscle rather than entrapping the muscle. In the absence of a Colibri-type forceps, these forceps can be used to manipulate the corneal tissue safely (**Figure 5.8**). Alternatives to forceps in manipulation of the globe are fixation sutures or blunt instruments such as a strabismus hook or a cotton tip applicator, pushed into the fornix to move the globe in the appropriate direction. Extreme caution should be exercised with all forms of globe manipulation if the cornea is weakened or perforated.

Needle holders

Because the suture material is a minimum of 5-0 in size and the needles are very small, a microsurgical needle holder that is easily manipulated with finger motion and does not damage the needle is necessary for corneal and conjunctival surgery. A variety of designs are available, with variations in whether they lock, the locking mechanism, and the size and shape of the jaws (**Figure 5.9**).

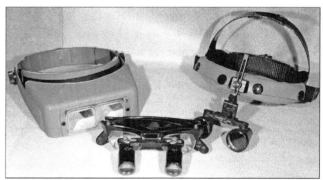

Figure 5.11 Magnification options for microsurgery. Left to right: Single-lens loupe, (foreground) Galilean loupes mounted on glasses frame, Galilean loupes mounted on headband. Single-lens loupe systems are inexpensive and provide magnification by allowing user to get closer to objects, thus innate magnification. The shorter working distances, however, make surgery difficult. The Galilean loupe system is composed of multiple lenses, so the surgeon can order loupes for a fixed magnification to be used at a fixed distance. Galilean loupes are expensive but are far superior to the single-lens loupe systems.

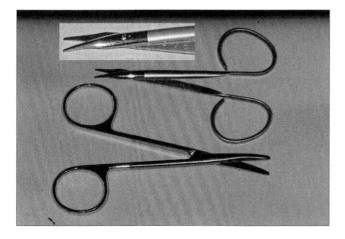

Figure 5.10 Scissors for ophthalmic surgery. Above, Steven's tenotomy scissors. Below, fine Metzenbaum scissors. Note insert, tips of tenotomy scissors are blunt, and noncutting sides of blades have "cut outs" that enhance blunt dissection of conjunctiva from Tenon's capsule.

The surgeon who only performs the occasional ocular surgery may prefer the locking needle holder. This instrument and the corneal forceps are the two most expensive instruments in a minor ophthalmic surgery pack for extraocular surgery.

Miscellaneous instruments

A muscle or strabismus hook is an inexpensive instrument that can be used for various manipulations of the globe and eyelids, as well as in enucleation (**Figure 5.12**). When performing an enucleation, the strabismus hook is used to hook the extraocular muscles by passing it posterior to the equator, where the muscle separates from the globe, and then coming forward to catch the muscle/tendon of insertion.

A cyclodialysis-type spatula is a general-purpose instrument. It can be used for performing lamellar dissection in a superficial keratectomy, sweeping anterior synechiae off the inner cornea with perforated ulcers, and removing fibrin membranes from the pupil and iris (**Figure 5.12**). It is rarely used as originally designed for performing the cyclodialysis procedure for glaucoma due to the poor success rate of the surgery.

Irrigation through a blunt lacrimal needle is used to control hemorrhage in the surgical field and keep the cornea moist. Lacrimal needles often have a malleable end to adjust the angle to the surgeon's preference.

A wide variety of scalpel blades for ophthalmic surgery are available (**Figure 5.13**), but most surgeons utilize only two types: a small curved blade and a small pointed blade. While specialized handles and blades (such as Beaver handles and blades) are preferred by some surgeons, the regular #15 and #11 Bard–Parker blades are quite satisfactory for most extraocular procedures. For delicate corneal/intraocular surgery, the 6400, 6500, and 6700 Beaver blades with Beaver system handle are superior to the larger, less refined Bard–Parker blades. Diamond knives are the ultimate for a sharp instrument.

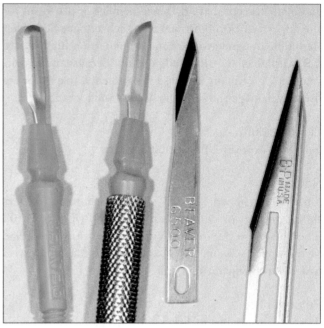

Figure 5.13 Scalpel blades used for ophthalmic surgery. Left to right: 6400 Beaver blade, 6700 Beaver blade with knurled, rounded Beaver handle, 6500 Beaver blade, and #11 Bard–Parker blade.

Sponges used in ophthalmic surgery can be either the common cotton-tipped applicators or cellulose sponges. If the globe is intact, cotton-tipped applicators are satisfactory and inexpensive. Cellulose sponges are preferred when the cornea is perforated or when performing intraocular surgery to avoid loose cotton fibers entering the eye and creating an inflammatory reaction (**Figure 5.14**).

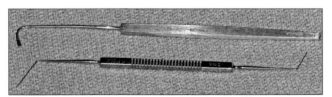

Figure 5.12 Strabismus hook and cyclodialysis spatula. Strabismus hook (above) may be used to push into conjunctival sac to rotate the globe and/or hook extraocular muscles. Cyclodialysis spatula may be used to tease iris and fibrin membranes off the cornea, for superficial keratectomies, and/or to dissect vitreous from posterior aspect of lens during intracapsular lensectomy.

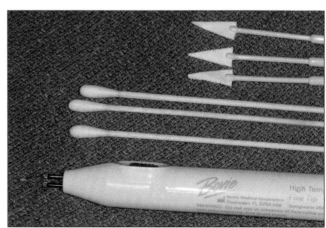

Figure 5.14 Methods for hemostasis in extraocular and corneal surgery. Cotton-tipped applicators are used if the eye is not open. The cellulose spears (top) are preferred if the globe is open to avoid leaving residual foreign material. Low-temperature battery cautery can control conjunctival, corneal, and iris bleeding.

Hemostasis

Hemostasis during ophthalmic surgery may be affected by sponging and clamping with hemostats, as in general surgery. Conjunctival and corneal hemostasis is usually affected with cotton-tipped applicators or with cellulose sponges if the eye is open. Cotton-tipped applicators should never be used for intraocular hemorrhage for the reasons listed previously. Alternative methods for hemostasis include gentle flushing with 1:10,000 epinephrine; flushing with an electrolyte solution; battery-powered, low-temperature cautery (**Figure 5.14**); or bipolar wet field cautery. Disposable, low-temperature cautery units are quite effective in controlling conjunctival, scleral, and corneal hemorrhage that continues despite flushing/use of dilute epinephrine. They can be reused if ethylene oxide sterilization is available.

A well-stocked surgery pack for extraocular and corneal surgery should include:

- Instruments as for extraocular surgery
- Wire eyelid speculums, pediatric and adult size
- Corneal forceps such as Colibri (or Castroviejo)*
- Microsurgical ophthalmic needle holders*
- Beaver blade holder or small handle for Bard–Parker blades
- Spatula such as a cyclodialysis or iris spatula
- Irrigation cannula
- Cellulose sponges

*Expensive instruments

Irrigation solution

The type of sterile electrolyte solution used for irrigation in extraocular and corneal surgery is not critical. Irrigating solutions used for prolonged intraocular surgery (greater than 15–20 minutes of irrigation) should be balanced for pH, buffered with bicarbonate, and contain glutathione and glucose. Most intraocular irrigation procedures take only a few minutes, and lactated Ringer's solution or Ringer's solution is as efficacious as the more expensive and unstable commercial intraocular irrigating solutions.[8,9]

Suture material

Suture material for lid skin should be 4-0 to 5-0 in size. Silk suture was the past gold standard, but some dogs develop suture abscesses and excess granulation if the suture is left in place for more than 7–10 days due to gamma globulin binding to the silk. Nylon or other monofilament/braided nonabsorbable suture, and even synthetic absorbable suture, can be used on the skin with good results. If difficulty is anticipated in suture removal because of location or temperament of the animal, synthetic absorbable sutures are indicated with the suture being left to extrude on its own. Braided absorbable sutures and monofilament sutures should be avoided in the skin if the ends may rub on the cornea. Fine (6-0 to 8-0) braided synthetic sutures should be used for basic corneal laceration repair and conjunctival flap placement procedures and allowed to extrude on its own. More sophisticated corneal surgeries (transplantations and transpositions) should only be performed by experienced microsurgeons, and ultrafine monofilament nonabsorbable sutures may be used in these instances. If the suture is to be buried in the lid, an absorbable suture 5-0 to 6-0 in size is usually used.

The general surgeon should have some ophthalmic suture on hand for corneal lacerations and perforated ulcers. The size and material type can vary somewhat with preference, but the needle should be a good quality, ophthalmic, reverse cutting or spatula needle. Use of an inappropriate needle when suturing the cornea results in excessive distortion and stress on the globe and inaccurate depth placement of the needle. Ophthalmic needles are very sharp and should be handled, with forceps, only on the shank, or they can be quickly blunted. The needle must be pushed far enough through the tissue so that, when pulled through, it can be grasped behind the point to avoid blunting the cutting edges.

Gut and collagen sutures should never be used on the cornea since the advent of newer synthetic absorbable sutures. Suture sizes used in the cornea vary from 6-0 to 10-0. Very fine nylon suture is the least reactive, but it has inherent difficulties in handling if the surgeon is not equipped (appropriate instruments and magnification); plus, removal of nonabsorbable sutures from the cornea/sclera usually requires a second anesthetic/heavy sedation procedure.

> Ophthalmic suture in the smaller sizes and with ophthalmic needles is very expensive; the general surgeon will want to be judicious as to the variety and sizes kept in stock. Synthetic braided absorbable suture (6-0 in size) with a spatula or reverse cutting needle should suffice for most uncomplicated conjunctival and corneal suturing, although the ophthalmologist may often use an 8-0 size in small animals and a 7-0 size in large animal corneal surgery.

Technique

In the healthy cornea, the needle entrance and exit from the incision or laceration should be 1 mm from the edge. The needle tip enters the cornea on a vertical plane. The needle should be sufficiently small enough in curvature to enter from this distance and exit deep in the incision edge. If the needle is not entered vertically, the bite may be very superficial, resulting in posterior gaping of the incision. If the needle does not have a steep curvature, it is difficult to place the suture deep in the cornea and have it exit the cornea at the incision. The side of the incision being sutured should be held with forceps to provide counter pressure to the force of driving the needle and to allow eversion of the edge of the incision to visualize the depth of the needle tract. The needle is passed as deep as possible, emerging under the forceps and just anterior to Descemet's membrane. The opposite side of the incision is then stabilized with the forceps, and the needle is pushed across the incision at the same depth that it emerged from on the other side. The suture is tied with a minimum of two loops on the first throw, and if nylon is used, three loops are recommended. A second and third throw of a single loop each is then placed. If 10-0 nylon is used, the ends can be cut short and the suture rotated to draw the knot into the suture tract. Larger sutures are cut close to the knot and left exposed.

When suturing edematous, friable tissue or incisions with excess tension, for additional holding capacity, the needle bite is usually extended to 2 mm from each edge. Synthetic absorbable suture should dissolve in about 3–5 weeks but may stimulate excessive vascularization. If this occurs, the sutures should be removed. Nylon suture larger than 10-0 is removed. Suture removal can many times be performed after appropriate sedation and application of topical anesthesia. In the nervous/intractable patient, short-acting general anesthesia may be necessary to safely remove nonabsorbable corneal sutures. Rather than using scissors, a fine-tipped blade should be used to cut the suture. Scissors are usually too large, and if the animal moves during the procedure, the suture is torn out rather than cut.

Storage and cleaning of instruments

The investment in and delicate nature of ophthalmic instruments dictate that care in cleaning and maintenance of instruments be emphasized. Cleaning of instruments is best performed with an ultrasonic cleaner. Alternatively, careful brushing, avoiding instrument contact and entanglement, and drying will prolong the life of the instruments. The hinges should be lubricated in "instrument milk" after each use. Instrument corrosion may occur if the instruments are not thoroughly cleaned, instrument milk is not used, the instruments are not dried, and contact with other instruments is allowed. Prior to using instruments lubricated in "instrument milk" in an open eye or for intraocular surgery, the instruments should

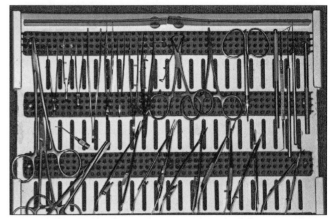

Figure 5.15 Microsurgical instrument delivery system. The soft plastic "pegs" support and separate the instruments; when combined with the aluminum casing of the tray, this system offers superior protection for expensive microsurgical instruments.

be thoroughly rinsed in saline or lactated Ringer's solution (LRS) as the instrument milk may cause severe sterile intraocular inflammation if deposited in the anterior chamber.

Instruments should be stored and sterilized so they are not in contact with adjacent instruments. Special instrument trays (**Figure 5.15**) and storage devices are available, but a simple container that has several narrow pockets sewn in it to hold the instruments can be made from a draping cloth. This can be doubled over, rolled up, and sterilized in a pack. Instruments with cutting edges and teeth should have the ends covered with tips that can either be bought commercially or made from silicone tubing. Damaged instruments can sometimes be repaired to new condition by the manufacturer, and this is usually cost effective.

Sterilization of metal ophthalmic instruments can be by any means if good technique is followed. If instrument milk is not used, instruments should be well dried before steam sterilization. Ethylene oxide sterilization is probably too expensive and toxic to be used in the usual practice environment. The standards for level of acceptable environmental contamination with ethylene oxide has been reduced, and since escaped ethylene oxide levels are difficult to monitor, ethylene oxide use is not worth the risk to personnel.

Improper use, storing, and cleansing of instruments often results in rusted, bent, or damaged tips and teeth of forceps and dull scissors.

POSTOPERATIVE CARE

Prevention of self-mutilation

Depending on the postoperative pain expected and the temperament of the animal, postoperative sedation and mechanical devices used to prevent self-trauma varies. In general, it is preferable to err on the side of caution rather than have sutures pulled out or the eye traumatized. When animals are recovering from anesthesia, it is often necessary to hold them or their head to prevent the eye being traumatized. Postoperative systemic analgesics and sedation may be used to minimize self-trauma, particularly in the very nervous animal. Mechanical devices, such as the Elizabethan collar in small animals or a protective full blinker cup in horses, are commonly used to prevent self-trauma after ocular and adnexal surgery. An alternative to commercial collars is a plastic bucket that has the bottom cut out, with the edge that is placed over the head padded and tied to a collar. This arrangement is preferred for dolichocephalic dogs or large dogs with short legs.

In patients who have had entropion surgery and have had extensive blepharospasm and are very "eye conscious," it is usually prudent to omit/minimize topical ocular therapy since any contact with the eyes will likely precipitate blepharospasm. When topical medications are administered postoperatively, the patient is held or observed for several minutes afterwards to prevent self-trauma.

> Attention to prophylactic measures regarding self-trauma by the patient pays great dividends that are intangible when successful.

Postoperative infection prophylaxis

Routine lid and conjunctival surgery is treated with a prophylactic topical, broad-spectrum bactericidal antibiotic for 5–7 days. Parotid duct transplantation is an inherently nonsterile surgery and is treated with a systemic, broad-spectrum bactericidal antibiotic immediately before and for 7–10 days postoperatively. Perforated ulcers and intraocular surgery should be treated more intensively with systemic antibiotics immediately before surgery, with systemic and topical postoperative antibiotics for 5–7 days.

The use of prophylactic antibiotics other than immediately before and after aseptic surgery is questionable, but the natural caution of the clinician with regard to postoperative infection is difficult to overcome.[10] In the case of surgery for a septic corneal condition, systemic and topical antimicrobials as well as periocular hygiene may be important for good long-term outcome as many of these cases may have the same infection periocularly that is seen in the cornea.

REFERENCES

1. Haskins, S., Munger, R., Helphrey, M. et al. 1981. Effect of acetazolamide on blood acid–base and electrolyte values in dogs. *Journal of the American Veterinary Medical Association* 179:792–796.
2. Parker, A. 1973. Blood pressure changes and lethality of mannitol infusions in dogs. *American Journal of Veterinary Research* 34:1523–1528.
3. Martin, C. 1971. The effect of topical vitamin A, antibiotic, mineral oil, and subconjunctival steroid on corneal epithelial wound healing in the dog. *Journal of the American Veterinary Medical Association* 159:1392–1399.
4. Sullivan, T.C., Hellyer, P.W., Lee, D.D., and Davidson, M.G. 1998. Respiratory function and extraocular muscle paralysis following administration of pancuronium bromide in dogs. *Veterinary Ophthalmology* 1:125–128.
5. Clutton, R., Boyd, C., Richards, L., and Schwink, K. 1988. Significance of the oculocardiac reflex during ophthalmic surgery. *Journal of Small Animal Practice* 29:573–579.
6. Roberts, S., Severin, G., and Lavach, J. 1986. Antibacterial activity of dilute povidone–iodine solutions used for ocular surface disinfection in dogs. *American Journal of Veterinary Research* 47:1207–1210.
7. Isenberg, S., Apt, L., and Yoshimieri, R. 1983. Chemical preparation of the eye in ophthalmic surgery. I. Effects of conjunctival irrigation. *Archives of Ophthalmology* 101:761–763.
8. Edelhauser, H., Gonnering, R., and Van Horn, D. 1978. Intraocular irrigating solutions. A comparative study of BSS plus and lactated Ringers solution. *Archives of Ophthalmology* 96:516–520.
9. Nasisse, M., Cook, C., and Harling, D. 1985. Response of the canine corneal endothelium to intraocular irrigation. *Proceedings of the Scientific Meeting of the American College of Veterinary Ophthalmology* 16:16–25.
10. Vasseur, P., Paul, H., Enos, L., and Hirsh, D. 1985. Infection rates in clean surgical procedures: A comparison of ampicillin prophylaxis vs a placebo. *Journal of the American Veterinary Medical Association* 187:825–827.

CHAPTER 6

ORBIT AND GLOBE

BERNHARD M. SPIESS

ANATOMY

The orbit, or enclosure for the eye and associated muscles, nerves, and vasculature, is the conical cavity outlined by the periorbita. The orbit is incompletely encased in bone laterally and ventrally in all domestic animals. The bones that form the orbit in the dog, the cat, and the cow are the frontal, lacrimal, zygomatic, maxilla, presphenoid, basisphenoid, and palatine bones (**Figures 6.1 and 6.2**). In the horse, the squamous portion of the temporal bone also contributes to the orbit. The horse and the cow have a complete bony orbital rim, whereas in the cat and the dog, the lateral orbital rim is formed by the orbital ligament (**Figures 6.1 and 6.2**).

The periorbita is modified periosteum that becomes thicker over the lateral and lateral–ventral orbit, where bone is lacking. The periorbita forms a cone with the point at the optic foramina and orbital fissure and the base at the orbital rim. The periorbita divides at the orbital rim where the superficial leaf continues as the periosteum of the facial and cranial bones, and the deep leaf continues into the lid as the orbital septum. In the orbit, the periorbita is separated from most of the bone and the periosteum by orbital fat. The periorbita reflects over the extraocular muscle and forms the muscular fascia or Tenon's capsule. The muscular fascia is divided into three layers: a thick superficial layer that originates from the orbital septum; a middle layer that attaches just posterior to the limbus of the globe and covers the extraocular muscles and attaches to the lateral aspect of the third eyelid; and a deep muscular layer that covers the deep surface of the rectus muscles and separates them from the retractor bulbi muscle.[2] The bulbar fascia or Tenon's capsule is located deep to the deep muscular fascia.

Circumferentially oriented smooth muscle is present in the periorbita, in the muscular fascia layers, and in the area of the dorsomedial wall of the orbit. Contraction of this smooth muscle produces exophthalmos and,

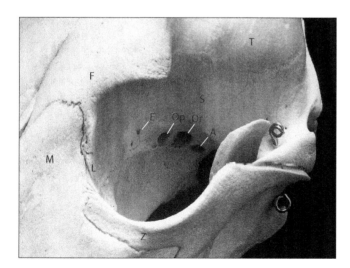

Figure 6.1 Skull of a mesaticephalic dog with the bones that form the orbit and the major foramina. (F: frontal; L: lachrymal; M: maxilla; S: sphenoid; T: temporal; Z: zygomatic; Op: optic foramen; Or: orbital fissure; E: ethmoidal foramen; A: rostral alar foramen.) (From Martin, C.L., and Anderson, B.G. 1981. In: Gelatt, K., editor. *Veterinary Ophthalmology*, 1st edition. Lea & Febiger: Philadelphia, PA, pp. 12–121.)

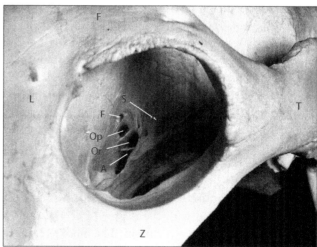

Figure 6.2 Equine orbital bones. (F: Frontal; L: Lacrimal; S: Sphenoid; T: Temporal; Z: Zygomatic; Op: Optic foramen; Or: Orbital fissure; E: Ethmoidal foramen; A: Rostral alar foramen.) (From Martin, C.L., and Anderson, B.G. 1981. In: Gelatt, K., editor. *Veterinary Ophthalmology*, 1st edition. Lea & Febiger: Philadelphia, PA, pp. 12–121.)

Table 6.1 **Orbital foramina and associated structures in domestic animals.**

FORAMEN OR FISSURES	PRESENCE IN DOMESTIC SPECIES	STRUCTURES ASSOCIATED WITH FORAMEN
Alar, rostral	Equine, canine, feline	Maxillary artery, maxillary nerve
Ethmoid (one or more)	All species	Ethmoidal nerve and vessels
Orbital	Equine, canine, feline	Abducens, ophthalmic trochlear, and oculomotor cranial nerves
Orbitorotundum	Bovine	Oculomotor, trochlear, maxillary, ophthalmic, and abducens cranial nerves
Optic	All species	Optic nerve, internal ophthalmic artery
Rotundum	Equine, canine, feline	Maxillary nerve
Supraorbital	Bovine, equine, canine, (variable feline)	Supraorbital nerve and vessels

conversely, loss of tone with sympathetic denervation produces enophthalmos.[3]

In the dog, the size of the orbit varies with the skull type and the size of the dog. Globe position in the orbit is dramatically affected by the skull type. The size of the orbit is also influenced by the presence or size of the globe during development. Early enucleation or microphthalmos may decrease the size of the orbit by up to 27% but can be partially prevented by placing an implant in the orbit.[4]

The foramina of the orbit in various domestic animals and the structures that traverse them are listed in **Table 6.1**. The periorbita attaches around the optic foramen and orbital fissure. The extraocular muscles and levator palpebrae muscle form a muscular cone that originates around the optic foramen. The optic nerve and internal ophthalmic artery and vein traverse the optic foramen. The retractor bulbi muscle originates from the margins of the orbital fissure. The oculomotor (III), trochlear (IV), and abducens (VI) cranial nerves, the ophthalmic division of the trigeminal (V) cranial nerve, the orbital vein, and the anastomotic artery traverse the orbital fissure (**Figure 6.3**).

The placement of the eye in the skull of animals is usually correlated with the dietary evolution. Carnivores, or hunting animals, have frontal eyes with an overlap of visual fields that give them good binocular vision for depth perception. Herbivores, or the hunted, have lateral placement of the eyes to give a wide field of vision with little or no blind spots, so that they can graze and watch for the hunters (**Figure 6.4**). The lateral placement of the eyes is also correlated with the degree of decussation of the optic nerve fibers at the chiasm. The more lateral the eye, the more complete the decussation, that is, 81% in horses, 83% in cattle, 89% in sheep, 88% in pigs, 75% in dogs, 65% in cats, and 50% in humans.[5] This translates functionally into variations in the pupillary light reflex (PLR). Animals with a high percentage of crossed fibers have minimal consensual light reflexes because the input is unequal to both eyes.

The size of the globe does not increase proportionately to the body size between or within species (**Table 6.2**). The ratio of eye weight to body weight in a small dog is 1:545 and in a large dog is 1:2,574.[7] The globe in the cat and the dog is somewhat spherical with the three perpendicular axes (anterior–posterior, vertical, transverse) being within 1 mm of each other. The globe of the cow, and less so the horse, is flattened in the anterior–posterior axis (**Figure 6.5**). See **Table 6.3** for the various globe dimensions of domestic animals.

The cornea of most domestic animals is slightly oblong or egg-shaped, with the longest axis horizontal and the narrow end temporal. The optic nerve enters the globe ventrotemporally. Two long posterior ciliary arteries leave

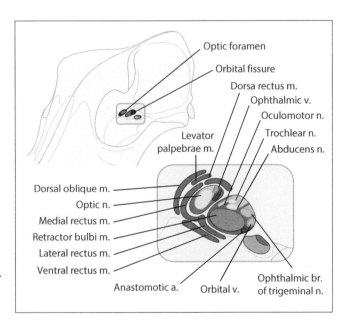

Figure 6.3 **Orbital apex of the dog illustrating structures passing through the optic foramen and orbital fissure, as well as extraocular muscle attachments. (From Martin, C.L., and Anderson, B.G. 1981. In: Gelatt. K., editor. *Veterinary Ophthalmology*, 1st edition. Lea & Febiger: Philadelphia, PA, pp. 12–121.) (br: Branch; m: Muscle; n: Nerve; v: Vein.)**

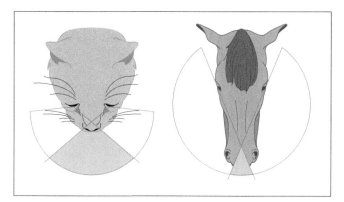

Figure 6.4 Visual fields of a cat compared to the horse. Note the frontal eye placement increases the binocular field with an attendant increase in depth perception in the cat. The horse, with lateral eye position and horizontally elongated pupil, can see threatening objects from behind without moving the head or the eyes. (From Coutler, D., and Schmidt, G. 1984. In: Swenson, M., editor. *Duke's Physiology of Domestic Animals*. Cornell University Press: Ithaca, NY, pp. 728–741.)

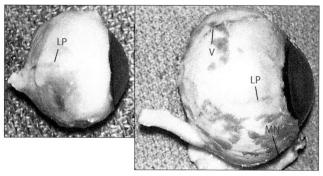

Figure 6.5 Lateral view of the canine and equine globe comparing the size of globe and the position of the optic nerve. (LP: Long posterior ciliary artery; V: Vortex vein; MN: Membrana nictitans.) (From Martin, C.L., and Anderson, B.G. 1981. In: Gelatt, K., editor. *Veterinary Ophthalmology*, 1st edition. Lea & Febiger: Philadelphia, PA, pp. 12–121.)

their course with the nerve at this point to course anteriorly in the sclera at 3 and 9 o'clock. These arteries are landmarks and guides in the orientation of an enucleated globe.

The sclera of domestic animals is very thin at the equator (0.5 mm [500 µm]) with little inherent rigidity. Consequently, the globe collapses when opened surgically and is difficult to prepare for histopathologic examination. The globe is relatively immobile in a vertical and horizontal plane in domestic animals compared with humans, but, unlike humans, animals can dramatically move the eye in an anterior–posterior direction. Domestic animals have, in addition to the four recti and two oblique muscles, a retractor bulbi muscle that draws the eye into the orbit for protection and passively allows the third eyelid to move across the globe (**Figure 6.6**).

VISION IN DOMESTIC ANIMALS

Humans have always been inquisitive as to how well or what animals see. This relates to humans being so visually oriented that they assume that animals live in the same sensory world. Many animals have a sensory world that is far expanded beyond that of humans. The most common questions that the veterinarian is asked regarding animal vision are related to color perception and visual acuity.

The puppy is not precocious, and it has incomplete development of the visual system, first evident in the physiologic ankyloblepharon that is present until 10–14 days postpartum. PLRs are present on opening of the lids, but they are sluggish and exhibit hippus (alternate dilating and constricting). The menace response and visual cliff reactions are not present until 4 weeks postpartum.[8]

Miller has written two excellent reviews[9,10] on the subject of animal vision, and readers are encouraged to explore these publications further. Many of the following comments are summarized from these articles. By necessity, veterinarians equate vision in animals based on their comparative human experience, and it is probably fair to say this does not do justice to the visual world of animals.

The dog obviously has a lower threshold for perception of light than humans based on the predominant rod retina, a rhodopsin characteristic of animals that function in dim light, and the presence of a tapetum. The tapetum, while enhancing light, also induces a scatter factor that decreases the resolution. Vision in dogs is thought to be sensitive to motion because of the predominance of rods in the retina and perhaps due to a horizontal visual streak. Dogs do not fuse individual flickers of light until 70 or more cycles/sec (Hz), and this is often given as the reason

Table 6.2 **Comparison of eye and body weight.**			
ANIMAL	**AVERAGE BODY WEIGHT (KG)**	**WEIGHT OF EYES (G)**	**RATIO**
Horse	500	100.8	1:4960
Cow	400–500	65.0	1:6923
Sheep	85	23.3	1:3648
Pig	75	19.0	1:3947
Dog (large)	36.55	14.2	1:2574
Dog (small)	4.7	8.6	1:545
Cat	2.9	10.9	1:267

Source: Translated from Bayer, J. 1914. *Angenheilkunde*. Braumueller: Vienna, p. 22. Measurements by Koschel.

Table 6.3 Dimensions of the globe in domestic animals (mm).

ANIMALS	A-P AXIS	VERTICAL AXIS	TRANSVERSE AXIS	RATIO		
	A	V	T	A:V	A:T	V:T
Horse	43.68	47.63	48.45	1:1.09	1:1.10	1:1.01
Mule	43.00	47.50	48.50	1:1.10	1:1.12	1:1.01
Cow	35.34	40.82	41.90	1:1.15	1:1.18	1:1.02
Calf	26.50	32.50	34.20	1:1.22	1:1.20	1:1.05
Sheep	26.85	30.02	30.86	1:1.11	1:1.15	1:1.02
Pig	24.60	26.53	26.23	1:1.08	1:1.06	1:0.99
Dog	21.73	21.34	21.17	1:0.98	1:0.97	1:0.99
Cat	21.30	20.60	20.55	1:0.97	1:0.96	1:0.99

Source: Translated from Bayer, J. 1914. *Angenheilkunde*. Braumueller: Vienna, p. 22.

most dogs do not watch television. Television is 60 Hz, and a dog would view it as individual frames rather than a fused picture.

The visual field of dogs varies between breeds, based on the length of the nose and how frontal the eyes are. The total visual field is 240–250°, with up to 60° binocular or overlap field. Visual acuity, the ability to discriminate between objects, requires that the object be focused on the retina. Most dogs tested are emmetropic, although myopia and hyperopia have been noted and may have some breed predisposition.[11] The visual acuity of the dog given in the familiar Snellen fractions is about 20/65–20/85 and varies significantly with the methodology employed. Accommodation in the dog is said to be only 2–3 D.

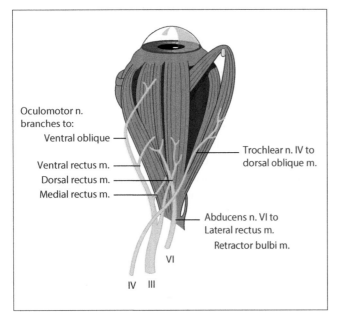

Figure 6.6 Dorsal view of the extraocular muscles and their innervation in a dog. (m: Muscle; n: Nerve.)

Dogs are like humans with deuteranopia (partial color blindness to red and green), discerning colors in the blue and yellow spectrum, and they are blind to the red/green colors.[12]

The cat tapetum is high in riboflavin, which produces the yellow color and tapetal fluoresence.[13] The amount of light reflected is a function of the color, with the yellow tapetum reflecting over 60% of the light and the green tapetum reflecting 50%.[14] The amount of light required for vision in the cat is 5.5–7× less than humans.[15] This is facilitated by the tapetum and a large cornea and pupil, which allow more light into the retina. Cats have a large binocular field of approximately 130°, with a total monocular field of 200° and a total field of view of 287°.[16] The cat has a large lens that is positioned deep in the eye to produce a small but concentrated image on the retina. The accommodative power of the cat has variably been reported as 4–11 D.[17,18] Anyone who has watched a cat follow an insect up a wall that was immediately in front of it would believe they have good accommodative powers. Surprisingly, visual discrimination in the cat is less than in the dog, being about 20/100,[19,20] but sensitivity to light is better. The color vision of cats has been variably reported but is probably partial, with weakness in distinguishing yellow from green.

Horses are functionally precocious when born, and their visual system reflects this compared to the dog. Foals have a menace response on average by 5 days postpartum, and all have PRLs on day 1.[21] Horses have been calculated as having visual acuities of 20/35[22] to 20/60.[23] Most horses are emmetropic, with equal amounts of very mild hyperopia and myopia found.[24] Because the horse has only about 1 D of accommodation, early theories of how the horse focused objects at different distances were based on a "ramp retina" theory. This was based on the shape of the equine globe (**Figure 6.5**) that was supposed to produce a different focal length for light at different angles, with axial light having the shortest focal length and ventral light (ground) having the longest focal length.[25] This theory was used to explain why horses move their head to view different objects. Sivak and Allen and Harman et al. discounted the ramp retina.[22,26] Harman et al., in evaluating head position, visual fields, and visual acuity of horses, found that binocular vision was present only in front and down the nose but not straight ahead with the nose down.[22] Thus, when grazing, the binocular vision is toward the ground with the peripheral vision giving a panoramic view of the lateral horizon. If an object of interest appears in the distance, horses raise their head to look down their nose at the object with binocular vision. Horses probably have dichromatic color vision and may lack the ability to see green.[27]

DISEASES OF THE ORBIT

Clinical signs

Diseases of the orbit produce signs by altering the volume of the orbit and/or the function of orbital structures. Alterations in the volume of the orbit produce either exophthalmos, enophthalmos, or deviation of the globe. An additional accompanying sign of exophthalmos may be either periocular or temporomandibular pain. Alterations in the function of orbital structures create signs as diverse as deviations in ocular alignment, blindness, disparities in pupil size and function, vascular congestion of the anterior segment, third eyelid prolapse, altered tear secretion, and hypoesthesia of the cornea (**Table 6.4**).

Exophthalmos

Exophthalmos is an increased prominence or protrusion of the globe and should be differentiated from buphthalmos and the conformational exophthalmos seen in animals with a shallow orbit and a large palpebral fissure. In most instances, this is not difficult, but measurements of the corneal diameter or ultrasonic measurements of the globe may be required to differentiate the two. Exophthalmos signifies a space-occupying orbital lesion, whereas buphthalmos is specific for glaucoma. Exophthalmos can be produced by a space-occupying lesion of the orbit or the retro-orbital space due to the incomplete bony orbit. Specifically, lesions of the muscles of mastication, the zygomatic salivary gland, and the adjacent soft tissues may produce exophthalmos.

Manifestations of exophthalmos are detected by observation and palpation. The relative prominence of the two globes can be compared by observing from a dorsal vantage point and comparing the position of the two corneal apexes (**Figure 6.7**). Previous alterations in one eye/orbit, such as enucleation or phthisis/microphthalmos, do not allow this comparison. Palpation is performed to

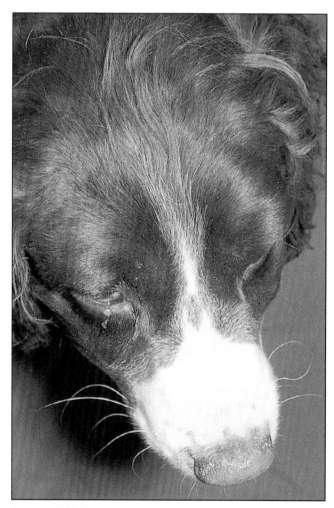

Figure 6.7 Examination for unilateral exophthalmos from the dorsal vantage point. There is some periocular swelling as well as mild exophthalmos. This dog has orbital hemorrhage from immune-mediated thrombocytopenia.

Table 6.4 **Signs of orbital disease.**

EXOPHTHALMOS OR ENOPHTHALMOS

- Prolapsed third eyelid.
- Deviations of the ocular axis (+/−).
- Periorbital swelling (+/−).
- Temporomandibular pain (+/−).
- Abnormal pupil size and function (+/−).
- Exposure keratitis (+/−).
- Blindness (+/−).
- Conjunctival hyperemia (+/−).
- Papilledema (+/−).
- Optic nerve atrophy (+/−).
- Orbital bruit (+/−).

determine the compressibility of the orbital contents. Compressibility is determined by pushing the eye into the orbit through the closed lids and determining the resistance to retropulsion (see Chapter 1, **Figure 1.4**). The degree of retropulsion is then compared between the two orbits.

> Orbital compressibility is an easy but frequently overlooked diagnostic test to confirm differences between the two orbits when evaluating an animal for exophthalmos.

Depending on the cause of the exophthalmos, additional signs of pain (ocular and on opening the mandible), ocular deviations or restrictions in movement, blindness, pressure striae in the fundus, prolapse of the third eyelid, and vascular congestion and swelling of the lids and conjunctiva may be present or may develop. **Table 6.5** presents the etiologies of exophthalmos. Further details are discussed with the specific diseases.

Diagnosis

Physical examination Physical examination of the mouth, sinuses, and teeth and history are very important in the workup of exophthalmos. Pain on opening the mouth and decreased retropulsion of the eye are typical of inflammatory disease. In larger dogs, deep palpation of the orbit may reveal a mass. Examination for ocular deviations or limitations of gaze may suggest the location of an orbital lesion. Masses within the muscle cone push the eye straight forward, and masses outside the muscle cone push the eye away from the mass. Vascular lesions are rare but produce unusual signs, such as an orbital bruit associated with an arteriovenous fistula[28] or intermittent exophthalmos dependent on head position associated with a venous aneurysm (varix).[29] Bilateral exophthalmos is relatively uncommon and is suggestive of a myositis of the muscles of mastication, a multicentric neoplasia, or systemic inflammatory/infectious disease.[30]

History The speed of onset and course are typically acute and short with inflammatory disease and hemorrhage and chronic with neoplasia. The response to prior therapy such as antibiotics or administration of systemic glucocorticoids may be important information. Information on relapse and pain should be obtained.

Radiography While noncontrast skull radiographs are routinely performed, it is, overall, a low-yield diagnostic test. Radiographs are examined for bone irregularities of the orbit, involvement of adjacent sinuses or nasal cavity, and tooth root lesions. Even when dramatic lesions from neoplastic invasion of the bony orbit are present, the changes on the radiographs are often subtle.

Orbitography Radiographs of the orbit utilizing contrast material of air or dye injected into the muscle cone or retroconal region may be helpful in defining an orbital lesion.[31] If the lesion cannot be localized by other techniques, then contrast orbital radiography may be indicated. However, excessive effort and money is often expended with these techniques, and a specific diagnosis is still not made.

Venograms and arteriograms Venograms of orbital veins via the angularis oculi vein, or arteriograms of the orbit by injecting the infraorbital artery, have been advocated for localizing and defining orbital lesions.[32,33]

Imaging techniques Magnetic resonance imaging (MRI) and computed tomography (CT) scans of the orbit have supplanted contrast radiographic procedures. They are the ideal noninvasive diagnostic techniques to evaluate the orbital contents and are now available in larger veterinary hospitals and clinics.[34–37]

Ultrasonography Ultrasonography is universally available in veterinary medicine and provides another practical and inexpensive imaging technique for detecting orbital lesions. Two-dimensional, real-time (B-mode) ultrasonography is useful in characterizing the lesions into discrete or nondiscrete and deforming or nondeforming lesions of the posterior globe.[38] In addition to transpalpebral and transcorneal imaging, orbital lesions should be imaged by a temporal approach, placing the probe laterally behind the orbital ligament.[39] The results of ultrasonography, like radiography, are

---

Table 6.5 Causes of exophthalmos.

- Orbital neoplasia: Primary or secondary
- Retro-orbital neoplasia: Bone, sinuses, nasal and oral cavity
- Orbital hemorrhage: Trauma, blood dyscrasia, clotting deficiencies
- Orbital cellulitis/abscess
- Retro-orbital cellulitis/abscess: Tooth root, zygomatic sialadenitis, foreign body
- Orbital edema: Trauma, immune-mediated?
- Orbital mucocele: Zygomatic origin
- Orbital cysts
- Arteriovenous fistula: Very rare
- Myositis of ocular muscles
- Myositis of muscles of mastication
- Mandibular hypertrophic osteoarthropathy in terriers

nonspecific in most cases, and the main advantage is localization of the lesion for future surgical exploration or guided-needle biopsies and fine-needle aspiration. Comparing ultrasonographic and histologic diagnoses in 116 eyes, satisfactory agreement was found for intraocular neoplasms and diseases of the lens, while inflammatory changes and retinal detachments showed relatively poor correlation.[40]

Fine-needle aspiration   Fine-needle aspiration (FNA) is inexpensive, rapid, and relatively safe and may yield a specific diagnosis. The main difficulty with this technique is the lack of certainty that the aspirated tissue is representative of the pathology. When FNA is positive, it usually eliminates the need for more extensive orbital surgery. In a series of fine-needle aspirates in 35 animals with exophthalmos, 34 were diagnostic.[41] However, in the author's own experience and that of others,[42] FNA has not been as successful in arriving at a specific diagnosis, and the cytologists often diagnose the type of neoplasia incorrectly. If lesions are observed on ultrasound, the FNA can be guided by ultrasound.

Orbital exploration   Exploratory orbital surgery is the main diagnostic modality for those cases that have not been diagnosed on cytology from FNA, have not responded to medical therapy, or are thought to be neoplastic. The surgical approach may vary depending on the animal's size and the location of the lesion. Animals with a large orbit and an anterior lesion may be explored and biopsied with a retrobulbar approach. Deep lesions with blind eyes may undergo enucleation or, if visual, a lateral orbitotomy.[43,44]

Laterality   Bilateral exophthalmos is usually due to systemic disease or myositis of the muscles of mastication or the extraocular muscles. Multicentric neoplasia, such as lymphosarcoma, may occasionally create bilateral exophthalmos in the dog and the cat, and orbital lymphosarcoma is well known in cattle.[45] Secondary or primary orbital neoplasia generally produces a unilateral, chronic, slowly progressing, nonpainful exophthalmos, but the author has observed neoplasia extending from the nose/frontal sinus region that extended into both orbits. Metastatic disease may occasionally involve both orbits, and bilateral orbital multilobular osteochondrosarcoma has been reported in the cat.[46]

Pain   While pain is typical of inflammatory lesions, milder degrees of discomfort in the periorbital region and temporomandibular joint may also be present with neoplasia. The presence of pain on opening the mouth should always be evaluated with exophthalmos. Granulomas and chronic walled-off abscesses may not have significant pain and are often referred to as pseudotumors, especially if idiopathic.[47,48] Cystic space-occupying lesions such as a mucocele are usually not painful.[49]

Ocular position   Ocular deviation usually points to the origin of the exophthalmos. Lesions in the muscle cone may restrict ocular movement and produce exophthalmos, blindness, and retinal pressure striae, but they usually do not produce an ocular deviation. The lesion is typically opposite to the direction of deviation.[50]

Onset   Sudden onset is typical of inflammatory lesions, but owners frequently underestimate the duration of exophthalmos with neoplasia.

Vision   Loss of vision with orbital disease is typically associated with involvement of the optic nerve and/or the chiasm with the orbital lesion. Bilateral blindness may result from chiasm involvement or, occasionally, from bilateral orbital disease. Retinal lesions may also contribute to blindness through retinal detachment or orbital lesions interfering with the retinal vascular system.

Lesion autonomy   For prognostic and diagnostic purposes, it may be helpful to determine whether structures surrounding the orbit are involved. Bone lysis is highly indicative of neoplasia, as is nasal and/or sinus involvement on radiographs.

Enophthalmos
Introduction/etiology
Enophthalmos, or a retraction of the globe into the orbit, must be differentiated from a decrease in globe size (microphthalmos, phthisis bulbi). This differentiation may be difficult because the globe may not be accessible to evaluate. The third eyelid is always prolapsed with enophthalmos. Entropion from loss of lid–globe support and ocular discharge are secondary events that may accompany enophthalmos. Causes of enophthalmos include:

- Extreme dehydration and cachexia: Will produce bilateral enophthalmos.
- Increased tone to extraocular muscles: Tetanus and strychnine poisoning produces enophthalmos by increased extraocular muscle (retractor) tone.
- Atrophy of orbital fat: Trauma to the orbit may result in post-traumatic atrophy of orbital fat and/or fibrosis of tissues causing restricted globe movement.

- Loss of periorbital lining: In the cat, a paradoxical syndrome of enophthalmos with orbital neoplasia may occur.[51] The enophthalmos is severe and may be confused with microphthalmos or phthisis bulbi. The enophthalmos is thought to be due to loss of the lateral–ventral periorbita, which essentially expands the orbit.
- Loss of retro-orbital muscle mass: Atrophy of the muscles of mastication is a relatively common cause of enophthalmos that may be unilateral or bilateral.

> Lesions that may be concurrent with orbital disease: periorbital lesions in the mouth, nasal cavity, sinuses, upper arcades, muscles of mastication; ocular lesions that may extend out of the globe such as neoplasia or infection.

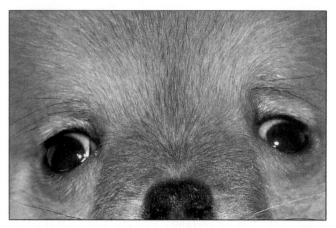

Figure 6.8 Lateral–ventral deviation of the eyes in a puppy with hydrocephalus due to expansion of the calvarium into the orbit.

Diagnosis

Important factors in the differentiation of the causes of enophthalmos are bilateral versus unilateral, the presence/absence of systemic signs, and the history.

Congenital orbital disease
Shallow orbits

The most common congenital abnormality of the orbit is a shallow orbit, usually observed in the brachycephalic breeds. Expansion of the orbit with growth depends on having a globe in the orbit and, consequently, if an eye is microphthalmic or enucleated early in life, the normal orbital size is not obtained.[4,52] A shallow orbit may also develop from congenital hydrocephalus, where the associated expansion of the calvarium encroaches on the orbit from the dorsomedial quadrant (**Figure 6.8**).

The significance of a shallow orbit depends on the degree of exophthalmos and consequent lagophthalmos. Animals with a shallow orbit are more susceptible to tear film problems, exposure keratitis, and traumatic injuries ranging from corneal abrasion to proptosis. A partial tarsorrhaphy (see Chapter 7) and ocular lubricants are utilized in both a proactive and reactive manner in animals with this conformation.

Extraocular muscle agenesis/hypoplasia

A congenital lack of most of the extraocular muscles was described in a miniature poodle. The patient was presented with a marked hypertropia in one eye that precluded vision and an esotropia in the opposite eye (**Figure 6.9**). On orbital exploration, only the medial rectus and the ventral oblique muscles were present. Excision of the medial rectus freed the globe, and the muscle was

diagnosed on histopathology to be hypoplastic.[53] A similar syndrome was observed in a goat kid (**Figure 6.10**).

Acquired orbital disease—inflammation
Orbital cellulitis/abscess, retro-orbital cellulitis/abscess
Introduction/etiology

Due to the incomplete bony orbit, the signs of inflammation inside the orbit are similar to retro-orbital inflammation, and the process may extend from one region to the other. Unless the cause of the space-occupying lesion is uncertain and surgical exploration is being considered, it is usually not important or possible

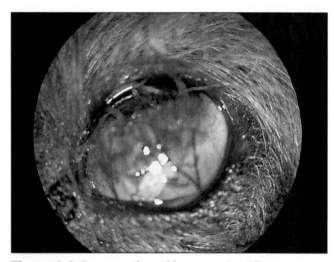

Figure 6.9 Severe unilateral hypertropia with excyclotropia that is fixed in position in a young dog. Surgical exploration revealed aplasia of all the extraocular muscles except the medial rectus and the ventral oblique, which were hypoplastic. The cornea is barely visible under the upper lid.

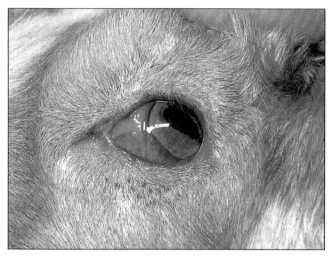

Figure 6.10 Young goat with congenital strabismus due to aplasia and hypoplastic extraocular muscles. The globe is immobile, needing forced duction or forceps to move the globe.

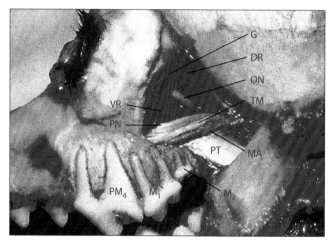

Figure 6.11 Dissected canine skull to illustrate the relationship of the upper dental arcade to the orbit. (G: Posterior globe; DR: Dorsal rectus muscle; ON: Optic nerve; VR: Ventral rectus muscle; TM: Maxillary branch of the trigeminal nerve; PN: Pterygopalatine nerve; MA: Maxillary artery; PT: Medial pterygoid muscle; PM₄: Maxillary fourth premolar tooth; M₁: Maxillary first molar tooth; M₂: Maxillary second molar tooth.) (From Ramsey, D.T. et al. 1996. *Journal of the American Animal Hospital Association* 32:215–224.)

to differentiate the two conditions. Most patients with orbital inflammation are presented in the acute cellulitis stage because of the dramatic signs. Abrams and Goodwin reported that 52% of canine cases of orbital cellulitis were presented during August and September.[54] The cause of the cellulitis was not established, which is frequently the case.

An important cause of orbital cellulitis is extension from an infected tooth root, nasal sinus, or zygomatic salivary gland (**Figure 6.11**).[55–57] A migrating plant foreign body, such as a grass awn, or penetration of a foreign body through the soft palate or posterior pharyngeal area are important and seasonal causes for retro-orbital cellulitis in many regions. When cellulitis is associated with extension from teeth or sinuses, or caused from a foreign body, it often responds to therapy, but relapse can occur if the primary cause is not removed. Direct inoculation into the orbit from a periocular injury through the lids or the conjunctiva may occur in both large and small animals.[58,59]

Orbital/retro-orbital inflammation is common in the dog and less common in other species. Most cases are due to bacterial infection, often anaerobic,[60,61] and respond promptly to antibiotics. However, mycotic etiologies have been described. Systemic mycoses such as *Cryptococcus* have been observed in the orbit of small animals and horses.[62,63] Cryptococcosis may be generalized or spread from local lesions in the adjacent sinuses and nasal cavity. Saprophytic fungi such as *Penicillium* spp. or *Aspergillus* spp. may rarely involve the orbit[64,65] and usually extend from the adjacent sinuses or from systemic involvement. An adult *Toxocara canis* worm has been reported as producing an acute orbital

cellulitis syndrome.[160] In many instances, the origin of the inflammation is not definitively determined.

Clinical signs
Orbital cellulitis typically has a sudden onset of unilateral protrusion of third eyelid, exophthalmos, and conjunctival swelling and hyperemia (**Figures 6.12 through 6.15**). If observed before exophthalmos is

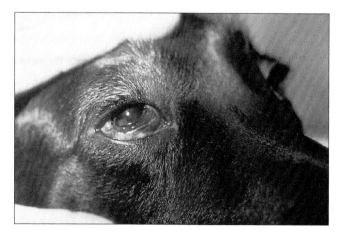

Figure 6.12 Early orbital cellulitis in a dog manifesting with prolapsed third eyelid, conjunctival hyperemia, mild mucopurulent exudation, and minimal periocular swelling. Easily misdiagnosed as conjunctivitis.

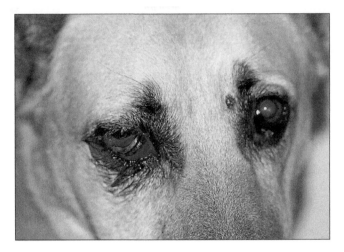

Figure 6.13 A dog with orbital cellulitis, with more dramatic signs of prolapsed third eyelid, conjunctival hyperemia, exophthalmos, and ocular discharge. Pain on opening the mouth will be evident.

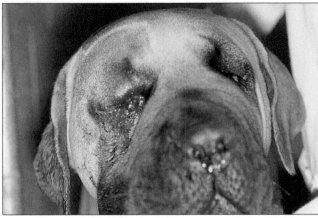

Figure 6.15 Extreme signs of orbital cellulitis in a dog with turgid swelling over the side and top of the head that on aspiration was purulent. The animal had received systemic prednisone. Anaerobes were cultured.

severe, it is likely to be misdiagnosed as conjunctivitis (**Figure 6.12**). Ocular discharge is generally present and begins as a serous discharge that rapidly develops to a mucoid to mucopurulent discharge. Retropulsion of the globe is decreased, with varying degrees of periocular swelling. The periocular swelling may migrate over the top of the head and/or may become dependent when severe. One of the most dramatic signs is often the severe pain manifest on periocular palpation and on opening the mouth. The pain can be so severe that cervical disk disease has been confused with the condition. Fever, depression, and leukocytosis may occur in severe cases but is not universal.

Usually, heavy sedation or general anesthesia is necessary to inspect the posterior oral cavity, and swelling or a fistula may be present in the roof of the mouth behind the last molar (**Figure 6.16**). The salivary gland papilla and posterior upper teeth should also be inspected for obvious pathology. On occasion, some of the patients that have a zygomatic sialadenitis may have an inflamed papilla and altered salivary secretions (**Figure 6.17**). Depending on which tooth roots are infected, either orbital cellulitis or a fistula that opens under the eye may be seen. The latter is classical for infection of the lateral roots of the fourth upper premolar tooth (**Figures 6.18 through 6.20**).

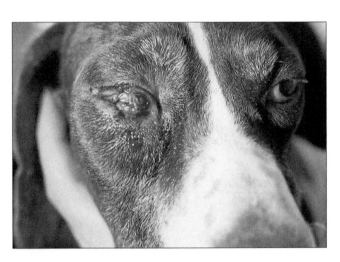

Figure 6.14 Moderately severe signs of orbital cellulitis in a dog with dramatic periocular swelling and prolapsed third eyelid. The globe is normal behind the third eyelid. The cause was a zygomatic sialadenitis (see Figure 6.17).

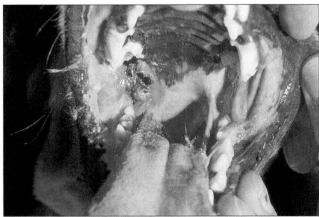

Figure 6.16 Examination of the mouth of a dog with orbital cellulitis under general anesthesia. Swelling and a fistula are present in the typical location behind the last upper molar.

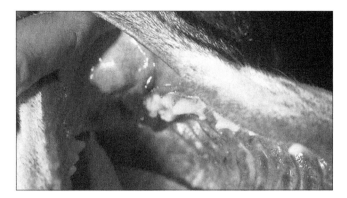

Figure 6.17 Inflamed zygomatic salivary gland papilla from the dog in Figure 6.14. Secretions were very viscous.

> Orbital cellulitis is a dramatic syndrome and is most common in the dog. It usually responds to systemic antibiotics, but a nidus for infection should be considered with relapsing conditions.

Diagnosis

Diagnosis of orbital cellulitis/abscess is made on the clinical signs of acute exophthalmos with pain, but differentiation from masticatory myositis may be difficult in the early stages. Diagnosing the cause of the cellulitis should involve inspection of the oral cavity for problems involving the upper molars, the last premolars, and the zygomatic papilla. If the area behind the last molars is swollen or has a fistula, careful probing may locate an abscess, and culturing may identify the infectious agent. Skull radiographs and ultrasound are particularly indicated in atypical cases or those that have relapsed.

Differential diagnosis

Differentials include other space-occupying orbital/retro-orbital masses. Neoplasia may exhibit pain, ocular discharge,

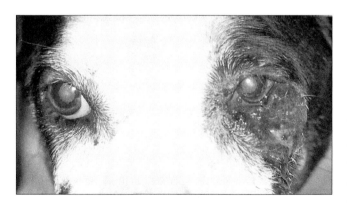

Figure 6.18 Chronic granulation under the eye from fistulation of an infected lateral root of the fourth upper premolar tooth.

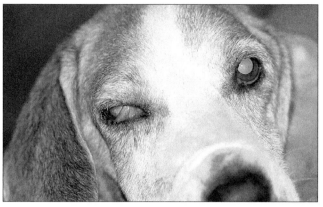

Figure 6.19 Aged beagle with exophthalmos, prolapsed third eyelid, and temporomandibular pain (note the muzzle). The edema below the eye is somewhat atypical for pure orbital cellulitis of this severity. Marked gum recession with root exposure is evident with several teeth of the upper arcade.

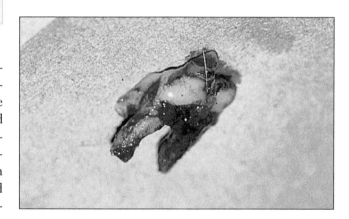

Figure 6.20 Fourth upper premolar from the dog in Figure 6.19. Note the black medial root.

and swelling but in general is nonpainful or not as acutely painful as inflammation (**Figure 6.21**). Fulminating panophthalmitis that extends into the orbit produces and mimics orbital cellulitis, but it has diffuse intraocular lesions and results in blindness (**Figure 6.22**).[161] A history of starting in the eye and later developing orbital signs, and the obvious intraocular pathology, should differentiate panophthalmitis from simple orbital cellulitis.

Orbital hemorrhage manifests as an acute space-occupying lesion, often with some degree of discomfort. If the hemorrhage does not dissect forward to the subconjunctival space, it may be confused with orbital cellulitis (**Figure 6.7**). Dicoumarol poisoning causing retrobulbar hemorrhage has at times been difficult to differentiate from cellulitis when the history is incomplete, and the hemorrhage does not dissect forward.

Early orbital cellulitis may have a similar presentation to acute masticatory myositis, with swelling and pain,

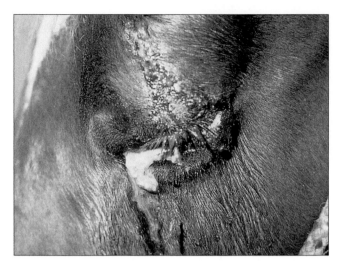

Figure 6.21 Horse with signs suggestive of orbital cellulitis (purulent ocular discharge, periocular swelling, decreased orbital retropulsion). FNA and biopsy behind the zygomatic arch diagnosed a squamous cell carcinoma.

except that myositis is typically bilateral. Cystic orbital lesions such as mucoceles will not have the acute pain or extensive periorbital involvement.

The main rule outs for orbital cellulitis/abscess are masticatory myositis, orbital neoplasia, orbital hemorrhage, and cellulitis as an extension of panophthalmitis.

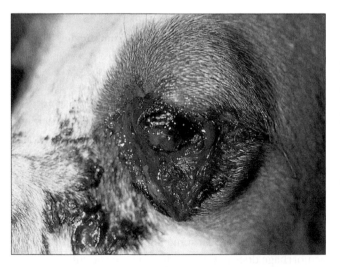

Figure 6.22 Hunting dog presented in the fall with an endophthalmitis presumed to be due to a plant foreign body. Despite systemic antibiotics, the process progressed through the sclera to involve the orbit within 24 hours. The dramatic ocular involvement differentiates this from a pure orbital cellulitis. Plant material (grass awns) was observed in the globe on histopathology with polarized light.

Therapy

Early in the disease, penicillin administered at a dose of 20,000–30,000 U/kg usually arrests and cures most uncomplicated cases of orbital cellulitis. Alternatively, other drugs that are effective against anaerobes, such as metronidazole, amoxicillin–clavulanate, chloramphenicol, and clindamycin, may be used. Due to the pain on opening the mouth, the injectable route is often used. In the author's experience, procaine penicillin has been more consistent in effecting a response than the broad-spectrum synthetic penicillins. Improvement is usually noted within 24–48 hours. If a relapse occurs, re-examination for a nidus of infection, such as an infected tooth root or a foreign body, is indicated. If skull radiographs were not performed initially, they are indicated at this time.

Because of the marked exophthalmos, lagophthalmos is frequently present, and the cornea may have to be protected by the liberal application of ointments.

Surgical drainage of the orbit by lancing the mucosa behind the last molar is often recommended for the treatment of orbital infection (**Figure 6.23**). However, since the procedure sets the resolution process back by about 48 hours, and the yield for finding an abscess is low, the author does not use drainage if the area is not swollen or discolored. If the area is swollen, drainage may be achieved by puncturing and probing with a blunt instrument such as a hemostat. A blade should not be used as the infraorbital artery may be incised. If the periorbital swelling is severe and has migrated over the head, and on needle aspiration the material is purulent, a Penrose drain

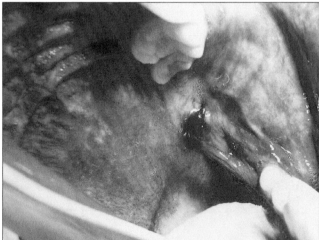

Figure 6.23 Lancing the soft area behind the last molar in a dog with orbital cellulitis. Probing should be with a blunt instrument. Sanguinopurulent material is draining from the opening, but often only blood is obtained if the area is not swollen.

is inserted. Obviously, if the source of the cellulitis is an infected tooth root, the tooth is extracted (**Figure 6.20**).

Eosinophilic (masticatory) myositis

Introduction/etiology

Eosinophilic myositis is best known for its acute involvement of the muscles of mastication. The pronounced muscle swelling impinges on the nonbony orbital wall, often producing dramatic ocular signs of exophthalmos, conjunctival hyperemia, third eyelid prolapse, and, occasionally, blindness from optic nerve involvement. The myositis may be more generalized than just the muscles of mastication, and the term polymyositis is more appropriate when this is evident. Masticatory muscles are predominantly type 2M fibers, whereas limb muscles contain types 1, 2A, and 2C fibers.[66,67] Eosinophilic myositis is predominantly found in large breeds of dogs, less than 4 years of age.[68] The syndrome was initially thought to affect primarily German shepherd dogs (GSDs) or GSD crosses, Weimaraners, Samoyeds, and Doberman pinschers, but it is not restricted to any breed.[67,68]

In the acute phase of the disease, the histopathologic findings are multifocal or diffuse plasmocytic, lymphocytic, macrophagic, and eosinophilic infiltration of the muscles with muscle necrosis.[67,68] The disease is suspected to be immune mediated, with selective reaction against the type 2M fibers,[67] and is characterized by recurrent, acute attacks that eventually result in muscle atrophy. The remission phase is variable, ranging from weeks to months. Blindness due to optic neuritis may also occur.[68–70]

Masticatory myositis has been reported in a horse as the main sign of nutritional selenium deficiency.[71] The signs were restricted to the masticatory muscles and eyes and were not generalized, perhaps because the horse had been restricted to a stall.

Clinical signs

Typically, masticatory myositis presents with bilaterally swollen, firm muscles of mastication, although early in the course, the swelling may be asymmetrical (**Figure 6.24**). The swelling is accompanied by trismus (difficulty in opening the mouth) and pain on opening the jaw. Peripheral lymphadenopathy may be present. On laboratory testing, peripheral eosinophilia is uncommon, but serum globulin and creatine kinase levels are often elevated.[68]

The exophthalmos with masticatory myositis may be dramatic and may produce a secondary exposure keratitis. Conjunctival vascular injection produces a red eye, and with exophthalmos, the condition may mimic glaucoma. The third eyelid is prolapsed from orbital pressure, and blindness that is later associated with optic nerve atrophy occasionally occurs.[68,69,72] If there are other signs of

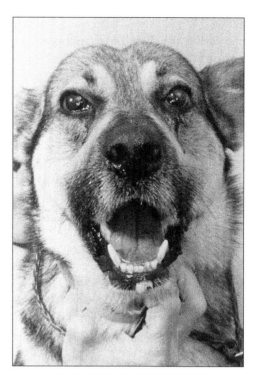

Figure 6.24 **Masticatory myositis evidenced by swollen temporal and masseter muscles and difficulty opening the mouth.**

muscular involvement, such as gait abnormalities, dysphagia, and profound weakness, polymyositis is probably present.[73]

The disease is characterized by recurrent attacks with each episode lasting 2–3 weeks. With repeated episodes, muscle atrophy develops and may result in enophthalmos with prolapse of the third eyelid, weight loss from the inability to eat, and loss of muscle mass of the head.

Diagnosis

The signalment and elevated serum creatine phosphokinase (CPK) during the acute phase (>200 IU/L) are very suggestive of the diagnosis of masticatory myositis. Elevations of CPK can be due to other insults to the muscles, such as trauma and medication injections. Elevated levels of the muscle enzymes CPK, aspartate aminotransferase, or lactic dehydrogenase have been variable in polymyositis, and normal levels do not rule out the diagnosis.[73]

A muscle biopsy with mononuclear inflammation and eosinophils is the most definitive test, but negative findings may occur due to sampling error since the inflammation may be patchy. Phagocytosis of necrotic myofibers is the most common histopathologic finding.[67]

Electromyography is not widely available in practice, but it may give additional evidence of myositis or polymyositis.

Therapy

Treatment during the acute phase is systemic predniso-lone at anti-inflammatory doses. Once the swelling and acute signs disappear, the dose is halved for a period of 2–3 weeks, and if remission is maintained, it is halved until a maintenance dose of 5–10 mg every other day is obtained. Therapy should be continued for several months and the animal monitored frequently for relapses. The emphasis is on control rather than on a cure. Alternatively, concurrent systemic prednisolone and azathioprine may be given[68]; after 3–4 weeks, the prednisolone is tapered off leaving a maintenance therapy of azathioprine.

Some of the worst cases of orbital cellulitis and absces-sation the author has observed had been misdiagnosed as masticatory myositis and had received immunosuppres-sive doses of prednisone (**Figure 6.15**). These cases were life threatening, were managed by experienced clinicians, and had undergone electromyography; such cases empha-size the importance of muscle biopsies to make a diagnosis of masticatory myositis when presented with an atypical clinical syndrome.

> Masticatory myositis and orbital cellulitis may be difficult to differentiate in the prodromal phase, and, unfortunately, their therapies are diametrically opposed.

Prognosis

The prognosis may be good if adequate glucocorticoid or other immunosuppressive therapy is administered early, at appropriate doses, for an adequate period of 3–4 weeks and then tapered gradually.[68] Client education is crucial to emphasize the importance of treating any relapses promptly.

Extraocular myositis

Introduction/etiology

A syndrome of myositis restricted to the extraocular muscles has been reported in the young (usually <1 year) Golden retriever, GSD, and Doberman pinscher.[74] About 30% of the patients had a recent, stressful event associated with the onset of the signs. The earliest sign is conjunctival hyperemia that develops into a nonpainful bilateral exoph-thalmos and apparent lid retraction (**Figure 6.25**). Vision is affected in 17% of cases, with funduscopic lesions of vascular tortuosity, focal retinitis, and papilledema that is reversible with therapy.[75] The intraocular pressure (IOP) may be mildly elevated. Repeated episodes may result in strabismus and mild enophthalmos.

Histopathologic examination of the extraocular muscles is characterized by a mononuclear infiltrate of

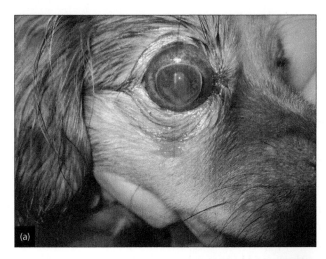

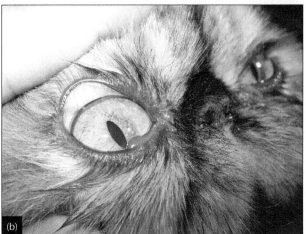

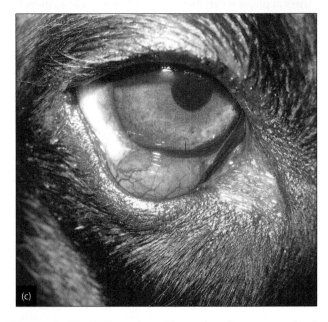

Figure 6.25 (a) Ventral strabismus in a dog as a result of restrictive myositis. (b) Orbital fat prolapse in a cat. Note the swelling of the dorsal bulbar conjunctiva. (c) Orbital fat prolapse in a dog. Note the swelling of the ventral bulbar conjunctiva.

T-lymphocytes in the extraocular muscle bellies, with the retractor muscle being spared.[74,75] The masticatory muscles are normal clinically and histopathologically.

Therapy
The condition was initially reported as responsive to a short course of systemic anti-inflammatory doses of glucocorticoids.[74] Ramsey et al. reported poor response to therapy when less than 1.1 mg/kg every 12 hours of prednisone was administered and a 57% relapse rate if the dose was tapered before 3 weeks.[75] Recurrences occurred in 81% of the dogs and may have been related to stress.

Restrictive extraocular myositis
Introduction/etiology
Restrictive extraocular myositis presents as a rapidly acquired, severe strabismus in young dogs of large breeds. It may be unilateral or bilateral. Reported breeds have been the Irish wolfhound, Shar Pei, Akita, Golden retriever, and dalmatian.[76] No relationship was found with masticatory myositis or generalized polymyositis. Restrictive extraocular myositis may be the end result of acute extraocular myositis as described in the Golden retriever, but the breeds involved, variation in clinical signs, and laterality make it unlikely. Histopathology is characterized by muscle fibrosis, myonecrosis, and mononuclear inflammation.

Clinical signs
Restrictive myositis presents as a rapidly developing strabismus in the ventral to ventromedial direction, and enophthalmos in young adult large breeds. Forced duction tests (forceps applied to the globe to move it) are positive or restricted when the globe is abducted or sursumducted (elevated). Limited serology for immune-mediated disease, infectious agents, antibodies against 2M fibers, and muscle enzymes are normal.[76]

Therapy
To date, therapy has been surgical resection of the affected extraocular muscles (ventral and medial rectus, ventral oblique) with good results, although enophthalmos persists. If the patient presents with acute signs, potent systemic anti-inflammatory therapy such as azathioprine and glucocorticoids would be indicated. However, the former seldom occurs.

Trauma (orbital fractures, hemorrhage, and edema)
Introduction/etiology
Blunt orbital trauma may result in fractures of the bones of the orbit or orbital rim. Swelling, crepitus, pain, and exophthalmos are usually present with acute fractures.

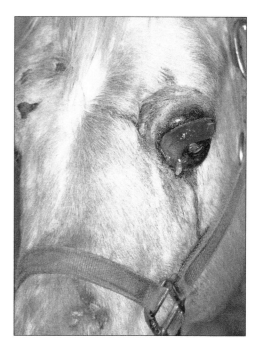

Figure 6.26 Head trauma in a horse resulting in bilateral fractures of the supraorbital process of the frontal bone. Severe chemosis and periocular swelling make it difficult to examine the eye. The eye is deviated ventrally, but it is normal. The fractured process was elevated, and the swelling resolved.

Chronic fractures may not have pain and crepitus. In the horse, fractures of the supraorbital process are relatively common (**Figure 6.26**). Fracture of the medial portion of the supraorbital process or the lacrimal bone may damage the paranasal sinuses, resulting in epistaxis, and it is a possible source for orbital sepsis.[77] Occasionally, severe orbital hemorrhage may occur secondary to trauma.

Shearing injuries to the optic nerve as it passes through the optic foramen may result in blindness. In the dog, the most common source of optic nerve injury secondary to trauma is associated with proptosis of the globe. In the horse, traumatic optic nerve injuries usually occur from a blow to the poll and involve the region of the optic nerve traversing the optic canal[78] or the chiasm.

The cat frequently develops orbital trauma associated with multiple fractures of the head (palatine, mandibular) from automobile accidents. The resultant exophthalmos often results in severe lagophthalmos and may require a temporary tarsorrhaphy for protection.

Diagnosis
Diagnosis of traumatic orbital disease is made on the history and associated contusions and abrasions and by radiography. Oblique radiographic views are often necessary to demonstrate fractures due to the complex anatomy of the region.

Therapy

Therapy is directed at protecting the cornea if exposure keratitis develops from proptosis or palpebral nerve paralysis. Medical therapy is indicated in the acute case to relieve swelling and may consist of cold compresses (for the first 24 hours) followed by warm compresses, systemic glucocorticoids, and dimethyl sulfoxide (DMSO). A tarsorrhaphy may be necessary to protect the cornea.

Repair of fractures should be performed if bony displacement is significant.

Orbital mucocele

Introduction/etiology

In the dog, a mucocele may rarely develop from the zygomatic salivary gland and extend into the orbit. Only one case has been reported in the cat[79] and the ferret.[80] Most cases in the literature have had obvious trauma,[81,82] although they may also develop spontaneously.[79,83] The presentation has been quite varied.

Clinical signs

Orbital mucoceles are presented with nonpainful exophthalmos, or enophthalmos, depending on which direction the mucocele is pushing the globe. Dissection of the mucocele behind the eye produces exophthalmos, and if dissection occurs forward to the orbital rim, it may push the globe caudally into the orbit. The location of the mucocele is variable and may present as a fluctuant swelling in the lower conjunctival cul-de-sac or on the top of the head (**Figure 6.27**).[83] Accompanying the orbital mucocele, a ranula-like swelling may be present along the duct in the mouth.

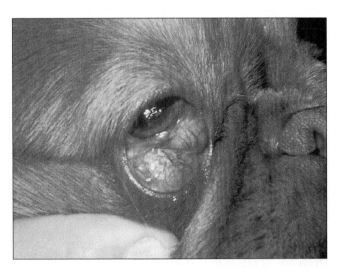

Figure 6.27 A dog with a zygomatic mucocele presenting as a fluctuant nonpainful swelling under the lower lid. The mucocele extended into the orbit, and there was also a ranula-like swelling in the oral vestibule.

Optic neuropathy and corneal ulcerations may occur as complications.

Diagnosis

The mucocele must be differentiated from other periocular cystic lesions and prolapse of orbital fat. Aspiration of the cyst may disclose a "honey-like material," but orbital cysts associated with nasal adenocarcinomas can have a similar consistency. The diagnosis is facilitated if an oral swelling involving the zygomatic duct located over the last molar is present. Sialography of the zygomatic salivary gland is the most definitive method of diagnosis.

Therapy

If the zygomatic duct is swollen in the mouth, marsupialization may be curative,[83] but most cases have had the cyst and the zygomatic salivary gland excised through an orbitotomy.[82,162]

Orbital neoplasia

Introduction/etiology

Neoplasia of the orbit is rather common in small animals and may be classified as primary or secondary. Secondary neoplasia may arise from distant metastasis, multicentric neoplasia, or extension from contiguous structures. While the incidence of orbital neoplasia increases with age, many are presented in the dog in young (2- to 3-year-old) animals.

Cattle have a unique syndrome of bilateral orbital involvement with lymphosarcoma, which is relatively rare in other species. This produces a gradually developing unilateral or bilateral exophthalmos. The cow usually has involvement of other lymph nodes and target organs, and the globe is not involved except secondarily from exposure (**Figure 6.28**). Most animals die within 6 months.[45]

Orbital lymphosarcoma also occurs in young dogs and is typically very fulminating. The eyes are normal unless exposure keratitis develops (**Figure 6.29**).

In the dog, almost all orbital neoplasms are malignant (91%–95%) and 75%–82% are primary orbital tumors. The typical dog is purebred, female, and middle-aged (8 years old).[42,84,85] Large breeds are overrepresented in the author's experience.

Over 18 tumor types have been reported from the orbit. Primary neoplasia originates from orbital bone, muscle, lacrimal gland, and neural, vascular, fat, and connective tissue. Osteosarcoma, fibrosarcoma, multilobular osteosarcoma (chondroma rodens), meningioma, glioma, rhabdomyosarcoma, squamous cell carcinoma, and adenocarcinoma may occur as primary neoplasms, with connective tissue tumors predominating.[42,84,85] Orbital cellulitis may be confused with neoplasia because both conditions may exhibit pain on opening the mouth and be

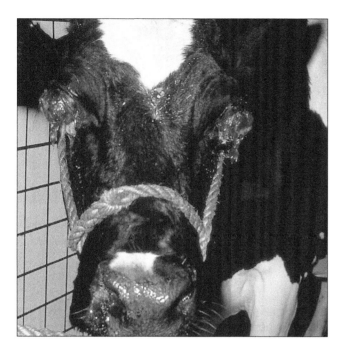

Figure 6.28 Bilateral lymphosarcoma of the orbit in a cow, producing marked exophthalmos and a secondary exposure keratitis. (Courtesy of Dr. W. Rebhun [deceased] of Ithaca, NY.)

transiently responsive to antibiotics. Thirty-six percent of orbital tumors had signs that were suggestive of cellulitis.[42] Case reports abound on a variety of orbital tumors but with relatively few series of cases. A few unique tumor types are discussed in detail below.

> Approximately 90% of orbital tumors are malignant, and about one-third mimic orbital cellulitis with exophthalmos and some degree of pain.

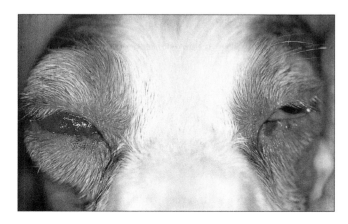

Figure 6.29 Bilateral orbital lymphosarcoma in a young Brittany spaniel. The eyes were normal except for exposure keratitis. Exophthalmos is more severe in one eye. Generalized peripheral lymphadenopathy was present.

Multilobular osteosarcoma

Multilobular osteosarcoma is a dramatic but infrequent orbital tumor that has had multiple case reports. Historically, synonyms for the tumor have varied, creating confusion and implying the tumor was benign. Synonyms have included parosteal osteoma, multilobular osteoma, chondroma rodens, and calcifying aponeurotic fibroma.[86] While multilobular osteosarcoma may initially be benign, follow-up examinations indicate that 58% develop metastases by 14 months, and this percentage increases if the tumor is incompletely excised. The lesions develop from the membranous bones of the skull, that is, mandible, maxilla, or cranium. The histologic feature is nodules that have a cartilaginous or osteoid core, surrounded by fibrous tissue. Plain radiographs are often suggestive of the diagnosis and demonstrate multiple lobules of tumor, which contain calcium. In one report, the overall median survival rate was 22 months.[86]

Canine orbital meningioma Canine orbital meningioma is a relatively benign tumor that arises within the muscle cone, so it typically produces exophthalmos without strabismus. Patients with meningiomas frequently have visual complaints (60%) and fundus lesions from involvement of the optic nerve (35%). Bilateral blindness may occur from invasion of the cranial vault and involvement of the chiasm. The tumors are epithelioid (meningotheliomatous), and the majority contain bone or cartilage metaplasia.[87]

Canine lobular orbital adenoma Headrick et al.[163] described a benign lobular tumor of lacrimal or salivary gland origin. The mass most commonly presented as a subconjunctival and, less frequently, as a space occupying orbital mass (i.e., exophthalmos, third eyelid protrusion, decreased retropulsion). Recurrences were common after surgical excision or even enucleation, but metastasis was not documented.

Feline orbital tumors Feline orbital tumors have similar characteristics to the dog—age group (8.9 years old) and malignancy (90%)—but secondary (71%) and epithelial (67%) orbital tumors predominate. All primary orbital tumors in one report were mesenchymal,[88] and the mean survival time was 1.9 months. Enophthalmos was present in 24% of the cats, and fine-needle aspirates (FNAs) were diagnostic in only 45% of the patients. Enophthalmos is unique to orbital neoplasia in the cat.[51,88]

> The short survival time of cats with orbital neoplasia is in large part due to early euthanasia.

Orbital tumors in the horse

Orbital tumors in the horse are rare and are usually secondary tumors. Orbital extension of ocular or eyelid squamous cell carcinoma and lymphosarcoma are most common.[89] Case reports of a variety of equine orbital tumors exist without giving a clear picture of tumor frequency and malignancy. Tumors reported from the equine orbit include melanoma,[90] adenocarcinoma, glioma,[91] multiple osteoma,[92] neuroepithelial tumor,[93] and lipoma.[94]

Paraganglioma   Paraganglioma is a unique orbital tumor that has been described in the horse.[94,95] It arises from the neuroendocrine system and in the orbit is thought to arise from the ciliary ganglion.[95] Paraganglioma may invade the orbit from the nasal cavity and sinuses.[96] It appears to be slow growing but may metastasize or invade the cranial cavity through the optic foramen.[94] Systemic hypotension and severe hemorrhage may be complications during surgical resection.[97]

Clinical signs

Orbital neoplasia typically presents with a unilateral, non-painful, slowly progressive exophthalmos with decreased retropulsion of the globe. Metastases or, more commonly, multicentric or secondary neoplasia from the sinuses or nasal cavity, may be bilateral (**Figure 6.29**). Some degree of pain may be present from inflammation; Hendrix and Gelatt[42] reported that 36% of dogs with orbital neoplasia had signs of pain, ocular discharge, and at least a transient response to antibiotics, mimicking orbital cellulitis. The third eyelid is prolapsed, and if the lesion is outside the muscle cone, a strabismus is present (**Figure 6.30**). Lesions outside the muscle cone and anterior in the orbit may be able to be palpated near the orbital rim. Lesions

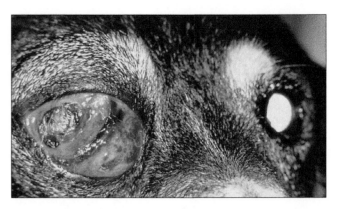

Figure 6.31 A dog with a meningioma producing marked proptosis of the globe. Severe exposure keratitis developed, and the eye was blind.

within the muscle cone, such as meningiomas, are likely to produce visual problems due to involvement of the optic nerve (**Figure 6.31**). Papilledema may be present early in the disease (**Figure 6.32**), and optic nerve atrophy results later if the neoplasia is impinging on the optic nerve. Pressure striae and indentation of the globe may be visible on ophthalmoscopy (**Figure 6.33**).

An enophthalmos syndrome has been observed in cats with the extension of a fibrosarcoma and squamous cell carcinoma into the orbit. The enophthalmos is profound and is not due to pushing of the eye into the orbit; rather, it is due to loss of the lateral periorbita from an unknown

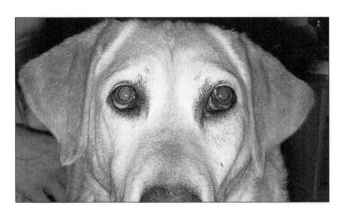

Figure 6.30 A dog with a multilobular osteosarcoma involving the ventral and ventromedial left orbit. Note the prolapsed third eyelid, dorsolateral strabismus, and swelling below the left eye that was very firm.

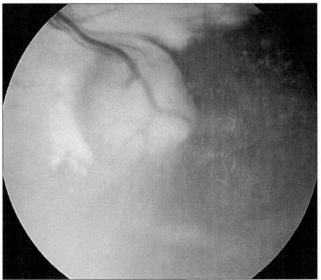

Figure 6.32 A dog with severe papilledema produced by an orbital mass that was diagnosed as a carcinoma on FNA. A very advanced renal carcinoma was also diagnosed and removed. It was not possible to determine whether the orbital lesion was a metastatic lesion or a primary lesion. Severe asteroid hyalosis obscures fine detail.

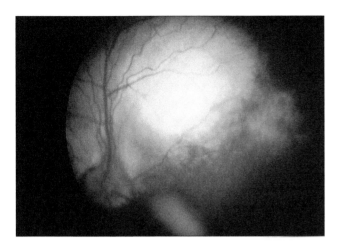

Figure 6.33 Canine fundus that is indented due to orbital involvement with a multilobular osteosarcoma. Most of the dorsal fundus is pushed inward.

mechanism. The loss of periorbita essentially expands the orbital space, and the eye sinks into the expanded space (**Figure 6.34**).

Diagnosis

A slowly progressive exophthalmos with minimal pain is highly suggestive of orbital neoplasia. Localization of the lesion in preparation for exploratory surgery is by deep orbital palpation, the direction of ocular deviation, ultrasound, radiography, and CT or MRI scans. Orbital neoplasia is characterized on ultrasonography by margins of the lesions being delineated, usually hypoechoic,

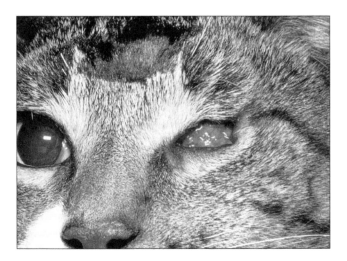

Figure 6.34 A cat with enophthalmos associated with a fibrosarcoma that was present over the frontal sinus (shaved area) and invaded the orbit. The mass was not pushing the eye into the orbit but was associated with a loss of lateral periorbita that expanded the orbit. The globe was normal on enucleation.

homogeneous, and often indenting the globe. The presence of mineralization of the lesion was indicative of neoplasia.[164]

Radiographs of the skull are taken to help define the composition of the neoplasia and to determine whether bony lysis has occurred and whether the adjacent structures, such as the nasal and frontal sinus cavities, may be the source of the neoplasia. FNA should be attempted if the location of the lesion is known. Because of questions on interpretation of the cytology, an excisional biopsy is often still required for diagnosing the type of tumor. For a definitive diagnosis, orbital exploration and biopsy are performed.

In medium to large-size dogs with adequate orbit size and with lesions outside the muscle cone, the author usually uses a transpalpebral approach to the quadrant in which the lesion is localized. In patients in which the lesion cannot be localized, the lesion is in the muscle cone, or, in small dogs and cats, with minimal space in the orbit to manipulate, a more extensive lateral orbitotomy with resection of the zygomatic arch is indicated.[43,44]

Therapy

The literature has concentrated on tumor types and clinical signs, with few reports of the results of therapy. Despite the malignant nature of these tumors, it is not uncommon to obtain survival rates of 6–12 months with combined surgical and radiation therapies. Hendrix and Gelatt reported 86% survival at 6 months of dogs following therapy.[42] However, further analysis was impossible due to the small numbers of patients in each therapy group.

Excision Due to the malignant nature of most orbital tumors, excision is not curative but debulks the lesion and provides a diagnosis. Primary orbital tumors that are isolated may respond to orbital exenteration. Exenteration of the orbit rather than enucleation is indicated for neoplasia and involves removal of the globe and orbital contents. Technically, exenteration is performed by stripping the periorbita from the bone, staying outside the orbit with the surgical dissection until the apex is ligated and excised. As usually performed, exenteration is not complete but is a transpalpebral enucleation with excision of the extraocular muscles (**Figure 6.35**). In horses, cats, and some dogs, if a wide skin excision is made around the lids, the amount of loose skin that can be mobilized over the exenterated orbit is very limited. A flap dissected over the course of the caudal auricular artery on the lateral cervical region and transposed forward over the orbit has been utilized with some success. The most common problem was distal flap necrosis, which required a revision surgery.[165]

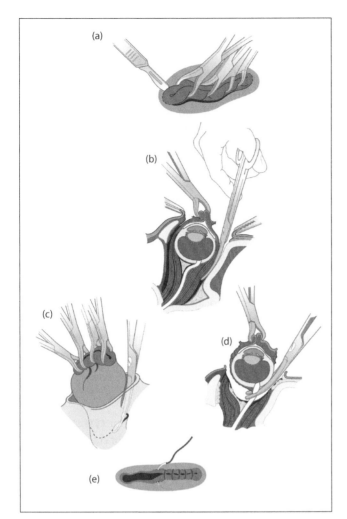

Figure 6.35 Modified transpalpebral exenteration of the orbit. The eyelids are closed with towel forceps or sutured with a continuous suture, and the skin is incised with a blade or electrosurgical scalpel (a). Scissors extend the dissection through the orbital septum into the orbit and remain external to the conjunctiva and muscle cone if neoplasia is present. If orbital neoplasia is present, the dissection is more liberal, with the muscles transected further back in the orbit rather than on the globe (b, c). Transection of the optic nerve. The optic nerve may be crushed with a snare device, an enucleation scissors, or with a hemostat, and cut rostrally to the hemostat or simply cut (d). Two-layer closure of orbital muscles and fascia and the superficial closure of the skin (e).

Enucleation and exenteration often result in a sunken appearance over the orbit (**Figure 6.36**), and attempts to improve this appearance are important to make it a more acceptable procedure to the owner. Suturing the muscle layer under the skin as a barrier to sinking has limited success. The use of a temporalis muscle flap to fill the orbit has been described but is a relatively involved procedure.[98]

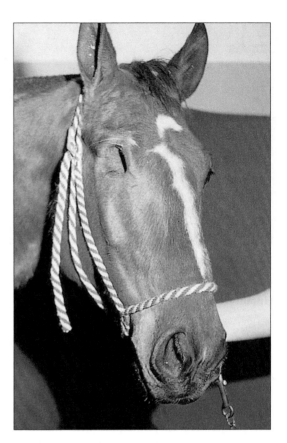

Figure 6.36 An example of extreme depression of the skin covering the orbit after enucleation in a horse.

Temporalis muscle flaps have also been used to close bony defects of the calvarium from neoplastic destruction and frontal sinus defects.[99] Synthetic meshes have also been used to cover the orbital opening and to prevent collapse of the surface.

The use of an orbital prosthesis after evisceration is questionable considering the high degree of malignancy of these tumors.

Chemotherapy Chemotherapy with doxorubicin resulted in remission of an undifferentiated orbital sarcoma of 7 months.[100] Data on protocols for chemotherapy of orbital neoplasia and success rates are lacking.

Radiation therapy Data are also lacking for the results of deep radiation therapy, or the combination of exenteration and radiation therapy, for malignant orbital lesions. Despite this, the author advocates a combination of surgical debulking or excision with deep radiation therapy.

In general, the prognosis for orbital neoplasia is grave but depends on the type of neoplasia. In the author's experience, patients have survived for up to 1 year with malignant lesions such as mucinous carcinoma, with no specific therapy.

Miscellaneous diseases of the orbit
Emphysema (pneumatosis)
Introduction/etiology

Accumulation of air in the enucleated orbit is a relatively rare complication of enucleation in the brachycephalic breeds. Air enters the orbit via the nasolacrimal duct. Due to a high positive pressure in the nasal cavity, air is apparently forced up the nasolacrimal duct and maintains the patency of one or both cut lacrimal canaliculi. Increased pressure within the nasal cavity may occur associated with exercise and mastication, producing a bellows effect in the nasal cavity and forcing air up the nasolacrimal duct.[101,102]

Clinical signs

The orbit becomes obviously distended and is nonpainful and compressible (**Figure 6.37**). Needle aspiration of the swelling reveals only air. The amount of distention may periodically get worse or improve, depending on physical activity.

Diagnosis

Diagnosis of orbital emphysema is by needle aspiration. Radiology may rule out a fracture into the sinuses as a source of the air.

Therapy

Treatment has involved exploration of the orbit and ligation of the canaliculus, if visible, or of the nasolacrimal sac in the nasolacrimal fossa.

Orbital cysts
Introduction/etiology

Cysts may arise in the orbit either as congenital malformations or acquired following trauma, surgery,

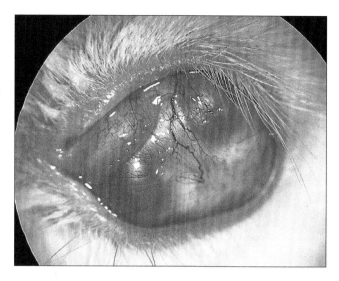

Figure 6.38 **Congenital bilateral cystic eye in a rabbit.**

inflammation, parasites, or neoplasia. Congenital anomalies that may be associated with cyst formation are microphthalmos and dermoids (**Figure 6.38**).[103,166] Acquired cysts following trauma may be a mucocele originating from the zygomatic salivary gland (**Figure 6.27**),[49,101] dacryops (a lacrimal cyst from the orbital lacrimal gland or the gland of the third eyelid) (see section Lacrimal cyst, Chapter 9),[104] or a hematic cyst from hemorrhage. An orbitonasal cyst has been described in a domestic shorthaired cat.[105]

Retrobulbar hydatid cysts may be a rare cause for a chronic, space-occupying lesion in horses and mules.[106]

Mucinous carcinomas originating from the nose or frontal sinus may invade one or both orbits, producing cystic space-occupying lesions (**Figure 6.39**).[49]

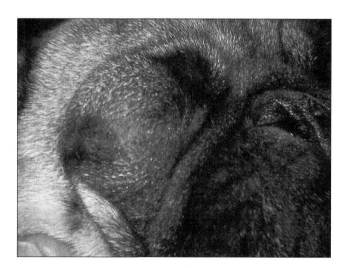

Figure 6.37 **Orbital emphysema in a pug. The enucleated orbit was distended with air, and the distention would recur after aspiration. The condition increased in severity following exercise or excitement.**

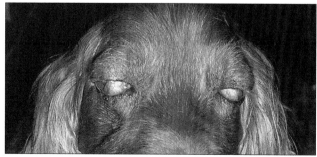

Figure 6.39 **Bilateral exophthalmos associated with a mucinous carcinoma of the frontal sinus in a dog. The neoplasia invaded both orbits and eroded through the top of the frontal sinus, producing a small fluctuant swelling dorsocaudal to the eyes. On FNA of the orbit, a thick tenacious material similar to a mucocele was aspirated. The dog lived for 1 year after cobalt therapy.**

Clinical signs

Cysts in the orbit present as slowly enlarging, nonpainful, space-occupying lesions with exophthalmos. The condition is usually unilateral (**Figures 6.27, 6.38, and 6.39**).

Diagnosis

Diagnosis of a cystic lesion is based on the clinical signs, needle aspiration of the orbit, ultrasonography, and CT scans. The presence of bony and nasal cavity changes on radiology may differentiate the malignant origin of cysts from a benign cyst.

> CT scans or MRI have become the gold standard for diagnosing and localizing orbital masses.

Cytology may help to determine the cause of the cyst but can be inconclusive. For instance, in the author's laboratory, cytology failed to differentiate between a neoplastic cyst and a zygomatic mucocele.

Therapy

Surgical excision of the cyst (except those associated with microphthalmos) is the preferred method of treating benign forms of orbital cysts. Aspiration and intralesional injection of oxytetracycline has been used as a sclerosing method for decreasing secretions. This produces acute inflammatory signs and should be used with caution.[107]

Orbital fat prolapse

Prolapse of orbital fat has been described in dogs, cats, and horses; it appears to be rare, however, with only a few cases reported in each species.[108,109] Orbital fat is separated from the subconjunctival space by Tenon's capsule. In humans, senile weaknesses of Tenon's capsule are responsible for herniation of orbital fat. The cause of orbital fat prolapse in animals, however, is unknown. In horses, resection of the nictitating membrane may predispose to orbital fat prolapse, and it is recommended to suture the conjunctiva to prevent this.

Prolapsed fat presents as conjunctival swelling in the dorsolateral or ventral fornix of the eye (**Figure 6.25**). Inflammatory reactions or ocular discharge are lacking. The swelling is easily movable and usually nonprogressive, but enophthalmos and protrusion of the nictitating membrane have been described as well. The diagnosis can be made based on fine-needle aspirates of adipose tissue.

If necessary, orbital fat prolapse can be treated surgically by excision of the prolapsed fatty tissue and suturing the conjunctiva to the episcleral tissue to prevent recurrences. Excessive removal of orbital fat should be avoided as enophthalmos may develop. The prognosis is good, and recurrences have not been described.

Cavernous sinus and orbital apex syndromes

Neurologic deficits of clusters of nerves that innervate orbital and facial structures occasionally are noted. The cavernous sinus syndrome refers to multiple nerve impairment involving the oculomotor (III), trochlear (IV), abducens (VI) cranial nerves, and the ophthalmic and maxillary division of the trigeminal (V) cranial nerve. These cranial nerves course through the cavernous sinus, and lesions in this area can affect all of them. The ocular signs include complete ophthalmoplegia or inability to move the eye, dilated pupil, ptosis, and hypalgesia of the cornea and eyelids. Vision should be present. The cause of the cavernous sinus syndrome is a mass lesion, and in the dog and the cat, it may be either inflammatory or neoplastic in nature.[110] Confirmation of the location of the lesion is by MRI or CT scans. The prognosis is guarded.

The orbital apex syndrome involves structures exiting the optic foramen and orbital fissure. The cranial nerves and function affected are: the optic (II, vision), oculomotor (III, ophthalmoplegia, dilated pupil), trochlear (IV, rotation of globe), abducens (VI, retracts eye, lateral movement), and the ophthalmic division of the trigeminal (V, sensory to cornea). Note that the maxillary division of CN V is intact. Masses at the apex of the orbit are the usual cause.

Steroid-induced exophthalmos in calves

In Holstein calves, administration of dexamethasone (30 μgm/kg every 12 hours subcutaneously from 3 days of age) was noted to produce a progressive, bilateral exophthalmos 28 days after injection. The condition was produced by deposition of retrobulbar fat and did not affect the health of the globe.[167] This is unlikely to be found as a clinical syndrome.

Sclerosing pseudotumors in cats
Introduction/etiology

A relatively rare syndrome of fibrous tissue infiltration of the orbit has been described in the cat. It follows a very slow insidious course and results in exophthalmos. The syndrome has been resistant to therapy, resulting in enucleation and/or euthanasia in all the cases. No cause was determined on histopathology of the globe and the orbit, although three of seven cats had a history of respiratory infection and had gingival hyperplasia. Six of seven cats were domestic shorthairs with no sex predilection.[102a]

Clinical signs

A slow, progressive exophthalmos develops in one eye, and in several weeks or months, the second eye also becomes involved. The globe resists retropulsion and has reduced mobility, the third eyelid may lose mobility, and the cornea develops a secondary exposure keratitis. Blindness may develop from optic nerve involvement, retinal detachment, or corneal complications. Titers, blood work, and histopathology have not revealed a cause.

Therapy

To date, the syndrome has not responded to therapy and, indeed, continues to progress to the second eye. Therapy has consisted of anti-inflammatory doses of glucocorticoids, radiation therapy, and antibiotics. Alternative immunosuppressive doses of glucocorticoids and alternative immunosuppressants may be indicated.

DISEASES OF THE GLOBE

Congenital

Microphthalmos

Introduction/etiology

Microphthalmos is a congenitally small eye. Microphthalmos includes a wide variety of anomalies such as a globe barely reduced in size with normal intraocular structures, a marked reduction in size of the globe with numerous intraocular anomalies, and a clinical anophthalmos in which no globe is present (**Figures 6.40 and 6.41**). Most cases of clinical anophthalmos are extreme examples of microphthalmos, with dysplastic ocular remnants in the orbit on serial sectioning.

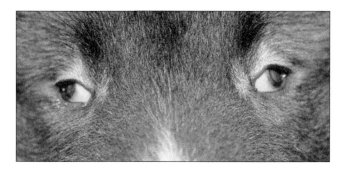

Figure 6.40 **Moderately severe bilateral microphthalmos in a puppy, with lateral strabismus.**

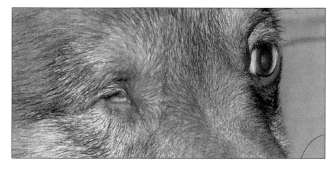

Figure 6.41 **Unilateral clinical anophthalmos in a puppy.**

The eye may or may not be visually functional with microphthalmos. Associated intraocular anomalies include cataract, persistent pupillary membranes, uveal colobomas, retinal detachment, retinal dysplasia, orbital cyst, and goniodysgenesis. Inbreeding dogs with color dilute genes (merle genes) and blue eyes often results in microphthalmos with multiple ocular anomalies.[111,112] In the Australian shepherd dog, the trait is simple recessive.[113] Although microphthalmos occurs in the horse and the cat, there are no described inherited syndromes as in the dog and the cow. Guernsey calves have a syndrome of microphthalmos with cardiac and tail defects that are thought to be recessively inherited.[114] Hereford cattle have a recessively inherited syndrome of microphthalmos, muscular dystrophy, and hydrocephalus,[115] and shorthorn cattle have an inherited syndrome of microphthalmos.[116] A possible dominant trait has been reported, resulting in microphthalmos in half of the offspring of a Hereford bull.[117] Despite several known inherited syndromes, most cases of anophthalmos–microphthalmos in calves have no demonstrable genetic basis.[118] In utero infection with bovine viral diarrhea virus may produce microphthalmos, cataract, retinal and optic nerve lesions, and cerebellar disease.[119]

- Inherited syndromes: Australian shepherd dog,[112] Akita,[120] St. Bernard,[121] collie, Doberman pinscher,[122,123] Cavalier King Charles Spaniel,[124] Old English sheepdog, Bedlington terrier,[125] Sealyham terrier,[126] miniature schnauzer,[127] and soft coated Wheaten terrier.[128] (See section Retinal dysplasia, Chapter 14, and section Congenital cataracts, Chapter 13.)
- Teratogenic drugs: Griseofulvin administered to pregnant queens produces cyclopia or anophthalmos and multiple neurologic, skeletal, and digestive tract malformations.[129]
- In utero viral infection: Bovine viral diarrhea virus may produce microphthalmos among many other ocular lesions if present between 76–150 days of gestation.[119]
- Many cases of microphthalmos are sporadic and without a known cause.[118]

Clinical signs

Microphthalmos may be unilateral or bilateral. The degree of reduction of globe size is usually obvious when it is unilateral, but mild decreases that are bilateral may not be so obvious. In milder forms, the condition is compatible with vision, but microphthalmos is often blinding due to the multiple ocular anomalies.

Therapy

None.

Anterior segment dysgenesis

Introduction/etiology

Anterior segment dysgenesis refers to a congenital syndrome observed in various breeds of horse such as the Rocky Mountain, Kentucky saddle, mountain pleasure, Morgan, ponies, miniature breeds, and American saddlebred. It is a syndrome with varying degrees of manifestation depending on the coat color. The trait is dominant with incomplete penetrance that manifests only with the dominant silver dapple locus that imparts a chocolate coat with a flaxen or white mane. Black horses are protected.[57]

Clinical signs

The basic lesion with anterior segment dysgenesis is ciliary body cysts that are manifested in the temporal region (see Chapter 11). Some of the horses with cyst manifestation may have peripheral retinal detachments, retinal dysplasia, and arcuate lines of retinal pigmented epithelium proliferation from previous retinal detachments. The homozygous individual with a flaxen mane can have, in addition, varying degrees of multiple ocular anomalies, consisting of cornea globosa (see Chapter 11), goniodysgenesis and synechiae, nuclear cataracts, posteroventral luxated lens, miotic pupil, iris stromal hypoplasia, large palpebral fissures, and microphthalmos.[57]

Therapy

Therapy is limited to genetic counseling of breeding to black stallions.

Strabismus

Introduction/etiology

Deviations of the normal visual axis are common in brachycephalic and toy breeds, Siamese cats, and cattle. The condition is often inherited, although strabismus may be acquired. In the Siamese cat, strabismus is typically an esotropia and is associated with the albino gene (**Figure 6.42**). Various albino animals may have an increased number of optic nerve fibers decussating at the optic chiasm from the temporal retina. This results in abnormal retinotopic projections to the lateral geniculate and occipital cortex.[130–132] The strabismus is thought to be a compensatory mechanism and develops in the first 6 months of life in the Siamese cat.[133] A fine pendular nystagmus may be associated with the strabismus.

Congenital hypoplasia or aplasia of the extraocular muscles may, rarely, be responsible for dramatic ocular deviations, and these conditions have been observed in the dog and the goat (**Figures 6.9 and 6.10**).[53]

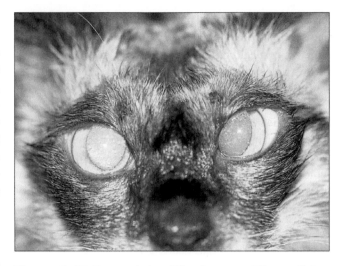

Figure 6.42 **Esotropia in a Himalayan cat. The condition is associated with an increased percentage of fibers from temporal retina crossing at the chiasm.**

Convergent strabismus with or without exophthalmos is an inherited trait in Jersey and shorthorn cattle[134] and is observed less frequently in Ayrshire, Holstein–Friesian,[135] and brown Swiss cattle (**Figure 6.43**).[114] Strabismus may occasionally be observed in the horse, with the Appaloosa most commonly affected with a hypertropia.[136,137] Strabismus in the Appaloosa horse has also been associated with night blindness.[138]

Bilateral exotropia with hypotropia (eyes are deviated down and out) is commonly associated with congenital hydrocephalus due to enlargement of the calvarium and encroachment on the dorsomedial orbit (**Figure 6.8**). Ocular deviations after replacement of a proptosed globe are

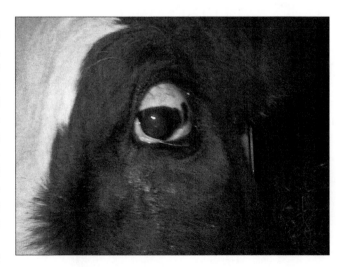

Figure 6.43 **Microphthalmos and esotropia present bilaterally in a Holstein cow. A pendular nystagmus was present. The condition was genetic.**

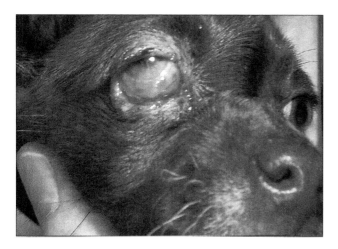

Figure 6.44 A dog with typical postproptosis strabismus in a dorsolateral direction. Note the irritation to the ventromedial globe and cornea.

common. The most common deviation is an exotropia–hypertropia (dorsolateral) (**Figure 6.44**), although the deviation may occur in any direction (**Figure 6.45**). The deviation usually results from avulsion of the ventral and medial rectus muscles or, possibly, nerve damage. The deviation moderates over a period of 4–8 weeks but does not return to normal.

Therapy

In most strabismus cases, no therapy is attempted. The strabismus in Siamese cats has not responded to surgical correction. Severe deviations associated with trauma may be treated by anchoring sutures or medial tarsorrhaphies to improve the appearance and protect the cornea. If forced duction tests indicate limitations of movement, surgery can be performed on the limiting muscles to weaken them by recession or removal of the muscle insertions.[53,136]

Acquired conditions of the globe
Phthisis bulbi

Phthisis bulbi is a shrunken disorganized globe usually resulting from massive intraocular pathology. Cyclitic membranes or inflammatory membranes that stretch across the globe between the ciliary body are usually present and result in ciliary body detachment and marked hypotony. A yellow–white corneal opacification, cataract, and retinal detachment are usually present (**Figure 6.46**). The eye is nonfunctional and in veterinary medicine is often not removed due to the owner's objection to the appearance of an enucleated orbit. The danger of having a nonfunctional eye with opaque media is that subsequent intraocular neoplasia may arise and not be recognized until very late. In the cat, the increased recognition of intraocular sarcomas after trauma and severe intraocular disease is an argument for the enucleation of phthisical eyes (**Figure 6.47**). Other problems related to phthisis are appearance, subtle discomfort, and poor lid–globe apposition that results in entropion and chronic ocular discharge.

Microphthalmos and phthisis bulbi may be difficult to differentiate if the animal's history is not available. Diffuse corneal opacity is more typical of phthisis bulbi.

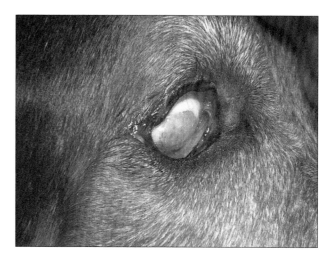

Figure 6.46 A dog with phthisis bulbi after cyclocryotherapy for glaucoma. Note the dense corneal opacity and the mismatching of the globe size to third eyelid and palpebral fissure. These features help to differentiate phthisis from microphthalmos.

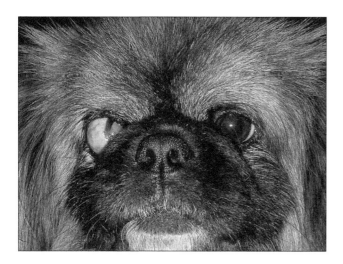

Figure 6.45 A dog with severe esotropia as the result of a prior proptosed globe.

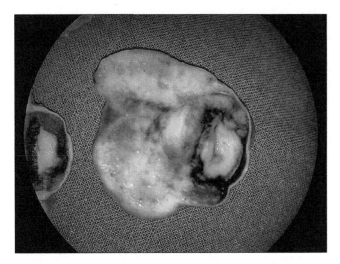

Figure 6.47 Intraocular chondrosarcoma that fills the vitreous cavity in a cat. Sarcomas such as these have been related to past trauma and inflammation and typically are advanced by the time they are detected because they arise in blind eyes with opaque media.

The easiest solution to phthisis is the implantation of an orbital prosthesis at the time of enucleation. Silicone orbital prostheses have been applied in dogs, cats, birds (**Figure 6.48**), and horses. Commercial methyl methacrylate orbital prostheses have been successful in the dog, but a significant failure rate has occurred in cats due to an accumulation of orbital fluid.[139]

> Cats should have phthisical eyes enucleated to avoid ocular sarcomas later in life.

The size of implant that the orbit can accommodate varies with head conformation in the dog. Often the leading edge of the implant will be shaved flat. The horse usually accommodates a 40- to 47-mm diameter sphere and the dog a 20- to 22-mm sphere, unless it is a brachycephalic dog where 14–16 mm is recommended.[139,140] In the short term, orbital prosthesis is a significant improvement over enucleation. However, with time, some prostheses may be pushed forward by orbital granulation, resulting in a questionable cosmetic improvement.

Proptosis (prolapse) of the globe

Proptosis of the globe out of the orbit with subsequent entrapment by the lids is a common traumatic event in the dog and the cat. Two forms of trauma are associated with proptosis: Car accidents and dogfights. In extremely brachycephalic dogs, simply grasping the skin over the back of the neck may result in proptosis. Since the trauma necessary to cause proptosis in a cat or mesaticephalic

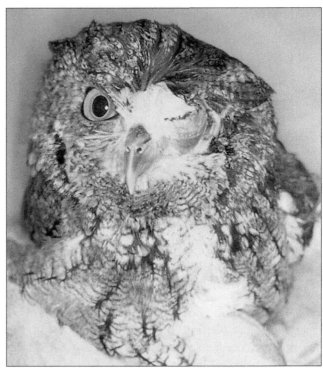

Figure 6.48 Screech owl with an orbital prosthesis after enucleation.

dog is much more than in a brachycephalic dog, the attendant injuries to the globe are usually more severe in the cat and longer nosed dogs. Since proptosis is indicative of head trauma, many patients have significant neurologic signs.

> It is rare to preserve vision in a proptosed globe in a cat or a dolichocephalic dog.

Clinical signs

Proptosis is obvious and often grotesque, but evaluation of other ocular signs is important for prognostic purposes (**Figure 6.49**). A variety of pupil abnormalities may be present in the affected eye but are not important in evaluating visual function. If the direct PLR is present, this is a good sign. The pupil of the affected eye may be dilated from oculomotor nerve paralysis or constricted. Marked constriction may result from an antidromic axonal reflex of the ophthalmic branch of cranial nerve V due to corneal pain or traumatic uveitis (see Chapters 10 and 11). The important pupillary reaction for evaluating vision is often the consensual reaction; a defect in the opposite eye indicates retinal/optic nerve injury and a poor prognosis for vision.

The extraocular muscles, especially the medial rectus, are usually torn and are responsible for the strabismus that

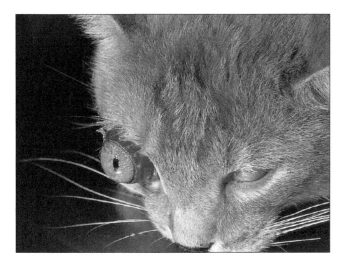

Figure 6.49 Proptosed globe in a cat. Note the miotic pupil.

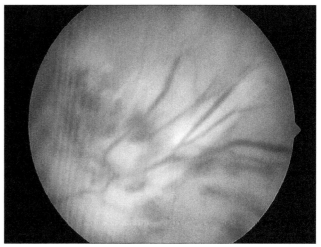

Figure 6.50 Avulsion of the optic nerve and retinal vessels associated with a proptosis of the globe in a young Doberman pincher. The optic disc is swollen, retinal hemorrhages are present, retinal vessels contain only residual blood and are incompletely filled, and the retina has become white and opaque from infarction.

is a common complication of proptosis. Three or more torn extraocular muscles have been cited as an unfavorable prognostic indicator,[141] but this is difficult to ascertain in practice. Conjunctival tears are common, and the cornea appears dry and covered with mucus and hair. Superficial ulceration is common.

If the fundus can be visualized, severe damage may be observed associated with avulsion of the optic nerve and retinal vessels. This presents in the acute stage with large, white, ischemic areas of retina; bloodless blood vessels; and papilledema (**Figure 6.50**). Later, the tapetal coloration may be lost, or if present, it is hyperreflective with a lack of retinal blood vessels, and a gray–white atrophied optic disc is present.

Intraocular hemorrhage usually occurs with severe intraocular damage, such as a ruptured globe, and indicates a poor prognosis (**Figure 6.51**). An important prognostic sign is the IOP; specifically, if the globe is very soft, it usually indicates that it is ruptured. The rupture is usually posterior and not visible, although vitreous may herniate through conjunctival lacerations (**Figure 6.52**).

> A very soft proptosed globe probably has a posterior rupture and will become phthisical.

Diagnosis

The diagnosis is obvious, but the prognosis should be determined for sight and appearance. Ultrasound may help in detecting posterior globe ruptures.

Prognosis

Gilger et al. reported retention of vision in only 27% of dogs with proptosis, with a better prognosis for brachycephalic dogs.[141] No cats retained vision after proptosis.

The prognosis is considered based on two outcomes, vision and cosmetic appearance. If the prognosis for both is poor, then enucleation is recommended, as the eye will remain problematic.

Therapy

Neurologic signs, if present, frequently preclude expedient management of the proptosis. Patients with severe neurologic signs and proptosed globes often need to wait for 1–3 days to stabilize before administration of general anesthesia. However, the prognosis for the proptosed globe in these patients is usually grave, and enucleation is indicated.

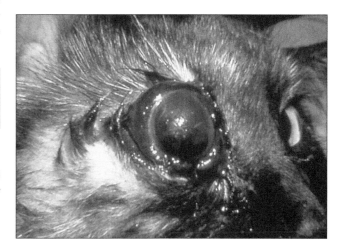

Figure 6.51 Proptosed globe in a cat with intraocular hemorrhage. Marked hypotony was present on palpation of the globe.

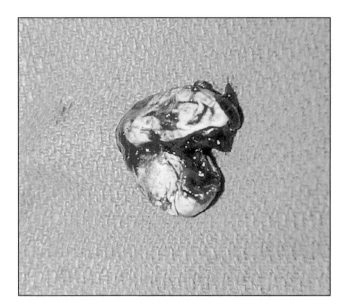

Figure 6.52 Posterior rupture of the globe enucleated from Figure 6.51.

> General rule: You can always remove the globe, but you cannot put it back, so try to salvage most globes for cosmetic purposes, even if the animal is likely to be blind.

Enucleation

The eye should be enucleated if:

- The owner is pragmatic: The globe after replacement requires ongoing chronic postoperative care, and if the eye is blind, some owners do not appreciate the expense and the effort.
- The eye is very soft: It will be neither functional nor cosmetic, as the eye will become phthisical.
- The globe is dangling from a few muscles.
- There is significant intraocular blood present, which usually indicates that the globe is ruptured.

Replacement of the globe Most owners will want to try and salvage the eye whether it is functional or not. The lid margins must be lifted up and over the equator of the globe while simultaneously pushing on the globe (**Figures 6.53 and 6.54**). This maneuver usually requires general anesthesia. The main difficulty occurs when only the edge of the folded over lid is grasped, rather than the lid margins. The lid margins can be rolled out by placing hemostats parallel and near the rolled over edge and then rolling the hemostats. Another method is to "leap-frog" or alternately grasp with two pair of forceps until the lid margin is reached. Once each lid margin is elevated and everted

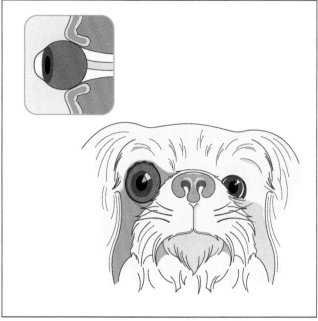

Figure 6.53 Illustration of proptosis and how the rolled lid entraps the globe when caught posterior to the equator.

outward, the globe is pushed into the orbit, and the lid margins are released as they pass the equator of the globe. At this time, torn conjunctiva and avulsed muscles can be sutured if they can be found.

A tarsorrhaphy is placed with an everting suture pattern (see Chapter 7, **Figure 7.43**) and tied firmly so that

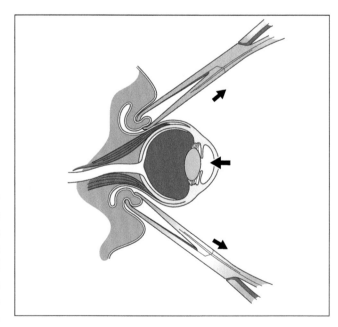

Figure 6.54 Illustration of replacement of a globe following proptosis. Note that the lid margins must be rolled out and away from the globe, while simultaneously pushing on the globe to replace the globe in the orbit.

when the swelling subsides the sutures do not rub on the cornea. Steroids should not be injected into the orbit, and systemic steroids should only be used cautiously because of the danger of corneal ulceration. Orbital swelling improves quickly, and the main justification for using steroids is for treating traumatic optic neuritis. Injection of systemic mannitol may also be justified for this reason but not for simply replacing the globe. Neuroprotective therapy in the form of calcium channel blockers is indicated for minimizing collateral nerve damage from ischemia (see Chapter 12). The tarsorrhaphy should be in place for 2 weeks as most cases have inadequate tear function and lagophthalmos. Upon removal of the sutures, the cornea should be observed for keratoconjunctivitis sicca (KCS) over the next several days. Corneal ulceration is a common problem after removal of the tarsorrhaphy, and supplemental artificial tears are often needed for several weeks.

Strabismus with the eye directed up and out is common and slowly improves over 4–6 weeks in most cases. A strabismus usually remains but is milder than the original deviation and acceptable cosmetically. The medial cornea often develops ulcerations due to the exposure that the dorsolateral strabismus produces, and a medial canthoplasty is helpful for protection and for cosmetic purposes (see Chapter 7, **Figure 7.37**).

> Client education is critical with proptosed globes because of the frequency of long-term sequelae that require therapy, despite the globe being visually nonfunctional.

Trauma
Perforating and penetrating ocular injuries
A perforating injury to the globe is one that enters and exits the globe, while a penetrating injury is one that enters without exiting. Perforating injuries to the globe with BB (air gun) shot and pellets are common and are quite devastating to the function of the eye. The corneal injury frequently seals uneventfully, but damage to the lens, vitreous hemorrhage, and retinal detachment are common accompanying lesions. Vitreous hemorrhage is important as it often leads to subsequent retinal detachment with contraction of the clot (**Figure 6.55**).

> The size of the corneal defect with perforating missiles and injuries has no prognostic value for vision. The smallest corneal defect may result in blinding sequelae.

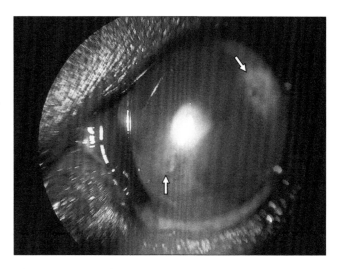

Figure 6.55 Multiple BB shot corneal perforations (arrows) that occurred in both eyes. Despite the self-sealing nature of the injuries, the prognosis is very guarded for sight.

Larger pellets and BB shot injuries may mimic acute corneal ulcers with or without iris prolapse, but they should be differentiated for prognostic purposes (see Chapter 10). While infection is uncommon, sterile inflammation may be overwhelming. The initial traumatic inflammation may be controlled, but 2–3 weeks or later, another more severe inflammatory reaction occurs due to phacoclastic uveitis. Penetrating injuries from sticks and porcupine quills may or may not be obvious, depending whether they are retained in the eye.

Diagnosis
The history of a peracute onset of the injury or perhaps knowledge of the injury, as in hunting dogs, is important to stimulate diagnostic testing. Typically, malicious injuries have a history of the dog being let out for a couple of hours and returning with a perforated cornea. The perforating injury should be differentiated from an acute perforating corneal ulcer. With metallic missiles, this is easily accomplished with radiographs of the skull. Ultrasound can also be utilized to determine the extent of ocular injuries and to locate the foreign body more precisely. Nonmetallic penetrating foreign bodies, if not visible, are most easily diagnosed with ultrasonography.[61]

> Peracute corneal perforations should not be confused with complicated corneal ulcers. Skull radiographs are indicated to find a metallic foreign body.

Prognosis

Before initiating therapy, consideration should be given to the three objectives of maintaining function, comfort, and cosmesis. The prognosis is dependent on the extent of injury to specific ocular tissue, whether the lens is damaged and the extent of damage (**Figure 6.56**), the presence of significant vitreous hemorrhage, and the size of any exit wound. Small BB shot perforating through the peripheral cornea and not hitting the lens is compatible with good cosmesis, although the prognosis for function may be guarded. Larger pellet injuries have more concussive force and are rarely compatible with saving function and cosmesis. Infection is uncommon with metallic foreign bodies, although severe inflammation is common. Penetrating injuries from cat claws, sticks, and porcupine quills are more likely to be infected, although not as often as one might anticipate.

A perforating injury through the lens, with significant vitreous hemorrhage, signals an eye that has a high probability of developing overwhelming inflammation, as well as losing function from a detached retina. A penetrating injury is less likely to have both anterior segment and posterior segment considerations for prognosis. The type of metal retained affects the tissue reaction; lead is relatively nonreactive as an insoluble carbonate envelope develops that isolates the metal from surrounding tissue.[142]

Therapy

The objectives of therapy are to maintain function, limit inflammation, prevent or treat infection, and maintain a comfortable eye. The decision to treat may be based not only on the prognosis but also on prognostic uncertainties and an owner who is adamant in wanting to save the eye. Any leaking corneal defect or iris prolapse should be repaired, but many small lesions are self-sealing. Traumatic inflammation should be treated first, and this usually subsides within 2 weeks with anti-inflammatory therapy given both topically and systemically. Anti-inflammatory therapy may have to be given for an extended period of time. Concurrent topical and systemic antibiotics are administered for 7–10 days, and topical atropine administered to control ocular pain and to maintain a pupil. Lead foreign bodies such as BB shot and pellets in the orbit or globe are not removed, as they are well tolerated,[142] and the surgical trauma involved usually far outweighs the benefit of removal.

With penetrating injuries (without posterior segment lesions), the lens should be removed to prevent phacoclastic uveitis if the lens capsule has a tear larger than 2 mm.[143] Phacoclastic uveitis usually manifests 2–3 weeks after the injury, just as traumatic uveitis is resolving. While lens extraction can be performed, posterior segment injuries often preclude a visually functional eye, so it is an expensive surgery to save an eye just for cosmetic purposes.

In humans, vitrectomies are routinely performed for removal of vitreous hemorrhage, to prevent subsequent retinal detachment, and to remove any metallic foreign bodies. The best timing for vitrectomy is still debated. The use of both intravitreal and IV antibiotics with open globe injuries is also debated.[144] As veterinary ophthalmologists develop the skills and instrumentation for performing vitrectomies, such procedures may become routine in managing these types of injuries. It should be emphasized that even with procedures involving lensectomy, vitrectomy, and suturing the sclera, or combination surgery, the prognosis for vision is very poor.

Ruptured globe

Blunt trauma to the globe may cause it to rupture either posteriorly or anteriorly. Ruptures of the globe from blunt trauma in the dog and the cat are usually posterior and associated with proptosis of the globe. In the horse, ruptures are usually observed in the cornea and adjacent sclera and are due to throwing the head and hitting an object or rearing over and hitting the floor (**Figure 6.56**). An anterior rupture is accompanied by iris prolapse, and it may mimic a laceration or, occasionally, a perforated ulcer.

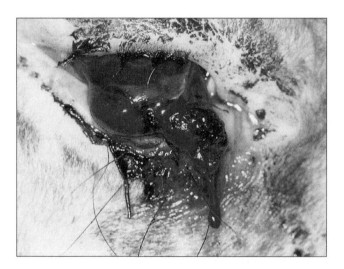

Figure 6.56 Horse that had suffered blunt trauma to the eye resulting in a rupture across the entire corneal diameter. The lens was expelled at the time of injury.

It is important to differentiate between these conditions, as lacerations and ulcerations have a relatively good prognosis for retaining vision, whereas ruptured globes have a very poor prognosis and usually result in phthisis.

Methods for differentiating laceration from rupture have been discussed in the equine literature, but incomplete historical data is not helpful.[145] (See section Ruptured globe, for more details.)

Diagnosis

Differentiating a ruptured globe from a laceration is facilitated if the history is complete or there is further evidence of blunt trauma to the head. Injuries of the cornea that cross the limbus are usually ruptures. In horses, only approximately 4/24 of cases that had wounds crossing the limbus were successfully managed.[145] Ultrasonography may identify an absence of the lens, retinal detachment, and perhaps vitreous hemorrhage in rupture, features which are not typical for the usual laceration. Surgical exploration of a rupture usually reveals the lens is missing or the lens capsule is ruptured.

Therapy

If the diagnosis of a ruptured globe is certain, enucleation or evisceration with implantation of a silicone sphere is recommended to minimize expense and pain. Evisceration carries the risk of extruding the prosthesis, but most are retained, and the procedure prevents phthisis bulbi. Enucleation should be the procedure of last resort. Enucleation may be performed with a transpalpebral, subconjunctival, or lateral approach. The transpalpebral approach (**Figure 6.35**) usually removes more orbital tissue than the other approaches and all the conjunctival tissue, and thus, it has fewer complications of postoperative accumulation of secretions. If the ocular surface is infected or neoplastic, the transpalpebral approach minimizes the risk of carrying infection or seeding of neoplastic cells deeper into the orbit. The method has two major disadvantages: most surgeons simply excise until the globe is free, with little attempt at retaining orbital tissue to minimize a postoperative shrunken appearance; and the skin and orbicularis oculi muscle often bleed profusely if electrocautery is not used.

The subconjunctival approach eliminates bleeding from the skin and orbicularis muscle while performing the enucleation and is usually more clear and distinct in dissection, but it may not remove all the potential secreting membranes (**Figure 6.57**). In animals with a tight globe–orbit relationship, such as the cat, or buphthalmos, dissection is more difficult. The lid margins and the third eyelid with its gland are excised before suturing the orbit closed (**Figure 6.57**).

Complications of enucleation include factors that made the procedure necessary, such as infection or neoplasia, as well as complications that are specific to the procedure. Postsurgical infection is usually managed with systemic

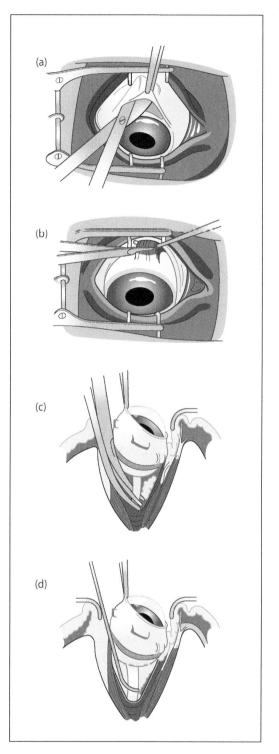

Figure 6.57 Subconjunctival approach to enucleation. Incision and blunt dissection of conjunctiva from the globe, for 360° (a). Individual extraocular muscles are lifted up with a strabismus hook and excised with tenotomy scissor (b). After the extraocular muscles have been excised from the globe, the optic nerve is crushed either with a Kelly forceps and then cut with scissors, or a tonsil/enucleation snare is passed over the globe and used to crush/cut the nerve (c, d). *(Continued)*

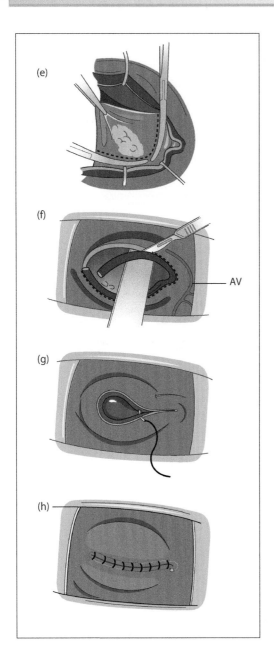

(e)

(f)

AV

(g)

(h)

Figure 6.57 (Continued) After the globe is removed, the third eyelid is excised after placing forceps at the base and ligating (e). The lid margins are removed with special attention given to the medial canthus. The medial canthal ligament can be cut to loosen the skin from the skull and make it easier to dissect (f). Note the proximity to the angularis oculi vein (AV). An orbital prosthesis can be placed, and the orbit closed in a deep layer of muscle and fascia, and a superficial skin closure performed (g, h).

antibiotics. When contamination is present or suspected at the time of enucleation, flushing the orbit with antibiotics such as crystalline penicillin and utilizing preoperative, intraoperative, and postoperative systemic antibiotics is usually successful. Seton stitches or drainage tubes are used on rare occasions.

A common complication of enucleation is excessive orbital hemorrhage, with a swollen orbit after surgery. This can be treated with initial cold compresses, followed with warm compresses after 24 hours. The condition usually resolves without incident, although serum may be expelled if the incision is disrupted. Increased attention to hemostasis minimizes bleeding, for example, using an electroscalpel on the skin and the muscle, ligating the base of the third eyelid before excising, and crushing the optic nerve before cutting.

In the cat, the surgeon should be cautious of how much forward traction is placed on the globe during enucleation to avoid optic chiasm damage. Cats have become blind in the contralateral eye after enucleation because of such damage.[146]

In the cat, a large globe and a small orbit make enucleation more difficult; pulling the globe forward for exposure may avulse the optic chiasm.

An additional common complication of enucleation is orbital retention of sterile serous secretions that subsequently drain from the medial canthus. Removal of all the conjunctival surfaces and the third eyelid is performed to try to prevent postoperative secretions, but most surgeons do not remove the orbital lacrimal gland; some patients continue to have orbital secretions that presumably are from this gland. In most instances, the drainage is tolerated. Therapy for chronic orbital drainage includes 95% ethanol injected into the orbit,[147] orbital exploration for any remaining conjunctiva, and excision of the orbital lacrimal gland.

In some very complicated cases that require enucleation, the eyelids and the periorbital skin may not be viable for use in covering the orbit, either because of infection or neoplasia. The cat, the horse, and some small breeds of dog have very little mobile skin surrounding the eye compared to the average and large breeds of dog. In these instances, flaps of axial pattern skin grafts can be used to cover the avascular bed of the enucleated orbit. Axial flaps based on the distribution of the superficial temporal artery[148,149] and the caudal auricular artery[150] have been used successfully to close the orbit after enucleation.

The most common complication of enucleation is cosmetic: a sunken orbit. (See section Enucleation, Chapter 12 for methods to minimize this objectionable appearance.) An alternative to enucleating a ruptured globe is evisceration together with a silicone sphere implantation (see section Ocular evisceration, Chapter 12). These cases have an increased risk of extrusion of the sphere through the ruptured cornea, but the implant prevents phthisis from occurring.

The repair of the rupture can be performed by excising uveal tissue and suturing the fibrous tunic as for a laceration, but the most of these eyes will become phthisical, and the cornea will be opaque. Medical therapy consists of glucocorticoids (systemically), prostaglandin inhibitors, and antibiotics.

Inflammation of the globe

Panophthalmitis/endophthalmitis

Panophthalmitis refers to inflammation that involves all tissues of the eye, that is, fibrous (cornea and sclera), uveal, and neurosensory (retina). The vitreous is also involved. The inflammatory process may be either sterile or septic, with the latter being most common. The infectious agent may originate either from hematogenous routes or be external in origin, such as from penetrating injuries or from a perforating corneal ulceration. Most of the time these processes produce an endophthalmitis (involvement of the inner tunic), but if overwhelming infection occurs, the entire thickness of the globe may become involved, and inflammation may extend into the orbit. Blindness and pain are the devastating end result, and the course is often very rapid.

Fungi are not an uncommon cause of panophthalmitis/endophthalmitis, and inflammation may be due to systemic fungi, hematogenous saprophytic fungi, or fungi inoculated into the eye from penetrating injuries. Viruses that produce vasculitis, such as malignant catarrhal fever in the cow and feline infectious peritonitis (FIP) in the cat, may produce a panophthalmitis. Bacteria are the most common causes of panophthalmitis, and the most feared form is postsurgical infection. While accurate statistics are not available for large numbers of cases in veterinary medicine, in human intraocular surgery, endophthalmitis occurs in about 0.1% of patients. One would expect endophthalmitis postsurgically to be higher in veterinary medicine, and the horse may be most susceptible. Millichamp and Dziezyc reported four cases in 34 cataract surgeries.[151] The most common causes of bacterial endophthalmitis in man[152] and animals[151] are Gram-positive organisms.

Occasionally, infection may occur due to contamination of surgical instruments outside the surgical arena, and when this occurs, it usually produces clusters of infections. Most bacterial infections arise from the patient's bacterial flora. Considering the high incidence of culture-positive aqueous humor (24%)[153] that occurs during canine and human cataract surgery, the incidence of infection appears to be very small. The prevalence of intraoperative positive cultures has not been affected by perioperative scrubbing[154] or antibiotics given by any route and does not appear to affect the postoperative outcome.

Clinical signs

Panophthalmitis/endophthalmitis is characterized by ocular pain, marked conjunctival and episcleral injection, corneal edema with neovascularization, hypopyon and/or hyphema, pupillary constriction, and a hazy vitreous if visible. Marked decrease in vision or blindness is present. If the process has become a panophthalmitis, it has passed through the sclera, and the conjunctiva is very chemotic, the lids are hot and tender, and decreased orbital retropulsion is present, appearing as orbital cellulitis. The rapidity of the development of signs varies depending on the virulence of the organism. In veterinary medicine, typically the signs develop peracutely in a period of 12–24 hours. In humans, postoperative infection is often associated with low virulence organisms, and signs may not develop for weeks or months after surgery. Because of the pain involved, the animals may manifest systemic signs such as depression, colic, and leukocytosis.

Diagnosis

If endophthalmitis is suspected, bold, rapid, definitive action is necessary. Aqueous and vitreous humor centesis is necessary to identify rapidly the organism on cytology and for culture and sensitivity testing.

Therapy

Intraocular antibiotics should be administered at the time of ocular centesis, with caution exercised over the dose and form of drug utilized. The vitreous is the most difficult tissue to clear of bacteria, so intravitreal injections are preferred. The data on safe antibiotic dosage should be verified by experimental work, as toxicity of drugs or preservatives is of real concern. The choice of antibiotics has varied over the years, based on the acquisition of bacterial resistance to drugs. In general, a drug, or combination of drugs, is used that has both a Gram-positive and Gram-negative spectrum of activity and be bactericidal. Historically, gentamicin with a cephalosporin was recommended, but because of drug resistance and drug toxicity, amikacin has replaced gentamicin, and second- and third-generation cephalosporins are used. Vancomycin has been advocated because of its effectiveness against resistant staphylococci. The trend today is to inject intravitreally with 0.4%/0.1 mL vancomycin and a third-generation cephalosporin such as ceftazidime 2.25 mg/0.1 mL.[155] These two drugs are incompatible and must be injected with separate syringes.

Intraocular antibiotics are now universally accepted for the treatment of endophthalmitis, but it remains controversial whether concurrent antibiotics given by other routes such as subconjunctival[156] or systemic are beneficial.[152,157] Despite the evidence that they are not of additional benefit, they remain in widespread use because of the catastrophic nature of the disease. If the process has become a panophthalmitis with orbital involvement, systemic therapy is warranted.

A routine component of treating endophthalmitis in humans is vitrectomy.[152] The removal of the vitreous removes a burden of infection that is difficult to reach through any route of therapy except intravitreal injection. Vitrectomies also remove the inflammatory cells that perpetuate inflammation and produce inflammatory membranes that result in retinal detachment. To date, vitrectomies have not been commonly performed in the treatment of acute endophthalmitis, except for equine recurrent uveitis.[158]

Additional therapy for endophthalmitis/panophthalmitis includes intraocular injections of tissue plasminogen activator (tPA) to break up clots, topical atropine for pain, systemic nonsteroidal anti-inflammatory drug (NSAID) therapy, hot-packing the lids, and cleansing the ocular surface.

The prognosis remains very guarded for most cases of established endophthalmitis treated without surgery. Even when treated aggressively, the eye remains inflamed long after it is sterile, as judged by cultures and cytology. Panophthalmitis cases usually need enucleation, but selecting the appropriate time can be a difficult decision. When the field is septic, the author prefers to decrease the inflammation or have it resolved, and this may necessitate a delay of several days.

Miscellaneous
Head shaking in horses

Head shaking in the horse can be a serious fault that results in a dysfunctional animal. A variety of causes have been proposed, but removal of potential causes has generally not been successful. The onset of head shaking is usually noted in the spring, and the condition becomes chronic. Photic head shaking is a specific type that is induced by exposure to sunlight and can be stopped by blindfolding and a dark environment.[159] Exercise also stimulates head shaking. Head shaking is usually in a vertical manner and is often accompanied by snorting. The condition may spontaneously improve, only to recur the following spring. Animals develop avoidance behavior of natural light. The cause is unknown, but it is compared to photic sneezing in man. Interaction between the optic nerve and cranial nerve V are postulated to produce vasodilatation in the nose, or stimulation of the sensory nerves in the nose, to stimulate the snorting and head shaking. Therapies including anti-inflammatories, analgesics, melatonin, and sedatives have been unsuccessful. Cyproheptadine, a H-1 histamine and serotonergic blocking agent, was successful in treating 71% of a small cohort of horses at 0.3 mg/kg every 12 hours orally.[159]

CLINICAL CASES

CASE 1

A 5-year-old Persian cat is presented several days after enucleation of the left eye with massive swelling of the surgical site.

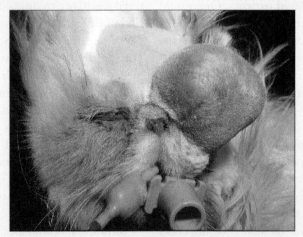

Q: What is your clinical diagnosis?

Answer:
Postoperative orbital emphysema

CASE 2

A 2-year-old mixed breed dog is presented with a protruding right eye.

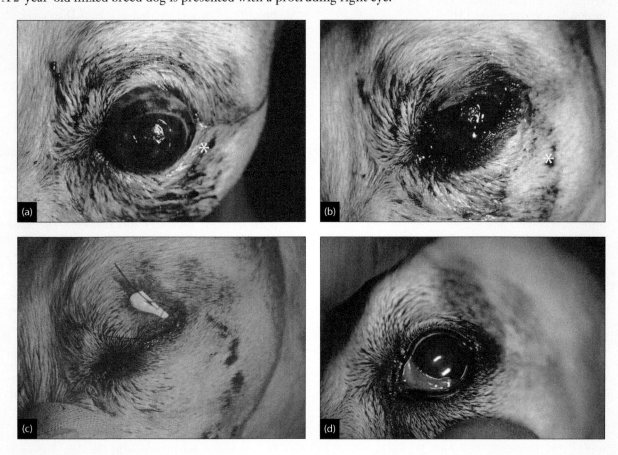

Q1: What is your clinical diagnosis?
Q2: What is the prognosis for vision?

Answers:

1. Proptosis of the right globe
2. The prognosis for vision is usually poor.

REFERENCES

1. Martin, C.L., and Anderson, B.G. 1981. Ocular anatomy. In: Gelatt, K., editor. *Veterinary Ophthalmology*, 1st edition. Lea and Febiger: Philadelphia, PA, pp. 12–121.
2. Constantinescu, G., and McClure, R. 1990. Anatomy of the orbital fascia and the third eyelid in dogs. *American Journal of Veterinary Research* 51:260–263.
3. McClure, R. 1974. The distribution and action of the smooth muscle tissue in the periorbital membrane in the dog. *Anatomy Record* 178:406.
4. Kennedy, R. 1965. The effect of early enucleation on the orbit. *American Journal of Ophthalmology* 60:277–306.
5. Herron, M., Martin, J., and Joyce, J. 1978. Quantitative study of the decussating optic axons in the pony, cow, sheep, and pig. *American Journal of Veterinary Research* 39:1127–1129.
6. Coutler, D., and Schmidt, G. 1984. The eye and vision. In: Swenson, M., editor. *Duke's Physiology of Domestic Animals*. Cornell University Press: Ithaca, NY, pp. 728–741.
7. Bayer, J. 1914. *Angenheilkunde*. Braumueller: Vienna, p. 22.
8. Fox, M. 1963. Postnatal ontogeny of the canine eye. *Journal of the American Veterinary Medical Association* 143:968–974.
9. Miller, P.E., and Murphy, C.J. 1995. Vision in dogs. *Journal of the American Veterinary Medical Association* 207:1623–1634.
10. Miller, P.E. 2000. *A Limited Review of Feline and Equine Vision*. Bill Magrain Basic Science Course for Veterinary Ophthalmologists: Raleigh, 2, pp. 1–11.

11. Murphy, C.J., Zadnik, K., and Mannis, M.J. 1992. Myopia and refractive error in dogs. *Investigative Ophthalmology and Visual Science* 33:2459–2463.

12. Neitz, J., Geist, T., and Jacobs, G.H. 1989. Color vision in the dog. *Visual Neuroscience* 3:119–125.

13. Elliott, J.H., and Futterman, S. 1963. Fluorescence in the tapetum of the cat's eye. *Archives of Ophthalmology* 70:137–140.

14. Weale, R.A. 1953. The spectral reflectivity of the cat's tapetum measured *in situ. Journal of Physiology* 212:30–42.

15. Gunter, R. 1951. The absolute threshold for vision in the cat. *Journal of Physiology* 114:8–15.

16. Duke-Elder, S. 1958. The perception of space in the eye in evolution. In: Duke-Elder, S. (ed.), *System of Ophthalmology* vol. 1. CV Mosby: St. Louis, MO, pp. 666–707.

17. Vakkur, G.J., and Bishop, P.O. 1963. The schematic eye in the cat. *Vision Research* 3:357–381.

18. Vakkur, G.J., Bishop, P.O., and Kozak, W. 1963. Visual optics in the cat, including posterior nodal distance and retinal landmarks. *Vision Research* 3:289–314.

19. Wassle, H. 1971. Optical quality of the cat eye. *Vision Research* 11:995–1006.

20. Blake, R., Cool, S.J., and Crawford, M. 1974. Visual resolution in the cat. *Vision Research* 14:1211–1216.

21. Enzerink, E. 1998. The menace response and pupillary light reflex in neonatal foals. *Equine Veterinary Journal* 30:546–548.

22. Harman, A.M., Moore, S., Hoskins, R., and Keller, P. 1999. Horse vision and an explanation for the visual behaviour originally explained by the "ramp" retina. *Equine Veterinary Journal* 31:384–390.

23. Murphy, C.J., Neitz, J., and Ver Hoeve, J.N. 1999. Temporal and spatial vision in the horse. *Proceedings of the Scientific Meeting of the American College of Veterinary Ophthalmologists* 30:75.

24. Stuhr, C.M., Abrams, G., Bullimore, M., and Murphy, C.J. 1999. The normal refractive state of the equine. *Proceedings of the Scientific Meeting of the American College of Veterinary Ophthalmologists* 30:74.

25. Nicolas, E. 1930. *Veterinary and Comparative Ophthalmology.* J & W Brown: London.

26. Sivak, J.G., and Allen, D.B. 1975. An evaluation of the "ramp" retina of the horse eye. *Vision Research* 15:1353–1356.

27. Pick, D.F., Lovell, G., Brown, S., and Dail, D. 1994. Equine color perception revisited. *Applied Animal Behavioral Science* 42:61–65.

28. Rubin, L., and Patterson, D. 1965. Arteriovenous fistula of the orbit in a dog. *Cornell Veterinarian* 55:471–481.

29. Millichamp, N.J., and Spencer, C.P. 1991. Orbital varix in a dog. *Journal of the American Animal Hospital Association* 27:56–60.

30. Koch, S. 1969. The differential diagnosis of exophthalmos in the dog. *Journal of the American Animal Hospital Association* 5:229–237.

31. Ackerman, N., and Munger, R. 1979. Intraconal contrast orbitography in the dog. *American Journal of Veterinary Research* 40:911–918.

32. Gelatt, K., Guffy, M., and Boggess, T. 1970. Radiographic contrast techniques for detecting orbital and nasolacrimal tumors in dogs. *Journal of the American Veterinary Medical Association* 156:741–746.

33. Lee, R., and Griffiths, I.R. 1972. A comparison of cerebral arteriography and cavernous sinus venography in the dog. *Journal of Small Animal Practice* 12:225–238.

34. Lecouteur, R., Fike, J., Scagliotti, R., and Cann, C. 1982. Computed tomography of orbital tumors in the dog. *Journal of the American Veterinary Medical Association* 180:910–913.

35. Borofffka, S.A., and Voorhout, G. 1999. Direct and reconstructed multiplanar computed tomography of the orbits of healthy dogs. *American Journal of Veterinary Research* 60:1500–1507.

36. Daniel, G.B., and Mitchell, S.K. 1999. The eye and orbit. *Clinical Techniques in Small Animal Practice* 14(3): 160–169.

37. Dennis, R. 2000. Use of magnetic resonance imaging for the investigation of orbital disease in small animals. *Journal of Small Animal Practice* 41:145–155.

38. Morgan, R. 1989. Ultrasonography of retrobulbar diseases of the dog and cat. *Journal of the American Animal Hospital Association* 25:393–399.

39. Stuhr, C., and Scagliotti, R. 1996. Retrobulbar ultrasound in the mesaticephalic and dolichocephalic dog using a temporal approach. *Veterinary and Comparative Ophthalmology* 6:91–99.

40. Gallhoefer, N.S., Bentley, E., Ruetten, M., Grest, P., Haessig, M., Kircher, P.R., Dubielzig, R.R., Spiess, B.M., and Pot, S.A. 2013. Comparison of ultrasonography and histologic examination for identification of ocular diseases of animals: 113 cases (2000–2010). *Journal of the American Veterinary Medical Association* 243(3):376–388.

41. Boydell, P. 1991. Fine needle aspiration biopsy in the diagnosis of exophthalmos. *Journal of Small Animal Practice* 32:542–546.

42. Hendrix, D.H., and Gelatt, K.N. 2000. Diagnosis, treatment, and outcome of orbital neoplasia in dogs: A retrospective study of 44 cases. *Journal of Small Animal Practice* 41:105–108.

43. Slatter, D.H., and Abdelbaki, Y. 1979. Lateral orbitotomy by zygomatic arch resection in the dog. *Journal of the American Veterinary Medical Association* 175:1179–1182.

44. Gilger, B.C., Whitley, D.R., and McLaughlin, S.A. 1994. Modified lateral orbitotomy for removal of orbital neoplasms in two dogs. *Veterinary Surgery* 23:53–58.

45. Rebhun, W. 1982. Orbital lymphosarcoma in cattle. *Journal of the American Veterinary Medical Association* 180:149–152.

46. Cottrill, N.B., Carter, J.D., Pechman, R.D., Dubielzig, R.R., and Waldron, D.R. 1987. Bilateral orbital parosteal osteoma in a cat. *Journal of the American Animal Hospital Association* 23:405–408.

47. Dziezyc, J., and Barton, C.L. 1992. Exophthalmia in a cat caused by an eosinophilic infiltrate. *Progress in Veterinary & Comparative Ophthalmology* 2:91–93.

48. Miller, S., van der Woerdt, A., and Bartick, T. 2000. Retrobulbar pseudotumor of the orbit in a cat. *Journal of the American Veterinary Medical Association* 216:356–358.

49. Martin, C., Kaswan, R., and Doran, C. 1987. Cystic lesions of the periorbital region. *Compendium on Continuing Education for the Practicing Veterinarian* 9:1021–1029.

50. Spiess, B.M., and Pot, S.A. 2013. Diseases and surgery of the canine orbit. In: Gelatt, K.N., Gilger, B.C., and Kern, T.J., editors. *Veterinary Ophthalmology*. Wiley-Blackwell: Ames, IA. 2:793–831.

51. Pentlarge, V.W., Powell-Johnson, G., Martin, C.L. et al. 1989. Orbital neoplasia with enophthalmos in a cat. *Journal of the American Veterinary Medical Association* 195:1249–1251.

52. Sarnat, B.G., and Shanedling, P.D. 1970. Orbital volume following evisceration, enucleation, and exenteration in rabbits. *American Journal of Ophthalmology* 70:787–799.

53. Martin, C.L. 1978. Strabismus associated with extraocular muscle agenesis in a dog. *Journal of the American Animal Hospital Association* 14:486–489.

54. Abrams, K., and Goodwin, C. 1996. Seasonal influence of inflammatory orbital disease in dogs in the northwest United States. *Proceedings of the Scientific Meeting of the American College of Veterinary Ophthalmologists* 27:87.

55. Simison, W.G. 1993. Sialadenitis associated with periorbital disease in a dog. *Journal of the American Veterinary Medical Association* 202:1983–1985.

56. Grahn, B., Szentimrey, D., Battison, A., and Hertling, R. 1995. Exophthalmos associated with frontal sinus osteomyelitis in a puppy. *Journal of the American Animal Hospital Association* 31:397–401.

57. Ramsey, D.T., Marretta, S.M., Hamor, R.E. et al. 1996. Ophthalmic manifestations and complications of dental disease in dogs and cats. *Journal of the American Animal Hospital Association* 32:215–224.

58. Koch, S., and Buell, B.E. 1970. Medial orbital abscess in a Collie dog. *Journal of the American Veterinary Medical Association* 156:1905–1906.

59. Brightman, A.J., McLaughlin, S.A., Brogdon, J.D., Ream, V.B., and Szajerski, M.E. 1985. Intraorbital foreign body in the dog: A case report. *Veterinary Medicine* 80:45–48.

60. Collins, B.K., Moore, C.P., Dubielzig, R.R., and Gengler, W.R. 1991. Anaerobic orbital cellulitis and septicemia in a dog. *Canadian Veterinary Journal* 32:683–685.

61. Grahn, B.H., Szentimrey, D., Pharr, J.W., Farrow, C.S., and Fowler, D. 1995. Ocular and orbital porcupine quills in the dog: A review and case series. *Canadian Veterinary Journal* 36:488–493.

62. Scott, E.A., Duncan, J.R., and McCormack, J.E. 1974. Cryptococcosis involving the postorbital area and frontal sinus in a horse. *Journal of the American Veterinary Medcial Association* 165:626–627.

63. Rebhun, W.C., and Edwards, N.J. 1977. Cryptococcosis involving the orbit of a dog. *Veterinary Medicine/Small Animal Clinician* 72:1447–1450.

64. Peiffer, R.L., Belkin, P.V., and Janke, B.H. 1980. Orbital cellulitis and pneumonitis by *Penicillium* spp. *in a cat*. *Journal of the American Veterinary Medical Association* 176:449–450.

65. Willis, M.A., Martin, C.L., and Stiles, J. 1999. Sino-orbital aspergillosis in a dog. *Journal of the American Veterinary Medical Association* 214:1644–1647.

66. Shelton, G.D., Bandman, E., and Cardinet, G.H. 1985. Electrophoretic comparison of myosins from masticatory muscles and selected limb muscles in the dog. *American Journal of Veterinary Research* 46:493–498.

67. Shelton, G.D., Cardinet, G.H., and Bandman, E. 1987. Canine masticatory muscle disorders: A study of 29 cases. *Muscle Nerve* 10:753–766.

68. Gilmour, M., Morgan, R.V., and Moore, F.M. 1992. Masticatory myopathy in the dog: A retrospective study of 18 cases. *Journal of the American Animal Hospital Association* 28:300–306.

69. Glauberg, A., and Beaumont, P. 1979. Sudden blindness as the presenting sign of eosinophilic myositis: A case report. *Journal of the American Animal Hospital Association* 15:609–611.

70. Lescure, F. 1985. Myosite des masticateurs et cecite chez le chien. *Revue de Médicine Vétérinaire* 136:761–776.

71. Step, D.L., Divers, T.J., Cooper, B., Kallfelz, F.A., Karcher, L.F., and Rebhun, W.C. 1991. Severe masseter myonecrosis in a horse. *Journal of the American Veterinary Association* 198:117–119.

72. Lescure, F. 1983. La rubeose de l'iris chez le chat son traitement par l'acetate de methyl prednisolone. *Revue de Médicine Vétérinaire* 134:527–531.

73. Kornegay, J., Gorgacz, E., Dawe, D., Bowen, J., White, N., and Debuysscher, E. 1980. Polymyositis in dogs. *Journal of the American Veterinary Medical Association* 176:431–438.

74. Carpenter, J., Schmidt, G., Moore, F., Albert, D., Abrams, K., and Elner, V. 1989. Canine bilateral extraocular polymyositis. *Veterinary Pathology* 26:510–512.

75. Ramsey, D.T., Hamor, R.E., Gerding, P.A., and Knight, B. 1995. Clinical and immunohistochemical characteristics of bilateral extraocular polymyositis of dogs. *Proceedings of the Scientific Meeting of the American College of Veterinary Ophthalmologists* 26:130–132.

76. Allgoewer, I., Blair, M., Basher, T. et al. 2000. Extraocular muscle myositis and restrictive strabismus in ten dogs. *Veterinary Ophthalmology* 3:21–26.

77. Caron, J., Barber, S., Bailey, J., Fretz, P., and Pharr, J. 1986. Periorbital skull fractures in five horses. *Journal of the American Veterinary Medical Association* 188:280–284.

78. Martin, C., Kaswan, R., and Chapman, W. 1986. Four cases of traumatic optic nerve blindness in the horse. *Equine Veterinary Journal* 18:133–137.

79. Speakman, .AJ., Baines, S.J., Williams, J.M., and Kelly, D.F. 1997. Zygomatic salivary cyst with mucocele formation in a cat. *Journal of Small Animal Practice* 38:468–470.

80. Miller, P.E., and Pickett, J.P. 1989. Zygomatic salivary gland mucocele in a ferret. *Journal of the American Veterinary Medical Association* 194:1437–1438.

81. Knecht, C., Slusher, R.K., and Guibor, E. 1969. Zygomatic salivary cyst in a dog. *Journal of the American Veterinary Medical Association* 155:625–626.

82. Schmidt, G.M., and Betts, CW. 1978. Zygomatic salivary mucoceles in the dog. *Journal of the American Veterinary Medical Association* 172:940–942.

83. Martin, C. 1971. Orbital mucocele in a dog. *Veterinary Medicine/Small Animal Clinician* 66:36–38.

84. Gross, S., Aguirre, G., and Harvey, C. 1979. Tumors involving the orbit of the dog. *Proceedings of the Scientific Meeting of the American College of Veterinary Ophthalmologists* 10:229–240.

85. Kern, T. 1985. Orbital neoplasia in 23 dogs. *Journal of the American Veterinary Medical Association* 186:489–491.

86. Straw, R.C., LeCouteur, R.A., Powers, B.E., and Withrow, S.J. 1989. Multilobular osteochondrosarcoma of the canine skull: 16 cases (1978–1988). *Journal of the American Veterinary Medical Association* 195:1764–1769.

87. Mauldin, E.A., Deehr, A.J., Hertzke, D., and Dubielzig, R.R. 2000. Canine orbital meningiomas: A review of 22 cases. *Veterinary Ophthalmology* 3:11–16.

88. Gilger, B.C., McLaughlin, S.A., Whitley, R.D., and Wright, J.C. 1992. Orbital neoplasms in cats: 21 cases (1974–1990). *Journal of the American Veterinary Medical Association* 201:1083–1086.

89. Rebhun, W., and Piero, F. 1998. Ocular lesions in horses with lymphosarcoma: 21 cases (1977–1997). *Journal of the American Veterinary Medical Association* 212:852–854.

90. Beech, J. 1983. Retrobulbar melanoma in a horse. *Equine Veterinary Journal Supplement* 2:123–124.

91. Finn, J.P., and Tennant, B.C. 1971. A cerebral and ocular tumor of reticular tissue in a horse. *Veterinary Pathology* 8:458–466.

92. Richardson, D.W., and Acland, H.M. 1983. Multilobular osteoma (chondroma rodens) in a horse. *Journal of the American Veterinary Medical Association* 182:289–291.

93. Bistner, S., Campbell, J., Shaw, D., Leininger, J.R., and Ghobrial, H.K. 1983. Neuroepithelial tumor of the optic nerve in a horse. *Cornell Veterinarian* 73:30–40.

94. Basher, A.W., Severin, G.A., Chavkin, M.J., and Fran, A.A. 1997. Orbital neuroendocrine tumors in three horses. *Journal of the American Medical Veterinary Association* 210:668–671.

95. Goodhead, A.D., Venter, I.J., and Nesbit, J.W. 1997. Retrobulbar extra-adrenal paraganglioma in a horse and its surgical removal by orbitotomy. *Veterinary and Comparative Ophthalmology* 7:96–100.

96. van Maanen, C., Klein, W.R., and Dik, K.J. 1996. Three cases of carcinoid in the equine nasal cavity and maxillary sinuses: Histologic and immunohistochemical features. *Veterinary Pathology* 33:92–95.

97. Miesner, T. et al. 2009. Extra-adrenal paraganglioma of the equine orbit: Six cases. *Veterinary Ophthalmology* 12(4):263–268.

98. Tomlinson, J., and Presnell, K. 1981. Use of the temporalis muscle flap in the dog. *Veterinary Surgery* 10:77–79.

99. Bentley, J., Henderson, R., and Simpsons, S. 1991. Use of a temporalis muscle flap in reconstruction of the calvarium and orbital rim in a dog. *Journal of the American Animal Hospital Association* 27:463–466.

100. Schoster, J., and Wyman, M. 1978. Remission of orbital sarcoma in a dog using doxorubicin therapy. *Journal of the American Veterinary Medical Association* 172:1101–1103.

101. Martin, C. 1971. Orbital emphysema: A complication of ocular enucleation in the dog. *Veterinary Medicine/Small Animal Clinician* 66:986–989.

102. Bedford, P. 1979. Orbital pneumatosis as an unusual complication to enucleation. *Journal of Small Animal Practice* 20:551–555.

103. Walde, I., Hittmair, K., Henninger, W., and Czedik-Eysenberg, T. 1997. Retrobulbar dermoid cyst in a Dachshund. *Veterinary and Comparative Ophthalmology* 7:239–244.

104. Harvey, C., Koch, S., and Rubin, L. 1968. Orbital cysts with conjunctival fistula in a dog. *Journal of the American Veterinary Medical Association* 153:1432–1435.

105. Zemljic, T. et al. 2011. Orbito-nasal cyst in a young European short-haired cat. *Veterinary Ophthalmology* 14(Suppl 1):122–129.

106. Barnett, K., Cottrell, B., and Rest, J. 1988. Retrobulbar hydatid cyst in the horse. *Equine Veterinary Journal* 20:136–138.

107. Pickett, J. 1987. Intracystic injection of tetracycline for cystodesis of an intraorbital cyst in a dog. *Proceedings of the Scientific Meeting of the American College of Veterinary Ophthalmologists* 18:18.

108. Boydell, P. et al. 1996. Orbital fat prolapse in the dog. *Journal of Small Animal Practice* 37(2):61–63.

109. Gelatt, K.N. 1970. Herniation of orbital fat in a colt. *Veterinary Medicine Small Animal Clinic* 65(2):146.

110. Theisen, S.K., Podell, M., Schneider, T., Wilkie, D., and Fenner, W. 1996. A retrospective study of cavernous sinus syndrome in four dogs and eight cats. *Journal of Veterinary Internal Medicine* 10:65–71.

111. Lucas, D. 1954. Ocular associations of dappling in the coat colour of dogs. *Journal of Comparative Pathology* 64:260–266.

112. Gelatt, K.N., and McGill, L.D. 1973. Clinical characteristics of microphthalmia with colobomas of the Australian Shepherd Dog. *Journal of the American Veterinary Medical Association* 162:393–396.

113. Gelatt, K., Powell, G., and Huston, K. 1981. Inheritance of microphthalmia with coloboma in the Australian Shepherd Dog. *American Journal of Veterinary Research* 42:1686–1690.

114. Rebhun, W. 1979. Diseases of the bovine orbit and globe. *Journal of the American Veterinary Medical Association* 175:171–175.

115. Urman, J.K., and Grace, O.D. 1964. Hereditary encephalomyopathy: A hydrocephalus syndrome in newborn calves. *Cornell Veterinarian* 54:230–249.

116. Leipold, H., Gelatt, K., and Huston, K. 1971. Multiple ocular anomalies and hydrocephalus in grade beef Shorthorn cattle. *American Journal of Veterinary Research* 32:1019–1026.

117. Kaswan, R., Collins, L., Blue, J., and Martin, C. 1987. Multiple hereditary ocular anomalies in a herd of cattle. *Journal of the American Veterinary Medical Association* 191:97–99.

118. Leipold, H., and Houston, K. 1968. Congenital syndrome of anophthalmia–microphthalmia with associated defects in cattle. *Pathologica Veterinaria* 5:407–418.

119. Bistner, S., Rubin, L., and Saunders, L. 1970. The ocular lesions of bovine viral diarrhea-mucosal disease. *Veterinary Pathology* 7:275–286.

120. Laratta, L., Riis, R., Kern, T., and Koch, S. 1985. Multiple congenital ocular defects in the Akita dog. *Cornell Veterinarian* 75:381–392.

121. Martin, C., and Leipold, H. 1974. Aphakia and multiple ocular defects in Saint Bernard puppies. *Veterinary Medicine/Small Animal Clinician* 69:448–453.

122. Arnbjerg, J., and Jensen, O. 1982. Spontaneous microphthalmia in two Dobermann puppies with anterior chamber cleavage syndrome. *Journal of the American Animal Hospital Association* 18:481–484.

123. Lewis, D., Kelly, D., and Sansom, J. 1986. Congenital microphthalmia and other developmental ocular anomalies in the Dobermann. *Journal of Small Animal Practice* 27:559–566.

124. Narfstrom, K., and Dubielzig, R. 1984. Posterior lenticonus, cataracts, and microphthalmia: Congenital ocular defects in the Cavalier King Charles Spaniel. *Journal of Small Animal Practice* 25:669–677.

125. Rubin, L. 1968. Hereditary of retinal dysplasia in Bedlington Terriers. *Journal of the American Veterinary Medical Association* 152:260–262.

126. Ashton, N., Barnett, K., and Sachs, D. 1968. Retinal dysplasia in the Sealyham Terrier. *Journal of Pathology and Bacteriology* 96:269–272.

127. Rubin, L., Koch, S., and Huber, R. 1969. Hereditary cataracts in Miniature Schnauzers. *Journal of the American Veterinary Medical Association* 154:1456–1458.

128. van der Woerdt, A., Stades, F.C., van der Linde-Sipman, J.S., and Boeve, MH. 1995. Multiple ocular anomalies in two related litters of Soft Coated Wheaten Terriers. *Veterinary and Comparative Ophthalmology* 5:78–82.

129. Scott, F.A.D., Schultz, R., Bistner, S., and Riis, R. 1975. Teratogenesis in cats associated with griseofulvin therapy. *Teratology* 11:79–86.

130. Creel, D. 1971. Visual system anomaly associated with albinism in the cat. *Nature* 231:465–466.

131. Hubell, D., and Wiesel, T. 1971. Aberrant visual projections in the Siamese cat. *Journal of Physiology* 218:33–62.

132. Guillery, R., Casagrande, V., and Oberdorfer, M. 1974. Congenitally abnormal vision in Siamese cats. *Nature* 252:195–199.

133. Blake, R., and Crawford, M. 1974. Development of strabismus in Siamese cats. *Brain Research* 77:492–496.

134. Holmes, J., and Young, G. 1957. A note on exophthalmos with strabismus in Shorthorn cattle. *Veterinary Record* 69:148–149.

135. Julian, R.J. 1975. Bilateral divergent strabismus in a Holstein calf. *Veterinary Medicine/Small Animal Clinician* 70:1151.

136. Gelatt, K., and McClure, J. 1979. Congenital strabismus and its correction in two Appaloosa horses. *Journal of Equine Medicine and Surgery* 3:240–244.

137. Lavach, J. (ed.) 1990. Orbit, sinuses, and eyeball. In: *Large Animal Ophthalmology*. CV Mosby: Philadelphia, PA, p. 232.

138. Rebhun, W.C., Loeu, E.R., and Riis, R.C. 1984. Clinical manifestations of night blindness in the Appaloosa horse. *Compendium on Continuing Education for the Practicing Veterinarian* 6:103–106.

139. Nasisse, M., Van, E.E.R., Munger, R., and Davidson, M. 1988. Use of methyl methacrylate orbital prosthesis in dogs and cats: 78 cases (1980–1986). *Journal of the American Veterinary Medical Association* 192:539–542.

140. Provost, P., Ortenburger, A., and Caron, J. 1989. Silicone ocular prosthesis in horses: 11 cases (1983–1987). *Journal of the American Veterinary Medical Association* 194:1764–1766.

141. Gilger, B.C., Hamilton, H.L., Wilkie, D.A., van der Woerdt, A., McLaughlin, S.S., and Whitley, R.D. 1995. Traumatic ocular proptosis in dogs and cats: 84 cases (1980–1993). *Journal of the American Veterinary Medical Association* 206:1186–1190.

142. Schmidt, G., Dice, P., and Koch, S. 1975. Intraocular lead foreign bodies in four canine eyes. *Journal of Small Animal Practice* 16:33–39.

143. Davidson, M., Nasisse, M., Jamieson, V., English, R., and Olivero, D. 1991. Traumatic anterior lens capsule disruption. *Journal of the American Animal Hospital Association* 27:410–414.

144. Mittra, R.A., and Mieler, W.F. 1999. Controversies in the management of open-globe injuries involving the posterior segment. *Survey of Ophthalmology* 44:215–225.

145. Lavach, J.D., Severin, G.A., and Roberts, S.M. 1984. Lacerations of the equine eye: A review of 48 cases. *Journal of the American Veterinary Medical Association* 184:1243–1248.

146. Stiles, J., Buyukmihci, N.C., Hacker, D.V., and Canton, D.D. 1993. Blindness from damage to optic chiasm. *Journal of the American Veterinary Medical Association* 202:1192.

147. Janig, C.J., and Hornblass, A. 1986. Treatment of postenucleation orbital cysts. *Annals of Ophthalmolmogy* 18:191–193.

148. Smith, M.M., Shults, S., Waldron, D.R., and Moon, M.L. 1993. Platysma myocutaneous flap for head and neck reconstruction in cats. *Head and Neck* 15:433–439.

149. Fahie, M.A., and Smith, M. 1997. Axial pattern flap based on the superficial temporal artery in cats: An experimental study. *Veterinary Surgery* 26:86–89.

150. Smith, M.M., Payne, J.T., Moon, M.L., and Freeman, L.E. 1991. Axial pattern flap based on the caudal auricular artery in dogs. *American Journal of Veterinary Research* 52:922–925.

151. Millichamp, N.J., and Dziezyc, J. 2000. Cataract phacofragmentation in horses. *Veterinary Ophthalmology* 3:157–164.

152. Group, E.V.S. 1995. Results of the endophthalmitis vitrectomy study: A randomized trial of immediate vitrectomy and of intravenous antibiotics for the treatment of postoperative bacterial endophthalmitis. *Archives of Ophthalmology* 113:1479–1496.

153. Taylor, M.M., Kern, T.J., Riis, R.C., McDonough, P.L., and Erb, H.N. 1995. Intraocular bacterial contamination during cataract surgery in dogs. *Journal of the American Veterinary Medical Association* 206:1716–1720.

154. Beigi, B., Westlake, W., Mangelschots, E., Chang, B., Rich, W., and Riordan, T. 1997. Perioperative microbial contamination of anterior chamber aspirates during extracapsular cataract extraction and phacoemulsification. *British Journal of Ophthalmology* 81:953–955.

155. Roth, D.B., and Flynn, H.W. 1997. Antibiotic selection in the treatment of endophthalmitis: The significance of drug combinations and synergy. *Survey of Ophthalmology* 41:395–401.

156. Jaanus, SD. 1996. Prevention of postoperative infection: Limits and possibilities. *British Journal of Ophthalmology* 80:681–682.

157. Davis, J.E. 1996. Intravenous antibiotics for endophthalmitis. *American Journal of Ophthalmology* 122:724–726.

158. Fruhauf, B., Ohnesorge, B., Deegen, E., and Boeve, M. 1998. Surgical management of equine recurrent uveitis with single port pars plana vitrectomy. *Veterinary Ophthalmology* 1:137–151.

159. Madigan, J.E., Kortz, G., Murphy, C., and Rodger, L. 1995. Photic headshaking in the horse: 7 cases. *Equine Veterinary Journal* 27:306–311.

160. Laus, J.L. et al. 2003. Orbital cellulitis associated with Toxocara canis in a dog. *Veterinary Ophthalmology* 6:333–336.

161. Tova, M.C., and Gomezi, M.A. 2005. Orbital cellulitis and intraocular abscess caused by migrating grass in a cat. *Veterinary Ophthalmology* 8:353–356.

162. Bartoe, J.T. 2007. Modified lateral orbitotomy for vision-sparing excision of a zygomatic mucocele in a dog. *Veterinary Ophthalmology* 10:127–131.

163. Headrick, J.F. et al. 2004. Canine lobular orbital adenoma: A report of 15 cases with distinctive features. *Veterinary Ophthalmology* 7:47–51.

164. Boroffka, S.A. et al. 2007. Assessment of ultrasonography and computed tomography for the evaluation of unilateral orbital disease in dogs. *J Am Vet Med Assoc* 230:671–680.

165. Stiles, J. et al. 2003. Use of a caudal auricular axial pattern flap in three cats and one dog following orbital exenteration. *Veterinary Ophthalmology* 6:212–226.

166. Munoz, E. et al. 2007. Retrobulbar dermoid cyst in a horse: A case report. *Veterinary Ophthalmology* 10:394–397.

167. Townsend, WM. et al. 2003. Dexamethasone-induced exophthalmos in a group of Holstein calves. *Veterinary Ophthalmology* 6:265–268.

CHAPTER 7

EYELIDS

J. PHILLIP PICKETT

INTRODUCTION

The dog has the highest incidence of eyelid disease due to the wide variation in conformation that has been bred into the species. Also, in this species many dermatoses with eyelid involvement may involve the face. The dog will be considered the model for discussion, unless otherwise noted.

The opening of the eyelids is termed the palpebral fissure and is usually somewhat almond shaped. The conformation varies between individuals and breeds of dogs, depending on the size and depth of the orbit, globe size in relation to orbit size, and the amount of redundant facial skin.

Anatomy
Skin

The skin of the eyelids is typically thin and loosely adherent to the underlying tissue to facilitate movement. This looseness may result in subcutaneous edema or hemorrhage accumulation from relatively minor trauma such as rubbing. In mammals, the upper eyelid is the most mobile. In most birds and some reptiles, the lower lid is the most mobile. Dorsomedially (at the medial point of the brow), there is located a group of tactile hairs, innervated by a branch of the ophthalmic branch of the trigeminal nerve, termed the supraorbital pili.

Muscles
Orbicularis oculi muscle

The orbicularis oculi muscle is a superficial facial sphincter muscle and is the only muscle that contributes significantly to closure of the palpebral aperture (**Figure 7.1**). Beginning from the lid margin, it may be divided into the pretarsal, preseptal, and orbital zones. It consists mainly of type 2 fast twitch muscle fibers, which are involved in initiating contractions of rapid and short duration (blinking).[1]

When making surgical incisions into the eyelid, the orbicularis oculi muscle is encountered immediately under the skin. Motor innervation is via the palpebral branch of cranial nerve VII. The orbicularis oculi muscle is involved in the efferent arm of the palpebral reflex (tapping the lids results in blinking), the corneal reflex (touching the cornea results in a blink), the glabellar reflex (tapping the frontal bone between the eyes results in a blink), the dazzle reflex (quickly shining a bright light towards the eye results in blinking), and the menace response (a threatening motion to the head results in blinking). The orbicularis oculi muscle is a strong muscle that is responsible for the severe blepharospasm seen with ocular pain. It is anchored medially by the medial palpebral (canthal) ligament, a palpable structure connecting the medial commissure of the palpebral fissure to the lacrimal bone (**Figure 7.2**). The lateral palpebral ligament is poorly developed in many dogs and connects the lateral commissure of the eyelids to the orbital ligament.

Levator anguli oculi medialis muscle

This muscle is a superficial facial muscle that helps to elevate the medial upper lid. Motor innervation is by cranial nerve VII.

Retractor angularis oculi lateralis muscle

The retractor angularis oculi lateralis muscle is a superficial facial muscle that draws the lateral canthus laterally, thus acting as a lateral canthal ligament (**Figure 7.2**). Motor innervation is by cranial nerve VII.

Malaris muscle

The malaris muscle is also a superficial facial muscle, and the palpebral portion depresses the lower lid (**Figure 7.1**). Motor innervation is by cranial nerve VII.

Levator palpebrae superioris

The levator palpebrae superioris muscle is the only striated muscle of the eyelid that originates from within the orbit above the optic foramen. It is the main skeletal muscle that elevates the upper lid (**Figure 7.3**). Motor innervation is by cranial nerve III.

Müller's muscle

Müller's muscle originates from the dorsal surface of the levator palpebrae superioris muscle to the upper lid and from the ventral rectus muscle to the lower lid. It is a smooth muscle that inserts in the lids and third eyelid and

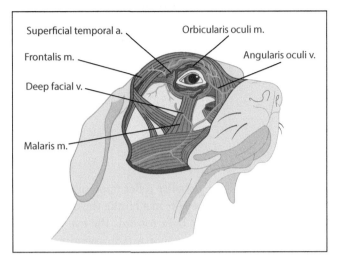

Figure 7.1 **Gross anatomy of the eyelids and surrounding muscles, nerves, and vessels of the dog. (a: Artery; m: Muscle; v: Vein.)**

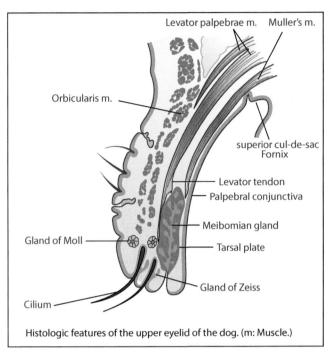

Histologic features of the upper eyelid of the dog. (m: Muscle.)

keeps them tonically retracted (**Figure 7.3**). Innervation is by sympathetic fibers traveling in the nasociliary branch of the ophthalmic division of cranial nerve V.

Fascia

The periosteum of the orbit (periorbita) divides at the orbital rim to reflect as periosteum on the cranial and facial bones and continues as a fascial sheath into the lids to join the tarsus. This fascial sheet in the lids is termed the orbital septum, and it provides an important barrier separating the orbit from the superficial lid. Lacerations in the orbital septum may allow infection to penetrate the orbit. Weak areas or voids in the orbital septum may allow prolapse of intraorbital contents (fat) into the palpebral, third eyelid, or bulbar subconjunctival spaces.

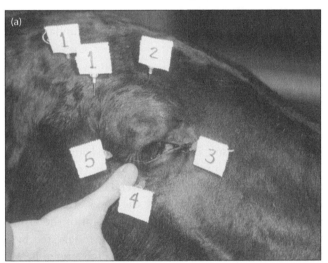

Figure 7.3 **(a) Landmarks for nerve blocks of the eyelid in a horse. 1. Palpebral nerve, branch of CN VII. Nerve may be blocked high (where nerve crosses dorsal-most point of zygomatic arch) or low (as nerve passes over zygomatic arch adjacent to supraorbital fossa). 2. Frontal nerve, branch of CN V. Nerve may be blocked as it exits supraorbital foramen. 3. Infratrochlear nerve, branch of CN V. Nerve may be blocked dorsal and ventral to the trochlear notch, bony prominence on the lacrimal bone. 4. Zygomatic nerve, branch of CN V. Nerve can be blocked with a line block along the lateral aspect of the ventral orbital rim. 5. Lacrimal nerve, branch of CN V. Nerve can be blocked along lateral one-third aspect of the dorsal orbital rim.**

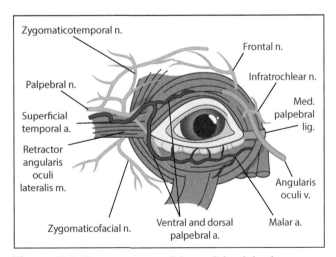

Figure 7.2 **Gross anatomy of the eyelids of the dog. (a: Artery; lig: Ligament; m: Muscle; n: Nerve; v: Vein.)**

Nerves

Sensory

The sensory innervation to the eyelids is entirely by cranial nerve V (trigeminal). The sensory nerves emerge around the orbital margin and can be blocked with injectable anesthetic agent by a ring or a line block or at specific sites of emergence (**Figure 7.2**). In the horse, localization and local anesthesia of the four main sensory nerves allows for surgical manipulations to be performed in the standing animal[2] with appropriate sedation (**Figure 7.3a**).

Maxillary division of trigeminal nerve
- Zygomaticotemporal nerve (termed lacrimal nerve in the horse): Sensory to the lateral dorsal lid.

Ophthalmic division of trigeminal nerve
- Infratrochlear nerve: Sensory to the medial canthus, medial dorsal and ventral lid.
- Frontal (supraorbital) nerve: Sensory to the middle portion of the upper lid.
- Zygomaticofacial nerve (termed zygomatic nerve in the horse): Sensory to the lateral ventral lid.

Motor

Oculomotor (III)

The oculomotor nerve supplies motor (somatic efferent) fibers to the levator palpebrae superioris muscle, as well as to all the extraocular muscles except the dorsal oblique, retractor bulbi, and lateral rectus muscles. The oculomotor nerve also supplies parasympathetic fibers (visceral efferent) to the iris and ciliary smooth muscles, Müller's muscle, and smooth muscle in the third eyelid and periorbita.

Facial (VII)

The facial nerve supplies the superficial facial muscles involving the lid, that is, orbicularis oculi, malaris, and levator anguli oculi medialis muscles.

Sympathetic fibers

Sympathetic fibers, via the trigeminal nerve branches, supply smooth muscle in the lids (Müller's muscle), third eyelid, and the lacrimal glands.[3,4]

> The orbicularis oculi muscle closes the eyelids and is innervated by cranial nerve VII; the levator palpebral (skeletal) and Müller's muscle (smooth) elevate the upper eyelid and are innervated by cranial nerve III and by sympathetic fibers, respectively.

Ligaments

Medial and lateral canthal ligaments

This is a well-developed collagenous structure that originates from medial fibers of the orbicularis oculi muscle and inserts on the orbital rim of the lacrimal bone. A comparable lateral ligament does not exist, but lateral fascial attachments and the retractor angularis oculi lateralis muscle keep the palpebral aperture almond shaped rather than circular (**Figure 7.2**). In mesaticephalic broad-based canine skulls, the lateral canthal ligament may be more developed and misdirected medially, producing tension on the lateral canthus that may result in involution (lateral entropion).[5]

Blood vessels

Superficial temporal artery

The superficial temporal artery (a branch of the external carotid artery) courses with the palpebral nerve 1 cm (0.4 in) dorsal to the zygomatic arch and terminates in the lateral superior and inferior palpebral arteries (**Figure 7.2**). Caution is required when injecting a local anesthetic to block the palpebral nerve to avoid intra-arterial injection.

Malar artery

The malar artery originates ventrally inside of the orbit from the infraorbital artery (the continuation of the maxillary artery). It supplies medial periocular structures such as the eyelid, third eyelid, and nasolacrimal duct and anastomoses with the lateral inferior palpebral artery (**Figure 7.2**).

Angularis oculi vein

The angularis oculi vein is a branch of the facial vein. It passes superficial to the medial canthal ligament to enter the dorsal orbit (**Figures 7.1 and 7.2**), where it becomes the dorsal ophthalmic vein. The ophthalmic vein provides the major venous drainage of the orbit, and it courses through the orbital fissure to join the cavernous sinus. The ophthalmic vein does not contain valves, and blood may flow either towards the face or the cavernous sinus.[6] Septic processes involving this vein may spread to the cranial cavity, and accidental cutting or puncture of this vein during enucleation, placement of subpalpebral lavage systems in horses, or third eyelid gland repositioning procedures in dogs may result in profuse hemorrhage. The vein is readily accessible percutaneously or with a surgical cut down; prior to more advanced imaging modalities (MRI/CT), injection of radiographic contrast material into the vein enabled the orbital veins, space-occupying lesions of the orbit, and the base of the brain (for pituitary tumors) to be studied.[7]

Exuberant dissection in the dorsal medial eyelid and orbit frequently transects the angularis oculi vein and results in marked venous hemorrhage.

Lid margins

Surgery frequently involves the lid margin and accurate reconstruction is essential for cosmetic and functional considerations. Important landmarks are discussed.

Cilia

The cilia are tactile organs present in three to four rows near the margin of the upper lid only in the dog (**Figure 7.3**). The cat is often said not to have true cilia, but, in fact, they are present in the upper lid, although much less well developed than in the dog. The horse, cow, New World camelids, and other domestic species have well-developed cilia on both the upper and lower eyelids. The dog has numerous problems with cilia, while cilia problems are relatively rare in other species.

Lid trough

A trough or furrow runs the length of the lid on the middle of the lid margin. The meibomian glands (tarsal glands) open into this trough and are observed as 30–40 pinpoint white orifices (depressions) on each lid margin. The trough serves as a surgical landmark ("gray line") for procedures that involve lid splitting or halving. This trough also serves to help maintain the precorneal tear film meniscus, and when this trough is disrupted, especially on the lower lid, tear spillage onto the lower lid/face may occur.

Tarsus (tarsal plate)

The tarsus (tarsal plate) is a fibrous plate that runs parallel to the lid margin and contains the embedded meibomian glands. The tarsus gives some rigidity to the lids, but in domestic animals, the tarsus is poorly developed compared to humans, resulting in relatively "floppy" lids (**Figure 7.3**).

Meibomian glands

The meibomian (tarsal) glands are large sebaceous glands that can be viewed through the palpebral conjunctiva as white parallel streaks near the lid margin (**Figure 7.3**). Secretion from the meibomian glands provides nutrition to the cornea and forms the lipid layer of the precorneal tear film, which prevents evaporation and spilling of tears onto the face. Alterations in secretion may produce lid and corneal pathology. The glands may undergo metaplasia to become hair follicles, producing a hair that emerges on the lid margin (distichia) or directly extends through the palpebral conjunctiva to rub on the cornea (ectopic cilium).

Glands of Zeiss

The glands of Zeiss are sebaceous glands located at the base of the cilia and they open into the follicle of the cilia (**Figure 7.3**).

Glands of Moll

The glands of Moll are rudimentary sweat glands that are located at the base of the cilia and open onto the lid margin and the follicle of the cilia (**Figure 7.3**).

Glands of Krause and Wolfring

Some texts refer to the glands of Krause and Wolfring (seen in man) as accessory lacrimal glands, but they have not been demonstrated in the dog and the cat.

Conjunctiva

The conjunctiva that lines the eyelids is termed the palpebral conjunctiva. It is composed of stratified squamous epithelium and is more tightly adherent to the underlying tissues over the tarsal plate. Towards the fornix, the epithelium is stratified columnar and has more goblet cells. The conjunctiva reflects onto the globe at the fornix to become the bulbar conjunctiva.

Lacrimal punctum

In the dog, the cat, the horse, and the cow, a single lacrimal punctum exists on the conjunctival surface of each lid, about 1–2 mm from the lid margin. The orifices are slit-like (horizontally oriented in the lower lid and more vertically oriented in the upper) and about 5 mm from the medial canthus in the lower lid and 7–8 mm from the medial canthus in the upper lid. The edges of the puncta are usually identified at the medial most aspect of the tarsal plate. Not all species have two puncta: The rabbit has one large ventral punctum that is present in the ventral cul-de-sac away from the lid margin.

PHYSIOLOGY

Function of the eyelids

- Protect the ocular surfaces (cornea, bulbar and palpebral conjunctiva, and inferior and superior cul-de-sacs) from the entrance of foreign particles.
- Aid in removing surface ocular foreign particles by blinking.
- Distribute the precorneal tear film and aid in propulsion of tears toward the lacrimal puncta. The palpebral fissure closes in a zipper-like fashion,

starting at the lateral canthus and closing toward the medial canthus.

- Removal of visual stimuli for sleeping.
- Contain glands that contribute to the tear film and, therefore, are of importance in optics and nutrition of the cornea.
- Cilia and vibrissae are important tactile organs.

Blinking

Reflex blinking

- Tactile, that is, corneal, glabellar, and palpebral reflexes, are examples of tactile reflex blinking.
- Optical: The dazzle reflex is the induction of a blink in response to a strong light. It is used to evaluate the intactness of the lower visual system. In humans, the dazzle reflex is frequently accompanied by sneezing ("photic sneeze reflex").

The menace response occurs when the sudden presentation of a threatening object to the eye stimulates a blink. It is not considered a true reflex because it involves input from the cerebral cortex. The pathway for the menace response is somewhat vague, but it involves the visual pathways as well as the motor cortex, cerebellum, and facial nerve (see Chapter 1, Figure 1.66). The auditory response occurs when a loud noise produces a blink.

The menace response may not be present until 7–10 days after birth in foals and 4 weeks (or more) after birth in puppies. Conditions other than blindness (e.g., dementia, coma, postictal seizure episode, drug therapy) can interfere with the menace response.

Spontaneous blinking

Spontaneous blinking occurs without obvious stimuli. The rate of blinking varies greatly between species and under varying environmental influences. Blinking may occur unilaterally or bilaterally. The cat blinks less frequently than most other species (1–5 blinks/5 min[8], 2 blinks/min[9]), with half of these being incomplete. The dog blinks about 3/min[8] to 14/min[10], with most of them incomplete. Horses blink 5–20/min, cattle 5/min, and pigs 10/min. This normal infrequent blinking may explain the higher tear production and increased ability to tolerate facial paralysis in many animals compared to humans.

DISEASES OF THE EYELIDS

Congenital diseases

Ankyloblepharon

The dog and the cat are born with a physiologic ankyloblepharon that lasts for 10–15 days. The ankyloblepharon

may open prematurely with no adverse reaction, or an exposure keratitis may develop.[11,12] The corneal pathology may be related more to an accompanying lack of lacrimal secretion and palpebral reflexes than to premature opening. If signs of keratitis develop, either a temporary tarsorrhaphy should be performed utilizing local anesthesia or copious amounts of ocular lubricants used to protect the cornea.

In the dog, a persistent ankyloblepharon associated with pulmonary edema has been reported to be associated with feeding raw eggs to the dam. It was postulated that avidin was responsible for this syndrome, as it corrected with cooking the eggs.[13] Ankyloblepharon may be seen in premature foals and should be allowed to separate on its own to avoid exposure keratitis problems.

If neonatal conjunctivitis occurs, the ankyloblepharon may be detrimental due to retention of exudates (**Figure 7.4**). If exudate or swelling is present, the lids should be opened digitally or by gently spreading a hemostat at the medial canthus followed by topical antibiotics. Corneal perforation is the most severe sequela of this syndrome. Cultures of the exudate in dogs often yield a mixed bacterial infection. In the cat, neonatal infection with feline herpesvirus is frequently the cause of neonatal ophthalmia.[14]

Coloboma

Introduction/etiology

A coloboma is a fissure or notch-like defect of the lid, the iris, the ciliary body, the lens, or the posterior segment. Small notch-like defects are common in the upper middle to medial eyelid of certain lines of dogs of varying breeds. These defects have very minor esthetic significance but no functional significance. Rarely seen

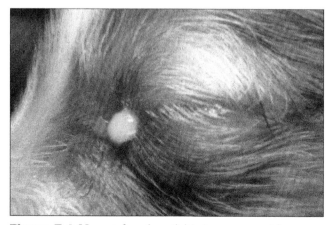

Figure 7.4 Neonatal conjunctivitis in a puppy with physiologic ankyloblepharon. Note the outward bulging of the eyelids with the purulent exudate leaking from the medial canthus.

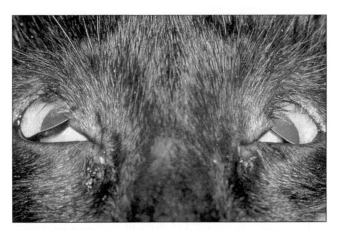

Figure 7.5 Young adult cat with bilateral eyelid agenesis or colobomas. Note trichiasis but relatively normal corneas.

in horses, these minor upper and lower lid notches are equally insignificant. The most notable colobomatous defect of the lids is agenesis of the upper eyelid, observed in kittens (**Figure 7.5**). This condition is part of a syndrome termed multiple ocular colobomas (MOC) that has been observed in snow leopards in zoos, the domestic cat, and a captive Texas cougar.[15] Usually an individual kitten is presented, but an entire litter may be involved with variable manifestations within the litter, from minor defects in the upper lateral lids to severe microphthalmos.[16] The most common lesion of MOC is a bilateral lack of the lateral two-thirds of the upper eyelid. The cause is unknown, and to date, attempts to prove a genetic link in the snow leopard have failed.[17,18] There are no reports in the domestic cat to support a genetic cause for either MOC or lid colobomas.

Clinical signs

- Young kitten with lower lid blepharospasm, globe retraction, and third eyelid protrusion.
- Bilateral defect of upper lids involving the temporal two-thirds of the lid. The normal lid margin is missing, usually resulting in the facial hairs being misdirected toward the cornea (trichiasis). Varying degrees of malformation may be observed in a litter, from mild thinning of the lateral canthus to a large defect in the upper lid (**Figure 7.5**).
- Variable amounts of keratitis are present under the defect.
- Persistent pupillary membrane is the most common associated defect observed in individual kittens; occasionally iris colobomas, cataract, and lens subluxation are noted.
- Colobomas of the optic nerve and peripapillary region[14,19] (see Chapter 14).

- Multifocal retinal dysplasia (see Chapter 14).
- Microphthalmia is the most severe manifestation of MOC.

Course

The blepharospasm often abates with time; consequently, as the cat gets older and is a better candidate for surgery, the necessity to treat is often not as urgent. In this author's hands, removing the frictional irritation (trichiasis) with cryosurgery early on (as early as 4–6 weeks of age) many times results in a comfortable cat with no need for additional surgical therapy.

Diagnosis

A young cat is usually presented with trichiasis, and upon detailed examination, the normal mucocutaneous junction of the lid margin is missing, and the normal curvature of the upper lid is deviated dorsally. A full ophthalmic examination should be performed to look for other colobomatous defects.

Therapy

Due to the diminutive size of most patients when initially presented with MOC, they are not good candidates for definitive surgery because of mechanical and anesthetic difficulties. As stated previously, cryosurgery to remove trichiasis under chemical sedation may yield an economical, good long-term result. A variety of surgical procedures have been devised for correction. Definitive surgery is usually postponed until 5–6 months of age.

Pedicle graft A rotating pedicle skin graft from the lower lid, with or without conjunctival grafting, may be used to fill the coloboma (**Figure 7.6**).[20,21] Dr. Martin developed a skin flap technique that rotates the flap down from the forehead, rather than from the lower lid, because of the danger of creating ectropion in the lower lid. This approach also ensures the direction of the hair is away from the globe (**Figure 7.7**).

Cutler–Beard procedure The Cutler–Beard procedure (**Figure 7.8**) gives excellent results, but the eye is covered for several weeks, which is a major disadvantage since agenesis is a bilateral disease.[22] A sliding H-plasty technique (**Figure 7.8a**) where skin from above the upper eyelid is slid ventrally and lined with palpebral conjunctiva from the lower lids[23] also works well, but it has the same disadvantages of having the operated globe covered for several weeks, as is the case with the Cutler–Beard technique.

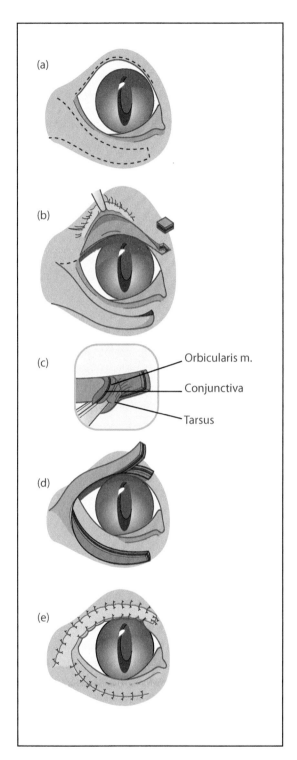

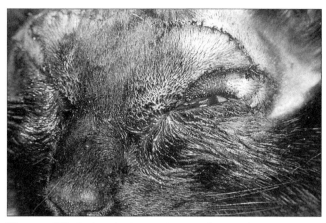

Figure 7.7 Patient in Figure 7.5—24 hours after surgery, with a rotating pedicle graft from the upper forehead and a rotating pedicle conjunctival graft from the lower conjunctival sac.

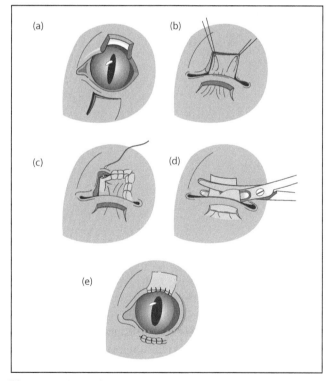

Figure 7.6 Rotating a pedicle flap from the lower lid to fill a colobomatous upper eyelid in a cat. The lid is split into skin and conjunctiva, and a pedicle flap is outlined from the lower lid (a). The canthus is cut to allow rotation and squaring of the tip of the pedicle and minimize ischemia (b). The layers are transposed, leaving conjunctiva (c). Transposition (d). Sutured pedicle and donor area (e). (Modified from Roberts, S.R., and Bistner, S.I. 1968. *Modern Veterinary Practice* 49:40–43.[20]) (m: Muscle.)

Figure 7.8 Cutler–Beard two-stage procedure for repair of eyelid defects. The procedure can be reversed for lower lid defects but may create a mild ptosis. A full-thickness lid pedicle from the opposite lid is created, leaving a bridge of normal lid approximately 5-mm wide (a). The pedicle is placed and sutured in two layers; this is left to heal for 6 weeks (b, c). The pedicle is cut after healing; because it is under tension, the cut should be about 1 mm from the continuation of the adjacent lid margin (d). The cut conjunctiva is sutured to the skin in a continuous pattern, to form a new mucocutaneous border (e).

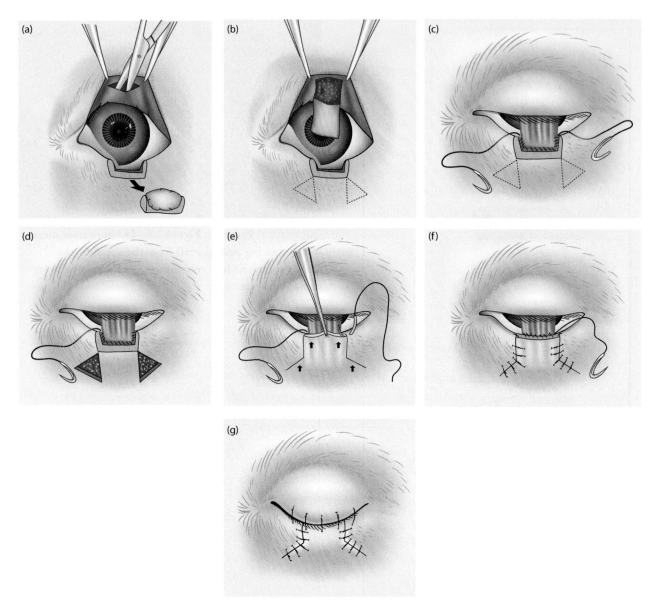

Figure 7.8a Sliding H-plasty technique for correction of eyelid agenesis or closure of a large full-thickness eyelid deficit. Following full-thickness excision of lid, or following splitting the skin from the globe in the case of eyelid agenesis, palpebral conjunctiva from the opposite lid is split from the lid stroma (a). The initial incision parallel to the lid margin begins just caudal to the base of the meibomian glands (a). Once the conjunctiva is free from the underlying lid stroma, a conjunctival fornix based flap is freed with the two parallel incisions (perpendicular to the lid margin) being made slightly wider than the void to be filled on the opposite lid (b). The freed conjunctival pedicle flap is sutured to the conjunctiva of the excision/agenesis site with a continuous suture pattern of fine, absorbable suture (c). Two skin thickness incisions are extended from the edges of the excision/agenesis site in a slightly diverging manner (d). These incisions should be two to three times the length of the void to be filled. At the ends of these incisions, two Burow triangles are excised in the skin (the sides of the triangles should be the length of the void to be filled) (b and d). The skin flap and areas around the triangles are undermined to allow the tissue to be easily moved. The flap is advanced, skin-to-skin is sutured at the corners of the flap/lid margin (e), the Burow triangles are closed (f), and the remainder of the skin incisions closed with simple interrupted non-absorbable suture (dead space may be closed with fine, buried absorbable suture). The skin flap edge is sutured to the conjunctival flap with fine absorbable suture in a running pattern such that the suture does not penetrate the conjunctival flap and abrade the underlying cornea while the grafts are healing (f). Temporary tarsorrhaphy sutures over stents (see Figure 7.45 in this chapter) immobilize the tissues during the healing phase (g). At 3–4 weeks post-op, the skin sutures and temporary tarsorrhaphy sutures are removed, and the conjunctival bridge is cut between the intact lid margin and the reconstructed eyelid margin.

Cryoepilation Cryoepilation of the offending cilia is a rapid, easy alternative to extensive plastic surgery and can be performed on the very young kitten. This removes the trichiasis but does not correct the defect or protect the globe. A double freeze-thaw technique is utilized, and care must be taken to not aggressively freeze the sclera, potentially causing damage to underlying intraocular structures (choroid, retina, ciliary body).

Subdermal collagen injection with a modified Stades procedure to relieve trichiasis Wolfer described the injection of bovine subdermal collagen into the lid immediately above the eyelid coloboma, followed weeks later by lid splitting and removal of 1 cm (0.4 in) of skin the length of the coloboma.[24] The remaining bulbar conjunctiva was then mobilized and sutured about one-third of the distance across the wound bed that was created, with the remainder left to granulate. The relative simplicity of the procedure facilitated its use in young kittens. The result of relieving trichiasis but not correcting the lid deficit is similar to the results of cryosurgery.

Lip commissure to eyelid transposition technique Whittaker et al. described a technique of transposing the ipsilateral lip commissure (with skin, mucosa, a mucocutaneous junction, and muscle) to the lateral canthus/upper lid void that resulted in complete protection of the globe as well as a mobile lid in some cases[25] (**Figure 7.8b**).

Dermoid
Introduction/etiology
A dermoid is a choristoma or congenital misplacement of tissues that is not normal to the location. The misplacement involves dermal elements of skin, hair, glandular tissue, and fat. Dermoids involving the eyelids may be an extension from extensive dermoids of the cornea and conjunctiva or an isolated island of tissue, usually near the lid margin. Dermoids have been observed in both the dog and the cat, where inheritance has been suggested but not defined in the Burmese cat (**Figure 7.9**), dachshund, St. Bernard, and GSD.[26,27] A bilateral syndrome has been found in Hereford calves, and pedigree analysis suggests either a recessive or a polygenic trait for the condition.[28] Martin observed very large dermoids on the cornea of calves, and these dermoids reflected onto the eyelids (**Figure 7.10**). This author has seen dermoids of the lids, third eyelids, and corneas in Hereford cross and Holstein calves.

Clinical signs
- Tufts or masses on the lid margin or lateral canthus with hair that often extends onto the conjunctival surfaces and cornea.

- Hairs on the lid may point toward the eye and produce epiphora, blepharospasm, and keratitis (**Figure 7.9**).

Therapy
Therapy is surgical excision and repair of the defect (see section Eyelid neoplasia, Therapy). If the lesion extends to the cornea, a superficial keratectomy can remove this portion of the lesion.

Diseases of the cilia
Diseases of the cilia are very common in the dog but relatively rare in other species. Most of the conditions are probably inherited, but they have not been studied in enough detail to determine the mode of inheritance.

Distichia
Introduction/etiology
Distichiasis is the presence of an additional row of lashes on the lid margin. The original proposed pathogenesis was that distichia originated from metaplastic meibomian glands (closely related to hair follicles embryologically) and emerged on the lid margin (or through the palpebral conjunctiva in the case of ectopic cilia). Alternatively, Raymond-Letron et al. proposed, after studying histologic sections in dogs, that abnormal hair follicles are located close to the meibomian glands and envelop the follicle, and the hair reaches the surface via the path of least resistance, which is the duct of the meibomian gland.[29] While most distichia are thought to be developmental, they may not be observed in the young puppy but can manifest later in the growing dog. Distichia have also been hypothesized to arise due to chronic inflammatory irritation to the meibomian glands and so may arise later in life.[30] The lashes can be stout or fine, few or numerous (**Figure 7.11**). Distichiasis is very common in many breeds of dogs such as the American (75%+ incidence) and English Cocker Spaniel, Shih Tzu, English bulldog, Pekingese, toy and miniature poodle, Shetland sheepdog, Cavalier King Charles spaniel, Siberian husky, and Golden retriever (for a comprehensive list of eyelid disorders felt to be of genetic origin, please see **Table 7.1** at the end of this chapter). The mode of inheritance is undetermined but has been postulated as dominant with irregular penetrance.[31]

Clinical signs
- Most animals with distichia are asymptomatic, and therapy is not recommended simply because they are present.
- Mild signs include epiphora and nonulcerative keratitis.
- Severe cases of distichiasis may present with blepharospasm and ulcerative keratitis.

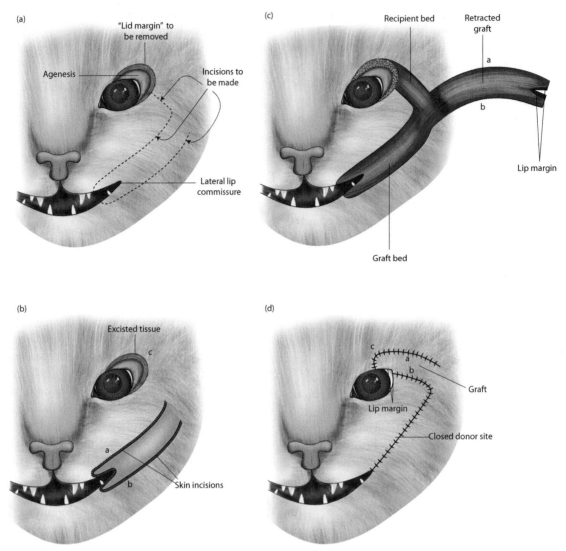

Figure 7.8b Lip commissure to lid transposition for repair of feline eyelid agenesis (a). Skin around the agenesis site is to be freshened to allow receipt of the graft from the lateral commissure of the lips (a). The flap to be moved is outlined as well as the bridging incision in the skin to allow the graft to be transposed to the lateral lids (a). The skin around the agenesis site is removed, and the skin incision for the graft is made (b). At the level of the lip commissure, the incision is full thickness (skin, muscle, and mucous membrane) for 2–3 centimeters and then becomes only skin thickness for the remainder of the graft (b). The graft is retracted (c), and the connecting bridge skin excision is made and undermined to create the recipient bed for the graft (c). The graft is sewn in place with the upper "lip" becoming the upper "lid" at site "c," and the lower "lip" becomes the lower "lid/lateral canthus" (d). Fine absorbable suture may be used to close dead space around the recipient bed and under the graft. The skin is closed with simple interrupted sutures of non-absorbable material. The lateral lip commissure area is closed in two layers with absorbable and non-absorbable suture material.

Diagnosis

Diagnosis of distichiasis is made by observing the presence of hairs on one or more lid margins. Magnification is often necessary to observe the fine hairs. Examination against different backgrounds (such as cornea and sclera) may make the hairs more visible. If distichia contact the ocular surface, they become covered in a "dewdrop" of tears or mucus (which can be accentuated with application of fluorescein stain), and this may highlight their presence. If a hair is observed, it is important to determine that it is rubbing on the cornea and is in the corresponding location to be associated with the corneal pathology. Plucking out the distichia should then relieve the signs. Milder manifestations of distichiasis, such as epiphora, may have many causes; most dogs with distichia are asymptomatic. Consequently, it is important to establish cause and effect. If in doubt as to the significance of the distichia, plucking with relief of signs can confirm their

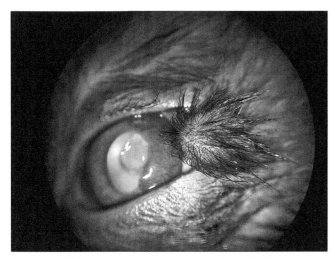

Figure 7.9 Dermoid at the lateral canthus of a Burmese cat. Note corneal ulceration and neovascularization.

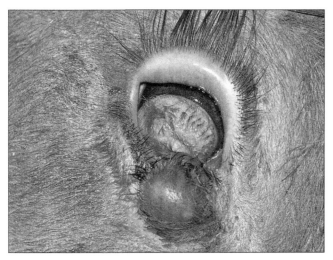

Figure 7.10 Massive dermoid on the cornea, extending across the conjunctival sac to the lids, in a calf. The lesion was bilateral and was surgically removed.

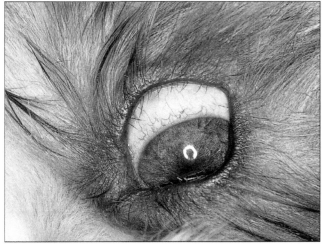

Figure 7.11 Marked distichia of both lids, but only visualized well in the photo of the upper lid of a Shih Tzu.

role in producing the signs. *Plucking of distichia is not a definitive therapy as regrowth (sometimes of even thicker, more irritating hairs) inevitably occurs.*

> Distichiasis is one of the most common eyelid lesions observed in dogs, but it produces appreciable signs in only a small percentage of affected animals. The challenge is not in diagnosing distichiasis but to attribute ocular signs accurately to the condition to avoid unnecessary surgery.

Therapy

A wide variety of surgical therapies have been used over the years, with many having significant complications. The most common complication of surgery is regrowth of hairs. Preliminary to performing any of the procedures, the meibomian glands should be expressed by squeezing against a firm plate or the handle of an instrument or with an untoothed forceps. This procedure pushes hidden hairs out of the meibomian orifice; these hairs would otherwise remain overlooked and be considered regrowth later.[31–33]

Surgical resection Surgical procedures involving the lid margins, such as lid splitting and tarsoconjunctival resection (**Figure 7.12**), are currently out of favor with most ophthalmologists due to the risk of postoperative deformities of the eyelid margins and regrowth of hairs. Tarsoconjunctival resection performed on the upper lid removes most of the supporting tissue for the normal cilia, resulting in their collapse onto the cornea. In the past, a special lid plate was designed to facilitate lid-splitting surgery.[34]

Resection of the meibomian glands with their distichia from the conjunctival surface was a preferable method by Martin because it spared the lid margin (**Figure 7.12d**). A strip of tissue 2–3 mm in width was removed from the conjunctival side that included the involved meibomian glands.[33,35] Martin used this method combined with cryotherapy for extensive numbers of distichia over the length of the lid. This author has found this procedure to be complicated by cicatricial entropion and disruption of the lid trough (especially of the lower lid) with secondary tear film instability and epiphora.

Electrolysis Electrolysis is an old therapy for removing unwanted hairs. It involves passing a fine needle into each individual meibomian gland/hair follicle to supposedly destroy the follicle with an electric current (**Figures 7.13 and 7.14**). This is a very tedious procedure when the hairs are numerous. The strength of the

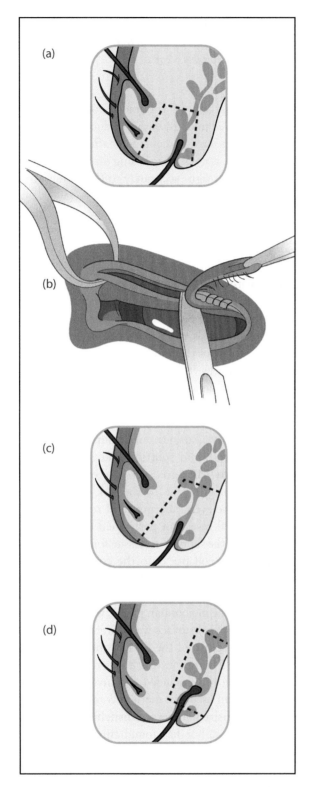

(a)

(b)

(c)

(d)

Figure 7.12 Various lid-splitting techniques devised for distichia removal. True lid splitting with both incisions on the lid margin (a, b). Modification with only one lid margin incision (c). Tarsoconjunctival resection is the safest procedure (d). Lid-splitting procedures are currently out of favor by most veterinary ophthalmologists due to the potential for postoperative lid margin deformities.

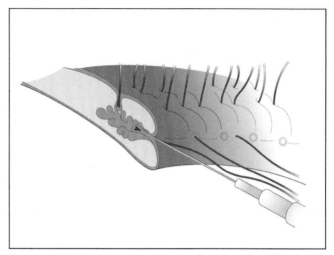

Figure 7.13 Electrolysis of distichia.

current is critical to destroy the hair follicle without causing excessive destruction of the lid. Recurrences are frequent when battery-operated electrolysis needles are used. If the power supply is of higher strength (surgical electrocautery unit), it is very easy to apply excessive current, resulting in lid margin deformities and scarred depigmented foci on the lid margin (**Figure 7.15**). This author has seen a high incidence of postelectrolysis ectopic cilia in patients that preoperatively did not have ectopic cilia.

Electrocautery Electrocautery from the conjunctival side[36] running parallel to the lid margin has been advocated for distichia. This incision transects the base of the hair follicle, allowing the hair to be easily plucked (**Figure 7.16**). As was the case with surgical resection techniques, regrowth

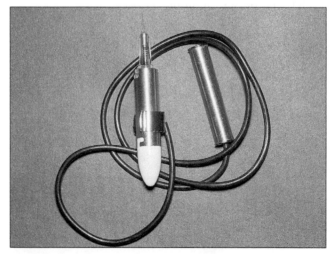

Figure 7.14 Battery-operated electrolysis unit. This method is prone to regrowth of hairs but does not disfigure the lid as much as surgical unit electrocautery.

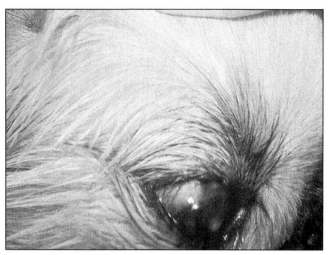

Figure 7.15 Lid margin deformities and depigmentation secondary to aggressive surgical unit electrocautery for distichiasis. Chronic epiphora resulted from damage to the eyelid margins.

of hairs may be frequent, and deformation of the lid margins with chronic secondary epiphora is common.

Cryosurgery The germinal epithelium of hair follicles and melanocytes are most susceptible to injury from freezing, thus providing a noninvasive, rapid technique that is more effective than electrolysis. Nitrous oxide units are used to obtain a tissue temperature of –25°C (–13°F) without sloughing. A chalazion clamp can be placed over the area of freezing to facilitate eversion and to decrease the blood flow to ensure an adequate freeze. This author prefers not to use a chalazion clamp on small dogs with very thin eyelids to avoid excessive tissue damage from

excessive freezing. The probe is placed on the palpebral conjunctiva over the base of the meibomian glands and activated until the ice ball reaches the trough on the lid margin (**Figure 7.17**). The author routinely treats the area with a double freeze-thaw technique. The hairs are removed after freezing. Freezing can occur over the lacrimal canaliculi without apparent damage to function.[37–39]

The postoperative swelling with cryotherapy is usually mild/moderate and transient. A topical corticosteroid is administered after freezing unless the condition is accompanied by corneal ulceration. Systemic nonsteroidal anti-inflammatory drugs help decrease postoperative swelling and pain. Depigmentation of lid margins usually occurs post freezing, but most dogs regain the pigment over several weeks. Overzealous cryosurgical treatment (freezing too long per site, more than two times per site, or use of much colder liquid nitrogen units) can result in excessive sloughing of lid margins with damage to the meibomian glands and the lid trough, resulting in postoperative epiphora due to tear film instability. One advantage of cryosurgery over other techniques of distichia removal is that regrown hairs are usually finer, less bristly, and depigmented; so, if hairs regrow, they may not cause clinical signs in patients.

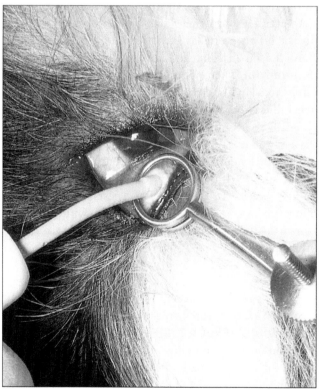

Figure 7.17 Cryothermy to the meibomian gland region, utilizing a chalazion clamp to position and restrict blood flow, to treat distichia in a dog. Freezing is suspended when the ice ball reaches the middle of the lid margin. This can be performed over the lacrimal puncta without injury.

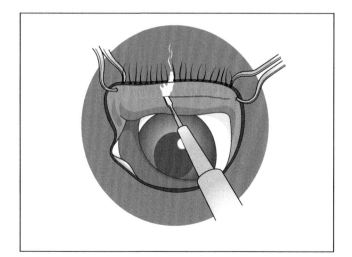

Figure 7.16 Electrocautery used to cut across the base of the cilia. Distichia may easily pluck out but often regrow. (Courtesy of Dr. R. Riis, Cornell Veterinary College, Ithaca, NY.)

Carbon dioxide laser The carbon dioxide (CO_2) laser has been used for distichia removal but is very tedious to use and has the potential for excessive tissue damage. The laser beam is directed over each offending hair follicle and activated to coagulate the tissue. The CO_2 laser, while expensive, has become available in practice. The author has no experience with the use of the CO_2 laser for distichia, only with its complications (scarred lid margins, cicatricial entropion).

Plucking Plucking of distichia is tedious, requires a pair of nontoothed forceps with good apposition, and is only a temporary measure since regrown hairs are ultimately bristlier than the hairs originally plucked. Before performing definitive surgery, plucking is useful to ascertain whether hairs are responsible for the clinical signs.

> All forms of distichia therapy may have some regrowth of hairs in some patients.

Adventitious, ectopic, or aberrant cilia

Introduction/etiology
In the dog, cilia frequently grow aberrantly through the conjunctiva toward the globe. The cilia may be either fine or bristly, are characteristically very short, 2–5 mm from the lid margin, and are usually in the upper lid (**Figure 7.18**). There are usually one or two cilia, although rarely an island of cilia may be present. Ectopic cilia are generally associated with distichia, as the cilia appear clinically to arise from the base of the meibomian glands (base of the tarsal plate) just like distichia. The condition was originally described in the boxer[34,40] and is most commonly seen by this author in the Shih Tzu and English bulldog breeds. In the Shih Tzu, "nests" of cilia resembling tiny dermoids may be seen along with individual hairs as early as 8 weeks of age. Ectopic cilia are rare in other species.[41]

Clinical signs
Blepharospasm and varying degrees of a focal, usually ulcerative keratitis are characteristic because the cilium is short and stiff (**Figure 7.18**). The history is often one of acute onset in a young dog. The ulcer may be vertically linear, following the path of the lid across the cornea while blinking.

Diagnosis
Aberrant cilia are often overlooked and consequently misdiagnosed because the lid margin must be adequately everted to observe the palpebral conjunctival surface, and

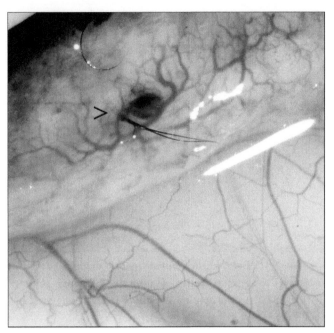

Figure 7.18 Aberrant/ectopic cilia (arrow) in the upper palpebral conjunctiva of a dog. The cilia arise from the base of the tarsal plate. Note the chemotic, hyperemic palpebral and bulbar conjunctiva. Dorsal to the ectopic cilium is a distichia arising from the lid margin.

adequate magnification (5–10×) is critical to visualize the very short cilium. The location of the cilium is suspected by the location of the ulcer. A small elevation or depigmented spot is often present where the hair emerges. Topical application of fluorescein dye may delineate the cilia by staining mucous that adheres to the cilia.

> Magnification of 5–10× is usually necessary to visualize the short hairs. It is very easy to overlook aberrant/ectopic cilia as the cause of a nonhealing ulcer.

Therapy
While this can be the most difficult of the cilia problems to diagnose, it can be the easiest to treat. The therapy for aberrant cilia is excision of a block of conjunctiva/tarsus/meibomian gland, utilizing a chalazion clamp to fixate the region and maintain hemostasis (**Figure 7.19**). D'Anna et al. utilized a 2- to 3-mm dermal punch to remove the aberrant cilia and follicle.[42] Surgery is usually successful, although new hairs or regrowth may occur due to incomplete excision. CO_2 laser coagulation or cryosurgery of the excision area may help reduce the incidence of regrowth if the hair follicle is not completely excised. The corneal ulcer usually heals rapidly after removal of the cilia.

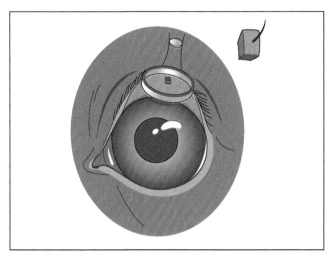

Figure 7.19 Removal of aberrant cilium utilizing chalazion forceps for immobilization and hemostasis.

Trichiasis
Introduction/etiology
Trichiasis occurs when normally placed hair follicles or cilia are abnormally directed toward the cornea, causing frictional irritation. Trichiasis may be congenital or acquired from lid scarring or from entropion. Congenital trichiasis (a rare disorder) may be unilateral or bilateral, involves the upper lid, and is usually found in small breeds of dogs (**Figure 7.20**). Acquired trichiasis may be due to redundant skin over the head pushing down on the upper lid, such as in the Shar Pei, Chow Chow, Neapolitan mastiff, bulldog, hounds such as the bloodhound, and St. Bernard (see section Ptosis). In all species, lacerations of the lid that are not properly repaired may result in trichiasis (see section Lacerations). Entropion in all species

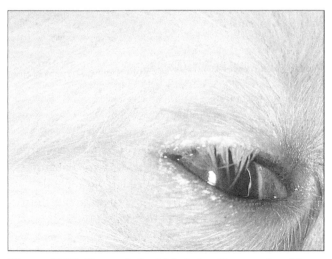

Figure 7.20 Congenital trichiasis in a Pomeranian. Note the collapsed eyelashes on the cornea. The condition was bilateral.

is significant because of the trichiasis that it produces. In brachycephalic breeds of dogs (and cats), medial trichiasis due to medial entropion or nasal fold trichiasis is common.

Clinical signs
- Epiphora is the mildest sign.
- Blepharospasm and keratitis, either ulcerative or nonulcerative, are the usual significant signs.
- In congenital trichiasis, the cilia of the lateral two-thirds of the upper lid are collapsed on the cornea due to laxity of the tarsus, but the lid is not rolled inward.

Therapy
Trichiasis following scarring or from laceration may require excision/reconstruction, advancing pedicle grafts, or rotating pedicle flaps to correct the lid defect as well as to correct the trichiasis.

Trichiasis/entropion due to excessive skin folds over the top of the head is difficult to manage. Correction usually requires massive resection of skin folds over the head and, perhaps, anchoring sutures to the underlying periosteum or fascia (see sections Entropion and Ptosis). Stades described a technique for removal of lid skin and upper lid cilia, allowing the area to heal by granulation (**Figure 7.21**).[43,44] While this procedure removes the cilia, it has the esthetic disadvantage of a wound healing by second intention.

Congenital trichiasis of the upper lid has been treated similarly to entropion by excision of adjacent skin (Hotz–Celsus procedure), but this may relapse. Cryotherapy has been a rapid and effective alternative method for destroying the hair follicles and their offending hairs.

Trichomegaly
Trichomegaly (long eyelashes) is observed in the American Cocker Spaniel and Shih Tzu. The cilia are normally placed but of such extreme length that they fall forward over the eye (**Figure 7.22**). However, no ocular irritation occurs with the syndrome, and thus no therapy is required.

Macroblepharon (euryblepharon)
Introduction/etiology
Occasionally, macroblepharon (enlarged palpebral fissure) is unilateral, but typically it is bilateral in various breeds of hounds, St. Bernards, mastiffs, Newfoundlands, Bernese mountain dogs, and spaniels, where it is associated with lower lid ectropion and often lateral canthal/upper and lower lid entropion (**Figure 7.23**). In breeds with taut skin, such as brachycephalics, ectropion is not present, but varying degrees of exposure keratitis and proptosis of the globe is more likely (**Figure 7.24**). Stades et al. measured

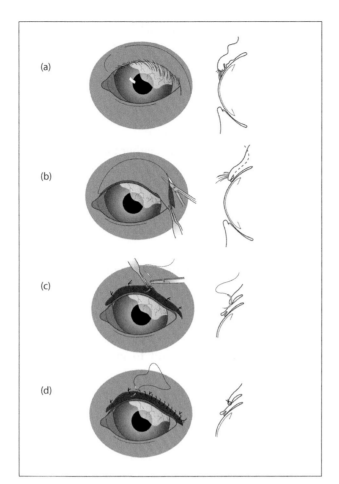

Figure 7.21 Stades method for correction of trichiasis and ptosis. Preoperative appearance with skin folds (a). A lid splitting incision is made 0.5–1 mm external to the meibomian gland orifices to remove the lash follicles; a second incision follows the dorsal orbital rim (b). The superior wound margin is positioned with interrupted sutures to the palpebral subcutis just superior to the base of meibomian glands (c), and then with continuous suture (d). The remaining area granulates and contracts. (From Stades, F.C. 1987. *Journal of the American Animal Hospital Association* 23:603–606.[43])

the palpebral length in dogs and cats and found a mean of 32.7 ± 4.2 mm for dogs and 27.8 ± 2.7 mm for cats.[45] In general, breeds with longer palpebral fissures are predisposed to entropion, but individuals with entropion do not have longer fissures than normal individuals of the same breed. In the sphinx cat, macroblepharon with entropion has been observed.

Clinical signs
- Excessively large palpebral fissure that is most evident when the skin over the head is pulled taut and the lateral canthus is retracted towards the ear.

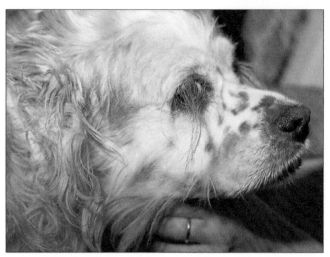

Figure 7.22 Trichomegaly in an American Cocker Spaniel. The appearance is rather dramatic, but few pathological signs are produced.

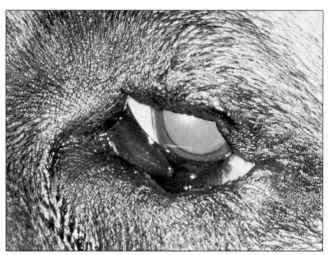

Figure 7.23 Macroblepharon with ectropion and entropion in a mastiff.

- Ectropion and perhaps lateral canthal/ upper and lower lid entropion due to lack of lateral canthal support and tarsus laxity.
- Conjunctivitis due to exposure.
- In the brachycephalic breeds, varying degrees of ulcerative or nonulcerative keratitis may develop from exposure with lagophthalmos and macroblepharon. A shallow orbit combined with a large palpebral fissure predisposes to proptosis with minimal effort, such as with restraint from the nape of the neck.

Diagnosis
Diagnosis is by visual inspection while retracting the lateral canthus laterally.

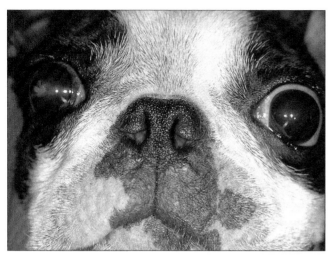

Figure 7.24 Macroblepharon in a Boston terrier with increased amounts of exposed globe. Corneal scarring and pigmentation is evident in the right eye.

Therapy
Conservative Antibiotic/glucocorticoid preparations are used to control the conjunctivitis but only with caution in brachycephalic breeds due to propensity for corneal ulcerations. Daily rinsing with eyewash of debris from the inferior cul-de-sacs in large breed dogs helps reduce conjunctivitis. Ocular lubricants (viscous drops or ointments) are administered to protect the ocular surface in brachycephalic breeds.

Canthoplasty Lateral canthoplasty is performed in brachycephalic breeds to protect the cornea (**Figure 7.25**).[46] Alternatively, a medial canthoplasty may be performed to shorten the fissure and obliterate medial entropion (see section Entropion). If medial entropion is not a problem, lateral canthoplasty may be preferred because of the esthetics.

Ectropion correction Procedures to shorten the lids must also provide lateral traction on the lid/skin to avoid a shortened lid that still droops (see section Ectropion).

Microblepharon or blepharophimosis
Introduction/etiology
A small palpebral fissure in the absence of microphthalmos is observed bilaterally in several breeds of dog. Breeds such as the Collie, Shetland sheepdog, Pomeranian, Chow Chow, Shar Pei, Kerry blue terrier, English bull terrier, and other small terrier breeds are typically affected. The condition rarely produces clinical signs.

Clinical signs
• Little if any exposed bulbar conjunctiva or sclera even with manipulation of the lids.

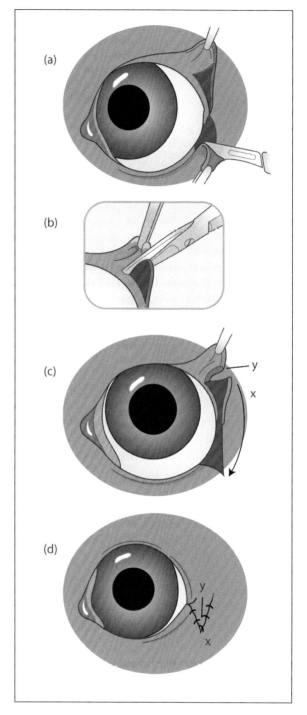

Figure 7.25 Lateral canthoplasty using a halving technique for strength. Triangles of skin and conjunctiva of equal size are removed from opposite lids. The length of the triangle along the lid margin is equal to the amount of shortening desired. The upper lid is incised along xy. xy is transposed and sutured to the tip of the triangle in the lower lid (c). The full-thickness cut upper lid is transposed down to form the new lateral canthus, and the remaining cut surfaces are sutured. This technique provides a broader healing area than cut lid margins and, thus, is less prone to dehiscence.

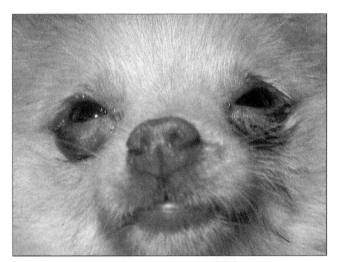

Figure 7.26 Blepharophimosis in a Pomeranian. The dog appears blepharospastic due to small fissures. Marked epiphora was present due to tight lid–globe conformation resulting in a small lacrimal lake. Enlargement of the palpebral fissures relieved the epiphora.

- Tight lid–globe conformation, which may result in a limited lacrimal lake and resultant epiphora (**Figure 7.26**).
- Globe may appear small because of limited exposure.
- Entropion is the most serious sequela and usually results in significant corneal pathology because of the tight lid–globe conformation.

Diagnosis

The diagnosis is usually by inspection, but microblepharon may be overlooked as the predisposing cause for entropion.

Therapy
- No therapy is necessary for most animals with minimal signs.
- Chronic epiphora may be treated medically with low-dose tetracycline or tylosin orally to lessen the tear staining. This medical therapy does not reduce the epiphora. A partial permanent lateral canthotomy[47] may help reduce the tight lid-globe conformation and reduce epiphora.
- Surgical removal of the third eyelid gland may enlarge the lacrimal lake, but risks predisposing the patient to keratoconjunctivitis sicca (KCS) and is, therefore, not recommended.
- Entropion should be corrected; this may require creation of a lateral canthal ligament to evert the lateral canthus (see section Entropion).

Entropion

Introduction/etiology

Entropion is a rolling of the eyelid inward toward the eye. It is a very common condition in dogs and is less common

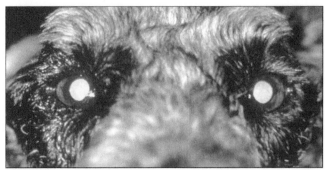

Figure 7.27 Enophthalmos associated with chronic masticatory myositis. Note the bilateral lower lid entropion and marked tear staining of the lower lids and periocular facial hair.

in the cat, the horse, and the cow. It is considered familial in the dog, but the genetics are unknown.[48] It is probably a combination of inherited conformation and exciting environmental influences, and thus it does not behave as a simple autosomal trait. In large animals, it is most common in neonates. In sheep, it is reported to be inherited.[49,50]

The tarsus/tarsal plate in domestic animals is poorly developed and lacks the rigidity found in humans. In addition, the lids are supported by the globe, so that in animals (particularly dogs) with "deep-set" eyes, or in conditions of ocular pain where the retractor bulbi muscle retracts the globe into the orbit, this support is lost or is minimal. A loss of orbital mass or ocular mass (phthisis bulbi) may also be responsible for loss of lid support, resulting in entropion (**Figure 7.27**). Without the internal support to the lid and with the additional loss of support from the globe, contraction of the orbicularis oculi muscle causes the lid to roll inward.

Entropion involving the lateral canthus in mesaticephalic breeds with broad heads may also be associated with a lateral canthal ligament that is misdirected in a more medial direction. Entropion is seen commonly in the lateral half of the lower lid. However, it may extend to the lateral third of the upper lid in the St. Bernard, bulldog, boxer, Chow Chow, Kerry blue terrier, Rottweiler, and in spaniels, retrievers, and pointers (**Figure 7.29**). Entropion associated with ocular pain can occur in any breed. Entropion of the medial lower lid and, less frequently, of the upper medial lid is seen commonly in the miniature and toy poodle, Pekingese, pug, English bulldog, Shih Tzu, Ihasa Apso, Cavalier King Charles spaniel, and Maltese. Heavy, lax facial skin can result in the upper lids rolling over the corneal surface in breeds with this conformation (bloodhound, Neapolitan mastiff, and Shar Pei).

Entropion can be classified as conformational, spastic, or cicatricial.

Conformational   Conformational entropion is often called congenital, although entropion is not usually present at birth. Entropion in the horse and the sheep is usually present in neonates and involves the lower lid. The Shar Pei typically has entropion of very early onset. Environmental influences are also present, as most patients have a period of normalcy before the entropion is noted. Early intervention by counteracting the spastic component may halt the process and avoid definitive surgery.

Conformational features that predispose to entropion are redundant folds over the head (see section Ptosis), deep-set eyes that do not support the lids, wide head conformation in mesaticephalic breeds that alters the direction of the tension of the lateral canthal ligament, and a personality trait of excessive guarding of the eyes or blepharospasm with pain on ocular manipulation.

Spastic   Spastic entropion is secondary to a painful ocular condition such as corneal ulcer. Most conformational entropions are normal for weeks to months after birth before becoming manifest and are probably initiated by conditions such as conjunctivitis that stimulate blepharospasm. A vicious cycle of pain and blepharospasm occurs that, once it is well established in conformationally predisposed animals, is not relieved by removing the pain. Almost all entropions in cats begin as a spastic entropion that, if allowed to remain, becomes permanent. Topical anesthetic relieves the pure spastic entropion and allows the surgeon to estimate the spastic component for surgical evaluation.

Cicatricial   Cicatricial entropion may occur secondary to injury with scarring and contracture.

Clinical signs
Mild   Epiphora and conjunctivitis, often associated with excessive conjunctival lymphoid follicles, is typical (**Figure 7.28**). It is possible that conjunctivitis is the initiating factor in many instances, as conjunctivitis is usually present in both eyes, and entropion may be present in only one eye (thus entropion did not cause the conjunctivitis). Dogs with lower lid entropion may protect the cornea by retracting the globe and prolapsing the third eyelid. Epiphora produces altered pigmentation of the inverted lid margin. Varying degrees of blepharospasm are usually present.

Modest   Blepharospasm (moderate), corneal ulcer, or focal superficial keratitis with scarring, pigment, and neovascularization are present (**Figure 7.29**). Secondary bacterial infection may occur with mucopurulent ocular discharge, rather than epiphora.

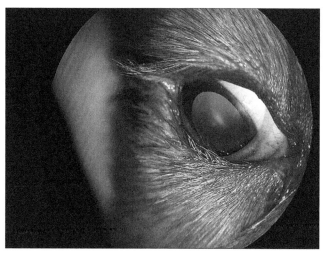

Figure 7.28 Entropion of the lower lid in an 8-week-old Irish setter puppy. No corneal lesions have yet developed due to the third eyelid and deep orbit.

Severe   Extreme blepharospasm and, usually, a severe keratitis are present, although the cornea may be hard to evaluate until the animal is anesthetized. Blepharospasm may even persist after topical or general anesthesia.

Diagnosis
Blepharospasm with absence of the normal hairless zone of the lid margin against the cornea is diagnostic. The facial hairs extend to the apparent lid margin (**Figures 7.28 and 7.29**). The head should be examined unrestrained, as manipulation of the head, facial skin, and lids usually precipitate or exaggerate blepharospasm in many dogs. The head is supported by lifting under the mandible without touching the side or top of the head. The animal should

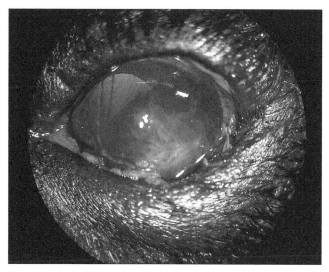

Figure 7.29 Entropion of the lower lateral lid and lateral canthus in a Rottweiler. Note the ventrotemporal corneal neovascularization, fibrosis, and pigmentation.

be examined in an elevated position (exam table) with the head parallel to the floor before and after the application of topical anesthetics.

Therapy

Everting mattress sutures   Most patients that are temporized by placing everting mattress sutures in the eyelid later require definitive surgery unless presented in the early, purely spastic phase of the disease. The objective is to relieve the primary condition (corneal ulcer, conjunctivitis) and to stop the pain–spasm cycle. Spastic entropion, acute-onset entropion, and entropion in the neonate and young animal of all species may be treated by placing two to three fine nylon sutures in a vertical or horizontal mattress pattern in the skin of the appropriate lid (**Figure 7.30**).[51] This has become routine in Shar Pei puppies. In many instances, this may be curative or at least relieves the problem until the puppy grows to the point of being suitable for a more definitive procedure. The everting effect of the sutures often only lasts a few weeks, but new sutures can be placed periodically if necessary. Surgical staples have also been utilized in place of everting sutures; however, their placement must be very meticulous to avoid contact with the corneal surface.

Martin described utilizing temporary tarsorrhaphy sutures in 2- to 3-week-old puppies to remedy frictional irritation and spasm, but the puppy could not see if the condition was bilateral. The sutures often only remained in place for 2–3 days but usually were successful in abating the spastic entropion.

Fornix-based sutures   Williams used a suture pattern to temporarily evert lids with entropion that was a modification of the Quickert–Rathbun technique utilized in humans.[52] A double-armed 4-0 polyglycolic acid suture was placed beginning from the conjunctival side at the fornix and passed in the lid to exit the skin just external to the lid margin. When both needles were passed, this created a horizontal mattress pattern that was tied on the skin adjacent to the lid margin. Williams only used the technique with lower lid entropion. The technique would be best with spastic and mild entropion that may self-correct once the blepharospasm is relieved.

Subcutaneous injection   Agents such as penicillin have been injected subcutaneously adjacent to the entropion in sheep and foals. Injection of approximately 1 mL of penicillin everts the lid margin away from the globe and may break the pain–blepharospasm cycle. Injection of more irritating substances, such as mineral oil or liquefied paraffin, results in a foreign body granuloma with subsequent permanent depigmented alopecia and is not recommended.

Removal of skin   Established entropion requires surgical correction. Various procedures have been devised, but most patients respond to the simple removal of an ellipse of skin and, possibly, of underlying orbicularis muscle (Hotz–Celsus procedure) adjacent to the entropion (**Figure 7.31**). The amount of skin removed and the length of the incision is a judgment decision. A general rule of thumb is that the incision closest to the lid margin is at the level of the hair line, and the second incision is at the level of the hair/skin altered pigmentation with the maximum amount of skin removed usually being no more than 5–6 mm at the widest part of the ellipse. Removal of underlying orbicularis muscle is certainly not harmful but is not necessary. A smooth tapering of the incision both medial and lateral to the area of enrolling gives a smooth, cosmetic appearance postoperatively. If only a short length of lid is affected, correction using a Y–V procedure may minimize a secondary ectropion (**Figures 7.32a and b**). The Hotz–Celsus procedure can be combined with lateral full-thickness wedge excision of the lid margin to tighten up the lower lid (**Figure 7.33**).[53] This would seem most appropriate in dogs with entropion associated with slack or floppy eyelids. A modification of Bigelbach's technique for lateral canthal entropion/lower lid ectropion correction[54] is another technique that uses skin excision for entropion correction (see section Ectropion).

Creation and cutting of lateral canthal ligaments   In patients where the lateral canthus is rolling inward, "prosthetic" lateral canthal ligaments can be fashioned from the orbicularis muscle[55] (**Figure 7.34**) or from buried absorbable or nonabsorbable suture (**Figure 7.35**).[56] Utilizing the orbicularis muscle or absorbable suture, the initial tautness produced may be lost over several weeks/months.

A tenotomy of the overdeveloped lateral canthal ligament has been advocated to release the inward rolling lateral canthus (**Figure 7.36**). Any remaining entropion of the lower and upper lid is repaired by skin excision and/or the macroblepharon is shortened.[5] This procedure may give good results and is not as laborious as creating the canthal ligaments.

Skin excision with tarsal pedicles   Elliptical skin excision with the creation of tarsal pedicles that are anchored in pockets away from the lid margin is a method used to minimize a recurrence of entropion.[57] The principle is similar to the lateral canthal ligaments procedure, except the tarsal pedicle tags are smaller, and the tension is perpendicular to the lid margin.

Medial canthoplasty   Medial entropion in brachycephalics is most easily treated by performing a medial

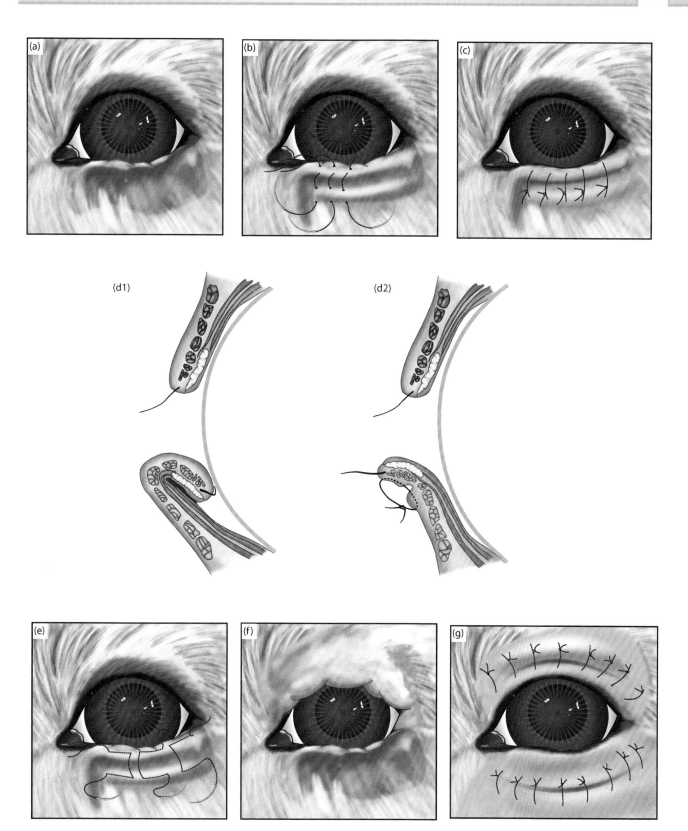

Figure 7.30 Placement of everting vertical or horizontal mattress sutures to treat spastic entropion or to allow growth of the animal before performing a definitive procedure. Often such sutures are combined with a Hotz–Celsus procedure (Figure 7.31) to counteract initial blepharospasm from surgery and medications.

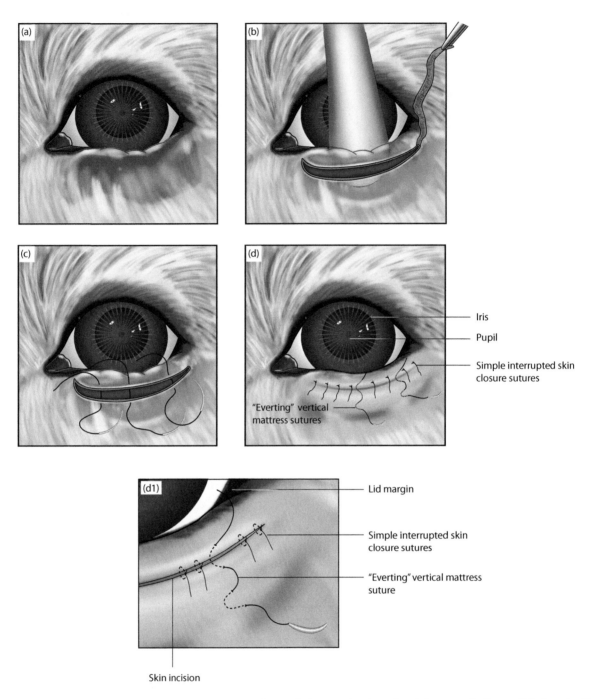

(a)

(b)

(c)

(d)

— Iris

— Pupil

— Simple interrupted skin closure sutures

"Everting" vertical mattress sutures

(d1)

— Lid margin

— Simple interrupted skin closure sutures

— "Everting" vertical mattress suture

Skin incision

Figure 7.31 Hotz–Celsus procedure for correction of lower lid entropion in a dog. The use of a Jaeger lid plate facilitates scalpel incisions, and excision of orbicularis muscle is optional. The incision closest to the lid margin is just within the hairline. The second incision should at least be to the level of altered coloration of the skin/hair (not to usually exceed 5–6 mm). Temporary everting sutures may be used to prevent spasm and frictional irritation from sutures while the surgical wound is healing.

canthoplasty (**Figure 7.37**).[58–60] If treated by routine skin excision, entropion usually recurs in the brachycephalic breeds because of the redundant skin in this region. Medial canthoplasty simply obliterates the lid region that had the entropion. Owners must be forewarned that the appearance may be modestly altered (**Figure 7.38**).

Lateral canthal tenotomy Mesaticephalic breeds with involution of the lateral canthus, usually in combination with entropion of the lower lid, may respond to lateral canthal tenotomy by itself or, more commonly, in conjunction with lid shortening or lid eversion (**Figure 7.36**). After transection of the lateral canthal ligament, the size

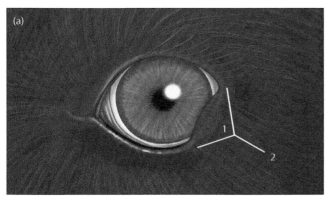

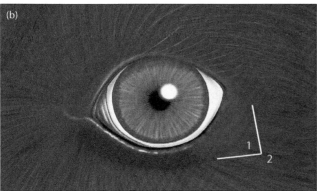

Figure 7.32 Y–V procedure for entropion correction. This technique is indicated for entropion involving a short length of the lid and avoids overcorrection of adjacent normal lid. Initial skin incision is in the shape of a "Y" (a). Following undermining of peri-incisional skin, the skin closure is in the shape of a "V" (b).

and the position of the lids are evaluated to determine what additional steps are needed. Frequently, lid shortening or eversion may also be necessary.

> No one surgical procedure is effective for all patients with entropion. A detailed study of the conformation while the patient is as relaxed as possible is necessary to select the most appropriate technique and location for surgery.

Ectropion

Introduction/etiology

Ectropion is eversion of the lower lid. It is common in dogs but rare in other animals. There are four forms: Conformational, transient, cicatricial, and paralytic.

Conformational Dogs such as hounds, setters, spaniels, retrievers, bulldogs, and boxers are usually affected (**Figure 7.39**). In some breeds, such as hounds, a degree of ectropion is considered normal. In heavy-faced giant breeds

(St. Bernard, mastiff, Newfoundland) a combination of macropalpebral fissure, lateral canthal entropion, medial lower lid ectropion, and a "notch" in the tarsus of the medial upper lid is common and sometimes considered desirable ("pagoda eye" or "diamond eye") (**Figures 7.23 and 7.39 upper image**).

Transient Hunting breeds, such as retrievers and setters, may exhibit intermittent ectropion that becomes manifest late in the day, after exercise, or when the animal is relaxed. This is a subtype of conformational ectropion.

Cicatricial Ectropion may occur secondary to scar contracture in the lid. This form is usually unilateral and is relatively rare (**Figure 7.40**). Unfortunately, the most common cause is iatrogenic overcorrection from entropion surgery.

Paralytic Paralytic ectropion may occur from facial/palpebral nerve paralysis.

Therapy

While ectropion is common, therapy directed towards the primary problem is relatively infrequently requested. Medical treatment of the associated conjunctivitis with daily flushing of debris from the cul-de-sacs with eyewash and judicious use of topical antibiotic–corticosteroid preparations is the most frequent form of therapy.

Surgical correction should be postponed until about 6 months of age or when adult conformation is obtained, as some animals improve with growth. A modification of the Kuhnt–Szymanowski procedure has given good results in cases of moderate ectropion (**Figure 7.41**).[61] A variety of other procedures usually succeed in shortening the palpebral fissure but do not usually correct the slack lid margin. Ectropion that is localized to a notch in the middle of the lid can be repaired by simple excision of the notch and shortening of the lid (see full-lid-thickness resection for excision of eyelid mass, **Figure 7.74**). The most difficult ectropion to correct is associated with marked redundancy of heavy, loosely adherent skin over the head and lateral face with the previously mentioned macropalpebral fissure, lateral entropion, medial lower lid ectropion, and the tarsus notch of the medial upper lid margin ("pagoda eye"). A modification of Bigelbach's[54] combined tarsorrhaphy-lateral canthoplasty technique[62] with "prosthetic" lateral canthal ligaments can shorten the macropalpebral fissure, reduce the ectropion, and correct the lateral canthal entropion in one procedure (**Figures 7.39a,b, and 7.42**).

> Relatively few patients with ectropion undergo surgical correction unless it is accompanied by entropion.

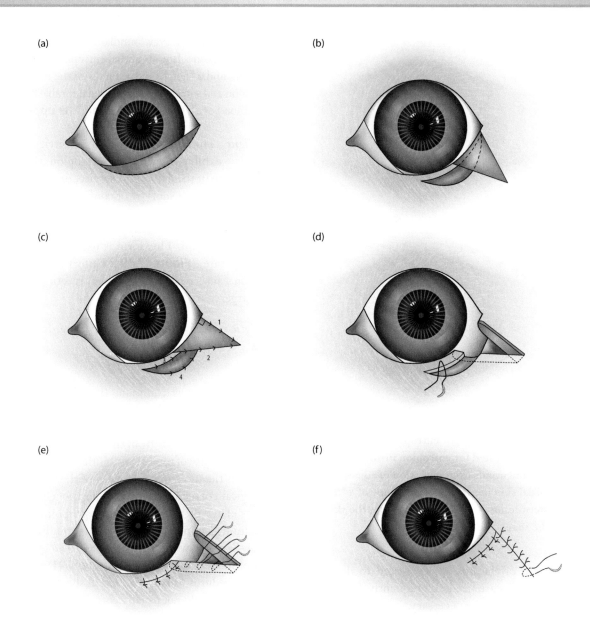

Figure 7.33 Diagram of a combined Hotz–Celsus procedure and a lateral eyelid wedge resection to correct entropion and macropalpebral fissure. (a) Lower eyelid entropion of lateral and middle lid. (b) Superimposed diagram of Hotz–Celsus procedure and lateral eyelid wedge resection technique skin incisions. (c) Modification of skin incisions with numbers indicating order and directions in which incisions are to be made. (d) Following excisions for modified Hotz–Celsus/eyelid wedge resection. (e) Hotz–Celsus skin incision portion closed first followed by split-thickness closure of deep layers of wedge resection. (f) Following completion of lateral wedge resection with two-layer closure.

A V–Y blepharoplasty is specific and successful with modest amounts of cicatricial ectropion. The V–Y plasty is not recommended for other types of ectropion (**Figure 7.43**).

Large nasal folds
Introduction/etiology
Nasal fold problems are overdiagnosed as the cause of corneal disease in Pekingese and other brachycephalic breeds. Careful examination of the medial lids behind the nasal fold often reveals the problem as a medial entropion. Both factors may be present and producing corneal disease (**Figure 7.44**).

Clinical signs
- Mild: Epiphora.
- Modest: Chronic superficial keratitis with a pigmented wedge of the medial bulbar conjunctiva and cornea.
- Severe or acute signs: Ulcerative keratitis of the medial cornea.

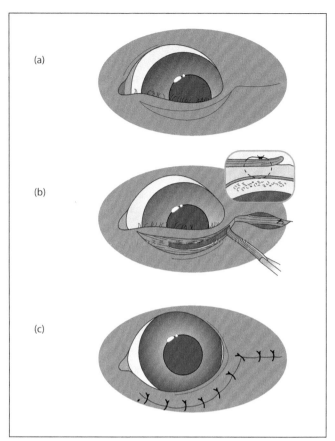

(a)

(b)

(c)

Figure 7.34 **Modified Wyman's lateral canthoplasty in a dog. Strips of orbicularis muscle are fashioned and sutured under tension to the zygomatic bone periosteum to pull the lateral canthus outward. It is currently rarely performed as other procedures are superior. There is a marked tendency for overcorrection, and the ligaments usually do not maintain contraction for more than a few weeks.**

Signs may occur from multiple causes such as medial entropion, distichiasis, and lagophthalmos due to shallow orbits. Pekingese may have all these conditions, so sometimes it is difficult to know which of the conditions is producing the problem.

Diagnosis
Diagnosis depends on demonstration that the nasal fold hairs are rubbing on the area of pathology and that a medial lower lid entropion is not behind the fold.

Therapy
Conservative In mild cases or in show dogs, applying ointments to make the hairs lie flat is all the owners may allow.

Surgical excision Excision may meet with owner resistance, as this is an expected part of the breed conformation. Complete excision is performed by cutting at the base of the nasal fold and suturing the cut edges. Cut suture ends should not be directed toward the eye. Incomplete excision is a better cosmetic solution, but if the eyes are extremely prominent, this may not be sufficient to reduce contact with hair. Medial canthoplasty (**Figure 7.37**) may help protect the medial cornea from frictional irritation as well as correct medial entropion. Aggressive cryodestruction of offending hairs on the nasal folds may help, but resulting poliosis (white hair) and vitaligo (white skin) and alopecia may be cosmetically displeasing.

Lagophthalmos
Introduction/etiology
Lagophthalmos is an inability to close the eyelids completely. In animals, due to the presence of a third eyelid, lagophthalmos may be tolerated reasonably well, but the cornea over time is likely to develop secondary exposure problems. Lagophthalmos can be congenital or acquired.

Congenital lagophthalmos is common in Pekingese and other brachycephalic breeds due to very shallow orbits. The eyes are often so prominent that the lids are unable to close completely unless an added facial effort to blink is made.

Lagophthalmos because of facial/palpebral nerve paralysis is a common isolated symptom in the American Cocker Spaniel, and it occurs with inner ear disease in all breeds.[63] In this study,[63] facial nerve paralysis was deemed idiopathic in 75% of dogs and 25% of cats. One study[64] showed 88% of hypothyroid dogs presented for neurological deficits had a lack of palpebral and corneal reflexes due to facial paralysis. In the horse, most cases of facial nerve paralysis are far enough peripheral (halter injuries) that they do not involve the lids. Guttural pouch disease may cause facial paralysis in the horse. Exophthalmos from increased orbital mass, such as a tumor, inflammation, hemorrhage, and edema, can cause lagophthalmos.

Diagnosis
Lagophthalmos is demonstrated by being able to touch the cornea without eliciting a total blink or eliciting only a partial blink. With chronicity, most animals probably also have decreased corneal sensation. The clinician must differentiate between lagophthalmos due to a lack of motor innervation, cranial nerve V paralysis, and a lack of sensation to the eyelids and/or cornea when testing the palpebral and corneal reflexes.

Clinical signs
Signs of lagophthalmos are ulceration, pigmentation, or scarring of the cornea. Owners may report that the animal sleeps with the eyes partially open.

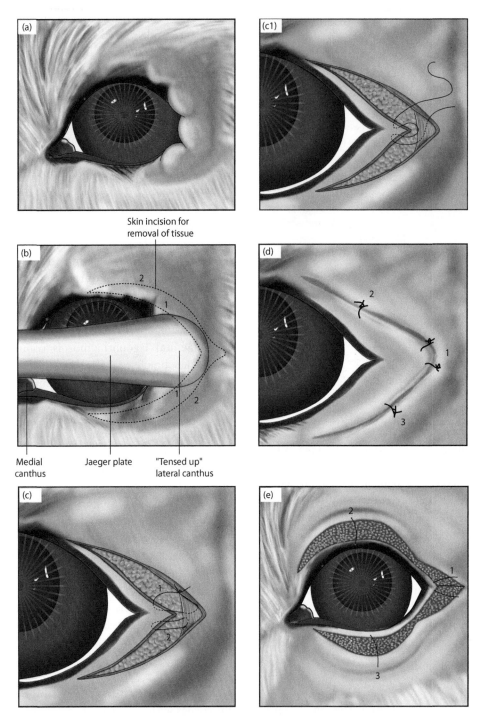

Figure 7.35 "Arrowhead" technique for correction of lateral canthal entropion with or without formation of "prosthetic" lateral canthal ligaments to retract canthus in loose-skinned dogs. (a) Lateral canthal entropion with lateral upper lid and lower lid entropion as well, left eye. (b) "Tensing" of the lateral canthus skin is accomplished by placing a Jaeger lid plate in lateral conjunctival cul-de-sac and lifting while surgeon tenses lid skin with thumb and index finger and makes skin incisions in order numbered (incisions closest to lid margins are ~ 2 mm from lid margin, second incisions are based on how much skin needs to be removed to correct entropion). (c) and (c1) Either 4-0 or 5-0 monofilament nylon or polydioxanone is used to retract the tips of the tarsus/tarsal plates laterally by anchoring the suture to the periosteum of the zygomatic arch or the orbital ligament. (d) The skin is closed with simple interrupted sutures beginning with closure of the lateral aspect of the incision followed by closure of the upper and lower skin incisions. (e) In the case of more involved upper and lower eyelid entropion, the upper and lower skin incisions may be extended across the span of the lids as traditional Hotz–Celsus entropion corrections along with the lateral canthoplasty.

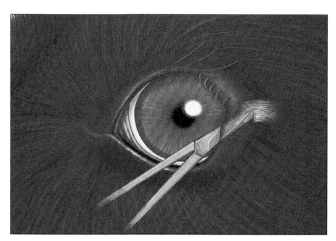

Figure 7.36 Lateral canthal tenotomy performed in a dog by cutting the taut band through the conjunctival surface. Additional lid shortening, Hotz–Celsus procedure, or a lateral canthal "arrowhead" technique may need to be performed, depending on the conformation.

Therapy

Lagophthalmos secondary to facial/palpebral nerve paralysis usually does not require therapy unless the animal is also very exophthalmic. Frequent use of lubricating artificial tears or ointments may be adequate to protect the exposed cornea. A partial permanent lateral tarsorrhaphy (**Figure 7.25**) may be necessary for cases of permanent facial nerve paralysis.

Lagophthalmos from exophthalmos due to orbital space-occupying lesions may require a temporary tarsorrhaphy (**Figure 7.45**) until the orbital lesion is resolved. If the tarsorrhaphy needs to be in place for more than 2–3 days, stents may need to be used to prevent sutures tearing through the lid margins.

Congenital lagophthalmos in the brachycephalic breeds can benefit from either lateral or medial canthoplasty to prevent multiple bouts of ulceration and decrease the risk of proptosis of the globe. Lateral canthoplasty gives better cosmetic results than medial canthoplasty (**Figure 7.25**) If medial entropion or trichiasis is also a problem, medial canthoplasty is indicated.

Artificial tear preparations or lubricants are often administered in addition to all the previously listed surgical procedures.

Ptosis

Introduction/etiology

Ptosis is an inability to elevate the upper eyelid to a normal degree. Ptosis may be acquired or congenital and due either to pathology of the muscles that elevate the lid (levator palpebrae or Müller's muscle) (**Figure 7.46**),

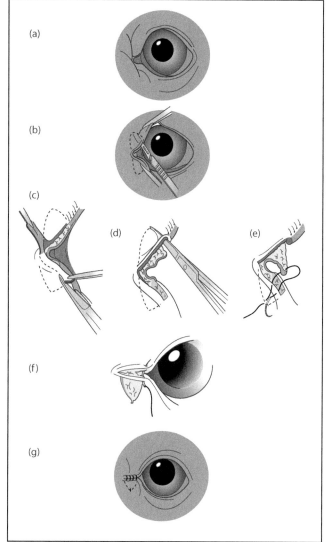

Figure 7.37 Pocket flap medial canthoplasty used to shorten the palpebral fissure and obliterate medial entropion and lacrimal caruncle trichiasis in the dog (a). The lid is split along the length to be shortened (b). Damage to the lower lacrimal canaliculus must be avoided (by passing a catheter if necessary). A strip of lid margin is removed (c). The inner half of the upper lid is cut along the border (d). The upper triangle is rotated into the lower pocket by a suture placed at the tip of the triangle (e). The cut lid margins are sutured (f). The final appearance (g). The large healing surfaces of lids that have been split create stronger adhesions than simple edge-to-edge closure alone.

disease of the peripheral nerves or central nervous system (CNS; oculomotor or sympathetic fibers or centers), or redundant skin over the head weighing down the upper lid (**Figure 7.47**).

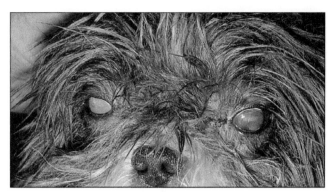

Figure 7.38 Lhasa Apso with bilateral medial canthoplasties, performed for keratitis of the medial cornea from entropion and trichiasis. Note that the eyes will appear further apart.

The most common cause of ptosis is weight of redundant skin, and this is seen in St. Bernards, Neapolitan mastiffs, English bulldogs, Chow Chows, Shar Peis, and hounds.

Clinical signs

If ptosis is associated with neurologic disease, it may be accompanied by either a dilated or a constricted pupil. With sympathetic denervation (Horner's syndrome), the pupil is miotic (**Figure 7.46**); with central oculomotor denervation, if the parasympathetic fibers are affected, the pupil is dilated. With peripheral oculomotor denervation to the levator palpebrae, ventral deviation of the globe may be seen. Generalized muscular atrophy/dystrophy may occasionally be a cause of ptosis.

Diagnosis

The palpebral fissure should be carefully examined for symmetry and to eliminate the presence of blepharospasm. A neurologic and physical examination should be performed, and function of other extraocular muscles and pupil should be evaluated.

Therapy

The treatment for ptosis is usually not specific except for redundant skin problems (see sections Entropion and

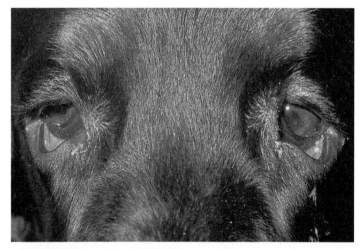

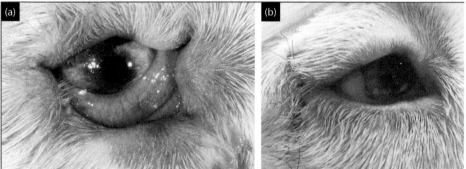

Figure 7.39 (upper image) Conformational ectropion in a Gordon Setter. Note the palpebral conjunctivitis. (a) and (b) "Pagoda eye" in a young Clumber spaniel. Note the lateral canthal entropion, the tendency for lower lid ectropion, and the "notch" of the medial aspect of the upper lid. When the lateral canthus was stretched laterally, notable macropalpebral fissure was present. Presurgery (a) and post-Bigelbach technique (b).

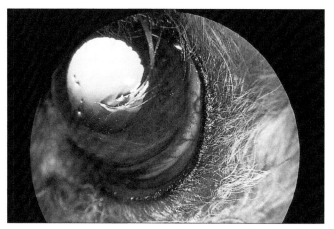

Figure 7.40 Cicatricial ectropion in a miniature poodle several months following trauma to the lower lid. The condition was unilateral.

Trichiasis). Excision of facial skin folds (stellate rhytidectomy[65]) requires a laborious job of suturing, but if adequate amounts of skin are removed, it results in significant improvement (**Figure 7.48**). A technique of creating a sling of mersilene mesh that is anchored to the periosteum of the skull to elevate the upper lid has given excellent results in the dog (**Figures 7.49 and 7.50**).[66–68] While this requires acquiring the mesh and runs the increased risk of infection (burying a foreign body), the excellent results obtained make it an attractive alternative to skin fold excision for owners who are insistent on retaining the forehead folds.

Acquired diseases
Blepharoedema
Introduction/etiology
Blepharoedema is usually a sign rather than a disease. The skin of the lid is thin and loose to allow mobility, resulting in dramatic subcutaneous edema with minimal insult.

Bilateral blepharoedema may be caused by an immune-mediated process, such as angioedema from hypersensitivity to insect bites/stings, vaccines (**Figure 7.51**), systemic medications, or food. Trauma, whether self-inflicted or external in origin, is a common cause of blepharoedema. The combination of ocular hypersensitivity with mast cell degranulation and self-inflicted trauma from rubbing is common in the horse.

Venomous insect and snakebites and topical chemicals such as surgical scrubs may produce chemically induced blepharoedema. Infectious causes of periocular and orbital inflammation are common causes of blepharoedema.

Clinical signs
Blepharoedema is usually unilateral with trauma, bee stings, and periorbital cellulitis and bilateral with allergic

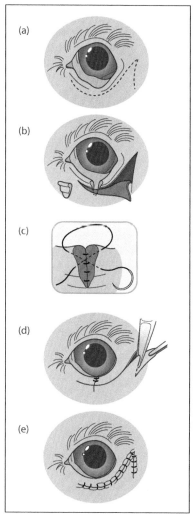

Figure 7.41 Modified Kuhnt–Szymanowski technique for ectropion correction. The lids are studied to estimate the amount of shortening. A skin incision is made 3 mm from, and parallel to, the lid margin from the lateral one-half to three-quarters of the lower lid (a). The incision curves dorsolaterally to a point 1–1.5 cm beyond the lateral canthus, following the natural curve of the lower lid. The skin flap is undermined from the orbicularis muscle, and the amount of estimated shortening is made by removing a triangular shaped piece of lid margin from the middle of the lower lid (b). The tarsoconjunctival layer is sutured with 6-0 synthetic absorbable suture in a simple continuous pattern. The lid margin is closed in a figure-of-eight pattern to avoid suture ends rubbing the cornea (c). The previously dissected skin flap is now made taut, the excess skin excised, and the skin sutured (d, e).

angioedema and many forms of blepharitis. Associated signs are often of importance in differential diagnosis: Exophthalmos, dermatitis elsewhere, edema of the muzzle, and perhaps urticaria on the body with angioneurotic edema.

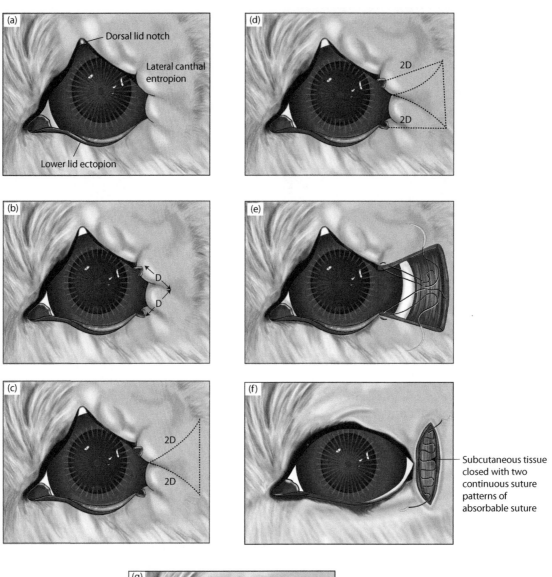

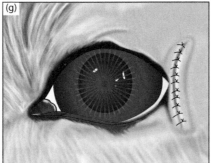

Figure 7.42 (a) Modification of Bigelbach's technique to correct lateral canthal entropion/lower lid ectropion ("pagoda eye"). Upper and lower lids are notched to indicate length of lid margins to be resected to correct macropalpebral fissure, distance **D** **(b)**. While tensing the lateral canthal tissue, sweeping skin incisions that roughly follow the curvature of the lid margins begin at the lateral canthus and extend a distance of two times distance **D**. The distal ends of these skin incisions are connected with a skin incision **(c)**. Using a Jaeger lid plate and scissors or scalpel, the full thickness of the lids is cut at the previously notched sites extending to the tips of the skin incisions **(d)**. After removal of the full-thickness lid pieces and triangular skin excision, the tarsal plates dorsally and ventrally are retracted laterally and sutured to the orbital ligament using 5-0 monofilament nylon or polydioxanone suture **(e)**. The lid stroma is closed to the subcuticular tissue with a continuous suture pattern of synthetic absorbable suture followed by skin closure with simple interrupted monofilament nylon **(f and g)**.

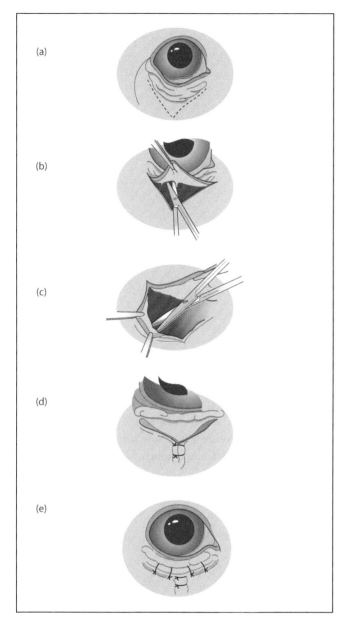

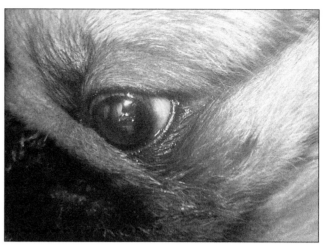

Figure 7.44 Trichiasis from large nasal folds in a Pekingese.

Figure 7.43 V–Y correction of cicatrical ectropion (a). Dissection of scar tissue (b). Mobilization of adjacent skin (c). Suturing the V incision without incorporating original incised lid skin pushes the skin toward the eye (d). The final appearance (e).

Therapy

Allergic blepharoedema is usually treated with systemic steroids and/or antihistamines, although most patients improve spontaneously. Cases of anaphylaxis with accompanying airway obstruction may also require systemic epinephrine. Trauma and acute inflammation (post surgical) often benefit from initial cold compresses in the first 12–24 hours, followed later by warm compresses. Blepharoedema secondary to infection should be specifically treated. Elizabethan collars to prevent self-trauma in small animals, or face masks in the horse, may be beneficial.

Blepharitis

Introduction/etiology of blepharitis

Blepharitis is a common syndrome, but it is often ignored if it is part of a more generalized dermatitis, unless secondary corneal disease occurs. Blepharitis may be diffuse or focal and acute or chronic. Examples of focal blepharitis are hordeolums, chalazions, and focal pyogranulomas. An external hordeolum ("stye") is an infection of the Zeis or Moll glands on the outside of the lid. This is much more common in human medicine. Some veterinary ophthalmologists refer to a stye as an acute abscessation of one or more meibomian glands (internal hordeolum) of the eyelid (**Figure 7.52**). A chalazion (internal hordeolum) is considered by some to be more of a chronic lipid granuloma, caused by meibomian gland contents being liberated into the adjacent tissue after blockage of drainage ducts/orifice. Focal pyogranulomas and furunculosis (**Figures 7.53 and 7.54**) are deep infections of the hair follicles of the skin and lashes.[69,70]

The causes of blepharitis are similar to and as varied as the causes of dermatitis in general. Many forms of dermatitis with a potential for generalized involvement or systemic implications have a propensity to begin with, or selectively involve, the eyelids.

Parasites

Mites: Demodectic mange in the dog (**Figure 7.55**) and the cat, notoedric mange in the cat, and sarcoptic mange in the dog and the cow produce a dry, scaly dermatitis that often involves the eyelids. Demodectic mange is typically nonpruritic, while notoedric and sarcoptic mange are intensely pruritic. Secondary infections with bacteria may produce a moist dermatitis and self-trauma.

(a)

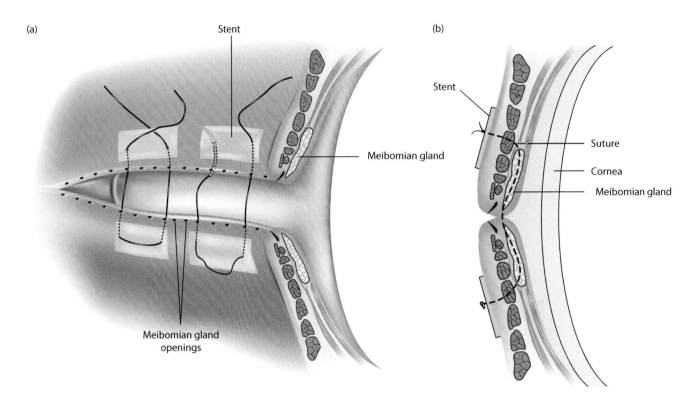

(b)

Figure 7.45 Proper placement of temporary tarsorrhaphy sutures over stents. Frontal view of suture placement with suture passing through stent, through lid to exit margin, through margin of second lid and stent, and then back in a horizontal mattress pattern (a). Cross section of temporary tarsorrhaphy suture placement (b). Note suture entering and exiting at meibomian gland orifices. Pieces of sterilized large rubber bands make satisfactory stents.

Cuterebra *larvae*: *Cuterebra* fly larvae are normal subcutaneous parasites of rodents, but on occasion, they are found in the lids, the conjunctiva, and the eye of the cat and the dog (**Figure 7.56**).[71,72] The fly lays eggs along rodent paths and burrows where hunting cats might become exposed. The subcutaneous larvae stimulate a

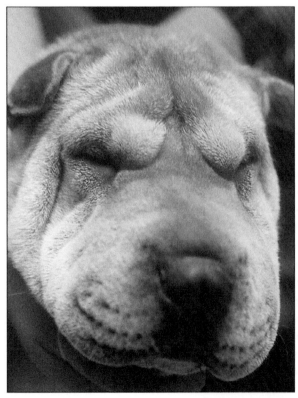

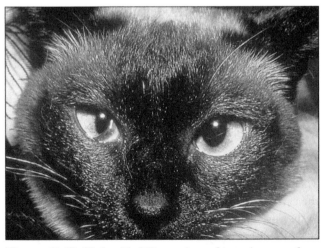

Figure 7.46 Right-sided Horner's syndrome in a cat after cleansing the ear canals. Note the modest ptosis, prolapse of the third eyelid, and miosis.

Figure 7.47 Ptosis in a Shar Pei, secondary to redundant skin over the forehead.

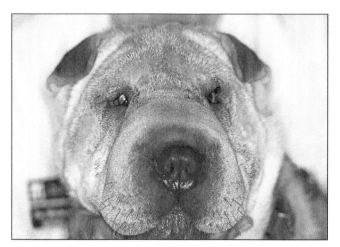

Figure 7.48 The dog in Figure 7.47 after facial fold removal and entropion surgery of the lower lids.

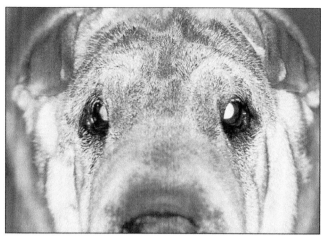

Figure 7.50 Shar Pei that has had bilateral frontal sling surgery. Note the folds over the head are retained. Overcorrection can produce lagophthalmos.

severe reaction and a burrowing hole, within which the larvae can be visualized, if present.

Habronema *larvae:* In the warmer months, *Habronema* larvae may produce typical chronic medial canthal/lid margin lesions, lesions around the lips, and lesions on the ventral midline and prepuce in the horse ("summer sores"). These lesions are usually an erosive/proliferative lesion with yellow caseated or calcified particles ("sulfur granules") and involve the lids, the conjunctiva, and the third eyelid (**Figure 7.57**).[73] The larvae are carried by *Musca domestica* (housefly). Since ivermectin kills the

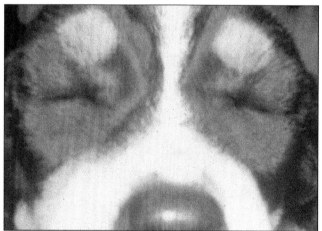

Figure 7.51 Bilateral angioedema in a puppy after vaccination.

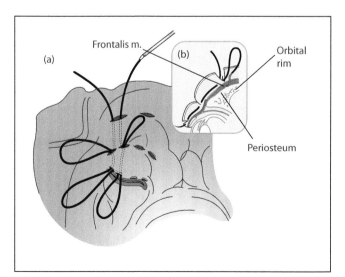

Figure 7.49 Ptosis correction utilizing a mersilene sling. Five small stab incisions are made in the skin (a), and the strip of mersilene that is attached to a straight needle is passed from one incision to the next and finally anchored to the temporal bone periosteum (b). Usually two slings are needed per lid. (m: Muscle.)

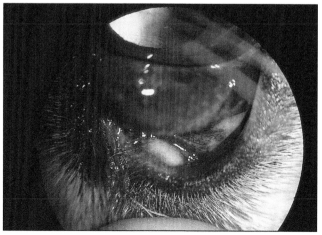

Figure 7.52 Internal hordeolum (stye) in a dog. It is a small acute abscess of the meibomian glands.

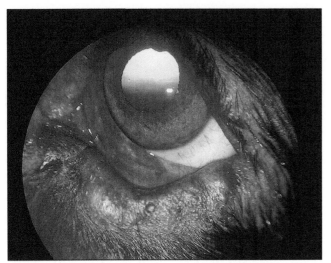

Figure 7.53 Multiple pyogranulomas in an English springer spaniel. The history was compatible with an atopic dog. The dog responded initially to systemic antibiotics and steroids but required low-dose steroids to keep the condition from recurring.

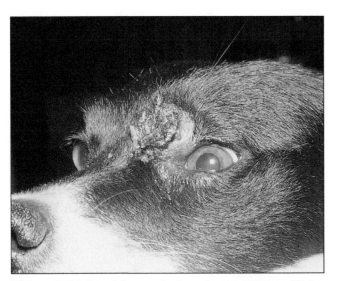

Figure 7.54 Local furunculosis or deep pyoderma of hair follicles in a dog. Onset was rapid, and while the condition responded to antibiotics, several days of therapy were necessary.

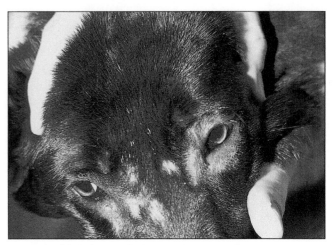

Figure 7.55 Periocular demodectic mange in a dog. The condition was localized to the head.

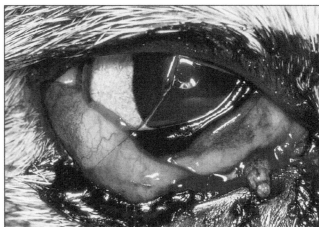

Figure 7.56 *Cuterebra* sp. larva visible near the medial lower lid margin of a cat. Note the severe conjunctival reaction. (Courtesy of Dr. J. Stiles, Purdue Veterinary College.)

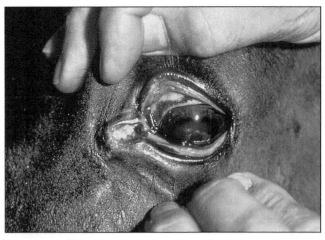

Figure 7.57 *Habronema* sp. infestation of the medial canthus of a horse. Note the yellow caseous material and the erosive nature of the lesion.

Habronema larvae, lesions have become a rarity with contemporary routine deworming programs.

Viruses In the cat, feline herpesvirus 1 (FHV-1) has been implicated in producing an ulcerative facial and nasal dermatitis with an eosinophilic/neutrophilic inflammatory response. Holland et al. were able to detect FHV-1 DNA in polymerase chain reaction (PCR) assays of skin biopsies from all cats suspected of having herpes dermatitis, and they found FHV-1 DNA in only 1 of 17 biopsies from cats with nonherpetic dermatitis and no instance in 21 biopsies from cats with no dermatitis.[74]

Bacteria   Facial pyodermas frequently involve the eyelids. In adult dogs, focal or generalized bacterial blepharitis can be secondary to bacterial infection of eyelash follicles or meibomian glands, bite wounds, clipper burns, and "spilling over" from bacterial conjunctivitis (**Figure 7.58**). In intact free-roaming cats, the most common cause of bacterial blepharitis is bite wounds (**Figure 7.59**).

Chronic blepharitis and keratoconjunctivitis may be associated with staphylococcal infection and meibomian gland dysfunction in humans and possibly in dogs and cats. A proposed mechanism of action is that keratin plugs block the meibomian orifices, providing the environment for the bacterial flora to thrive. The bacteria then produce lipases that hydrolyze lipids to toxic free fatty acids[75] that leach into the surrounding tissue, resulting in lipogranulomatous blepharitis. This may be a contributing underlying etiology for feline lipogranulomatous conjunctivitis (see Chapter 8, section Lipogranuloma).

Fungi and yeasts   Dermatophyte lesions may be limited to the periocular region or can be part of a generalized infection in all species. The appearance of the lesions is quite variable, but a dry, alopecic, scaly lesion is common (**Figure 7.60**). Most cases of localized dermatomycosis are self-limiting in the dog and the cat. Dermatomycosis has zoonotic potential. Periocular *Malassezia* spp. infection is seen mostly in the dog as dark, greasy malodorous debris staining the periocular hair and skin. This is one of the many causes of "poodle epiphora" and usually accompanies cases of chronic epiphora.

Protozoa   In the dog, the most common ocular lesion with *Leishmania infantum* is a scaly blepharitis or periocular alopecia (**Figure 7.61**). Pena et al. reported that 24% of all dogs with leishmaniasis had ocular lesions; the most common ocular lesion was either periocular alopecia or blepharitis (52%).[76] The appearance of blepharitis varied from dry, scaly lesions to diffusely thickened lesions that were hyperemic or ulcerated. Focal nodular granulomas may occur in the eyelids. Most reported cases of leishmaniasis have a history of being in the Mediterranean region, but a New World form of leishmaniasis due to *L. chagasi* has been reported in North, Central, and South America. The dog is a reservoir for the parasite, which is transmitted by sandflies.[77,78]

Burns   Sunlight on nonpigmented eyelid skin and mucocutaneous junctions produces sunburn in all species, and chronic exposure may eventually result in squamous cell carcinoma (SCC). Therapeutic deep radiation for nasal and brain tumors often results in blepharitis and hair loss from surface burns (**Figure 7.62**).

Lye, acids, and fire may induce facial and eyelid burns (**Figure 7.63**). Contracture of the eyelids in the healing phase often becomes a major complication of chemical and thermal burns.

Seborrhea/keratinization disorders   Generalized primary or secondary seborrhea in the dog, and idiopathic facial dermatitis and primary seborrhea of Persian cats, can be associated with blepharitis in addition to other typical clinical signs. In Persian cats with idiopathic facial dermatitis, a black, waxy material becomes adherent to the hairs of the face and variable amounts of underlying dermatitis are present. Otitis externa is often present, and *Malassezia* spp. yeast may be isolated from about half of the patients.[79]

Immune-mediated skin diseases   A range of immune-mediated diseases, from allergy to autoimmune diseases, may be characterized by facial dermatosis.[80]

Juvenile pyoderma: Juvenile pyoderma/cellulitis ("puppy strangles," juvenile sterile granulomatous dermatitis) is an excellent example of pyoderma with an affinity for the eyelids. It usually presents in puppies less than 4 months of age as an acute, severe, deep pyoderma that is usually restricted to the head (lids, face, pinnae, and submandibular lymph nodes). Although some cases may be contaminated with bacteria (*Staphylococcus* spp.), the underlying cause and pathogenesis of the disorder is unknown. Heritability (increased incidence in some breeds) and dramatic response to glucocorticoid therapy suggests an underlying immune dysfunction.[81]

In the early stages puppies may be presented with only swelling or pustules of the lids (**Figure 7.64**), but within days, the pyoderma may extend to the ears and the muzzle. The lesions become moist and purulent, and the submandibular lymph nodes become markedly enlarged. Affected puppies may be anorexic, lethargic, and/or febrile. Usually only one animal in the litter is involved. Occasionally, puppies develop a more generalized pyoderma.

Atopic blepharitis: Atopic blepharitis is typically associated with generalized pruritus, rubbing of the eyes, otitis, and licking of the feet. It may be accompanied by conjunctivitis. Most affected dogs begin to show clinical signs between 1–3 years of age. Predisposed breeds include the Shar Pei, West Highland white terrier and other terrier breeds, Lhasa Apso, Shih Tzu, Golden retriever, and Labrador retriever.

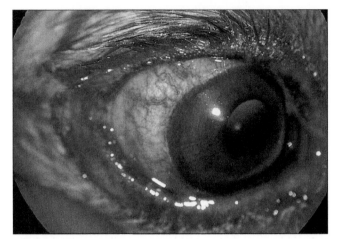

Figure 7.58 Acute bacterial infection of the lids in a dog that resulted from "spilling over" from a bacterial conjunctivitis.

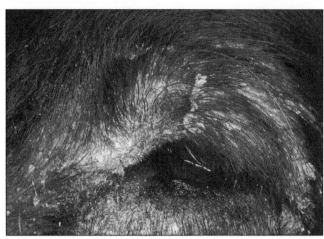

Figure 7.61 Scaly dermatitis in a dog with leishmaniasis. (Courtesy of Dr. S. Pizzirani, Florence, Italy.)

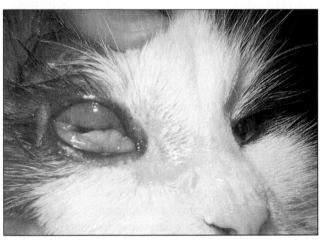

Figure 7.59 Cat with a bite wound abscess in the upper eyelid. The abscess is draining into the conjunctival sac. Note the bite wound just below the practitioner's thumb.

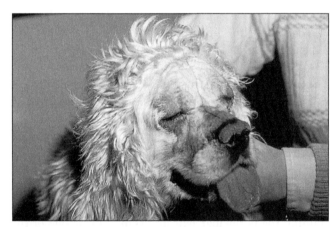

Figure 7.62 Radiation-induced alopecia and dermatitis in a dog after teletherapy for nasal neoplasia.

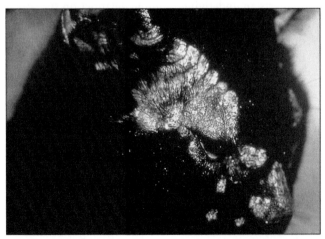

Figure 7.60 Cat with *Microsporum* dermatomycosis, characterized by dry, scaly dermatitis. (Courtesy of Prof. M. Lorenz, College of Veterinary Medicine, Oklahoma State University.)

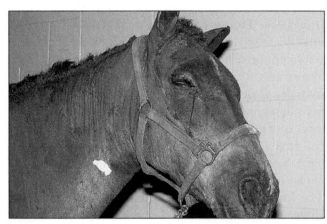

Figure 7.63 Severe burns over the upper lid of a horse, with diffuse, less severe burns over the entire body. The eyelid lesions contracted with time producing marked distortion.

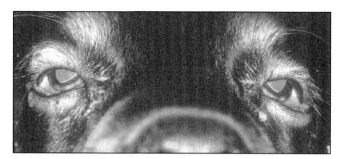

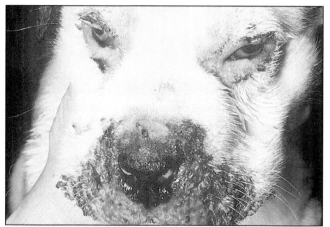

Figure 7.64 Juvenile pyoderma ("puppy strangles") in a 12-week-old Gordon Setter (top). Note the bilaterally symmetrical firm, granulomatous eyelid swelling. The puppy at the bottom has the ulcerative periocular and muzzle granulomatous lesions as well as granulomatous lesions of the submandibular lymph nodes.

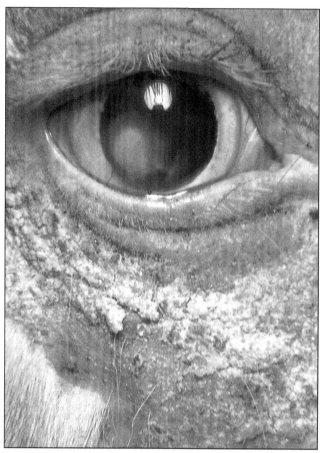

Figure 7.65 Contact hypersensitivity to topical medications utilized to treat corneal lesions in a horse. Note the periocular pattern of distribution, especially the inferior lid and face ventral to the eye.

Drug eruption: Immune-mediated reactions to drugs may occur from systemically administered drugs or from contact sensitivity to topical drugs. Both forms of exposure to sensitizing drugs may produce blepharitis and facial dermatitis. The topical exposure is limited to the lids and the face (**Figure 7.65**), whereas systemic drugs produce bilateral lids lesions and more generalized dermatologic lesions (**Figure 7.66**).

> Drug hypersensitivity should be suspected whenever there is a worsening of the ocular condition once therapy has commenced.

Eosinophilic plaque: In the cat, lesions of the eosinophilic granuloma complex may manifest on the lids and precede skin lesions at other sites.[82] These lesions usually reflect underlying hypersensitivity (flea allergy, atopy, food allergy).

Pemphigus complex: The autoimmune skin diseases of pemphigus vulgaris, pemphigus vegetans,

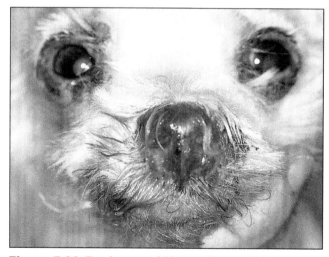

Figure 7.66 Erythema multiforme (Stevens–Johnson syndrome) in a dog with skin reactions to systemically administered sulfa drugs for a septicemia. (Courtesy of Dr. L. Medleau, Department of Small Animal Medicine, University of Georgia.)

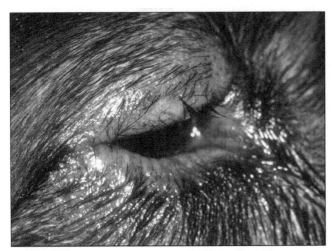

Figure 7.67 Mucocutaneous lesions in a dog due to pemphigus vulgaris. The 2-year-old Irish setter also had lesions of the lips, vulva, anus, and interdigital areas.

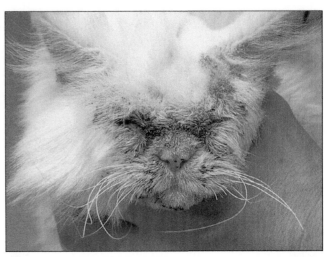

Figure 7.68 Presumed discoid lupus erythematosus in a cat. The cat was positive on LE preparation and negative on immunostaining of skin biopsies for pemphigus. The condition responded to oral anti-inflammatory doses of corticosteroids. Discoid lupus erythematosus appears similar to idiopathic facial dermatitis of the Persian cat.

pemphigus foliaceus, pemphigus erythematosus, and bullous pemphigoid are often accompanied by facial dermatosis and eyelid involvement in the dog and the cat (depigmentation, erosions, crusting).[80,82–86] Pemphigus vulgaris, pemphigus vegetans, and bullous pemphigoid are characterized clinically by involvement of the mucocutaneous junctions (**Figure 7.67**). The pemphigus complex is characterized by autoantibodies against epithelial intercellular cement substance.

Discoid and systemic lupus erythematosus: The immune-mediated diseases of lupus erythematosus may occur as discoid lupus erythematosus, a local disease limited to the skin, or systemic lupus erythematosus (SLE), which is a multiorgan disease with skin involvement in 30%–60% of cases. The lesions in both conditions are frequently a facial dermatosis with eyelid involvement (depigmentation, erosions, crusting) (**Figure 7.68**). Systemic lupus erythematosus has an increased incidence in the collie, Shetland sheepdog, and GSD.[80,85] Pathogenesis of skin lesions in the lupus disorders involves antinuclear antibodies that bind to keratinocytes to cause cytotoxic injury and cytokine release, resulting in attraction of lymphocytes and further epithelial damage.

Uveodermatologic syndrome: Uveodermatologic syndrome, or Vogt–Koyanagi–Harada-like (VKH-like) syndrome, produces skin lesions characterized by vitiligo (skin depigmentation) and poliosis (whitening of hair), which preferentially involve the eyelids, the lips, the nose, the foot pads, and the scrotum of young adult dogs (mean age 2.8 years).[87] In occasional cases, the skin changes may be generalized.[88]

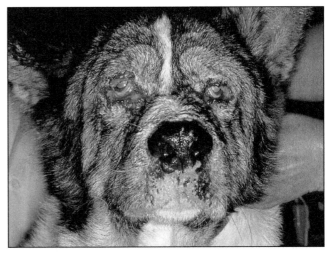

Figure 7.69 Uveodermatologic syndrome in an Akita. Note the moist erosive dermatitis with depigmentation of the lids and the muzzle/lips.

> The skin lesions of uveodermatologic syndrome usually occur after ocular lesions that typically manifest as a bilateral panuveitis.

While the eyelid lesions are characterized by depigmentation, some cases progress to a more erosive, crusting dermatitis (**Figure 7.69**). VKH-like syndrome has been reported in a variety of breeds, but the Akita represents 80% of reported cases.[88]

Reactive cutaneous and systemic histiocytosis: Non-neoplastic (as compared to histiocytic sarcoma) proliferative disorders of perivascular dermal dendritic antigen-presenting cells, these diseases may present as infiltrating nodules, plaques, crusts, and/or depigmented areas within the skin and subcutaneous tissues, including the lids. Systemic histiocytosis is differentiated by its peripheral lymph node and organ involvement.[89] Systemic histiocytosis was first described in the Bernese mountain dog, and a polygenetic mode of inheritance has been proven.[90] The genetic disorder was subsequently documented in Rottweilers, Irish wolfhounds, Golden retrievers, and Labrador retrievers.

Clinical signs of blepharitis
Blepharitis lesions vary with the cause, chronicity, modification with therapy, and amount of self-trauma. Alopecia, crusts, edema, hyperemia, cicatrization, keratitis, and conjunctivitis are common signs.

Diagnosis of blepharitis
Historical data and other clinical findings, including the age, breed, environment, distribution of lesions, presence or absence of pruritus, and course and response to therapy, are often important clues to the specific cause.

> Skin scrapings and cytology should be performed on most cases of blepharitis to detect causative organisms such as parasites, bacteria, and fungi.

Cultures should supplement cytology when bacterial or fungal causes are suspected. Biopsy of *Habronema* lesions typically reveals granulation tissue with collagenolysis, eosinophils, mast cells, and neutrophils. Larval elements may not be seen on biopsy. If fine-needle aspirate of intralesional mast cell accumulation is obtained, mast cell tumor may be misdiagnosed.[73]

Serologic tests are available for diagnosing exposure to *Leishmania*, but they can cross-react with *Trypanosoma*-positive dogs.[91] Actinic/radiation/chemical-induced or heat-induced burns are diagnosed based on history, lesion distribution, and histopathologic findings.

Keratinization disorders are diagnosed by characteristic histopathology and clinical findings. Primary seborrhea is diagnosed only after all causes of secondary seborrhea have been ruled out (allergies, infection, parasites, endocrine disease, nutritional disorders).

For dogs with symptoms compatible with atopy, intradermal skin testing may indicate the offending allergen(s). Drug eruptions are diagnosed by establishing a temporal relationship of lesion development to drug administration and resolution of symptoms with drug discontinuation. Common topically applied ophthalmic medications inducing hypersensitivity reactions with chronic use include aminoglycoside antibiotics (neomycin and gentamicin), dorzolamide, atropine, and corn oil-based compounded cyclosporine preparations. Eosinophilic plaques are diagnosed by characteristic histopathologic findings. Autoimmune skin diseases are diagnosed by biopsy with characteristic histopathology. Immunostaining may demonstrate characteristic immunoglobulin deposition.

Histologic findings in uveodermatologic syndrome include pigmentary incontinence and a lichenoid infiltration with histiocytes, plasma cells, multinucleated giant cells, and lymphocytes. Response to immunosuppressive therapy is a common means of making a provisional diagnosis.

Characteristic histologic findings and breed predisposition are diagnostic for systemic and reactive cutaneous histiocytosis.

Therapy for blepharitis
Mites Mitocides are often used topically, but care should be taken to avoid the conjunctiva/corneal surfaces. Demodectic mange is usually self-limiting in a young dog. If limited to a few local regions such as the periocular area, specific therapy is usually unnecessary. If the condition becomes generalized, treatment options include amitraz dips, oral ivermectin (except in herding breeds),[92] or oral milbemycin. Topical avermectin and milbemycin products may be used periocularly with success.

Habronema Therapy consists of mechanical expression and debridement of irritating granules in the lesion. Systemic ivermectin (0.2 mg/kg) kills the larvae[93] with perilesional reaction to the dying larva necessitating topical or intralesional injection of glucocorticoid. Fly control and routine deworming with an avermectin product is important to prevent reinfestation.

Bacteria If infection is superficial, therapy consists of topical antibiotic; if the infection is deep, systemic antibiotics are usually required (**Figure 7.70**). Autogenous or commercially available bacterins historically have been helpful in recurrent or resistant cases,[94] but they are uncommonly used today.

Chalazions are treated by incision and curettage through the conjunctival side. Tissue should be sent for histopathology as neoplasia may mimic a chalazion. Acute internal hordeolum is treated by lancing from the conjunctival surface with topical antibiotic administration

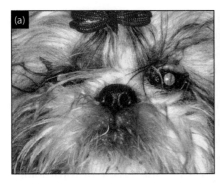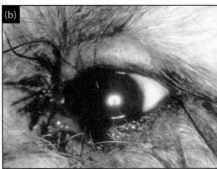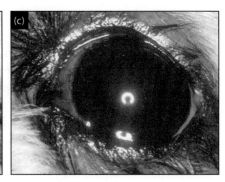

Figure 7.70 Bilateral blepharitis in a Lhasa Apso with atopic skin disease and *Staph* spp. hypersensitivity (a). Close-up of left eye, showing periocular alopecia and hyperemia with firm thickening of upper lid due to chalazia (b). Left eye 3 weeks after symptomatic therapy (trimming hair and warm, moist compresses), systemic antibiotic therapy, and judicious systemic corticosteroid therapy (c).

until healed. Chronic meibomian gland dysfunction should be treated with frequent warm, moist compresses and gentle manual expression or with diluted baby shampoo to remove keratin plugs from the orifices along with low-dose systemic tetracycline antibiotic to inhibit bacterial lipase production.[75]

Focal pyogranulomas have been treated in a variety of ways including systemic antibiotics, systemic glucocorticoids, intralesional antibiotics, curettage of lesions, staphylococcal vaccine, and tetracycline/niacinamide therapy. The latter combination is postulated to have immunomodulatory properties, and it has been used to treat dogs with focal granulomas and with episcleritis/scleritis. Tetracycline and niacinamide are administered at a dose of 250–500 mg of each drug every 8 hours, and dose frequency is gradually reduced once a response is observed.[70,95,96] Supportive therapy consists of removal of scabs with warm moist gauze, hot packing for 15 minutes every 8–12 hours, and expressing and treating infections of meibomian glands or lash follicles.

Fungi In dogs, localized disease may be self-limiting or may be treated with topical antifungal agents. It is important to not get topical antifungal products on the corneal/conjunctival surfaces as many products have a high percentage of alcohol. Compounded topical miconazole solutions used to treat equine fungal keratitis are safe and effective for periocular dermatomycosis. Dogs with generalized or multifocal disease, and cats, are treated with a combination of topical and systemic antifungal medications (griseofulvin 50 mg/kg daily [should not be used in pregnant animals or breeding males], ketoconazole 5–10 mg/kg/day, or itraconazole 5–10 mg/kg/day). Dilute bleach cleaning (1:10) of the immediate environment is indicated to prevent spread and reinfection[97] as long as it does not contact cornea/conjunctival surfaces.

Leishmaniasis Leishmaniasis therapy has traditionally used pentavalent antimony compounds administered until clinical remission is noted. The relapse rate is high (75%)[98] unless therapy is maintained on a long-term intermittent dose of allopurinol 20 mg/kg daily for 1 week once a month.[99]

Burns Exposure to the most intense sun should be limited by housing the animal during the day, use of UV protectant fly masks in horses, and using chemical sunscreens if necessary. Tattooing may be attempted[100] but needs periodic retreatment.

Chemical and thermal burns are treated acutely by copious cool water lavage. Affected skin should then be kept clean of exudate and debris with gentle daily lavage. Daily topical application of silver sulfadiazine cream can prevent secondary bacterial infection and speed healing of injured skin. Reconstructive surgery may be needed to correct scarring/lid contracture.

Seborrhea/keratinization disorder Antiseborrheic shampoos are indicated, but care should be taken to avoid contact with the eyes. In severe cases, steroids or retinoids may be helpful.

Immune-mediated Atopic blepharitis can be treated with topical steroids, oral antihistamines, systemic cyclosporine, or intermittent oral glucocorticoids. Desensitization in an atopic animal is an adjunct or alternative to systemic glucocorticoids when the offending allergen is known.[101]

Drug eruption/hypersensitivity is treated by withdrawal of the causative drug, with or without immunosuppressive medication, if lesions do not spontaneously improve within 2–3 weeks of withdrawing treatment.

Eosinophilic granuloma complex in cats is commonly treated with intermittent injectable or oral glucocorticoids.

Refractory lesions may respond to chlorambucil, gold salts, or radiation therapy. Cats with recurrent or refractory lesions should be evaluated and treated for underlying hypersensitivity disorder (flea allergy, atopy, food allergy).

Autoimmune diseases are usually treated with systemic immunosuppressive doses of glucocorticoids that may be combined with azathioprine, cyclosporine, cyclophosphamide, or chlorambucil in severe cases.[83,86,102] After remission is induced, drugs are slowly tapered over several months to the lowest dose that controls the disease. Glucocorticoids alone are inadequate in about 50% of pemphigus disease cases.[103] Refractory cases may respond to gold salts[83,103,104] or cyclosporine.

Discoid lupus erythematosus may also be successfully treated with tetracycline and niacinamide, and dogs with localized disease may benefit from topical administration of glucocorticoids or compounded cyclosporine. Uveodermatologic syndrome is usually treated initially with a combination of systemic glucocorticoids and azathioprine, cyclosporine, or leflunomide in addition to topical ophthalmic glucocorticoids and atropine. After remission is induced, drugs are slowly tapered over several months to the lowest dose of systemic drug(s) that controls the disease.

Lacerations

Lacerations of the eyelids are somewhat common in all species. In the dog and the cat, lid lacerations are usually the result of fighting, accidents in the field in working dogs, or automobile accidents. In large animals, lid lacerations are usually caused by barbed wire or a nail (or hook) in the stall. Lacerations should not be dismissed as not worth the trouble to suture, as they may become quite disfiguring if not treated. The usual sequela is a lid margin notch/defect that allows spillage of tears or cicatrization, which may result in entropion, ectropion, or trichiasis that progress to a secondary keratitis. Lacerations are of two main types:

- Perpendicular to the lid margin. Even small nicks in the lid margin may remain as notches due to the orbicularis oculi muscle separating the edges (**Figure 7.71**). This opposing tension must be considered when repairing the lid or removing masses from the eyelid.
- Parallel to the lid margin. Lacerations of this type often consist of a very narrow pedicle of skin that is tempting to excise (**Figure 7.72**). It is important to remember that the pedicle contains the normal mucocutaneous junction of the lid. A common sequela to excision of this pedicle is for trichiasis to develop months later (**Figure 7.73**). This type of

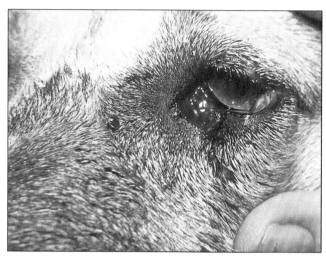

Figure 7.71 Lid laceration in the lower medial canthal area of a dog, perpendicular to the lid margin. Note the separation of the wound edges with exposure of the underlying third eyelid due to orbicularis oculi tension.

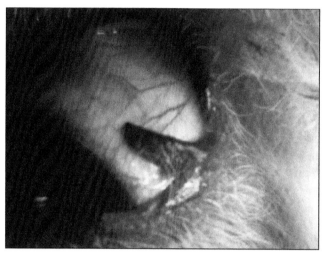

Figure 7.72 Lid laceration in a dog parallel to the margin, with a narrow tag containing the lid margin. These tags should always be sutured back in place.

laceration does not have the opposing muscle tension pulling it apart.

Clinical signs

The signs of lacerations are usually obvious, but the globe should be examined for corneal ulcerations or penetrating/perforating wounds of the cornea or sclera.

Therapy

Lacerations should be repaired as soon as possible as chronicity makes the edges indurated and thicker, detracting from the ultimate cosmetic appearance. Typically, a significant amount of debris and hair must be removed from the wound. When preparing the site for surgery,

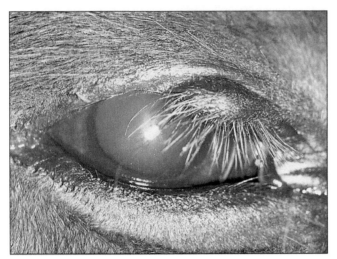

Figure 7.73 Sequela of excision of a lid tag from a parallel laceration of the upper lid margin in a horse. Note the acquired margin defect/coloboma laterally, trichiasis of the remaining cilia medially, and small hairs touching the cornea at the mucocutaneous junction laterally.

if clipping of adjacent hair is done, sterile lubricant gel coated scissors should be used, and the wound may be filled with sterile lubricant gel to trap the hair. The gel with the hair can then be removed from the wound. Minimal debridement is recommended because most tags of tissue remain viable.

Lacerations perpendicular to the lid margin should have at least two layers of sutures placed to minimize the dehiscing force of the orbicularis muscle.[105] A continuous layer of 5-0 to 6-0 braided synthetic absorbable suture (polyglycolic acid and others) is placed in the tarsus and the subconjunctival stroma, with the knots tied within the tissue so the cornea is not irritated. Braided or monofilament 4-0 to 5-0 suture is suitable for the muscle–skin layer in small animals. In the horse (or even very large, thick-lidded dogs), some horizontal mattress absorbable sutures may be used to appose the orbicularis muscle prior to skin closure. Extra care should be taken to appose the lid margin accurately, as this is the most obvious functional/cosmetic landmark. If the margin is not smooth, the suture must be repositioned until the margin is in apposition, as it will not self-correct. In situations where there is excessive tension on a perpendicular laceration repair, or the closed tissue is friable, placing a temporary tarsorrhaphy suture on either side of the laceration closure site can "splint" the wound until the area heals. It is also important to develop a strategy to avoid the suture ends from rubbing on the cornea (see **Figure 7.74** for methods).[106] Topical and systemic antibiotics, as well as tetanus prophylaxis in horses, are typical postoperative therapy.

The temptation to excise pedicles of lid that contain the mucocutaneous junction (lid margin) should be resisted, and the pedicles should be sutured back in place. Most even, thin pedicles will remain viable enough to preserve the normal lid margin.

Eyelid neoplasia in the dog

Lid neoplasia is very common in the dog, but fortunately, >75% are benign. Sebaceous adenomas, papillomas, and melanocytomas account for about 82% of lid tumors, and more than one type may occur in an individual. The most common tumor arises from the meibomian gland and, depending on the differentiation, can be termed as sebaceous hyperplasia, sebaceous adenoma, adenocarcinoma, epithelioma, or basal cell tumor (**Figures 7.75 through 7.77**). The average age for developing lid neoplasia is approximately 8 years, and breeds such as the boxer, poodle, English springer spaniel, and American Cocker Spaniel have a higher incidence than the hospital population. While <25% of lid tumors are malignant, metastasis is rare.[107] In the author's experience, the exception is aggressively growing mast cell tumors of the lid (**Figure 7.78**) and melanomas involving the lid margin/palpebral conjunctiva. The aggressive mast cell tumor (histologic grade III or high grade based on cellular anaplasia and high mitotic figure counts[108,109]) probably has the worst lid tumor prognosis in the dog. Fortunately, mast cell tumor of the lid is not common. They are usually of a low-grade malignancy potential and are easily diagnosed with fine-needle aspirates (**Figure 7.79**). Melanocytomas on the external lid surface (flat or pedunculated with a small base) are typically benign, whereas melanomas of the lid margin extending into the palpebral conjunctiva have a higher incidence of being malignant based on biological activity (local lymph node metastasis) and histologic morphology (high mitotic figure counts). Other lid tumors occasionally observed are squamous cell carcinoma (SCC), fibroma and fibrosarcoma, and histiocytoma.[107,110,111] Two lid tumors typically occur in young dogs, viral papilloma (**Figure 7.80**) and histiocytoma (**Figures 7.81 and 7.82**), and they are unique in that they develop rapidly and usually regress spontaneously. Viral papillomas of the lid may occur concurrently with oral papillomas. The papilloma is usually typical in appearance with a pedunculated, cauliflower appearance. Surgical manipulation may result in multiple papillomas occurring, and they may involve the conjunctiva and cornea as well as the eyelids.[112] The histiocytoma is typically a broad-based, elevated red lesion with a relatively smooth surface (**Figure 7.81**).

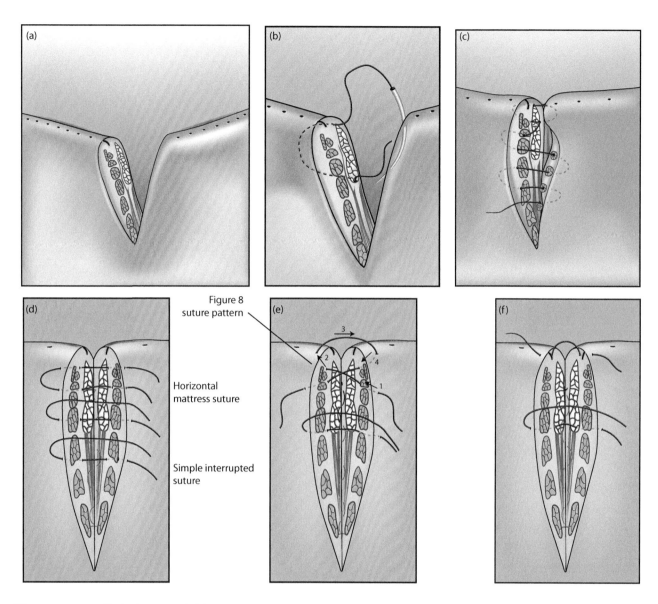

Figure 7.74 Full-thickness eyelid laceration repair. Frontal/cross-section view of laceration (a). Proper placement of a fine, synthetic, absorbable suture apposes the cut edges of the tarsus. Knot is buried in the stromal tissue (b). A continuous suture pattern apposes the conjunctiva/muscle tissues. Suture should not pass through the conjunctiva to prevent frictional irritation to the cornea (c). If the lid is very thickened (large dog or horse), additional horizontal mattress sutures may be used to appose the orbicularis muscle further. *Methods used to close skin/lid margin*: Horizontal mattress followed by simple interrupted sutures (d), cruciate or "figure-of-eight" margin pattern followed by simple interrupted sutures (e), and simple interrupted (f) followed by further simple interrupted sutures. In each case, the suture tags are left long, and with each subsequent suture placement, the previous suture tags are incorporated in the subsequent suture's knot, thereby "tying back" the suture tags to minimize suture rubbing on the cornea and enhance suture removal once healed.

Systemic histiocytosis of Bernese mountain dogs produces multiple cutaneous nodules over the body, with the eyelids being one of the common sites.[113]

Eyelid neoplasia in the cat

Eyelid neoplasia is relatively uncommon in the cat.[114] The most common lid tumor of the cat is SCC.[114,115] The lesion is associated with actinic radiation and usually occurs in pale skin, white-furred cats. The location is usually on the lower lid near the medial canthus, and most are initially erosive (**Figure 7.83**) followed by deep tissue infiltration. Early on, local metastasis does not appear to be common, but inappropriate diagnosis and treatment allows for local metastasis as well as regional lymph node metastasis. Neoplasms of the feline lids (listed in order of incidence from a retrospective study[116]) are: SCC, mast cell tumor

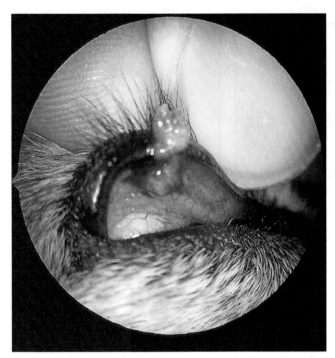

Figure 7.75 Eyelid sebaceous adenoma in a dog. Note the cauliflower appearance. The site of origin can be followed to the conjunctival side of the lid.

(**Figure 7.83**), hemangiosarcoma, adenocarcinoma, apocrine hidrocystoma (**Figure 7.83**), peripheral nerve sheath tumor, lymphoma, and hemangioma. Additional described feline eyelid tumors include papilloma, basal cell tumor, fibroma/fibrosarcoma, and xanthoma.[115] In the cat, cutaneous mast cell tumors are usually benign.[117–119] Berger and Scott and Molander-McCrary et al. found no correlation with biologic behavior and histologic grading of the tumor, while Wilcock et al. divided mast cell tumors into two subtypes based on these two characteristics.[117–119] Wilcock et al. found that 76% (65/85) were

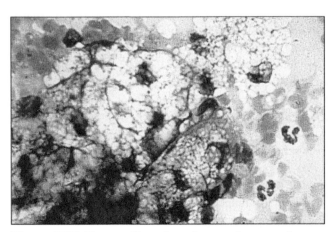

Figure 7.76 Fine-needle aspirate from a sebaceous adenoma in a dog. Several vacuolated sebaceous epithelial cells are present, with fewer basophilic reserve cells (Wright's stain).

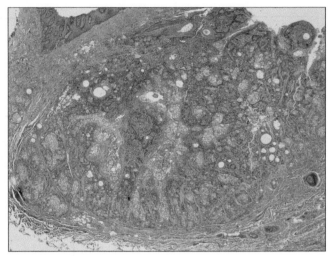

Figure 7.77 Meibomian gland adenoma, eyelid, dog. The tumor is well demarcated, encapsulated, and composed of multiple lobules of cells with sebaceous and basal differentiation. (Courtesy of Dr. Thomas Cecere, Department of Biomedical Sciences and Pathology, VA–MD College of Veterinary Medicine, Virginia Tech.)

solitary, discrete nodules with mild atypia that behaved benignly, although seven in this group had more anisocytosis and mitotic activity and spread or recurred within 3 months following excision.[117] A second morphologic form with histiocytic-looking mast cells that were often multiple nodules occurred predominantly in young Siamese cats and often regressed spontaneously over 2 years. In another study of 33 cases of feline periocular mast cell tumors,[120] tumors considered of low-grade malignancy had a low rate of recurrence even when incomplete surgical margins were noted on histologic evaluation.

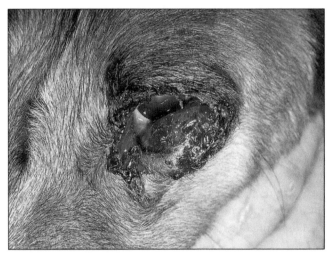

Figure 7.78 Mast cell tumor that developed very rapidly in a dog. The dog was euthanized shortly after presentation due to systemic complications of disseminated mastocytosis. The tumor is easily diagnosed by fine-needle aspiration.

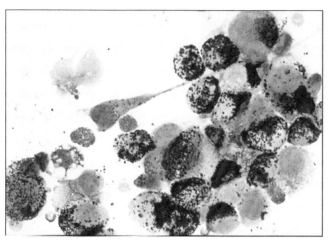

Figure 7.79 Fine-needle aspirate from a mast cell tumor in a dog, with large round cells with nuclear and cytoplasmic pleomorphism. The cytoplasm contains basophilic cytoplasmic granules typical of mast cells. A few eosinophils are present.

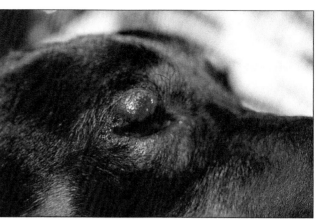

Figure 7.81 Histiocytoma of the upper lid of a young adult dog. Rapid onset; hairless, nonulcerated, smooth, broad-based lesion; and young age are indicators of histiocytoma, and diagnosis is confirmed by fine-needle aspiration. The lesion regressed spontaneously.

Eyelid neoplasia in the horse

Squamous cell carcinoma

Eyelid neoplasia in the horse and the cow is less common than in the dog. SCC is the most common tumor of the eye and the adnexa in horses, and the eyelid is the least common site (approximately 23% of cases) compared to the third eyelid/medial canthus (approximately 28%) or limbus (approximately 28%).[121–123] It is usually found on the lower lid or medial canthal region (**Figures 7.84 and 7.85**). Ultraviolet radiation is believed to be the major predisposing factor for SCC (along with geographic influence of decreased latitude, increased altitude, and increased mean annual solar radiation exposure).[124] About 16% of ocular SCCs are bilateral. The incidence increases with age, with the mean age ranging from 9 to 12 years. In one study, males were twice as likely to be affected as females, and the gelding was five times more susceptible than the stallion.[124] However, another study found no gender predisposition difference.[125] The draft horse and the Appaloosa are at greater risk, as are horses with white, cremello, and palomino hair colors.[121,123,124,126,127] The author sees a higher incidence of SCC in Tennessee walking horses and Haflingers compared to the hospital population.

Despite the well-known predisposition for SCC in older color dilute horses, it is not unusual to observe SCC in heavily pigmented horses such as bays and in young adult horses of any coat color.

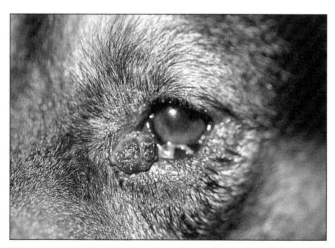

Figure 7.80 Viral-induced papilloma in a young Rottweiler dog. Papillomas were also present in the mouth. All lesions regressed of their own accord over a month's time.

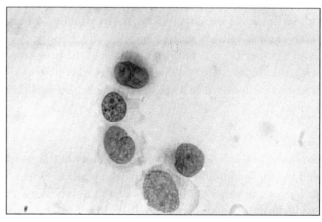

Figure 7.82 Fine needle aspirate of a histiocytoma in a dog. A monopopulation of large cells with an oval, hyperchromatic nuclei and abundant cytoplasm typical of histiocytes can be seen (Wright's stain).

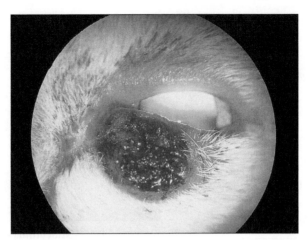

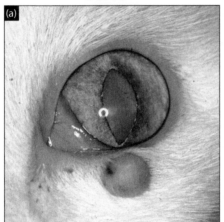
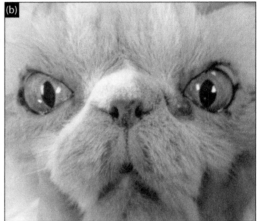

Figure 7.83 (Top) Squamous cell carcinoma of the lower eyelid in a white cat. A slowly progressive, proliferative erosive lesion in a white-furred cat is a typical presentation. (a) Cutaneous mast cell tumor of the lower lid of an old cat. Surgical excision with closure consisting of a semicircular flap was incomplete; however, long-term follow-up failed to reveal tumor recurrence. (b) Apocrine hidrocystoma of the left lower lid in a Persian cat. Partial-thickness excision, curettage, and cryosurgery resulted in good cosmetic result with no recurrence.

SCC has a high recurrence rate (>30%)[123] but a late and low metastatic rate. Local metastasis is usually to adjacent ocular/adnexal tissues, orbital tissues, and periorbital bone. More distal metastasis is usually to local lymph nodes, salivary glands, and the lung. Reports vary as to whether the site of origin influences the prognosis, with one report citing a higher recurrence/dissemination rate with eyelid SCC than from the third eyelid or limbus.[124]

Sarcoid

Sarcoids are the second most common tumor of the eyelid and the most common equine tumor in general. Sarcoids in horses and other equidae are believed to be caused by bovine papilloma virus (BPV).[128–130] Prior to the most recent scientific studies implicating BPV, early reports[131] did not demonstrate a predilection for breed, sex, or coat color. Unlike most neoplasia, sarcoids are much more likely to be found in young horses.

A genetic predisposition has been reported and related to the equine leukocyte antigen.[132–135] There is reported predisposition of sarcoid in the American quarter horse, Appaloosa, and Arabian breeds.[135,136] When found periocularly, the lesions are proliferative, may have erosions, and may infiltrate into deeper adnexal/periorbital structures (**Figures 7.86 and 7.87**). Knottenbelt and Kelly described six forms of periocular sarcoids and correlated the type with response to various therapies administered over a 25-year period.[137] Occult sarcoid presented with periocular alopecia or altered hair color and had small subdermal nodules or plaques. Verrucose sarcoids had alopecia and hyperkeratosis of the periocular region, with varying amounts of ulceration of the surface and subdermal nodules. Nodular sarcoids were either a well-defined solid nodule or multiple nodules with an intact skin (Type A), or nodules with varying amounts of skin ulceration (Type B). Fibroblastic sarcoids were either pedunculated (Type A) or broad-based (Type B) and were proliferative,

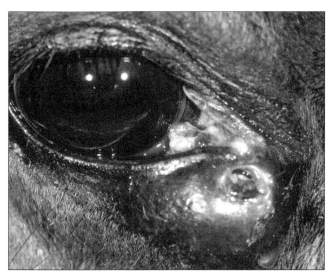

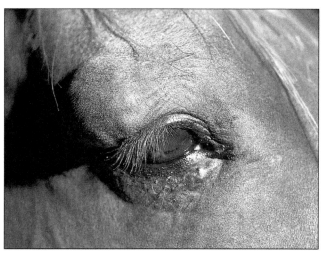

Figure 7.84 Squamous cell carcinoma of the lower lid and medial canthus in a horse. Aggressive surgical debulkment, liquid nitrogen cryosurgery, and repeated intralesional injections of 5-fluorouracil resulted in no recurrence for 2 years post-treatment; however, 2+ years post-treatment, the horse died from pulmonary metastasis.

Figure 7.86 Equine nodular sarcoid (Type A) of the lateral upper lid. The lesion is firm and had infiltrated eyelid musculature and orbital rim periosteum and could therefore be termed "malignant."

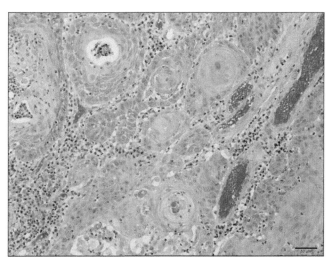

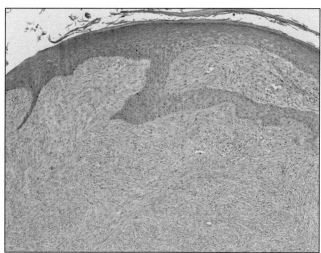

Figure 7.85 Equine ocular squamous cell carcinoma. Cords and islands of neoplastic squamous epithelial cells infiltrate into the surrounding lid stroma. Neoplastic cells occasionally exhibit progressive central keratinization ("keratin pearls"). (Courtesy of Dr. Thomas Cecere, Department of Biomedical Sciences and Pathology, VA–MD College of Veterinary Medicine, Virginia Tech.)

Figure 7.87 Sarcoid, eyelid, horse. Raised, firm, multinodular mass adjacent to the eyelid. The mass has two components: (1) Hyperplastic epidermis, forming branching rete pegs, and (2) a densely cellular population of fibroblasts that expands the dermis and abuts the overlying epidermis. (Courtesy of Dr. Thomas Cecere, Department of Biomedical Sciences and Pathology, VA–MD College of Veterinary Medicine, Virginia Tech.)

with diffuse ulceration. Mixed sarcoids had characteristics of two or more types, while a malignant sarcoid was one that had grown rapidly and infiltrated deeply into the adjacent tissues and orbit. Lesions may be found on either the upper or lower lids and/or canthal regions. While sarcoids may be locally invasive and frequently recur after therapy, they have no tendency for distal metastasis.[138] About one-third of horses with sarcoid may undergo spontaneous regression unrelated to any specific clinical parameter or equine leukocyte antigen type.[133,139]

Biopsy of equine lid sarcoids should be followed quickly by definitive therapy, since they may become more aggressive with surgical manipulation.[137]

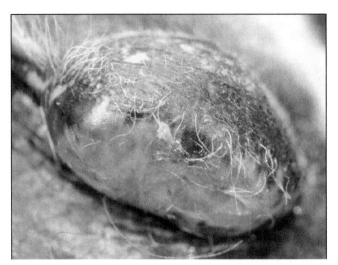

Figure 7.88 Eyelid melanoma of the entire upper eyelid margin in an aged Arabian mare. The mare had masses of perianal and perivulvar melanomas as well.

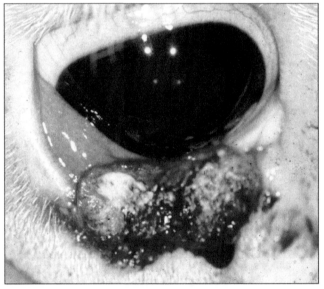

Figure 7.89 Typical appearance of a squamous cell carcinoma of the eyelid in a Hereford cow.

Other tumors described as arising from the equine lid include melanoma (**Figure 7.88**), mast cell tumor, lymphosarcoma, schwannoma, and papilloma.[121,140–142]

Eyelid neoplasia in the cow

SCC of the eye and adnexa is a significant economic disease in cattle. It is found most frequently in the Hereford, Hereford crosses, Simmental, and shorthorn breeds, although it has been observed in a variety of other breeds. The eyelids are the least common site for involvement, accounting for only about 12%–15% of cases (**Figure 7.89**).[143] The etiology is multifactorial, with ultraviolet light and genetic predisposition being crucial.[144,145]

The amount of periocular pigmentation may be associated with neoplasia.[146,147] The corneal limbus is the most frequent site of involvement in the cow (see Chapter 10). Bovine papilloma virus may cause benign papillomatosis of the external lids and conjunctival surfaces.

Diagnosis

A tentative diagnosis of eyelid neoplasia is usually made on appearance and confirmed by biopsy and histopathologic evaluation of the lesion.

Therapy

The appropriate therapy for eyelid neoplasia varies with the type and extent of the tumor, history of previous therapy, systemic health, and resources available. As most lid tumors in the dog are benign or slow to metastasize, the most common complication is local regrowth. In most instances of benign canine lid tumors, there is no clear evidence that one form of therapy is superior to another; selection of a particular modality is based on familiarity and what is available to the clinician. In the cat, lid tumors have more potential to be malignant (e.g., squamous cell carcinoma), and more initial aggressive therapy is warranted to prevent localized/distal metastasis with subsequent loss of life. In large animals, aggressive neoplasia is also more common than in the dog, but economic factors may play a role in selection of treatment modalities.

Surgical excision Excision is a common form of lid tumor therapy in general veterinary practice, mainly because it does not require instrumentation beyond that available to most practitioners. A commonly used technique is the full-thickness wedge resection excision. The average dog has enough length of lid to accommodate the removal of one-quarter to one-third of full-thickness lid/margin using this technique without permanent cosmetic blemish or loss of function. Toy dogs with small palpebral fissures, cats, and horses may not tolerate more than one-quarter of the lid length being removed and primarily closed without noticeable cosmetic/functional defect. When excising the mass, incision through the lid must be perpendicular to the lid margin, with the two incisions medial and lateral to the tumor being parallel past the level of the tarsus/tarsal plate. The remainder of the full-thickness excision through the lid skin, the stroma, and the conjunctiva should taper to the depth of the cul-de-sac to ensure a smooth closure without bunching of the tissue following closure. This is best performed with the aid of a Jaeger lid plate and scalpel through the skin and the orbicularis muscle and a fine scissor through the palpebral conjunctiva. Closure is similar to an eyelid laceration (**Figure 7.74**). In the case

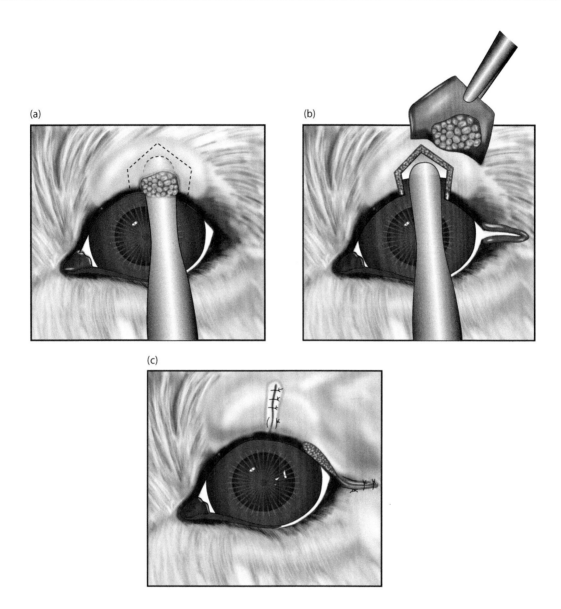

(a)

(b)

(c)

Figure 7.90 Wedge resection of an eyelid mass using principles of parallel incisions through the tarsal plate and a releasing lateral canthotomy as mentioned in the text. The excision site tapers to the depth of the cul-de-sac for a smoother closure and postop appearance (a and b), the incision is closed in two layers as was the case for an eyelid laceration closure (c), and the lateral canthotomy (b) allows the excised lid to be closed primarily without excess tension. The lateral canthotomy site is closed in two layers without trying to oppose the medial edges (c). The edge of the lateral canthotomy on the excised lid can heal by second intention.

where the area of excised lid is greater than what can be closed without loss of function or disfigurement, a lateral canthotomy may be performed to allow the remaining lid tissue to be slid medially while the primary excision site is closed (**Figure 7.90**). In the case where more lid margin must be excised than can easily be closed (50+% of the lid in most dogs), a semicircular flap technique[148] may be used to close the void (**Figure 7.91**). The author has successfully closed defects of up to 50% in cats and horses (**Figure 7.92**) and up to 65% of upper lid defects in dogs using this technique.

A wide variety of intricate plastic procedures have been advocated for repair of large defects, but most all have the disadvantage of not having a normal lid margin, which may result in trichiasis at a later date.[149–153] The Cutler–Beard ("bucket-handle") procedure can be used to fill a variety of defects along the length of the upper or lower lids (**Figure 7.8**).[154] This procedure can give good cosmetic results, but the major disadvantage is that it is a two-stage procedure requiring two anesthetic episodes (as is the case with many other plastic procedures such as the sliding H-plasty skin/conjunctiva flap previously

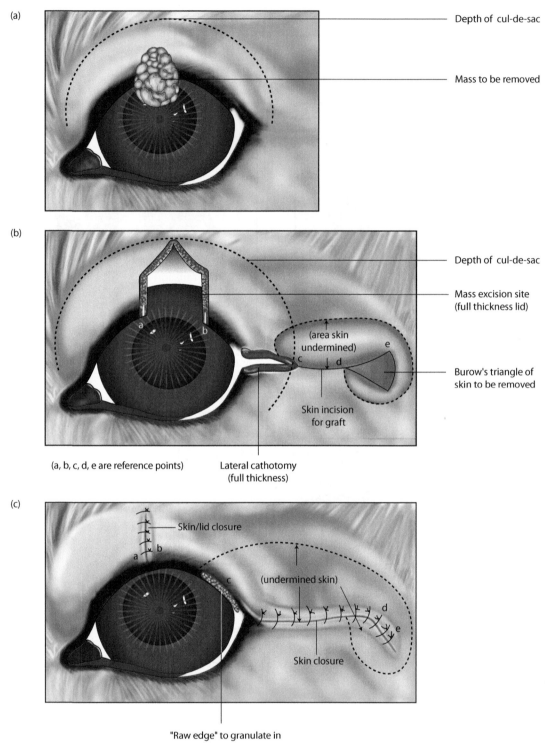

(a)

Depth of cul-de-sac

Mass to be removed

(b)

Depth of cul-de-sac

Mass excision site
(full thickness lid)

(area skin
undermined)

Burow's triangle of
skin to be removed

Skin incision
for graft

(a, b, c, d, e are reference points)   Lateral cathotomy
(full thickness)

(c)

Skin/lid closure

(undermined skin)

Skin closure

"Raw edge" to granulate in

Figure 7.91 Semicircular flap to fill in a large eyelid void following large mass (a) removal. Following excision of the lid mass, a lateral canthotomy is performed (b), and a sweeping skin incision is made beyond the canthotomy. This curved skin incision should approximate a mirror image of the curve of the pathological lid, and the length of the skin incision should be 2–3 times the length of the lid margin excision. A Burow's triangle is cut through the skin at the end of the semicircular skin incision, with the three sides of the triangle being the length of the lid margin excision. The skin flap and the area surrounding the Burow's triangle are undermined. The lid margin excision site is closed in two layers (c), followed by sliding the canthotomy site and undermined skin towards the mass excision site. The Burow's triangle is closed, and the subcutaneous dead space under the advanced flap is reduced with buried fine absorbable sutures. The skin incision is closed to the new lateral canthus, and the remaining "raw edge" of the lateral canthotomy is allowed to heal by second intention.

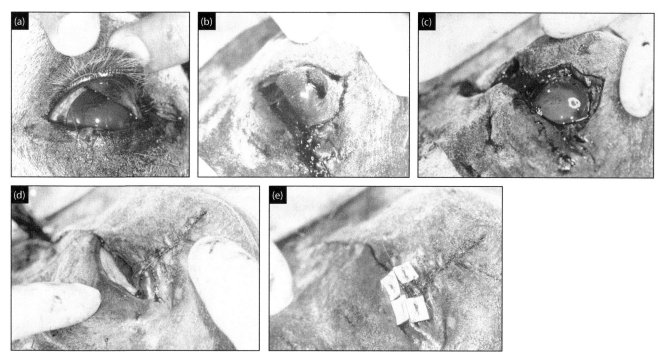

Figure 7.92 Solitary pigmented mass involving approximately half of the width of the upper eyelid in an Arabian cross mare (a). "Housetop" full-thickness excision of the intrastromal eyelid melanoma with incisions being perpendicular to tarsal plate and then tapering to the upper palpebral fornix (b). A semicircular skin flap was raised beyond the lateral canthus (c). The tumor excision site was closed in multiple layers (d). The semicircular flap was closed, leaving the "lid margin" from the semicircular flap to heal by second intention, and the excision site was "splinted" using temporary tarsorrhaphy sutures over rubber band stents (e). A protective blinker was used to prevent self-trauma while the surgical site healed. In 2 weeks, the skin sutures were removed. Despite moderate ptosis of the upper lid due to removal of most of the levator palpebrae muscle, the reconstructed lid functioned to protect the globe, and the horse was visual from the eye and was safe to trail ride.

described to repair feline eyelid agenesis, **Figure 7.8a**). A procedure that does not involve a two-step approach is the lip commissure to lid transposition technique previously described for repair of eyelid agenesis (**Figure 7.8b**); however, this technique is somewhat limited to repair of voids of the lateral canthus/lateral lids in small animal species.

Rather than try to master and remember a wide variety of plastic techniques that are rarely utilized, it is probably more pragmatic for the practitioner to be familiar with a rather simple technique such as the semicircular flap technique and leave more advanced reconstruction to a specialist.

Surgical resection of equine lid neoplasia can present a challenge because of the lack of mobile skin. This combined with a high recurrence rate with sarcoids (35%–50%)[133] makes surgical resection one of the least desirable forms of eyelid neoplasia therapy in the horse. In the cow, partial-thickness sliding H-blepharoplasty techniques[155] may be used for excision of SCC, but in this author's hands, the incidence of tumor regrowth is high. The use of partial-thickness excision/debulkment followed by liquid nitrogen cryosurgery or radiofrequency hyperthermia results in a lower incidence of tumor regrowth than excision alone, and the resulting function of the lid and cosmetic results are usually adequate.

Cryotherapy Cryotherapy is a rapid, rather imprecise means of treating many tumors. When dealing with potentially malignant tumors, thermocouples should be implanted to ensure adequate tissue freezing (–20°C for most tumors but a target temperature of –30°C for SCC). Therapy may be performed under adequate sedation/local anesthetic, which has advantage in the aged small animal and large animals. Roberts and Severin reported that the rate of tumor recurrence in the dog after surgical excision and cryotherapy was similar, although the mean recurrence time after cryotherapy was 7.4 months versus 28.3 months for surgery.[111] The intense cold of liquid nitrogen (–196°C) has advantage over the less intense cold (–98°C) of nitrous oxide when dealing with neoplasia. Nitrous oxide is only deliverable through a closed system/probe, but liquid nitrogen is capable of being delivered via closed probe or as a spray of the cryogen directly onto the neoplastic tissue.

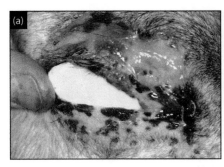
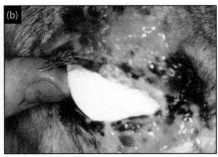
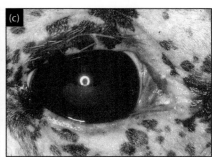

Figure 7.93 Liquid nitrogen cryosurgery to treat an eyelid margin SCC in an Appaloosa. Following local nerve blocks and sedation, a lubricated Styrofoam insulator (piece of a disposable coffee cup) is positioned to protect the globe. Petrolatum is applied to the normal lid tissue for protection from the sprayed cryogen (a), and the mass is debulked with scalpel. The liquid nitrogen is sprayed onto the debulked mass area until core temperature reaches −30°C. The area is allowed to thaw slowly and is then frozen a second time ("double freeze-thaw technique") (b). The area is allowed to heal by second intention. Weeks later, the granulated lid margin is smooth and tumor free (c). Long-term follow-up revealed no tumor regrowth.

Nitrous oxide units are uniformly more expensive than smaller, handheld liquid nitrogen delivery units. Liquid nitrogen, while usually more cumbersome to maintain and administer, has demonstrated its effectiveness in treating a variety of neoplasms, especially SCC in all species (**Figure 7.93**).[156,157] Tarwid et al. have described cryotherapy as one of the more effective therapies for equine sarcoid, although Knottenbelt and Kelly found a high rate of recurrence with cryotherapy and a transformation to a more aggressive sarcoid.[138,137,179]

Surgical debulking of the tumor should precede cryotherapy. Despite sloughing of frozen tissue, the lid is usually able to maintain its architecture without the need for secondary reconstructive surgery, especially when treating meibomian gland tumors in dogs and SCC in large animals.

Hyperthermic therapy The use of heat to kill neoplastic cells became readily available with the advent of a commercial unit designed to treat SCC in cattle (**Figure 7.94**). Hyperthermic therapy is based on the observation that neoplastic cells are killed by temperatures of 41–45°C. It provides a rapid means of therapy and requires a minimum of technical skills. The results of treating SCC with cryotherapy and hyperthermic therapy are very similar.[158,159] In cattle, 90% of squamous cell tumors regressed, and the site remained free of tumor for over 1 year. The lesions should be aggressively debulked prior to therapy as penetration of tumor-killing radiofrequency waves into tissue is very superficial, and multiple therapies to totally cover the residual tumor mass must be used. Hyperthermic therapy has also been successful in treating equine sarcoid after debulking. Ford et al. reported a 91% success rate with hyperthermia in 10

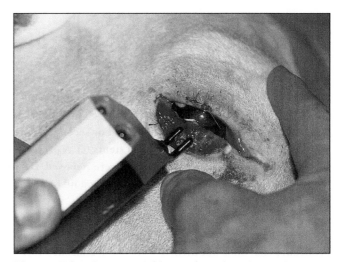

Figure 7.94 Commercial hyperthermia unit treating a squamous cell carcinoma of the lower lid in a horse, after debulking the lesion. The tissue is heated to 50°C (122°F) between the probes, and treatment time is typically 30 seconds per site. Multiple sites must be treated to cover the total tumor mass.

equidae involving 13 sarcoids.[160] The initial therapy was a combination of debulking and hyperthermia treatment, and hyperthermia was repeated at 2- to 4-week intervals, with a minimum of five therapies.

Radiation therapy Radiation therapy is not readily available, but it is a very effective therapy for SCC in all species and equine sarcoid. Brachytherapy, or the implantation of encapsulated radioactive materials, has been used extensively in malignant lid tumors of all species. Brachytherapy is more likely to prevent local recurrence and results in better cosmetic results than surgery alone. Compared to radiation teletherapy, it requires fewer anesthetic episodes. In the horse, brachytherapy with iridium-192 resulted in 87% lesion-free for sarcoid and 82% for SCC at 1 year. At 5 years, 74% and 64% were lesion-free for sarcoid and SCC, respectively.[161] Knottenbelt and Kelly had almost 100% success with treating equine sarcoids with brachytherapy.[137] Temporary implants utilized are usually iridium-192 or cesium-137. The seeds are gamma radiation emitters and require that the animal be isolated from human exposure until the seeds are subsequently removed. Disadvantages are the relative unavailability and cost of the implants and radiation exposure to the radiologist during implantation.[162,163] Beta radiation (strontium-90) is often used for treating superficial SCC (cornea or bulbar conjunctiva) in all species after debulking.

> Brachytherapy, while not widely available in practice, is statistically one of the most successful means of managing difficult lid tumors such as equine sarcoids, aggressive SCC of all species, and canine mast cell tumors.

Chemotherapy Chemotherapy is rarely performed in the dog due to the relatively benign nature of most lid tumors, the variety of other treatment modalities that are usually successful, and the lack of responsive tumors. Chemotherapy for lid neoplasia in the dog is rarely utilized, apart from palliative glucocorticoid chemotherapy for mast cell tumors. The injection of deionized sterile water in some mast cell tumors has been effective in cats and dogs, resulting in lysis of cells and shrinkage of lesions.[164]

In the horse, intralesional cisplatin in sesame oil (1 mg/mL given every 2 weeks for four treatments) has been successful in treating periocular sarcoid and SCC. One-year relapse-free rates were 87% for sarcoid and 65% for SCC.[165] When cisplatin intratumoral injections were combined with surgical debulking for SCC and sarcoid in the horse, the relapse interval was 41 months. The concurrent use with surgery did not interfere with wound healing.[166] In a comparison between intralesional cisplatin injections versus intralesional bleomycin injection to treat equine eyelid SCC, cisplatin injection had a 91% success rate at 1 year versus 78% bleomycin success rate.[167] Cisplatin injections are appropriate to use on eyelid lesions but not on globe lesions due to toxicity to the cornea. The clinician should be cautious with intralesional injections of toxic preparations such as cisplatin, since the drug frequently leaks or oozes out of the surface of the tumor, or if the lesion is dense, the syringe may blow off the needle, exposing the clinician to the drug.

Implantation of cisplatin beads with or without surgical debulkment and additional therapies resulted in resolution of 84% of sarcoid cases for 2 years follow-up and 55% of SCC cases for 2 years follow-up.[168] These 3-mm diameter 7% cisplatin in a biodegradable calcium sulfate and dextran sulfate polymer beads are now commercially available (http://www.wedgewoodpetrx.com) in the United States. The beads are embedded into tumor masses, one bead every 1.5 cm (large masses are aggressively debulked prior to bead implantation). Horses are followed up every 30 days, and re-implanted if the tumor mass is still present. The author has had excellent results with the treatment of sarcoids using this protocol, but treatment of SCC has been less reliable.

5-fluorouracil (5-FU) has been used topically for SCC and equine sarcoids with some success. Knottenbelt and Kelly reported a 35%–66% success rate with occult and verrucose sarcoids, with two different forms of topical 5-FU.[137] Injection of a 5% solution of 5-FU into sarcoids and SCC has anecdotally been reported as being successful in resolving these tumors. The author has been somewhat successful with multiple injections 2–4 weeks apart in the case of sarcoids, but once injections are discontinued in the case of SCC, the tumors tend to recur.

Immunotherapy Immunotherapy has been used for both SCC in cattle and equine sarcoid. While bovine SCC has been somewhat responsive, the immunostimulant used was a mycobacterium cell wall fraction, which had the disadvantage of turning the animals into tuberculin reactors.[169] A phenol–saline extract of bovine SCC also produced regression of lesions when injected intramuscularly.[170] Regrowth may occur and be resistant to further immunization.

Oral cimetidine may be used as an immunomodulator for eyelid tumors. It has been reported as a treatment for cutaneous equine melanoma and in humans to treat ocular papillomatosis.[171] It would seem most logical to use immunomodulation to hasten resolution in conditions that have a normal involution, such as canine histiocytomas and papillomas in all species.[172]

Immunotherapy has been most popular in the treatment of equine sarcoid, although it has also been successful in treating a SCC that had not responded to cryotherapy.[173] Due to the large size of many of the lid lesions, regression rather than resection is desirable. Immunotherapy utilizing intralesional bacillus of Calmette and Guérin (BCG) or BCG cell wall fraction in oil has had a high cure rate. The use of the cell wall fraction lessens the chance of anaphylaxis. The tumor is usually saturated or given about 1 mL/cm³ at 2- to 3-week intervals until regression is complete. Multiple therapies are needed, and swelling, necrosis, and exudation at the injection site can be expected, with the most reaction occurring after the second injection. A 93% cure rate has been obtained if used in periocular sarcoids <7 cm (2.7 in) in diameter.[174–176] The evaluation of sarcoid treatment in the horse is confused by the relatively high incidence of spontaneous regression with these tumors.

Photodynamic therapy   Injection of a photosensitizing agent into a neoplasm or injecting it systemically and then exciting the chemical with the appropriate light wavelength has been on the periphery of clinical application for several years. The principles of photodynamic therapy (PDT) in the treatment of equine periocular tumors have been described.[177] Recently, comparison between SCC cases treated with debulkment and cryo-surgery versus debulkment and PDT revealed 100% suc-cess in resolving SCC in 10 horses with PDT (minimum

follow-up 25 months).[178] This methodology shows great promise in the treatment of SCC in the horse. Confounding factors for the routine use of this therapy include costs of the photosensitizing agent (verteporfin) and the LED continuous wave laser excitation unit operat-ing at 688 nm wavelength.

> The most important point to emphasize to owners of all species with SCC is that because of the underly-ing genetic predisposition for SCC, the long-term outcome of therapy is not cure but control. While the present lesion may be cured, the probability for new lesions in the same or opposite eye is significant, and periodic examinations for the life of the patient are critical to initiate treatment at an early stage.

CLINICAL CASES

CASE 1

A 9-year-old F/S Labrador retriever presented for a slow growing black pedunculated mass of the lid mar-gin. With occasional self-trauma, the mass bled but otherwise did not appear to cause the patient any irri-tation/pain. When the eyelid was everted, the mass appeared to originate from the bulbar surface of the lid (as in **Figure 7.75**). A tentative diagnosis of meibomian adenoma was made, and under heavy sedation, the mass was debulked, and the remaining tissue frozen using a double freeze-thaw technique with a closed probe liq-uid nitrogen cryo unit (as in **Figure 7.17**). Topical anti-biotic ointment was used to treat the excision site until the site healed via second intention. Initial vitaligo of the surgical site was noted; this re-pigmented within 6 months. No recurrence was seen with a 3+-year follow-up. Histopathological assessment confirmed the mass to be a benign adenoma (as in **Figure 7.77**). Additional treatment options could have included full-thickness wedge resection of the mass (as in **Figure 7.90**) or sur-gical debulkment and CO$_2$ laser ablation.

CASE 2

A 10-month-old Shih Tzu presented with a sudden onset of blepharospasm and a corneal ulceration of the dorsal cornea. Historically, the patient had epiphora and occasional blepharospasm during the 7 months that

the owner had owned the puppy. Application of topical anesthetic partially resolved the blepharospasm, and a vertically linear fluorescein positive area of superficial corneal ulceration was identified on the affected eye. Numerous distichia were noted on the upper and lower lid margins in both eyes (as in **Figure 7.11**). Eversion of the lids revealed an ectopic cilium of the upper eye-lid in the ulcerated eye (as in **Figure 7.18**). Under gen-eral anesthesia, the ectopic cilium and the surrounding tissue was removed with a 4-mm punch biopsy using a chalazion clamp for stabilization. The remaining lid margins were double freeze-thaw treated with a closed probe nitrous oxide cryosurgical unit applied to the bul-bar surface of the lids, over the base of the meibomian glands (as in **Figure 7.17**). Following cryosurgery, the distichia were plucked with flat, fine forceps. Post cryosurgery, there was moderate blepharoedema that resolved in 5 days with warm, moist compresses and use of oral NSAIDs. Some distichia regrew over a 6-month period, but they were fine and less pigmented than the original distichia. The patient showed no sign of bleph-arospasm or epiphora once the surgical sites healed, and there was no recurrence of the ectopic cilia or cor-neal ulceration. Additional treatment options could have included electrolysis of the distichia follicles (as in **Figures 7.13 and 7.14**), electrocautery of the base of the meibomian glands (as in **Figure 7.16**), or lid split-ting for removal of the tarsal plate/meibomian glands (as in **Figure 7.12**). Nitrous oxide cryosurgical ablation of the hair follicles was chosen in this case due to the small patient size, the involvement of the entire lid margins, upper and lower lids, in each eye, and concern for postoperative lid scarring and instability of precorneal tear film following surgery. In this case, despite minor regrowth of fine distichia, the patient experienced no ectopic cilia regrowth or recurrent blepharospasm.

CASE 3

A 2-year-old M/N Clumber spaniel was presented for chronic ocular discharge, recurrent corneal ulcerations, and a history of unsuccessful entropion correction surgery, bilaterally. Clinically, the patient had lateral canthal entropion, some lower lid entropion with a dramatic spastic component that only partially corrected with application of topical anesthetic, and a "notch" in the medial aspect of the upper eyelid ("Pagoda eye" or "diamond eye," **Figure 7.39a**). Retraction of the lateral canthus to straighten the upper and lower lids revealed macropalpebral fissures, bilaterally (palpebral fissures approximately 38 mm). A lid shortening/entropion correcting combination surgical procedure (Bigelbach's technique, **Figure 7.42**) was performed bilaterally, with resulting improvement of lid carriage and resolution of the frictional irritation to the cornea from the entropion (**Figure 7.39b**). Other surgical treatments could have included an "arrowhead" technique (**Figure 7.35**), a modified Wyman's lateral canthoplasty (**Figure 7.34**), a lateral canthal tenotomy (**Figure 7.36**) and Hotz–Celsus procedure (**Figure 7.31**), or a modified Kuhnt–Szymanowski (**Figure 7.41**) procedure. Since the patient had a macropalpebral fissure and lax skin about the face as well as the entropion/ "diamond eye" configuration, it was felt that the Bigelbach technique would best correct all problems with one surgical episode. Two-year follow-up showed good resolution of clinical signs and a comfortable patient.

CASE 4

A 6-year-old F/S Lhasa Apso presented for chronic blepharitis and self-trauma to the face/eyelids. The patient historically had atopic skin disease and was on intermittent antihistamines, corticosteroids, and a hypoallergenic diet. Clinically, the patient had firm swelling of the eyelids with some dried periocular crusts, alopecia, and dermal hyperemia as well as some chalazia (**Figure 7.70a,b**). Schirmer tear test (STT) values were decreased, bilaterally. Gentle expression of some of the chalazia yielded exudate that was culture positive for *Staphylococcal* species. The crusted periocular hairs were trimmed; the areas were treated symptomatically with warm, moist compresses, t.i.d. Systemic antibiotics (based on culture and sensitivity results) were used for 6 weeks along with a tapering dose of systemic corticosteroids. Topical antibiotic and cyclosporine were used while the patient was being treated with systemic antibiotics. To prevent self-trauma, an Elizabethan collar was used. At the 3-week recheck, the lid swelling and hyperemia were significantly reduced (**Figure 7.70c**), and the patient was much more comfortable and not attempting self-trauma. STT values had increased to the normal range. By 6 weeks, the patient was being treated with only topical cyclosporine and was comfortable. Long term, the patient underwent allergy testing and an attempt at desensitization, which failed. Systemic cyclosporine was eventually used long-term to control the patient's atopic skin disease.

CASE 5

An aged Arabian cross mare was presented for a dark, intrastromal mass (melanoma/melancytoma) of the right upper eyelid. No other melanomas were identified on physical examination. The mass was within the eyelid stroma and involved approximately half of the length of the upper eyelid (**Figure 7.92a**). The owner wished to retain the globe as the horse was still used for trail riding, and she did not feel that the horse would be sound to ride if the eye were to be removed because of the lid tumor. Under general anesthesia, the mass was removed using a "housetop" wedge resection (**Figure 7.90**) of the mass with a semicircular flap (**Figure 7.91**) to help close the large void (**Figure 7.92b–e**). Once healed, the reconstructed upper lid had moderate ptosis due to removal of most of the levator palpebrae muscle, but the reconstructed lid protected the globe adequately, and the patient could see and was sound to ride. During a 5-year follow-up, there was no recurrence of the mass. Other treatment options for this mare could have included debulkment of the mass and systemic use of cimetidine, a Cutler–Beard two-stage procedure (**Figure 7.8**), or a sliding H-plasty technique (**Figure 7.8a**). A desire by the owner to completely excise the mass, preferably with only one surgical procedure, was the reason the semicircular flap was selected for this case. Since melanomas are seldom sensitive to chemotherapeutic agents such as cisplatin, 5-fluorouracil, bleomycin, or immunostimulants drugs such as BCG, medical therapy was not chosen. Melanomas also tend to not respond to radiofrequency hyperthermia or cryosurgery.

Table 7.1 Genetic predisposition: Eyelids.

Dermoids

- Canine—Dachshund, Saint Bernard, German shepherd dog
- Feline—Burmese
- Cattle—Hereford

Distichiasis

- Canine—American and English Cocker Spaniel, Shih Tzu, English bulldog, Pekingese, toy and miniature poodle, Shetland sheepdog, Cavalier King Charles spaniel, Siberian husky, Golden retriever

Trichiasis

- Canine—Shar Pei, Chow Chow, English bulldog, bloodhound, Neapolitan mastiff, Newfoundland, Pomeranian, miniature and toy poodle, brachycephalic breeds (medial and nasal fold trichiasis)
- Ectopic cilia—Boxer, Shih Tzu, English bulldog, Golden retriever

Macroblepharon

- Canine—Saint Bernard, Mastiff, Newfoundland, Bernese mountain dog, American Cocker Spaniel, some retriever breeds
- Feline—Sphinx

Microblepharon

- Collie, Shetland sheepdog, Pomeranian, chow chow, Shar Pei, Kerry blue terrier, English bull terrier, Bedlington terrier

Entropion
Medial

- Canine—Miniature and toy poodle, Pekingese, pug, Shih Tzu, Lhasa Apso, English bulldog, Maltese, Cavalier King Charles spaniel
- Feline—Persian, brachycephalic breeds

Lower lid

- Canine—Retrievers, pointers, spaniels
- Equine—American quarter horse
- Sheep—Rambouillet

Lateral canthal

- Canine—Chow Chow, Shar Pei, Saint Bernard, Mastiff, Rottweiler, English bulldog, bloodhound

Upper lid

- Canine—Neapolitan Mastiff, bloodhound

Ectropion

- Hounds, setters, retrievers, spaniels, English bulldog, Saint Bernard, boxer, mastiff, Newfoundland

Lagophthalmos

- Canine—Brachycephalic breeds (Boston terrier, Shih Tzu, Cavalier King Charles spaniel, Pekingese)
- Feline—Persian

Atopic blepharitis

- West Highland white terrier, Shar Pei, Lhasa Apso, Shih Tzu, miniature and toy poodle, Golden retriever, Labrador retriever

Uveodermatologic syndrome

- Akita, Siberian husky, Samoyed, Shetland sheepdog

Systemic histiocytosis

- Bernese mountain dog, Rottweiler, Irish wolfhound, Golden retriever, Labrador retriever

Ocular squamous cell carcinoma

- Feline—White skinned/white coat cats
- Equine—Appaloosa, draft breeds, Tennessee walking horse, Haflinger, and paint, pinto, and palomino coat color

Sarcoid

- American quarter horse, Appaloosa, Arabian

REFERENCES

1. Miller, W., and Braund, K. 1991. Morphologic and histochemical features of the normal canine orbicularis oculi muscle. *Progress in Veterinary and Comparative Ophthalmology* 1:150–154.

2. Gilger, B.C., and Stoppini, R. 2011. Equine ocular examination: Routine and advanced diagnostic techniques. In: Gilger, B.C., editor. *Equine Ophthalmology*, 2nd edition. Elsevier/Saunders: St. Louis, MO, pp. 11–13.

3. Thomas, J.W. 1961. The nerve supply to the nictitating membrane of the cat. *Journal of Anatomy* 95:371–785.

4. Powell, C. 1988. Innervation to the canine lacrimal glands. *Masters thesis*, University of Georgia, Athens, GA, USA, pp. 1–17.

5. Robertson, B.F., and Roberts, S.M. 1995. Lateral canthus entropion in the dog, Part I. *Veterinary Comparative Ophthalmology* 5:151–156.

6. Miller, M., Christensen, G., and Evans, H. 1964. The venous system. In: *Anatomy of the Dog*. WB Saunders: Philadelphia, PA, p. 393.

7. Lee, R., and Griffiths, I.R. 1972. A comparison of cerebral arteriography and cavernous sinus venography in the dog. *Journal of Small Animal Practice* 12:225–238.

8. Gum, G. 1991. Physiology of the eye. In: Gelatt, K., editor. *Veterinary Ophthalmology* 2nd edition: Lea & Febiger: Philadelphia, PA, p. 124.

9. Carrington, S.D., Bedford, P.G., Guillon, J.P., and Woodwards, E.G. 1987. Polarized light biomicroscopic observations on the pre-corneal tear film. 3. The normal tear film of the cat. *Journal of Small Animal Practice* 28:821–826.

10. Carrington, S.D., Bedford, P.G., Guillon, J.P., and Woodward, E.G. 1987. Polarized light biomicroscopic observations on the pre-corneal tear film. 1. The normal tear film of the dog. *Journal of Small Animal Practice* 28:605–622.

11. Aguirre, G., and Rubin, L.F. 1970. Ophthalmitis secondary to congenitally open eyelids in a dog. *Journal of the American Veterinary Medical Association* 156:70–72.

12. Gelatt, K.N. 1974. Premature eyelid opening and exposure keratitis in a puppy. *Veterinary Medicine/Small Animal Clinician* 69:863.

13. McCuiston, W.R. 1965. Pulmonary edema and persistent ankyloblepharon in puppies. *Veterinary Medicine/Small Animal Clinician* 60:1206–1207.

14. Nasisse, M.P. 1991. Feline ophthalmology. In: Gelatt, K.N., editor. *Veterinary Ophthalmology* 2nd edition: Lea & Febiger: Philadelphia, PA, pp. 529–575.

15. Cutler, T.J. 2002. Bilateral eyelid agenesis repair in a captive Texas cougar. *Veterinary Ophthalmology* 5:143–148.

16. Martin, C., Stiles, J., and Willis, M. 1997. Feline colobomatous syndrome. *Veterinary and Comparative Ophthalmology* 7:39–43.

17. Gripenberg, U., Blomqvist, L., Pamilo, P. et al. 1985. Multiple ocular coloboma (MOC) in snow leopards (*Panthera uncia*). Clinical report, pedigree analysis, chromosome investigations, and serum protein studies. *Hereditas* 102:221–229.

18. Schaffer, E., Wiesner, H., and von Hegel, G. 1988. Multiple oculare kolobome (MOC) mit persistierender pupillarmembran beim schneeleopard (*Panthera uncia*). *Tieraztl Prax* 16:87–91.

19. Bellhorn, R.W., Barnett, K.C., and Henkind, P. 1971. Ocular colobomas in domestic cats. *Journal of the American Veterinary Medical Association* 159:1015–1021.

20. Roberts, S.R., and Bistner, S.I. 1968. Surgical correction of eyelid agenesis in the feline. *Modern Veterinary Practice* 49:40–43.

21. Dziezyc, J., and Millichamp, N. 1989. Surgical correction of eyelid agenesis in a cat. *Journal of the American Animal Hospital Association* 25:513–516.

22. Doherty, M.J. 1973. A bridge-flap blepharorrhaphy method for eyelid reconstruction in the cat. *Journal of the American Animal Hospital Association* 9:238–241.

23. Gelatt, K.N., and Gelatt, J.P. 2001. Surgery of the eyelids. In: Gelatt, K.N. and Gelatt, J.P., editors. *Small Animal Ophthalmic Surgery: Practical Techniques for the Veterinarian*. Butterworth-Heinemann: Boston, MA, pp. 121–122.

24. Wolfer, J.C. 2002. Correction of eyelid coloboma in four cats using subdermal collagen and a modified Stades technique. *Veterinary Ophthalmology* 5:269–272.

25. Whittaker, C.J.G., Wilke, D.A., Simpson, D.J., Deykin, A., Smith, J.S., and Robinson, C.L. 2010. Lip commissure to eyelid transposition for repair of feline eyelid agenesis. *Veterinary Ophthalmology* 13:173–178.

26. Koch, S.A. 1979. Congenital ophthalmic abnormalities in the Burmese cat. *Journal of the American Veterinary Medical Association* 174:90–91.

27. Brandsch, H., and Schmidt, V. 1981. Erbanalytische untersuchungen zum dermoid des auges beim hund. *Veterinary Medicine* 37:305–306.

28. Barkyoumb, S., and Leipold, H. 1984. Nature and cause of ocular dermoids in Hereford cattle. *Veterinary Pathology* 21:316–324.

29. Raymond-Letron, I., Bourges-Abella, N., Rousseau, T. et al. 2012. Histologic features of canine distichiasis. *Veterinary Ophthalmology* 15:92–97.

30. Lawson, D.D. 1973. Canine distichiasis. *Journal of Small Animal Practice* 14:469–478.

31. Halliwell, W.H. 1967. Surgical management of canine distichia. *Journal of the American Veterinary Medical Association* 150:874–879.

32. Gelatt, K.N. 1969. Resection of cilia-bearing tarsoconjunctiva for correction of canine distichia. *Journal of the American Veterinary Medical Association* 155:892–897.

33. Campbell, L.H. 1977. Conjunctival resection for the surgical management of canine distichiasis. *Journal of the American Veterinary Medical Association* 171:275–276.

34. Bedford, P.G.C. 1971. Eyelashes and adventitious cilia as causes of corneal irritation. *Journal of Small Animal Practice* 12:11–17.

35. Long, R. 1991. Treatment of distichiasis by conjunctival resection. *Journal of Small Animal Practice* 32:146–148.

36. Riis, R.C. 1982. Basal Meibomian gland cautery: A surgical technique for distichiasis. *Proceedings of the American College of Veterinary Ophthalmology and International Society of Veterinary Ophthalmology*, Lake Tahoe, NV, USA, pp. 88–93.

37. Chambers, E.D., and Slatter, D.H. 1984. Cryotherapy (N²O) of canine distichiasis and trichiasis: An experimental and clinical report. *Journal of Small Animal Practice* 25:647–659.

38. Liu, D., Natiella, J., Schaefer, A., and Gage, A. 1984. Cryosurgical treatment of eyelids and lacrimal drainage ducts of the Rhesus monkey. *Archives of Ophthalmology* 102:934–939.

39. Wheeler, C.A., and Severin, G.A. 1984. Cryosurgical epilation for the treatment of distichiasis in the dog and cat. *Journal of the American Animal Hospital Association* 20:877–884.

40. Helper, L.C., and Magrane, W.G. 1970. Ectopic cilia of the canine eyelid. *Journal of Small Animal Practice* 11:185–189.

41. Hacker, D.V. 1989. Ectopic cilia in a Siamese cat. *Companion Animal Pracitice* 19:29–31.

42. D'Anna, N., Guerriero, A., Guandalini, A., and Sapienza, J.S. 2007. Use of a dermal biopsy punch for removal of ectopic cilia in dogs: 19 cases. *Veterinary Ophthalmology* 7:343–347.

43. Stades, F.C. 1987. A new method for surgical correction of upper eyelid trichiasis–entropion: Operation method. *Journal of the American Animal Hospital Association* 23:603–606.

44. Stades, F.C., and Boeve, M.H. 1987. Surgical correction of upper eyelid trichiasis–entropion: Results and follow-up in 55 eyes. *Journal of the American Animal Hospital Association* 23:607–610.

45. Stades, F.C., Boeve, M.H., and van der Woerdt, A. 1992. Palpebral fissure length in the dog and cat. *Progress in Veterinary and Comparative Ophthalmology* 2:155–161.

46. Kaswan, R.L., Martin, C.L., and Doran, C.C. 1988. Blepharoplasty techniques for canthus closure. *Companion Animal Practice* 2:6–8.

47. Gelatt, K.N., and Gelatt, J.P. 2001. *Small Animal Ophthalmic Surgery, Practical Techniques for the Veterinarian.* Butterworth-Heinemann: Boston, MA, pp. 112–113.

48. Rubin, L. 1989. *Inherited Eye Diseases in Purebred Dogs.* Williams and Wilkins: Baltimore, MD.

49. Littlejohn, A. 1954. Entropion in newborn lambs. *Veterinary Record* 66:211.

50. Crowley, J., and McGloughlin, P. 1963. Hereditary entropion in lambs. *Veterinary Record* 75:1104.

51. Lenarduzzi, R.F. 1983. Management of eyelid problems in Chinese Shar Pei puppies. *Veterinary Medicine/Small Animal Clinician* 78:548–550.

52. Williams, D.L. 2004. Entropion correction by fornix-based suture placement: Use of the Quickert-Rathbun technique in ten dogs. *Veterinary Ophthalmology* 7:343–347.

53. Read, R.A., and Broun, H.C. 2007. Entropion correction in dogs and cats using a combination Hotz–Celsus and lateral eyelid wedge resection: Results in 311 eyes. *Veterinary Ophthalmology* 10:6–11.

54. Bigelbach, A. 1996. A combined tarsorrhaphy-canthoplasty technique for the repair of entropion and ectropion. *Veterinary and Comparative Ophthalmology* 6:220–224.

55. Wyman, M. 1971. Lateral canthoplasty. *Journal of the American Animal Hospital Association* 7:196–201.

56. Pickett, J.P. 2015. Surgery of the eyelids. In: Bojrab, M.J., Waldron, D.R., and Toombs, J.P., editors. *Current Techniques in Small Animal Surgery* 5th edition: Teton New Media: Jackson, WY, pp. 150–151.

57. Wyman, M., and Wilkie, D.A. 1988. New surgical procedure for entropion correction: Tarsal pedical technique. *Journal of the American Animal Hospital Association* 24:345–349.

58. Jensen, H.E. 1979. Canthus closure. *Compendium on Continuing Education for the Practicing Veterinarian* 10:735–741.

59. Moore, C.P. 1982. Multiple indications for pocket-flap canthotomy in the canine. In: *Proceedings of the American College of Veterinary Ophthalmology and International Society of Veterinary Ophthalmology*, Lake Tahoe, NV, USA, pp. 69–73.

60. Pickett, J.P. 2015. Surgery of the eyelids. In: Bojrab, M.J., Waldron, D.R., and Toombs, J.P., editors. *Current Techniques in Small Animal Surgery* 5th edition: Teton New Media: Jackson, WY, pp. 151–154.

61. Munger, R.J., and Carter, J.D. 1984. A further modification of the Kuhnt–Szymanowski procedure for correction of atonic ectropion in dogs. *Journal of the American Animal Hospital Association* 20:651–656.

62. Pickett, J.P. 2015. Surgery of the eyelids. In: Bojrab, M.J., Waldron, D.R., and Toombs, J.P., editors. *Current Techniques in Small Animal Surgery* 5th edition: Teton New Media: Jackson, WY, pp. 150–152.

63. Kern, T., and Erb, H. 1987. Facial neuropathy in dogs and cats: 95 cases (1975–1985). *Journal of the American Veterinary Medical Association* 191:1604–1609.

64. Jaggy, A., Oliver, J., Ferguson, D.C. et al. 1994. Neurological manifestations of hypothyroidism: A retrospective study of 29 dogs. *Journal of Veterinary Internal Medicine* 8(5):328–336.

65. Stuhr, C.M., Stanz, K., Murphy, C.J., et al. 1997. Stellate rhytidectomy: Superior entropion repair in a dog with excessive facial skin. *Journal of the American Animal Hospital Association* 33:342–345.

66. Elder, M. 1993. Mersilene mesh and fascia lata in brow suspension: A comparative study. *Ophthalmology Surgery* 24:105–108.

67. Kirschner, S. 1995. Modified brow sling technique for the upper lid entropion. *Proceedings of the Scientific Meeting of the American College of Veterinary Ophthalmologists* 25, Newport, RI, USA, pp. 68–69.

68. Willis, M., Martin, C., Stiles, J., and Kirschner, S. 1999. Brow suspension for treatment of ptosis and entropion in dogs with redundant facial skin folds. *Journal of the American Veterinary Medicial Association* 214:660–662.

69. Barrie, K.P., and Parshall, C.J. 1979. Eyelid pyogranulomas in four dogs. *Journal of the American Animal Hospital Association* 14:433–437.

70. Sansom, J., Heinrich, C., and Featherstone, H. 2000. Pyogranulomatous blepharitis in two dogs. *Journal of Small Animal Practice* 41:80–83.

71. Rosenthal, J.J. 1975. *Cuterebra* infestation of the conjunctiva in a puppy. *Veterinary Medicine/Small Animal Clinician* 70:462–463.

72. Harris, B.P., Miller, P.E., Bloss, J.R., and Pellitteri, P.J. 2000. Ophthalmomyiasis interna anterior associated with *Cuterebra* spp. in a cat. *Journal of the American Veterinary Medical Association* 216:352–355.

73. Rebhun, W., Mirro, E., Georgi, M., and Kern, T. 1981. Habronemic blepharoconjunctivitis in horses. *Journal of the American Veterinary Medical Association* 179:469–472.

74. Holland, J.L., Outerbridge, C.A., Affolter, V.K., and Maggs, D.J. 2006. Detection of feline herpesvirus 1 DNA in skin biopsy specimens from cats with or without dermatitis. *Journal of the American Veterinary Medical Association* 229:1442–1446.

75. Dougherty, J., McCulley, J., Silvany, R., and Meyer, D. 1991. The role of tetracycline in chronic blepharitis. *Investigative Ophthalmology and Visual Science* 32:2970–2975.

76. Pena, M.T., Roura, X., and Davidson, M.G. 2000. Ocular and periocular manifestation of leishmaniasis in dogs: 105 cases (1993–1998). *Veterinary Ophthalmology* 3:35–41.

77. Kontos, V.J., and Koutinas, A.F. 1993. Old world canine leishmaniasis. *Compendium on Continuing Education for the Practicing Veterinarian* 15:949–959.

78. Slappendel, R.J., and Ferrer, L. 1998. Leishmaniasis. In: Greene, C., editor. *Infectious Diseases of the Dog and Cat* 2nd edition: WB Saunders: Philadelphia, PA, pp. 450–458.

79. Bond, R., Curtis, C.F., Ferguson, E.A., Mason, I.S., and Rest, J. 2000. An idiopathic facial dermatitis of Persian cats. *Veterinary Dermatology* 11:35–11.

80. Miller Jr., W.H. 1979. Canine facial dermatoses. *Compendium on Continuing Education for the Practicing Veterinarian* 1:640–649.

81. Miller, W.H., Griffin, C.E., and Campbell, K.L. 2013. Miscellaneous skin diseases. In: Miller, W.H., Griffin, C.E., and Campbell, K.L., editors. *Muller and Kirk's Small Animal Dermatology* 7th edition: Elsevier Mosby: St. Louis, MO, pp. 708–710.

82. Latimer, C., and Dunstan, R.W. 1987. Eosinophilic plaque involving eyelids of a cat. *Journal of the American Animal Hospital Association* 23:649–653.

83. Manning, T.O., Scott, D.W., Kruth, S.A., Sozanski, M., and Lewis, R.M. 1980. Three cases of canine pemphigus foliaceus and observations on chrysotherapy. *Journal of the American Animal Hospital Association* 16:189–202.

84. Scott, D.W., Miller Jr., W.H., Lewis, R.M., Manning, T.O., and Smith, C.A. 1980. Pemphigus erythematosus in the dog and cat. *Journal of the American Animal Hospital Association* 16:815–822.

85. Walton, D.K., Scott, D.W., Smith, C.A., and Lewis, R.M. 1981. Canine discoid lupus erythematosus. *Journal of the American Animal Hospital Association* 17:851–858.

86. Caciolo, P.I., Nesbitt, G.H., and Hurvitz, A.I. 1984. Pemphigus foliaceus in eight cats and results of induction therapy using azathioprine. *Journal of the American Animal Hospital Association* 20:571–577.

87. Morgan, R.V. 1989. Vogt–Koyanagi–Harada syndrome in humans and dogs. *Compendium on Continuing Education for the Practicing Veterinarian* 11:1211–1218.

88. Herrera, H.D., and Duchene, A.G. 1998. Uveodermateological syndrome (Vogt–Koyanagi–Harada-like syndrome) with generalized depigmentation in a Dachshund. *Veterinary Ophthalmology* 1(1):47–51.

89. Miller, W.H., Griffin, C.E., and Campbell, K.L. 2013. Neoplastic and non-neoplastic tumors. In: Miller, W.H., Griffin, C.E., and Campbell, K.L., editors. *Muller and Kirk's Small Animal Dermatology*. 7th edition: Elsevier Mosby: St. Louis, MO, pp. 819–820.

90. Padgett, G.A., Madewell, B.R., Keller, E.T. et al. 1995. Inheritance of histiocytosis in Bernese mountain dogs. *Journal of Small Animal Practice* 36:93–98.

91. Vercammen, F., Berkvens, D., Le Ray, D., and Vervoort, J. 1997. Development of a slide ELISA for canine leishmaniasis and comparison with four serological tests. *Veterinary Record* 153:328–330.

92. Medleau, L. 1994. Using ivermectin to treat parasitic dermatoses in small animals. *Veterinary Medicine* 89:770–774.

93. Bridges, E. 1985. The use of ivermectin to treat genital cutaneous habronemiasis in a stallion. *Compendium on Continuing Education for the Practicing Veterinarian* 7:S94–S97.

94. Chambers, E.D., and Severin, G.A. 1984. Staphylococcal bacterin for treatment of chronic staphylococcal blepharitis in the dog. *Journal of the American Veterinary Medical Association* 185:422–425.

95. White, S.A., Rosychuch, R.A.W., Reinke, S.I., and Pardis, M. 1992. Use of tetracycline and niacinamide for treatment of autoimmune skin disease in 31 dogs. *Journal of the American Veterinary Medical Association* 200:1497–1500.

96. Rothstein, E., Scott, D.W., and Riis, R.C. 1997. Tetracycline and niacinamide for the treatment of sterile pyogranuloma/granuloma syndrome in a dog. *Journal of the American Animal Hospital Association* 33:540–543.

97. Moriello, K.A. 1996. Treatment of feline dermatophytosis. *Feline Practice* 24:32–37.

98. Lester, S.J., and Kenyon, J.M. 1996. Use of allopurinol to treat visceral leishmaniasis in a dog. *Journal of the American Veterinary Medical Association* 209:615–617.

99. Ginel, P.J., Lopez, L.R., and Molleda, M.M.J. 1998. Use of allopurinol for maintenance of remission in dogs with leishmaniasis. *Journal of Small Animal Practice* 39:271–274.

100. Gionfriddo, J.R., Severin, G.A., Schou, E., and Woodward, S. 2009. Tattooing of the equine eyelid: A retrospective study. *Journal of Equine Veterinary Science* 29:82–86.

101. Scott, D.W. 1981. Observations on canine atopy. *Journal of the American Animal Hospital Association* 17:91–100.

102. Miller, W.H., Griffin, C.E., and Campbell, K.L. 2013. Autoimmune and immune-mediated dermatoses. In: Miller, W.H., Griffin, C.E., and Campbell, K.L., editors. *Muller and Kirk's Small Animal Dermatology* 7th edition: Elsevier Mosby: St. Louis, MO, pp. 435–438.

103. Scott, D.W., Manning, T.O., Smith, C.A., and Lewis, R.M. 1982. Observations on the immunopathology and therapy of canine pemphigus and pemphigoid. *Journal of the American Veterinary Medical Association* 180:48–52.

104. Ihrke, P.J.J., Stannard, A.A., Ardans, A.A., and Griffin, C.E. 1985. Pemphigus foliaceus in dogs: A review of 37 cases. *Journal of the American Veterinary Medical Association* 186:59–60.

105. Rebhun, W.C. 1980. Repair of eyelid lacerations in horses. *Veterinary Medicine/Small Animal Clinician* 75:1281–1284.

106. Schoster, J.V. 1988. Surgical repair of equine eyelid lacerations. *Veterinary Medicine/Small Animal Clinician* 83:1042–1049.

107. Krehbiel, J.D., and Langham, R.F. 1975. Eyelid neoplasms of dogs. *American Journal of Veterinary Research* 36:115–119.

108. Patnaik, A.K., Ehler, W.J., and MacEwen, E.G. 1984. Canine cutaneous mast cell tumor: Morphologic grading and survival time in 83 dogs. *Veterinary Pathology* 21:469–474.

109. Kiupel, M., Webster, J.D., Bailey, K.L. et al. 2011. Proposal of a 2-tier histologic grading system for canine cutaneous mast cell tumors to more accurately predict biological behavior. *Veterinary Pathology* 48:147–155.

110. Barrie, K., Gelatt, K.N., and Parshall, C.P. 1982. Eyelid squamous cell carcinoma in four dogs. *Journal of the American Animal Hospital Association* 18:123–126.

111. Roberts, S., and Severin, G. 1986. Prevalence and treatment of palpebral neoplasms in the dog. *American Veterinary Medical Association* 10:1355–1359.

112. Collier, L.L., and Collins, B.K. 1994. Excision and cryosurgical ablation of severe periocular papillomatosis in a dog. *Journal of the American Veterinary Medical Association* 204(6):881–883.

113. Moore, P. 1984. Systemic histiocytosis of Bernese Mountain Dogs. *Veterinary Pathology* 21:554–563.

114. McLaughlin, S.A., Whitley, R.D., Gilger, B.C. et al. 1993. Eyelid neoplasia in cats: A review of demographic data (1979–1989). *Journal of the American Animal Hospital Association* 29:63–67.

115. Williams, L.W., Gelatt, K.N., and Gwin, R.M. 1981. Ophthalmic neoplasms in the cat. *Journal of the American Animal Hospital Association* 17:999–1008.

116. Newkirk, K.M., and Rohrbach, B.W. 2009. A retrospective study of eyelid tumors from 43 cats. *Veterinary Pathology* 46:916–927.

117. Wilcock, B., Yager, J., and Zink, M. 1986. The morphology and behavior of feline cutaneous mastocyctomas. *Veterinary Pathology* 23:320–324.

118. Buerger, R., and Scott, D. 1987. Cutaneous mast cell neoplasia in cats: 14 cases (1975–1985). *Journal of the American Veterinary Medical Association* 190:1440–1444.

119. Molander-McCrary, H., Henry, C., Potter, K., Tyler, J., and Buss, M. 1998. Cutaneous mast cell tumors in cats: 32 cases (1991–1994). *Journal of the American Animal Hospital Association* 34:281–284.

120. Montgomery, K.W., Van der Woerdt, A., Aquino, S.M. et al. 2010. Periocular cutaneous mast cell tumors in cats: Evaluation of surgical excision (33 cases). *Veterinary Ophthalmology* 13:26–30.

121. Lavach, J., and Severin, G. 1977. Neoplasia of the equine eye, adnexa, and orbit: A review of 68 cases. *Journal of the American Veterinary Medical Association* 170:202–203.

122. Dugan, S.J., Roberts, S.M., Curtis, C.R. et al. 1991. Prognostic factors and survival of horses with ocular/adnexal squamous cell carcinoma: 147 cases (1979–1988). *Journal of the American Veterinary Medical Association* 198:298–303.

123. Schwink, K. 1987. Factors influencing morbidity and outcome of equine ocular squamous cell carcinoma. *Equine Veterinary Journal* 19:198–200.

124. Dugan, S., Curtis, C., Roberts, S., and Severin, G. 1991. Epidemiologic study of ocular/adnexal squamous cell carcinoma in horses. *Journal of the American Veterinary Medical Association* 198:251–256.

125. King, T.C., Priehs, D.R., Gum, G.G. et al. 1991. Therapeutic management of ocular squamous cell carcinoma in the horse: 43 cases (1979–1989). *Equine Veterinary Journal* 23:449–452.

126. Strafuss, A. 1976. Squamous cell carcinoma in horses. *Journal of the American Veterinary Medical Association* 168:61–62.

127. Junge, R., Sundberg, J., and Lancaster, W. 1984. Papillomas and squamous cell carcinomas of horses. *Journal of the American Veterinary Medical Association* 185:656–659.

128. Martens, A., DeMoor, A., and Ducatelle, R. 2001. PCR detection of bovine papilloma virus DNA in superficial swabs and scrapings from equine sarcoids. *The Veterinary Journal* 161:280–286.

129. Chambers, G., Ellsmore, V.A., O'Brien, P.M. et al. 2003. Association of bovine papilloma virus with the equine sarcoid. *Journal of General Virology* 84:1055–1062.

130. Nasir, L., and Reid, S.W. 1999. Bovine papillomaviral gene expression in equine sarcoid tumours. *Virus Research* 61(2):171–175.

131. Ragland, W.L., Keown, G.H., and Spencer, G.R. 1970. Equine sarcoid. *Equine Veterinary Journal* 2:2–11.

132. Lazary, S., Gerber, H., Glatt, P.A., and Straub, R. 1985. Equine leucocyte antigens in sarcoid-affected horses. *Equine Veterinary Journal* 17(4):283–286.

133. Brostrom, H., Fahlbrink, E., Dubath, M.L., and Lazary, S. 1988. Association between equine leucocyte antigens (ELA) and equine sarcoid tumors in the population of Swedish halfbreds and some of their families. *Veterinary Immunology Immunopathology* 19(3–4):215–223.

134. Mohammed, H.O., Rebhun, W.C., and Antczak, D.F. 1992. Factors associated with the risk of developing sarcoid tumors in horses. *Equine Veterinary Journal* 24:165–168.

135. Bronstrom, H. 1995. A clinical and epidemiological study in relation to equine leucocyte antigens (ELA). *Acta Veterinaria Scandinavica* 36:223–236.

136. Piscopo, S.E. 1999. The complexities of sarcoid tumors. *Equine Practice* 21:14–18.

137. Knottenbelt, D.C., and Kelly, D.F. 2000. The diagnosis and treatment of periorbital sarcoid in the horse: 445 cases from 1974 to 1999. *Veterinary Ophthalmology* 3:169–191.

138. Tarwid, J., Fretz, P., and Clark, E. 1985. Equine sarcoids: A study with emphasis on pathologic diagnosis. *Compendium on Continuing Education for the Practicing Veterinarian* 7:S293–S300.

139. Studer, U., Marti, E., Stornetta, D., Lazary, S., and Gerber, H. 1997. The therapy of equine sarcoid with a non-specific immunostimulator: The epidemiology and spontaneous regression of sarcoids. *Schweiz Arch Tierheilkd* 139(9):385–391.

140. Altera, K., and Clark, L. 1970. Equine cutaneous mastocytosis. *Pathologia Veterinaria* 7:43–45.

141. Murphy, C., Lavoie, J.P., Groff, J., Hacker, D., Pryor, P., and Bellhorn, R.W. 1989. Bilateral eyelid swelling attributable to lymphosarcoma in a horse. *Journal of the American Veterinary Medical Association* 194:939–942.

142. Giuliano, E.A. 2011. Equine ocular adnexal and nasolacrimal disease. Gilger, B.C., editor. In: *Equine Ophthalmology* 2nd edition: Elsevier Saunders: Marlland Heights, MO, p. 162.

143. Monlux, A., Anderson, W., and Davis, C. 1957. The diagnosis of squamous cell carcinoma of the eye (cancer eye) in cattle. *American Journal of Veterinary Research* 28:5–34.

144. Anderson, D.E., and Badzioch, M. 1991. Association between solar radiation and ocular squamous cell carcinoma in cattle. *American Journal of Veterinary Research* 52:784–788.

145. Tsujita, H., and Plummer, C.E. 2010. Bovine ocular squamous cell carcinoma. *Veterinary Clinics of North America-Food Animal Practice* 26:511–529.

146. Anderson, D., Lush, J., and Chambers, D. 1957. Studies on bovine ocular squamous carcinoma ("cancer eye"). II. Relationship between eyelid pigmentation and occurrence of cancer eye lesions. *Journal of Animal Science* 16:739–746.

147. Nishimura, H., and Frisch, J. 1977. Eye cancer and circumocular pigmentation in *Bos taurus* and crossbred cattle. *Australian Journal of Experimental Agriculture and Animal Husbandry* 17:709–711.

148. Pellicane, C.P., Meek, L.A., Brooks, D.E., and Miller, T.R. 1994. Eyelid reconstruction in five dogs by the semicircular flap technique. *Veterinary and Comparative Ophthalmology* 4:93–103.

149. Gelatt, K.N. 1967. Blepharoplastic procedures in horses. *Journal of the American Veterinary Medical Association* 151:27–44.

150. Gelatt, K.N., and Blogg, J.R. 1969. Blepharoplastic procedures in small animals. *Journal of the American Animal Association* 5:67–78.

151. Blanchard, G.L., and Keller, W.F. 1976. The rhomboid graft flap for the repair of extensive ocular adnexal defects. *Journal of the American Animal Hospital Association* 12:576–580.

152. Munger, R.J., and Gourley, I.M. 1981. Cross-lid flap for repair of large upper eyelid defects. *Journal of the American Veterinary Medical Association* 178:45–48.

153. Hamilton, H.L., Whitley, R.D., McLaughlin, S.A., and Swaim, S.F. 1999. Basic blepharoplasty techniques. *Compendium on Continuing Education for the Practicing Veterinarian* 21:946–953.

154. Cutler, N., and Beard, C. 1955. A method for partial and total upper lid reconstruction. *American Journal of Ophthalmology* 39:1–7.

155. Welker, B., Modransky, P.D., Hoffsis, G.F., Wyman, M.W., Rings, D.M., and Hull, B.L. 1991. Excision of neoplasms of the bovine lower eyelid by H-blepharoplasty. *Veterinary Surgery* 20:133–139.

156. Farris, H., and Fraunfelder, F. 1976. Cryosurgical treatment of ocular squamous cell carcinoma of cattle. *Journal of the American Veterinary Medical Association* 168:213–216.

157. Holberg, D., and Withrow, S. 1979. Cryosurgical treatment of palpebral neoplasms: Clinical and experimental results. *Veterinary Surgery* 8:68–73.

158. Grier, R., Brewer, W.J., and Theilen, G. 1980. Hyperthermic treatment of superficial tumors in cats and dogs. *Journal of the American Veterinary Medical Association* 177:227–232.

159. Kainer, R., Stringer, J., and Lueker, D. 1980. Hyperthermia for treatment of ocular squamous cell tumors in cattle. *Journal of the American Veterinary Medicial Association* 176:356–360.

160. Ford, M.M., Champagne, E.S., Giuliano, E.A., Galle, L.E., Kramer, J., and Moore, C.P. 2002. Radiofrequency hyperthermia as a treatment for equine periocular sarcoids: Ten cases. *(Abstract) Veterinary Ophthalmology* 5:290.

161. Theon, A.P., and Pascoe, J.R. 1995. Iridium-192 interstitial brachytherapy for equine periocular tumours: Treatment results and prognostic factors in 115 horses. *Equine Veterinary Journal* 27(2):117–121.

162. Banks, W., and England, R.A. 1973. Radioactive gold in the treatment of ocular squamous cell carcinoma of cattle. *Journal of the Veterinary Medical Association* 163:745–748.

163. Turrel, J., and Koblik, P. 1983. Techniques of afterloading iridium-192 interstitial brachytherapy in veterinary medicine. *Veterinary Radiology* 24:278–283.

164. Grier, R., Kigurardo, G., Schaffer, C., Pedrosa, B., Myers, R., Merkley, D.F., and Touvenelle, M. 1991. Mast cell destruction by deionized water. *American Journal Veterinary Research* 51:1116–1120.

165. Theon, A.P., Pascoe, J.R., Carlson, G.P., and Krag, D.N. 1993. Intratumoral chemotherapy with cisplatin in oily emulsion in horses. *Journal of the American Veterinary Medical Association* 202(2):261–267.

166. Theon, A., Pascoe, J., and Meagher, D. 1994. Perioperative intratumoral administration of cisplatin for treatment of cutaneous tumors in Equidae. *Journal of the American Veterinary Medical Association* 205:1170–1176.

167. Theon, A.P., Pascoe, J.R., Madigan, J.E. et al. 1997. Comparison of intratumoral administration of cisplatin versus bleomycin for treatment of periocular squamous cell carcinoma in horses. *American Journal of Veterinary Research* 58:431–436.

168. Hewes, C.A., and Sullins, K.E. 2006. Use of cisplatin-containing biodegradeable beads for treatment of cutaneous neoplasia in equidae: 59 cases (2000–2004). *Journal of the American Veterinary Medical Association* 229:1617–1622.

169. Kleinschuster, S., Rapp, H., Green, S., Bier, J., and Kampen, K. 1981. Efficacy of intratumorally administered mycobacterial cell walls in the treatment of cattle with ocular carcinoma. *Journal of the National Cancer Institute* 67:1165–1171.

170. Hoffman, D., Jennings, P., and Spradbrow, P. 1981. Immunotherapy of bovine ocular squamous cell carcinomas with phenol–saline extracts of allogeneic carcinomas. *Australian Veterinary Journal* 57:159–162.

171. Shields, C.L., Lally, M.R., Singh, A.D., Shields, J.A., and Nowinski, T. 1999. Oral cimetidine (Tagamet) for recalcitrant, diffuse conjunctival papillomatosis. *American Journal of Ophthalmology* 128:362–364.

172. Goetz, T.E., Ogilvie, G.K., Keegan, K.G., and Johnson, P.J. 1990. Cimetidine for treatment of melanomas in three horses. *Journal of the American Veterinary Medical Association* 196:449–452.

173. McCalla, T., Moore, C., and Collier, L.A. 1992. Immunotherapy of periocular squamous cell carcinoma with metastasis in a pony. *Journal of the American Veterinary Medical Association* 200:1678–1681.

174. Wyman, M., Rings, M., Tarr, M., and Alden, C. 1977. Immunotherapy in equine sarcoid: A report of two cases. *Journal of the American Veterinary Medical Association* 171:449–451.

175. Murphy, J., Severin, G., Lavach, J., and Helper, D. 1979. Immunotherapy in ocular equine sarcoid. *Journal of the American Veterinary Medical Association* 174:269–272.

176. Lavach, J., Sullins, K., Roberts, S., Severin, G. et al. 1985. BCG treatment of periocular sarcoid. *Equine Veterinary Journal* 17:445–448.

177. Giuliano, E.A., Ota, J., and Tucker, S.A. 2007. Photodynamic therapy: Basic priciples and potential uses for veterinary ophthalmologists. *Veterinary Ophthalmology* 10:337–343.

178. Giuliano, E.A., Johnson, P.J., Delgado, C. et al. 2014. Local photodynamic therapy delays recurrence of equine periocular squamous cell carcinoma compared to cryo therapy. *Veterinary Ophthalmology* 17S1:37–45.

179. Joyce, J. 1975. Cryosurgery for removal of equine sarcoids. *Veterinary Medicine/Small Animal Clinician* 70:200–203.

CHAPTER 8

CONJUNCTIVA AND THIRD EYELID

BERNHARD M. SPIESS

ANATOMY AND PHYSIOLOGY

The conjunctiva is a thin mucous membrane that lines the posterior surface of the lids (palpebral conjunctiva) and reflects forward at the fornix or recess onto the globe (bulbar conjunctiva). In animals lower than primates, it is also reflected over a cartilage and glandular tissue to form the membrana nictitans, or third eyelid in the medial–ventral cul-de-sac. Depending on the location, the epithelium of the conjunctiva is either stratified columnar or stratified squamous, and it is continuous with the corneal epithelium (**Figure 8.1**).[1] The stem cells of the palpebral conjunctiva (rabbit) are located at the mucocutaneous junction and migrate toward the fornix.[2] Presumably, the stem cells for the bulbar conjunctiva reside at the limbus with the corneal stem cells.

Perilimbal pigment is present to a variable degree in most animals. The presence of conjunctival pigment is a protecting factor for development of squamous cell carcinomas, which are stimulated by ultraviolet (UV) radiation. The conjunctival melanocytes migrate into the cornea with corneal neovascularization, resulting in the corneal pigmentation observed in an inflamed cornea.[3]

Tenon's capsule (or fascia) of the globe becomes intimately involved with the overlying conjunctiva about 2–3 mm posterior from the limbus and is heaviest over the rectus muscle insertions dorsally and ventrally. This is clinically evident as the most difficult dissection area when performing conjunctival flap surgery.

The epithelium contains goblet cells that contribute to the mucin layer of the tear film. The mucin allows an aqueous solution to spread over a hydrophobic lipid corneal epithelium (**Figure 8.1**). The concentration of goblet cells varies with the area examined, and in the dog, they are most numerous in the lower medial fornix and are least numerous on the bulbar conjunctiva.[4] The female dog has a greater density of goblet cells than the male. A lack of goblet cells results in a specific form of keratoconjunctivitis sicca (KCS).[5,6] The nerve supply of the conjunctiva is the long ciliary nerve (ophthalmic division of cranial nerve V).

The third eyelid is well developed in domestic animals, while in higher primates, it is a vestigial structure, the plica semilunaris. It functions as a protective mechanism that is very active in grazing animals and birds and is a source of tears. The movement of the third eyelid across the globe consists of a passive component and an active component, the latter being found in birds and, perhaps, cats. The passive movement is produced when the globe is retracted into the orbit by the retractor bulbi muscle, which results in pressure on the base of the third eyelid pushing it forward. Any condition that increases the orbital volume pushes on the base of the third eyelid, and any decrease in orbital volume may cause the globe to sink into the orbit and push on the base of the third eyelid.

Birds lack a retractor bulbi muscle but have a very active third eyelid that is pulled from the dorsonasal quadrant across the eye by the pyramidalis muscle, which originates from the posterior globe.[7] The cat has been reported to have an active component of protrusion of the third eyelid due to slips of skeletal muscle that originate from the lateral rectus muscle and insert near the free margin.[8] Innervation is supplied by cranial nerve VI. These slips of skeletal muscle were not confirmed by Nuyttens and Simoens,[9] but they did report nine smooth muscle slips that attach to the third eyelid; four protract and four retract the third eyelid, and one has an unknown function. These smooth muscles are part of a fibroelastic plate that originates in the levator, medial, ventral, and lateral rectus muscles.

Similar dissections have not been reported for other domestic animals, but most appear to have smooth muscle that retracts the third eyelid tonically. Innervation of the smooth muscle of the third eyelid in the dog[10] and the medial side of the third eyelid in the cat[11] is by sympathetic fibers arriving via the infratrochlear nerve, a branch of the ophthalmic division of the trigeminal nerve (cranial nerve V). The smooth muscle in the ventral aspect of the third eyelid in the cat is innervated by sympathetic fibers carried by the zygomatic branch of the maxillary division of cranial nerve V.[11] Denervation results in protrusion of the third eyelid in Horner's syndrome.

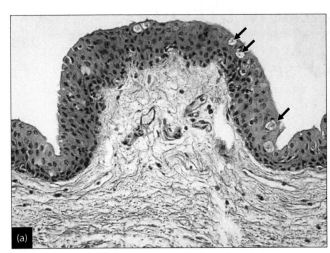
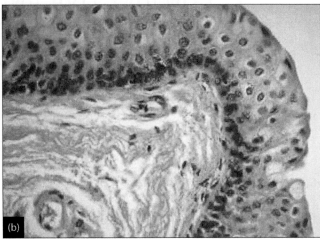

Figure 8.1 (a) Bulbar conjunctiva of a dog near the fornix, consisting of stratified squamous epithelium with scattered goblet cells in the epithelium. Note the loose stroma under the epithelium (H&E). (b) Bulbar conjunctiva of a dog that has melanocytes scattered throughout the basal aspect of the epithelium. The pigment is observed clinically, and in large animals, it is protective for development of squamous cell carcinoma.

The third eyelid varies among species, but in general, it consists of a T-shaped hyaline cartilage skeleton that is covered with conjunctiva and has a gland enveloping the base (**Figure 8.2**). This gland is one of two lacrimal glands for each eye and is often referred to erroneously as the Harderian gland. The true Harderian gland is deeper in the orbit than the third eyelid gland and is found only in certain domestic animals such as the rabbit, the cow, and the pig.[12] These animals, therefore, have two glands associated with the third eyelid. The secretions of the mammalian Harderian gland have a high lipid content.[13]

A cluster of lymphoid follicles is found on the bulbar surface of the third eyelid in most animals (**Figure 8.2**). These frequently become hyperplastic and hypertrophied with chronic antigenic stimulation. The margin of the third eyelid is usually pigmented, but individuals may lack pigmentation in one or both eyes. Animals with nonpigmented conjunctival surfaces are more prone to ocular irritation and neoplasia. In cattle, periocular pigmentation has a heritability factor of 0.53 (about the same as lid pigmentation), increases with age, and is protective for squamous cell carcinoma.[14,15]

EXAMINATION OF THE CONJUNCTIVA

Diffuse light and magnification

The various conjunctival surfaces should be examined for hyperemia, chemosis, follicular development, type and quantity of exudation, mechanical factors, and involvement of other ocular or adnexal structures.

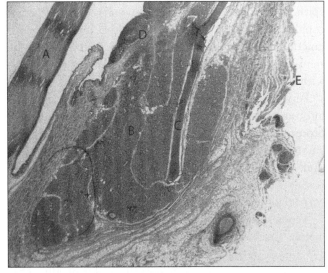

Figure 8.2 Histologic section of a normal canine third eyelid. (A) Cornea; (B) gland of the third eyelid; (C) cartilage; (D) lymphoid follicles; (E) palpebral surface.

Microbiologic culture

If cultures are indicated, swabs should be taken before instilling topical anesthetics due to the bactericidal action of the preservatives and before applying rose bengal stain due to its virucidal action.[16] Swabs should be plated immediately or placed in transport medium.

Schirmer tear test (STT)

An STT should be performed in most cases of red eye to evaluate for quantitative tear deficiencies. It must be performed before instilling topical drops. Keratoconjunctivitis sicca (KCS) is a commonly overlooked cause of chronic conjunctivitis.

Conjunctival scraping

Conjunctival scrapings obtained with a spatula, a cotton bud, or a cytology brush, and stained with either Giemsa or a quick stain for cytology and Gram stain for bacterial population, are frequently helpful in making a specific etiologic diagnosis (**Table 8.1**). If indirect fluorescent antibody (IFA) staining is to be performed, such as in the diagnosis of herpesvirus or chlamydia, prior use of topical fluorescein should probably be avoided. Conflicting evidence exists as to whether prior staining of the cornea and the conjunctiva with fluorescein results in false-positive results with IFA staining.[17,18]

Double eversion of the lids and third eyelid

Eversion of the lids is indicated, particularly in refractory conjunctivitis and with refractive ulcerative keratitis, to make sure contributing mechanical factors such as an aberrant hair or a foreign body are not overlooked.

Table 8.1 Cellular responses associated with conjunctivitis.	
DISEASE	**CELLULAR RESPONSE**
Acute bacterial conjunctivitis	Predominantly neutrophils, few mononuclear cells, many bacteria, degenerating epithelial cells
Chronic bacterial conjunctivitis	Predominantly neutrophils, many mononuclear cells, degenerate or keratinized epithelial cells, goblet cells, bacteria may or may not be seen, mucus, fibrin
Feline herpes viral conjunctivitis	Neutrophils and mononuclear cell numbers depend on stage of infection
Feline mycoplasmal conjunctivitis	Predominantly neutrophils, fewer mononuclear cells, basophilic coccoid or pleomorphic organisms on cell membranes
Feline chlamydial conjunctivitis	Predominantly neutrophils, mononuclear cells in subacute cases are increased in number, plasma cells, basophilic cytoplasmic inclusions early in the disease
Keratoconjunctivitis sicca	Epithelial cells keratinized, goblet cells, mucus, neutrophilic response marked if there is infection, bacteria
Canine distemper	Varies with stage of disease: Early: Giant cells, mononuclear cells; later: Neutrophils, goblet cells, and mucus. Infrequent cellular inclusions
Allergic conjunctivitis	Eosinophils, neutrophils may be marked, basophils possible

Lacrimal outflow

Chronic epiphora or a mucopurulent conjunctival discharge, usually unilateral, may occur with obstruction of the lacrimal outflow system and thus must be differentiated from conjunctivitis.

Meibomian glands

The meibomian glands may be the site of residual or persistent infection that extends to the conjunctiva or the source of irritating lipid breakdown products (see section Blepharitis, Chapter 7) resulting in chronic conjunctivitis.

DISEASES OF THE CONJUNCTIVA: CONJUNCTIVITIS

Introduction/etiology

Conjunctivitis is the most commonly diagnosed ocular disease in general practice. Chronic conjunctivitis is frequently frustrating to treat, as the etiologic diagnosis is often presumptive and not based on laboratory results, and the response to therapy is often inconclusive. However, neither veterinary nor medical ophthalmologists are very successful in arriving at a definitive diagnosis with chronic conjunctivitis, despite exhaustive testing.[19–21]

Clinical signs

Hyperemia

Hyperemia of the conjunctiva is the hallmark of conjunctivitis and may vary in severity. Hyperemia of conjunctivitis should be distinguished from distension of selected conjunctival veins draining the episcleral and scleral veins. The latter is an important indicator of intraocular disease. The hyperemia of conjunctivitis is diffuse and more severe toward the fornix and not restricted to a few large veins (**Figure 8.3**). The hyperemia of conjunctivitis is usually located in the palpebral conjunctiva (**Figure 8.4**) but on occasion may involve all conjunctival surfaces (**Figure 8.3**).

Chemosis

Conjunctivitis of acute onset produces variable degrees of chemosis (edema). A mild-to-moderate degree of chemosis is manifested by thicker folds of dorsal bulbar conjunctiva forming when the lid is rubbed against the bulbar conjunctiva. The fluid retention, as well as the hyperemia of the bulbar conjunctiva, obscures the episcleral vessels and the underlying scleral venous plexus to a variable degree. Shar Peis often have the appearance of chemosis (**Figure 8.48**), presumably due to increased amounts of glycosaminoglycans (mucin) in the conjunctival stroma, similar to the subcutis (mucinosis).

Adverse reactions to topical medications produce dramatic chemosis with minimal inflammation (**Figure 8.5**).

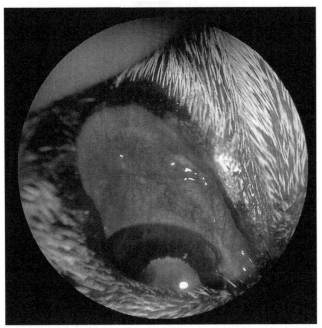

Figure 8.3 Diffuse hyperemia of the palpebral and bulbar conjunctiva in a dog with conjunctivitis associated with atopy.

Cyclopentolate, a topical mydriatic, is very predictable in producing marked chemosis in dogs.

Ocular discharge

The presenting complaint is usually ocular discharge. Ocular exudates may be minimal or absent, as observed in

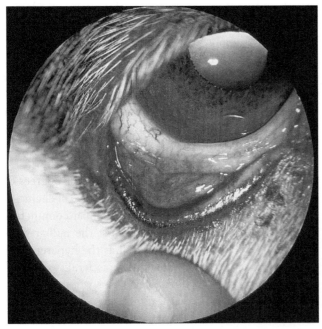

Figure 8.4 Typical appearance of conjunctivitis that preferentially involves the palpebral conjunctiva more than the bulbar conjunctiva. Note chemosis (folds in conjunctiva) and diffuse hyperemia.

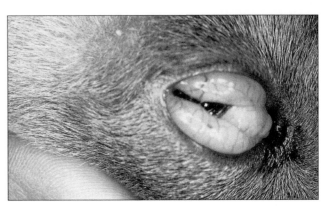

Figure 8.5 Marked chemosis without hyperemia in a cat. Chemosis of this degree without hyperemia is often due to topical medications or allergens.

cases of uncomplicated viral conjunctivitis and atopy. Mild inflammation results in a serous discharge from hypersecretion of the lacrimal glands due to irritation.

The next degree of severity of ocular discharge is excessive production of mucus. Small quantities of mucus are normal, and mucus has an important role in the tear film. Depending on the nature of the irritant, variable degrees of polymorphonuclear cell exudation may occur and, if severe, manifest as a purulent exudate. These frequently, but not invariably, are associated with a bacterial infection and are usually accompanied by excess mucus and thus become mucopurulent in nature. Certain breeds of cats such as the Persian, Himalayan, and Siamese are predisposed to a black, waxy discharge with conjunctivitis. The source is probably the meibomian glands, as it may still be present with KCS (**Figure 8.6**). This material may play a role in the black deposits found with corneal sequestrum.

Follicles

Lymphoid follicles may be present on the conjunctival surfaces in variable numbers. Follicles have a characteristic "cobblestone" appearance, and their numbers may not be fully appreciated until the lids are everted, and both surfaces of the third eyelid are examined. Follicular hyperplasia is frequently a nonspecific reaction to chronic conjunctival irritation (**Figure 8.7**). In the horse, they have been associated with *Onchocerca* spp. infestation, and in the cat, possibly with herpesvirus.

Pain

Pain or discomfort observed with conjunctivitis varies greatly with the type of conjunctivitis and the species. In humans, the discomfort of conjunctivitis is described as a "foreign body sensation on the eye." Cats with conjunctivitis frequently have some degree of blepharospasm,

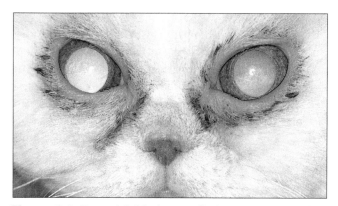

Figure 8.6 Brownish-black waxy discharge in a cat with chlamydial infection. Discharge is not specific for chlamydia but is unique in certain cats for any conjunctival irritation.

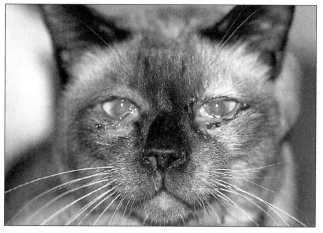

Figure 8.8 Mild ocular discomfort characteristic of cats with conjunctivitis. Note the mild blepharospasm with prominent third eyelid and ocular and nasal discharge. The conjunctivitis was due to herpesvirus infection.

whereas dogs often are oblivious to the condition (**Figure 8.8**). When blepharospasm is present, corneal pain should be ruled out by fluorescein staining before ascribing the pain to conjunctivitis.

Laterality

Most cases of conjunctivitis are bilateral, and when unilateral, unique conditions such as mechanical irritation from a foreign body or hair should be investigated. Some infectious conditions begin in one eye but usually spread to the opposite eye or have one eye more severely involved than the other. Herpetic conjunctivitis in cats may be unilateral.

Classification by etiology

The usual classification of various inflammatory diseases of the conjunctiva has been based on descriptive terminology

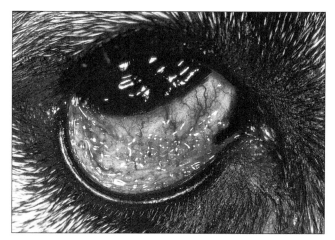

Figure 8.7 Marked follicle formation visible on the palpebral conjunctiva and palpebral surface of the third eyelid of a dog.

of the duration (acute and chronic) and type of exudate (mucoid and purulent). While this methodology makes it convenient to label or make a superficial diagnosis, it adds very little to our understanding of the etiology of conjunctivitis. It is preferable to classify inflammatory lesions by emphasizing the cause.

Viral conjunctivitis

Viruses are common etiologic agents of conjunctivitis in all domestic animals. Often, the conjunctivitis is among the least of the many signs produced in a particular viral disease and as such may be chosen to be ignored by the clinician. The diagnostic challenge occurs when the conjunctivitis is the main sign and represents either a prodromal or subclinical systemic syndrome.

Canine distemper

Introduction/etiology

Distemper seems to be almost invariably associated with some degree of bilateral conjunctivitis. The classical picture is a mucopurulent ocular discharge in association with other catarrhal signs. While the mucopurulent exudate is usually described as typical for distemper, this form is usually not purely viral, as secondary bacteria and a variable degree of tear deficiency promote the mucopurulent exudation. Distemper may also present as bilateral marked hyperemia of the conjunctiva, with a minimal seromucoid discharge (**Figure 8.9**). The animal's pharynx and tonsils may also be inflamed, and a mild fever of 39.5–40°C (102–104°F) may be present but no other systemic signs.

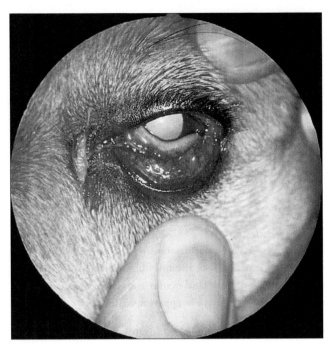

Figure 8.9 Distemper conjunctivitis in an apparently healthy young dog that was febrile when presented for vaccination. The palpebral conjunctiva was severely hyperemic bilaterally, and minimal exudation was present. Conjunctival scrapings are presented in Figure 8.10. Myoclonus developed within 1 month.

If observed early in the disease, conjunctival scrapings frequently may have distemper inclusion bodies in the cytoplasm of the epithelial cells (**Figure 8.10**). There is usually an absolute lymphopenia in the blood count, and the animal may develop other signs of distemper later.

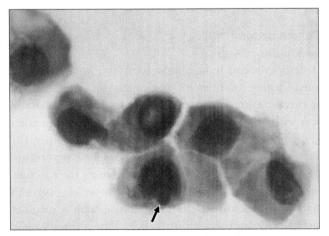

Figure 8.10 Conjunctival cytology from the case in Figure 8.9. A red cytoplasmic inclusion body is present (arrow) in the central epithelial cell (Schorr's stain).

Diagnosis

The diagnosis of distemper is usually based on history, accompanying systemic signs, intracytoplasmic inclusions in epithelial cells on conjunctival scrapings (**Figure 8.10**), and an absolute lymphopenia in the peripheral blood. A lack of inclusion bodies is not definitive as the peak observation period of inclusions is 7–11 days post inoculation, with a range of 5–21 days.[22] Thus, chronic distemper cases are often negative. Fluorescent antibody staining is more sensitive for detecting inclusions than routine cytology. A reverse transcription-polymerase chain reaction (RT-PCR) is available for detection of canine distemper virus DNA.[23]

Adenoviruses

Canine adenovirus type 1 (CAV-1) and canine adenovirus type 2 (CAV-2) both produce conjunctivitis. CAV-1 is the agent of infectious canine hepatitis, while CAV-2 is one of the etiologic agents of tracheobronchitis or "kennel cough." Both agents may be responsible for a bilateral conjunctivitis characterized by marked hyperemia and a serous to seromucous exudate.[24] The systemic signs may provide clues for differentiating the adenovirus infections from distemper, but it may be difficult to differentiate complicated tracheobronchitis from distemper.

Herpesvirus
Introduction/etiology
Cat
Conjunctivitis is present to a variable degree in all the feline viral respiratory syndromes. The herpesvirus, calicivirus, and reovirus groups have been isolated from the respiratory tract and the conjunctiva.[25] Serologic evidence indicates that herpesvirus and calicivirus are widespread in the cat population and account for most of the cases of infectious upper respiratory disease.[26] Reovirus appears to be an insignificant cause of feline conjunctivitis.[27] The prevalence of the varying viral causes has depended on the method of detection, with newer techniques utilizing polymerase chain reaction (PCR) being more sensitive than IFA, cultures, and serology. It has been suggested that the more severe forms of conjunctivitis are associated with herpesvirus (**Table 8.2**), but factors such as antigenic variants, individual immunity, potentiation by other viruses, and bacteria may all modify the disease so that considerable overlap occurs between clinical signs.[28]

Feline herpesvirus type 1 (FHV-1), the causative agent of feline rhinotracheitis, has a tropism for conjunctival and respiratory epithelium, where it replicates and produces necrosis. This is most severe in the young animal

Table 8.2 **Clinical differentiation of feline respiratory infection.**

	FVR	FVC	*CHLAMYDOPHILA* SPP.
Severity	Primary infection typically severe	Variably mild to moderate	Mild
Ocular symptoms	Conjunctivitis often prominent	Conjunctivitis mild to absent	Chronic and marked
Nasal discharge	Often profuse	Scanty to moderate	Scanty to moderate
Epithelial ulceration	Very occasionally tongue or pharynx	Very frequently tongue, also hard palate, external nares	Not associated
Coughing	Common	Rare, if ever	Rare, if ever

Source: From Povey, R. 1976. *Canadian Veterinary Journal* 17:93–100.

undergoing a primary infection.[29,30] It may also replicate in the corneal epithelium, producing ulceration, the most typical being a linear "dendritic" ulceration.[31,32] Following primary infection, latent infection for the life of the cat occurs in the trigeminal ganglion[33,34] and perhaps the corneal stroma[35–38] in about 80% of cats.[39] In young cats, infection with herpesvirus may produce severe conjunctivitis, and usually there are upper respiratory signs. Signs of conjunctivitis progress from seromucoid to mucopurulent in 4–5 days, and the discharge is often quite profuse (**Figures 8.8 and 8.11**).

In young kittens, the conjunctival surface is often ulcerated, with fibrinous exudation resulting in persistent symblepharon (**Figures 8.12 and 8.13**).[40] The resultant conjunctival adhesions may adhere to the cornea if it is concurrently ulcerated, create a permanent protrusion of the third eyelid from adhesions, or obliterate the lacrimal lake or lacrimal puncta in the lower medial conjunctival cul-de-sac, creating a chronic epiphora. Various degrees of keratitis may occur with herpesvirus,[31] but keratitis is

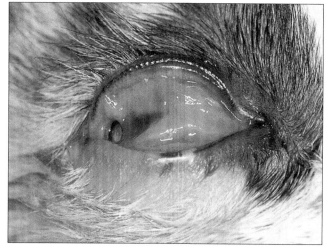

Figure 8.12 Marked fibrinous reaction in a kitten with herpesvirus conjunctivitis, resulting in symblepharon. The condition is bilateral.

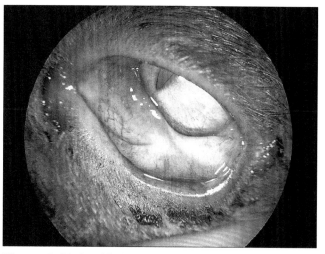

Figure 8.13 Symblepharon (adhesions of conjunctiva to the third eyelid). In the cat, these are usually associated with early herpesvirus infection as a kitten. This can result in epiphora from blockage of the lower puncta, normal tear flow in the lower conjunctival cul-de-sac, and a more prominent third eyelid.

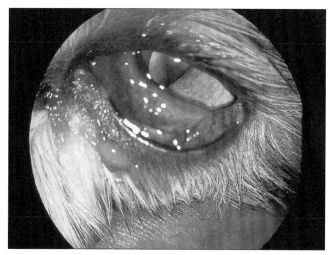

Figure 8.11 A cat with chronic bilateral seromucoid discharge associated with herpesvirus conjunctivitis.

not present with the other viral etiologies of the respiratory disease/conjunctivitis complex. The duration of the acute clinical signs is usually 10–14 days.[40] Adult cats frequently manifest chronic herpesvirus conjunctivitis unilaterally or bilaterally with minimal respiratory signs, and these represent the biggest diagnostic and therapeutic challenge.[20,21,41]

Dog

The herpesvirus responsible for neonatal puppy death produces a transient follicular genital infection in adult males and females, as well as a transient (4–5 days) conjunctivitis.[42] A herpesvirus was suspected in a syndrome of chronic follicular conjunctivitis and balanitis of dogs. The disease was produced after passage through tissue culture, but the agent was not isolated.[43] Later work by the same authors could not duplicate the transmissibility of the syndrome.[44] A follicular conjunctivitis associated with balanitis or vaginitis does exist, but an infectious cause has yet to be confirmed.

A keratopathy that was similar in appearance to a lipid keratopathy has been reported to be associated with herpesvirus but has not been confirmed.[45] While many ophthalmologists have suspected that a canine herpes syndrome exists in the adult dog due to the occasional dendritic ulcer and found it curious why the dog should be unique in not having an adult ocular herpes syndrome, Ledbetter et al. confirmed that indeed the adult dog does have an ocular herpes syndrome.[207] They reported on two dogs with dendritic corneal ulcers and isolated canine herpes type 1 (CHV-1) from the lesions. Both dogs were responsive to topical antiviral therapy. In recent years, several reports have documented the role of CHV-1 in keratoconjunctivitis.[46-49]

Horse

Equine herpesvirus 2 (EHV-2) may produce a keratoconjunctivitis (see Chapter 10), and viral arteritis may produce a conjunctivitis.[50-52] Viral conjunctivitis and keratouveitis may be observed with adenoviral infection in foals. The role of EHV-2 and EHV-5 in equine keratoconjunctivitis is controversial, however.[53]

Cow

Bovine herpesvirus 1, the cause of infectious bovine rhinotracheitis (IBR), may produce infectious pustular vulvovaginitis or respiratory signs and may involve the conjunctiva, to the extent that eye or ocular signs predominate.[54] Manifestation depends on the strain of virus. Conjunctival involvement typically produces elevated red plaques that are proliferations of lymphocytes, follicles, and white necrotic areas (**Figure 8.14**).[55,56] Ocular

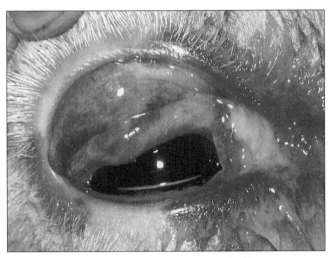

Figure 8.14 Marked conjunctivitis in a calf with respiratory and ocular disease due to infectious bovine rhinotracheitis. Note the marked chemosis and white areas coalescing in the conjunctiva. On histopathology, these represent infiltrations of lymphocytes and, possibly, surface necrosis. Multiple animals were involved, and other calves had keratitis and anterior uveitis.

involvement may be observed with respiratory signs and, in addition to conjunctivitis, consists of anterior uveitis and a nonulcerative keratitis that is characterized by peripheral edema that spreads centrally. Lesions may be either unilateral or bilateral. As with other herpesvirus infections, animals often become latent carriers and may become symptomatic when stressed.

IBR virus has also been isolated from goats with ocular lesions of conjunctivitis, keratitis, and respiratory disease.[57]

Diagnosis

A presumptive diagnosis of viral conjunctivitis may be made by observing conjunctivitis associated with typical systemic signs, exclusion of other etiologies, lack of response to antibiotics in a condition that is contagious, or a typical disease in that species. As diagnostic tests are not often widely available, and are expensive or ambiguous, clinical judgement is often relied upon for making a diagnosis of viral conjunctivitis (particularly herpesvirus).[20,41]

The main differential diagnosis of infectious conjunctivitis in cats is *Chlamydophila felis* (*Chlamydia psittaci*) infection. Sykes et al. correlated the clinical signs with the results of PCR testing for both Chlamydophila and feline herpesvirus and found that of cats with upper respiratory signs, 14% were positive for Chlamydophila, and 21% were positive for herpesvirus.[58] In cats with conjunctivitis, a history of recent exposure to other cats, sneezing, and acute signs were correlated with positive herpesvirus on PCR.

Cats with conjunctivitis and that were Chlamydophila-positive were younger cats (9 weeks–6 months), and there was a seasonal incidence in the summer.

Viral culture

Viral cultures from conjunctiva may be performed but are usually reserved for outbreaks with multiple animals. With herpesvirus infection, cultures are frequently negative because of the latent carrier state. Rose bengal is highly virucidal and should not be applied to the cornea before obtaining viral cultures.[16] Hickman et al. found in a herpesvirus outbreak in a colony of specific pathogen-free (SPF) cats that only 4% of the cats were actively shedding herpesvirus.[59] Upon activation of herpesvirus infection with glucocorticoid injections, 21% of previously negative cats shed the virus after one injection and an additional 12% after a second glucocorticoid injection. Maggs et al. found 11% of clinically normal cats were culture positive, which was markedly higher than in previous reports.[37,38,60-62]

Indirect fluorescent antibody staining and cytology

Inclusion bodies may be found with adenoviruses and distemper virus (**Figure 8.10**), but herpesvirus inclusions are not seen with routine cytologic processing.[63] Fixation for 1 hour in Bouin's solution retains herpesvirus inclusions.[64]

IFA staining is a more sensitive method of detecting viral antigen than routine cytologic examination. Prior application of fluorescein to the eye before taking samples for IFA may result in a false-positive test,[65] but this is controversial; reports in the human literature and the author's own experience indicate that prior fluorescein staining does not interfere with IFA interpretation.[17] Viral inclusions are often transient and present only early in disease. Thus, a negative result is inconclusive. IFA testing is positive in only about 20% of cats experimentally infected with herpesvirus,[41] and in the author's research and clinical experience, it is almost always negative.[37,38]

> Many ophthalmologists dismiss conjunctival cytology as a low-yield test for feline conjunctivitis; however, it is a quick and inexpensive method to diagnose Chlamydophila, mycoplasmal, and eosinophilic conjunctivitis.

Serology

Serologic testing is complicated by the widespread vaccination and ubiquitous nature of many of the viral agents. Maggs et al. found herpesvirus serology to be of no use in differentiating normal cats from diseased cats.[60]

Polymerase chain reaction

PCR testing for virus DNA may be overly sensitive when many cats are carriers for herpesvirus. The rate of positive herpesvirus on PCR testing of normal cats has varied from <1%[37,38] to 11%.[59,62,208] Vaccine virus DNA is also detected by PCR, decreasing the diagnostic sensitivity, and the various PCR assays published also have significantly variable detection rates.[209]

Therapy

Treatment of viral conjunctivitis with topical antibiotics is usually undertaken only if the disease is incorrectly diagnosed or thought to be complicated with bacteria. Topical antiviral agents are not effective against distemper virus or adenoviruses but are effective against the herpesvirus group. The efficacy of the various antiherpes agents varies, with reports indicating a decreasing sensitivity order of: Trifluridine > idoxuridine = ganciclovir > cidofovir = penciclovir > vidarabine > acyclovir = foscarnet.[205,210] Despite this, Williams et al. reported clinical improvement in feline herpes syndromes with topical 0.5% acyclovir given five times a day.[211] Similarly, topical 0.5% cidofovir every 12 hours in experimental herpes significantly decreased the severity of the clinical signs and viral shedding.[212] Cidofovir has the advantage of decreased frequency of dosing because of its long half-life in ocular tissues. While the course of the disease may be shortened with therapy, a cure is not produced due to the carrier status that many animals develop.

Immunization does not protect animals from most of the ocular manifestations of herpesvirus infection, nor does it have a known role in therapy, although anecdotal reports may suggest otherwise. Sykes et al. found previous vaccination history to have no statistical value in determining the cause of upper respiratory disease.[58] Interferon given intranasally or topically onto the eye has been used for therapy, although it has not been critically evaluated in clinical practice. Topical application of recombinant feline interferon omega (rFeIFN-omega) resulted in a dose-dependent expression of Mx protein, a marker of the biological response to rFeIFN-omega.[66] *In vitro* testing of feline herpesvirus to acyclovir was potentiated eightfold by the addition of alpha interferon at doses of 10–100 U.[67] However, no beneficial effects of treatment with rFeIFN-omega on the course of primary FHV-1 infection in cats could be documented in another study.[68]

L-lysine (500 mg every 12 hours orally) decreased the severity of herpesvirus-induced conjunctivitis in cats but did not alter the duration of the disease or the ability to isolate the virus. Lysine was administered 6 hours before inoculation with the virus; this raises the question of efficacy in the clinical situation, where therapy is initiated after the infection is established.[69] Maggs et al. tested the effectiveness of lysine in cats with upper respiratory infections and found the mean disease scores were higher.[213] FHV-1 DNA was more frequently detected, and the blood arginine levels were lower in the lysine-treated group. This study raises serious questions about the efficacy and potential side effects of using dietary lysine. Lysine may have a role in prophylaxis when administered daily in catteries, in multicat households, or when new animals are introduced.

The elimination of herpesvirus from catteries is best performed by PCR testing and culling of carriers. In an SPF colony, all cats with positive viral cultures of oral swabs before and 10 days after two injections of 5 mg/kg methylprednisolone acetate IM at 6-week intervals were culled from the colony. Despite these drastic measures, 23% of cats that were herpesvirus negative after two glucocorticoid injections were positive after a third injection.[59]

Prophylaxis

Prevention of viral conjunctivitis as well as other forms of infectious conjunctivitis should consist of segregation of animals by age, function, and health status and should be quarantined upon first acquisition. Immunization of new animals before introduction into the main herd or cattery, decreasing the concentration of animals, good ventilation, and avoiding fomite transmission by hand washing are important steps in minimizing outbreaks of infectious conjunctivitis. L-lysine (500 mg every 12 hours) may be administered to cats in quarantine and throughout the period of introduction into the household or colony to minimize signs if exposed to herpesvirus.

Chlamydophila felis

Introduction/etiology

The agent of feline pneumonitis has undergone various name changes, from *Miyagawanella felis* to *Chlamydia psittaci*; most recently, *Chlamydia psittaci* has been divided into four new species, *Chlamydophila felis*, *C. psittaci*, *C. abortus*, and *C. caviae*. These, respectively, primarily infect cats, birds, sheep, and guinea pigs.[70–72] *Chlamydophila* spp. are obligate intracellular Gram-negative bacteria that have a tropism for mucous membranes. There are two forms, the elementary body (infectious form) and the reticulate body (intracellular, metabolically active form).[73] Although mammalian strains are thought to have relatively low infectivity for humans, they should still be considered a zoonosis.[74,75] After reviewing the literature on human infections with *C. felis*, Browning concluded that of seven cases, only one case in an immune compromised patient could be definitely attributed to *C. felis*.[214]

Clinical signs

While *C. felis* was initially described as an agent for pneumonitis in cats, subsequent studies have indicated the conjunctiva and the nasal cavity are the primary sites of infection, with rare lower respiratory infection.[76–78] In a survey of feline conjunctivitis, *C. felis* were cultured in 30% of cases.[79] Utilizing PCR for both herpesvirus and *C. felis*, Sykes et al. found *C. felis* in 14% of cats with upper respiratory disease, and all had conjunctivitis.[58] Cats with conjunctivitis were as likely to be positive on PCR for herpesvirus as for *C. felis*; however, sneezing cats with conjunctivitis and cats with acute disease were 2.2× and 2.3× as likely to be herpesvirus positive, respectively.[58] No cats with upper respiratory disease without conjunctivitis were positive for *C. felis*; coinfection with *C. felis* and herpesvirus was uncommon, and 56% of cats with upper respiratory disease were negative for both agents. *C. felis* had a higher prevalence in young cats (5 weeks–9 months). Vaccination history was no help in differentiating the infectious agents involved in conjunctivitis and upper respiratory disease.[58]

The conjunctivitis of *C. felis* infection is usually the predominant sign and may be unilateral on initial examination, although it usually spreads to the opposite eye in 5–7 days.[63,80] In the early stages, the conjunctiva is chemotic, smooth, shiny, and a grayish-pink color. In the initial stages, the ocular discharge is serous, but within 2 days, the secretion becomes mucopurulent, and the conjunctiva becomes thick and more hyperemic (**Figure 8.15**). The ocular discharge is progressively reduced until only a scant or moderate mucopurulent exudate is present. In chronic cases, hyperplasia, hyperemia, and follicle formation may develop.

Untreated, the disease may run a prolonged course of several months.[76,77,80,81] Kittens born to carrier queens may manifest neonatal conjunctivitis before the physiologic ankyloblepharon separates. Isolation of the feline agent from humans with conjunctivitis indicates that it may have zoonotic potential.[74]

Chlamydophila spp. may also produce conjunctivitis and keratoconjunctivitis in the horse, the sheep, the goat, and the pig and may be associated with polyarthritis.[82,83] Keratitis may develop in these species, unlike the cat, where this has not been described or documented (**Figure 8.16**). Two serotypes of *Chlamydophila* have been described in cattle: Type 1 is responsible for abortion, genital infection, and enteric infections, and type 2 produces polyarthritis, polyserositis, keratoconjunctivitis, encephalomyelitis, and pneumonia. Transmission has been proposed as via oral, tick vectors, aerosol, and direct contact routes. With aerosol and direct contact exposure, the predominant signs are conjunctivitis and pneumonia. The manifestation of the

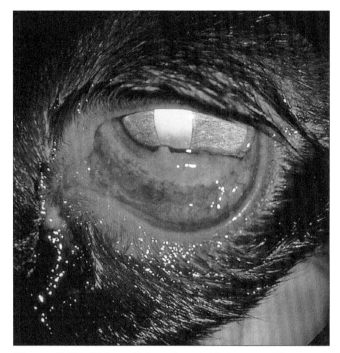

Figure 8.15 Chlamydial conjunctivitis in a cat. The condition was unilateral. Note hyperemia, glistening follicles, and seromucoid discharge. Inclusion bodies were found on cytology.

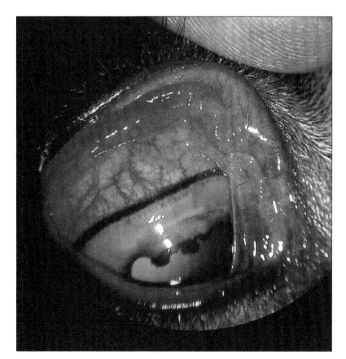

Figure 8.16 Chlamydial keratoconjunctivitis in a goat. Typical inclusion bodies were found on conjunctival cytology. The condition responded to topical tetracycline. Several young goats were involved.

disease is dependent on the virulence of the strain and the age and immunity of the animal.[84]

Diagnosis

Associated clinical signs vary with the species. Conjunctivitis is typically present in the young animal and is chronic, associated with a thickened, hyperemic conjunctiva. Conjunctival cytology contains primarily polymorphonuclear neutrophils (PMNs), but some lymphocytes are present as well. Cytoplasmic inclusion bodies in epithelial cells may be found as long as 50 days after infection but are most numerous in the first 2 weeks of the disease (**Figure 8.17**).[63] A history of possible exposure such as boarding, cat shows, veterinary hospitals, and introduction of new animals onto the premises indicates exposure. The diagnosis can be confirmed with a Chlamydiaceae real-time (RT) PCR.[85–87]

Therapy

Topical tetracyclines have been the traditional therapy for chlamydial infections. Animals usually respond well if treated early in the disease. The enigma lies in controlling the disease in catteries, herds, and hospitals because of the carrier state and short-lived immunity. The carrier state resides in the gastrointestinal tract, and consequently, treatment emphasis has shifted from topical to systemic tetracyclines.

Systemic doxycycline (5 mg/kg every 12 hours) for 3 weeks produced improvement in signs within 3 days of commencing treatment, and no relapse of disease was noted in experimental infection.[62] The author's personal experience with using systemic doxycycline in treating

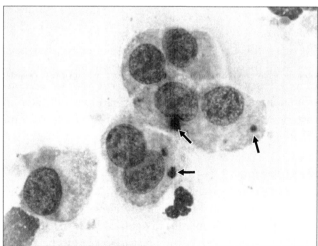

Figure 8.17 Chlamydial inclusions (arrows) in the cytoplasm of conjunctival epithelial cells of a cat (Wright's stain).

C. felis infection in a group of hospital blood donor cats has not been as successful, with relapses common. Dean et al. followed the clinical signs and presence of *C. felis* DNA with real-time PCR and found that at least a 28-day course of doxycycline was needed to eliminate the organism.[215] An alternative to twice daily systemic doxycycline therapy is azithromycin; azithromycin (5 mg/kg every 48 to 72 hours in the cat) is a long-acting macrolide similar to erythromycin that has proved efficacious against *C. felis*. Pradofloxacin and enrofloxacin are active against *C. felis* and *Mycoplasma* spp., but neither drug was as effective at clearing *C. felis* as doxycycline, resulting in more relapses.[216,217] Clavulanic acid–amoxicillin was successful in treating *C. felis* when given for 4 weeks.[218] While doxycycline has been taken as the "gold standard" for treating *C. felis*, alternative antibiotics may have fewer serious side effects.

> Oral doxycycline may be associated with esophageal strictures in cats, resulting in signs of regurgitation. Administering the drug with food or water may diminish the risk.[219]

Therapy should be continued for 10–14 days after clinical recovery, as relapse is common.[27] Cats with infectious conjunctivitis and/or respiratory signs that have a prolonged course or have relapsing episodes should be screened for immune suppression with feline leukemia virus (FeLV) or feline immunodeficiency virus (FIV).[88,89] Cats with *C. felis* and FIV infection shed *Chlamydophila* sp. for 270 days and have prolonged signs; dual infection accelerates the progression of FIV.[89]

Prophylaxis

Previous killed vaccines have been ineffective, but new, modified, live vaccines have demonstrated more efficacy.[90–92] An inactivated feline *C. felis* vaccine demonstrated immunity for 1 year.[93] Vaccination is indicated in catteries and in situations where increased exposure to other cats is present.

Mycoplasma

Introduction/etiology

As with mycoplasmal infections in other tissues and species, the role of mycoplasma in ocular disease of cats is not without controversy. A stress factor appears to be necessary in addition to the mycoplasma, as direct inoculation onto the conjunctiva does not produce the disease without prior cortisol administration.[63,94,95] Clinically, the mycoplasma may occur as a sequel to, or in conjunction with,

other viral upper respiratory diseases. The pure clinical picture is distinctive enough to help differentiate mycoplasmal conjunctivitis from Chlamydophila and viral conjunctivitis.[81]

Mycoplasma is a fastidious organism that is difficult to culture, and this may have contributed to the clinical impression over the last 25 years that it is not frequently associated with feline conjunctivitis. With the use of PCR testing, *Mycoplasma* DNA is once again being pushed to the forefront as a significant cause for feline conjunctivitis. Heather et al. detected *Mycoplasma* DNA in 9.6% of cats with conjunctivitis, FHV-1 DNA in 6.7%, and *C. felis* in 3.2%.[220]

Clinical signs

Feline mycoplasmal conjunctivitis is characterized by an initial unilateral, serous-to-mucopurulent exudate that usually extends to the opposite eye within 7 days. Conjunctival hyperemia is severe on all conjunctival surfaces, with modest-to-marked chemosis, papillary hypertrophy, and blepharospasm (**Figure 8.18**). In 4–10 days, the response moderates with less hyperemia, loss of papilla, pale conjunctiva with thickening and induration, increased mucopurulent exudation and, in some cases, a pseudodiphtheritic membrane. The disease is self-limiting, having a course of about 30 days with little change throughout the duration.

Mycoplasma is also a significant ocular pathogen in sheep and goats. In addition to an infectious conjunctivitis, ocular lesions of keratitis[96] and anterior uveitis may be produced, as well as mastitis, pleuropneumonia, and arthritis.

In cattle, *Mycoplasma bovoculi* and *Ureaplasma diversum* have been isolated from herds with conjunctivitis. When

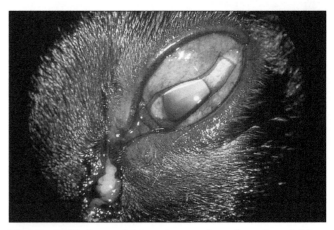

Figure 8.18 **A cat with acute mycoplasmal conjunctivitis. Marked chemosis and ocular discharge are present, mycoplasma organisms were cultured, and the conjunctival cytology was positive for mycoplasma (Figure 8.19).**

inoculated experimentally, the organisms produce a conjunctivitis syndrome of approximately 1 month's duration. During the syndrome, the signs vacillate between mild and severe.[97,98]

In swine, an infectious conjunctivitis and keratoconjunctivitis syndrome without systemic signs has been attributed to mycoplasma.[99] Ocular mycoplasma syndromes in the horse and the dog have not been described.[100,101]

Diagnosis

Conjunctival cytology is the most practical method for diagnosing mycoplasma. Mycoplasma appear as coccoid to coccobacillary organisms in clusters, on or near the surface of the epithelial cell (**Figure 8.19**). The organisms should be differentiated from pigment granules in the epithelial cells. The inflammatory exudation cytology is completely polymorphonuclear.[63,94,95] The diagnosis can be confirmed by PCR.[102,103]

Therapy

The course of the disease can be shortened to 4–5 days with the use of topical tetracyclines, chloramphenicol, gentamicin, fluoroquinolones, or erythromycin preparations.

Bacterial conjunctivitis

Introduction/etiology

Bacterial conjunctivitis is more important in the dog than the cat (excluding mycoplasmal conjunctivitis).[20] Cultures are readily obtained, but the difficulty lies in interpretation of the results, assuming satisfactory collection techniques have been observed. Urban et al. isolated bacteria from 91% of conjunctiva of clinically normal dogs.[104] Other studies utilizing different techniques yielded bacterial growth from 72%–94% of cultures from the conjunctiva of normal dogs (**Table 8.3**).[105–108] The incidence

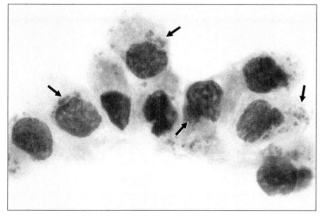

Figure 8.19 **Mycoplasma organisms on conjunctival epithelial cells of the cat in Figure 8.18; mycoplasma was also cultured from the conjunctival cul-de-sac.**

of isolates in normal eyes varies between breeds, and as one might expect, there is some correlation of isolates to lid conformation.[104] The normal flora is predominantly Gram-positive (**Table 8.3**). In the dog, streptococci, staphylococci, and diphtheroids are the predominant isolates from both normal animals and those with conjunctivitis. Thus, some clinical judgment must be made as to the significance of positive cultures.[109–112]

Compared to dogs, cats have a relatively sterile conjunctiva with bacterial isolates reported in 34%–67% of conjunctival swabs from normal cats (**Table 8.4**).[94,113,114]

The horse conjunctival sac has a predominantly Gram-positive resident flora with *Corynebacterium* spp., *Staphylococcus epidermidis*, *Bacillus cereus*, and hemolytic and nonhemolytic *Streptomyces* being most prevalent.[115] In the horse, *Streptococcus* sp. (44%), *Staphylococcus* spp. (24%), and *Pseudomonas* spp. (14%) were isolated from the conjunctiva and cornea of animals with extraocular disease.[116] Nutritionally variant streptococci have been shown to be a significant cause of equine corneal ulcers, and their significance in extraocular infections is unknown. Cultures may be negative as these organisms do not grow on the usual liquid or solid media unless the medium includes thiol-containing compounds and B,[5] or has an additional organism growing that produces these compounds.[18]

The virulence and number of organisms are factors in infection, and so is the individual's resistance, such as immunoglobulin level and local or systemic stress. Examples of stress may be local trauma, ultraviolet radiation, and concurrent systemic or local disease. Since the animal's defenses are important, it is not surprising to find that many dogs with bacterial conjunctivitis may have the following concurrent problems: Generalized seborrhea, pyoderma, otitis externa, lip fold infections, distemper, ectropion, entropion, trauma, and KCS. Depending on the host's predisposing factors, the infection may only be controlled rather than cured; a course of antibiotics, even if given for a prolonged period, may only improve the ocular condition transiently.

Acute bacterial conjunctivitis

Clinical signs

The signs of acute bacterial conjunctivitis are usually associated with sudden onset of a dramatic purulent ocular discharge, marked diffuse conjunctival hyperemia, and moderate chemosis (**Figure 8.20**). The infection may extend onto the eyelids, producing an acute moist blepharitis.

Diagnosis

Diagnosis of acute bacterial conjunctivitis is usually made on clinical signs and conjunctival cytology. Culture and antibiotic sensitivity testing is performed to confirm and

Table 8.3 **Isolation of bacteria from the conjunctival sac of clinically normal dogs (%).**

ORGANISM	BISTNER ET AL. (1969)[105]	URBAN ET AL. (1972)[104]	HACKER ET AL. (1979)[107]
Staphylococcus spp. (total)	70.0	70.7	59.0
Coagulase-positive	24.0	44.7	NR
Coagulase-negative	46.0	55.3	NR
Streptococcus spp. (total)	6.0	43.3	NR
Nonhemolytic	NR	12.0	51.0
α-hemolytic	4.0	34.0	5.0
β-hemolytic	2.0	7.3	3.0
Corynebacterium spp. (total)	75.0	30.0	NR
Undifferentiated	NR	11.3	NR
C. psuedodiphtheriticum	NR	9.3	NR
C. xerosis	NR	12.7	NR
Neisseria spp. (total)	NR	26.0	NR
Undifferentiated	NR	4.0	NR
N. catarrhalis	NR	8.7	NR
N. pharyngitidis	NR	4.0	NR
N. sicca	NR	3.3	NR
N. caviae	NR	2.7	NR
N. lactamicas	NR	2.7	NR
N. flavescens	NR	2.7	NR
Pseudomonas spp.	NR	14.0	NR
Moraxella spp.	NR	6.7	NR
Bacillus spp.	12.0	6.0	18.0

NR: not reported.

guide the therapy, especially if an immediately favorable response is not obtained. Conjunctival scraping and Gram staining are rapid methods to aid in the selection of antibiotic.

The head in general should be examined, as the early stages of acute orbital cellulitis or retrobulbar infections frequently mimic acute purulent conjunctivitis. Differentiation between simple acute purulent conjunctivitis and endophthalmitis or panophthalmitis with accompanying purulent exudation may be made by the lack of active intraocular inflammation with conjunctivitis. Predisposing factors such as conjunctival foreign bodies, blocked nasolacrimal duct, and entropion should be eliminated.

Therapy

Initial specific therapy is usually a broad-spectrum topical antibiotic. Most animals respond well in 3–5 days. In the horse, many strains of streptococci are resistant to the usual triple antibiotic or aminoglycoside preparations, and chloramphenicol, erythromycin, or ciprofloxacin

Table 8.4 **Bacteria isolated from normal cats.**

LOCATION	ORGANISM	%
Conjunctiva	*Staphylococcus albus*	16.3
	S. aureus	10.4
	Mycoplasma spp.	5.0
	M. felis[a]	–
	Bacillus spp.	2.9
	α-hemolytic streptococci	2.5
	Corynebacterium spp.	1.3
Lids	*S. albus*	13.8
	S. aureus	8.8
	α-hemolytic streptococci	1.7
	Bacillus spp.	1.7
	Escherichia coli	0.4

Source: Adapted from Campbell, L. et al. 1973. *Feline Practice* 3:10–12.
[a] Five *Mycoplasma* isolates were lost prior to identification.

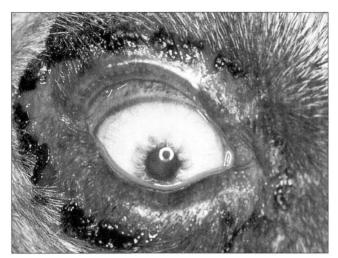

Figure 8.20 Acute unilateral bacterial conjunctivitis in a Weimaraner.

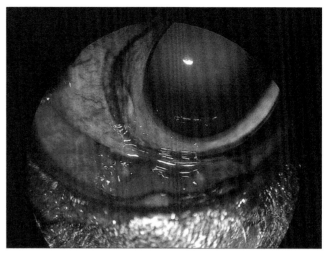

Figure 8.21 A dog with chronic staphylococcal pyoderma and chronic bilateral severe conjunctivitis. Note the thickened conjunctiva with follicles and possibly pyogranuloma.

preparations are more appropriate. In resistant or relapsing cases, specific antibiotics are chosen based on culture and antibiotic sensitivity testing. Cleansing the eye of exudate with a collyrium and soaking the crusts off the lid margins are important supportive measures.

Chronic bacterial conjunctivitis

Clinical signs
Exudation varies from mucoid to mucopurulent, and the conjunctiva is thickened, hyperemic, and has redundant folds. Some degree of follicular hyperplasia is usually present, and the process frequently extends to the dermis, resulting in depigmentation of the lid margins. The condition is often bilateral and may be associated with obvious disease in other organs (skin, ear) or poor lid conformation (**Figure 8.21**). Spaniels, St. Bernards, bulldogs, and hounds are frequently affected with chronic bacterial conjunctivitis. If allowed to go unchecked, a superficial keratitis eventually develops. Occasionally, a marginal corneal ulceration may develop that is thought to be a hypersensitivity reaction to the toxins produced with staphylococcal conjunctivitis. Tear production often decreases with chronicity, and this contributes to the conjunctivitis by keeping the surface debilitated (**Figure 8.22**).

Diagnosis
A STT should always be performed when examining chronic conjunctivitis. If the STT has only been performed late in the disease, it may not be possible to determine whether the KCS is primary or secondary. Despite this uncertainty, therapy must be directed at the tear deficiency to effect an improvement (see Chapter 9). An additional important differential diagnosis for chronic unilateral bacterial conjunctivitis is dacryocystitis.

Blockage of the nasolacrimal duct results in stagnation of tears and bacterial infection that refluxes back into the conjunctival sac (see Chapter 9). Differentiation is based on the results of nasolacrimal duct flushing. Culture and antibiotic sensitivity testing are usually performed if prior antibiotic therapy has been unsuccessful.

Therapy
Specific therapy should consist of controlling systemic or other local disease processes (ectropion, KCS, otitis) and administration of antibiotic or antibiotic–steroid preparations based on culture and antibiotic sensitivity tests. The medication may need to be continued at a low frequency

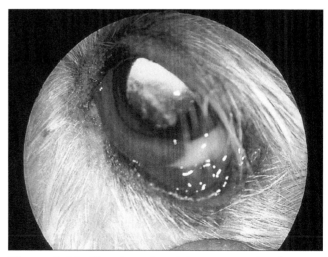

Figure 8.22 Chronic conjunctivitis associated with sicca. The conjunctiva is hyperemic, indurated, and has mucopurulent exudation.

indefinitely or given intermittently as the signs dictate. In many cases of keratoconjunctivitis, the importance of control rather than cure should be emphasized to the owner, and vigorous treatment kept for use in the more "acute" exacerbations. Supportive therapy consists of cleansing the eye with collyrium.

Mycotic conjunctivitis

Introduction/etiology

Mycotic agents are a rare cause of conjunctivitis in the dog and the cat, although *Nocardia* spp., fungi, or yeast have been isolated in 17% of cultures from eyes with chronic conjunctivitis.[109] The significance of finding mycotic elements in the conjunctiva is unknown, as in normal animals, 22% of dogs, 40% of cats, 95% of horses, and 100% of cows culture positively for fungi.[117] This study was performed in a subtropical climate and in a building whose ventilation system was contaminated with fungi, and thus, it may not be representative of other environments. Other studies have found fungal isolates from normal conjunctiva in dogs (12%[108]) and hospitalized and stabled horses (55% and 83%, respectively[115]). The environment was significant in determining the presence of transient flora such as fungi but did not influence the bacterial isolates.[115] In the horse, 53% of the isolates were *Cladosporium* spp. or *Alternaria* spp. In a recent study from Europe, 92% of normal horses showed fungal growth from at least one eye. The most common fungal genera were *Alternaria*, *Eurotium*, *Rhizopus*, and *Cladosporium*. *Aspergillus* spp. and *Penicillium* spp. were isolated frequently, while no *Fusarium* spp. was found.[118]

Animals with mycotic conjunctivitis or keratitis often have a history of treatment with a variety of topical antibiotics or antibiotic–steroid preparations that resulted in temporary improvement and then remained static or regressed (**Figure 8.23**). The horse has a unique susceptibility to fungal infections of the cornea after traumatic breaks in the epithelium. Primary fungal conjunctivitis is rare, even in the horse.

Diagnosis

Diagnosis is initially established by conjunctival cytology and is confirmed by culture (**Figure 8.24**).

Therapy

A variety of antifungal antibiotics are available, but few are marketed for ophthalmic use. Natamycin is the only available topical ophthalmic antifungal preparation and, based on sensitivity testing, is the most effective.[115] The lack of widespread availability and the expense of natamycin

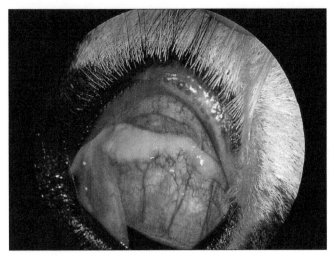

Figure 8.23 Calf with a pseudomembrane adhered to conjunctiva. Cytology and culture demonstrated *Mucor* sp. The calf had systemic mucormycosis with joint and pulmonary signs.

limit its use (see section Fungal, Chapter 10). Intravenous miconazole preparations are well tolerated and are effective as topical ophthalmic preparations, but they have been removed from the market in the United States and must be compounded by a specialty compounding pharmacy. Itraconazole with DMSO[119] and IV fluconazole have also been used topically for fungal keratitis. Topical silver sulfadiazine and other antifungal agents used on other mucous membranes are often used in place of natamycin. Common fungal isolates from healthy horses and horses with keratomycosis demonstrated the best susceptibility to voriconazole (Vfend®, Pfizer).[118]

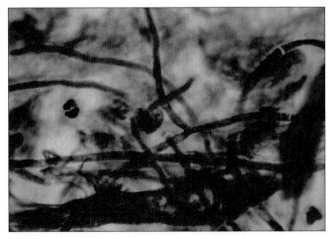

Figure 8.24 Cytology slide of a corneal scraping of a horse with keratomycosis. Note the parallel walls, the septae, and the branching of the fungal hypae.

Parasitic conjunctivitis

Introduction/etiology

Thelazia is a genus of nematode worms that has been recovered from a variety of domestic and wild animals and is usually associated with mild conjunctival irritation. The parasite is widespread in North America, although it is not recognized as producing signs very often. The worms reside within the ducts of the lacrimal glands and on the conjunctival surface. Larvae are released into the tears and ingested by the intermediate host (thought to be *Musca autumnalis*), which transmits it after the larvae develop into the third stage.[120] *Thelazia callipaeda* is thought to be transmitted by *Phortica* flies.[121]

In dogs, *Thelazia callipaeda* has been identified as a frequent cause of conjunctivitis in cattle, dogs, and cats in southern Europe.[122-125]

In cattle, in one postmortem study the highest incidence was in 3- to 4-year-olds, with a 53% infection rate.[126] A similar age predilection was found in younger horses in Kentucky, with a prevalence of 45% in 3-year-olds and 50% in 4-year-olds, with an overall prevalence of 43% for 1- to 4-year-old horses.[127] Other equine studies also indicate the highest incidence is in young horses <1–3 years old.[128,129]

In birds, *Philophthalmus gralli*, a trematode, has been described in the conjunctival sac. The freshwater snail is the intermediate host.[130]

Clinical signs

Infection may be unilateral or bilateral. In cattle, most animals are unilaterally affected, whereas in the horse, most are bilaterally affected. The signs do not seem to be correlated with the worm burden, and most animals are asymptomatic. Signs usually consist of epiphora and conjunctivitis, but conjunctival nodules may be produced by the worms and, rarely, conjunctival cysts and keratitis.[131]

Therapy

Mechanical removal with forceps or flushing the worms out if they are numerous has been the standard recommendation. Most systemic anthelmintics have not been efficacious,[132] but topical application of doramectin (poured on the skin) is effective against eyeworms and other gastrointestinal and pulmonary worms.[133]

Bianciardi and Otranto successfully treated dogs with *Thelazia callipaeda* infestation with a single dermal application of imidacloprid 10% and moxidectin 2.5%.[221] The moxidectin appeared to be the effective agent in the combined product, as imidacloprid by itself was not effective.

KCS-related conjunctivitis

Reduced tear production should be investigated as a cause for all conjunctivitis patients not exhibiting obvious epiphora. STT values below 12–15 mm/min are often associated with variable degrees of conjunctivitis, and the condition may be acute or chronic, unilateral, or bilateral. Varying degrees of mucoid to mucopurulent discharge is typical of KCS-associated conjunctivitis. With chronicity, the hyperemia involves all conjunctival surfaces, and the tissues are thickened. (See Chapter 9 for a detailed discussion of KCS.)

Allergic-/immune-mediated conjunctivitis

Introduction/etiology

Allergic conjunctivitis is probably overdiagnosed as it is often based solely on history and response to steroid therapy.

Clinical signs

The response of the conjunctiva to an allergen is usually a serous discharge and moderate-to-intense hyperemia (**Figure 8.4**). Chemosis, while occasionally dramatic, is usually mild. Pruritus is often present from mast cell degranulation involving the eye and is not expected with most infectious etiologies. Inflammation of the pharynx, gums, and ear canals, a serous rhinitis, and more generalized dermatologic allergic manifestations may be concurrent, and a seasonal incidence may be present.

Topical medicaments are possible antigens, and a sudden increase in ocular irritation after medicating the eye may be indicative of a drug allergy. This should be differentiated from reactions to drugs, which are irritating, as well as from the vasodilatation and reactive hyperemia, which may occur with many of the autonomic drugs.

Diagnosis

Diagnosis of immune-mediated conjunctivitis is frequently presumptive, relying on response to cortisone therapy, history, and accompanying systemic signs. Conjunctival cytology may aid diagnosis with findings of eosinophils, lymphocytes, and plasma cells.

Therapy

If possible, the offending antigen is removed. The most common therapy is low doses of topical steroids if the problem is confined to the eyes, or systemic steroids if signs are more generalized. The least amount of drug, both in concentration and frequency of application, should be employed to control the disease. In mild cases, the use of topical antihistamines may be of value.

Mast cell granule stabilizers such as cromolyn sodium may be effective in treating allergic conjunctivitis; however, their cost and the fact that they are most effective when administered before exposure limits their widespread use. Topical cyclosporine is another alternative to topical glucocorticoids when treating conditions mediated via mast cells and eosinophils. In mice, topical cyclosporine therapy was as effective as topical glucocorticoids for the treatment of allergic conjunctivitis.[134] Topical nonsteroidal drugs have also reduced the signs of seasonal allergic conjunctivitis and are another alternative to glucocorticoids.[135,136]

Eosinophilic conjunctivitis of cats

Introduction/etiology

A condition in cats has been described, characterized by a chronic conjunctivitis that is accompanied by eosinophil and mast cell infiltration of the tissues and, in some cases, by a peripheral eosinophilia.[137] Pentlarge described five cats with this condition, and Allgoewer reported 12 cases.[137,138] This condition may be a variant of eosinophilic keratitis that is associated with herpesvirus; three of the five cats in the Pentlarge series had keratitis. In addition, Larocca reported a case with concurrent herpesvirus and eosinophilic conjunctivitis that developed a dendritic ulcer when glucocorticoid therapy was initiated.[139] The 12 cases in the Allgoewer series, however, had no keratitis, and herpesvirus was not detected by PCR from Schirmer tear strips, although some saliva and nasal swabs were positive (test performed on 8/12). All palpebral conjunctival biopsies (from 6/12) were negative for herpesvirus on electron microscopy. The animals in this series were older (mean 7.2 years) than in the other two series (mean 4 years). All the animals in the Allgoewer and Larocca series had significant blepharitis of the lower lid.

Clinical signs

A severe conjunctivitis is present, involving the bulbar and palpebral conjunctiva of one or both eyes and often months in duration (**Figure 8.25**). The third eyelid conjunctiva may also be affected. Conjunctival papillae develop that produce a granular or cobblestone surface. Modest blepharospasm is often present, and minor amounts of superficial keratitis may develop with chronicity. An erosive blepharitis with depigmentation and swelling may be present involving the lower lid and canthal regions.

Tear production may be decreased with chronicity but is normalized with appropriate therapy. Marked conjunctival chemosis is thought to obstruct the lacrimal ductules.

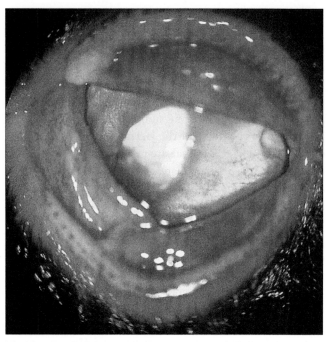

Figure 8.25 Chronic unilateral eosinophilic conjunctivitis in a cat. The condition was diagnosed by conjunctival cytology and responded to topical glucocorticoids. (Courtesy of Dr. V. Pentlarge, Athens, GA.)

Diagnosis

Diagnosis is based on conjunctival cytology or biopsy that has numerous eosinophils and mast cells or mast cell granules. If decreased STT values are present, they may mislead the clinician into misdiagnosing a primary KCS. Presumptive evidence is based on the response to glucocorticoid therapy and lack of response to antibiotic therapy.

Therapy

- Topical glucocorticoids given frequently initially and then tapered down for indefinite duration maintenance therapy.
- Topical inhibitors of mast cell degranulation, such as cromolyn sodium or lodoxamide, may also be indicated as well as topical cyclosporine.
- Artificial tears if KCS is present and until it is resolved with the reduction of swelling.
- Topical antiviral therapy should be considered if a keratitis is present or develops with the use of glucocorticoid therapy.

Actinic-related conjunctivitis

All species with lightly pigmented lid margins and lack of pigmentation of the third eyelid are predisposed to solar blepharitis and conjunctivitis, that if chronic may result in squamous cell carcinoma (SCC) formation. Similarly, patients with SCC characteristically have a moderate-to-severe conjunctivitis that is more diffuse than simple mechanical irritation would produce. The reason for this is not clear, but it may be due to factors liberated from the neoplasm.

Lipogranuloma
Introduction/etiology

White nodular lesions of one or both eyes have been described in older cats. The lesion may be single or multiple and involve one or both eyes, and it is associated with conjunctivitis (**Figure 8.26**). Read and Lucas described the condition in 21 eyes of 13 cats and found a mean age of 11 years and a preference for involvement of the palpebral conjunctiva of the lower lid.[140] On histopathology, the lesion is a lipogranuloma, but the source of the lipids is unknown. Potential sources are the meibomian glands, adipose tissue in the conjunctiva, systemic hyperlipidemia, or exogenous lipids from medications.[141] Read and Lucas postulated that the lipids originate from the meibomian glands because of their consistent location near the lid margin and inclusion of ruptured meibomian glands in some of the biopsies. The relative high frequency in Australia and in lighter pigment animals may indicate UV radiation may have a contributing role.

Therapy

Curettage of lesions from the conjunctival side and topical glucocorticoids has been curative. Since the cause is not known, a thorough ocular and systemic examination should be performed.

Ligneous conjunctivitis
Introduction/etiology

Ligneous conjunctivitis is a rare form of chronic membranous conjunctivitis. Currently, it is usually found in the Doberman pinscher. The signs are very dramatic, chronic, and resistant to conventional therapy. The cause is unknown, but the disease has systemic implications as oral, respiratory, and renal disease may also be present. On histopathology, the conjunctival blood vessel endothelium has multilaminar basement membranes, suggesting increased permeability. A thick, amorphous, hyaline-like membrane is present in the substantia propria of the conjunctiva and contains T-lymphocytes.[142] In humans, it has recently been linked to a familial deficiency of plasminogen.[143]

The deficiency of plasminogen results in disruption of the fibrinolytic pathway. This allows fibrin to accumulate, with minor trauma due to impaired proteolysis, and the surface is arrested at the granulation stage. Johnstone et al. described a 7-month-old Golden retriever with ligneous conjunctivitis that repeatedly had low circulating plasminogen levels that responded to systemic fresh frozen plasma and surgical resection but not to topical fresh frozen plasma.[222] Torres et al. described a case in a Yorkshire terrier that was moderately responsive to topical cyclosporine, tacrolimus, and glucocorticoids.[223]

Clinical signs

Ligneous conjunctivitis is characterized by bilateral, marked, firm swelling of the conjunctival surfaces (including third eyelid) with gray membranes covering the surface (**Figure 8.27**). The membranes are firmly adherent, and attempts to peel them off result in hemorrhage. The cornea eventually becomes involved with pannus formation, but it is often surprisingly healthy considering the

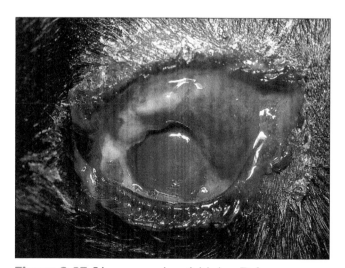

Figure 8.27 Ligneous conjunctivitis in a Doberman pinscher. Note the dramatic swelling of the conjunctiva that was firm with a relatively normal cornea. The dog also had oral and skin lesions and eventually developed a keratitis. The condition was nonresponsive to topical therapies.

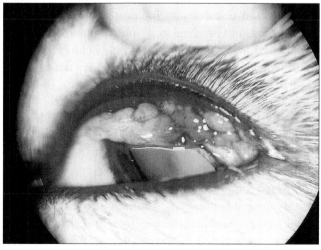

Figure 8.26 Unilateral lipogranuloma in a cat.

dramatic conjunctival lesions. Systemic signs relating to the oral cavity and the respiratory and/or urinary system may be present.

Diagnosis

Diagnosis of ligneous conjunctivitis is made by the dramatic signs of a thick membranous conjunctivitis occurring in a Doberman pinscher. Biopsy of the lesion confirms the nature of the membranes.

Therapy

Ligneous conjunctivitis has been resistant to conventional conjunctivitis therapy. The most successful therapy has been systemic prednisolone and azathioprine, with topical cyclosporine. In humans, an infant was successfully treated with IV lys-plasminogen.[143] The Golden retriever with a plasminogen deficiency described previously responded to IV fresh frozen plasma but not to topical plasma. The half-life of plasminogen is about 24 hours, so daily IV injections of fresh frozen plasma were given. In addition to surgical debridement, topical fresh frozen plasma, tissue plasminogen activator, topical cyclosporine, heparin, and corticosteroids were administered. Cessation of the systemic fresh frozen plasma resulted in relapse of signs. However, the frequency of administration and the cost and availability of fresh frozen plasma limit this modality of therapy.

Conjunctivitis secondary to physical irritation

Introduction/etiology

Conjunctivitis due to irritation is usually mild to modest in severity, with a serous to mucoid exudation. The factors for irritation can be endogenous or exogenous. Endogenous sources are usually aberrant anatomic relationships such as trichiasis, distichiasis, entropion, ectropion, exophthalmos, lagophthalmos, and nasal folds. The cornea may be involved, with an ulcerative or superficial keratitis. Exogenous factors may be foreign bodies of various forms, from fiberglass to plant awns. Dust and wind are common irritants. Hunting dogs that are frequently in the water may have problems with their eyes and ears throughout the working season.

Diagnosis

Diagnosis is based mainly on history and exclusion of other causes. Endogenous irritations are often obvious on detailed examination. Exogenous sources of irritation are usually bilateral unless due to a foreign body.

Therapy

Removal of the source of irritation is usually curative, although a topical antibiotic–steroid preparation is usually used if corneal ulceration is not present.

Differential diagnosis of causes of conjunctivitis

In general, serous-to-mucoid discharge of acute duration is suggestive of an irritant, allergic, or viral cause and not a bacterial cause. Chronic serous-to-mucoid discharge is generally the same etiology, although bacterial components are probably emerging as contributing factors. If the discharge is mucopurulent, this suggests definite bacterial association or complications; in addition, the status of the tear secretion should be evaluated.

The cause of conjunctivitis is determined by the history, conjunctival cytology and culture, STT, and detailed examination of the eye and the adnexa. Mechanical factors such as distichiasis must be evaluated based on whether their presence correlates with the location and the extent of signs. Entropion may cause conjunctivitis or be produced by conjunctival irritation; therefore, both eyes should be evaluated.

Differential diagnosis of conjunctivitis from other ocular disease

Conjunctivitis is the most common ocular diagnosis in practice, but it is important to avoid overdiagnosing it and undertreating a more serious intraocular syndrome. Conjunctivitis produces a "red eye," and the emphasis is usually on differentiating it from other conditions that produce conjunctival hyperemia. Conjunctivitis must be differentiated from anterior uveitis and glaucoma. Scleritis and episcleritis are also important diseases that may mimic conjunctivitis. Differentiation of intraocular disease from conjunctivitis is important but is usually not difficult in most instances if the clinician looks beyond the hyperemic conjunctiva (**Table 8.5**). The error of not observing is much more common than observing and not correctly interpreting signs.

Uncomplicated conjunctivitis does not involve the interior of the eye; therefore, signs such as anisocoria, appreciable variation of ocular tension, anterior chamber flare, and decreased visual acuity indicate intraocular disease. The cornea is not involved in simple conjunctivitis, but in complicated or chronic cases, a keratoconjunctivitis may be present. Thus, clarity of the cornea may not be a differentiating factor between intraocular disease and complicated conjunctivitis.

Pain is quite variable in all the categories, and if present with conjunctivitis, corneal ulceration should be looked for with fluorescein stain. Patients with conjunctivitis often do not exhibit pain, but when present, pain is mild to modest and in humans is described as "like having sand or grit in the eye(s)." Anterior uveitis, especially of acute onset, has appreciable pain, but in chronic cases, pain may not be noted. Glaucoma has variable amounts of pain ranging from severe to not appreciable. Ocular pain

Table 8.5 **Differential diagnosis of conjunctival hyperemia.**

	ANTERIOR UVEITIS	CONJUNCTIVITIS	GLAUCOMA
Conjunctiva	Not thickened; episcleral vessels easily seen	Thick, folded, and hyperemic; episcleral vessels concealed	Not thickened
Conjunctival vessels	Selective injection of large	Diffuse injection of conjunctival vessels, usually palpebral	Selective injection of large conjunctival vessels
Secretion or discharge	Often serous	Serous to mucopurulent	Often serous
Pain	Moderate (acute)	None to slight	Subtle, behavior changes
Photophobia	Moderate	Mild	Slight
Cornea	Variable degree of edema	Clear	Variable degree of edema
Pupil size	Small, sluggish, irregular, or fixed	Normal	Dilated, moderate to complete, fixed
Pupillary light response	Poor	Normal	Absent
Intraocular pressure	If uncomplicated will be low	Normal	Elevated

may not only be manifested locally by blepharospasm and retraction of the globe in the orbit but also by changes in behavior such as excessive sleeping or lethargy, rubbing the eye on the ground, and worsening of temperament. Ocular discharge of variable character may be found with all three conditions.

Conjunctival vascular injection or congestion is present in both conjunctivitis and intraocular disease. The pattern of vascular congestion varies on close examination. In conjunctivitis, the palpebral conjunctiva is most commonly hyperemic, and the bulbar conjunctiva, when involved, is most severely hyperemic near the fornix, decreasing toward the limbus (**Figure 8.28**). The hyperemia of conjunctivitis is diffuse, involving even small caliber vessels.

In glaucoma and anterior uveitis, deep congestion is very noticeable just posterior to the limbus in the episcleral vessels and scleral venous plexus that lie under the conjunctiva. The conjunctival vessels, which are engorged, are the numerous veins that drain the deeper scleral veins (**Figure 8.29**). The conjunctiva between the draining veins is not diffusely hyperemic, as would be expected with conjunctivitis. Episcleritis/scleritis has a similar selective large conjunctival venous engorgement, and in addition, the episclera is thickened to nodular, obscuring the scleral veins (**Figure 8.30**). Episcleritis/scleritis often involves the peripheral cornea with a rim of edema and neovascularization. An anterior uveitis may be present with deep scleritis.

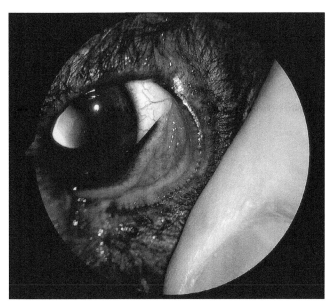

Figure 8.28 Diffuse conjunctival hyperemia, primarily of the palpebral conjunctiva, that is typical of most cases of atopic conjunctivitis in dogs.

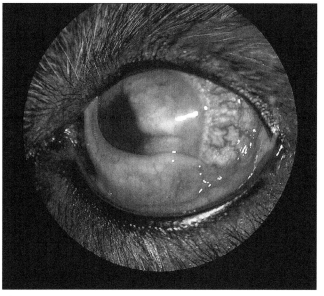

Figure 8.29 Selective conjunctival injection of the large vessels and the deeper episcleral vessels in a dog with secondary glaucoma (lymphosarcoma related). This vascular pattern is typical of intraocular disease.

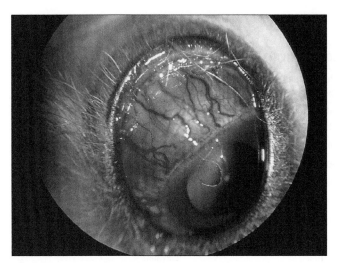

Figure 8.30 A dog with selective vascular injection with thickening of the episcleral tissue typical of episcleritis. Note the thin peripheral rim of corneal edema and early neovascularization.

The pupil is a sensitive indicator of the presence of intraocular disease. Unilateral intraocular disease produces anisocoria. In general, glaucoma dilates the pupil, and anterior uveitis contracts the pupil. Prior drug therapy, synechiae, iris atrophy, and denervation may alter the pupil. No change is expected with simple conjunctivitis.

Principles of therapy

When treating routine superficial infections of the eye such as conjunctivitis, it is a good principle to use an antibiotic or a combination of antibiotics, which are not generally administered systemically. This decreases the possibility of sensitizing the patient to a drug, which may have some value in future systemic administration. Also, the indiscriminate use of potent antibiotics is more likely to result in resistant strains of bacteria and, as a result, may eliminate future effectiveness in systemic therapy

Topical therapy is adequate in most instances, and the frequency and the duration of therapy varies depending on the severity and the chronicity of the infection. Most simple cases of acute bacterial conjunctivitis respond to therapy every 6–8 hours for 7–10 days, whereas chronic cases may require an intermittent or continuous low-frequency therapy for prolonged periods of time if the underlying cause cannot be determined or removed.

TRAUMA-ASSOCIATED CONDITIONS

Subconjunctival hemorrhage

Introduction/etiology

Subconjunctival hemorrhage is a common, often dramatic lesion, but is of little consequence. However, it signals that

possible ocular trauma has occurred or systemic disease may be present. Both eyes and the head should be examined for other evidence of trauma and a good physical examination carried out for clues of systemic disease. Owners often presume trauma when they observe hemorrhage, and unless the trauma has been observed, or there is other evidence such as abrasions of the head, it is often best to rule out other etiologies and diagnose trauma by exclusion.

In neonatal foals, 8% may have subconjunctival hemorrhage, usually in the dorsal conjunctiva. The presence of subconjunctival hemorrhage is related to foaling difficulty and is more common in multiparous mares that foal more rapidly. The hemorrhage resolves spontaneously and has no long-term implications.[144]

Causes of subconjunctival hemorrhage include:

- Trauma: Subconjunctival hemorrhage most commonly originates from direct trauma, but choking injuries creating elevated intravascular pressure in the head may produce subconjunctival hemorrhage.
- Blood dyscrasias and bleeding or clotting deficiency: Due to neoplasm, toxin, infection, or autoimmune origin.
- Vasculitis: May be either infectious, immune-, or neoplastic-mediated.

Clinical signs

A variable amount of blood is present under the bulbar conjunctiva; this can be either unilateral or bilateral. Depending on the duration of the hemorrhage, the color ranges from bright red (acute) to blue-green (reabsorbing stage). The hemorrhage(s) may be petechial or be flat with little conjunctival elevation. In severe cases, the conjunctiva is elevated (**Figures 8.31–8.33**). Occasionally,

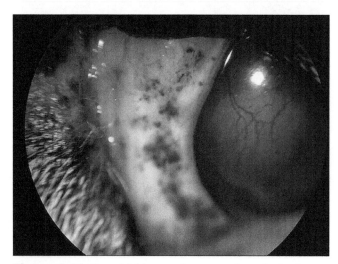

Figure 8.31 Petechial hemorrhages on the palpebral surface of the third eyelid in a dog with immune-mediated thrombocytopenia.

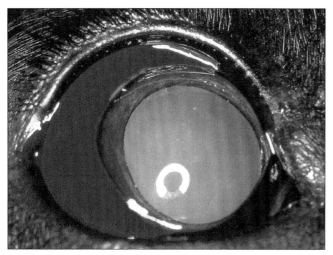

Figure 8.32 Acute, diffuse subconjunctival hemorrhage in a puppy with a strangulation injury.

retro-orbital hemorrhage may dissect rostrally to the subconjunctival space and present with additional signs of anterior displacement of the globe, decreased retropulsion of the globe, and prolapse of the third eyelid.

Diagnosis

A definite history of observed trauma or other evidence of trauma to the head should be present rather than assumed. Alternatively, trauma is diagnosed by exclusion by performing a complete ocular and physical examination and searching for additional evidence of bleeding or coagulation defects. When trauma is the cause of subconjunctival hemorrhage, it is a warning that other ocular structures may have been disrupted, and a complete ocular examination of both eyes should be performed for accurate prognosis.

Therapy

Specific therapy for hemorrhage is not given unless the underlying etiology is treatable. Cold compresses may be given in the peracute stage. Trauma to the lids and the conjunctiva may be a destabilizing stress to the host's mucous membranes, and a secondary bacterial conjunctivitis may develop and need treatment with antibiotics. Most cases of traumatic origin do not require any therapy, although antibiotics are often administered as a placebo to satisfy the owner.

Lacerations

Most lacerations confined to the conjunctiva and less than 0.5–1 cm will probably heal rapidly without suturing. If the conjunctival insertion of the third eyelid is torn, suturing is frequently necessary, as the tissues do not remain in apposition. If suturing is necessary, 6-0 absorbable sutures are utilized.

Subconjunctival prolapse of orbital fat

Either congenital defects, senile weakness, or traumatic rupture of the orbital septum may allow orbital fat to prolapse under the conjunctiva. This presents as dorsal or ventral, smooth, nonirritating swelling. The condition may be unilateral or bilateral, and it has been observed more often in large animals than in the dog or the cat. In cattle, subconjunctival orbital fat is commonly observed dorsally when the dorsal lid is retracted, and the eye is rolled ventrally. In the horse, the author has repeatedly observed prolapse of orbital fat after third eyelid excision for SCC (**Figure 8.34**). The condition may be surgically corrected by excision and suturing the orbital septum or ignored.

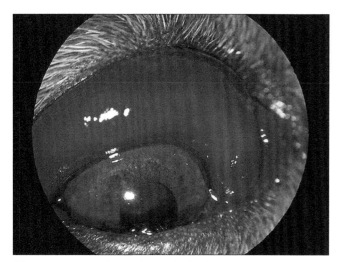

Figure 8.33 A dog with marked subconjunctival hemorrhage due to dicoumarol poisoning. Retrobulbar hemorrhage had dissected anteriorly into the subconjunctival space.

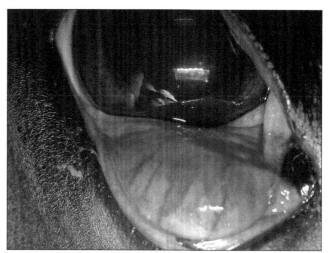

Figure 8.34 Prolapsed orbital fat in the lower conjunctival cul-de-sac of an older horse. The third eyelid was rudimentary or had been excised (possibly for squamous cell carcinoma). The owner had just purchased the horse, so no history was available.

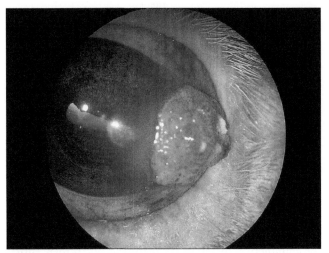

Figure 8.35 Squamous cell carcinoma on the temporal limbus of a cow. This is the most common site of occurrence of SCC in cattle. Note the lack of periocular and lid pigmentation.

Neoplasia

Neoplasia of the conjunctival surface is most common in the horse and the cow and is discussed further with third eyelid and corneal neoplasia. The most common neoplasm of the conjunctiva in large animals is SCC (**Figure 8.35**). The occurrence of SCC in general is thought to be related to ultraviolet (UV) radiation and genetic susceptibility that in part is related to periocular and eyelid pigmentation.[145–147] In susceptible herds, the incidence of SCC was >50% in cattle over 7 years of age.[147] Clearly, advising on genetic selection must be an important factor in treating herds with SCC. On a molecular basis, mutations of the p53 tumor suppression gene have been implicated in UV-related skin cancers. The p53 tumor suppressor gene monitors the genome and regulates the cell cycle, delaying DNA replication if DNA is damaged. Mutant p53 may result in uncontrolled cell growth and selection of malignant clones.[148] Overexpression of the p53 gene has been demonstrated in SCC of the horse, the cow, the cat, and the dog.[148,149]

As SCCs have a strong genetic and environmental component, it is best to explain to the owners that SCC is a treatable but not a curable disease. The individual lesion may be cured, but new lesions are likely to develop elsewhere. Periodic rechecks are critical.

Lymphoma in the horse and the cow may produce a bilateral conjunctival infiltration that manifests as chemosis or swelling without significant redness (**Figure 8.36**).

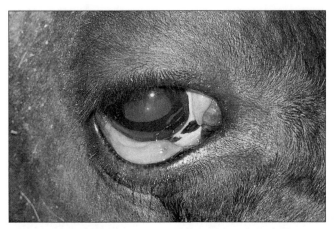

Figure 8.36 A Holstein cow with conjunctival swelling due to lymphosarcoma that mimics chemosis. Note the lack of hyperemia and tearing. The condition was bilateral, and peripheral lymphadenopathy was present.

In one study of lymphoma in the horse, the eye and the adnexa were involved in 20% of cases, and infiltration of the conjunctiva was the most common ocular lesion.[150] On physical examination, a marked lymphadenopathy is usually present that associates the conjunctival swelling with lymphoma, but the ocular lesion may precede overt systemic involvement.[150,151]

Mast cell tumors involving conjunctival surfaces have been observed by the author in the dog, the cat, and the horse (**Figure 8.37**). Subconjunctival masses in the dog are chronic and apparently benign, in that they respond to surgical excision.[152,224] Conjunctival mast cell tumors and hemangiosarcomas may in general be more benign in behavior than their respective type in other locations, but they still deserve to be treated aggressively and followed closely.

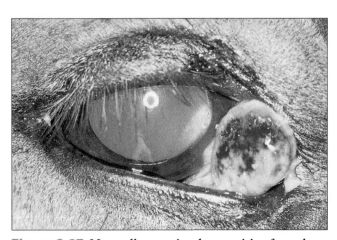

Figure 8.37 Mast cell tumor in a horse arising from the palpebral conjunctiva. It was treated by excision and beta radiation therapy.

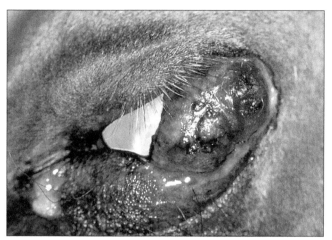

Figure 8.38 Conjunctival melanoma invading the cornea in a horse. The lesion had previously been resected, and it relapsed after further resection and adjunctive diode laser therapy.

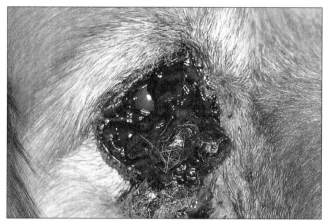

Figure 8.40 Massive conjunctival melanoma that had previously been excised in an elderly mixed breed dog. Enucleation was performed.

Conjunctival melanoma is fortunately infrequent, since it is probably the most aggressive form of melanoma that arises from ocular tissue. In the horse, melanoma of the conjunctiva has rarely been reported, so insufficient data on malignancy are available (**Figure 8.38**).[153,225] Conjunctival melanomas frequently involve the cornea by the time of presentation and must be differentiated from epibulbar melanoma that is progressing into the cornea and intraocular melanoma that has penetrated the sclera. Canine and feline conjunctival melanoma is locally aggressive and may metastasize.[154–156] The third eyelid is the most common location for conjunctival melanoma of the dog (**Figures 8.39 and 8.40**). Recurrence after surgical excision is common, and the preferred therapy appears to be surgical excision followed by cryotherapy.

Conjunctival vascular tumors are most common in the dog and the horse. The vascular lesions may range from small areas of telangiectasia (angiokeratoma) to hemangioma and hemangiosarcoma. Angiokeratoma is a small, localized, red, raised lesion that does not progress and may be found on the conjunctiva or third eyelid (**Figure 8.41**).[157,158] Hemangiomas and hemangiosarcomas arise from the temporal limbal region and the third eyelid, perhaps reflecting the relationship to solar radiation exposure (**Figure 8.42**). In the horse, hemangioma has been reported[159] but is uncommon. Lesions are usually hemangiosarcomas and should be considered malignant; they frequently metastasize to the regional lymph nodes (**Figure 8.43**).[160,161] Hemangiosarcomas should be treated by enucleation rather than excision. Wide excision is usually not possible, and hemangiosarcomas appear resistant to adjunctive therapy of radiation, cryotherapy, chemotherapy, or immunotherapy. Murphy et al. reported bilateral hemangioma in a dog.[162] Conjunctival hemangioma and hemangiosarcoma may recur in the dog, but metastasis has not been reported.[162,163,226] The author has

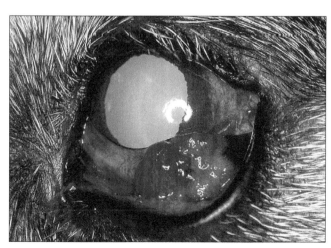

Figure 8.39 Conjunctival melanoma arising from the third eyelid in a 13-year-old dog.

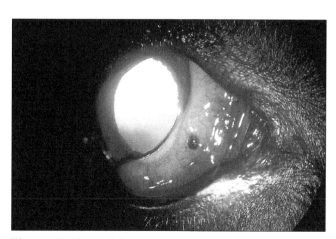

Figure 8.41 Angiokeratoma in a 9-year-old mixed breed dog.

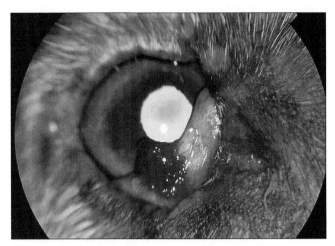

Figure 8.42 Hemangioma of the third eyelid in an 11-year-old Brittany.

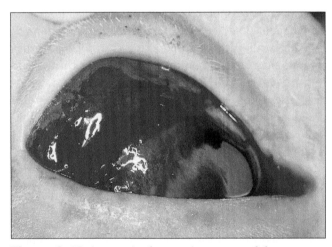

Figure 8.43 Aggressive hemangiosarcoma of the temporal conjunctiva in an elderly white horse. The prognosis is guarded.

noted very aggressive canine conjunctival hemangiosarcomas on histopathology specimens that invaded the globe, and thus not all would appear to be benign in behavior. Therapy should be wide excision, and if this is not possible, enucleation.

MISCELLANEOUS CONJUNCTIVAL DISEASES

Ectopic lacrimal gland tissue

Ectopic lacrimal gland tissue has been described under the dorsal conjunctiva and involving the cornea of a 4-month-old German shepherd dog (GSD).[164] Excisional biopsy was curative.

Inclusion cysts

Inclusion cysts in the conjunctiva have been reported in the dog.[162] They appear as smooth, relatively small, cystic

structures that are diagnosed and treated by excisional biopsy. The cause is unknown, although trauma and therapy with ointments have been suggested.

Conjunctival overgrowth

A condition of progressive covering of the cornea by an overgrowth of bulbar conjunctiva may be observed in rabbits. The dwarf or dwarf-cross rabbit may be predisposed. The conjunctiva is not adherent and consists of a fold of redundant bulbar conjunctiva that progressively covers the cornea over several weeks. Simple excision usually results in regrowth. The cause is unknown, and therapy has consisted of excision combined with topical cyclosporine.[165] Allgoewer et al. reported on six dwarf rabbits with the syndrome treated successfully with six radial incisions around the circumference of the overgrowth and then retracted with six transpalpebral sutures.[227] The sutures were placed from the external lid into the fornix and then into the central extent of the overgrown conjunctiva, back out through the lid, and tied. The sutures were left in place for 3 or more weeks. No recurrences were noted.

CONGENITAL DISEASES OF THE THIRD EYELID

Eversion

Eversion of the third eyelid is a sporadic and benign condition found in developing large breed dogs. In the German shorthair pointer, it is thought to be inherited as a recessive trait, but the inheritance is unknown in other breeds.[166] The deformity has been postulated to be due to either unequal growth rates of the two conjunctival surfaces or a primary deformity of the cartilage. Everted cartilage has been described as a genetic deformity seen in the Burmese cat, but it is not clear whether it develops with growth (as in the dog), due to the variation in ages at presentation.[167]

Clinical signs
Everted cartilage manifests as either unilateral or bilateral scrolling forward of the free margin of the third eyelid (**Figure 8.44**). A serous ocular discharge is usually present, and initially, the conjunctival surface is very hyperemic. The condition persists indefinitely, although in some instances it improves spontaneously with growth. Chronic cases develop pigmentation of the surface and become less noticeable.

Diagnosis
Identification of the free margin of the everted cartilage and demonstration of the scrolling may be performed

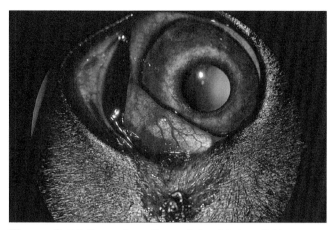

Figure 8.44 Everted cartilage of the third eyelid in a young Great Dane. A scrolling forward of the free margin is present, and the gland is not visible. A seromucoid discharge is present.

with forceps. Occasionally, eversion of the cartilage may be combined with a prolapsed gland. The main differential diagnosis is prolapse of the gland of the third eyelid, which is more common.

Therapy
If the dog is 3–4 months of age, it may be advisable to wait for spontaneous improvement and treat the ocular irritation with topical steroids. Most cases do not improve spontaneously, and surgical correction is necessary to make a cosmetic improvement. Surgery consists of removing the bent portion of the cartilage through the bulbar conjunctiva, while preserving the pigmented free margin[168,169] and then suturing as a third eyelid flap to the upper lid or globe during the healing process. The placement of the third eyelid over the globe allows the tissues to heal with a normal curvature rather than allowing the free margin to be loose and floppy. A very elegant method has recently been published, in which the deformation of the cartilage is corrected by thermal cautery.[170] The major advantage of this procedure is that the cartilage is not incised or excised.

Coloboma
A notch defect that bisects the third eyelid has been observed in the horse and the dog. The defect is bilateral and occurs with other congenital ocular anomalies such as corneal dermoids and coloboma of the optic nerve. The defect results in a reduced protective capability. Improvement can be made cosmetically by making an incision along the coloboma and suturing the opposing edges. The third eyelid gland may be prolapsed with the defect and may need reducing.

Nonpigmented margin
Introduction/etiology
The free margins of one or both third eyelids may be non-pigmented. This condition is often associated with other albinoid features such as blue irises, white hair, and pink skin.

Clinical signs
The lack of a pigmented border to the third eyelid is usually most obvious when it is unilateral and the contrast between the two eyes is noted (**Figure 8.45**). Patients often present for ocular irritation due to the obvious pinkness, but this may be more apparent than real. The nonpigmented conjunctiva is more prone to actinic radiation and, perhaps, carcinoma. Bilateral large corneoconjunctival dermoids associated with bilateral dermoids of the nasal planum were reported in an Angus/Hereford calf. The dermoids in both sites contained ectopic glandular tissue.[228]

Diagnosis
Diagnosis is by observation.

Therapy
Usually, symptomatic treatment of the conjunctivitis is given in the form of low-dose topical steroids or a decongestant. Tattooing of the third eyelid margin is not necessary or permanent in most instances.

Dermoid
Dermoids involving the conjunctiva may be restricted to the conjunctiva or involve the cornea and/or the eyelid. The condition is usually recognized by finding a raised island of hairs, and this is easily removed (**Figure 8.46**)

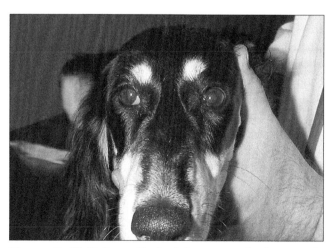

Figure 8.45 Unilateral lack of pigment on the free margin of the third eyelid in a Saluki. The asymmetrical pink tissue draws the observer's eye to that side of the head.

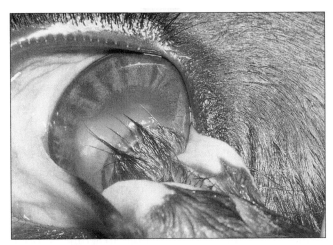

Figure 8.46 A dermoid in an Aberdeen Angus calf involving the third eyelid and cornea.

Table 8.6 **Breed predispositions to diseases of the conjunctiva and nictitating membrane.**

CONJUNCTIVAL DISEASE	PREDISPOSED BREED
Ligneous conjunctivitis	Doberman pinscher[142,143]
Eversion of the nictitans	German shorthair pointer[166]
Dermoids	Burmese cat
	German shepherd
	Saint Bernard
	Dachshund
	Cattle[171–174]
Prolapse of the gland of the third eye lid	American Cocker Spaniel
	English Bulldog
	Boston terrier
	Lhasa Apso
	Shih Tzu
	Beagle
	Pekingese
Plasma cell conjunctivitis	German shepherd (crosses)[183]

(see Chapter 10). Dermoids are sporadic and relatively uncommon. They are reported to be inherited in the Burmese cat and, perhaps, the GSD, Saint Bernard, and dachshund, and in cattle.[171–174]

ACQUIRED DISEASES OF THE THIRD EYELID

Prolapse of third eyelid gland (cherry eye)

Introduction/etiology

Prolapse of third eyelid gland is a disease of young dogs, from 4 weeks to 2 years of age. Cats rarely exhibit the condition,[175] apart from the Burmese.[167,171,174] A unilateral or bilateral prolapse of the gland may appear as a red mass in the medial canthus. The prolapse is sudden in onset, but it may regress once or twice for a few days, and finally, it returns to remain for the animal's life. Certain breeds such as the American Cocker Spaniel, English bulldog, Boston terrier, Lhasa Apso, Shih Tzu, beagle, and Pekingese are more prone to develop the condition (**Table 8.6**). These are largely the same breeds that are prone to develop KCS. The etiology is unknown, and there is disagreement as to whether inflammation predisposes the animal to prolapse. Dugan et al. found only mild surface inflammation associated with prolapse in the beagle.[176] The histologic features in the gland may vary between breeds predisposed to KCS and those not predisposed, such as the beagle. Severin, without evidence, suggested that the condition is due to weak fibrous structures that normally hold the gland in place.[177]

Under certain circumstances, cherry eye may appear to be infectious. Several dogs housed in proximity may develop the condition, and, occasionally, a febrile patient with depression, tonsillitis, and partial anorexia may develop a cherry eye. Usually there is no history of systemic involvement.

Protrusion of the gland of the third eyelid is occasionally observed in older animals, and these animals should be investigated for orbital disease using the history and a physical examination. Cherry eye has been observed in dogs after orbital cellulitis and in dogs with orbital neoplasia.

Clinical signs

Sudden development of a red mass at the medial canthus is the most dramatic sign (**Figures 8.47 and 8.48**). Acute cases often have a mucopurulent discharge and may have reduced tear production.[176] Chronic cases develop pigmentation of the conjunctival surface, and

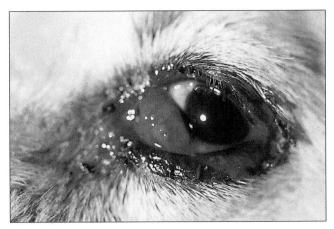

Figure 8.47 Prolapsed gland of the third eyelid in a young American Cocker Spaniel. The condition was bilateral. Note the mucopurulent exudate that can accompany a transient sicca or secondary bacterial infection.

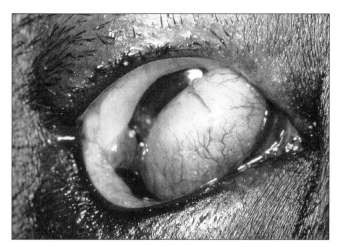

Figure 8.48 Very large prolapsed gland of the third eyelid in a Shar Pei. Note the puffy conjunctiva that is typical of this breed.

the gland becomes less noticeable. Corneal ulceration rarely develops as a complication. Usually there are no deleterious effects to the eye except for the risk of developing KCS.

Diagnosis

Diagnosis of a prolapsed third eyelid gland is made by observation of a red mass protruding over the free margin of the third eyelid.

Therapy

Initial treatment with a topical antibiotic/steroid preparation may appear transiently to cause the gland to become replaced. Prolapse may occur two or three times, and eventually the gland remains prolapsed.

Excision Although not recommended by veterinary ophthalmologists, excision of the gland is still practiced by some general practitioners. Excision is not the preferred method used by veterinary ophthalmologists, as patients that have been treated by glandular excision and subsequently develop KCS are frequently observed. Morgan et al. found that 48% of 27 eyes treated by glandular excision developed KCS within 0.5–6 years of surgery.[178] In dogs that had the gland replaced, 14% developed KCS, and 42% developed KCS if the gland remained prolapsed. When only the high-risk breeds for KCS were evaluated, 59% developed KCS with excision of the gland, 17% with gland replacement, and 75% when no treatment was given.

Repositioning the gland Because of the risk of KCS, various techniques have been developed for replacing and anchoring the gland in a more correct anatomic position.

A desirable technique should not only reposition the gland but also spare the ducts on the bulbar surface. Moore et al. investigated the location of the ducts of the third eyelid gland and found multiple ducts all exited onto the posterior surface with the lymphoid follicles.[179] Thus, any technique that debrides the posterior surface to create adhesions may obliterate the ducts. Tacking the gland to the orbital rim (**Figures 8.49 and 8.50**) gives good results if the gland is well anchored to the orbital rim.[180,181] The modification of Stanley and Kaswan allows easier placement of the critical orbital rim anchor.

Anchoring techniques are relatively difficult to perform and may fail if incorrectly performed. The risk of infection is probably higher when a monofilament suture is buried. Postoperatively, dogs with large palpebral fissures may have the third eyelid more prominent.

Pocket technique on the bulbar surface of the third eyelid (**Figure 8.51**) Two parallel incisions into the bulbar conjunctival surface on either side of the prolapsed gland are created, and the bases of these incisions are joined with a simple continuous suture. When the suture is tightened, the gland is forced ventrally. The knots may be tied on the outside surface by taking a preliminary bite at the beginning and at the end of the suture pattern on the outside surface. The two incisions should not connect; this avoids formation of a retention cyst. This technique was 94% successful in one study.[178] The most common complications are recurrence, a corneal ulcer from the suture knots, and a retention cyst (**Figure 8.52**). The author has seen a recurrence of prolapse 1–2 years after replacement, and the surgical adhesions were still in place.

Unfortunately, all the surgical techniques for gland replacement may have the complication of re-prolapse. Some breeds such as the English bulldog, Shar Pei, and Neapolitan mastiff are more prone to this complication.

Follicular conjunctivitis of the third eyelid

Introduction/etiology

Follicular conjunctivitis occurs primarily in dogs. Some forms of conjunctivitis have a pronounced follicular reaction, and the third eyelid is preferentially involved due to hyperplasia of the normal follicles on the bulbar surface. The cause is unknown but is generally considered to be due to chronic antigenic stimulation in the dog. In the cat (*Chlamydophila felis*, herpesvirus), the horse (*Onchocerca*

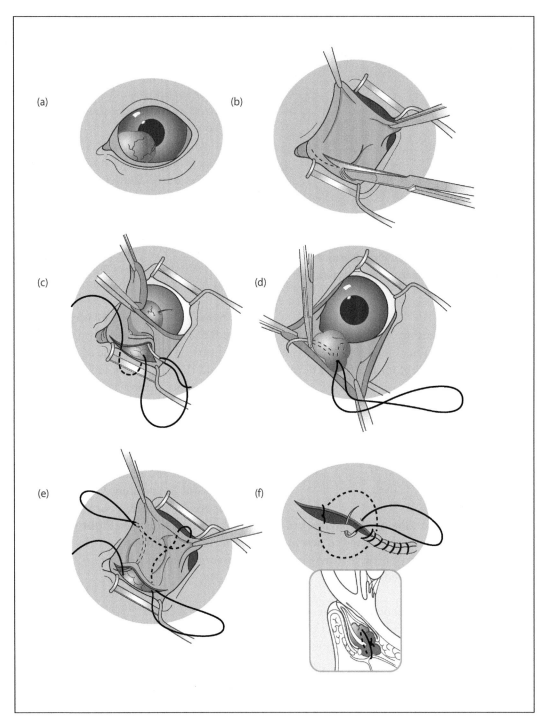

Figure 8.49 Tacking of the prolapsed gland to the orbital rim in a dog. This requires general anesthesia. Prolapsed gland of third eyelid (a). Scissors are used to cut the fornix of the conjunctiva in front of the third eyelid (b). A 1-0 or 2-0 monofilament suture with a cutting needle is used to place the anchoring portion of the suture to the periosteum of the rim of the orbit (c). This is the most critical step and may be guided by a finger on the skin side. If anchored correctly, the suture is very firm when tugged. The needle is then passed from the outer surface of the third eyelid to the inner side, emerging on the top and to one side of the prolapsed gland. The needle is then passed back into the hole so that little if any exposed suture is present, and the needle is passed across to the opposite side of the top of the gland (d). The needle is then redirected back into the tract and down to emerge in the original incision and tied (e). Cross section of the third eyelid with gland pulled down and anchored to the rim of the orbit (f).

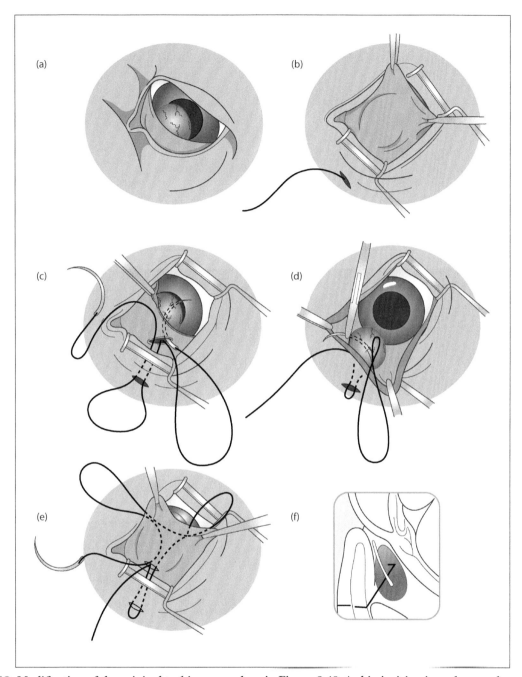

Figure 8.50 Modification of the original tacking procedure in Figure 8.48. A skin incision is made over the medial ventral orbital rim (a, b), and the suture is anchored to the periosteum (c). The orbital rim is closer to the skin in larger dogs, and it is easier to place the anchoring bite from this vantage point than from the conjunctival fornix. The remaining suture pattern is similar to the original procedure (d–f).

spp.), and cattle (herpesvirus), infectious agents may be responsible. Follicular formation in the horse is typically perilimbal.

Any chronic antigenic stimulation to the conjunctival surfaces is thought to be capable of initiating follicular hyperplasia. Other mucous membranes such as the prepuce or the vagina may have similar proliferations. A herpesvirus has been discounted as an etiology in the dog.[43,44]

Clinical signs

Dogs are usually presented with a serous ocular discharge, hyperemia, and, in addition, marked follicular hyperplasia on both conjunctival surfaces of the third eyelid and often the remaining conjunctiva (**Figure 8.53**). Some dogs may have blepharospasm, and the lids may appear thickened in extreme cases. The author has observed multiple pyogranulomas restricted to the inner third eyelid of the dog that

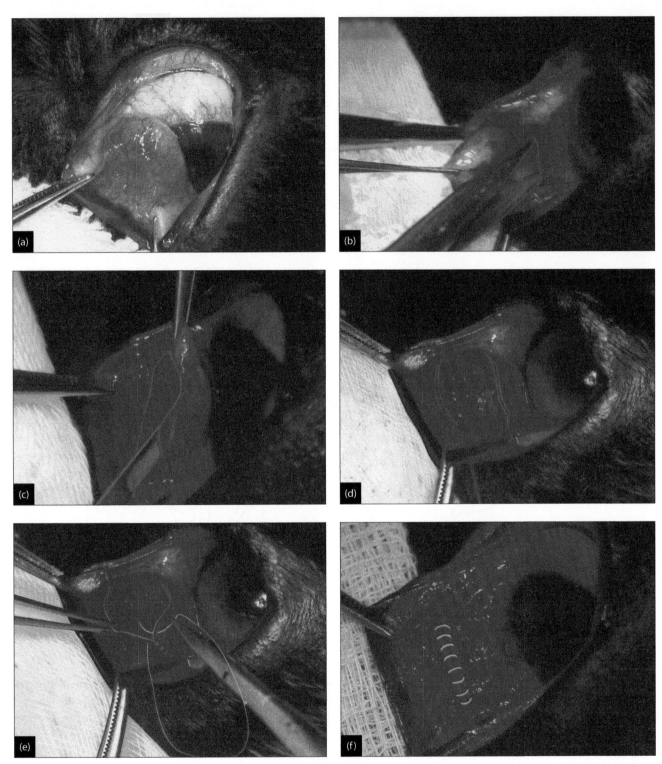

Figure 8.51 Pocket procedure for replacing the third eyelid gland of a dog. Third eyelid everted with prolapsed gland (a). A conjunctival incision through the bulbar surface near the fornix (b). A second parallel incision adjacent to lymphoid follicles made with a blade and avoiding transection of the cartilage (c). Two parallel incisions that do not meet (d). A simple continuous suture of 6-0 absorbable suture (e). A bite is taken and a knot tied on the palpebral face before penetrating to the bulbar face. Cut conjunctival edges can be opposed or bites taken at the bottom of incisions and apposed. The completed running suture with knot tied on palpebral side to avoid corneal irritation (f).

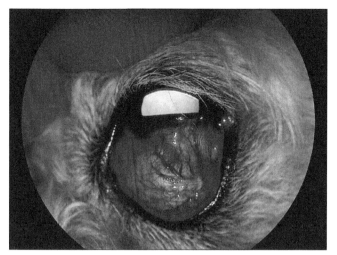

Figure 8.52 Cyst formation 2 years after a pocket procedure for a prolapsed gland in a dog. It was treated by opening the cyst from the bulbar side and allowing drainage. The gland remained in place.

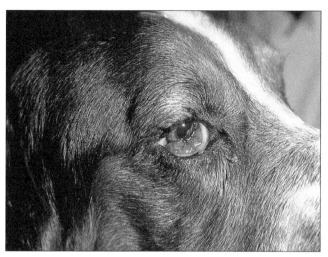

Figure 8.54 Chronic conjunctivitis of the third eyelid that involved both eyes in a dog. Excisional biopsy revealed pyogranuloma of unknown cause.

mimicked severe follicular conjunctivitis (**Figure 8.54**). The cause was unknown, but excision was curative.

Diagnosis

Careful observation of the conjunctival surfaces, including both sides of the third eyelid, may reveal numerous, small, raised, lymphoid follicles. Determination of the cause of the hyperplasia is based on history and is usually presumptive.

Therapy

Most cases respond well to topical corticosteroids and frequent irrigation and cleansing of the conjunctival

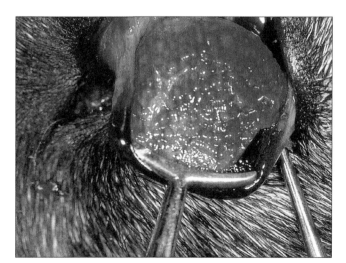

Figure 8.53 Marked follicular hyperplasia and hypertrophy of the normal patch of follicles on the bulbar surface of the third eyelid of a dog.

fornices.[182] In nonresponsive cases, excessive follicles may be carefully abraded with a gauze sponge. Aggressive surgical removal of follicles or the use of caustic agents such as copper sulfate should be avoided.

Plasma cell conjunctivitis

Introduction/etiology

GSD, GSD crosses, and collie types may develop a bilateral pinkish-gray nodular infiltration of the margin of the third eyelid that produces a thickening and loss of the pigmented margin. Some, but not all, of these dogs may eventually develop pannus or an immune-mediated keratitis. On cytology/histology, the infiltration is found to be due to plasma cells, and thus, the condition is thought to be immune mediated. The course of the disease is chronic.[183]

Clinical signs

Plasma cell conjunctivitis manifests as a bilateral thickening of exposed third eyelids with a gray-pink infiltrate (**Figure 8.55**). A serous-to-seromucoid ocular discharge accompanies the infiltration. Plasma cell conjunctivitis may occur with chronic superficial keratoconjunctivitis.

Therapy

The most important and least practical therapy is to change the environment. Hospitalization can result in noticeable improvement in some cases. Topical or subconjunctival steroids only produce a very modest response. Similarly, β-radiation therapy can improve the condition, but often topical glucocorticoids are still necessary. Topical 0.2% cyclosporine every 12 hours gives excellent

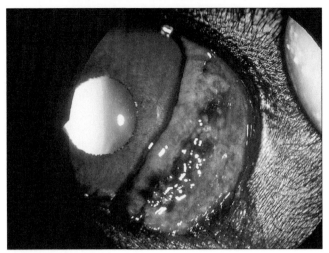

Figure 8.55 Plasma cell conjunctivitis of the third eyelid in a German shepherd dog. Note the roughened gray surface with depigmentation of the margin of the third eyelid. The condition is bilateral.

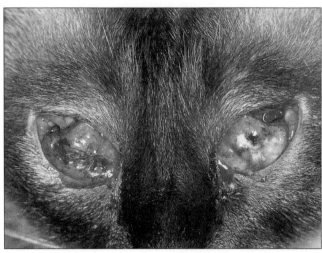

Figure 8.56 Granulomatous inflammation of both third eyelids in a cat that was due to *Cryptococcus neoformans*. No other ocular or systemic lesions were noted, and the condition responded well to topical and systemic antifungal therapy.

clinical and histopathologic improvement over 6 weeks. Therapy is presumed to be needed indefinitely.

Eosinophilic granuloma

In the cat, eosinophilic granuloma involves various ocular and adnexal tissues including the eyelids, the cornea, the conjunctiva, the orbit, and the third eyelid.[184] Third eyelid involvement is characterized by bilateral large red masses that are attached to the palpebral surface of the third eyelid. The lesions are covered with foci of white caseous material. An allergic cause has not been determined, and excision followed by topical glucocorticoid therapy is curative. Herpesvirus testing would be prudent, as Nasisse et al. found that 76% of feline eosinophilic keratitis patients were positive on PCR testing for FEV-1.[185]

INFECTIOUS CAUSES OF INFLAMMATION OF THE THIRD EYELID

The infectious causes of conjunctivitis, previously discussed in the cat, usually involve the third eyelid. When the third eyelid is protruded, due to discomfort, it may appear to be the predominant conjunctival surface that is involved. *Cryptococcus neoformans* produced marked bilateral granulomatous reactions in the third eyelid of a cat without intraocular lesions (**Figure 8.56**).[186] No other systemic signs were present or developed, even though the cat had antigenemia, and the condition responded to systemic itraconazole.

LACERATIONS OF THE THIRD EYELID

Lacerations involving the cartilage, even if they are very small, need suturing, or they may leave a permanent cosmetic defect. Larger lacerations involving the conjunctival attachments should have two layers of absorbable suture to minimize dehiscence (**Figure 8.57**).

FOREIGN BODIES OF THE THIRD EYELID

Foreign bodies, usually from plant material, can lodge behind the third eyelid, creating a refractive ulcerative keratitis

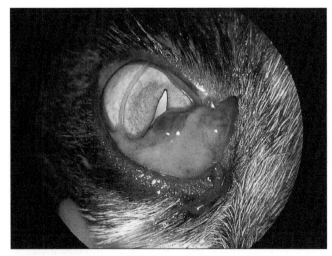

Figure 8.57 A cat with a large laceration of the conjunctival attachment of the third eyelid from fighting. Sutured with a two-layer closure.

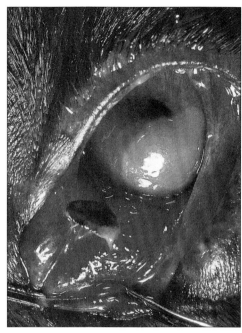

Figure 8.58 A dog with a plant foreign body behind the third eyelid that had created a superficial corneal ulcer. Note the amount of corneal neovascularization which correlates with the duration of injury. (Courtesy of Dr. M. Wyman.)

until they are discovered and removed (**Figure 8.58**). The condition is usually unilateral but may be bilateral and is common in areas with a hot dry season. Retained foreign bodies are important in the differential diagnosis of infectious keratoconjunctivitis in cattle in the dry summer of the western United States.

> Any nonhealing ulcer, nonresponsive keratitis, or persistent blepharospasm should prompt eversion of the third eyelid to look for a foreign body or a source of physical irritation. The longer the interval between presentation and diagnosis, the more embarrassment it can cause.

Protrusion of the third eyelid
Introduction/etiology
The lay term for a protruding third eyelid is "haws." The causes of a protruding third eyelid are numerous, but in most cases, the cause becomes readily apparent if a logical algorithm is followed. When searching for the cause of a protruded third eyelid, the following should be considered:

- Decreased orbital mass: Dehydration and emaciation with loss of orbital fat or volume is bilateral, but traumatic atrophy may be unilateral. The eyes become enophthalmic and the third eyelid protrudes.
- Decreased ocular mass: Microphthalmos and phthisis bulbi, which may be bilateral or unilateral.
- Increased orbital mass: Inflammation, neoplasia, or hemorrhage. These are usually unilateral, although multicentric neoplasia such as lymphoma may produce bilateral disease.
- Sympathetic denervation: Horner's syndrome, which also has miosis and ptosis and is usually unilateral. Key–Gaskell syndrome in cats is a generalized dysautonomia and is bilateral.[187,188] Key–Gaskell has been described in the United Kingdom and parts of Europe. The cause is unknown.
- Ocular pain from the cornea, iris, or conjunctiva causes the globe to be retracted into the orbit, resulting in protrusion. The causes of pain may be unilateral or bilateral.
- Increased extraocular muscle tone: If systemic, such as with tetanus or strychnine and mycotoxin poisoning, the condition is bilateral. If associated with extraocular muscle fibrosis and contracture, it may be unilateral.
- Idiopathic: Diagnosis by exclusion. A bilateral syndrome occurs in the cat that lasts 6–8 weeks and may be associated with intestinal parasites or gastrointestinal malfunction. A Toro virus-like particle was isolated from 14% of cats with watery diarrhea, which preceded a protruding third eyelid.[189] Some of the cats appeared to have decreased anal sphincter tone. The disease lasted for more than 4 weeks in about half of the cases but could not be reproduced by transmitting the virus to kittens. Further work is needed to define the role of this or other viruses in producing these symptoms.

> The protrusion of the third eyelid is a sensitive indicator of changes in orbital/ocular mass and ocular pain.

Therapy
The cause of the protrusion should be defined and treated. Therapy with topical sympathomimetics (epinephrine or phenylephrine every 6–8 hours) can improve idiopathic cases and those due to denervation.

A surgical procedure has been devised for correcting a protruding third eyelid that involves shortening the eyelid, but this is usually not necessary. The procedure involves removing a full-thickness piece of the third eyelid parallel to the free margin and above the gland. The width of the excision is the amount of "shortening," and the defect is sutured in two layers. The margin can also be shortened by removing a V-shaped piece at one end.[190] The third eyelid should not be removed for benign conditions.

Cysts in the third eyelid

Cysts may develop in the base of the third eyelid and have previously been described as a complication of other disease/surgery: *Thelazia* spp. infestation in a calf and surgical replacement of a prolapsed third eyelid gland with the pocket technique (**Figure 8.51**). Spontaneous cysts may occasionally be observed in the dog, presumably from blockage of the ducts of the third eyelid gland.[191,192] They are easily recognized as cysts by their smooth surface and, if necessary, by fine-needle aspiration (**Figure 8.59**). Excision is curative.

Neoplasia of the third eyelid

Tumors of the third eyelid and conjunctiva are relatively rare in the dog and the cat, whereas they are the most common tumors of the horse and the cow. Neoplasms arising from the conjunctival surfaces are SCC, papilloma, angiokeratoma, hemangioma, hemangiosarcoma, fibrosarcoma, melanoma, lymphoma, adenoma, and adenocarcinoma.

Neoplasia of the conjunctival surfaces is most common in large animals and commonly originates from the third eyelid and the conjunctiva near the limbus. SCC of the third eyelid (**Figure 8.60**) is rare in small animals.[193] In the cat, SCC is most frequent in the white-furred cat and usually involves the mucocutaneous junction of the lid. SCC must be differentiated from the more benign lesions of papilloma and pseudoepitheliomatous hyperplasia.[194] In

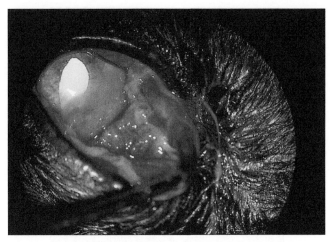

Figure 8.60 Squamous cell carcinoma at the base of the third eyelid in a cat. Note this cat is heavily pigmented.

the cow, the third eyelid accounts for 7%–15% of ocular and lid SCC, and it is the most common site of origin of ocular SCC in the horse (**Figure 8.61**) (see section Corneal tumors, Chapter 10).

If diagnosed early, excision of the free margin of the third eyelid with the involved tumor is the treatment of choice and is relatively simple. When extension occurs to adjacent conjunctival and corneal surfaces, excision is more difficult. If the tumor extends deep into the orbit, the prognosis is guarded.

Vascular lesions of the conjunctival surfaces of the third eyelid include telangiectasia, angiokeratoma, hemangioma, and hemangiosarcoma (**Figures 8.41–8.43**).[195,196] Angiokeratomas are benign superficial telangiectasia that appear as small, red, raised lesions that are differentiated from hemangiomas on histopathology (**Figure 8.41**). Angiokeratoma has dilated vascular spaces

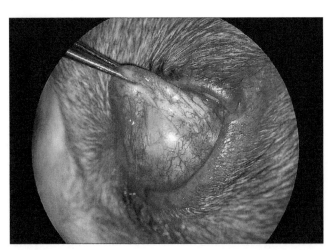

Figure 8.59 Blue cyst (dacryops) at the base of the third eyelid in a young Shetland sheepdog. It was treated by excision.

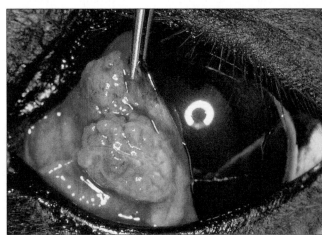

Figure 8.61 Squamous cell carcinoma of the third eyelid in a horse. The third eyelid is the most common site for SCC in the horse. It was treated by excision and beta radiation therapy of the excisional margin.

with hyperplastic epithelium.[157] Pirie et al. reported on 108 canine conjunctival vascular tumors that were comprised of 70 hemangiomas and 38 hemangiosarcomas.[226] The most common site was the third eyelid and the temporal bulbar conjunctiva, with a breed predisposition for outdoor working breeds. UV radiation was thought to be contributory due to a predisposition in nonpigmented and exposed sites, breeds most likely to be outdoors, and high UV light states. Excision or excision with cryotherapy appeared curative, but a retrospective pathologic study in a centralized pathology laboratory had inherent deficiencies in evaluating clinical outcomes.

Pirie et al. reported on eight cases of vascular tumors of the conjunctiva in cats; the third eyelid was the most common site.[229] Older neutered male domestic shorthaired cats predominated. No metastases were recorded at the time of excision, and only two cases (hemangiosarcomas) required repeat surgery. Since only two of the eight cases were hemangiosarcomas, there is not enough evidence to support a good prognosis. UV radiation was thought to be a contributing factor based on location of lesions and patients originating from high UV states, although the environment of the patients was known in only three cases.

Papillomas may occur as one or more lobulated lesions near the mucocutaneous borders of the lids and involve the conjunctiva and the cornea. Young and old dogs have been presented with the disease. Young animals may have oral papillomas, and the disease may be associated with a viral etiology (**Figure 8.62**).[197–200]

In a series of 12 conjunctival melanomas in the dog, 83% arose from the third eyelid, 75% were in females, and the Weimaraner had a breed predisposition.[156] Metastatic rates were 17%–33% depending on the criteria used. The recurrence rate was 55% after surgical excision, reflecting

the difficulty in obtaining wide excision (**Figures 8.38–8.40**). Fewer reports are available for the cat, but a malignant potential has been documented.[201,202]

Adenocarcinomas may arise from the third eyelid gland in all species, but they appear to be relatively rare, with most of the reports being in the dog. The tumor frequently recurs due to incomplete removal, and it may metastasize to lymph nodes and lungs in the dog and the cat.[203,204] Therapy is total removal of the third eyelid.

Fibrosarcomas have also been reported in the third eyelid, and clinically they may look like SCCs.[206] Systemic lymphoma may involve the third eyelid of the dog and the cat, but extranodal lymphoma has also been recorded with no evidence of systemic involvement (**Figures 8.63 and 8.64**).[230–232] Incomplete excision results in regrowth. In the author's experience, the disease has been associated in the

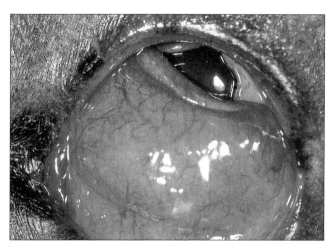

Figure 8.63 Lymphoma that was restricted to the third eyelid of a dog.

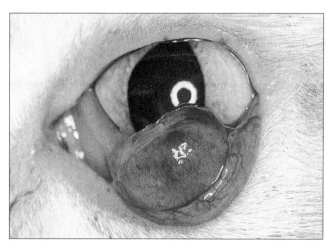

Figure 8.64 Lymphoma nodule involving the third eyelid of a cat that was FeLV- and FIV-negative and had no systemic signs. The lymphoma recurred quickly after simple excision. Excision and systemic chemotherapy was successful for over 1 year until lost to follow-up.

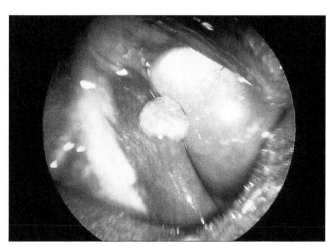

Figure 8.62 Viral papilloma on the margin of the third eyelid of a young Shar Pei. A papilloma was also present in the oral cavity.

cat with FeLV-negative animals. Therapy has been excision and systemic chemotherapy despite the lack of obvious systemic neoplasia.

Clinical signs

An obvious mass or a roughened area is observed on the conjunctival surface of the third eyelid. Mild cases may have only epiphora with a mildly "irritated" surface.

Diagnosis

Cytology or biopsy of the lesion can be performed if the diagnosis is not obvious. SCC in large animals is so characteristic that excisional biopsy and adjunctive therapy are often given at the same time.

Therapy

The mass or the entire third eyelid should be excised if the lesion is extensive. Neoplasia is one of the few indications for complete excision of the third eyelid; keratitis may be a sequel of such treatment. Additional therapy, if indicated by type of tumor and/or incomplete excision, may include cryotherapy, beta radiation, brachytherapy, or chemotherapy depending on the availability and reported sensitivity of the neoplasm.

CLINICAL CASES

CASE 1

An 8-year-old spayed female border collie is presented for a red mass at the lateral limbal conjunctiva of the left eye. The lesion has been present for 3–4 months.

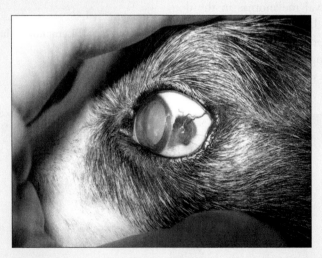

Q1: Name three possible clinical diagnoses.
Q2: How would you treat this lesion?

Answers:

1. Hemangioma/hemangiosarcoma; foreign body granuloma, parasitic granuloma
2. Surgical excision with wide margins followed by cryotherapy

CASE 2

A 12-year-old spayed female Persian cat is presented for swelling of the dorsal bulbar conjunctiva of the right eye.

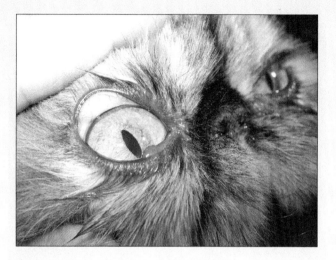

There is no hyperemia of the conjunctiva, no blepharospasm or discharge.

Q1: What is the most likely clinical diagnosis?
Q2: How would you treat this condition?

2. Resection of prolapsed fat and closure of the orbital septum

1. Orbital fat prolapse

Answers:

CASE 3

A 13-year-old male Golden retriever is presented for lobulated mass on the palpebral face of the nictitating membrane of the right eye. The mass has been present for several months.

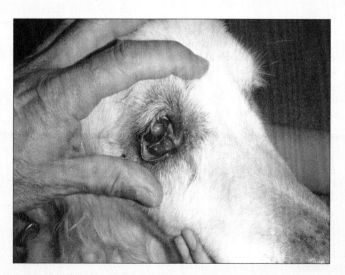

Q1: What is your clinical diagnosis?
Q2: What is your diagnostic/therapeutic approach?

2. Excisional biopsy followed by cryotherapy

1. (Malignant) melanoma of the third eyelid

Answers:

CASE 4

A 2-year-old rabbit is presented for a lesion in the right eye.

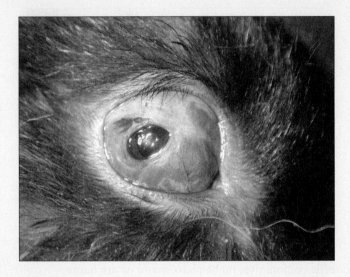

Q: What is your clinical diagnosis?

Conjunctival overgrowth

Answer:

REFERENCES

1. Martin, C., and Anderson, B. 1981. Ocular anatomy. In: Gelatt, K., editor. *Veterinary Ophthalmology.* Lea & Febiger: Philadelphia, PA, pp. 12–121.
2. Wirtschafter, J.D., Ketcham, J.M., Weinstock, R.J., Tabesh, T., and McLoon, L.K. 1999. Mucocutaneous junction as the major source of replacement palpebral conjunctival epithelial cells. *Investigative Ophthalmology and Visual Science* 40:3138–3146.
3. Bellhorn, R., and Henkind, P. 1966. Superficial pigmentary keratitis in the dog. *Journal of the American Veterinary Medical Association* 149:173–175.
4. Moore, C.P., Wilsman, N., Nordheim, E., Majors, L., and Collier, L. 1987. Density and distribution of canine conjunctival goblet cells. *Investigative Ophthalmology and Visual Science* 28:1925–1932.
5. Moore, C., and Collier, L. 1990. Ocular surface disease associated with loss of conjunctival goblet cells in dogs. *Journal of the American Animal Hospital Association* 26:458–465.
6. Cullen, C.L., Njaa, B.L., and Grahn, B.H. 1999. Ulcerative keratitis associated with qualitative tear film abnormalities in cats. *Veterinary Ophthalmology* 2:197–204.
7. Duke-Elder, S. editor. 1958. The eyes of birds. In: *Systems of Ophthalmology: The Eye in Evolution.* Mosby: St Louis, MO, pp. 234–427.
8. Rosenblueth, A., and Bard, P. 1932. The innervation and functions of the nictitating membrane in the cat. *American Journal of Physiology* 100:537–544.
9. Nuyttens, J., and Simoens, P. 1995. Morphologic study of the musculature of the third eyelid in the cat (*Felis catus*). *Laboratory Animal Science* 45:561–563.
10. Powell, C. 1988. Autonomic innervation of the canine lacrimal glands. *Master's thesis*, University of Georgia.
11. Thompson, J.W. 1967. The nerve supply to the nictitating membrane of the cat. *Journal of Anatomy* 95:371–385.
12. Prince, J., Diesem, C., Eglitis, L., and Ruskell, G., editors. 1960. The orbit and ocular adnexa. In: *Anatomy and Histology of the Eye and Orbit in Domestic Animals.* CC Thomas: Springfield, IL, pp. 3–12.
13. Sakai, T., and Yohro, T. 1981. A histological study of the Harderian gland of Mongolian gerbils, *Meriones meridianus. Anatomy Record* 200:259–270.
14. Anderson, D.E. 1991. Genetic study of eye cancer in cattle. *Journal of Heredity* 82:21–26.
15. Nishimura, H., and Frisch, J. 1977. Eye cancer and circumocular pigmentation in *Bos taurus* and crossbred cattle. *Australian Journal of Experimental Agricultural Animal Husbandry* 17:709–711.
16. Roat, M., Romanowski, E., Araullo-Cruz, T., and Gordon, J. 1987. The antiviral effects of rose bengal and fluorescein. *Archives of Ophthalmology* 105:1415–1417.
17. Vrabec, M., and McCanna, P. 1988. The effect of topically applied fluorescein on fluorescent monoclonal antibodies in the diagnosis of chlamydial conjunctivitis. *Annals of Ophthalmology* 20:421–423.
18. Da Silva Curiel, J., Murphy, C., Jang, S., and Bellhorn, R. 1990. Nutritionally variant streptococci associated with corneal ulcers in horses: 35 cases (1982–1988). *Journal of the American Veterinary Medical Association* 197:624–626.

19. Jackson, W.B. 1993. Differentiating conjunctivitis of diverse origins. *Survey of Ophthalmology* 38(Supplement):91–104.

20. Nasisse, M., Guy, J., and Stevens, J. 1993. Clinical and laboratory findings in chronic conjunctivitis in cats: 91 cases (1983–1991). *Journal of the American Veterinary Medical Association* 203:834–837.

21. Stiles, J. 1995. Treatment of cats with ocular disease attributable to herpesvirus infection: 17 cases (1983–1993). *Journal of the American Veterinary Medical Association* 207:599–603.

22. Fairchild, G., Wyman, M., and Donovan, E. 1967. Fluorescent antibody technique as a diagnostic test for canine distemper infection: Detection of viral antigen in epithelial tissues of experimentally infected dogs. *American Journal of Veterinary Research* 28:761–768.

23. Martellaa, V., Eliaa, G., Lucentea, M.S., Decaroa, N., Lorussoa, E., Banyaib, K., Blixenkrone-Møllerc, M. et al. 2007. Genotyping canine distemper virus (CDV) by a hemi-nested multiplex PCR provides a rapid approach for investigation of CDV outbreaks. *Veterinary Microbiology*, 122(1–2):32–42.

24. Swango, L., Wooding, W., and Binn, L. 1970. Comparison of the pathogenesis and antigenicity of infectious canine hepatitis virus and the A26/61 virus strain (Toronto). *Journal of the American Veterinary Medical Association* 156:1687–1699.

25. Scott, F., Kahn, D., and Gillespie, J. 1970. Feline viruses: Isolation, characterization, and pathogenicity of a feline reovirus. *American Journal of Veterinary Research* 31:11–20.

26. Ardley, R., Gaskell, R., and Povey, R. 1974. Feline respiratory viruses: Their prevalence in clinically healthy cats. *Journal of Small Animal Practice* 15:579–586.

27. Gaskell, R.M. 1993. Upper respiratory disease in the cat (including chlamydia): Control and prevention. *Feline Practice* 21:29–34.

28. Povey, R. 1976. Feline respiratory infections: A clinical review. *Canadian Veterinary Journal* 17:93–100.

29. Hoover, E.A., Rohovsky, M.W., and Griesmer, R.A. 1970. Experimental feline viral rhinotracheitis in the germ-free cat. *American Journal of Pathology* 58:269.

30. Nasisse, M., Guy, J., Davidson, M., Sussman, W., and Fairley, N. 1989. Experimental ocular herpesvirus infection in the cat. *Investigative Ophthalmology and Visual Science* 30:1758–1768.

31. Bistner, S., Carlson, J., Shively, J., and Scott, F. 1971. Ocular manifestations of feline herpesvirus infection. *Journal of the American Veterinary Medical Association* 159:1223–1237.

32. Roberts, S., Dawson, C., Coleman, V., and Togni, B. 1972. Dendritic keratitis in a cat. *Journal of the American Veterinary Medical Association* 161:285–288.

33. Gaskell, R.M., Dennis, P.E., Goddard, L.E. et al. 1985. Isolation of feline herpesvirus from the trigeminal ganglia of latently infected cats. *Journal of General Virology* 66:391–394.

34. Nasisse, MP., Davis, B.J., Guy, J.S., Davidson, M.G., and Sussman, W. 1992. Isolation of feline herpesvirus 1 from the trigeminal ganglia of acutely and chronically infected cats. *Journal of Veterinary Internal Medicine* 6:102–103.

35. O'Brien, W.J., and Taylor, J.L. 1989. The isolation of herpes simplex virus from rabbit corneas during latency. *Investigative Ophthalmology and Visual Science* 30:357–364.

36. Kaye, S.B., Lynas, C., Patterson, A., Risk, J.M., McCarthy, K., and Hart, C.A. 1991. Evidence for herpes simplex viral latency in the human cornea. *British Journal of Ophthalmology* 75:195–200.

37. Stiles, J., McDermott, M., Bigsby, D. et al. 1997. Use of nested polymerase chain reaction to identify feline herpesvirus in ocular tissue from clinically normal cats and cats with corneal sequestra or conjunctivitis. *American Journal of Veterinary Research* 58:338–342.

38. Stiles, J., McDermott, M., Willis, M., Roberts, W., and Greene, C. 1997. Comparison of nested polymerase chain reaction, virus isolation, and fluorescent antibody testing for identifying feline herpesvirus in cats with conjunctivitis. *American Journal of Veterinary Research* 58:804–807.

39. Gaskell, R.M., and Povey, R.C. 1977. Experimental induction of feline viral rhinotracheitis virus re-excretion in FVR recovered cats. *Veterinary Record* 100:128–133.

40. Spiess, B. 1985. Symblepharon, pseudopterygium and partielles ankyloblepharon als folgen feliner herpes keratokonjunktivitis. *Kleintier Praxis* 30:149–154.

41. Nasisse, M.P., and Weigler, B.J. 1997. The diagnosis of ocular feline herpesvirus infection. *Veterinary and Comparative Ophthalmology* 7:44–51.

42. Hill, H., and Mare, C. 1974. Genital disease in dogs caused by canine herpesvirus. *American Journal of Veterinary Research* 35:669–672.

43. Jackson, J., and Corstvet, R. 1975. Transmission and attempted isolation of the etiologic agent associated with lymphofollicular hyperplasia of the canine species. *American Journal of Veterinary Research* 36:1207–1210.

44. Jackson, J., and Corstvet, R. 1980. Study of nictitating membranes and genitalia of dogs with reference to lymphofollicular hyperplasia and its cause. *American Journal of Veterinary Research* 41:1814–1822.

45. Keller, W., Hinz, R., and Blanchard, G. 1972. Experimentally produced canine herpetic keratitis. *Proceedings of the Scientific Meeting of the American College of Veterinary Ophthalmologists* 3:2–7.

46. Ledbetter, E.C., Marfurt, C.F., Dubielzig, R.R. 2013. Metaherpetic corneal disease in a dog associated with partial limbal stem cell deficiency and neurotrophic keratitis. *Veterinary Ophthalmology* 16(4):282–288.

47. Ledbetter, E.C. 2013. Canine herpesvirus-1 ocular diseases of mature dogs. *New Zealand Veterinary Journal* 61(4):193–201.

48. Ledbetter, E.C. et al. 2012. Frequency of spontaneous canine herpesvirus-1 reactivation and ocular viral shedding in latently infected dogs and canine herpesvirus-1 reactivation and ocular viral shedding induced by topical administration of cyclosporine and systemic administration of corticosteroids. *American Journal of Veterinary Research* 73(7):1079–1084.

49. Gervais, K.J. et al. 2012. Acute primary canine herpesvirus-1 dendritic ulcerative keratitis in an adult dog. *Veterinary Ophthalmology* 15(2):133–138.

50. McChesney, A., England, J., and Rich, L. 1973. Adenoviral infection in foals. *Journal of the American Veterinary Medical Association* 162:545–549.

51. Thein, P., and Bohm, D. 1976. Aeiologie und kinik einer virusbedingten keratokonjunktivitis beim fohlen. *Zentralblatt fuer Veterinaermedizin Reihe B* 23:507–519.

52. Collinson, P., O'Rielly, J., Ficorilli, N., and Studdert, M. 1994. Isolation of equine herpesvirus type 2 (equine gamma herpesvirus 2) from foals with keratoconjunctivitis. *Journal of the American Veterinary Medical Association* 205:329–331.

53. Sonderegger, F., Pot, S., Walser-Reinhardt, L., Hässig, M., and Spiess, B.M. 2013. The prevalence of DNA of

EHV-2 and EHV-5 in horses with keratoconjunctivitis and clinically normal horses in Switzerland. *Pferdeheilkunde* 29(4):457–459.

54. Cook, N. 1998. Combined outbreak of the genital and conjunctival forms of bovine herpesvirus 1 infection in a UK dairy herd. *Veterinary Record* 143:561–562.

55. Abinati, F., and Plumer, G. 1961. The isolation of infectious bovine rhinotracheitis virus from cattle affected with conjunctivitis: Observations on the experimental infection. *American Journal of Veterinary Research* 22:13–17.

56. Rebhun, W., Smith, J., Post, J., and Holden, H. 1978. An outbreak of the conjunctival form of infectious bovine rhinotracheitis. *Cornell Veterinarian* 68:297–307.

57. Mohanty, S., Lillie, M., Corselius, N., and Beck, J. 1972. Natural infection with infectious bovine rhinotracheitis virus in goats. *Journal of the American Veterinary Medical Association* 160:879–880.

58. Sykes, J.E., Anderson, G.A., Studdert, V.P., and Browning, G.F. 1999. Prevalence of feline *Chlamydia psittaci* and feline herpesvirus-1 in cats with upper respiratory tract disease. *Journal of Veterinary Internal Medicine* 13:153–162.

59. Hickman, J., Reubel, G., Hoffman, D., Morris, J., Rogers, Q., Pedersen, N. 1994. An epizootic of feline herpesvirus type 1 in a large specific pathogen-free cat colony and attempts to eradicate the infection by identification and culling of carriers. *Laboratory Animal* 28:320–329.

60. Maggs, D.J., Lappin, M.R., Reif, J.S. et al. 1999. Evaluation of serologic and viral detection methods for diagnosing feline herpesvirus 1 infection in cats with acute respiratory tract or chronic disease. *Journal of the American Veterinary Medical Association* 214:502–507.

61. Harbour, D.A., Howard, P.E., and Gaskell, R.M. 1991. Isolation of feline calicivirus and feline herpesvirus from domestic cats 1980–1989. *Veterinary Record* 128:77–80.

62. Sykes, J.E., Studdert, V.P., and Browning, G.F. 1999. Comparison of the polymerase chain reaction and culture for the detection of feline *Chlamydia psittaci* in untreated and doxycycline-treated experimentally infected cats. *Journal of Veterinary Internal Medicine* 13:146–152.

63. Cello, R. 1971. Clues to differential diagnosis of feline respiratory infections. *Journal of the American Veterinary Medical Association* 158:968–973.

64. Plotkin, J., Reynaud, A., and Okumoto, M. 1971. Cytologic study of herpetic keratitis. *Archives of Ophthalmology* 85:597–599.

65. Da Silva Curiel, J., Nasisse, M., Hook, R., Wilson, H., Collins, B., and Mandell, C. 1991. Topical fluorescein dye: Effects of immunofluorescent antibody test for feline herpesvirus keratoconjunctivitis. *Progress in Veterinary and Comparative Ophthalmology* 1:99–104.

66. Bracklein, T. et al. 2006. Activity of feline interferon-omega after ocular or oral administration in cats as indicated by Mx protein expression in conjunctival and white blood cells. *American Journal of Veterinary Research* 67(6):1025–1032.

67. Weiss, R. 1989. Synergistic antiviral activities of acyclovir and recombinant human leukocyte (alpha) interferon on feline herpesvirus replication. *American Journal of Veterinary Research* 50:1672–1677.

68. Haid, C. et al. 2007. Pretreatment with feline interferon omega and the course of subsequent infection with feline herpesvirus in cats. *Veterinary Ophthalmology* 10(5):278–284.

69. Stiles, J., Townsend, W.M., Rogers, Q.R., and Krohne, S.G. 2002. Effect of oral administration of L-lysine on conjunctivitis caused by feline herpesvirus in cats. *American Journal of Veterinary Research* 63:99–103.

70. Herring, A.J. 1993. Typing *Chlamydia psittaci*: A review of methods and recent findings. *British Veterinary Journal* 149:455–475.

71. Sykes, J.E. 2001. Feline upper respiratory tract pathogens: *Chlamydophila felis*. *Compendium on Continuing Edication for the Practicing Veterinarian* 23:231–240.

72. Becker, A. et al. 2007. Intensively kept pigs pre-disposed to chlamydial associated conjunctivitis. *Journal of Veterinary Medicine - Series A* 54(6):307–313.

73. Wyrick, P.B., and Richmond, S.J. 1989. Biology of chlamydiae. *Journal of the American Veterinary Medical Association* 195:1507–1516.

74. Schachter, J., Ostler, H.B., and Meyer, K.F. 1969. Human infection with the agent of feline pneumonitis. *Lancet* 1:1063–1065.

75. Schachter, J. 1989. Chlamydial infections: Past, present, future. *Journal of the American Veterinary Medical Association* 195:1501–1506.

76. Hoover, E., Kahn, D., and Langloss, J. 1978. Experimentally induced feline chlamydial infection (feline pneumonitis). *American Journal of Veterinary Research* 39:541–547.

77. Shewen, P., Povey, R., and Wilson, M. 1978. Feline chlamydial infection. *Canadian Veterinary Journal* 19:289–292.

78. Bart, M.F., Guscetti, F., Zurbriggen, A., Popischil, A., and Schiller, I. 2000. Feline infectious pneumonia: A short literature review and a retrospective immunohistological study on the involvement of *Chlamydia* spp. and distemper virus. *Veterinary Journal* 159:220–230.

79. Willis, J. 1988. Prevalence of *Chlamydia psittaci* in different cat populations in Britain. *Journal of Small Animal Practice* 29:327–339.

80. Cello, R. 1967. Ocular infections in animals with PLT (*Bedsonia*) group agents. *American Journal of Ophthalmology* 2:244–248.

81. Campbell, L., and Otis, B. 1983. Ocular changes associated with mycoplasmal, chlamydial, and herpesvirus infections in the cat. *Modern Veterinary Practice* 64:529–531.

82. Hopkins, J., Stephenson, E., Storz, J., and Pierson, R. 1973. Conjunctivitis associated with chlamydial polyarthritis in lambs. *Journal of the American Veterinary Medical Association* 163:1157–1160.

83. Rogers, D.G., Andersen, A.A., Hogg, A., Nielsen, D.L., and Huebert, M.A. 1993. Conjunctivitis and keratoconjunctivitis associated with chlamydiae in swine. *Journal of the American Veterinary Medical Association* 203:1321–1323.

84. Idtse, F. 1984. Chlamydia and chlamydial diseases of cattle: A review of the literature. *Veterinary Medicine/Small Animal Clinician* 79:543–550.

85. Sibitz, C. et al. 2011. Detection of Chlamydophila pneumoniae in cats with conjunctivitis. *Veterinary Ophthalmology* 14(Suppl 1):67–74.

86. Richter, M. et al. 2010. *Parachlamydia acanthamoebae* in domestic cats with and without corneal disease. *Veterinary Ophthalmology* 13(4):235–237.

87. Rampazzo, A. et al. 2003. Prevalence of *Chlamydophila felis* and feline herpesvirus 1 in cats with conjunctivitis in northern Italy. *Journal of Veterinary Internal Medicine* 17(6):799–807.

88. Bech-Nielsen, S., Fullton, R.W., Downing, M.M., and Hardy, W.D. 1981. Feline infectious peritonitis and viral respiratory diseases in feline leukemia virus infected cats. *Journal of the American Animal Hospital Association* 17:759–765.

89. O'Dair, H., Hopper, C., Gruffydd-Jones, T., Harbour, D., and Waters, H. 1994. Clinical aspects of *Chlamydia psittaci* infection in cats infected with feline immunodeficiency virus. *Veterinary Research* 134:365–368.

90. Mitzel, J., and Strating, A. 1977. Vaccination against feline pneumonitis. *American Journal of Veterinary Research* 38:1361–1363.

91. Shewen, P., Povey, R., and Wilson, M. 1980. A comparison of the efficacy of a live and four inactivated vaccine preparations for the protection of cats against experimental challenge with *Chlamydia psittaci*. *Canadian Journal of Comparative Medicine* 44:244–251.

92. Gill, M., Beckenhauer, W., and Thurber, E. 1987. Immunogenicity and efficacy of a modified live feline chlamydia vaccine. *Norden News* summer:26–30.

93. Wasmoen, T., Chu, H.J., Chavez, L., and Acree, W. 1992. Demonstration of one-year duration of immunity for an inactivated feline *Chlamydia psittaci* vaccine. *Feline Practice* 20:13–16.

94. Campbell, L., Fox, J., and Snyder, S. 1973. Ocular bacteria and mycoplasma of the clinically normal cat. *Feline Practice* 3:10–12.

95. Campbell, L., Synder, S., Reed, C., and Fox, J. 1973. *Mycoplasma felis*-associated conjunctivitis in cats. *Journal of the American Veterinary Medical Association* 163:991–995.

96. Dagnall, G.J. 1993. Experimental infection of the conjunctival sac of lambs with *Mycoplasma conjunctivae*. *British Veterinary Journal* 149:429–435.

97. Rosenbusch, R.F., and Knudtson, W.U. 1980. Bovine mycoplasmal conjunctivitis: Experimental reproduction and characterization of the disease. *Cornell Veterinarian* 70:307–320.

98. Argue, B., Chousalkar, K.K., and Chenoweth, P.J. 2013. Presence of *Ureaplasma diversum* in the Australian cattle population. *Australian Veterinary Journal* 91(3):99–101.

99. Rogers, D., Frey, M., and Hogg, A. 1991. Conjunctivitis associated with a mycoplasma-like organism in swine. *Journal of the American Veterinary Medical Association* 198:450–452.

100. Rosendal, S. 1982. Canine mycoplasmas: Their ecologic niche and role in disease. *Journal of the American Veterinary Medical Association* 180:1212–1214.

101. Rosendal, S. 1986. Detection of antibodies to *Mycoplasma felis* in horses. *Journal of the American Veterinary Medical Association* 188:292–294.

102. Tasker, S. et al. 2003. Use of a PCR assay to assess the prevalence and risk factors for *Mycoplasma haemofelis* and "*Candidatus Mycoplasma haemominutum*" in cats in the United Kingdom. *The Veterinary Record* 152(7):193–198.

103. Criado-Fornelio, A. et al. 2003. Presence of *Mycoplasma haemofelis*, *Mycoplasma haemominutum* and piroplasmids in cats from southern Europe: A molecular study. *Veterinary Microbiology* 93(4):307–17.

104. Urban, M., Wyman, M., Reins, M., and Marraro, V. 1972. Conjunctival flora in clinically normal dogs. *Journal of the American Veterinary Medical Association* 161:201–206.

105. Bistner, S.I., Roberts, S.R., and Anderson, R.P. 1969. Conjunctival bacteria: Clinical appearances can be deceiving. *Modern Veterinary Practice* 50:45–47.

106. McDonald, P.J., and Watson, A.D.J. 1976. Microbial flora of normal canine conjunctiva. *Journal of Small Animal Practice* 17:809–812.

107. Hacker, D.V., Jensen, H.E., and Selby, L.A. 1979. A comparison of conjunctival culture techniques in the dog. *Journal of the American Animal Hospital Association* 15:223–225.

108. Gerding, P.A., Cormany, K., Weisiger, R., and Kakoma, I. 1993. Survey and topographic distribution of bacterial and fungal microorganisms in eyes of clinically normal dogs. *Canine Practice* 18:34–38.

109. Verwer, M., and Gunnink, J. 1968. The occurrence of bacteria in chronic purulent eye discharge. *Journal of Small Animal Practice* 9:33–36.

110. Stone, A., and Schrock, J. 1972. Bacterial conjunctivitis in the dog: Preliminary findings. *Journal of the American Animal Hospital Association* 8:10–12.

111. Murphy, J., Lavach, J., and Severin, G. 1978. Survey of conjunctival flora of dogs with clinical signs of external eye disease. *Journal of the American Veterinary Medical Association* 172:66–68.

112. Gerding, P.A., McLaughlin, S.A., and Troop, M.W. 1988. Pathogenic bacteria and fungi associated with external ocular diseases in dogs: 131 cases (1981–1986). *Journal of the American Veterinary Medical Association* 193:242–244.

113. Gerding, P.A., Cormany, K., Weisiger, R., and Kakoma, I. 1993. Survey and topographic distribution of bacterial and fungal microorganisms in eyes of clinically normal cats. *Feline Practice* 21:20–23.

114. Espinola, M.B., and Lilenbaum, W. 1996. Prevalence of bacteria in the conjunctival sac and on the eyelid margin of clinically normal cats. *Journal of Small Animal Practice* 37:364–366.

115. Moore, C. 1988. Prevalence of ocular microorganisms in hospitalized and stabled horses. *American Journal of Veterinary Research* 49:773–777.

116. McLaughlin, S., Brightman, A., Helper, L., Manning, J., and Tomes, J. 1983. Pathogenic bacteria and fungi associated with extraocular disease in the horse. *Journal of the American Veterinary Medical Association* 182:241–242.

117. Samuelson, D., Andresen, T., and Gwin, R. 1984. Conjunctival fungal flora in horses, cattle, dogs, and cats. *Journal of the American Veterinary Medical Association* 184:1240–1242.

118. Voelter-Ratson, K. et al. 2013. Evaluation of the conjunctival fungal flora and its susceptibility to antifungal agents in healthy horses in Switzerland. *Veterinary Ophthalmology* 17(Suppl 1):31–36.

119. Ball, M., Rebhun, W., and Gaarder, J. 1997. Evaluation of itraconazole–dimethyl sulfoxide ointment for treatment of keratomycosis in nine horses. *Journal of the American Veterinary Medical Association* 211:199–203.

120. Barker, I. 1970. *Thelazia lacrymalis* from the eyes of an Ontario horse. *Canadian Veterinary Journal* 11:186–189.

121. Magnis, J. et al. 2010. Local transmission of the eye worm *Thelazia callipaeda* in southern Germany. *Parasitology Research* 106(3):715–717.

122. Sargo, R. et al. 2014. First report of *Thelazia callipaeda* in red foxes (Vulpes vulpes) from Portugal. *Journal of Zoo & Wildlife Medicine* 45(2):458–460.

123. Motta, B. et al. 2014. Epidemiology of the eye worm *Thelazia callipaeda* in cats from southern Switzerland. *Veterinary Parasitology* 203(3–4):287–293.

124. Pimenta, P. et al. 2013. Canine ocular thelaziosis caused by *Thelazia callipaeda* in Portugal. *Veterinary Ophthalmology* 16(4):312–315.

125. Caron, Y. et al. 2013. *Thelazia callipaeda* ocular infection in two dogs in Belgium. *Journal of Small Animal Practice* 54(4):205–208.

126. Ladouceur, C., and Kazacos, K. 1981. Eye worms in cattle in Indiana. *Journal of the American Veterinary Medical Association* 178:385–386.

127. Lyons, E., Tolliver, S., Drudge, J., Swerczek, T., and Crowe, M. 1986. Eyeworms (*Thelazia lacrymalis*) in one- to four-year-old thoroughbreds at necropsy in Kentucky (1984–1985). *American Journal of Veterinary Research* 47:315–316.

128. Lyons, E., Drudge, J., and Tolliver, S. 1980. Age distribution of horses in Kentucky infected with the eye worm *Thelazia lacrymalis*. *Journal of the American Veterinary Medical Association* 176:221–223.

129. Robertson, J.T., and Johnson, F.M. 1980. Age distribution of horses in Kentucky infected with the eye worm *Thelazia lacrymalis*. *Journal of the American Veterinary Medical Association* 176:221–223.

130. Greve, J., and Harrison, G. 1980. Conjunctivitis caused by eye flukes in captive-reared ostriches. *Journal of the American Veterinary Medical Association* 177:909–910.

131. Miller, P., and Campbell, B. 1992. Subconjunctival cyst associated with *Thelazia gulosa* in a calf. *Journal of the American Veterinary Medical Association* 201:1058–1060.

132. Lyons, E., Drudge, J., and Tolliver, S. 1981. Apparent inactivity of several antiparasitic compounds against the eyeworm *Thelazia lacrymalis* in equids. *American Journal of Veterinary Research* 42:1046–1047.

133. Marley, S., Illyes, E., and Keller, D. 1999. Efficacy of topically administered doramectin against eyeworms, lungworms, and gastrointestinal nematodes of cattle. *American Journal of Veterinary Research* 60:665–668.

134. Whitcup, S., Chan, C., Luyo, D., Bo, P., and Li, Q. 1996. Topical cyclosporine inhibits mast cell-mediated conjunctivitis. *Investigative Ophthalmology and Visual Science* 37:2686–2693.

135. Tinkellman, D.G., Rupp, G., Kaufman, H., Pugely, J., and Schultz, N. 1993. Double-masked, paired-comparison clinical study of ketorolac tromethamine 0.5% ophthalmic solution compared with placebo eyedrops in the treatment of seasonal allergic conjunctivitis. *Survey of Ophthalmology* 38:133–140.

136. Notivol, R., Martinez, M., and Bergamini, M.V. 1994. Treatment of chronic nonbacterial conjunctivitis with a cyclo-oxygenase inhibitor or a corticosteroid. *American Journal of Ophthalmology* 117:651–656.

137. Pentlarge, V. 1991. Eosinophilic conjunctivitis in five cats. *Journal of the American Animal Hospital Association* 27:21–28.

138. Allgoewer, I., Schaffer, E., Stockhaus, C., and Vogtlin, A. 2001. Feline eosinophilic conjunctivitis. *Veterinary Ophthalmology* 4:69–74.

139. Larocca, R. 2000. Eosinophilic conjunctivitis, herpesvirus, and mast cell tumor of the third eyelid in a cat. *Veterinary Ophthalmology* 3:221–225.

140. Read, R.A., and Lucas, J. 2001. Lipogranulomatous conjunctivitis: Clinical findings from 21 eyes in 13 cats. *Veterinary Ophthalmology* 4:93–98.

141. Kerlin, R.L., and Dubielzig, R.R. 1997. Lipogranulomatous conjunctivitis in cats. *Veterinary and Comparative Ophthalmology* 7:177–179.

142. Ramsey, D., Ketringn, K., Glaze, M., and Render, J. 1996. Ligneous conjunctivitis in four Doberman Pinschers. *Journal of the American Animal Hospital Association* 32:439–447.

143. Schott, D., Beck, P., Liermann, A. et al. 1998. Therapy with a purified plasminogen concentrate in an infant with ligneous conjunctivitis and homozygous plasminogen deficiency. *New England Journal of Medicine* 339:1679–1686.

144. Munroe, G. 1999. Subconjunctival haemorrhages in neonatal thoroughbred foals. *Veterinary Record* 144:279–282.

145. Anderson, D., Lush, J., and Chambers, D. 1957. Studies on bovine ocular squamous cell carcinoma ("cancer eye"). II. Relationship between eyelid pigmentation and occurrence of cancer eye lesions. *Journal of Animal Science* 16:739–746.

146. Bailey, C.M., Hanks, D.R., and Hanks, M.A. 1990. Circumocular pigmentation and incidence of ocular squamous cell tumors in *Bos taurus* and *Bos indicus* x *Bos taurus* cattle. *Journal of the American Veterinary Medical Association* 196:1605–1608.

147. Den Otter, W., Hill, G., Klein, W. et al. 1995. Ocular squamous cell carcinoma in Simmental cattle in Zimbabwe. *American Journal of Veterinary Research* 56:1440–1444.

148. Sironi, G., Riccaboni, P., Mertel, L., Cammarata, G., and Brooks, D. 1999. p53 protein expression in conjunctival squamous cell carcinomas of domestic animals. *Veterinary Ophthalmology* 2:227–231.

149. Teifke, J.P., and Lohr, C.V. 1996. Immunohistochemical detection of p53 overexpression in paraffin wax-embedded squamous cell carcinoma of cattle, horses, cats, and dogs. *Journal of Comparative Pathology* 114:205–210.

150. Rebhun, W., and Piero, F. 1998. Ocular lesions in horses with lymphosarcoma: 21 cases (1977–1997). *Journal of the American Veterinary Medical Association* 212:852–854.

151. Joyce, J. 1973. Chemosis associated with malignant lymphoma in a heifer. *Veterinary Medical/Small Animal Clinician* 68:33–34.

152. Johnson, B., Brightman, A., and Whiteley, H. 1988. Conjunctival mast cell tumor in two dogs. *Journal of the American Animal Hospital Association* 24:439–442.

153. Hamor, R., Ramsey, D., Wiedmeyer, C., Gerding, P., Knight, B., and Whiteley, H. 1997. Melanoma of the conjunctiva and cornea in a horse. *Veterinary and Comparative Ophthalmology* 7:52–55.

154. Cook, C.S., Rosenkrantz, W., Peiffer, R.L., and MacMillan, A. 1985. Malignant melanoma of the conjunctiva in a cat. *Journal of the American Veterinary Medical Association* 186:505–506.

155. Patnaik, A., and Mooney, S. 1988. Feline melanoma: A comparative study of ocular, oral, and dermal neoplasms. *Veterinary Pathology* 25:105–112.

156. Collins, B.K., Collier, L., Miller, M., and Linton, L. 1993. Biologic behavior and histologic characteristics of canine conjunctival melanoma. *Veterinary and Comparative Ophthalmology* 3:135–140.

157. Buyukmihci, N. 1981. Canine conjunctival angiokeratomas. *Journal of the American Veterinary Medical Association* 178:1279–1282.

158. George, G., and Summers, B.A. 1990. Angiokeratoma: A benign vascular tumour of the dog. *Journal of Small Animal Practice* 31:390–392.

159. Vestre, W.A., Turner, T.A., and Carlton, W.W. 1982. Conjunctival hemangioma in a horse. *Journal of the American Veterinary Medical Association* 180:1481–1482.

160. Moore, P.F., Jacker, D.V., and Buyukmihci, N.C. 1986. Ocular angiosarcoma in the horse: Morphological and immunohistochemical studies. *Veterinary Pathology* 23:240–244.

161. Crawley, G.R., Bryan, G.M., and Gogolewski, R.P. 1987. Ocular hemangioma in a horse. *Equine Practice* 9:11–13.

162. Murphy, C.J., Bellhorn, R.W., and Buyukmihci, N.C. 1989. Bilateral conjunctival masses in two dogs. *Journal of the American Veterinary Medical Association* 195:225–227.

163. Mughannam, A.J., Hacker, D.V., and Spangler, W.L. 1997. Conjunctival vascular tumors in six dogs. *Veterinary and Comparative Ophthalmology* 7:56–59.

164. Regnier, A., Magnol, J., and Servantie, J. 1986. Corneal and subconjunctival ectopic lacrimal glands in a dog. *Canadian Practice* 13:12–14.

165. Roze, M., Ridings, B., and Lagadic, M. 2001. Comparative morphology of epicorneal conjunctival membranes in rabbits and human pterygium. *Veterinary Ophthalmology* 4:171–174.

166. Martin, C., and Leach, R. 1970. Everted membrana nictitans in German Shorthaired Pointers. *Journal of the American Veterinary Medical Association* 157:1229–1232.

167. Albert, R., Garrett, P., Whitley, R., and Thomas, K. 1982. Surgical correction of everted third eyelid in two cats. *Journal of the American Veterinary Medical Association* 180:763–766.

168. Gelatt, K. 1972. Surgical correction of everted nictitating membrane in the dog. *Veterinary Medicine/Small Animal Clinician* 67:291–292.

169. Kuhns, E. 1977. Correction of eversion of the membrana nictitans in the dog. *Veterinary Medical/Small Animal Clinician* 72:411–417.

170. Allbaugh, R.A., Stuhr, C.M. 2013. Thermal cautery of the canine third eyelid for treatment of cartilage eversion. *Veterinary Ophthalmology* 16(5):392–395.

171. Koch, S.A. 1979. Congenital ophthalmic abnormalities in the Burmese cat. *Journal of the American Veterinary Medical Association* 174:90–91.

172. Brandsch, H., and Schmidt, V. 1982. Erbanalytische untersuchungen zum dermoid des auges beim hund. *Monutshelte fur Veterinarmedizin* 37:305–306.

173. Barkyoumb, S., and Leipold, H. 1984. Nature and cause of ocular dermoids in Hereford cattle. *Veterinary Pathology* 21:316–324.

174. Christmas, R. 1992. Surgical correction of congenital ocular and nasal dermoids and third eyelid gland prolapse in related Burmese kittens. *Canadian Veterinary Journal* 33:265–266.

175. Schoofs, S. 1999. Prolapse of the gland of the third eyelid in a cat: A case report and literature review. *Journal of the American Animal Hospital Association* 35:240–242.

176. Dugan, S., Severin, G., Hungerford, L., Whiteley, H., and Roberts, S. 1992. Clinical and histologic evaluation of the prolapsed third eyelid gland in dogs. *Journal of the American Veterinary Medical Association* 201:1861–1867.

177. Severin, G., editor. 1995. Third eyelid. In: *Severin's Veterinary Ophthalmology Notes*, 3rd edition. American Animal Hospital Association, Fort Collins, Colorado, p. 214.

178. Morgan, R., Duddy, J., and McClurg, K. 1993. Prolapse of the gland of the third eyelid in dogs: A retrospective study of 89 cases (1980–1990). *Journal of the American Animal Hospital Association* 29:56–60.

179. Moore, C., Frappier, B., and Linton, L. 1996. Distribution and course of ducts of the canine third eyelid gland: Effects of two surgical replacement techniques. *Veterinary and Comparative Ophthalmology* 6:258–264.

180. Kaswan, R., and Martin, C. 1985. Surgical correction of third eyelid prolapse in dogs. *Journal of the American Veterinary Medical Association* 186:83.

181. Stanley, R., and Kaswan, R. 1994. Modification of the orbital rim anchorage method for surgical replacement of the gland of the third eyelid in dogs. *Journal of the American Veterinary Medical Association* 205:1412–1414.

182. Glaze, M.B. 1991. Ocular allergy. *Seminars in Veterinary Medicine and Surgery (Small Animal)* 6(4):296–302.

183. Teichert, G. 1966. Plasmazellulare infiltration des dritten augenlides beim hund. *Berliner und Muenchner Tieraerztliche Wochenschrift* 79:499.

184. Keil, S., Olivero, D., McKeever, P., and Moore, F. 1997. Bilateral nodular eosinophilic granulomatous inflammation of the nictitating membrane of a cat. *Veterinary and Comparative Ophthalmology* 7:258–262.

185. Nasisse, M., Glover, T., Moore, C., and Weigler, B. 1998. Detection of feline herpesvirus-1 DNA in corneas of cats with eosinophilic keratitis or corneal sequestration. *American Journal of Veterinary Research* 59:856–858.

186. Martin, C., Stiles, J., and Willis, M. 1996. Ocular adnexal cryptococcosis in a cat. *Veterinary and Comparative Ophthalmology* 6:225–229.

187. Rochlitz, I. 1984. Feline dysautonomia (the Key–Gaskell or dilated pupil syndrome): A preliminary review. *Journal of Small Animal Practice* 25:587–598.

188. Sharp, N., Nash, A., and Griffiths, I. 1984. Feline dysautonomia (the Key–Gaskell syndrome): A clinical and pathological study of forty cases. *Journal of Small Animal Practice* 25:599–615.

189. Muir, P., Jones, T., and Howard, P. 1990. A clinical and microbiological study of cats with protruding nictitating membranes and diarrhoea: Isolation of a novel virus. *Veterinary Research* 127:324–330.

190. Peruccio, C. 1981. Surgical correction of prominent third eyelid in the dog. *California Veterinarian* 4:24–27.

191. Latimer, C., Wyman, M., Szymanski, C., and Werling, K. 1983. Membrana nictitans gland cyst in a dog. *Journal of the American Veterinary Medical Association* 183:1003–1005.

192. Martin, C., Kaswan, R., and Doran, C. 1987. Cystic lesions of the periorbital region. *Compendium on Continuing Education for the Practicing Veterinarian* 9:1021–1029.

193. Lavach, J., and Snyder, S. 1984. Squamous cell carcinoma of the third eyelid in a dog. *Journal of the American Veterinary Medical Association* 184:975–976.

194. Peiffer, R., and Johnston, S. 1976. Pseudoepitheliomatous hyperplasia of the membrana nictitans in a dog. *Veterinary Medicine/Small Animal Clinician* 71:636–637.

195. Hargis, A., Lee, A., and Thomassen, R. 1978. Tumor and tumor-like lesions of perilimbal conjunctiva in laboratory dogs. *Journal of the American Veterinary Medical Association* 173:1185–1190.

196. Peiffer, R., Duncan, J., and Terrell, T. 1978. Hemangioma of the nictitating membrane in a dog. *Journal of the American Veterinary Medical Association* 172:832–833.

197. Hare, C., and Howard, E. 1977. Canine conjunctivocorneal papillomatosis: A case report. *Journal of the American Animal Hospital Association* 13:688–690.

198. Bonney, C., Koch, S., Dice, P., and Confer, A. 1980. Papillomatosis of conjunctiva and adnexa in dogs. *Journal of the American Veterinary Medical Association* 176:48–51.

199. Bonney, D., Koch, S., Confer, A., and Dice, P. 1980. A case report: A conjunctivocorneal papilloma with evidence of a viral etiology. *Journal of Small Animal Practice* 21:183–188.

200. Sansom, J., Barnett, K.C., Blunden, A.S., Smith, K.C., Turner, S., and Waters, L. 1996. Canine conjunctival papilloma: A review of five cases. *Journal of Small Animal Practice* 37:84–86.

201. Schaeffer, E.H., Pfleghaar, S., Gordon, S., and Knoedlseder, M. 1994. Maligne nickhauttumoren bei hund und katze. *Tieraerztl Praxis* 22:382–391.

202. Roels, S., and Ducatelle, R. 1998. Malignant melanoma of the nictitating membrane in a cat. *Journal of Comparative Pathology* 119:189–193.

203. Wilcock, B.P., and Peiffer, R.L. 1988. Adenocarcinoma of the gland of the third eyelid in seven dogs. *Journal of the American Veterinary Medical Association* 193:1549–1550.

204. Kkomaromy, A.M., Ramsey, D.T., Render, J.A., and Clark, P. 1997. Primary adenocarcinoma of the gland of the nictitating membrane in a cat. *Journal of the American Animal Hospital Association* 33:333–336.

205. Nasisse, M.P., Guy, J.S., Davidson, M.G., Sussman, W., and De Clercq, E. 1989. *In vitro* susceptibility of feline herpesvirus-1 to vidarabine, idoxuridine, trifluridine, acyclovir, or bromovinyl deoxyuridine. *American Journal of Veterinary Research* 50:158–160.

206. Buyukmihci, N. 1975. Fibrosarcoma of the nictitating membrane in a cat. *Journal of the American Veterinary Medical Association* 167:934–935.

207. Ledbetter, E.C. et al. 2006. Corneal ulceration associated with naturally occurring canine herpesvirus-1 infection in two adult dogs. *Journal of the American Veterinary Medical Association* 229:376–384.

208. Volopich, S. et al. 2005. Cytologic findings snd feline herpesvirus DNA and *Chlamydophila felis* antigen detection rates in normal cats and cats with conjunctival and corneal lesions. *Veterinary Ophthalmology* 8:25–32.

209. Maggs, D.J., Clarke, H.E. 2005. Relative sensitivity of polymerase chain reaction assays used for detection of feline herpesvirus type 1 DNA in clinical samples and commercial vaccines. *American Journal of Veterinary Research* 66:1550–1555.

210. Maggs, D.J., Clarke. H.E. 2004. In vitro efficacy of gannciclovir, cidofovir, penciclovir, foscarnet, idoxuridine, and aciclovir against feline herpesvirus type 1. *American Journal of Veterinary Research* 65:399–403.

211. Williams, D.L. et al. 2005. Efficacy of topical aciclovir for the treatment of feline herpetic keratitis: Result of a prospective clinical trial and data from in vitro investigations. *Veterinary Record* 157:254–257.

212. Foentenelle, J.P. et al. 2008. Effect of topical ophthalmic application of cidofovir on experimentally induced primary ocular feline herpesvirus-1 infection in cats. *American Journal of Veterinary Research* 69:289–293.

213. Maggs, D.J. et al. 2007. Effects of dietary lysine supplementation in cats with enzootic upper respiratory disease. *Journal of Feline Medicine and Surgery* 9:97–108.

214. Browining, G.F. 2004. Is Chlamydophila felis a significant zoonotic pathogen? *Australian Veterinary Journal* 82:695–696.

215. Dean, R. et al. 2005. Use of quantitative real-time PCR to monitor the response of Chlamydophila felis infection to doxycycline treatment. *Journal of Clinical Microbiology* 43:1858–1864.

216. Hartmann, A.D. et al. 2008. Efficacy of pradofloxacin in cats with feline upper respiratory tract disease due to Chlamydophila felis of Mycoplasma infections. *Journal of Veterinary Internal Medicine* 22:44–52.

217. Berhardt, N. et al. 2006. Pharmacokinetics of enrofloxacin and its efficacy in comparison with doxycycline in the treatment of Chlamydophila felisd infection in cats with conjunctivitis. *Veterinary Record* 159:591–594.

218. Sturgess, C. et al. 2001. Controlled study of the efficacy of clavulanic acid-potentiated amoxycillin in the treatment of Chlamydia psittaci in cats. *Veterinary Record* 149:73–76.

219. Germann, A.J. et al. 2005. Oesophegal strictures in cats associated with doxyxcline therapy. *Journal of Feline Medicine and Surgery* 7:33–41.

220. Heather, L. et al. 2007. Prevalence of feline herpesvirus 1, Chlamydophila felis, and Mycoplasma spp. DNA in conjunctival cells collected from cats with and without conjunctivitis. *American Journal of Veterinary Research* 68:643–648.

221. Bianciardi, P., Ottranto, D. 2005. Treatment of dogs with thelaziosis caused by Thelazia callipaeda (Spirurida, Thelaziidae) using a topical formulation of imidacloprid 10% and moxidectin 2.5%. *Veterinary Parasitology* 129:89–93.

222. Johnstone, N.S. et al. 2008. Ligneous conjunctivitis secondary to a congenital plasminogen deficiency in a dog. *Journal of the American Veterinary Medical Association* 232:715–721.

223. Torres, M.D. et al. 2006. Ligneous conjunctivitis in a dog: A case report. *Proceedings of American College of Veterinary Ophthalmology (San Antonio)* 37:25.

224. Barsotti, G. et al. 2007. Primary conjunctival mast cell tumor in a Labrador retriever. *Veterinary Ophthalmology* 10:60–64.

225. Moore, C.P. et al. 2000. Conjunctival malignant melanoma in a horse. *Veterinary Ophthalmology* 3:201–206.

226. Pirie, C.G. et al. 2006. Canina conjunctival hemangioma and hemagiosarcoma: A retrospective evaluation of 108 cases (1989–2004). *Veterinary Ophthalmology* 9:215–226.

227. Allgoewer, I. et al. 2008. Aberrant conjunctival stricture and overgrowth in the rabbit. *Veterinary Ophthalmology* 11:18–22.

228. Brudenall, D.K. et al. 2008. Bilateral corneaconjunctivals dermoids and nasal choristomas in a calf. *Veterinary Ophthalmology* 11:202–206.

229. Pirie, C.G., Dubielzig, R.R. 2006. Feline conjuctival hemangioma and hemangiosarcoma: A retrospective evaluation of eight cases (1993–2004). *Veterinary Ophthalmology* 9:227–231.

230. Radi, Z.A. et al. 2004. B-cell conjunctival lymphoma in a cat. *Veterinary Ophthalmology* 7:413–415.

231. Vascellari, M. et al. 2005. Unicentric extranodal lymphoma of the upper eyelid conjunctiva in a dog. *Veterinary Ophthalmology* 8:67–70.

232. Holt, E. et al. 2006. Extranodal conjunctival Hodgkin's-like lymphoma in a cat. *Veterinary Ophthalmology* 9:141–144.

CHAPTER 9

LACRIMAL APPARATUS

J. PHILLIP PICKETT

The lacrimal system is divided into secretory and excretory components. The secretory components consist of the orbital lacrimal gland, the third eyelid gland, and the glands and secretory cells of the eyelids. Cows, pigs, birds, and rodents have an additional deeper gland in the third eyelid, the Harderian gland,[1] the secretions of which are high in lipids.[2] In general, the Harderian gland is absent from terrestrial carnivores and primates. The excretory components of the lacrimal system consist of a lacrimal punctum on each eyelid (in most domestic species), a lacrimal canaliculus draining the punctum into the rudimentary lacrimal sac, and the nasolacrimal duct (**Figure 9.1**).

ANATOMY AND PHYSIOLOGY

The orbital lacrimal gland and the third eyelid gland are mixed, seromucoid, compound tubuloacinar glands. The glandular tubules contain serous granules, and the acini contain sialomucin granules on histochemistry and ultrastructural studies (**Figure 9.2**).[3] In the third eyelid gland, peripheral acini contain large amounts of lipids and no striated ducts (**Figure 9.3**).

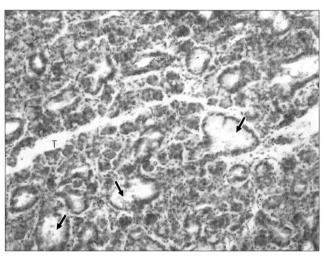

Figure 9.2 Normal canine third eyelid gland with acini granules staining positive for alcian blue (arrows) that indicates sialomucin; the tubules (T, structures with lumen) do not stain as they contain serous granules. (Alcian blue pH 2.5, nuclear fast red counterstain, ×200.)

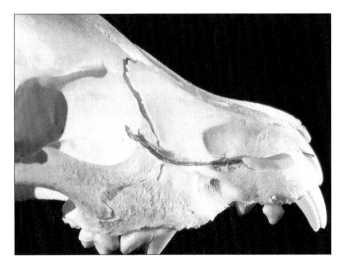

Figure 9.1 **Cast of nasolacrimal duct in a sculptured skull of a dog. Note the lack of a distinct lacrimal sac, the proximal bone encased portion passing through the lacrimal and maxillary bones, and the proximity to the root of the upper canine tooth.**

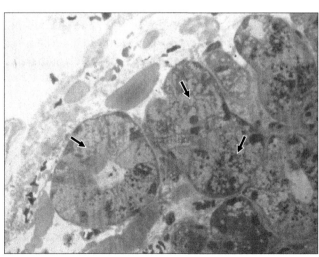

Figure 9.3 Peripheral lobules of a canine third eyelid gland containing acini with lipids (arrows). (1 μm section, toluidine blue stain.)

The ultrastructure of the normal equine lacrimal gland[4] is similar to that of the dog, as are the lacrimal glands of sheep and goats.[5] In the dog and the cat, the gland of the third eyelid surrounds the base of the cartilage of the third eyelid, and the orbital lacrimal gland is flattened and lies in a fold of periorbita beneath the dorsolateral orbital rim and the orbital ligament. Based on extirpation of glands and measuring the decrease in tear production, Gelatt et al. determined that in the dog approximately 62% of tear secretion is produced by the main lacrimal gland and 35% by the third eyelid gland, although either gland alone can supply adequate tears to maintain surface ocular health in a normal eye.[6] Helper et al. observed that in the dog a 5%–23% decrease in tear production occurred with removal of the lacrimal gland, and a 29%–57% decrease occurred with removal of the third eyelid gland.[7] Saito et al. showed that following third eyelid gland removal, reflex tearing was decreased 26% at 3–7 months; however, reflex tear measurements were normal 1 year post third eyelid gland removal.[8] In the cat, the orbital lacrimal gland contributes 13%–46% of aqueous tears, and the third eyelid gland contributes approximately 25% of the tears.[9] These percentages are misleading, as they do not consider the compensatory increase of tears by the remaining gland over time.

In the past, it has been stated that removal of only one of the two main aqueous tear producing glands does not produce a sufficient decrease in tears to produce disease.[6,10] However, later studies[8,11] reveal that deleterious effects on basal tear production, tear film break up time, and corneal epithelial health occur following removal of third eyelid glands in dogs. Removal of both the orbital lacrimal gland and the third eyelid gland results in keratoconjunctivitis sicca (KCS) in the dog[7] and the cat. Precorneal tear film mucus is produced by conjunctival goblet cells as well as the lacrimal and third eyelid gland. Accessory lacrimal glands are limited to the small glands of Zeis and Moll in the eyelids. No comparable accessory lacrimal glands to the glands of Krause and Wolfring seen in man have been demonstrated in the dog and the cat.

> Although removal of one of the two main lacrimal glands may not result in significant decrease in aqueous tear production quantity in a normal eye, deleterious effects on basal tearing and tear quality may be seen. Removal of an aqueous tear-producing gland in a breed predisposed to keratoconjunctivitis sicca may accelerate the onset of disease and may leave the stigma of an iatrogenic cause with the owner.

Sexual dimorphism in lacrimal gland morphology exists in a variety of species, with males having a greater mass of acinar tissue.[12] This gender difference also translates into functional differences and may partially explain the effect of gender and neutering on the incidence of KCS.[13]

The lacrimal glands secrete a slightly alkaline (8.05 ± 0.26, canine, 7.84 ± 0.30, equine[14]), protein-poor, isotonic serous fluid with a small component of mucin.[15] The secretion of the aqueous phase is the result of passive osmotic drawing of water into the lumen from active secretion of electrolytes, typical of most exocrine glands. The tears lubricate the corneal surface, providing a smooth, regular surface that enhances the optical properties of the cornea. Tears also mechanically cleanse the conjunctival sac and function in the nourishment of the cornea and the conjunctiva. A variety of growth factors, antibacterial substances, and proteases have been isolated from human and animal species' tears. Forty to sixty different proteins have been isolated from human tears, and many others are species specific. These tear proteins include pre-albumin or specific tear albumin (STP), albumin, immune globulins (IgA, IgG, IgE, IgD, and IgM), metal carrying proteins, complement, other inflammatory mediators, histamine, plasminogen activator substance, prostaglandins, proteases, lysozyme, beta-lysin, lactoferrin, and interferon. Lysozyme is one of the most important of the proteins in primates accounting for 15%–30% of the total protein but is absent or present in only very low levels in non-primates. Lysozyme has mucolytic and antibacterial activity for Gram positive bacteria while beta lysine is active against Gram negative organisms. The total antibacterial action of tears in humans is much greater than the lysozyme antibacterial activity alone.[199] The concentration of the various proteins, and thus their importance, may vary with species.

Although the tear film consists mainly of water, it is not a homogenous solution. In man, the axial tear film thickness is 3.4 ± 2.6 µm thick.[17] Traditionally, the tear film has been described as consisting of three layers (**Figure 9.4**). The inner layer is a hydrophilic mucin, a mixture of glycoproteins probably secreted mainly by the goblet cells but also by the lacrimal glands. The mucin contributes to the glycocalix on the surface of the epithelium and makes the naturally hydrophobic epithelium wettable. The mucus also protects the epithelium from bacteria and other noxious agents. The second and most voluminous layer is aqueous, secreted by the lacrimal glands. The thin outer layer of lipids is secreted by the meibomian glands in the lid margins and increases surface tension and retards evaporation.[18] Recent concepts of the tear film mucous layer favor a transition of mucus from the mucus-rich corneal side extending into the aqueous phase, resulting in a bilaminar model of aqueous–mucin and lipid.[19]

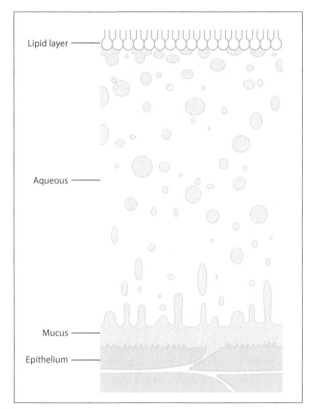

Figure 9.4 **Trilaminar structure model of the normal tear film.**

The third eyelid gland and the lacrimal gland are under dual autonomic control. The third eyelid gland receives parasympathetic fibers that originate in the facial nerve (nucleus intermedius) but arrive via a branch of the infratrochlear nerve (ophthalmic division of the trigeminal nerve).[20] The parasympathetic fibers of the orbital lacrimal gland originate similarly to those of the third eyelid but reach the gland via the lacrimal nerve, a branch of the ophthalmic division of the trigeminal nerve (**Figure 9.5**).[21,22] Parasympathetic stimulation increases the lacrimal flow rate and electrolyte content, and adrenergic stimulation controls the macromolecular content of the secretion. In the cat and the rabbit, excess adrenergic stimulation may noticeably decrease both reflex and basal tear secretion. The control of goblet cell mucus production is not well understood but is felt to be controlled by histamine, immune complexes, mechanical action, muscarinic and adrenergic stimulation, as well as stimulation by neuropeptides.[23–26] A mucus-stimulating factor has been demonstrated to be present in normal human tears and absent from individuals with various dry eye syndromes.[27]

Tears pool ventrally within the recess of the conjunctival sac in the medial canthus, forming a lacrimal lake. Drainage proceeds into the lacrimal canaliculi through the lacrimal puncta. In the dog, the lower punctum is normally

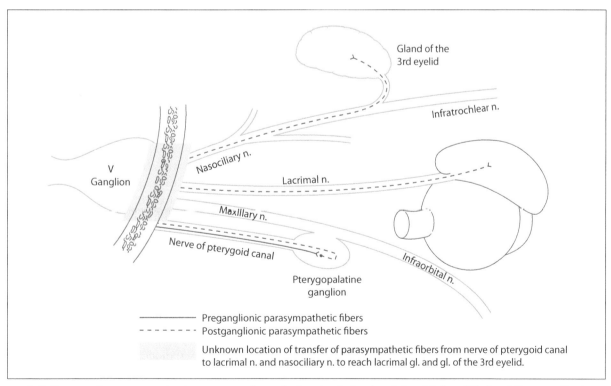

Figure 9.5 **Proposed parasympathetic nerve supply to the lacrimal gland and the third eyelid gland. Preganglionic nerve fibers leave the skull via the pterygoid canal nerve, synapse in the pterygopalatine ganglion, return in the pterygoid canal nerve, and distribute to ophthalmic nerve branches. (n: Nerve.) (From Powell, C. 1988. *Autonomic innervation of the canine lacrimal glands.* Master's thesis, University of Georgia, pp. 1–77.)**

situated about 5 mm from the medial canthus and 1–2 mm from the mucocutaneous margin within the palpebral conjunctiva. The dorsal punctum is similarly situated 5–8 mm from the medial canthus in the dorsal lid. In the dog, the cat, the horse, and the cow, the palpebral puncta are located just medial to the end of the tarsal plate. The rabbit has only a single large ventral punctum (located in the inferomedial conjunctival fornix) and canaliculus.

The canaliculi converge in a vestigial lacrimal sac encased within the depression of the lacrimal bone. The nasolacrimal duct carries tears from the lacrimal sac to the anterior end of the nasal vestibule. The lacrimal canaliculi, the lacrimal sac, and the nasolacrimal duct have a stratified columnar epithelium.[5] The nasolacrimal duct consists of a proximal portion encased within the lacrimal and maxillary bones and a distal membranous portion. The bone-encased portion is narrower and often has constrictions in various species (**Figures 9.1 and 9.6**).[28,29] The nasal puncta in the horse are found in the inferomedial floor of the nasal vestibule. In the dog and the cat, the nasal puncta are located on the inferolateral floor of the nasal vestibule. In cattle and camelids, the nasal puncta are located dorsolaterally over the alar cartilage. Imperfections may occur in the distal nasolacrimal duct of individual dogs and cats, with the result that drainage may occur posteriorly into the nasopharynx. These variations are particularly common in brachycephalic breeds. In brachycephalic cats, the distal nasolacrimal duct is deviated dorsally under the root of the canine tooth.[30] This deviation may explain why brachycephalic dogs and cats have epiphora while still having a patent nasolacrimal duct system when mechanically flushed from lid to nose.

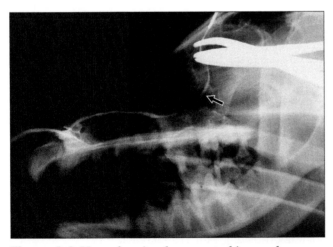

Figure 9.6 **Normal canine dacryocystorhinography performed by injection of an aqueous contrast material. Note the ventral curvature of the proximal half (arrow) and how narrow the lumen is through the bony portion in the maxillary bone.**

DISEASES OF THE LACRIMAL SYSTEM

Most diseases of the lacrimal system can broadly be categorized into problems of decreased tear production, increased tear production, obstruction of the outflow system, and abnormal masses.

Keratoconjunctivitis sicca

Introduction/etiology

Commonly called "dry eye" or xerophthalmia, KCS can be defined as a progressive inflammatory condition of the cornea and the conjunctiva caused by a lack of tears. The deficiency is usually in the aqueous phase, but deficiencies in mucin have been recognized in the dog and the cat.[31–33] A deficiency of the precorneal tear film is commonly encountered in small animal practice. In a 1976 survey of 14 veterinary colleges, approximately 0.4% of the general hospital population had KCS.[34] Updated analysis (1991) of a similar database showed an increase in prevalence to 1.52%.[13] Newer still data (1996) indicated incidence of KCS in dogs at 0.9%.[35] These changes in frequency of diagnosis of KCS in the dog probably represent an increased awareness as well as changes in breed popularity over the years.

With loss of the nutritive and protective functions of the tears, a spectrum of acute and chronic corneal and conjunctival lesions is produced. In the acute to subacute patient, the epithelium of the cornea is thinned to three to four layers, with loss of the basal layer. In the acute disease, epithelium develops keratinization and subepithelial inflammatory cell infiltration. The epithelium with chronicity becomes thickened, develops rete pegs, contains pigment granules, and is keratinized. The anterior corneal stroma develops extensive neovascularization and mononuclear inflammatory cell infiltration. There is a decrease in the number of goblet cells in the conjunctival epithelium.[36] Short-term studies in the cat indicate that the epithelial changes of decreased goblet cell density and squamous metaplasia are not associated with decreased tear film but with the infiltration of subepithelial lymphocytic inflammatory infiltration, whatever the cause.[37] Lim and Cullen found a clinical correlate for this, in that cats with conjunctivitis from a variety of causes had decreased tear break-up times.[33] There was no relationship between the Schirmer tear test (STT) and the conjunctivitis in this study. Kern et al. were unable to demonstrate decreased goblet cell numbers on scanning electron microscopy in a subacute experimental model.[38]

Most reports indicate no apparent sex predisposition in most breeds, apart from the West Highland white terrier, which has a marked female predominance.[34,39] Neutering of either the male or the female dog increases the predisposition to KCS. Because more females are neutered

(3.4×) than males, statistically older female dogs develop KCS more often than do older male dogs.[13] The effect of neutering on KCS prevalence is not noted until animals are 10 years of age.[13] Androgens have an effect on lacrimal gland size and function and on autoimmunity and may inhibit an endogenous tear suppresser such as prolactin. The incidence of KCS is higher in older dogs (7–9 years at onset).[13] Sanchez et al. presented contemporary statistics for "idiopathic" KCS as reflected in Scotland and found that 58% of the cases were comprised of four breeds: English Cocker Spaniel, West Highland white terrier, Cavalier King Charles spaniel, and Shih Tzu.[40] These numbers were not matched against a hospital-based population and, therefore, are somewhat relative. All cases were bilateral disease or progressed to bilateral disease. The disease in the two brachycephalic breeds presented at an earlier age and was more rapidly referred due to a more acute syndrome, often with corneal ulcerations and upper eyelid trichiasis. The West Highland white terrier and English Cocker Spaniel had a female predisposition and a more chronic course.

English Bulldogs, Cocker Spaniels, and Dachshunds are predisposed to KCS, often with concurrent generalized skin disease. The West Highland white terrier and miniature schnauzer have a high incidence of KCS independent of skin disease. Helper reported highest incidence of KCS (in order of frequency of occurrence) in English bulldogs, West Highland white terriers, pugs, Yorkshire terriers, American Cocker Spaniels, Pekingese, miniature schnauzers, and English Cocker Spaniels.[35] In exophthalmic breeds, lagophthalmos often complicates a deficiency of tears, causing the KCS lesions to be more pronounced. Even when STT values are only slightly reduced, dry spots and exposure keratitis develop easily with lagophthalmos. In some breeds, such as the pug and Pekingese, melanocyte activity is particularly intense, and severe pigmentary keratitis is common in conjunction with decreased tear production. (See **Table 9.1** for incidence of KCS in specific canine breeds.)

A variety of causes or conditions are known to be associated with KCS. The most common etiology of KCS is a (probable) genetically based autoimmune adenitis, often with systemic ramifications[40,41] Response to therapy with immunomodulators supports immune-mediated lacrimal/third eyelid gland adenitis as the most common cause of KCS in the dog.[42–44]

Congenital alacrima Congenital KCS occurs occasionally as an extreme dryness (STT = 0 in most cases) and is many times unilateral. It is most commonly observed in small breeds[36] (**Figure 9.7**). Herrera et al. reinforced this clinical picture by reporting on 16 Yorkshire terriers

BREED	RELATIVE POPULATION (%)	RELATIVE INCIDENCE
American Cocker Spaniel	2.8	6.76
Boston terrier	0.76	3.89
Bulldog	0.64	20.12
Chihuahua	1.09	1.31
Dachshund	2.96	1.48
Doberman pinscher	3.20	0.15
German shepherd dog	7.60	0.57
Lhasa Apso	0.56	16.56
Miniature schnauzer	1.91	3.93
Mixed breed	27.09	0.82
Pekingese	0.99	6.31
Pug	0.4	7.87
Shih tzu	0.27	4.02
Yorkshire terrier	0.64	5.33
West Highland white terrier	0.39	18.36

Table 9.1 **KCS breed distribution (597,516 cases).**

with early onset of a unilateral profound KCS.[45] Biopsy of the lacrimal gland region was attempted on one dog without success, indicating either a lack of a lacrimal gland or a technical problem. None of the cases responded to cyclosporine therapy. Barnett reported on a syndrome in the Cavalier King Charles spaniel that was well known in the breeding fraternity, but not the veterinary profession, of congenital bilateral KCS associated with a curly coat.[46] The signs began as early as 10 days of age, often with corneal ulceration. With maturity, the hair became coarse, pruritus developed, and the skin became hyperkeratotic on the ventral abdomen and on the paws and nail beds, with distortion of the nails. On necropsy, the

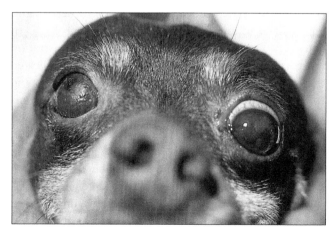

Figure 9.7 **Congenital lack of tears in a Chihuahua.** This is typically observed in small breeds and is commonly unilateral. Note the profound dryness.

orbital and third eyelid lacrimal glands were normal on light microscopy. This author has seen a higher incidence of congenital alacrima in beagles, miniature dachshunds, and miniature pinschers than other breeds, with the disorder being bilateral (especially in miniature pinschers) with some frequency. This occurrence may reflect a local breed-related incidence.

Neurologic KCS may be observed in animals with facial nerve palsy of central origin or occurring in the very proximal nerve before branching of the parasympathetic fibers in the petrous temporal bone.[47] Denervation of the parasympathetic fibers in the lacrimal nerve may also occur from damage such as proptosis in the dog and cat. Ruskell reported that in primates, serous secretory cells in the lacrimal glands require cholinergic innervation, whereas mucus-secreting cells are autonomous.[48] Trauma to cranial nerve VII with neurologic sequelae is the usual cause of KCS in the horse.[49,50] Dysautonomia (generalized lack of sympathetic or parasympathetic innervation) has been described as a cause of KCS in cats.[51–53]

Drug induced Atropine, phenazopyridine, anesthesia, 5-aminosalicylic acid, and sulfonamides can cause transient or permanent KCS in the dog, depending on how long the drug has been used.[54–61] The toxicity of phenazopyridine varies with species, and the lacrimal gland is unaffected in the cat, the rabbit,[62] or humans. Atropine- and anesthesia-induced KCS[63] is usually transient but may last for several days when combined with other postoperative complications. Topical atropine applied to one eye decreased the STT value in both eyes for up to 5 weeks in normal dogs.[64] In testing various sedative combinations, xylazine and butorphanol caused the most profound decrease in reflex Schirmer I value (6 mm), but the duration until recovery was not reported.[65]

Sulfonamide-induced KCS is frequently permanent, especially with long-term therapy and chronic KCS. In one study, KCS secondary to sulfonamide administration was permanent in 77% of dogs.[58] Another study indicated that dogs <12 kg were at increased risk of developing KCS.[66] KCS may develop after only a few doses of sulfonamide; in one study, most animals developed KCS within the first week of therapy,[66] while in another study, KCS was found only after long-term therapy.[67] The mechanism for toxicity is not completely understood but may be due to a T-cell-mediated response to proteins haptenated by oxidative sulfonamide metabolites.[68] Animals administered sulfonamide long term for conditions such as cystitis and colitis should be monitored frequently for decreased tear production. If STT values decrease while a dog is undergoing sulfonamide therapy, immediate discontinuation of the drug may allow recovery of the lacrimal tissue without subsequent permanent KCS. No association was found between the type of sulfonamide used, dosage, or duration of therapy and the prognosis for recovery from KCS.[67]

Beta-blockers such as timolol have been reported in human ophthalmology to reduce tear secretion and produce KCS symptoms in a small group of patients,[69] but similar findings have not been reported in veterinary medicine. Oral etodolac (EtoGesic®) has been associated with KCS in dogs.[70,71] In a retrospective report by Klauss et al., dogs administered oral etodolac for less than 6 months prior to diagnosis of KCS were 4.2 times more likely to experience complete resolution of KCS following discontinuation of etodolac than were dogs treated for 6 months or longer.[71]

Viral infection Distemper virus can cause a unilateral or bilateral acute lacrimal adenitis and severe xerophthalmia (STT < 5 mm/min).[72,73] Corneal ulceration with descemetocele formation frequently occurs. Sicca due to distemper usually resolves spontaneously in 6–8 weeks if the animal recovers systemically. Histopathologic lesions are marked glandular degenerative changes associated with a mononuclear and neutrophilic cellular infiltration. Despite the marked morphologic changes, glandular function usually recovers.[72] Experimentally, transient KCS has been reported in cats with FHV-1 infection. Cause of the decreased STT values (attributable to glandular or ductule damage) is unknown.[74]

Obstruction of the lacrimal ductules Obstruction due to chemosis or conjunctival cicatrization, especially in cats with chronic FHV-1 infections,[75] can cause transient or permanent sicca. Decreased STT values are frequent in cats with marked conjunctival swelling and are often transient.[74] Likewise, many dogs with secondary bacterial conjunctivitis may improve STT values with appropriate antibiotic therapy and reduction of conjunctival swelling and hyperemia. Vitamin A deficiency with squamous metaplasia of the ducts is a cause of KCS in turtles, but it is thought to be an unlikely etiology of canine KCS.[36,76] Vitamin A deficiency in rats does not alter the volume of tears, but it does alter the composition of tears as a result of marked changes in secretory granule development.[77] *Leishmania* infection in the dog may produce KCS in 2.8% of infected animals. Naranjo et al. described the lacrimal gland pathology in dogs with leishmaniasis as a granulomatous to pyogranulomatous inflammation localized around the distal lacrimal ducts.[78] The organisms were found in this region as well. The pathogenesis of KCS may be due to ductal blockage as well as meibomian gland dysfunction, as the meibomian glands were also commonly infiltrated.

Removal of the third eyelid gland Controversy exists between ophthalmologists and general practitioners as to whether it is contraindicated to remove a prolapsed third eyelid gland ("cherry eye") or to remove the third eyelid gland for the treatment of epiphora. For KCS to occur, the orbital lacrimal gland must be damaged, as removal of the third eyelid gland does not lead to sicca.[6,7,9] While the normal dog can tolerate removal of the third eyelid gland, it is prudent to avoid surgical excision for benign conditions in those breeds predisposed to KCS. In breeds predisposed to cherry eye, 47% developed KCS after glandular excision, compared to 17% with glandular repositioning (see Chapter 8).[79]

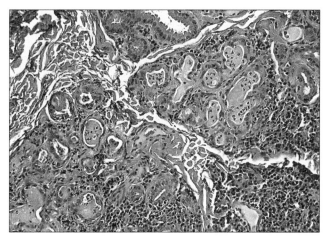

Figure 9.8 Extensive mononuclear adenitis with acinar atrophy and interstitial fibrosis. (H&E ×150.)

> KCS associated with third eyelid gland removal is not immediate but usually has a delayed onset of months or years. This delay may explain the diversity of opinion between ophthalmologists and general practitioners regarding third eyelid gland removal. In some circles, removal of the third eyelid gland in a dog, for reasons other than neoplasia, is considered veterinary medical malpractice.

Autoimmune-mediated adenitis Evidence for an autoimmune cause of KCS was found in histology from a series of 25 third eyelid glands or main lacrimal glands dissected from dogs with chronic KCS undergoing parotid duct transplant. The most common lesion was multifocal mononuclear cell infiltration with varying degrees of fibrosis (**Figures 9.8 and 9.9**). In about 50% of the biopsies, the morphologic changes were mild to modest and were not so disruptive as to explain the lack of glandular function, despite the chronicity and absolute deficiency of tears (**Figure 9.10**).[80,81] On serum electrophoresis, the beta-2 fraction of gamma globulin was elevated in 90% of KCS cases. Antinuclear antibodies and rheumatoid factor titers were elevated in 42% and 50%, respectively, of KCS cases.[82,83] A probable immune-mediated KCS has also been described in the horse, in which the histopathologic response is predominantly eosinophilic adenitis.[84–87] The author has seen some equine cases of bilateral eosinophilic keratoconjunctivitis that have concurrently suffered from absolute xerophthalmia (STT = 0) that failed to respond to topical immunomodulation but did respond to systemic corticosteroid therapy.[88]

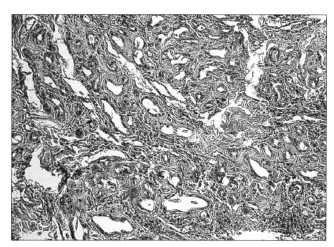

Figure 9.9 Advanced fibrotic changes with acinar loss in a third eyelid gland from a dog with sicca. This gland may not improve with therapy. (H&E ×150.)

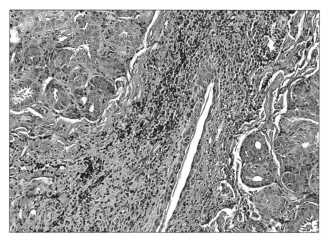

Figure 9.10 Modest mononuclear inflammation of the third eyelid gland with intact acini in a dog with chronic KCS. This type of gland would be expected to respond to therapy. (H&E ×150.)

Endocrine and other disease Hyperadrenocorticism, hypothyroidism, diabetes mellitus, demodectic mange, and systemic lupus erythematosus have been empirically associated with canine keratoconjunctivitis sicca. In one study, decreased STT values were seen in dogs with hyperadrenocorticism, hypothyroidism, and diabetes mellitus compared to control dogs without endocrinopathies.[89] In one study, 29% of canine KCS cases had other diseases related to immunologic disorders, and 32% had chronic refractory skin diseases.[82] Peruccio reported a 20% incidence of hypothyroidism in dogs with KCS as evidenced by a low T3 and T4.[90] Hypothyroidism and KCS are probably associated through a multiglandular autoimmune phenomenon, as hypothyroidism does not cause KCS when experimentally induced.[91,92] Dryness of the nasal and oral mucous membranes occurs in 10%–30% of KCS cases and should be evaluated before performing parotid duct transposition. Dogs[93] and cats[94] with multiglandular involvement and circulating autoantibodies have signs resembling Sjögren's syndrome in man.

Senile atrophy Although age of onset for many cases of canine KCS is high,[13] it is unknown whether age-related lacrimal/third eyelid gland atrophy exists in the dog as a cause of KCS.

Irradiation Irradiation for cancer therapy near the eyes may result in glandular damage. Although irradiation is an uncommon cause of KCS, in patients undergoing radiation therapy, it is quite common. Megavoltage therapy of nasal and paranasal lesions resulted in ocular complications in 75% of patients, of which 25% developed KCS.[95] Supervoltage or cobalt-60 irradiation of the head region resulted in 84% of patients developing ocular lesions, of which 35% were KCS.[96]

Retrograde infection into the lacrimal glands Chronic conjunctivitis with retrograde infection ascending the lacrimal ductules has historically been blamed as a cause of KCS. In most instances, it was not known whether the conjunctivitis was caused by, or produced, the KCS. Retrograde infection is not thought to be a significant cause of KCS in the dog, based on the absence of infectious agents on histopathology of the glands.[81]

Androgen deficiency Androgens have a significant modifying effect on the morphology and the function of the lacrimal gland. Androgen therapy of mouse models of Sjögren's syndrome (autoimmune adenitis) suppresses the lymphocytic inflammation in the lacrimal gland and improves the lacrimal function.[97] It has been theorized that an androgen deficiency causes an atrophy of lacrimal gland

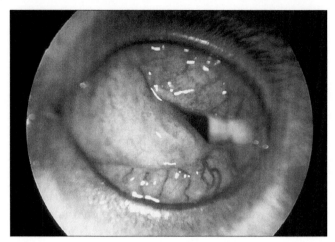

Figure 9.11 **Cat with marked conjunctival chemosis associated with ocular herpesvirus infection that resulted in a lack of tears. The tear secretion returned when the chemosis decreased.**

acini that triggers an autoimmune response.[98] Sullivan et al. were unable to produce either lacrimal gland inflammation or a decrease in function by castrating mice, rabbits, and guinea pigs, examining mice with dysfunctional androgen receptors, or examining men treated with antiandrogen therapy.[99]

Causes in the cat
The causes of KCS in the cat are not well documented, but conjunctival chemosis may be the cause for obstruction of the lacrimal ductules, as evidenced by rapid improvement in STT values with resolution of the chemosis (**Figure 9.11**). Ocular herpesvirus infection is thought to be responsible for KCS in the cat, although it is unknown whether the virus affects the gland or simply produces chemosis that may in turn cause obstruction.[74] Scarring of the lacrimal ductules in cats with chronic KCS or symblepharon from previous FHV-1 infections may cause KCS. Neurologic disease, whether traumatic, infectious, or neoplastic, may be associated with KCS in the cat. Trauma to the orbit such as proptosis frequently results in KCS for about 8–12 weeks. Feline dysautonomia is a rare systemic disorder that may result in marked xerophthalmia along with other clinical signs.[51-53]

Clinical signs in the dog
Severity of signs varies with the species. The dog typically has the most dramatic signs, while in the cat, signs are often minimal, even with an absolute lack of aqueous tears. The horse is intermediate in the severity of signs.

Approximately 70% of KCS cases in the dog eventually become bilateral. The eyes may be sequentially or simultaneously involved.

Pain

Initially, corneal dryness is painful and may be associated with blepharospasm. Chronic cases usually do not exhibit blepharospasm due to hyperkeratinization of the corneal epithelium with decreased corneal sensation, but there seems to be individual and breed differences as to the manifestation of pain. The cornea of brachycephalic breeds is less sensitive than that of other breeds,[100] so many brachycephalic dogs may show minimal signs of pain as compared to other breeds.

In the author's experience, very acute onset of KCS produces more dramatic signs of pain and corneal ulceration versus a more chronic disorder. Acute-onset KCS seems to have a greater chance for spontaneous remission over a short (8–12-week) period versus a more chronic disorder.

Conjunctivitis

The bulbar and palpebral conjunctivae are usually intensely hyperemic and thickened. Mucoid to mucopurulent material is usually abundant in the conjunctival folds and fornices (**Figure 9.12**).

Ocular discharge

Mucin, produced by conjunctival goblet cells, is not dispersed because of the lack of an aqueous tear phase and, therefore, accumulates in varying degrees as tenacious "ropey' filaments. Mucin production is decreased in KCS as the goblet cell density decreases. Cellular exudation from secondary bacterial infection produces a mucopurulent discharge (**Figures 9.13 and 9.14**). In animals with severe tear deficiencies, this exudate, on culture, often contains

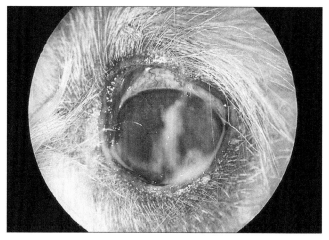

Figure 9.13 West Highland white terrier with tenacious, copious exudate from KCS. The third eyelid gland had previously been removed.

heavy growths of coagulase-positive staphylococci, beta-hemolytic streptococci, coliforms, and *Pseudomonas* spp.[101,102] Interestingly, in one study, bacterial growth post parotid duct transplant was more consistent and heavier, and the flora more pathogenic than before surgery.[102]

Keratitis

Multifocal punctate or central corneal ulceration (**Figure 9.15**) is common in the acute phase of KCS and may progress rapidly to stromal malacia and descemetoceles. In chronic KCS, the cornea develops a dull irregular appearance with neovascularization, fibrosis, and pigmentation. The corneal epithelium becomes hypertrophic. Pigment is deposited in patches or can become so dense that the cornea loses all transparency, and blindness ensues (**Figure 9.16**). In the cat, chronic ulceration may lead to corneal sequestrum formation (**Figure 9.17**).

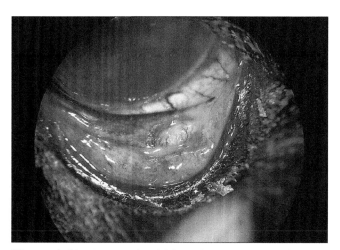

Figure 9.12 Hyperemic, thickened conjunctiva with tenacious exudate in conjunctival folds characteristic of KCS.

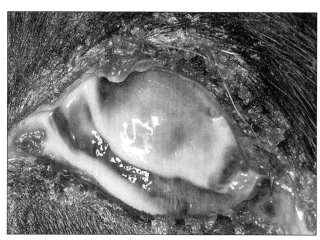

Figure 9.14 Extensive tenacious mucopurulent exudate with KCS.

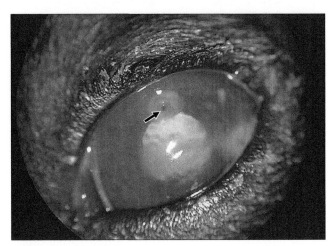

Figure 9.15 Small descemetocele (arrow, dark spot) in a Boston terrier with acute KCS. Note the tenacious discharge on the cornea and the dull surface.

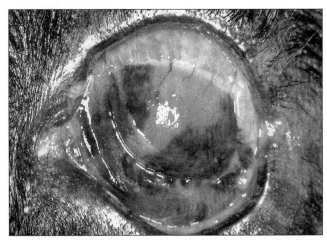

Figure 9.16 Same eye as Figure 9.14 after cleansing. Note the thickened conjunctiva, extensive corneal pigmentation, and gray scarring of the cornea.

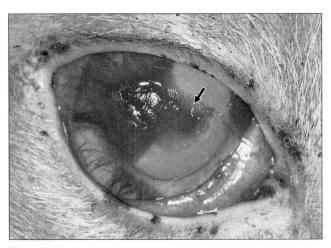

Figure 9.17 Cat with trauma-induced KCS that is forming a corneal sequestrum (arrow) in an ulcer bed.

Mucin deficiencies

Mucin deficiencies in the tear film are characterized by recurrent corneal ulceration, chronic keratoconjunctivitis, normal STT values, and a lack of ocular discharge. The tear film break-up time (TFBUT) is less than 5–10 seconds (normal canine 20+ seconds,[103] normal feline 12–21 seconds[104]), and on conjunctival biopsy, a deficiency of goblet cells with mononuclear inflammation is present.[31,32,105] In the case reports of mucin deficiencies, the condition has often been temporary and may reflect the fact that many causes for conjunctivitis produce a reduction in the tear break-up time and decreases in conjunctival goblet cells appear to be due to nonspecific conjunctival inflammation.

Clinical signs in the cat

The signs of KCS in the cat are usually much subtler than in the dog. The diagnosis is based on multiple low STT values and clinical signs. Cats may have very labile STT values, and one low reading is not diagnostic for KCS. KCS in the cat is characterized more by conjunctivitis with blepharospasm and less often with keratitis. Discharge is typically scant and mucoid. The conjunctivitis is characterized by hyperemia, chemosis, and thickened folds. KCS may be responsible for chronic nonhealing axial ulcers that develop a corneal sequestrum in the ulcer bed.

Clinical signs in the horse

KCS is rare in the horse. Painful blepharospasm is usually noted along with a lackluster corneal surface and occasionally axial corneal ulceration. Ocular discharge varies from mild mucoid (neurogenic cases) to moderate/severe mucoid to mucopurulent (inflammatory induced).

Diagnosis

Historically, KCS has been among the most commonly misdiagnosed ophthalmic diseases. Bacterial conjunctivitis and recurrent idiopathic corneal ulcers are commonly mistaken diagnoses made in cases of KCS. Misdiagnosed cases treated frequently with any topical ophthalmic preparation usually show transient improvement, falsely reinforcing the clinician's confidence in the original diagnosis. Virtually all topical medications wet the eye and add lubrication and, therefore, have some therapeutic benefit. A high degree of suspicion for KCS should be held for any recurrent conjunctivitis, keratitis, or corneal ulceration. Even though the cornea may not appear dry, a STT should be performed as a routine part of the anterior segment ophthalmic examination. The diagnosis should be based on multiple functional abnormalities, as has been suggested in human medicine.[106]

A diagnosis of KCS is made when a decrease in STT value occurs with mucopurulent keratoconjunctivitis, corneal inflammation, ulceration, or pigment deposition. The STT value in a normal dog is usually 16–24 mm/min, whereas in KCS cases, the STT value is typically <10 mm/min, with the majority <5 mm/min on repeated trials. In climates with low humidity, the acceptable level for STT readings before signs are observed is often increased due to tear loss from increased evaporation. Atropinization can cause transient dryness for 2–6 days post therapy. Fear-induced sympathetic stimulation also leads to sporadic low values, particularly in cats.

Inconsistencies have been demonstrated in STT values due to different papers used by different manufacturers[107] and the design of the strip.[108] Day-to-day variations in STT values as large as 5–9 mm in 17% and 10–21 mm in 6% of normal young beagles have been demonstrated.[109] Berger and King were unable to demonstrate significant variations in day-to-day measurements but did find differences in week-to-week values and between dogs of different sizes.[110] Large breeds of dogs had greater Schirmer I and II readings than small breeds of dogs. These differences in STT values must be considered when test results do not correlate to clinical signs.

> While variations occur in STT values of normal dogs, they are usually not of such magnitude that they would result in an error of diagnosis. KCS is diagnosed by correlating clinical signs with STT values, and as with any laboratory test, STT should be repeated when results do not correlate with clinical signs.

Mucin deficiency is diagnosed by the presence of a decreased tear film break-up time (TFBUT) and on biopsy of the medial ventral palpebral conjunctiva to examine for goblet cells. The TFBUT is evaluated by instilling fluorescein onto the cornea and examining it with a cobalt blue filter while keeping the animal from blinking. Tear film breakup is recognized by focal dark spots in the fluorescein film. The TFBUT is recorded as the time from last blink to the presence of the first dark spots. Values <10 seconds are low, and when combined with a STT value of >12 mm/min, they are suggestive of a mucin deficiency.[31,32] Because the TFBUT is not routinely performed in practice, this is probably an underdiagnosed condition.

Rose bengal staining of the cornea and the conjunctiva is suggestive but not specific for KCS. Rose bengal stains the epithelial surface when it is not protected by mucin (see Chapter 1).

Therapy

Medical therapy Medical therapy is the mainstay of therapy for KCS and should always be attempted for 2–3 months to evaluate whether the KCS is transient or permanent and whether the patient is responsive to medications.

Drugs that increase aqueous tear production

Topical calcium-dependent calcineurin/T-helper cell activation inhibitors Over the past 25 years, topical cyclosporine has become the gold standard for treating canine KCS. The original protocol of a 1%–2% solution every 12 to 24 hours gave remarkable results and quickly became the main form of therapy for KCS. The response to topical therapy usually seen is an increase of aqueous tear production and decreased corneal scarring. The response is often very rapid, but some cases may require 4–6 weeks of therapy to respond. Initial recommendation was that both eyes be treated, even if the KCS was unilateral. Most clinicians now only treat the affected eye. In general, the therapy controls but does not cure the problem; when therapy is withdrawn, the STT values decrease again in most cases of canine immune-mediated lacrimal adenitis.

The main form of KCS that appears responsive to cyclosporine is the immune-mediated lacrimal adenitis ("idiopathic") form. In an initial study, a statistically significant improvement in the glandular pathology after cyclosporine therapy was not demonstrated, although a trend towards improvement in histopathology lesions and regeneration of glandular lobules was identified.[111] In a subsequent study, decreased numbers of lymphocytes seen histologically and decreased CD8+ lymphocytes (T-helper cells) seen immunohistochemically were noted in the third eyelid gland tissue in treated dogs versus control dogs. In addition, signs of increased secretory activity were noted histologically in the treated dogs.[112] KCS associated with acute infection with distemper virus, glandular trauma, neurogenic KCS, and advanced glandular fibrosis usually does not respond to cyclosporine. KCS associated with systemic sulfonamide or systemic etodolac therapy usually does not respond when the loss of tears has been profound.[71,113,114]

Topical cyclosporine is thought to work in two distinct ways: A lacrimomimetic effect (stimulating tear secretions, minor effect in canine KCS) and an anti-inflammatory effect on the gland (major effect in canine KCS) and ocular surface. The lacrimomimetic effect may occur by releasing neurotransmitters such as substance P from sensory nerve endings in the lacrimal gland.[115] The anti-inflammatory effect on the lacrimal and third eyelid glands results in restoration of normal glandular health and structure, thus allowing normal production and secretion of aqueous tears.[111,112,116] The anti-inflammatory effect on the ocular surface may produce clinical improvement without an increase in tear production. The quality of the tears produced on stimulation by cyclosporine is similar to normal tears, without the decrease in secretory IgA that occurs with reflex tearing. Dogs with KCS that are treated with cyclosporine have a decrease in their tear IgG levels because of the anti-inflammatory effect on the re-establishment of the blood–tear barrier.[19]

Cyclosporine also has a direct beneficial effect on the conjunctival cells that have been altered by the induction of KCS. Moore et al. induced KCS in dogs with bilateral excision of both lacrimal glands and found that topical 2% cyclosporine rescued and maintained the quantity of mucin in the goblet cells, despite an ongoing deficiency in aqueous tears.[117] This resulted in less conjunctivitis and less mucoid discharge.

In patients with a STT value of 2 mm, all dogs responded to cyclosporine therapy with an increased STT value of at least 5 mm/min, whereas if the STT value was 0 mm/min, 36% of the patients failed to respond at all. Subsequent studies have reported a 75%–82% success rate of significantly increasing aqueous tear production, and a 1% solution was found to be as effective as a 2% solution.[42,43] Corneal pathology improved with cyclosporine therapy even in those patients that did not have improved tear production. Duration of KCS, gender, and breed had no affect on the outcome. The only factor that correlated with outcome was the initial STT value.

Localized adverse effects noted with 1%–2% compounded solutions to date have been ocular irritation and blepharitis, probably due to the vehicle or alcohol in the initially used homemade preparations. Compounding pharmacy-made aqueous preparations and mineral oil or coconut oil vehicle preparations free of alcohol have a much lower incidence of surface irritation than corn oil vehicle (incidence of corn hypersensitivities with chronic use is high) and alcohol-containing homemade preparations. After topical application of a 2% solution of cyclosporine, barely detectable blood levels are present, and depression of a lymphocyte proliferation test occurs, which may indicate a depressed cell-mediated immunity.[118] In dogs, chronic KCS treated with topical immunosuppressive therapy may also be a risk factor for the rare development of corneal squamous cell carcinoma.[119]

Cyclosporine is commercially available as a 0.2% ophthalmic ointment, and in most cases, but not all, this has been as successful as a 1%–2% compounded solution.[44] Topical application of 0.2% cyclosporine ointment is not detectable in the blood with current assay techniques. The vehicle used for the commercially available ointment product has been reported to maximize the bioavailability of the active drug.[120]

Tacrolimus (also a calcineurin inhibitor) suppresses T-cell activation and is 10–100× more potent on a weight basis than cyclosporine. As tacrolimus utilizes different cell receptors, it has been effective in some cases of KCS that were resistant to cyclosporine.[121] Tacrolimus has been compounded as a 0.02%–0.03% solution or ointment for topical treatment of KCS. With topical tacrolimus therapy, Chambers et al. obtained a 96% success rate, although the severity of cases treated was not stipulated.[122] Berdoulay et al. administered 0.02% aqueous solution of tacrolimus to dogs naïve to tear stimulation therapy, and in 85% of those with tear production less than 10 mm responded, with a mean increase of 7.5 mm/min.[123] In dogs with a marginal tear production of 11–15 mm/min, 25% responded with an increase of 2.7 mm/min. Dogs that had been on 1% cyclosporine responded to tacrolimus with a mean increase 2.8 mm/min, and 27% responded with an increase greater than 5 mm/min. Of the dogs that were unresponsive to 1%–2% cyclosporine, 51% had an increase in tear production of 5 mm/min or better on tacrolimus. Systemic effects were not noted, and only one dog was noted to rub his eyes after topical tacrolimus administration. Topical therapy with 1% tacrolimus aqueous solution was reported to increase STT values in dogs refractory to a variety of lacrimomimetic agents.[124] In this preliminary study, variable improvement of STT from 0 to >10 mm/min was reported, with improvement of keratitis being noted, even in those patients who did not respond with a measurable increase in STT.

In two clinical studies in KCS dogs comparing yet another calcineurin inhibitor, pimecrolimus 1% in corn oil, with 0.2% cyclosporine ointment, dogs on pimecrolimus responded on average with 4 mm/min more tears than those on cyclosporine[125,126] Pimecrolimus was also effective in treating superficial keratitis.

Initial uncomplicated KCS therapy usually consists of topical artificial tears every 6 hours with topical cyclosporine or tacrolimus, every 8 hours or every 12 hours; the artificial tear supplementation is discontinued as improvement is noted. If the patient is very responsive, cyclosporine or tacrolimus may be decreased in frequency or occasionally discontinued after several weeks or months; however, in most cases, calcineurin inhibitor therapy is usually assumed to be lifelong.

Pilocarpine Pilocarpine may be used for its acetylcholine-like action in stimulating lacrimal gland secretion. This is especially true for cases of neurogenic KCS due to lack of nervous stimulation of aqueous tear secretion due to CNVII damage. For an average 25-lb (12-kg) dog, one to two drops of 2% pilocarpine placed in food and given every 12 hours is initially recommended.[127] If no improvement in the STT value occurs, the dose can be increased by increments of one drop at a time. If hypersalivation, vomiting, or diarrhea occur, the medication should be stopped until signs abate and then reinstituted at a lower dosage. Bradycardia is a possible side effect of systemic use of pilocarpine, and pilocarpine may aggravate a pre-existing heart block. In cases where adverse side effects of systemic pilocarpine are seen, topical dilute (0.125%–0.25%) solutions of pilocarpine may be tried. Although topical application of pilocarpine has not been shown to increase tear production in the normal dog,[128] in dogs with neurogenic KCS, the restoration of normal aqueous tear production may be seen with pulsed (every 8 hours) topical administration. Pilocarpine as a commercially available topical 2% solution is quite acidic (pH = 3–5), and it is quite irritating; however, when diluted 1:15 or 2:15 (final concentration 0.125%–0.25%) with saline-based artificial tears (pH = 6–7) the resulting mixture is much more readily tolerated. Pilocarpine use has been supplanted by calcineurin inhibitor immunomodulating drugs, but on occasion, a dog that does not respond to topical cyclosporine may respond to oral or even topical pilocarpine.

Artificial tears Artificial tears are symptomatic therapy for dry eye and are used to replace the wetting action of the natural tears. They should be used as often as possible. Solutions should be used every 2–4 hours or, minimally, every 6 hours. Petrolatum-based ointments or highly viscous artificial tear preparations are used at night or when frequent administration is impossible. If a pet is kept indoors, particularly as a "lap" dog, frequent administration of eye drops may be an acceptable symptomatic therapy. Topical artificial tear application does not deal with the underlying cause of KCS; therefore, their use alone should be only in those cases where calcineurin inhibitors and pilocarpine have failed to restore tear production to a more normal level. Usually, artificial tear therapy alone fails to control the progression of sight-threatening lesions due to the client's inability or reluctance to treat the eyes as often as necessary.

Artificial tear solutions vary in pH, osmolarity, and individual tolerance to preservatives, wetting agents, and other components. Methylcellulose and polyvinyl alcohol increase surface tension and retard evaporation. Polyvinylpyrrolidone (PVP) increases the ability of the solution to adhere to the hydrophobic cornea and, therefore, gives a longer TFBUT. Viscoelastic agents such as hyaluronic acid and chondroitin sulfate have been used as components of tear substitutes. These substances enhance tear film stabilization and help reduce evaporation of the precorneal tear film. Because frequent administration of artificial tears in animals is often difficult, use of the more viscous viscoelastic agent containing products is warranted. Many companies make multiple concentrations of viscoelastic agents, with the higher concentration products being used as the frequency of administration potential goes down. Tear film osmolarity has been found to be hyperosmolar in human KCS patients compared to normal patients. This hyperosmolarity has been suggested as a cause of the pathology of the surface epithelium and as being responsible for the symptoms of discomfort.[129] As a result, hypo-osmolar tear substitutes have been recommended in man. If an owner can administer artificial tears on an hourly to bihourly basis, use of hypo-osmolar tear supplements would be recommended. Otherwise, the use of more viscous products is warranted due to the less frequent administration capability for most animals. In man, benzalkonium chloride, methylparathimerosal, and chlorobutanol are common preservatives in artificial tears, and chronic topical use may result in hypersensitivity to these preservatives. For this reason, "preservative-free" artificial tears are made for the human market and may be needed for those animals that develop hypersensitivities to these commonly used preservatives. Saline alone is not a substitute for a quality commercially available artificial tear supplement. Saline may act to rinse the mucin and oily portions for the tear film off the surface of the cornea/conjunctiva, thereby leaving the ocular surfaces totally unprotected once the saline evaporates.

Topical dilute serum (20% serum, 80% saline) has been advocated in the treatment of Sjögren's syndrome in humans.[130] This provides various substances that the tears would normally supply and that have a positive trophic effect on epithelial surfaces. *In situ* upregulation of mucin was also demonstrated. Topical dilute serum may therefore have special benefits for mucin tear deficiencies (e.g., brachycephalic breeds of cats) and deserves further study.

Additional symptomatic care *Antibiotics* Surface ocular overgrowth with normal commensal as well as atypical pathologic bacteria is commonly seen with long standing KCS.[102] Bacterial nonulcerative keratoconjunctivitis can be treated with topical antibiotics when necessary. In the case of ulcerative keratitis, aggressive topical antibiotic therapy should be instituted due to the tendency for KCS patients to develop proteolytic enzyme corneal stromal degradation. Cytology and/or culture and sensitivity should guide the clinician towards the choice of appropriate antimicrobial therapy. In the case of chronic KCS where multiple topical antibiotics have been previously used, culture and sensitivity and use of a novel initial topical antibiotic are recommended, as the incidence of antibiotic resistance is high in such cases.

Through the years, this author has seen many instances in his university-based referral hospital where dogs have been treated by the referring veterinarian with topical calcineurin inhibitors alone with little resultant improvement in aqueous tear production. In some cases, exuberant surface bacterial infection was successfully treated with appropriate topical antibiotic therapy with resultant decrease of conjunctival inflammation and restoration of normal aqueous tear production. For this reason, this author routinely uses topical antibiotic therapy in conjunction with calcineurin inhibitor therapy as his initial treatment for new cases of KCS seen with purulent ocular discharge.

Glucocorticoids If no active corneal ulceration is present, corneal neovascularization and/or conjunctivitis may be improved with short-term (7–10 days) use of topical glucocorticoids, every 8–12 hours. A fluorescein dye uptake test is mandatory prior to glucocorticoid usage because many cases of KCS have recurrent corneal ulcerations. Continued topical use of glucocorticoids is contraindicated because of the potential for resistant bacterial strain appearance and concern for complications should corneal ulceration occur.

Mucolytic agents: Acetylcysteine—Mucolytic agents are used to break up tenacious discharge in cases of excessive mucous accumulation. The agent commercially available is 10% and 20% acetylcysteine in single-use vials, and it should be diluted to 2%–4% to decrease irritation and avoid epithelial toxicity.[131] It can be used as often as every 2 hours. Acetylcysteine has a short shelf life once it is opened and requires refrigeration once opened. Once diluted in saline-based artificial tears, acetylcysteine should not be used for more than 30 days even with refrigeration. Combination preparations of additional topical agents (antibiotic and/or pilocarpine) in artificial tear carrier can be used effectively if care is taken to use only those ingredients necessary for each individual patient.

Keratoconjunctivitis "cocktails" In the 1970s, Severin developed a "keratoconjunctivitis sicca solution" that he recommended for use in dogs with KCS.[132] The original solution contained antibiotic (for surface bacterial infection), pilocarpine (to enhance aqueous tear production through parasympathetic stimulation), acetylcysteine (to help disperse mucoid discharge from the ocular surface), and a saline-based artificial tear as a carrier. This author has for three decades successfully used modifications of Severin's original "KCS solution" as symptomatic therapy for KCS-afflicted dogs. For the case of potential neurogenic KCS (very low STT [0–5 mm/min] in conjunction with a dry ipsilateral nare), the author begins therapy with a cocktail of 14-mL saline-based artificial tears with 2 mL of either 10% gentamicin sulfate or 2 mL of 10%

chloramphenicol succinate, 2 mL of 20% acetylcysteine, and 2 mL of 2% ophthalmic pilocarpine. Choice of antibiotic is based on cytology/Gram stain (gentamicin for Gram-negative rods predominating, chloramphenicol for Gram-positive cocci predominating). Once the bacterial infection abates, continued use of a similar solution (artificial tear base, acetylcysteine, and pilocarpine minus the antibiotic) is used if the tear production increases with pilocarpine usage. If tear production does not improve with use of the pilocarpine, this is discontinued, as the pilocarpine can be quite irritating when applied to the eye. If a patient has most likely immune-mediated lacrimal adenitis with secondary surface ocular infection and thick mucoid discharge, a "sicca cocktail" of artificial tears, antibiotic, and acetylcysteine is used in conjunction with topical calcineurin inhibitors until the bacterial infection is controlled. In cases where tear production never regains normal levels, and thick, mucoid discharge is constantly present, a cocktail of artificial tears and acetylcysteine (final concentration 2%) can be used indefinitely to help clean adherent mucus and reduce irritation. All of these "cocktails" must be refrigerated, as was the case with the acetylcysteine cocktail described previously.

Topical or systemic androgens While androgen receptors have been demonstrated in the nuclei of epithelium of the lacrimal gland, the conjunctiva, the cornea, the meibomian glands, the lens, and in the retinal pigment epithelium (RPE) in humans and laboratory animals, the significance of their role is largely unknown.[133] As previously discussed, androgen deficiency may produce acinar epithelial death that may trigger an immune-mediated inflammatory response.[98] At this time, there are no findings in domestic species that are afflicted with KCS that would indicate that androgen therapy is indicated in the treatment of these disorders.

Therapy of keratoconjunctivitis sicca in the cat Immune-mediated lacrimal adenitis that is so commonly seen in the dog is not seen in the cat. Sulfonamide-induced KCS has not been described in the cat. The most common cause of KCS in the cat is due to scarring of conjunctiva/lacrimal ductules secondary to previous surface ocular infections (e.g., FHV-1 infection). Neurogenic KCS occurs in the cat, usually secondary to trauma to the head/orbit. Dysautonomia is an extremely rare cause of neurogenic KCS in North America.[51–53] Symptomatic therapy for KCS in the cat is usually limited to application of topical tear replacements, with the use of viscoelastic-containing artificial tears being recognized as being superior due to the inability to frequently treat. Cats appear to tolerate decreased tear production much better than do dogs. Parotid duct transposition has been performed in the cat, but their decreased salivation compared to a dog makes the procedure less optimal for absolute definitive treatment of the disorder.

Of a more common incidence is tear film qualitative disorders (deficits in precorneal mucin tear film). Although these cats have relatively normal STT values, their TFBUT times are extremely short (2.5 seconds versus normal TFBUT in cats at 12–21 seconds),[33] and clinical signs usually include axial corneal ulcerations and corneal sequestrum formation.[32] The use of topical cyclosporine to enhance goblet cell health and topical viscoelastic-containing tear supplements is indicated for these usually brachycephalic conformation cats.

Therapy of keratoconjunctivitis sicca in the horse Kerato conjunctivitis sicca in the horse is very uncommon, and few case reports have indicated that it may occur secondary to immune-mediated disease[85,87,88] or trauma.[49,50] Topical use of cyclosporine A and systemic dexamethasone have helped some immune-mediated cases. In the case of traumatic KCS, the author has rarely seen improvement with time. Most cases of equine KCS are treated symptomatically with artificial tear supplement drops and ointments, partial permanent tarsorrhaphies, or enucleation if the horse develops severe complications such as descemetoceles or perforated corneas. Parotid duct transposition has been performed in the horse with mixed results.[84,134]

Surgical therapy If medical therapy is unsuccessful after a period of at least 90 days in restoring a manageable state for the owner and the patient, a parotid duct transposition (PDT) may be indicated. With the advent of calcineurin inhibitor therapy and better artificial tear products that make medical management more successful, PDT is infrequently performed, but it still has its indications. Dogs with total congenital alacrima, totally medically unresponsive cases with progressive ocular pathology and impending vision loss, and cases where the owner cannot/ will not provide the necessary medical therapy to manage the disease are candidates for attempts at surgical management using the PDT. The basal salivation rate and the patency of the parotid duct should be evaluated prior to anesthesia. Application of a bitter substance to the tongue (1% atropine ophthalmic solution) usually induces copious salivation erupting from the parotid papilla located on the buccal mucosa above the upper carnassial tooth. Some dogs with xerophthalmia (neurogenic KCS cases and others) have concurrent xerostomia. If no saliva exits the parotid papilla with pharmacologic stimulation, successful PDT with restoration of "moisture" to the ocular surface may not occur. In general, PDT done by a practiced surgeon is 63%–90% successful.[135–138] Parotid duct transposition can

be performed in the cat, but it is technically more difficult, and the success rate is lower than in the dog in this author's experience.

There are basically two methods of performing PDT: (1) The original open method of exposing the duct over the side of the cheek and dissecting it free (**Figures 9.18 and 9.19**)[135]; and (2) the closed method of performing all of the dissection of the duct from the mouth, starting from the parotid papilla and working posteriorly.[139] The closed method is quicker in the hands of an experienced surgeon, but contamination from the mouth is probably greater, the dissection is more blind and incomplete, and constricting forces on the tunnel from the conjunctiva are not seen and relieved at the time of surgery. Variations of the open method involve the placement of the skin incision, the degree of prior dissection of the papilla from the mouth, the type of cannula placed in the papilla, and the placement of the papilla in the conjunctival cul-de-sac.

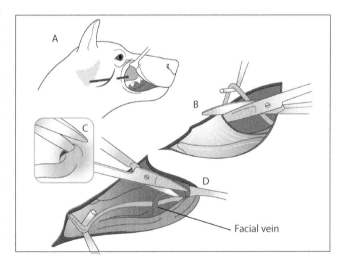

Figure 9.18 Open parotid duct transplantation. Before making the cheek incision, the duct is cannulated with 0 to 00 nylon suture and scissors used to dissect the papilla from the oral mucous membranes (A). An "open" J-shaped incision is made in the cheek with the horizontal member over the parotid duct. The duct may be palpated if cannulated or assumed to be at the level of the lateral commissure of the mouth (A). The superficial facial muscles are incised and the duct found on the surface of the masseter muscle between the dorsal and ventral buccal nerves. The duct is elevated and kept under moderate tension to show the fascial attachments, which are cut (B). The anterior dissection is more difficult because of the facial vein that crosses the duct; the duct burrows into the submucosa before forming the papilla (C, D). Once removed, the papilla is trimmed, and the duct is run between the fingers to unwind any twists that may have formed with the manipulations.

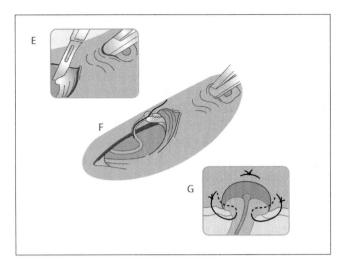

Figure 9.19 A tunnel is formed between the inferior cul-de-sac between the lower lid and the third eyelid, and the surgical site with a mosquito forceps (E). The papilla is pulled into the conjunctival sac (F). The papilla is sutured to the conjunctiva with 5–8 sutures of 7–0 polyglycolic acid (G). The original incision is closed in two layers. The mouth will need suturing if the defect created by removing the papilla is large.

Complications of PDT are many and include "epiphora" or spillage of saliva onto the face of varying degrees, lack of saliva flow due to prior sialoadenitis or neurogenic defect, twisting of the duct creating a stricture, cutting of the duct during surgery, transection of the duct before the papilla, infection of the surgery site, dilated duct over the zygomatic arch, postop sialoadenitis, blockage of the duct by a sialolith, and mineral deposits on the cornea and lid.[140–142] The second most common and most significant complication is mineral deposition from the saliva onto the cornea and the lids. Often this is mild, with modest dusting of the cornea with a white deposit (**Figure 9.20**). In severe instances, the opacity is plaque-like and very painful. The deposit may also accumulate on the lid margins and be felt as a very gritty material (**Figure 9.21**). Mild cases may respond to every 8-hour topical application of 1%–2% ethylenediaminetetraacetic acid (EDTA) solution (available from compounding pharmacies), but in severe cases, the only therapy to relieve the discomfort is partial or complete parotid duct ligation. The use of topical cyclosporine may help to reduce the keratitis induced by the mineralized saliva on the corneal surface. Feeding a reduced mineral/renal diet, tartar control diets, oral vitamin C supplementation, chronic oral tetracycline usage, and applying a teaspoon of powdered buttermilk to the food ration daily (Koch S., 2008, personal communication) are anecdotal treatments to reduce the mineral content of the parotid secretion.

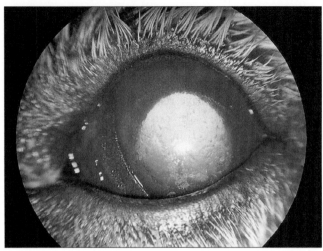

Figure 9.20 Fine white deposits on the cornea and the third eyelid of a dog after parotid duct transposition. The lesion is gritty and irritating when in high concentration and is thought to represent salivary mineral deposits.

When obstruction to the duct occurs, it is usually over the region of the zygomatic arch and may result from twisting, constriction of the tunnel created from the conjunctival cul-de-sac to the surgical site, or from external trauma to the duct over the bone (**Figure 9.22**). Obstruction at this site may be reversed by excision of the constriction, freeing the duct as much as possible, and resuturing the duct to the conjunctiva.[142]

Epiphora is present to some extent in all successful PDTs. Larger dogs with high salivary flow rates are most likely to have a pronounced epiphora. Brachycephalics may have nasal fold dermatitis from the chronic wetness, and others may develop a blepharitis on the lower lid. Partial

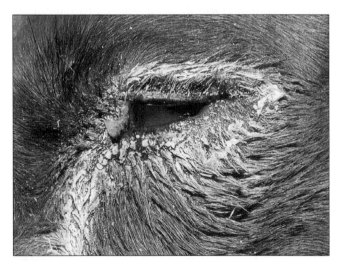

Figure 9.21 Severe mineral deposits on the lids of a dog after parotid duct transposition that resulted in severe pain with blepharospasm. The duct was ligated.

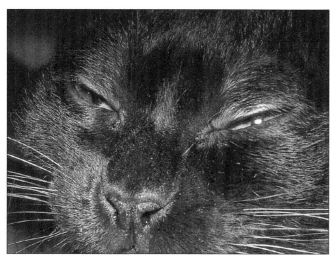

Figure 9.22 Burmese cat with a dilated parotid duct over the zygomatic arch that developed several weeks after parotid duct transposition.

ligation of the parotid duct may be attempted to reduce salivary flow, either at the time of the primary procedure in the larger breeds or as a secondary procedure.

Punctal occlusion Occlusion of the lacrimal puncta can help preserve the natural tears as well as preserve topical medications used in lubricating the eye. Occlusion may be performed by ligation, cautery, gelatin implants, or silicone plugs.[143] The improvement noted by this therapy is minimal.[144]

Episcleral cyclosporine implants for treatment of KCS Episcleral silicone matrix cyclosporine (ESMC) implants (1.9 cm length, 30% wt/wt cyclosporine in silicone; approximately 12 mg of cyclosporine loaded per implant) have been placed in the subconjunctival spaces in dogs with KCS that were (1) responsive to topical cyclosporine therapy or (2) not responsive to topical cyclosporine therapy.[145] In both groups evaluated, significant improvement in STT values, conjunctival hyperemia, corneal neovascularization, corneal opacity, and ocular discharge were noted with mean follow-up of 18 and 10.4 months, respectively. Further work was needed to determine duration of efficacy and optimal dose for cyclosporine. This repositol therapy may be of use for patients that are difficult for owners to treat and for KCS patients who have not responded to topical cyclosporine administration.

Prevention
- As discussed earlier, third eyelid gland removal is not recommended in breeds with a predisposition for KCS.
- Dogs placed on systemic sulfonamides and etodolac or topical mydriatics such as tropicamide or atropine should have a STT performed at frequent intervals to monitor tear production.

- Autoimmune dacryoadenitis probably has a genetic basis, and caution should be expressed with breeding from affected animals. It is not unusual to observe several generations of KCS in purebred dogs.

Anomalous nasolacrimal ducts

Supernumerary nasolacrimal ducts that open on the face below the eye have been described in brown Swiss cattle. The extra ducts originate from the proximal one-third of the duct. The condition is usually bilateral and does not produce significant signs. Hairless, pigmented areas may delineate the openings onto the face. The mode of inheritance has not been determined.[146] Additional types of anomalous openings of the nasolacrimal system from those described in brown Swiss cattle have been described in other breeds of cattle as well.[147,148]

Epiphora/lacrimation
Introduction/etiology
Epiphora refers to an abnormal flow of tears down the face. The term "epiphora" is often used to denote an obstructive cause of overflow, whereas "lacrimation" is used to denote an increased production of tears producing an overflow. Constant epiphora causes the hair and the skin around the medial canthus to be stained brown and often causes a moist dermatitis of the medial canthus (**Figure 9.23**). Epiphora/lacrimation can occur from an increased production of tears (usually due to ocular irritation), an obstruction to the outflow of tears, a wicking of tears onto the face from the hair, or from anatomic defects of the lower lid that permit "spillage" of the tears. Once reflex tearing or hypersecretion has been ruled out, obstructions of the lacrimal drainage system should be considered in the differential diagnosis of epiphora.

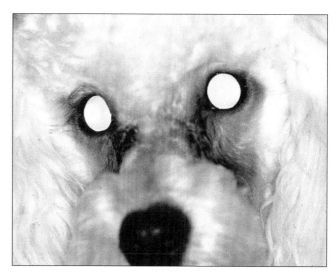

Figure 9.23 Severe bilateral epiphora ("poodle epiphora") in a miniature poodle. Mild medial entropion and medial canthal trichiasis were present.

Congenital atresia of the lacrimal punctum   Congenital imperforate lacrimal puncta occur mainly in the American Cocker Spaniel, Bedlington terrier, and Golden retriever[149] as well as miniature and toy poodles and Samoyeds. The lower punctum is usually involved (involvement of the upper lid punctum alone is usually asymptomatic), and the condition is usually unilateral (**Figure 9.24**). Usually there is a membrane only over the punctum opening, but rarely, the entire canaliculus may be lacking. Although uncommon, this author has occasionally seen apparent congenital palpebral lacrimal punctal atresia in otherwise healthy horses and cats with no clinical signs of epiphora.

Congenital atresia of the nasal end of the nasolacrimal duct   In the horse, the llama, and the alpaca, a syndrome of atresia of the distal end of the nasolacrimal duct may result in epiphora and, eventually, mucopurulent ocular discharge when dacryocystitis develops from the stagnant fluid that promotes bacterial/fungal overgrowth (**Figure 9.25**). The condition is usually unilateral and does not usually manifest the purulent discharge until 3–4 months after birth.[150–153]

Malplacement of the ventral punctum   In the dog, the ventral palpebral punctum may be improperly positioned in its relationship to the lid margin/lacrimal lake, so that tears are not readily drawn into the ventral canaliculus. Entropion of the medial lower lid that may both irritate the corneal/conjunctival surface and cause malposition of the lower punctum is a common cause of epiphora, especially in brachycephalic breeds as well as miniature poodles, bichons, and other toy breeds. Congenital displacement

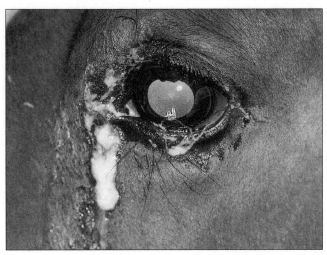

Figure 9.25 Unilateral mucopurulent discharge from the eye of a young horse. The condition was chronic. On examination of the nasolacrimal duct, the distal end was not patent, resulting in a blind-ended tube that became infected.

of the lacrimal puncta can be observed particularly in the American Cocker Spaniel.

Micropuncta   The lacrimal puncta may be very small in individual dogs and, while patent, be unable to handle the precorneal tear film outflow without epiphora.

Taut lid–globe conformation   In toy breeds, the lids are so taut against the globe (blepharophimosis) that it is probable that the lacrimal lake is small and access to the puncta is restricted (see Chapter 7). This may also play a role in the brachycephalic cat with epiphora.

Acquired symblepharon   Acquired adhesions of the conjunctiva in the region of the medial canthus and the puncta may obstruct the outflow of tears. This is a condition seen in cats with previous severe herpesvirus conjunctivitis and following trauma to this area (see Chapter 8).

Traumatic/surgical injury to the lower lid   Traumatic lacerations (or surgical manipulations such as medial canthoplasty) that either disrupt the continuity of the lid margin or disrupt the lower punctum or canaliculus may result in epiphora.

Wicking of tears   Wicking of tears onto the face may occur from long facial hairs (trichiasis) and breed-related medial entropion. Although medial trichiasis and excessively long hair of the lacrimal caruncle are usually more problematic, lateral canthal trichiasis may cause wicking/

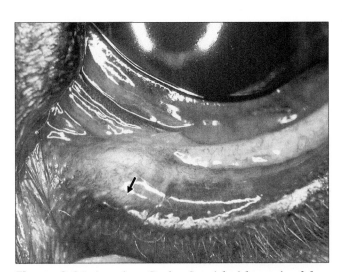

Figure 9.24 American Cocker Spaniel with atresia of the lower lacrimal punctum that was ballooned up (arrow) while irrigating through the upper punctum.

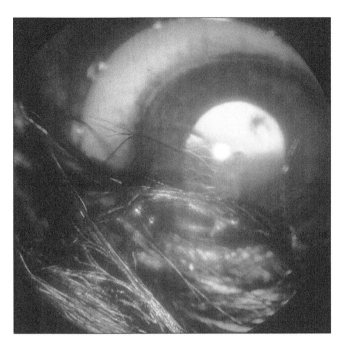

Figure 9.26 Shi Tzu with medial trichiasis due to medial entropion and nasal fold hairs with wicking of tears onto the face (epiphora). Also note the medial pigmentary keratitis.

epiphora as well. This is common in longhaired dogs such as the poodle, bichon, Shi Tzu, Maltese, and Lhasa Apso (**Figure 9.26**).

Hypersecretion of the glands Hypersecretion of tears may be due to irritation from glandular inflammation. Enlargement of the third eyelid gland (**Figure 9.27**), mononuclear inflammatory infiltration, squamous metaplasia of ducts, and cystic ducts have been observed

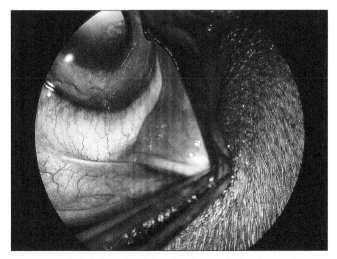

Figure 9.27 Adenitis of the third eyelid gland associated with epiphora. The gland is swollen, and the overlying conjunctiva is hyperemic with minimal follicular involvement.

in histopathology of the glands taken from dogs with epiphora.[154,155] Epiphora may be associated with swelling of the gland, decreasing the lacrimal lake, or increased production of tears due to irritation. However, it has been reported that in dogs with epiphora the tear production was only 10% above normal.[156,157]

Histologic hyperplasia and clinical enlargement of the nictitans gland was observed in a series of dogs with idiopathic epiphora.[158] The cause and effect were not clear, but removal of the gland improved epiphora, possibly by enlarging the lacrimal lake or decreasing the tear production. The postsurgical STT value was not significantly decreased from the presurgical STT value, indicating the improvement may not have been due to reduced tear production.

Reflex lacrimation

Ocular and periocular discomfort or pain Irritation can be from mechanical etiologies such as distichia, trichiasis, entropion, ectopic cilia, or foreign bodies. Atopic conjunctivitis often results in chronic epiphora, and brown staining may be present not only on the face but on the feet and flanks from licking. Pain associated with corneal ulceration is an obvious cause of reflex lacrimation, but it can also be noted with glaucoma and uveitis. Reflex lacrimation may occur without obvious ocular discomfort such as blepharospasm. Saito and Kotani found that 97% of small breeds of dogs with epiphora had an epitheliopathy, defined as epithelial staining with rose bengal and/or fluorescein.[159] Schirmer I values were normal, but the Schirmer II values were low, indicating an increase in reflex lacrimation. The authors postulated that a decrease in basal secretion was the cause of the epitheliopathy, and an increase in detached/exfoliated epithelial cells might interfere with tear outflow through the nasolacrimal ducts and also increase reflex lacrimation. In animals with epitheliopathy, breed (such as Shih Tzu and presumably other brachycephalics) had no correlation with lacrimation and Schirmer II tests.

Light and wind

Many individual dogs have epiphora outdoors but not while indoors. Obviously, environmental irritants can aggravate an individual animal's eyes, but dogs with this type of reflex lacrimation may have marked epiphora outside, irrespective of the weather or season. Excess lacrimation quickly subsides when sheltered. The Chow Chow, Shar Pei, and certain terrier breeds are predisposed.

Clinical signs

Epiphora and tear staining are usually visible at the medial canthus, but with lid defects or wicking of facial hairs, wetting and staining may occur anywhere along the length of the lid. The condition is often chronic, and, when associated with congenital defects such as atresia of the puncta, history of onset may date back to when the animal was young. Additionally, in animals with congenital defects, the palpebral puncta (especially the lower punctum) may not be visualized.

Additional signs associated with the cause of epiphora may be present, such as conformational defects (ectropion or entropion), inflammation (conjunctivitis or blepharitis), or pain. Signs of pain/blepharospasm of varying degrees may be associated with epiphora from reflex lacrimation but is not typical for epiphora from obstruction. Except for pain from dacryocystitis, obstructive nasolacrimal duct drainage disorders are not painful.

Diagnosis

In order to diagnose the cause of epiphora, the history should be evaluated, and a careful examination performed. It is easy to fall into the trap of trying to associate certain etiologies with breed (such as medial entropion/trichiasis in a brachycephalic breed of dog), without doing a thorough examination. Often, multiple etiologies are present in the same animal; the examination should not be curtailed when one possible etiology, such as distichia or conjunctivitis, is found.

On physical examination, the integrity of the lid margins (normal lower lid margin trough capable of holding a stable tear film on the ocular surface) and presence of conformational lid defects (entropion, ectropion, blepharophimosis) should be evaluated.

Causes of mechanical irritation (lash anomalies, lymphoid follicle hyperplasia, foreign bodies) and excess facial and caruncle hairs that may wick tear or cause frictional irritation should be looked for. Ocular inflammation or discomfort (disease such as glaucoma, anterior uveitis, or keratitis) should be ruled out as a cause of reflex over tearing. Presence or absence of normal puncta or their position should be evaluated. STTs may indicate an overproduction (higher than normal STT value compared to contralateral normal eye or compared to normal expected values for the species) versus impaired outflow (normal STT value), and fluorescein staining of the cornea may delineate minute defects of the epithelium that stimulate excessive lacrimation. Following placing a drop fluorescein on the bulbar surface, allow the dye to sit (without rinsing) on the ocular surface, and evaluate corneal tear film break-up time as well as where fluorescein may spill over onto the face (spillage at the medial canthus can mean obstructive disease or medial trichiasis/medial entropion, whereas fluorescein dye on the lower lid or lateral canthus may indicate entropion, ectropion, or trichiasis problems). In addition, visualization of fluorescein at the nostrils is indicative of a patent nasolacrimal duct. A lack of fluorescein in the nares

is not conclusive for impaired outflow, nor does a positive Jones test (or appearance of dye in the oropharynx) rule out obstruction of a single punctum.

Nasolacrimal duct irrigation is necessary in most cases of epiphora to demonstrate patency of puncta, the canaliculi, and the duct. This is a rather crude test and does not evaluate the possibility of a functional outflow deficiency that may be present despite an anatomically patent outflow system. Atresia is diagnosed by cannulation and infusion of fluid in one palpebral punctum, with the absence of flow out of the opposite punctum. A tenting of the conjunctiva at the site of the opposite punctum may be observed (**Figure 9.24**). Obstructions of the outflow system are usually further examined by contrast dacryocystorhinography (**Figures 9.6 and 9.28**) (see section Dacryocystitis).

Nasolacrimal irrigation is a minor procedure that can be performed in the horse and the dog under topical anesthesia (plus or minus sedation, depending on patient temperament). The same principles apply to duct cannulation as to venipuncture:

- Direct the catheter parallel to the course of the duct.
- Seat the catheter deeply in the duct.
- Keep the hand holding the syringe in contact with the animal's head to minimize the effects of head movements.

Since the dorsal canaliculus basically runs straight into the lacrimal sac versus the "bend" in the system as the lower canaliculus empties into the lacrimal sac, the upper punctum should be flushed first. If both the lid margin puncta and the main duct to the nasal punctum are patent, there is no need to attempt cannulation of the lower lid punctum (a procedure that usually results in more irritation to the patient).

Therapy

Treatment is specific for the etiology, if it can be found.

Medical therapy   Medical therapy for epiphora is either directed at reduction of inflammation and pain, if present, or reducing tear staining. Therapy aimed at reducing tear staining may involve just masking the tearing with grooming powders or trying to affect the stain itself (use of commercially available acetic acid/boric acid impregnated

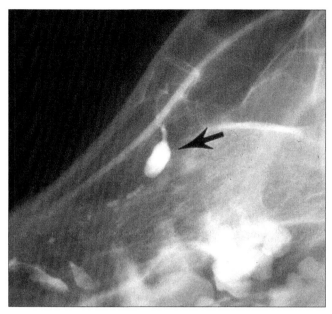

Figure 9.28 Contrast dacryocystorhinogram in a dog with chronic epiphora. Arrow denotes dilated region of nasolacrimal duct with failure of passage of contract material beyond the dilation.

wipes, hydrogen peroxide, or diluted chlorine bleach). If using cleansing/bleaching agents around the eye, it is imperative that caustic substances not make contact with the ocular surfaces. Systemic medical therapy directed at stain reduction has often been empirical, poorly documented, and controversial.

Tetracycline Low-dose tetracycline (50 mg/day/dog) can decrease the staining (and supposedly the wetness as well) of the face in many "idiopathic" cases of epiphora. The mechanism of action is not known, but since it does not decrease tear production in normal dogs, it is thought to interfere with the brown staining of the face.[160] Tetracycline should never be used in dogs prior to development of permanent dentition.

Metronidazole Low-dose metronidazole (100 mg per average dog for 10 days) has also been recommended for treating the tear staining of epiphora.[161] As with tetracycline, metronidazole does not decrease tear production or have a lacrimal toxic effect when given in high doses for short periods of time.[162] Some feel that metronidazole, as well as tetracycline, reduces the facial wetness.

Tylosin Low doses of tylosin have anecdotally claimed to reduce tear staining in dogs. Original tylosin-containing products marketed in the United States (Angels' Eyes™) have been replaced by "all natural" products containing no antibiotic.

After an initial trial period of 2–4 weeks, medical therapy with the previously listed antimicrobials may probably have to be given intermittently as needed to control the staining. Chronic, intermittent use of suboptimal doses of systemic antimicrobials may lead to bacterial drug resistance and is, therefore, not recommended by the author.

Surgical therapy Opening an atretic lacrimal punctum can be performed using topical anesthesia and appropriate manual/chemical restraint in lateral recumbency. The procedure consists of nicking or incising the area where the punctum is expected to be (or where the conjunctiva tents up when flushing) using a #11 Bard–Parker (or similar) blade (**Figure 9.29**). This is followed by insertion of a punctum dilator or fine scissor tip to distend the proximal end. Frequent digital massage of the area and topical antibiotic–corticosteroid drops are applied for several days to prevent the incision healing shut. If the punctum seals, the procedure can be repeated, and a nasolacrimal tube/ suture may be implanted for 2–3 weeks to ensure ultimate patency. In cases where the inferior punctum location is not apparent with flushing from the upper punctum, a pigtail lacrimal probe may be used to attempt cannulation of the canaliculi (upper canaliculus to lacrimal sac out through lower canaliculus) with placement of a suture stent until the area heals with a patent punctum.

Mechanical problems such as entropion, distichiasis, or excess hairs on the lacrimal caruncle can usually be surgically corrected. Multiple potential etiologies (i.e., distichia, conjunctivitis, medial entropion, wicking hairs) are often present in the same animal, and clinical judgment is necessary in assigning responsibility for the signs of epiphora.

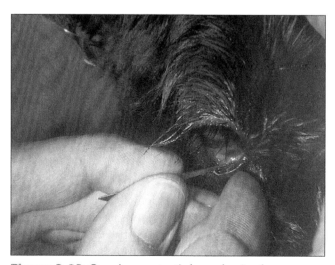

Figure 9.29 Opening an atretic lower lacrimal puncta in the right eye of a cocker spaniel with a #11 blade using topical anesthesia.

When in doubt as to the ultimate cause of epiphora, medical conditions should be treated first, followed by surgical therapy if epiphora is not corrected by medical therapy alone. A multipronged therapeutic approach (removal of a haired lacrimal caruncle, a Hotz–Celsus procedure to reduce medial entropion/lacrimal punctal malposition, and removal of facial trichiasis) may be attempted to correct the problem.

In dogs with no obvious cause for the epiphora, such as in many miniature poodles, bichons, Maltese, and so on, removal of the third eyelid gland has been advocated.[154] This may be an effective therapy, but the risk of contributing to KCS later in the animal's life is one that should be carefully considered and discussed with the owner. This author does not recommend excision of the third eyelid gland for treating epiphora.

Conjunctivorhinostomy has been advocated for surgical relief of epiphora. This consists of creating a permanent fistula between the medial–ventral conjunctival cul-de-sac and the nasal cavity or maxillary recess.[163,164] Although the surgery itself is not difficult, maintaining a stent in the hole created until a permanent mucosal lined fistula is formed requires prolonged restraint of the patient from rubbing at the eye (2–3 months). The procedure has not been as successful in the cat as in the dog. The labor/restraint to maintain the stent, risk of major intraoperative hemorrhage, and potential for failure (pet still has epiphora) preclude this as a form of treatment for epiphora, except for the exceptional case or demanding owner.

Another uncommonly performed procedure to drain tears from the lacrimal lake into the mouth is the conjunctivobuccostomy.[165] In this procedure, a tunnel from the inferior cul-de-sac to the upper fornix of the upper lip is created in the subcutaneous tissue. A long-term polyethylene catheter is placed from the inferior lid conjunctival fornix to the upper lip fornix until the tunnel becomes lined with a mucous membrane (2–3 months). As is the case with the conjunctivorhinostomy, this procedure is relatively easy to perform, but the aftercare as well as the potential for failure makes this a procedure only to be attempted for the very demanding owner.

Dacryocystitis

Introduction/etiology

Dacryocystitis is an inflammation of the lacrimal sac and the nasolacrimal duct. Dacryocystitis usually produces an obstruction or is caused by an obstruction to the lacrimal outflow system. It is a relatively uncommon condition but must be considered when persistent signs of epiphora, purulent ocular discharge, and conjunctival infection are present. Causes of dacryocystitis include:

- Congenital impatency of the inferior nasolacrimal duct/punctum (most commonly seen in horses, llamas, alpacas) (**Figures 9.25 and 9.30**).[150–153]
- Plant awns: Foreign bodies are the most common cause in arid climates during the dry seasons[166] and in outdoor dogs frequenting areas with tall grass crops.
- Facial bone fracture with occlusion of the nasolacrimal duct.
- Neoplasm of the nose, sinus, or bone that occludes the nasolacrimal duct.
- Aneurysmal dilation of the duct that allows fluid to pool **Figure 9.31**).[167]
- Periodontal disease of the upper premolars or canine teeth.

Clinical signs

Epiphora is present, usually chronic and unilateral in nature. Epiphora often changes to a chronic, unilateral, mucopurulent conjunctival discharge (**Figures 9.25 and 9.32**). The conjunctiva may or may not be significantly inflamed. The STT is normal, and the discharge responds transiently to topical antibiotics. Rarely, an acute abscessation produces swelling below the medial canthus (**Figure 9.33**).

Diagnosis

Application of fluorescein dye results in spillage of dye out over the medial canthus (indicating obstructive disease). Deep massage over the medial canthus may milk discharge from one or both palpebral puncta. Normograde irrigation of the nasolacrimal duct (small animals) through one of the lacrimal puncta may demonstrate an obstruction; reflux of a mucoid to mucopurulent material from the opposite punctum indicates a dacryocystitis

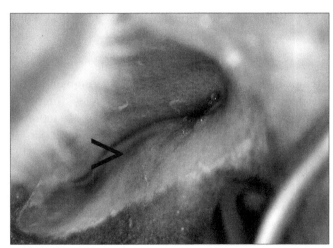

Figure 9.30 **Distension of nasolacrimal duct due to impatency of nasal punctum in a saddlebred filly (arrow).**

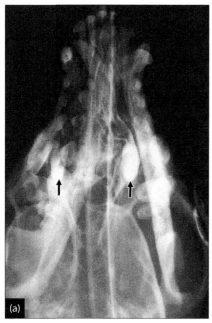

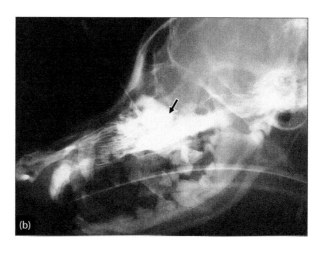

Figure 9.31 (a), (b) Dacryocystorhinogram of a Bichon Frise with a cystic lesion in the nasolacrimal duct resulting in persistent purulent exudate in the conjunctival cul-de-sac. The condition was cured with a rhinotomy and removal of the wall of the sac. Aberrant lacrimal gland was associated with the wall of the cyst, and the nasolacrimal duct was patent. Contrast material was injected into the left side, and cysts were visualized on both sides (arrows).

(**Figure 9.34**). Retrograde irrigation (large animals and large dogs) from the nasal punctum can flush debris/purulent material (and possibly the offending object) if the nasolacrimal duct is patent but temporarily obstructed.

The duct may have a temporary obstruction that may be relieved with forced irrigation. If flushing normograde, irrigation may expel the obstruction from the opposite punctum. If the obstruction is firm, the forced irrigation is painful and requires heavy sedation or general anesthesia. If general anesthesia in a large dog is necessary, attempt at retrograde irrigation should be made. Attempts at forced irrigation in a normograde manner may drive a foreign body deeper into the duct, making it more difficult to dislodge.

Dacryocystorhinography is indicated in most instances where the cause is not apparent, and the duct is impatent with forced irrigation (both normograde and retrograde). Dacryocystorhinography is performed by injecting a

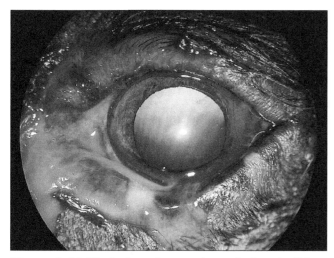

Figure 9.32 Marked purulent exudate caked on the lid margins and in the conjunctival cul-de-sac associated with obstruction of the nasolacrimal duct of a dog. The condition was unilateral.

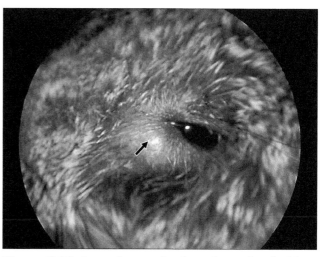

Figure 9.33 Acute abscessation (arrow) associated with dacryocystitis in a chinchilla.

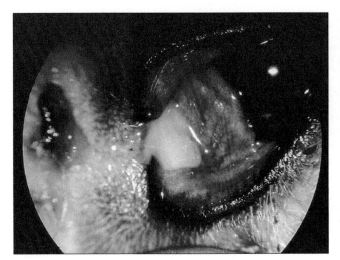

Figure 9.34 Reflux of purulent material out of the lower lacrimal punctum while flushing through the upper punctum of a dog. This indicates dacryocystitis.

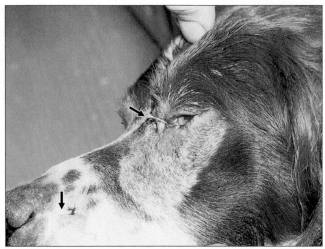

Figure 9.35 Polyethylene tube sutured in place for the treatment of dacryocystitis (arrow) in a dog. The tube will be left in place for >3 weeks.

radiopaque contrast material through a fine polyethylene or lacrimal catheter placed in one of the canaliculi, while occluding the opposite punctum to force the fluid nasally (**Figures 9.6, 9.28, and 9.31**).[168–170]

Therapy

Removing the cause of the obstruction is the basis of successful therapy but is not always possible. In horses, cattle, llamas (and in a few cases of large dogs) the author has been able to advance a 3.5-French polyethylene end-ported male canine urinary catheter from the nasal punctum to the palpebral puncta while flushing, thereby dislodging the offending foreign material. If the obstruction is removed, topical antibiotic/corticosteroid solutions, draining into the nasolacrimal ducts, may be used to treat any infectious agents and reduce mucosal swelling within the duct. Injection of antibiotic–corticosteroid solution directly into the duct may also be performed. While improvement may occur, it is usually transient, and repeat flushing and injections are necessary.

In most cases of dacryocystitis with obstruction relapse, a polyethylene or silicone tube should be placed in the nasolacrimal duct to maintain patency (**Figure 9.35**).[171] Antibiotic solutions based on culture and sensitivity results are applied topically, and the tube is left in place for 3–4 weeks to maintain patency while the mucosal surfaces heal. Many dogs do not tolerate the tube well, and restraining devices (Elizabethan collars) must be used to prevent premature removal.

If grass awns are likely to be the cause due to the season and incidence in the practice area, surgical exploration of the lacrimal sac can be performed.[172,173] Anecdotally, some

dogs with grass awn foreign bodies that cannot be totally removed may eventually "clear" as the herbaceous material breaks down in the duct. Repeated flushing of the duct on a weekly basis and symptomatic therapy with topical antibiotic-corticosteroid drops and flush sometimes result in restoration of patency and relief of the dacryocystitis over a couple month's period (Gratzek A. 1999. Personal communication).

In horses with osseous fibrosis/obstruction of the duct following fractures or localized osteomyelitis from dacryocystitis, the author has on occasion been able to pass a polyethylene 3.5-French canine urinary catheter with a stainless-steel wire stylet through the bony obstruction and into the maxillary sinus. Leaving the tubing in place for 8–10 weeks established a patent fistula from duct into sinus, resulting in adequate tear drainage and resolution of the dacryocystitis.

Cystic dilation of the duct (potentially congenital in the dog, see caniculops below) does not always produce obstruction to tear outflow but creates an area that has stagnant tears and secondary infection. Treatment is by performing a rhinotomy and either removing the cyst or opening it into the nose so that it can drain.[167,174,175]

Lacrimal cyst

Introduction/etiology

Lacrimal cysts (dacryops) are rare cystic dilations of the ducts or gland. They may be associated with the orbital lacrimal gland or the third eyelid gland.[176–182] A condition termed caniculops, a cystic dilation of the lacrimal canaliculus, may manifest under the medial canthus.[167,175,183–185] The condition has been reported in the dog, in one cat,[185] and the author has seen canaliculops in an Angus cross heifer.

The cause of dacryops or canaliculops is usually unknown. The reported incidence of canaliculops seems to be mostly in young, larger breed dogs, so a developmental anomaly of the embryologic formation of the nasolacrimal duct from surface ectoderm surrounded by deeper mesenchyme during development of the facial bones[186] seems possible. In man, dilation of the duct system weakened by inflammation is suspected.[187] Three of the reported cases have been in young basset hounds,[179,180] and three of the reported cases have been in Labrador retrievers,[182] suggesting a genetic developmental defect may occur in the duct system during embryogenesis and during early facial bone growth and maturation.

Clinical signs

Most lesions are recognized as cystic by their fluctuant nature, and this can be easily confirmed by centesis. The proximity of the cyst to one of the lacrimal glands is usually suggestive of the dacryops, but this may not always be obvious. Canaliculops lesions may exhibit acute pain and expansion due to hemorrhage within the cyst, and secondary bony malformations may occur around the cyst (**Figures 9.36 and 9.37**).[167,175,179,184,185]

Diagnosis

Dacryops is usually suggested by the clinical signs and location (cystic swelling of the medial canthal structures or third eyelid). Confirmation is via fine needle aspirate of cystic fluid and cytology, surgical biopsy, or surgical

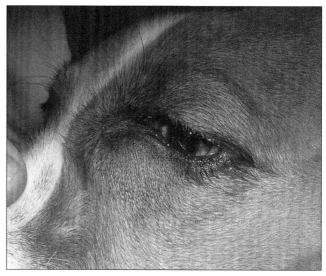

Figure 9.37 Dacryops or lacrimal cyst in a young basset hound. The condition was chronic, and the cyst had blood-tinged fluid. On exploration, the cyst was independent of the lacrimal sac but communicated with the gland of the third eyelid.

exploration and excision of the pathologic tissue. In the experience of Martin and others (including this author), nasolacrimal duct flushing is without enlargement of the cyst in a case of dacryops. Passage of fluid from the palpebral puncta to the nares with normograde nasolacrimal duct flushing may or may not occur. Injection of radiopaque dye into the cyst or through the nasolacrimal duct system followed by dacryocystorhinography does not demonstrate communication between the cyst and the nasolacrimal duct.[167,175,179,184,185]

Therapy

Careful dissection and excision of the cyst is curative. Since the canaliculi are usually within the cyst wall, accidental cutting of the canaliculus may necessitate suturing the duct over a stent,[184] allowing for patent healing of the transected duct. Methylene blue injected into the cyst may aid dissection. Bony projections from maxillary and lacrimal bone deformation may have to be smoothed down with a rongeur. Alternatively, the author sclerosed the walls of a canaliculops in a young heifer, following aspiration of cyst contents, via injection of tetracycline into the cyst. This resulted in shrinkage of the cyst and normal flow of tears through the nasolacrimal duct. The future use of polidocanol as a sclerosing agent to contract/fibrose these cystic structures may be an alternative to surgical excision as has become the case for intraorbital cysts.[188]

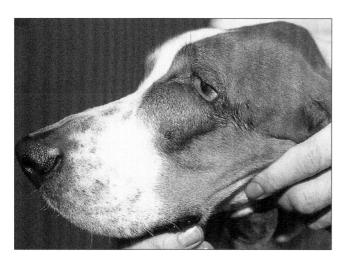

Figure 9.36 Canaliculops in a young basset hound that had produced secondary bony changes in the facial bones ventral to the cyst. No communication with the nasolacrimal duct or sac could be established.

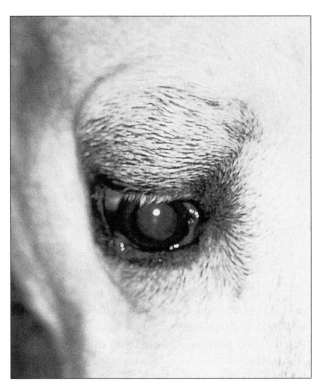

Figure 9.38 A cystadenoma of the lacrimal gland in a dog. The condition was treated with surgical excision and teletherapy.

Ectopic lacrimal gland(s)

Subconjunctival, corneal, and intraocular masses have been diagnosed on biopsy as ectopic lacrimal gland in the dog, the cow, and deer. Typically, the condition manifests itself in the young animal, but the signs may not be apparent until the lesion expands later in life.[189–191] Excision is successful when tissue is found on the ocular surface. In deer, microphthalmos masks the ectopic gland and is the predominant lesion.

Primary lacrimal gland tumor

Primary tumors arising from the lacrimal glands include adenoma (**Figure 9.38**)[192] and adenocarcinoma; they are relatively rare.[193–198] Treatment includes excision with or without radiation therapy. The prognosis is probably guarded for both diseases; however, prognosis with complete excision alone in the dog has been reported as good for long-term survival.[194] (For further information, see Chapter 8, Conjunctiva and Third Eyelid.)

A pseudotumor of granulation tissue protruding from the lower lacrimal punctum that took five attempts at excision has been reported in the dog.[16]

CLINICAL CASES

CASE 1

A 5-year-old F/S West Highland white terrier presented with a chronic history of mucopurulent ocular discharge that improved while being treated with various topical antibiotic/antibiotic–corticosteroid ointments and/or drops. The patient had atopic skin disease and was on systemic antihistamines, occasional systemic corticosteroids, and a hypoallergenic diet. Clinically, the patient had conjunctival hyperemia and mucopurulent discharge from both eyes (similar to **Figure 9.13**), no fluorescein stain retention, and STT values less than 10 mm/min in both eyes. Conjunctival scrapings showed neutrophilic inflammation with too numerous to count cocci bacteria in chains and clumps. Subsequent culture and sensitivity revealed heavy growth of *Staphylococcus* and *Streptococcus* species with moderate resistance to commonly used topical antibiotics (apart from chloramphenicol). Medical therapy was initiated as topical cyclosporine b.i.d. and topical "sicca mixture" (14 mL saline-based artificial tears, 2 mL of 20% acetylcysteine, and 2 mL of 10% chloramphenicol succinate), q.i.d. At 2-week recheck, the purulent discharge had abated, the conjunctival hyperemia was much improved, and the STT values were above 15 mm/min in both eyes. Chronic cyclosporine therapy kept the keratoconjunctivitis sicca in check. After attempting allergy testing and desensitization, the patient was eventually placed on oral cyclosporine for her atopic skin disease, which dramatically improved the dog's skin allergies. Serendipitously, the owner ran out of topical cyclosporine and discontinued its use for a few months before reporting that the dog's eyes did not seem "bad," even though the patient was no longer being treated with the topical cyclosporine. Repeat Schirmer tear testing showed that the dog's aqueous tear production was adequate despite not being treated with the topical cyclosporine. Although not common, this patient was able to control her atopic skin disease as well as her KCS with oral cyclosporine alone.

CASE 2

An 8-year-old American Cocker Spaniel presented for KCS that was unresponsive to topical cyclosporine use. The referring veterinarian had diagnosed KCS over a year prior to referral and had tried commercial topical cyclosporine as well as higher concentrations (1% and 2%) available from compounding pharmacies. Intermittent use of multiple topical antibiotics and antibiotic–corticosteroid combinations had somewhat kept the purulent discharge under control. None of the treatments had increased the patient's aqueous tear production substantially, however. Historically, the patient was deaf and had experienced numerous episodes of otitis externa/media during its lifetime as well as recurrent gastrointestinal disturbances (vomiting and diarrhea). Clinically, the patient was blepharospastic and had bilateral lackluster corneal/conjunctival surfaces, conjunctival hyperemia, mild pigmentary keratitis, and STT values in both eyes less than 5 mm/min. Both nares were clogged with dried mucoid crusts. Cultures of both ocular surfaces revealed overgrowth of *Staphylococcus*, *Streptococcus*, and *E. coli* species with moderate antibiotic resistance to commonly used topical antibiotics. Suspecting neurogenic KCS due to the history of otitis externa/media, the dried nares, and the lack of response to cyclosporine, a topical "sicca mixture" (14 mL saline-based artificial tears, 2 mL 20% acetylcysteine, 2 mL 10% chloramphenicol succinate, and 2 mL 2% pilocarpine) was used q.i.d. in both eyes in addition to the topical cyclosporine. At the 2-week recheck, ocular discharge was greatly improved, the dog appeared more comfortable/less blepharospastic, and STT values were greater than 15 mm/min in both eyes. Eventually, the patient was treated with a "sicca mixture" of artificial tears, acetylcysteine, and pilocarpine as well as the topical cyclosporine to help reduce corneal neovascularization and pigmentation. Although systemic pilocarpine could have been tried for the apparent neurogenic KCS, the dog had a history of gastrointestinal disorders that it was felt would best not be challenged with oral pilocarpine therapy. The patient responded favorably to the topical pilocarpine containing mixture, and the owner felt that the acetylcysteine helped remove tenacious discharge from the conjunctival fornices better than eyewash alone. Even though the topical cyclosporine alone did not help with the lack of tear production, once the tear production returned, the corneal scarring was improved, so cyclosporine use was continued to help keep the corneas clear of inflammatory changes such as neovascularization and pigmentation.

CASE 3

A 9-month-old F/S beagle presented with a history of recurrent eye infections since the owner purchased her at 3 months of age. The referring veterinarian diagnosed KCS and treated with topical cyclosporine and antibiotic ointment, and although the purulent discharge improved, the STT values in the afflicted eye remained 0 mm/min. After consultation, the referring veterinarian tried oral pilocarpine and increased the dose until the patient showed signs of toxicity (vomiting and diarrhea) with no improvement in aqueous tear production. On examination, the dog was blepharospastic and had mucoid discharge, no tear production, and mild neovascularization dorsolaterally in the afflicted eye. Topical anesthetic application partially resolved the blepharospasm. The naris on the ipsilateral side was moist. The other eye was normal. A tentative diagnosis of congenital KCS was made, and a parotid duct transposition (PDT) was performed. Two months following successful PDT, owner complaint was of facial wetting and dermatitis, accumulation of crusty debris on the periocular skin (as in **Figure 9.21**) and corneal surface, and blepharospasm. Surgery to constrict the parotid duct by partial ligation with a 5-0 monofilament nylon suture was successful in reducing the amount of saliva flowing from the papilla with less facial wetting. The owner was instructed to rinse the periocular hair with saline-based eyewash twice daily, and topical 1% EDTA solution and 1% cyclosporine drops (both from a compounding pharmacy) were used to chelate the mineral and help prevent accumulation on the corneal surface (EDTA) and reduce the mineral-induced keratitis (cyclosporine). This twice-a-day regimen was followed by the owner, and at the 2-year follow-up, the patient remained comfortable with minor periocular irritation. Other options for this case would have been frequent use of artificial tears and topical antimicrobials when bacterial overgrowth occurred. However, in this case, the dog was supposed to be a hunting dog, and frequent medication (more than twice daily) was not possible for the owner. Enucleation was also an option, but since the patient was visual (and young), the owner did not want to remove the eye.

CASE 4

A 7-month-old Saddlebred filly presented with a history of initial unilateral epiphora followed by copious purulent ocular discharge, all beginning at 3 months of age. Topical antibiotic ointment therapy by the referring veterinarian initially helped the purulent discharge but ultimately did no good. Clinically, the filly had copious mucopurulent discharge from the medial canthus with periocular dermatitis and alopecia (similar to **Figure 9.25**). The globe and the adnexa were otherwise normal. The contralateral eye was normal. Fluorescein dye passed from the ocular surface to the naris on the normal side but not on the contralateral side. The nasal punctum could be visualized in the ventral nasal vestibule on the normal side but not on the afflicted side. A distended bulge was seen in the nasal vestibule on the afflicted side (**Figure 9.30**), and when compressed, purulent material was expressed from the nasolacrimal puncta at the medial canthus. Cannulation of the palpebral nasolacrimal puncta and flushing of the duct with saline caused copious reflux of purulent debris from the inferior and superior palpebral punctae and re-distension of the cystic structure in the nasal vestibule. Congenital impatency of the nasolacrimal duct and secondary dacryocystitis was diagnosed, and under general anesthesia, a 5-French polyethylene canine urinary catheter was passed from the superior palpebral punctum to the nasal vestibule. The catheter could be palpated through the tissue overlying the nasal vestibule cyst. A scalpel was used to open a 3-cm incision, the catheter tip was pulled through and sutured to the nasal vestibule, and the edges of the incision were sutured open. The cannula was left in place for 3 weeks (sutured to the periocular skin at the medial canthus and to the nasal vestibule) and was then removed. This left a patent inferior punctum that did not close back over during a 1-year follow-up.

CASE 5

A 5-year-old M/N collie presented for purulent ocular discharge of 6 months' duration. The referring veterinarian had initially treated the patient with topical antibiotic ointment with minimal improvement of the discharge. Attempt at flushing the nasolacrimal duct by the referring veterinarian in a normograde fashion on the afflicted side was met with resistance and seemed painful to the patient, whereas the contralateral duct easily flushed with no apparent pain. Radiographs of the maxillary region of the skull by the referring veterinarian failed to reveal any bone density abnormalities. Clinically, both eyes and adnexa were normal with the only abnormality identified being the purulent discharge that drained from the inferior palpebral punctum. Dacryocystitis of undetermined etiology was tentatively diagnosed, and under general anesthesia, attempt at retrograde flushing of the duct was planned along with a possible dacryocystorhinogram (as in **Figure 9.6**) if the duct could not be flushed. A 3-French polyethylene canine urinary catheter was passed from the nasal punctum to a level approximately 4 cm from the medial canthus. At this point, passage of the catheter became difficult, and saline was flushed through the duct with force. A piece of grass awn, blood, and purulent debris were expelled from the inferior palpebral punctum, and the catheter was subsequently passed through to the inferior palpebral punctum. The catheter was sutured in place at the ocular and nasal ends and left for 2 weeks. Topical and systemic antibiotics were used while the catheter was in place, and a topical antibiotic–corticosteroid solution was used for 1 week after removal of the catheter. Apparently, the grass awn had passed normograde from the palpebral punctum into the nasolacrimal duct and had lodged in the constricted area where the duct passes through the maxillary bone. The foreign material and secondary bacterial infection had caused the obstruction of the duct drainage and the reflux of purulent material to the eye. The catheter was left in place following dislodgement of the foreign body so that the ulcerated duct would not heal closed following removal of the foreign body. A 1-year follow-up showed a patent nasolacrimal duct with no long-term complications. Had the foreign body not been expelled, weekly normograde flushing of the duct may have eventually yielded a patent duct once the vegetative material decomposed. Alternatively, the inflammation from the foreign body/infection could have caused permanent occlusion of the nasolacrimal duct with chronic dacryocystitis problems. The large size of the patient (40-kg collie) allowed for visualization of the nasal punctum. Had the patient been a small dog, a brachycephalic breed of dog, or a cat, visualization of the nasal punctum would have been much more difficult, and the outcome of the case may have been less rewarding.

GENETIC PREDISPOSITION, LACRIMAL SYSTEM

IMMUNE-MEDIATED KERATOCONJUNCTIVITIS SICCA

Canine—English bulldog, West Highland white terrier, Lhasa Apso, American Cocker Spaniel, pug, Pekingese, Cavalier King Charles spaniel, Yorkshire terrier, Shih Tzu, miniature Schnauzer, Boston terrier, miniature poodle, miniature dachshund

CONGENITAL ALACRIMA

Canine—Yorkshire terrier, Cavalier King Charles spaniel, miniature pinscher, beagle, miniature dachshund

EPIPHORA

Canine—Miniature and toy poodle, American Cocker Spaniel, Maltese, Bichon Frise, Papillion

Feline—Persian, brachycephalic breeds

CONGENITAL ATRESIA OF LACRIMAL PUNCTUM

Canine—American Cocker Spaniel, Bedlington terrier, Golden retriever, miniature and toy poodle, Samoyed

MALPLACEMENT OF VENTRAL PUNCTUM

Canine—Bichon Frise, miniature poodle, American Cocker Spaniel, toy breeds

DACRYOPS/CANALICULOPS

Canine—Basset hound, Labrador retriever

REFERENCES

1. Prince, J., Diesem, C., Eglitis, L., and Ruskell, G., editors. 1960. The orbit and adnexa. In: *Anatomy and Histology of the Eye and Orbit in Domestic Animals*. Charles C. Thomas: Springfield, IL, pp. 3–12.
2. Sakai, T., and Yohro, T. 1981. A histological study of the Harderian gland of Mongolian gerbils, Meriones meridianus. *Anatomy Record* 200:259–270.
3. Martin, C., Munnell, J., and Kaswan, R. 1988. The normal ultrastructure and histochemical characteristics of canine lacrimal glands. *American Journal of Veterinary Research* 49:1566–1572.
4. Orlandini, G., and Bacchi, A. 1977. Sulla ultrastruttura della ghiandola lacrimale negli equidi. *Archives Italian Anatomy and Embryology* 82:1–13.
5. Sinha, R., and Calhoun, L. 1966. A gross, histologic, and histochemical study of the lacrimal apparatus of sheep and goats. *American Journal of Veterinary Research* 27:1633–1640.
6. Gelatt, K.N., Peiffer Jr., R.L., Erickson, J.L., and Gum, G.G. 1975. Evaluation of tear formation in the dog, using a modification of the Schirmer tear test. *Journal of the American Veterinary Medical Association* 166:368–370.
7. Helper, L., Magrane, W., Koehm, J., and Johnson, R. 1974. Surgical induction of keratoconjunctivitis sicca in the dog. *Journal of the American Veterinary Medical Association* 165:172–174.
8. Saito, A., Izumisawa, Y., Yamashita, K., and Kotani, T. 2001. The effect of third eyelid gland removal on the ocular surface of dogs. *Veterinary Ophthalmology* 4:13–18.
9. McLaughlin, S., Brightman, A., Helper, L., Primm, N., Brown, M., and Greely, S. 1988. Effect of removal of the lacrimal and third eyelid glands on Schirmer tear tests in the cat. *Journal of the American Veterinary Medical Association* 193:820–822.
10. Helper, L. 1970. The effect of lacrimal gland removal on the conjunctiva and cornea of the dog. *Journal of the American Veterinary Medical Association* 157:72–75.
11. Saito, A., Watanabe, Y., and Kotani, T. 2004. Morphologic changes of the anterior corneal epithelium caused by third eyelid removal in dogs. *Veterinary Ophthalmology* 7:113–119.
12. Cornell-Bell, A., Sullivan, D., and Allansmith, M. 1985. Gender-related differences in the morphology of the lacrimal gland. *Investigative Ophthalmology and Visual Science* 26:1170–1175.
13. Kaswan, R., Salisbury, M., and Lothrop, C. 1991. Interaction of age and gender on occurrence of canine keratoconjunctivitis sicca. *Progress in Veterinary Ophthalmology and Comparative Ophthalmology* 1:93–97.
14. Beckwith-Cohen, B., Elad, D., Bdolah-Abram, T., and Ofri, R. 2014. Comparison of tear pH in dogs, horses, and cattle. *American Journal of Veterinary Research* 75:494–499.
15. Holly, F., and Lemp, M. 1977. Tear physiology and dry eyes. *Survey of Ophthalmology* 22:69–87.
16. Williams, D., Long, R., and Barnett, K. 1998. Lacrimal pseudotumour in a young Bull Terrier. *Journal of Small Animal Practice* 39:30–32.
17. Wang, J., Aquavella, J., Palakuru, J. et al. 2006. Relationship between central tear film thickness and tear menisci of the upper and lower eyelids. *Investigative Ophthalmology and Visual Science* 47:4349–4355.
18. Ehlers, N. 1965. The precorneal film: Biomicroscopical, histological, and chemical investigations. *Acta Ophthalmologica* 81:4–134.
19. Davidson, H.J., and Kuonen, V.J. 2004. The tear film and ocular mucins. *Veterinary Ophthalmology* 7:71–77.
20. Powell, C. 1988. *Autonomic innervation of the canine lacrimal glands*. Master's thesis, University of Georgia, pp. 1–77.
21. Bromberg, B. 1981. Autonomic control of lacrimal protein secretion. *Investigative Ophthalmology and Visual Science* 20:110–116.

22. Powell, C., and Martin, C. 1989. Distribution of cholinergic and adrenergic nerve fibers in the lacrimal glands of dogs. *American Journal of Veterinary Research* 50:2084–2088.

23. Chandler, J.W., and Gillette, T.E. 1983. Immunologic defense mechanisms of the ocular surface. *Ophthalmology* 90:585–591.

24. Corfield, A.P., Carrington, S.D., Hicks, S.J. et al. 1997. Ocular Mucins: Purification, metabolism, and functions. *Progress in Retinal and Eye Research.* 16:627–656.

25. Dartt, D.A., McCarthy, D.M., Mercer, H.J. et al. 1995. Localization of nerves adjacent to goblet cells in rat conjunctiva. *Current Eye Research* 14:993–1000.

26. Rios, J.D., Forde, K., Diebold, Y. et al. 2000. Development of conjunctival goblet cells and their neuroreceptor subtype expression. *Investigative Ophthalmology and Visual Science* 41:2127–2137.

27. Franklin, R., and Bang, B. 1980. Mucus-stimulating factor in tears. *Investigative Ophthalmology and Visual Science* 19:430–432.

28. Latimer, C., Wyman, M., Diesem, C., and Burt, J. 1984. Radiographic and gross anatomy of the nasolacrimal duct of the horse. *American Journal of Veterinary Research* 45:451–548.

29. Burling, K., Murphy, C., Da Silva Curiel, J., and Bellhorn, R. 1991. Anatomy of the rabbit nasolacrimal duct and its clinical implications. *Progress in Veterinary and Comparative Ophthalmology* 1:33–40.

30. Schueter, C., Budras, K.D., Ludewig, E. et al. 2009. Brachycephalic feline noses: CT and anatomical study of the relationship between head conformation and the nasolacrimal drainage system. *Journal of Feline Medicine and Surgery* 11:891–900.

31. Moore, C., and Collier, L. 1990. Ocular surface disease associated with loss of conjunctival goblet cells in dogs. *Journal of the American Animal Hospital Association* 26:458–465.

32. Cullen, C.L., Njaa, B.L., and Grahn, B.H. 1999. Ulcerative keratitis associated with qualitative tear film abnormalities in cats. *Veterinary Ophthalmology* 2:197–204.

33. Lim, C.C., and Cullen, C.L. 2005. Schirmer tear test values and tear film break-up times in cats with conjunctivitis. *Veterinary Ophthalmology* 8:305–310.

34. Helper, L. 1976. Keratoconjunctivitis sicca in dogs. *American Academy of Ophthalmology Otolaryngology* 81:624–628.

35. Helper, L.C. 1996. The tear film in the dog. Causes and treatment of diseases associated with overproduction and underproduction of tears. *Animal Eye Research* 15:5–11.

36. Aguirre, G., Rubin, L., and Harvey, C. 1971. Keratoconjunctivitis sicca in dogs. *Journal of the American Veterinary Medical Association* 158:1566–1578.

37. Johnson, B., Whiteley, H., and McLaughlin, S. 1990. Effects of inflammation and aqueous tear film deficiency on conjunctival morphology and ocular mucus composition in cats. *American Journal of Veterinary Research* 51:820–824.

38. Kern, T., Erb, H., Schaedler, J., and Dougherty, E.P. 1988. Scanning electron microscopy of experimental keratitis sicca in dogs: Cornea and bulbar conjunctiva. *Veterinary Pathology* 25:468–474.

39. Barnett, K. 1988. Keratoconjunctivitis sicca: Sex incidence. *Journal of Small Animal Practice* 29:531–534.

40. Sanchez, R.F., Innocent, G., Mould, J., and Billson, F.M. 2007. Canine keratoconjunctivitis sicca: Disease trends in a review of 229 cases. *Journal of Small Animal Practice* 48:211–217.

41. Giuliano, E.A. 2013. Diseases and surgery of the canine lacrimal secretory system. In: Gelatt, K.N., Gilger, B.C., and Kern, T.J., editors. *Veterinary Ophthalmology.* 5th edition. Wiley-Blackwell: Ames, IA, p. 920.

42. Morgan, R., and Abrams, K. 1991. Topical administration of cyclosporine for treatment of keratoconjunctivitis sicca in dogs. *Journal of the American Veterinary Medical Association* 199:1043–1046.

43. Olivero, D., Davidson, M., English, R., Nasisse, M., Jamieson, V., and Gerig, T. 1991. Clinical evaluation of 1% cyclosporine for topical treatment of keratoconjunctivitis sicca in dogs. *Journal of the American Veterinary Medical Association* 199:1039–1042.

44. Sansom, J., Barnett, K., Neumann, W., Schulte-Neumann, S., and Clerc, B. 1995. Treatment of keratoconjunctivitis sicca in dogs with cyclosporine ophthalmic ointment: A European clinical field trial. *Veterinary Record* 137:504–507.

45. Herrera, H.C., Weichler, N., Rodriguez Gomez, J., and Garcia de Jalon, J.A. 2007. Severe, unilateral, unresponsive keratoconjunctivitis sicca in 16 juvenile Yorkshire Terriers. *Veterinary Ophthalmology* 10:285–288.

46. Barnett, K.C. 2006. Congenital keratoconjunctivitis sicca and ichthyosiform dermatosis in the Cavalier King Charles Spaniel. *Journal of Small Animal Practice* 47:524–528.

47. Kern, T., and Erb, H. 1987. Facial neuropathy in dogs and cats: 95 cases (1975–1985). *Journal of the American Veterinary Medical Association* 191:1604–1609.

48. Ruskell, G. 1969. Changes in nerve terminals and acini of the lacrimal gland and changes in secretion induced by autonomic denervation. *Zellforsch Mikrosk Anatomy* 94:261–281.

49. Joyce, J., and Bratton, G. 1973. Keratoconjunctivitis sicca secondary to fracture of the mandible. *Veterinary Medicine/Small Animal Clinician* 68:619–620.

50. Spurlock, S., Spurlock, G., and Wise, M. 1989. Keratoconjunctivitis sicca associated with fracture of the stylohyoid bone in a horse. *Journal of the American Veterinary Medical Association* 194:258–259.

51. Sharp, N.J.H., Nash, A.S., and Griffiths, I.R. 1984. Feline dysautonomia (the Key-Gaskell syndrome): A clinical and pathological study of forty cases. *The Journal of Small Animal Practice* 25:599–615.

52. Cave, T.A., Knottenbelt, C., Mellor, D.J. et al. 2003. Outbreak of dysautonomia (Key-Gaskell syndrome) in a closed colony of pet cats. *The Veterinary Record* 153:387–392.

53. Kidder, A.C., Johannes, C., O'Brien, D.P. et al. 2008. Feline dysautonomia in the Midwestern United States: A retrospective study of nine cases. *Journal of Feline Medicine and Surgery* 10:130–136.

54. Bryan, G., and Slatter, D. 1973. Keratoconjunctivitis sicca induced by phenazopyridine in dogs. *Archives of Ophthalmology* 90:310–311.

55. Slatter, D., and Davis, W. 1974. Toxicity of phenazopyridine. *Archives of Ophthalmology* 91:484–486.

56. Slatter, D., and Blogg, J. 1978. Keratoconjunctivitis sicca in dogs associated with sulphonamide administration. *Australian Veterinary Journal* 54:444–446.

57. Vestre, W., Brightman, A., Helper, L., and Lowery, J. 1979. Decreased tear production associated with general anesthesia in the dog. *Journal of the American Veterinary Medical Association.* 174:1006.

58. Morgan, R., and Bachrach, A. 1982. Keratoconjunctivitis sicca associated with sulfonamide therapy in dogs. *Journal of the American Veterinary Medical Association* 180:432–434.

59. Arnett, B., Brightman, A., and Musselman, E. 1984. Effect of atropine sulfate on tear production in the cat when used with ketamine hydrochloride and acetylpromazine maleate. *Journal of the American Veterinary Medical Association* 185:214–215.

60. Collins, K., Moore, C., and Hagee, J. 1986. Sulfonamide-associated keratoconjunctivitis sicca and corneal ulceration in a dysuric dog. *Journal of the American Veterinary Medical Association* 189:924–926.

61. Barnett, K., and Hoseph, E. 1987. Keratoconjunctivitis sicca in the dog following 5-aminosalicyclic acid administration. *Human Toxicology* 6:377–383.

62. Slatter, D., Piek, J., and Costa, N. 1982. Lack of lacrimotoxicity to phenazopyridine in rabbits. *Journal of Veterinary Pharmacology and Therapeutics* 5:209–212.

63. Herring, I.P., Pickett, J.P., Champagne, E.S., and Marini, M. 2000. Evaluation of aqueous tear production in dogs following general anesthesia. *Journal of the American Animal Hospital Association* 36:427–430.

64. Hollingsworth, S.R., Canton, D.D., Buyukmihci, N.C., and Farver, T.B. 1992. Effect of topically administered atropine on tear production in dogs. *Journal of the American Veterinary Medical Association* 200:1481–1484.

65. Dodam, J.R., Branson, K., and Martin, D.D. 1998. Effects of intramuscular sedative and opioid combinations on tear production in dogs. *Veterinary Ophthalmology* 1:57–59.

66. Berger, S., and Scagliotti, R. 1995. A quantitative study of the effects of tribrissen on canine tear production. *Journal of the American Animal Hospital Association* 31:236–241.

67. Diehl, K., and Roberts, S. 1991. Keratoconjunctivitis sicca in dogs associated with sulfonamide therapy: 16 cases (1980–1990). *Progress in Veterinary and Comparative Ophthalmology* 1:276–282.

68. Trepanier, L.A. 2004. Idiosyncratic toxicity associated with potentiated sulfonamides in the dog. *Journal of Veterinary Pharmacology and Therapeutics* 27:129–138.

69. Van Buskirk, E.M. 1980. Adverse reactions from timolol maleate therapy. *Ophthalmology* 87:447–450.

70. Stiles, J. 2004. Warning of an adverse effect of etodolac. *Journal of the American Veterinary Medical Association* 225:503.

71. Klauss, G., Giuliano, E.A., Moore, C.P. et al. 2006. Canine keratoconjunctivitis sicca associated with etodolac administration. *Journal of the American Veterinary Medical Association* 230:541–547.

72. Martin, C., and Kaswan, R. 1985. Distemper-associated keratoconjunctivitis sicca. *Journal of the American Animal Hospital Association* 21:355–359.

73. de Almeida, D.E., Roveratti, C., Brito, F.L.C. et al. 2009. Conjunctival effects of canine distemper virus-induced keratoconjunctivitis sicca. *Veterinary Ophthalmology* 12:211–215.

74. Nasisse, M.P., Guy, J.S., Davidson, M.G. et al. 1989. Experimental ocular herpesvirus infection in the cat. Sites of virus replication, clinical features, and effects of corticosteroid administration. *Investigative Ophthalmology and Visual Science* 30:1758–1768.

75. Stiles, J. 2013. Feline ophthalmology. In: Gelatt, K.N., Gilger, B.C., and Kern, T.J., editors. *Veterinary Ophthalmology*. 5th edition: Wiley-Blackwell: Ames, IA, p. 1482.

76. Elkan, E., and Zwart, P. 1967. The ocular disease of young terrapins caused by vitamin-A deficiency. *Veterinary Pathology* 4:112–118.

77. Hayashi, K., Reddy, C., Hanninen, L., Wolf, G., and Kenyon, K. 1990. Pathologic changes in the exorbital lacrimal gland of the vitamin A-deficient rat. *Investigative Ophthalmology and Visual Science* 31:187–196.

78. Naranjo, C., Fondevilla, D., Leiva, M. et al. 2005. Characterization of lacrimal gland lesions and possible pathogenic mechanisms of keratoconjunctivitis sicca in dogs with leishmaniasis. *Veterinary Parasitology* 133:37–47.

79. Morgan, R., Duddy, J., and McClurg, K. 1993. Prolapse of the gland of the third eyelid in dogs: A retrospective study of 89 cases (1980–1990). *Journal of the American Animal Hospital Association* 29:56–60.

80. Moulimard, J. 1982. *Contribution a l'etude etiologique de la kerato conjonctivite seche chez le chien*. These pour le Doctorat Veterinaire, Ecole Nationale Veterinaire D'Alfort.

81. Kaswan, R., Martin, C., and Chapman, W. 1984. Keratoconjunctivitis sicca: Histopathologic study of nictitating membrane and lacrimal glands from 28 canine cases. *American Journal of Veterinary Research* 45:112–118.

82. Kaswan, R., Martin, C., and Dawe, D. 1985. Keratoconjunctivitis sicca: Immunological evaluation of 62 canine cases. *American Journal of Veterinary Research* 46:376–383.

83. Kaswan R., Martin C., Dawe D. 1983. Rheumatoid factor determination in 50 dogs with keratoconjunctivitis sicca. *Journal of the American Veterinary Medical Association* 183:1073–1075.

84. Wolf, E., and Merideth, R. 1981. Parotid duct transposition in the horse. *Journal of Equine Veterinary Science* 1:143–145.

85. Spiess, B., Wilcock, B., and Physick-Sheard, P. 1989. Eosinophilic granulomatous dacryoadenitis causing bilateral keratoconjunctivitis sicca in a horse. *Equine Veterinary Journal* 21:226–228.

86. Collins, K., Johnson, P., Moore, C., Collier, L., and Shaw, M. 1994. Immune-mediated keratoconjunctivitis sicca in a horse. *Veterinary and Comparative Ophthalmology* 4:61–65.

87. Reilly, L., and Beech, J. 1994. Bilateral keratoconjunctivitis sicca in a horse. *Equine Veterinary Journal* 26:171–172.

88. Sandberg, C.A., Herring, I.P., Schorling, J.J. et al. 2008. Ulcerative eosinophilic keratoconjunctivitis in three horses: Clinical course and characterization by electron microscopy. Abstracts: 39th Annual meeting of the American College of Veterinary Ophthalmologists. *Veterinary Ophthalmology* 11:413–429.

89. Williams, D.L., Pierce, V., Mellor, P. et al. 2007. Reduced tear production in three canine endocrinopathies. *Journal of Small Animal Practice* 48:252–256.

90. Peruccio, C. 1982. Incidence of hypothyroidism in dogs affected by keratoconjunctivitis sicca. *Proceedings of the American Society of Veterinary Ophthalmology and International Society of Veterinary Ophthalmology*, Las Vegas, NV, p. 47.

91. Miller, P., and Panciera, D. 1994. Effects of experimentally induced hypothyroidism on the eye and ocular adnexa of dogs. *American Journal of Veterinary Research* 55:692–697.

92. Dodds, W. 1997. Autoimmune thyroiditis and polyglandular autoimmunity of purebred dogs. *Canine Practice* 22:18–48.

93. Quimby, F., Schwartz, R., Poskitt, T., and Lewis, R. 1979. A disorder of dogs resembling Sjögren's syndrome. *Clinical Immunology and Immunopathology* 12:471–476.

94. Canapp, S.O., Cohn, L.A., Maggs, D.J. et al. 2001. Xerostomia, xerophthalmia, and plasmacytic infiltrates of the salivary glands (Sjogren's-like syndrome) in a cat. *Journal of the American Veterinary Medical Association* 218:59–65.

95. Roberts, S., Lavach, J., Severin, G., Withrow, S., and Gillette, E. 1987. Ophthalmic complications following megavoltage irradiation of the nasal and paranasal cavities in dogs. *Journal of the American Veterinary Medical Association* 190:43–47.

96. Jamieson, V., Davidson, M., Nasisse, M., and English, R. 1991. Ocular complications following cobalt-60 radiotherapy of neoplasms in the canine head region. *Journal of the American Animal Hospital Association* 27:51–55.

97. Sullivan, D.A., Wickham, L.A., Rocha, E.M., Kelleher, R.S., Silveir, L.A., and Toda, I. 1998. Influence of gender, sex steroid hormones, and the hypothalmic-pituitary axis on the structure and function of the lacrimal gland. *Advances in Experimental Medicine and Biology* 438:11–42.

98. Azzarolo, A.M., Mircheff, A.K., Kaswan, R.L. et al. 1997. Androgen support of lacrimal gland function. *Endocrine* 6:39–45.

99. Sullivan, D.A., Krenzer, K.L., Sullivan, B.D., Tolls, D.B., Toda, I., and Dana, M.R. 1999. Does androgen insufficiency cause lacrimal gland inflammation and aqueous tear deficiency? *Investigative Ophthalmology and Visual Science* 40:1261–1265.

100. Barrett, P., Scagliotti, R., Merideth, R., Jackson, P., and Alarcon, F. 1991. Absolute corneal sensitivity and corneal trigeminal nerve anatomy in normal dogs. *Progress in Veterinary and Comparative Ophthalmology* 1:245–254.

101. Salisbury, M.-A., Kaswan, R.L., and Brown, J. 1995. Microorganisms isolated from the corneal surface before and during topical cyclosporine treatment in dogs with keratoconjunctivitis sicca. *American Journal of Veterinary Research* 56(7):880–884.

102. Petersen-Jones, S. 1997. Quantification of conjunctival sac bacteria in normal dogs and those suffering from keratoconjunctivitis sicca. *Veterinary Comparative Ophthalmology* 7:29–35.

103. Moore, C.P., Willsman, N.J., Nordheim, E.V., and Majors, L.J. 1987. Density and distribution of canine conjunctival goblet cells. *Investigative Ophthalmology and Visual Science* 28:1925–1932.

104. Cullen, C.L., Lim, C., and Sykes, J. 2005. Tear film breakup times in healthy cats before and after anesthesia. *Veterinary Ophthalmology* 8:159–165.

105. Ralph, R. 1975. Conjunctival goblet cell density in normal subjects and in dry eye syndromes. *Investigative Ophthalmology and Visual Science* 14:299–302.

106. Taylor, H., and Louis, W. 1980. Significance of tear function test abnormalities. *Annals of Ophthalmology* 12:531–535.

107. Hawkins, E.C., and Murphy, C.J. 1986. Inconsistencies in the absorptive capacities of Schirmer tear test strips. *Journal of the American Veterinary Medical Association* 188:511–513.

108. van der Woerdt, A., and Adamcak, A. 2000. Comparison of absorptive capacities of original and modified Schirmer tear test strips in dogs. *Journal of the American Veterinary Medical Association* 216:1576–1577.

109. Hakanson, N., and Arnesson, K. 1997. Temporal variation in tear production in normal Beagle dogs as determined by Schirmer tear test. *Veterinary Comparative Ophthalmology* 7:196–203.

110. Berger, S.L., and King, V. 1998. The fluctuation of tear production in the dog. *Journal of the American Animal Hospital Association* 34:79–83.

111. Bounous, D., Carmichael, P., Kaswan, R., Hirsh, S., and Stiles, J. 1995. Effects of ophthalmic cyclosporine on lacrimal gland pathology and function in dogs with keratoconjunctivitis sicca. *Veterinary and Comparative Ophthalmology* 5:5–12.

112. Izci, C., Celik, I., Alkan, F. et al. 2002. Histologic characteristics and local cellular immunity of the gland of the third eyelid after topical administration of 2% cyclosporine for treatment of dogs with keratoconjunctivitis sicca. *American Journal of Veterinary Research* 63:988–694.

113. Kaswan, R., Salisbury, M., and Ward, D. 1989. Spontaneous canine keratoconjunctivitis sicca, a useful model for human keratoconjunctivitis sicca: Treatment with cyclosporine eye drops. *Archives of Ophthalmology* 107:1210–1216.

114. Kaswan, R., Salisbury, M., Ward, D., Martin, C., Ramsey, J., and Fischer C. 1990. Topical application of cyclosporine in the management of keratoconjunctivitis sicca in dogs. *Journal of the American Animal Hospital Association* 26:269–274.

115. Yoshida, A., Fujihara, T., and Nakata, K. 1999. Cyclosporin A increases tear fluid secretion via release of sensory neurotransmitters and muscarinic pathway in mice. *Experimental Eye Research* 68:541–546.

116. Tsubota, K., Saito, I., Ishimaru, N., and Hayashi, Y. 1998. Use of topical cyclosporine A in a primary Sjögren's syndrome mouse model. *Investigative Ophthalmology and Visual Science* 39:1551–1559.

117. Moore, C.E., McHugh, J.B., Thorne, J.G., and Phillips, T.E. 2001. Effect of cyclosporine on conjunctival mucin in a canine keratoconjunctivitis sicca model. *Investigative Ophthalmology and Visual Science* 42:653–659.

118. Gilger, B., Andrews, J., Wilkie, D., and Lairmore, M. 1996. Lymphocyte proliferation and blood drug levels in dogs with keratoconjunctivitis sicca receiving long-term topical ocular cyclosporine. *Veterinary Comparative Ophthalmology* 6:125–130.

119. Dreyfus, J., Schobert, C.S., and Dubielzig, R.R. 2011. Superficial corneal squamous cell carcinoma occurring in dogs with chronic keratitis. *Veterinary Ophthalmology* 14:161–168.

120. Fullard R.J., Kaswan R.M., Bounous D.I., Hirsch S.G. 1995. Tear protein profiles vs. clinical characteristics of untreated and cyclosporine-treated canine KCS. *Journal of the American Optometric Association* 66:397–404.

121. Hendrix, D.V.H., Adkins, E.A., Ward, D.A. et al. 2011. An investigation comparing the efficacy of topical ocular application of tacrolimus and cyclosporine in dogs. *Veterinary Medicine International* 2011:487592.

122. Chambers, L., Fischer, C., McCalla, T., Parshall, C., Slatter, D., and Yakley, B. 2002. Topical tacrolimus in treatment of canine keratoconjunctivitis sicca: A multicenter preliminary clinical trial. *Poster presentation at the Scientific Meeting of the American College of Veterinary Ophthalmologists*; Denver, CO.

123. Berdoulay, A., English, R.V., and Nadelstein, B. 2005. Effect of topical 0.02% tacrolimus aqueous suspension on tear production in dogs with keratoconjunctivitis sicca. *Veterinary Ophthalmology* 8:225–232.

124. Czepiel, T.M., Sapienza, J.S., and Strauss, R.S. 2015. Preliminary clinical findings in treating canine keratoconjunctivitis sicca with 1% tacrolimus aqueous solution.

Proceedings of the Scientific Meeting of the American College of Veterinary ophthalmologists; Coeur d' Alene, ID.

125. Nell, B., Walde, I., Billich, A. et al. 2005. The effect of topical pimecrolimus in keratoconjunctivitis sicca and chronic superficial keratitis in dogs: Results of an exploratory study. *Veterinary Ophthalmology* 8:39–46.

126. Ofri, R., Lambrou, G.N., Allgoewer, I. et al. 2009. Clinical evaluation of pimecrolimus eye drops for treatment of canine keratoconjunctivitis sicca: A comparison with cyclosporine A. *The Veterinary Journal* 179:70–77.

127. Rubin, L., and Aguirre, G. 1967. Clinical use of pilocarpine for keratoconjunctivitis sicca in dogs and cats. *Journal of the American Veterinary Medical Association* 151:313–320.

128. Smith, E., Buyukmihci, N.C., and Farver, T. 1994. Effect of topical pilocarpine treatment on tear production in dogs. *Journal of the American Veterinary Medical Association* 205:1286–1289.

129. Gilbard, J., Farris, L., and Santamaria, J. 1978. Osmolarity of tear microvolumes in keratoconjunctivitis sicca. *Archives of Ophthalmology* 96:677–681.

130. Tsubota, K., Goto, E., Fujita, H. et al. 1999. Treatment of dry eye by autologous serum application in Sjögren's syndrome. *British Journal of Ophthalmology* 83:390–395.

131. Thermes, F., Molon-Noblot, S., and Grove, J. 1991. Effects of acetylcysteine on rabbit conjunctival and corneal surfaces. *Investigative Ophthalmology and Visual Science* 32:2958–2963.

132. Severin, G.A., editor. 1996. Lacrimal apparatus. In: *Severin's Veterinary Ophthalmology Notes*. 3rd edition. DesignPointeTM Communications, Inc.: Fort Collins, CO, pp. 232–233.

133. Rocha, E.M., Wickham, L.A., da Silveira, L.A. et al. 2000. Identification of androgen receptor protein and 5 alpha-reductase mRNA in human ocular tissues. *British Journal of Ophthalmology* 84:76–84.

134. DeVries, J., Hackett, R., Kern, T. et al. 2013. Bilateral parotid duct transposition for keratoconjunctivitis sicca in a Connemara stallion. *Veterinary Ophthalmology* 16:303–311.

135. Lavignette, A. 1966. Keratoconjunctivitis sicca in a dog treated by transposition of the parotid salivary duct. *Journal of the American Veterinary Medical Association* 148:778–786.

136. Baker, G., and Formston, C. 1968. An evaluation of transplantation of the parotid duct in the treatment of keratoconjunctivitis sicca in the dog. *Journal of Small Animal Practice* 9:261–268.

137. Gelatt, K. 1970. Treatment of canine keratoconjunctivitis sicca by parotid duct transposition. *Journal of the American Animal Hospital Association* 6:1–12.

138. Schmidt, G., Magrane, W., and Helper, L. 1970. Parotid duct transposition: A follow-up study of 60 eyes. *Journal of the American Animal Hospital Association* 6:235–241.

139. Glen, J., and Lawson, D. 1971. A modified technique of parotid duct transposition for the treatment of keratoconjunctivitis sicca in a dog. *Veterinary Research* 88:210–213.

140. Harvey, C., and Koch, S. 1971. Surgical complications of parotid duct transposition in the dog. *Journal of the American Animal Hospital Association* 7:122–126.

141. Stanley, R. 1997. Failure of parotid duct transposition due to sialolith formation. *Veterinary and Comparative Ophthalmology* 7:126–127.

142. Betts, D., and Helper, L. 1977. The surgical correction of parotid duct transposition failures. *Journal of the American Animal Hospital Association* 13:695–700.

143. Startup, F. 1984. Intra-canalicular gelatin implants in lacrimal punctum surgery. *Journal of Small Animal Practice* 25:635–637.

144. Gelatt, K.N., MacKay, E.O., Widenhouse, C. et al. 2006. Effect of lacrimal punctal occlusion on tear production and tear fluorescein dilution in normal dogs. *Veterinary Ophthalmology* 9:23–27.

145. Barachetti, L., Rampazzo, A., Mortellaro, C. et al. 2015. Use of episcleral cyclosporine implants in dogs with keratoconjunctivitis sicca. *Veterinary Ophthalmology*. 18(3):234–241.

146. Heider, L., Wyman, M., Burt, J., Root, C., and Gardner, H. 1975. Nasolacrimal duct anomaly in calves. *Journal of the American Veterinary Medical Association* 167:145–147.

147. Wilke, D.A., and Rings, D.M. 1990. Repair of anomalous nasolacrimal duct in a bull by use of a conjunctivorhinostomy. *Journal of the American Veterinary Medical Association* 196:1647–1650.

148. van der Woerdt, A., Wilkie, D.A., and Gilger, B.C. 1996. Congenital epiphora in a calf associated with dysplastic lacrimal puncta. *Agricultural Practice* 17, 7–11.

149. Barnett, K. 1979. Imperforate and microlachrymal puncta in the dog. *Journal of Small Animal Practice* 20:481–490.

150. Lundvall, R., and Carter, J. 1971. Atresia of the nasolacrimal meatus in the horse. *Journal of the American Veterinary Medical Association* 159:289–291.

151. Latimer, C., and Wyman, M. 1984. Atresia of the nasolacrimal duct in three horses. *Journal of the American Veterinary Medical Association* 184:989–992.

152. Mangan, B.G., Gionfriddo, J.R., and Powell, C.C. 2008. Bilateral nasolacrimal duct atresia in a cria. *Veterinary Ophthalmology* 11:49–54.

153. Sandmeyer, L.S., Bauer, B.S., Breaux, C.B., and Grahn, B.H. 2011. Congenital nasolacrimal atresia in 4 alpacas. *Canadian Veterinary Journal*. 52(3):313–317.

154. Kerpsack, R., and Kerpsack, W. 1966. The orbital gland and tear-staining in the dog. *Veterinary Medicine/Small Animal Clinician* 61:121–124.

155. Loeffler, K., Branscheid, W., Rodenbeck, H., and Ficus, H. 1978. Histologische untersuchungen an nickhautdrusen von hunden mit vermehrtem tranenflub. *Kleintier Praxis* 23:215–220.

156. Roberts, S. 1962. Abnormal tear production in the dog. *Modern Veterinary Practice* 43:37–40.

157. Harrison, V. 1964. Clinical observations on epiphora. *Veterinary Record* 76:437.

158. Read, R., Dunn, K., Smith, K., and Barnett, K. 1996. A histological study of nictitans glands from dogs with tear overflow of unknown cause. *Veterinary Comparative Ophthalmology* 6:195–204.

159. Saito, A., and Kotani, T. 1999. Tear production in dogs with epiphora and corneal epitheliopathy. *Veterinary Ophthalmology* 2:173–178.

160. Thun, R., Abraham, R., and Helper, L. 1975. Effect of tetracycline on tear production in the dog. *Journal of the American Animal Hospital Association* 11:802–804.

161. Gale, V. 1976. Use of metronidazole in treating "tear staining' in the dog. *Veterinary Record* 98:14.

162. Filipek, M., and Rubin, L. 1977. Effect of metronidazole on lacrimation in the dog: A negative report. *Journal of the American Animal Hospital Association* 13:339–341.

163. Long, R. 1975. The relief of epiphora by conjunctivorhinostomy. *Journal of Small Animal Practice* 16:381–386.

164. Covitz, D., Hunziker, J., and Koch, S. 1977. Conjunctivorhinostomy: A surgical method for the control

of epiphora in the dog and cat. *Journal of the American Veterinary Medical Association* 171:251–255.

165. Gelatt, K.N., and Gelatt, J.P., editors. 2001. Surgery of the nasolacrimal apparatus and tear system. In: *Small Animal Ophthalmic Surgery, Practical Techniques for the Veterinarian.* Butterworth-Heinemann: Woburn, MA. p. 133.

166. Lavach, J., Severin, G., and Roberts, S. 1984. Dacryocystitis in dogs: A review of twenty-two cases. *Journal of the American Animal Hospital Association* 20:463–467.

167. van der Woerdt, A., Wilkie, D., Gilger, B., Smeak, D., and Kerpsack, S. 1997. Surgical treatment of dacryocystitis caused by cystic dilation of the nasolacrimal system in three dogs. *Journal of the American Veterinary Medical Association* 211:445–447.

168. Gelatt, K., Guffy, M., and Borgess, T. 1971. Radiographic contrast techniques for detecting orbital and nasolacrimal tumors in dogs. *Journal of the American Veterinary Medicine Association* 156:741–746.

169. Yakely, W., and Alexander, J. 1971. Dacryocystorhinography in the dog. *Journal of the American Veterinary Medicine Association* 159:1417–1421.

170. Gelatt, K., Cure, T., Guffy, M., and Jessen, C. 1972. Dacryocystorhinography in the dog and cat. *Journal of Small Animal Practice* 13:381–397.

171. Severin, G. 1982. Nasolacrimal duct catheterization in the dog. *Journal of the American Animal Hospital Association* 18:13–16.

172. Laing, E., Spiess, B., and Binnington, A. 1988. Dacryocystotomy: A treatment for chronic dacryocystitis in the dog. *Journal of the American Animal Hospital Association* 24:223–226.

173. Pope, E.R., and Champagne, E.S. 2001. Intraosseous approach to the nasolacrimal duct for removal of a foreign body in a dog. *Journal of the American Veterinary Medical Association* 218:541–542.

174. White, R.A.S. 1984. Endoscopic management of a cystic nasolacrimal duct obstruction in a dog. *Journal of Small Animal Practice* 25:729–735.

175. Lussier, B., and Carrier, M. 2004. Surgical treatment of recurrent dacryocystitis secondary to cystic dilation of the nasolacrimal duct in a dog. *Journal of the American Animal Hospital Association* 40:216–219.

176. Harvey, C., Koch, S., and Rubin, L. 1968. Orbital cysts with conjunctival fistula in a dog. *Journal of the American Veterinary Medical Association* 153:1432–1435.

177. Playter, R., and Adams, L. 1977. Lacrimal cyst (dacryops) in 2 dogs. *Journal of the American Veterinary Medical Association* 171:736–737.

178. Latimer, C., Wyman, M., Szymanski, C., and Werling, K. 1983. Membrana nictitans gland cyst in a dog. *Journal of the American Veterinary Medical Association* 183:1003–1005.

179. Martin, C., Kaswan, R., and Doran, C. 1987. Cystic lesions of the periorbital region. *Compendium on Continuing Education for the Practicing Veterinarian* 9:1021–1029.

180. Grahn, B.H., and Mason, R.A. 1995. Epiphora associated with dacryops in a dog. *Journal of the American Animal Hospital Association* 31:15–19.

181. Ota, J., Pearce, J.W., Finn, M.J. et al. 2009. Dacryops (lacrimal cyst) in three young Labrador retrievers. *Journal of the American Animal Hospital Association* 45: 191–196.

182. Delgado, E. 2013. Dacryops of the lacrimal gland of a dog. *Veterinary Ophthalmology* 16: 153–158.

183. Gerding, P. 1991. Epiphora associated with canaliculops in a dog. *Journal of the American Animal Hospital Association* 27:424–426.

184. Davidson, H.J., and Blanchard, G.L. 1991. Periorbital epidermoid cyst in the medial canthus of 3 dogs. *Journal of the American Veterinary Medical Association* 198:271–272.

185. Zemljic, T., Mateis, F.L., Venzin, C. et al. 2011. Orbitonasal cyst in a young European short-haired cat. *Veterinary Ophthalmology* 14(Suppl1):122–129.

186. Noden, D.M., and deLahunta, A. 1985. *The Embryology of Domestic Animals: Developmental Mechanisms and Malformations.* Williams & Wilkins: London.

187. Brownstein, S., Belin, M., Krohel, G., Smith, R.S., Condon, G., and Codere, F. 1984. Orbital dacryops. *Ophthalmology* 91:1424–1428.

188. Stuckey, J.A., Miller, W.W., and Almond, G.T. 2012. Use of a sclerosing agent (1% polidocanol) to treat an orbital mucocele in a dog. *Veterinary Ophthalmology* 15: 188–193.

189. Wyand, D.S., Lehav, M., and Albert, D.M. 1972. Intraocular lacrimal gland tissue with other ocular abnormalities occurring in a white-tailed deer. *Journal of Comparative Pathology* 82:219–221.

190. Linde-Sipman, V.D., and Klein, W.R. 1984. Ectopic lacrimal gland tissue in the globe of a cow. *Veterinary Pathology* 21:613–614.

191. Regnier, A., Magnol, J., and Servantie, J. 1986. Corneal and subconjunctival ectopic lacrimal glands in a dog. *Canadian Practice* 13:12–14.

192. Kirayama, K., Kagawa, Y., Tsuzuki, K. et al. 2000. A pleomorphic adenoma of the lacrimal gland in a dog. *Veterinary Pathology* 37:353–356.

193. Rebhun, W., and Edwards, N. 1977. Two cases of orbital adenocarcinoma of probable lacrimal gland origin. *Journal of the American Animal Hospital Association* 13:691.

194. Wilcock, B.P., and Peiffer, R.L. 1988. Adenocarcinoma of the gland of the third eyelid in seven dogs. *Journal of the American Veterinary Medical Association* 193:1549–1550.

195. Schaeffer, E.H., Pfleghaar, S., Gordon, S., and Knoedlseder, M. 1994. Maligne nickhauttumoren bei hund und katze. *Tieraerztl Praxis* 22:382–391.

196. Komaromy, A.M., Ramsey, D.T., Render, J.A., and Clark, P. 1997. Primary adenocarcinoma of the gland of the nictitating membrane in a cat. *Journal of the American Animal Hospital Association* 3:333–336.

197. Kunze, D.J., Schmidt, G.M., and Tvedten, H.W. 1979. Sebaceous adenocarcinoma of the third eyelid of a horse. *Veterinary Surgery* 3:452–455.

198. Mathes, R.L., Carmichael, K.P., Peroni, J., and Moore, P.A. 2011. Primary lacrimal gland adenocarcinoma of the third eyelid in a horse. *Veterinary Ophthalmology* 14:48–54.

199. Records, R. 2000. The Tear Film. In: Tasman, W. and Jaeger, E. editors. *Duane's Foundations of Clinical Ophthalmology* vol 2. Lippincott, Williams, and Wilkins: Philadelphia, pp. 1–22.

CHAPTER 10

CORNEA AND SCLERA

PHILLIP A. MOORE

ANATOMY AND PHYSIOLOGY

The cornea and the sclera comprise the fibrous tunic of the globe. The transitional zone between the cornea and the sclera is termed the limbus. In this area, the sclera superficially overlaps the cornea. This overlap is widest dorsal and ventrally. When the globe is viewed rostrally, the cornea is slightly horizontally elongated, especially in ungulates, and when viewed from the side, the cornea has a greater curvature than the sclera (**Figures 10.1 and 10.2**). The cornea of the dog has an average radius of curvature of 8.5 mm and varies from 13 to 17 mm in the horizontal axis and 12–16 mm in the vertical axis.[1,2] The cat cornea has an average radius of curvature of 8.6 mm, a horizontal axis of 17 mm, and a vertical axis of 16 mm.[3] Corneal measurements vary significantly in the horse, with the horizontal axis ranging from 28 to 34 mm and the vertical axis ranging from 23 to 27 mm.[1,4]

The corneal thickness of the cornea of the dog and the cat, unlike the cornea of humans, is often quoted as being thicker in the center than at the periphery.[4] However, early measurements were made postmortem. Modern measurement methods in the live animal confirm that the central cornea is slightly thinner than the periphery, as in humans. The central cornea of the dog is 0.62 mm (range 0.41–0.74 mm [410–740 μm]) and of the cat is 0.56 mm (560 μm).[5–7] In the dog, females have a thinner cornea than the males.[7] Moodie et al. studied the development of the feline curvature and corneal thickness from 9 weeks to 2 years of age and found that the thickness increased mainly during the first 4 months of life.[8] The corneal thickness increased from 0.379 mm at 9 weeks to 0.548 mm at 16 weeks and to 0.567 mm at 1 year or more. In the cat, an 8% increase in corneal thickness occurs diurnally and is associated with lid closure.[9]

The cornea not only serves to support and protect the interior ocular structures but has the unique property of being transparent. In the dog, the cornea produces 70% of the refraction (bending) of light rays. Almost 49 D of refraction occurs at the anterior corneal surface and −5.8 D at the posterior corneal surface, yielding a total refraction of 43 D.[2] In the cat, the refractive power decreases from 55 D in the kitten to 39 D at 1–2 years of age.[8] The cornea produces more refraction than the lens because refraction depends on the curvature of the surface and the difference in density of the two media.

The radius of curvature of the lens and cornea are similar. Light passes through air with a refractive index of 1, enters the cornea with a refractive index of 1.376, passes into the aqueous humor with a refractive index of 1.336, and finally into the lens with a refractive index of 1.42. Thus, the biggest difference in refractive index is between the air and the cornea. Therefore, more refraction occurs between the air and the cornea than between the aqueous humor and the lens.

The cornea is the transplant outer structure of the eye and is unique in its transparency. Anatomically, it is composed anteriorly of stratified squamous epithelium and its basal lamina, the central stroma, which comprises the major portion, and the posterior epithelium and its basal lamina (Descemet's membrane) (**Figure 10.3**). The posterior epithelium is a single cell layer and is often erroneously termed the endothelium, which has Descemet's membrane as an exaggerated basal lamina (**Figure 10.3**).

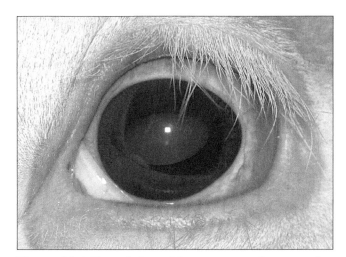

Figure 10.1 Frontal view of the cow cornea demonstrating the egg shape or elongated horizontal axis that is exaggerated in ungulates.

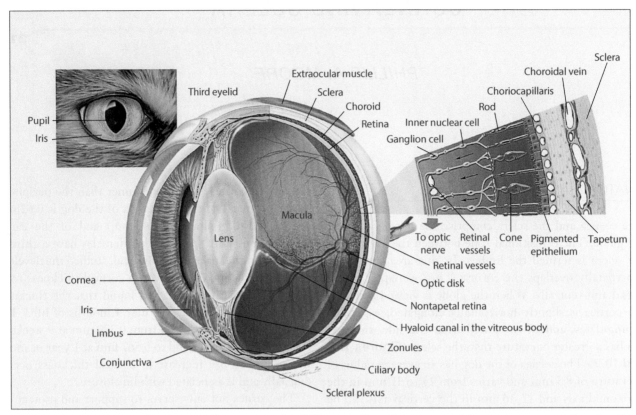

Figure 10.2 Illustration of a cat eye to demonstrate the different radius of curvature of the cornea compared to the globe and the relationships of the cornea and the sclera at the limbus.

The corneal epithelium in the dog and cat is 5–11 cells thick and has a turnover rate of approximately 7 days.[10] The flattened surface cells are polygonal and have numerous microvillae and microplicae (**Figure 10.4**) that are coated with a glycocalyx, which functions to stabilize the tear film.

The corneal stroma is 90% of the mass of the cornea and consists of parallel lamellae (bundles) of collagen fibers that extend across the entire diameter of the cornea (**Figure 10.3**). While the bundles are parallel to one another, they are not oriented in the same direction. The lamellae are most regular or parallel in the posterior stroma. The anterior subepithelial lamellae are more oblique to the surface, with more interweaving. This arrangement is responsible for the anterior stroma being more reflective when seen on biomicroscopy. Keratocytes, which are fibroblasts with branching processes, are scattered between the collagen lamellae.

The ground substance surrounding the collagen fibers is composed of proteoglycans, with the predominant glycosaminoglycan (GAG) being keratin sulfate. Dermatan sulfate is the other major GAG found in the stroma.[11] The GAGs act as anions and bind water. Keratin sulfate is most concentrated in the posterior cornea, whereas dermatin sulfate is concentrated in the anterior cornea.[12] The GAGs maintain corneal hydration and help to maintain the critical regular spacing of collagen fibers necessary for corneal transparency.

The cornea is richly supplied with sensory innervation from the long ciliary branches of the ophthalmic division of the fifth cranial nerve. The nerves are concentrated in the anterior stroma and penetrate the epithelium where they terminate as naked nerve endings. The corneal epithelium is the most densely innervated epithelium in the body.[11] The dog has an average of 12 nerve trunks[13] and the cat 19 nerve trunks[14] that enter the cornea. The nerve endings are sensitive to pain, pressure, and temperature. The dense concentration of nerve endings in the epithelium accounts for the severe pain observed with superficial epithelial loss, whereas a deep ulcer often does not exhibit the same degree of pain.[15]

Corneal sensitivity values measured with the Cochet–Bonnet anesthesiometer are similar for the dog, the cat, the horse, the cow, the sheep, and the goat.[16] Differences in corneal sensitivity depends on the area of cornea, skull type, age of the animal, health of the animal, and disease state of the eye. In dogs, the central cornea is more sensitive than the peripheral cornea.[13] A difference in corneal sensitivity is demonstrated between dog skulls. Brachycephalics dogs have decreased sensitivity compared to dolicocephalic and mesaticephalic breeds.[13] The central

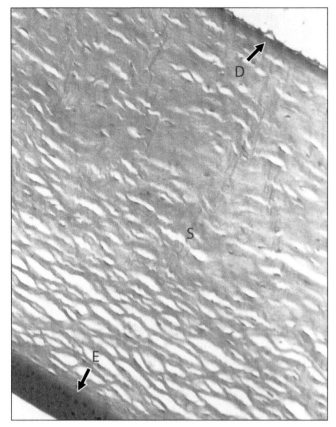

Figure 10.3 Normal histology of the canine cornea. The epithelium has a basal lamina, but there is no distinct Bowman's membrane (E). The majority of the cornea is stroma, composed of collagen fibers that traverse the cornea (S) without terminating. Descemet's membrane (D) abuts the deep stroma and is lined with a simple cuboidal epithelium.

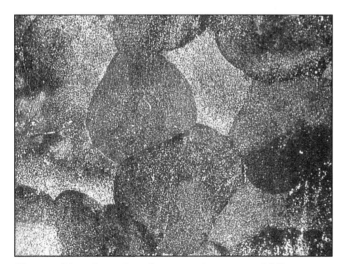

Figure 10.4 Scanning electron microscopy of feline corneal epithelium illustrating the light and dark polyhedral cells associated with the number of microplica on the surface (×480).

cornea is more sensitive than the peripheral regions in brachycephalic cats compared to domestic shorthaired (DSH) cats.[17] Dogs and cats are relatively more insensitive than other species tested.[13] In foals and cria, corneal sensitivity is greater than in the adult animal.[18,19] Sick foals, horses with pituitary pars intermedia dysfunction, and diabetic dogs have decreased corneal sensitivity compared to healthy animals of the same species.[18,20,21] In dogs with chronically elevated intraocular pressures, corneal sensitivity is decreased compared to the animal's normotensive contralateral eye.[22]

The sensory innervation has a positive trophic influence on the epithelium. Marfurt et al. investigated the anatomy and the neurochemistry of canine corneal nerves and confirmed that, as in other species, the anterior half of the stroma and epithelium is densely innervated with 14–18 radially oriented superficial nerves from the limbus that have repeated dichotomous branching.[23] The epithelium has dense leashes of nerves that are not oriented in a specific direction, unlike in some species. Marfurt et al. report that 99% of all the corneal nerves of dogs contained both substance P and calcitonin gene-related peptide, indicating their probable sensory function, while 30% contained tyrosine hydroxylase (TH). TH-positive nerves are concentrated in the stroma and are absent in the epithelium.[23] TH-positive nerves are thought to represent autonomic nerves, principally sympathetic nerves in the cornea. The neuropeptide substance P may stimulate DNA synthesis for epithelial healing; depletion of substance P slows epithelial healing.[24] Substance P, with insulin-like growth factor 1, stimulates corneal epithelial cell migration and adhesion but not mitosis in cell culture.[25]

> Any insult to the peripheral cornea and limbal region such as corneal incisions, lacerations, or lasering adjacent sclera for glaucoma may produce partial denervation of the cornea and loss of neurotrophic influences, resulting in slow-healing epithelial erosions.

Although it is not a true endothelium, the posterior layer of cells lining the cornea is usually referred to as the endothelium.[26] Its single layer of cells is usually hexagonal and lines the inner cornea (**Figure 10.5**). The endothelial cell count is 2700–2800/mm^2 for both the dog and cat and decreases with age.[6] While the endothelium is metabolically active, its mitotic activity is more questionable than the anterior epithelium. The regenerative capabilities vary with the species; minimal in the cat, good in the young

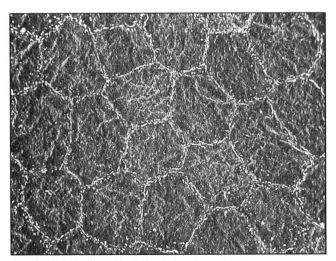

Figure 10.5 Scanning electron microscopy of equine corneal endothelium with the characteristic hexagonal shape of most of the cells (×1200).

dog.[27,28] Healing in the adult is mainly by cellular enlargement and migration rather than by mitosis. The posterior epithelium shows pleuripotenial capabilities with differentiation into the typical endodothelial cell, fibroblasts, or an epithelial cell type.[29] The epithelial cell type possesses desmosomal attachments and tonofilaments.

The basilar side of the posterior epithelium lies on the stroma and produces a modified basal lamina (Descemet's membrane) (**Figure 10.3**). It is produced throughout life and consequently is much thicker in the old animal than in the young animal. Although clinically it acts as an elastic membrane, it contains only fine fibrils that are predominantly type IV collagen.

The sclera is the major portion of the fibrous tunic; it does not have epithelial layers. The thickness varies considerably. It is thinnest at the equator and posterior pole of the globe and thickest over the base of the iris. The scleral collagen fibers branch and intermingle, and the fibers are fusiform in shape.[30] Elastic fibers are present in the sclera but are minimal in number. Cellular elements consist of scattered fibroblasts and melanocytes. The episclera is a thin collagenous and vascular layer on the outer surface of the sclera.

CORNEAL TRANSPARENCY

Several anatomic peculiarities contribute to corneal transparency:

- Smoothness of the epithelium aided by the tear film.
- Arrangement and size of the stromal collagen and GAGs. A lattice of collagen fibers is formed

that is regular and parallel. This is postulated to produce a mutual interference of light, which prevents the light from reflecting back to be visualized.[31] The small regular diameter of the collagen fibers is also thought to be important for corneal clarity.[32]

- Absence of blood vessels and pigment.
- Relative dehydration of the stroma.

HEALING OF CORNEAL WOUNDS

Epithelial healing

Epithelial wound healing is divided into three cellular phases: Migration, proliferation, and adhesion.

- Cell migration. Epithelial cells at the margin of a wound retract and become thicker within the first hour following trauma. Neutrophils from the tear film and fibrinous material are present in the epithelial defect within 1–3 hours. Hemidesmosomal attachments are dissolved around the edge of the wound, superficial cells are desquamated, and the leading edge of the wound decreases to a single cell layer. After a latent phase of 3–6 hours, sliding or cell migration occurs.[33] The cells flatten and increase their surface area by increasing cell volume with water.[34] Smaller defects are covered by a monolayer in this manner, which eventually thickens by cellular proliferation.
- Cell proliferation. Mitosis occurs, after a 24-hour delay, to re-establish the epithelial thickness. The stem cells for the corneal epithelium are located at the limbus.[35] The stem cells are long-lived cells that undergo mitosis and are responsible for cell replacement and tissue healing. They travel in a centripetal pattern from the limbus. If the healing is not accomplished by sheets of cells, the small groups of migrating cells form a whorl or vortex pattern.[34] Transient amplifying cells are produced by the stem cell, divide rapidly, and eventually differentiate into the terminally differentiated cell of the tissue. The amplifying cell of the corneal epithelium is the basal cell, and the superficial cells are the postmitotic and terminally differentiated cells.[34] Removal of the entire epithelium or removal of the limbal epithelium results in wound healing by conjunctival epithelium migrating over the cornea. Even lesions of the central corneal epithelium produce an increase in the mitotic rate of the conjunctival epithelium.[36] The conjunctival epithelium also produces goblet cells once on the cornea.

These goblet cells eventually undergo a process of transdifferentiation into corneal epithelial cells, which takes 6 weeks or more. If the cornea is vascularized, the transdifferentiation is retarded, with the epithelium retaining conjunctival characteristics.[37] Topical retinoids inhibit this transdifferentiation and are thought to be the blood-borne factor responsible for inhibition.[38]

- Cell adhesion. Although the epithelium regenerates rapidly, anchoring units are not formed until the defect is covered. If the basal lamina is intact, hemidesmosomes are formed within 1 week. If the basal lamina is removed, hemidesmosomes are much slower to regenerate (6–7 weeks). Consequently, the epithelium is susceptible to re-injury for a prolonged period when the basal lamina has been lost, as the epithelial attachment to the basal lamina is important for adhesion to the stroma.[39]

Stromal healing

Stromal healing initially involves the invasion of leukocytes from the tear film or the limbus within a matter of a few hours.[40] Within the first hour, keratocyte disintegration occurs at the margin of the wound, whereas beyond the margin the keratocytes undergo activation. Two to three days after the injury, the wound margin is filled with a mixture of keratocytes and fibroblast-type cells. Whether the fibroblasts are all transformed keratocytes or a mixture of transformed keratocytes and monocytes is controversial.[41] After 3–6 days, the fibroblasts invade the fibrin plug of the wound. The initial ground substance of the scar is dermatan sulfate, but by 15–30 days post trauma, keratin sulfate is detected, which indicates a transformation of fibroblasts to keratocytes. It takes up to 3 months to achieve normal levels of keratin sulfate.[42] The area of stromal healing is not transparent due to the disorganized and large collagen fibers. The tensile strength of the wound progresses slowly, with only 50% strength achieved by central corneal wounds in 100 days. A lack of epithelium over the stromal healing markedly decreases the tensile strength of the wound.[43]

Corneal scar formation and opacification

Epithelial healing may occur without scar formation, but when the stroma is damaged, the resultant fibroplasia with its disorganized stroma leaves some degree of residual scar. Clinically, scars are often described according to their size and density.

- A nebula is a small, very faint scar or opacity.
- A macula is a small but distinct white opacity.
- A leukoma is a large, dense, white opacity.
- An adherent leukoma is a dense white scar with an underlying adhesion of the iris to the cornea.

CORNEAL VASCULARIZATION

The cornea is normally devoid of vessels, but whether vascularization is inhibited by a factor (e.g., angiostatin) or is prevented by the compactness of the tissue is unknown. Conversely, many agents may stimulate vascularization, but their physiologic significance is often unknown. Hypoxia, neoplasia, and inflammation are frequent initiators of neovascularization. These events trigger angiogenic factors such as tumor angiogenic factor, fibroblast growth factor, transforming growth factor-β, platelet-derived growth factor, and vascular endothelial growth factor. Lymphokines produced by activated T-lymphocytes and prostaglandin (PG) E1 can produce corneal neovascularization.[44-46] Loss of compactness, i.e. corneal edema, is a factor but by itself is not sufficient to cause neovascularization.[47]

A variety of inhibitors of angiogenesis are known (angiostatin, endostatin, thrombostatin, platelet factor-4, fibronectin, and prolactin), but their interactions are complex and incompletely understood. Matrix metalloproteinases (MMPs) are enzymes that degrade the extracellular matrix, thereby allowing endothelial cell migration. Neutrophils are involved to some extent in most forms of corneal neovascularization. While leukopenic animals can develop neovascularization, the reaction is amplified by neutrophils.[48,49] Ocular vascular homeostasis is now thought to involve a balance between inhibitors and stimulators of neovascularization. Multiple mediators are probably responsible for varying phases of the process.[50]

Corneal neovascularization indicates keratitis (ulcerative or nonulcerative) or intraocular disease (e.g., uveitis and/or glaucoma).

- Superficial neovascularization: Long, branching corneal vessels may be seen with superficial ulcerative or nonulcerative keratitis.

- Focal deep neovascularization: Straight, nonbranching corneal vessels indicates a deep keratitis (ulcerative or nonulcerative).
- 360° deep neovascularization: Corneal vessels in a 360° pattern around the limbus may be seen with uveitis and/or glaucoma.

CORNEAL METABOLISM

The epithelium and the endothelium utilize most of the corneal oxygen and receive most oxygen from the atmosphere. Four sources of oxygen are:

- Aqueous humor—important for the endothelium.
- Limbal capillaries.
- Capillaries of the tarsus when the eyes are closed.
- Oxygen dissolved in the tear film layer. This is the most important source of oxygen.

Glucose is derived mainly from the aqueous humor and is metabolized via anaerobic glycolysis and the hexose monophosphate shunt.[11] The metabolic activity of the stroma is low.

CORNEAL TURGESCENCE

The normal cornea maintains a constant thickness. During the night when the lids are closed, a slight increase in thickness occurs due to the absence of evaporation of tears. The cornea is about 75%–80% water by weight, but it still has a marked affinity for more water. As a result, an excised piece of cornea immersed in solution becomes turgesced (swollen). Most of this swelling occurs in an anterior–posterior direction, with slight shortening of tangential length. The importance of turgesence is that it is always accompanied by a loss of transparency. The imbibition of water is due to the ground substance or GAGs in the stroma.

The normal cornea is in a deturgesced state. Any damage to or loss of epithelium produces localized edema, which is usually transient due to rapid epithelial regeneration. Endothelial damage, however, is far more serious, with marked and often permanent loss of transparency because of limited regenerative capacity of the endothelium.

The mechanism for maintaining corneal deturgescence in the endothelium and the epithelium is associated with a barrier function and a metabolic pump. The barrier consists of intercellular junctions which are leaky to water, but this is offset by active pumping out of water in the normal cornea (**Figure 10.6**). Conditions that damage

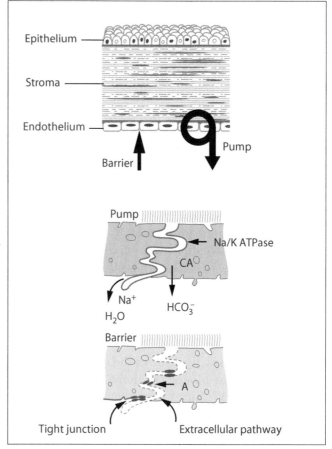

Figure 10.6 Illustration of the forces that control corneal hydration. The endothelium is an incomplete physical barrier to water from tight junctions at the lateral cell junctions. The intraocular pressure pushes water through these tight junctions, resulting in water having to be pumped back into the anterior chamber. The pumping of sodium and bicarbonate back into the aqueous humor osmotically draws water with them. (Reprinted with permission from Waring, G. et al. 1982. *Ophthalmology.* 89:531–590.)

the barrier cause the leak rate to exceed the pumping rate and result in stromal edema. The mechanisms by which water is pumped out of the cornea into the aqueous humor are incompletely understood. Prevalent theories emphasize the movement of water secondary to sodium and bicarbonate ion movement into the aqueous. A Na+/K+ ATPase metabolic pump is present on the lateral endothelial cell membrane and pumps Na+ ions into the aqueous humor, creating an osmotic gradient that draws water out of the stroma. Bicarbonate is also pumped into the aqueous humor under the influence of carbonic anhydrase (CA) and/or bicarbonate ATPase pump (**Figures 10.6 and 10.7**).[29] Surprisingly, topical or systemic carbonic anhydrase inhibitors (CAIs) do not cause corneal decompensation except on the rare occasion.

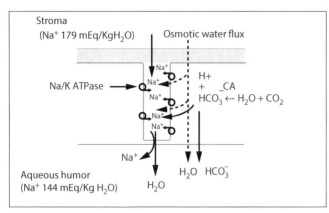

Figure 10.7 Proposed endothelial pump mechanisms that draw water out of the stroma into the aqueous humor. (Reprinted with permission from Waring, G. et al. 1982. *Ophthalmology.* 89:531–590.)

Corneal edema is blue–gray in appearance.

- Superficial corneal edema is focal in nature and typically is associated with loss of corneal epithelium and/or corneal neovascularization.
- Deep corneal edema is generalized in nature and has a cobblestone appearance. Deep corneal edema is typically associated with endothelial dysfunction (e.g., degeneration, uveitis, glaucoma or trauma).

DISEASES OF THE CORNEA

The cornea is easily visualized under magnification, enabling the clinician to examine the pathology and perform diagnostic tests. However, due to the limited response of the cornea to disease, many diseases affect the cornea similarly. One of the basic pathologic changes with corneal disease is a loss of clarity or opacification of the cornea. The types of opacity can be categorized on color; **Table 10.1** lists some of the most common causes for color changes in the cornea. The type of opacity, the depth of the lesion, and whether it is acquired or congenital may aid in making a diagnosis (**Table 10.2**).

CONGENITAL SUPERFICIAL NONINFLAMMATORY DISEASE

Puppy band keratopathy

Introduction/etiology
Puppy band keratopathy denotes a common benign condition that is often transient in neonatal puppies. The cause is

Table 10.1 **Common causes of color changes noted in the cornea**
White lesions: Edema, leukocytes, lipid, calcium, scar, infectious agents
Red lesions: Neovascularization, stromal hemorrhage, symblepharon, neoplasia
Pigmented lesions: Superficial benign melanin, sequestrum, uveal pigment (usually deep), pigmented neoplasia, dematiaceous fungi, exogenous pigment

Table 10.2 **Categorization of corneal lesions**
Congenital noninflammatory: Superficial and deep
Acquired noninflammatory: Superficial and deep
Nonulcerative inflammatory: Superficial and deep
Ulcerative: Superficial, deep, and perforated
Proliferative: Pseudotumors, congenital tumors, and acquired neoplasia

unknown but may be due to calcium in the diet. Histologic features are not known as the condition is benign. Roberts et al. report a central superficial white opacity in collie puppies due to an accumulation of a hematoxylin-staining, amorphous layer under the epithelium.[51] However, the central location and the appearance of the opacities in this study differed from the usual presentation. Puppy band keratopathy may affect all breeds of dog but is most often documented in breeds that are screened for genetic disease as puppies, that is, collie, English springer spaniel, and Sheltie.

Clinical signs
Puppy band keratopathy manifests with a faint, usually incomplete, superficial (subepithelial) hazy band in suckling puppies (**Figures 10.8 and 10.9**). The opacity is most commonly found adjacent to the medial and lateral limbal region and is usually self-correcting.

Diagnosis
Diagnosis is by the appearance of the cornea and the age of the puppy.

Therapy
No therapy is necessary.

Sclerocornea

Sclerocornea is a congenital corneal opacity at the limbal region. It is nonprogressive and occurs infrequently. Scleral-like tissue extends into the peripheral cornea and involves only a segment of the limbal circumference (**Figure 10.10**). The condition may be associated with

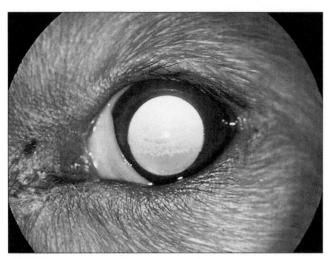

Figure 10.8 Puppy band keratopathy in a collie puppy visualized in retroillumination. Note that the lesions are faint and will spontaneously resolve.

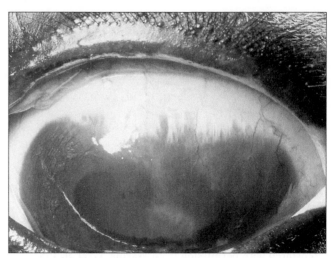

Figure 10.10 Scleralization of the dorsal cornea of a horse. The scleralization was most likely a congenital lesion. Acquired multifocal corneal scars with vascularization are also present.

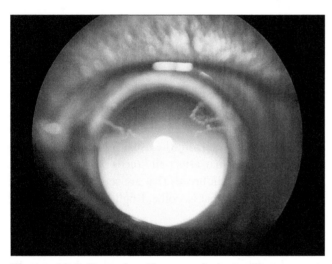

Figure 10.9 Puppy band keratopathy in a collie puppy that is typical of the extent of involvement. The faint superficial lesions are seen against the retroillumination of the tapetum and are typically adjacent to the limbus and do not form a complete band.

other congenital ocular lesions[52] and may be unilateral or bilateral. It has been observed in both the dog and horse.

CONGENITAL DEEP NONINFLAMMATORY DISEASE

Persistent pupillary membrane attachment (Peter's anomaly)

Introduction/etiology

This condition is associated with corneal opacification and embryonic aberrant persistent pupillary membrane (PPM) strands attached to the inner cornea. The condition is known to be inherited in some breeds such as the Basenji, Welsh corgi, and Chow Chow. In the Basenji, the condition is reported to be a dominant trait, but other studies indicate that in this breed the condition does not follow a simple dominant or recessive trait.[53–55] Peter's anomaly is observed less frequently in the cat. PPMs are commonly associated with eyelid agenesis or multiple ocular colobomas (MOC) in cats.

Clinical signs

Focal pigment deposits and/or a grayish-white opacity at Descemet's membrane are noted on examination. The lesions are usually axial, sparing the far peripheral cornea (**Figure 10.11**). Deep corneal lesions are reported to occur in 20% of Basenjis.[56] In young puppies, blindness may result from severe corneal edema, but the edema often improves with age, leaving a residual deep opacity at Descemet's level (**Figures 10.12 and 10.13**). PPMs are usually present but may break with age, making it more difficult to associate the deep corneal opacities to a specific etiology.

Diagnosis

The cause of the corneal opacity, whether pigmented, gray, or edematous, is obvious if associated with PPMs. Localization of the opacity to the Descemet's membrane, without an overlying stromal scar (indicating a perforating injury) or signs of prior intraocular inflammation in a young animal, is presumptive evidence of a PPM syndrome. Posterior polymorphous dystrophy may also produce white opacities at Descemet's membrane, but these are rare and relatively breed specific, and the

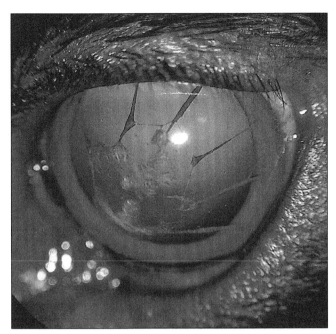

Figure 10.11 A dog with multifocal scars at Descemet's level with associated persistent pupillary membranes. The corneal lesions are both pigmented and white.

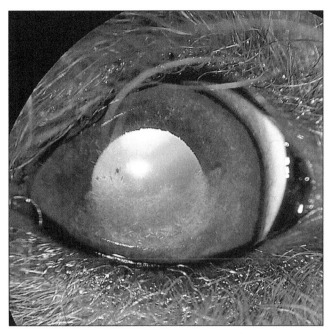

Figure 10.13 The appearance of the same dog in Figure 10.12 several months later after the edema has subsided. A deep white "scar" is residual at Desecemet's level.

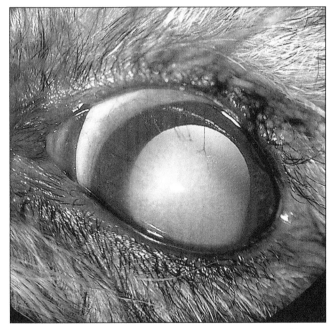

Figure 10.12 A more severe form of persistent pupillary membranes (PPMs) in a 10-week-old Welsh terrier puppy. The central cornea has deep, dense edema. PPM strands are visible at the periphery, which differentiates the edema from an infectious canine hepatitis reaction.

lesions are more diffuse. Historically, severe forms of infectious canine hepatitis with corneal edema were an important differential because both conditions presented in young animals.

The PPM syndrome with axial to paraxial "scars" is one of the most common causes of endothelial lesions in the dog. Diagnostic iridal strands are not present in many patients, and the diagnosis is presumptive based on lack of stromal scarring, breed involved, and age.

Therapy

No therapy is usually given or needed in most cases. A penetrating corneal graft can be performed in severe cases. Cutting the strands can improve the stromal edema, but given the spontaneous improvement in most cases, the benefit of surgery is questionable. Breeding affected dogs with corneal lesions is not recommended.

Posterior polymorphous dystrophy

Introduction/etiology

Posterior polymorphous dystrophy refers to a disease that has been observed in the American Cocker Spaniel and is characterized by multiple irregular-shaped opacities present at Descemet's membrane.[57] The condition is congenital and nonprogressive. It is thought to be inherited, with a suggested mode of a dominant or incomplete dominant trait. Histopathologic changes seen are focal endothelial necrosis and cell loss with fibrous metaplasia of the endothelial cells. Focal areas may be denuded of endothelial cells, with exposure of the Descemet's membrane.

Clinical signs

Bilateral, multiple, nonprogressive, grayish opacities are present in the deep cornea. The opacities are scattered over the entire posterior surface and vary from linear to vesicular in shape. There are no attachments of opacities to uveal tags or PPMs. No vision problems are noted.

Diagnosis

Diagnosis is made on the characteristic appearance and the location of opacities, the breed, and the lack of uveal attachments to the lesions.

Therapy

No therapy is needed. It is recommended to advise breeders that posterior polymorphous dystrophy is a suspected genetic disease.

Cornea globosa

Cornea globosa refers to a cornea that is large and protruding due to a large radius of curvature. The corneal diameter is not abnormal, and the globe itself is not enlarged, compared to buphthalmos. Cornea globosa is seen in horse with an inherited congenital ocular disorder referred to as MCOA syndrome (multiple congenital ocular abnormalities). This syndrome occurs at a high frequency in silver-colored horses, which is associated with mutations in the PMEL17 gene.[58,59] MCOA is seen in horses that are homozygous for the mutant allele and is reported in Rocky Mountain horses, Kentucky Mountain horses, Icelandic horses, American miniature horses, comtois horses, mixed breed ponies, and European Shetland and Deutsches classic ponies.[58–68] Quarter horses affected with hereditary equine regional dermal asthenia (HERDA) have a prominent cornea secondary to an increase in corneal curvature and corneal diameter.[69] In horses with globular corneas, the cornea is made more apparent with the presence of macropalpebral fissures (**Figure 10.14**).

ACQUIRED SUPERFICIAL NONINFLAMMATORY DISEASE

Calcific keratopathy/band keratopathy

Introduction/etiology

Calcific keratopathy refers to a deposition of calcium in the epithelium, the basal lamina, and the superficial stroma. Band keratopathy refers to a form of calcific keratopathy that follows the horizontal pattern of the palpebral fissure. Calcific keratopathy can be dystrophic in nature (associated with localized ocular inflammation) or metastatic (secondary to systemic hypercalcemia). Dystrophic changes can be associated with anterior surface disease, such as poor tear film quality or quantity, or intraocular disease, such as uveitis, glaucoma, or phthisis bulbi. Corneal calcification may also occur in old corneal scars. Older dogs may develop dystrophic calcium in the cornea that eventually sloughs, producing corneal ulcerations.[70,71] In the horse, rapid corneal calcification can occur after laser cyclophotocoagulation, but most cases are associated with chronic endogenous uveitis (**Figure 10.15**).[72,73] Metastatic changes have been reported with Cushing's disease in dogs[71,74] (**Figure 10.16**) and pituitary pars intermedia dysfunction (PPID) in horses.[73] Other causes of systemic hypercalcemia, such as neoplasia, hyperparathyroidism, pseudohyperparathyroidism, chronic renal disease, dietary intake, and hypervitaminosis D, are important considerations when investigating the cause of calcific keratopathy.

Although the dog and the horse are the most commonly affected species, calcific keratopathy is reported in several species. The mechanism of corneal calcification is unknown but increases in tissue pH associated with inflammation, and evaporation of tears are thought to be important.[75] Medications containing phosphates, such as topical steroid phosphates[76] and intracameral viscoelastic agents with phosphate buffers, have produced band keratopathy.[77]

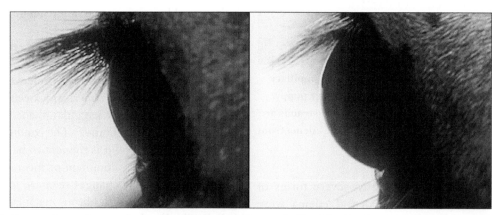

Figure 10.14 Comparison of corneal curvature in a normal horse (left) with a Rocky Mountain horse with cornea globosa (right). (Courtesy of Dr. D. Ramsey, Michigan State University.)

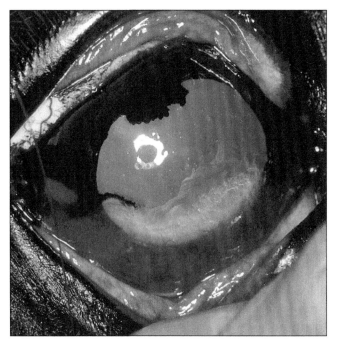

Figure 10.15 Band keratopathy in a horse after cyclophotocoagulation performed for glaucoma.

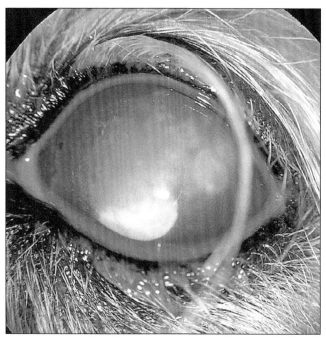

Figure 10.17 Band keratopathy in a dog with chronic uveitis. The patient was presented for acute pain from the ulcer that is stained with fluorescein. Note the foamy appearance; this is not as white or chalky as other examples of corneal calcification.

"moth-eaten" or a plaque-like white, granular lesion. The lesion feels gritty if scraped (**Figure 10.17**).

Depending on the cause of calcium precipitation, concurrent signs of uveitis, keratitis, or corneal scars may be present. As the calcium becomes dense and plaque-like, it may slough, producing an ulcer of variable depth with varying degrees of pain.

Diagnosis

A presumptive diagnosis of calcium deposition is usually made by the clinical appearance, but a definitive diagnosis can be obtained by biopsy (superficial keratectomy or corneal scraping).

Therapy

Complete excision with a superficial keratectomy, or removal of the epithelium and bathing the cornea with a 1%–3% ethylenediaminetetraacetic acid (EDTA) solution, are potential therapies. Diamond burr debridement is a safe and effective treatment for superficial disease.[78] Secondary deep corneal ulcerations, descemetocoeles, or perforations require surgical intervention. If the eyes are blind from intraocular disease, no therapy is usually warranted unless the condition is painful, or an ulcer is created by sloughing of the calcium. The advanced age and systemic disease may present a therapeutic dilemma when considering surgical therapy for a deep, slow-healing ulcer.

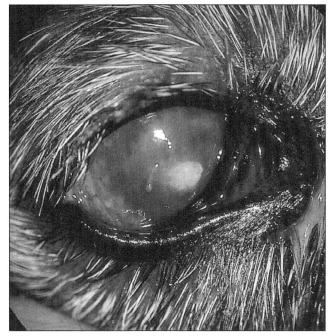

Figure 10.16 Axial dystrophic calcification in a dog with Cushing's disease. The lesions developed rapidly within several days.

Clinical signs

A grayish-white, very superficial opacity is present axial or periaxially and in a horizontal band extending across the cornea with band keratopathy. The degree of calcification is variable and does not extend to the limbus. Depending on the density of the calcium, it may appear as gray and

Superficial punctate keratopathy

Introduction/etiology

Superficial punctate keratopathy is a condition of unknown etiology usually seen in the Shetland sheepdog. It is characterized initially by brown, faint, superficial opacities that transform into multifocal grayish-white, superficial round or irregular rings 1–3 mm in diameter. It is observed in dogs as young as 4 months and may be a form of a corneal dystrophy.

Histologically, the lesions are limited to the epithelium and are composed of dyskeratotic cells and degenerate epithelial cells.[79,80] In the initial stages, there is no evidence of inflammation, but with chronicity, vascularization occurs. After months to years, the initial white opacities appear as crystalline or lipid deposits.

Clinical signs

Initially, bilateral brownish, circular maculae develop in the epithelium that progress to white maculae (**Figure 10.18**). No inflammatory signs, vascularization, or pain is present. Chronic cases may develop blepharospasm from corneal erosions. Symptomatic dogs have reduced Schirmer tear test (STT) values (10–12 mm), decreased tear film break-up time (BUT) of <10 seconds, and rose bengal stain retention. Vascularization is eventually stimulated when corneal erosions are present.

Diagnosis

Diagnosis is based on the clinical signs and the breed of dog. Superficial keratectomy can be used for biopsy purposes.

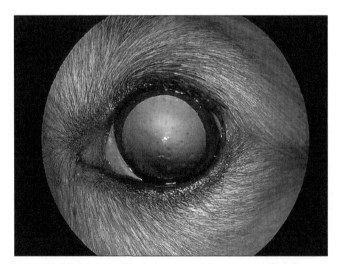

Figure 10.18 Macular keratopathy in a young Sheltie visualized in retroillumination. The lesions are multifocal, superficial, and brownish at this stage. They later evolved into white lesions.

Therapy

Artificial tears, hyperosmotic solutions, and soft contact lenses are recommended to protect the cornea. When vascularization is present but erosions are healed, topical corticosteroids, topical nonsteroidal anti-inflammatory drugs (NSAIDs), or topical cyclosporine are used to relieve mild discomfort.

Lipid keratopathy

Introduction/etiology

Lipid deposition at any or all depths of the cornea may be seen in a wide variety of dog breeds. The configuration, type of lipid, speed of progression, and age of onset varies with the breed and the disease. The condition is termed a lipid dystrophy if it is bilateral and presumed inherited, and a lipid degeneration if it is associated with systemic lipid abnormalities or previous corneal disease. Most lipid keratopathies seem to be local metabolic disturbances as hyperlipidemia and endocrinopathies are usually not present.[81,82] Breeds such as the Airedale, collie, Shetland sheepdog, Siberian husky, beagle, dachshund, Afghan hound, Cavalier King Charles spaniel, and German shepherd dogs (GSD) seem susceptible, but definite inheritance patterns are known in relatively few breeds.[83–86] Lipid dystrophy is reported to be a recessive trait in the Siberian husky.[87] In general, females are affected more commonly than males.[88]

In the author's experience, many dogs with lipid keratopathy have a history of receiving a coat conditioner, high-energy dog food, dry food with added oils and fat, or a fatty diet. The condition may manifest with a combination of dietary overload and a genetic intolerance to fat. Lipid keratopathy in the cat, in most instances, is secondary to previous corneal vascularization and is relatively infrequent.[89]

Systemic abnormalities that result in high blood lipids tend to produce a lipid keratopathy that is often more rapid in development and progressive. A familial lipid storage disease with corneal lipid accumulation in a peripheral circular ring adjacent to the limbus is reported in young fox terriers.[90] Lipids can accumulate in the cornea at the leading edge of raised corneal lesions, such as neoplasms and episcleritis, and in corneal lesions with previous vascularization. When corneal lipid accumulations are secondary to systemic or local ocular disease, the term lipid degeneration or keratopathy is preferred to dystrophy. Topical use of corticosteroids may also predispose many patients to corneal lipid deposition; their use in patients with pre-existing lipid keratopathy is avoided, if possible. If corticosteroids are required to treat an underlying condition such as inflammation, they are usually stopped, and topical nonsteroidals or immunomodulators, such as cyclosporine, are initiated if lipid deposition develops.

Clinical signs

Crystalline or white amorphous accumulations are present in one or both eyes. The texture of the lesion depends on the type of lipid deposited and the stage of the lesion. Cholesterol crystals are typically needle-like (**Figure 10.19**). Most cases are very superficial in nature, but lipids may accumulate at any level or throughout the full stromal thickness. The pattern varies with breed, cause, and chronicity of the condition (**Figure 10.20**). The condition is usually slowly progressive and rarely results in blindness. Often it will regress with long-term restriction of dietary fat.

If the condition is rapidly progressive or peripheral in location, a lipid profile is recommended and the adrenal, thyroid, pancreas, and liver metabolism evaluated to investigate for systemic lipid abnormalities (**Figures 10.21 and 10.22**). Vascularization usually develops with chronicity, but the lesion is not proportional to the vascularity (**Figures 10.21 and 10.22**).

Axial, superficial, oval, crystalline cholesterol deposits beginning in one cornea and eventually becoming a bilateral disease are a very common lesion in a wide variety of breeds on diets of >14% fat or given oral coat conditioners.

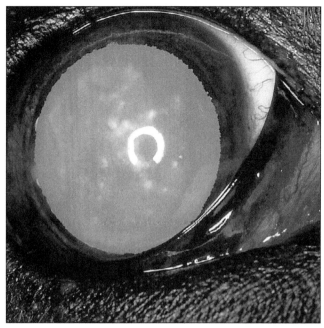

Figure 10.20 Multifocal diffuse superficial lipid accumulation in an English springer spaniel. The condition was bilateral. The lesions were rapidly progressive and were modified by fat restriction.

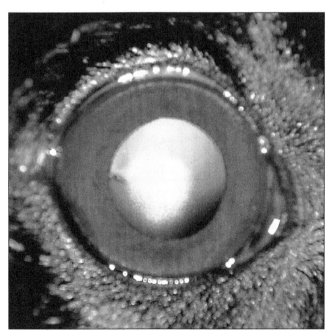

Figure 10.19 Axial superficial cholesterol crystals in a dog. These are usually bilateral and are a common form of dystrophy in several breeds. They can be modified by limiting the dietary fat.

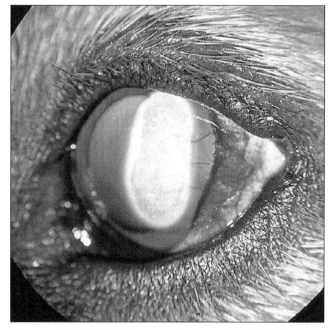

Figure 10.21 Lipid degeneration in a collie. The bitch had elevated cholesterol levels and had been on a high-energy diet for parturition and nursing. The lesion was surgically removed and, with dietary restriction, did not recur for the life of the dog.

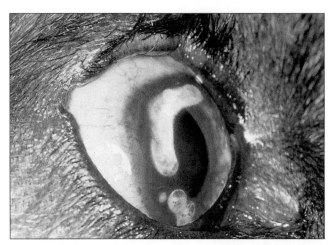

Figure 10.22 Arcus lipid degeneration in an Afghan hound with chronic hypothyroidism. This pattern of target-like rings of cholesterol accumulation has been noted in other Afghan hounds without known metabolic disorders.

Diagnosis

The crystalline appearance suggests the diagnosis, but keratectomy with histopathologic examination is necessary for confirmation. Calcium deposits may look very similar to lipids, and both may be present in lesions such as inflammatory scars.

Therapy

Therapy is often not needed due to the minimal opacity and slow, benign course of most cases. Restriction of dietary fat is recommended, and any systemic abnormality in lipid metabolism is controlled, for example, hypothyroidism. Superficial keratectomy can be performed in larger or progressive, superficial opacities. Following a superficial keratectomy, even if the underlying cause is not addressed, the cornea may remain clear postoperatively for extended periods.

Corneal lesions with metabolic storage disease

Introduction/etiology

Gangliosidosis G_{M1} and G_{M2}[91] and mucopolysaccaridosis types I and VI are reported to cause a cloudy cornea to develop in young cats.[92–97] Mucopolysaccharidosis types I and VII are also reported to be associated with a cloudy cornea in the dog.[96,97] The ocular lesions of these metabolic storage diseases may be overlooked because of the severity of the systemic neurologic signs. The corneal lesions are due to vacuolation of keratocytes and endothelium with GAGs. The lesions are throughout the full thickness of the corneal stroma.

Clinical signs

Bilateral, diffuse, hazy corneas are present that may be accompanied by blepharospasm, or the animal may hold the eyes partially closed. It is difficult to localize the haze because it is full thickness. Accompanying signs are related to the skeletal and neurologic systems.

Diagnosis

Neurologic and ophthalmic signs are suggestive of the diagnosis, as are histopathologic changes. Screening for mucopolysaccaridosis can be performed on urine samples dried on filter paper and stained with toluidine blue. Definitive diagnosis of the type of deficiency is made by measuring the lysosomal enzyme activities of leukocytes and fibroblasts.

ACQUIRED DEEP NONINFLAMMATORY DISEASE

Corneal endothelial dystrophy/ degeneration

Introduction/etiology

Endothelial dystrophy manifests as a slowly progressive corneal edema in one eye that eventually becomes bilateral. The Boston Terrier is predisposed, and the disease manifests mainly in older females. A variety of other breeds (poodle, Chow Chow, basset hound, Chihuahua, dalmatian) may develop the disease, but it is not restricted to females. In most cases, it appears to be a spontaneous senile degeneration of the endothelium. Pathologically, the endothelial cells are reduced in number, increased in size, bizarre in shape, and may have increased fibrillar deposition on Descemet's membrane.[98,99]

A hereditary corneal dystrophy in the Manx cat manifests with severe corneal edema resulting in epithelial bullae, but the endothelium is morphologically normal.[100] Mild, bilateral, axial, focal corneal edema develops at 4–5 months and slowly progresses. Late in the course, recurrent ulcerations develop secondary to ruptured bullae. A similar condition is reported in a domestic short-haired cat.[101] While the pathogenesis is not known, the endothelium appears to have at least a functional deficiency in the pump mechanism.

In cattle wormed with phenothiazine and allowed in the sunlight, a photosensitivity may develop that results in bilateral diffuse corneal edema. The edema is typically in the lower two-thirds of the cornea.[102] Animals on a low plane of nutrition may be more susceptible. Recovery may occur in 1 week if the animal is restricted indoors, or recovery may be prolonged to 2–3 months if kept on pasture. Ulcerations may occur secondary to the edema.

Diffuse corneal edema is reported in Doberman pinschers treated with long-term systemic tocainide for cardiomyopathy. The condition is reversible if recognized in the early stages (**Figure 10.23**) but is permanent at later stages.[103]

Clinical signs (dog)

A focal area of stromal edema is observed in one eye, often beginning temporally (**Figure 10.24**). Initially there is no inflammation in the cornea or in the eye, but most eyes develop significant conjunctival vascular injection. Edema slowly progresses over months to involve the entire cornea and eventually the second eye (**Figure 10.25**). Bullous keratopathy often develops as the severity of the corneal edema progresses. Epithelial bullae often develop from the increased water in the stroma collecting under and in the epithelium (**Figure 10.26**). The bullae frequently rupture, producing an acute superficial ulceration. The ulcer is often slow to heal due to the persistence of the corneal edema. Chronic edema combined with multiple ulcerative episodes results in vascularization and pigmentation of the cornea (**Figure 10.27**). The result is often blindness.

Cataracts frequently develop concurrently, but how they are related to the corneal edema is unknown.

Diagnosis

Diagnosis is by ruling out other causes of endothelial damage such as trauma, uveitis, luxated lens, PPMs, drug

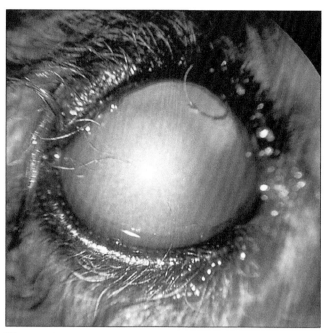

Figure 10.24 Deep stromal corneal edema from endothelial degeneration in a miniature poodle. The condition was initially unilateral but developed bilaterally and progressed rapidly within 12 months. Note the lack of inflammatory signs at this stage.

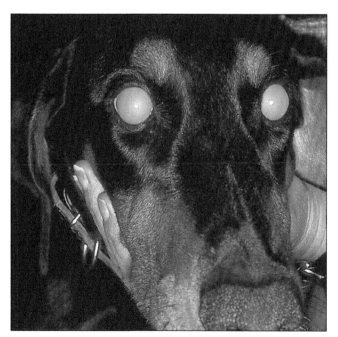

Figure 10.23 Doberman pinscher that was treated for a cardiomyopathy and developed diffuse bilateral deep corneal edema from tocainide toxicity.

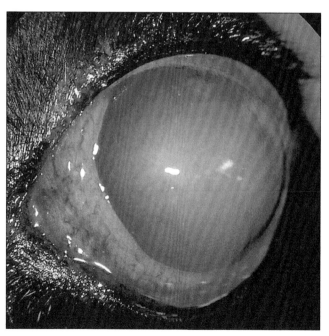

Figure 10.25 An 11-year-old Boston terrier with advanced, diffuse endothelial degeneration and accompanying deep corneal edema. A few bullae are present, and pigment is starting to invade the cornea dorsally.

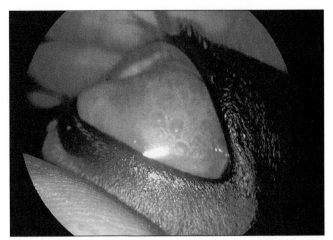

Figure 10.26 Boston terrier with advanced endothelial degeneration resulting in corneal edema with multiple bullae. The bullae rupture, producing acute, painful, ulcerative episodes that may result in the owner requesting enucleation or euthanasia.

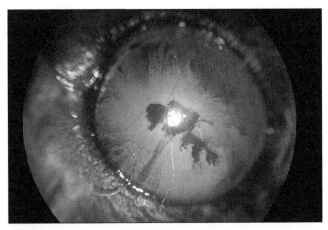

Figure 10.27 Miniature poodle with advanced stages of endothelial degeneration that has left the chronically edematous cornea vascularized and pigmented.

toxicity, or glaucoma. Biomicroscopy of the endothelium may reveal multiple holes in the endothelial sheet.

Therapy

Medical therapy is usually palliative, consisting of hypertonic salt solution (which draws water out of the cornea) and soft contact lenses. Hypertonic ointments or solutions have minimal effect on the corneal edema, but they reduce bullae formation and secondary ulceration. Soft lenses help reduce bullae rupture and ulcer formation, making the eyes more comfortable and the condition more acceptable to the owner.

Thermokeratoplasty (creating multiple burns in the cornea) with a low-temperature battery cautery is reported to produce corneal scarring that prevents recurrent

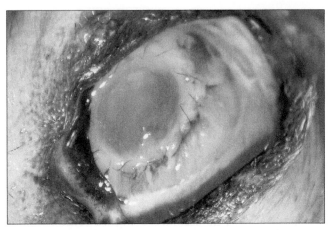

Figure 10.28 Full-thickness penetrating keratoplasty that was performed on the patient in Figure 10.24 later in development. The graft was rejected approximately 4 weeks later.

ulcerations and pain. The corneal fibrosis reduces the ability of the cornea to swell, and the corneal opacification may decrease.[104,105]

A Gundersen inlay conjunctival flap, following a peripheral superficial keratectomy, is suggested as a surgical alternative to chronic medical therapy in humans, dogs, and horses.[106–108] Corneal grafting may be attempted, but if performed late in the course, corneal vascularization can increase the chances of graft rejection (**Figure 10.28**). The concurrent development of cataracts often complicates the prognosis for vision.

Corneal collagen cross-linking is a less invasive surgical alternative for the treatment of symptomatic bullous keratopathy in dogs.[109,110] Collagen cross-linking is believed to result in compaction of the corneal stroma, decreasing the space for fluid accumulation. Although the procedure holds promise in the treatment of bullous keratopathy, its use in veterinary ophthalmology is currently limited.

Striate keratopathy

Striate keratopathy is usually due to breaks in Descemet's membrane and is usually the result of glaucoma. The condition manifests as curvilinear, often branching, double white lines that can be localized to Descemet's membrane with the slit lamp (**Figure 10.29**). Striae are described in the normal horse eye due to thinning of Descemet's membrane. It is important to rule out glaucoma before dismissing these lines as an innocent lesion.[111] In the horse, the signs of glaucoma may be very subtle, and the lack of readily available instruments to measure the intraocular pressure (IOP) makes glaucoma an underdiagnosed disease in the field. Acute corneal edema that follows the course of previous striae can be observed in the horse (**Figure 10.30**) and may be the first obvious

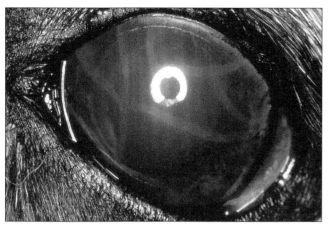

Figure 10.29 Striate keratopathy or multiple breaks in Descemet's membrane in an elkhound with glaucoma.

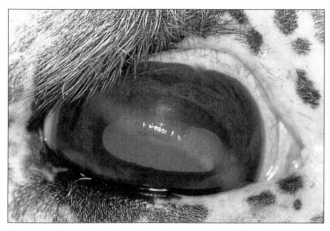

Figure 10.30 Acute striate keratopathy with overlying corneal edema in a horse. Multiple bullae are present in the edematous streak. Glaucoma was the cause of the striae, and edema was the first sign noted.

sign of glaucoma to the owner. Normal IOP at the time of examination does not rule out past elevation as being the cause for striate keratopathy. No therapy is given for the corneal lesions.

SUPERFICIAL NONULCERATIVE INFLAMMATORY DISEASE

Superficial keratitis

Introduction/etiology

Superficial keratitis may be unilateral or bilateral, and it is caused by a variety of agents. The condition may be focal or multifocal, or progressive and diffuse. There are many causes of superficial keratitis.

Mechanical

Hairs and foreign bodies are common causes of focal unilateral keratitis. Consideration is given to such factors in cases of unilateral keratitis, as the resulting keratitis is usually curable, and improvement will not occur until the cause is corrected. In grazing animals and working dogs, plant foreign bodies are a significant cause of keratitis in late summer and fall. If a chronic, unilateral, nonhealing keratitis is present, prompt reevaluation and a careful search for an embedded foreign body in the cornea, the conjunctiva, or behind the third eyelid (see Chapter 8, **Figure 8.58**) is warranted.

Infectious

Bacterial

Bacteria usually require breaks in the epithelium to become established, or they are carried into the stroma by a puncture wound. While bacterial keratitis is usually ulcerative, corneal abscessation from a puncture wound often no longer stains with fluorescein by the time of presentation. Abscessation is uncommon in the dog and the cat; when present, it is often in hunting dogs with punctures from plants and in cats with claw injuries from fighting.

Abscessation is most common in the horse and may be secondary to bacterial and/or fungal infections. Stromal abscesses occur more frequently in the temperate months of the year and more frequent in the spring and winter months in subtropical regions, the spring and fall months in the southeastern United States, and the spring and summer in more temperate regions.[112–115] An increase in frequency is reported in windier conditions.[116] Clinically, stromal abscesses may be superficial or very deep and may vary in size from a small pinpoint opacity to a more diffuse lesion. They present as a focal white, yellow, or pink, or diffuse yellow/white opacity. The color of the abscess is dependent upon the infectious organism and the type of inflammatory cells present.[112] Corneal vascularization is eventually very intense and is a necessary part of the healing process (**Figure 10.31**). Deep abscessation is often accompanied by a secondary anterior uveitis. Determining the organism in deep abscess is difficult since surface cultures are not representative, and the aqueous humor is usually sterile.[117]

Many corneal abscesses in the horse are due to fungal organisms. However, stromal abscess in horses can be secondary to Gram-positive or Gram-negative bacteria or associated with a mixed infection of bacteria and fungi.[112,118] Due to the difficulty in obtaining a representative sample for culture, it is recommended to treat all abscesses with both antifungal and antibacterial agents. In horses, following surgical removal of the abscess, fungal organisms can be identified by histopathology in only 47%–56% of the samples.[118–120] Henriksen et al. report fungi in 47.1% of the corneal samples submitted for histopathology, with

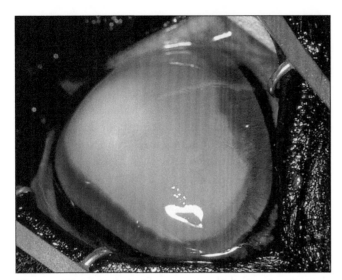

Figure 10.31 Relatively acute corneal abscess in a horse. Note the early but intense corneal neovascularization. The dense creamy opacity represents neutrophils, whereas the lighter corneal opacity is due to edema.

only 5.9% being positive by fungal culture.[112,120] Studies shows that bacteria are identified in only 12%–17.6% of histopathology samples.[112,118]

Moore et al. described a series of six cases of post-traumatic keratouveitis that were postulated to be sterile abscesses that required vascularization to heal.[121] The lack of positive cultures from the aqueous humor or tissue in three of the six horses indicate a sterile immune process due to corneal necrosis. A similar disease process is described by Brooks et al. with the lesions appearing pink in color.[122] Pink stromal abscess may represent a form of this disease process.[115,120] It is speculated that the lesion is inflamed cornea that started as a primary infection that is transformed to an immune-mediated process. Topical immunosuppressive medications are used with caution in these cases as they can cause more harm than good if the primary infection is still present. The author treats such abscesses as septic, unless a biopsy is obtained to confirm the diagnosis, and it is known that an infectious agent is not present.

A syndrome of granuloma formation in the cornea associated with an acid-fast bacterium has been described in the cat and is thought to be associated with feline leprosy.[123] Both diagnosis and therapy involved a superficial keratectomy. In Australia, 15 cats with granulomatous skin, subcuticular, ocular, and periocular lesions had a fastidious *Mycobacterium* that was difficult to culture, but numerous organisms were present on histopathology. Polymerase chain reaction (PCR) gene sequencing identified the organism as a member of the *Mycobacterium simiae*-related group, taxonomically related to the mycobacterium

that causes leproid granulomas in dogs.[124] Successful therapy included surgical debulking plus medical therapy. The nine-banded armadillo is used as an animal model for human leprosy as it is susceptible to *Mycobacterium leprae* without immune suppression. As in humans, armadillos may develop lepromatous corneal granuloma and anterior uveal lesions.[125]

In southern Florida, a disease characterized by multifocal small superficial macula (Florida spots) has been found in the dog and the cat; investigators have reported acid-fast bacteria present in the lesions on biopsy (**Figure 10.32**). Other investigators have found no organisms in the lesions. The lesions are not characterized by inflammation clinically or histopathologically, and they were previously assumed to be due to *Rhinosporidium* spp.[126,127] Florida spots are more common in cats than dogs. Histologically, they consist of abnormal collagen fibrils. The lesions do not respond to either steroids or antibiotics and do not progress in number of spots once the initial episode is over;[128] therefore, therapy is not recommended. Interestingly, humans in southern Florida also get nontuberculous mycobacterial keratitis that appears similar and is not responsive to antibiotics.[129]

Fungal

Fungal keratitis is most common in the horse. However, an increasing number of cases are reported in dogs and alpacas and is also reported in cats (**Figure 10.33**), rabbits, and cows.[130–136] *Aspergilla* spp. and *Fusarium* spp. are the most common fungal organisms identified in horses and alpacas,[133,137,138] where multiple different fungal species are identified in dogs with fungal keratitis. Dematiaceous

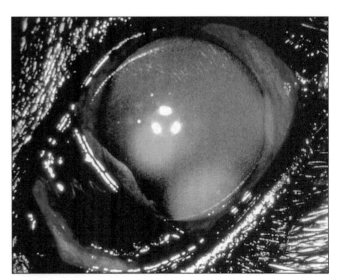

Figure 10.32 Two "Florida spots" in a dog. The opacities are white, stromal, with hazy borders, and there is no evidence of an inflammatory response.

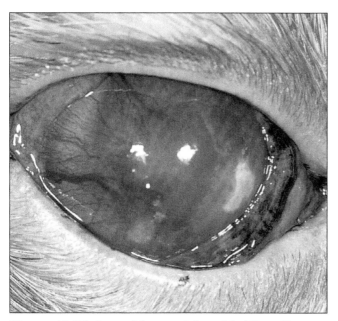

Figure 10.33 A cat with mycotic keratitis. The yellow-white opacities were mycotic plaques. The cat had been treated for months with a topical corticosteroid. Debridement and antifungal therapy instituted a rapid response.

fungi such as *Curvularia* spp. and *Cladosporium* spp. are uncommon infections but are unique in that they may produce a black pigmentation of the cornea.[139–141]

Fungal keratitis is usually preceded by corneal abrasion and treatment with an antibiotic or antibiotic–corticosteroid. In dogs and cats, fungal keratitis is more common in animals with high endogenous corticosteroids or that are immunocomprised.[142,143] The history is usually one of improving and then stabilizing or relapsing. Therefore, it is important to consider mycotic keratitis in animals with any corneal lesion that initially improves and then regresses, is characterized by plaques, and/or is antibiotic resistant. Mycotic keratitis is so common in the horse that the author avoids using glucocorticoids if possible for equine corneal disease and often treats simple abrasions and ulcers prophylactically with topical antifungal drugs as well as antibacterial drugs.

> Fungal keratitis typically responds initially to antibiotics and then regresses. Fungal keratitis should be suspected in any horse with keratitis and in any species that has been treated with immunosuppressive medication or that is systemically immunosuppressed.

In the mildest form, the patient is presented with epiphora and mild blepharospasm. On examination of the eye, the cornea has a faint to moderate superficial edema with characteristic subepithelial, multifocal white macula with hazy edges. The epithelium is loose, roughened, and easily removed (**Figure 10.34**). The previous application of topical corticosteroids may predispose to more chronic, deeper stromal lesions with more pronounced edema. Deeper lesions may develop surrounding furrows and slough, leaving deep to perforating lesions (**Figures 10.35 and 10.36**). The most severe form, with the worst prognosis, is the progressive stromal ulcer that often results in perforation (**Figure 10.37**).[144]

Some patients have a gritty plaque formation that is formed from a colony of organisms, often *Fusarium* spp. or *Aspergillus* spp. (**Figure 10.36**).[137] The predominant isolate may vary with the region and the environment. Fungi are frequently the cause of deep corneal abscessation at Descemet's membrane and seem to have an affinity for this location. The inaccessibility of the membrane makes clinical confirmation difficult (**Figure 10.38**). It is not uncommon through the course of mycotic keratitis to have complications with bacterial infection. Bacterial isolates may be identified in up to 30% of confirmed cases of equine fungal keratitis.[145] Two bacterial isolates are often (60%) present with 75% being Gram-positive bacteria. The course of the disease, even when specifically treated, is chronic, often lasting 6–8 weeks before the eye is "quiet" and comfortable.

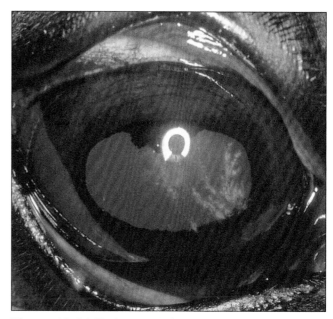

Figure 10.34 Early mycotic keratitis in a horse. The lesions are subepithelial, and no inflammatory response has been mounted. *Fusarium* spp. was subsequently cultured.

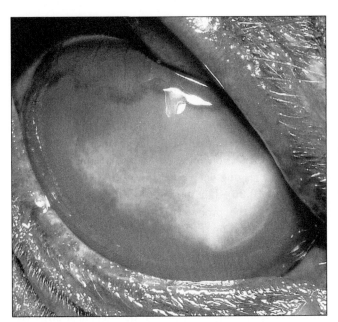

Figure 10.35 Mycotic keratitis in a horse that is more advanced than in the horse in Figure 10.34 but is still quite superficial. The lesion is subepithelial and requires vascularization in addition to antifungal therapy before it is healed.

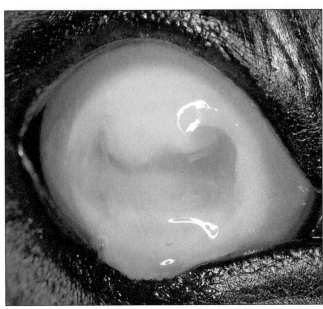

Figure 10.37 Rapidly melting corneal ulcer in a horse. Cultures and cytology were negative for bacteria, but an *Aspergillus* sp. was cultured. Note the massive neutrophilic response and malacic cornea ventrally.

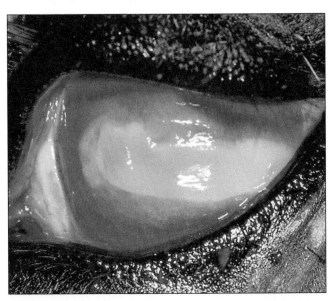

Figure 10.36 Mycotic plaque in a horse cornea due to *Fusarium* spp. Debridement of the plaque to reduce the fungal mass was performed repeatedly, in addition to topical antifungal therapy.

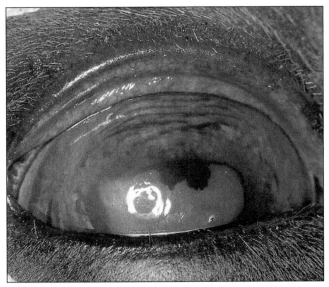

Figure 10.38 Focal opacity at Descemet's membrane adjacent to the flash artifact in a horse. Full-thickness keratoplasty "button" had fungal hyphae on histopathology.

Diagnosis of bacterial and fungal keratitis

Diagnosis is by corneal scraping for cytology and cultures, with emphasis placed on the cytology for directing the initial therapy (**Figure 10.39**). Cytology is pivotal in diagnosing fungal keratitis, except for deep stromal lesions, since culture requires >2 weeks for a definitive result. Massa

et al. report a positive result with infectious keratitis: 54% from cytology, 60% from culture, and 73% from both cytology and culture.[146] In the horse with corneal abscess, only 5.9%–12.5% of the cases are positive by routine culture.[112,115] However, specimens obtained during surgical intervention are positive by histopathology in 47%–56% of the samples.[112,120] A study by Zeiss et al. shows that nested PCR can be used to confirm cytology results, and nested

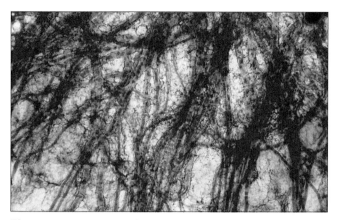

Figure 10.39 Corneal cytology from a horse with mycotic keratitis. The hyphae are more dense in this preparation than usual, and they may represent cytology from a fungal plaque.

PCR identifies more fungal organisms than culture in samples obtained from horses with fungal keratitis.[147] Although very limited in its use, due to expense of the equipment, confocal microscopy consistently detects fungal organisms *in vivo* in the cornea of horses with fungal keratitis.[131]

Therapy of bacterial and fungal keratitis

Therapy for bacterial keratitis is often fortified topical antibiotics every 4 hours. Removal of the epithelium may be performed to enhance antibiotic penetration. Deep abscessation often requires both systemic and topical antibiotics. In the horse, if treating without the benefit of cultures, more than one antibiotic is usually used. An antibiotic such as a cephalosporin that is effective against *Streptococcus* spp. is indicated. Compounding of topical antibiotics is often necessary as few commercial topical preparations are available for resistant organisms. The responsible agent is often not isolated, so antifungal therapy is indicated. Antifungal sensitivity testing to guide therapy is ideal, but the relative unavailability, cost, and time do not make it very practical.

A wide variety of drugs and methods have been used to treat fungal keratitis, which reflects the frustration involved. Natamycin is the only ophthalmic antifungal agent on the U.S. market, but it is not widely available, and it is very expensive. This has resulted in the use of a wide variety of nonophthalmic agents that have antifungal properties. Such agents include:

- Topical tincture of iodine or povidone–iodine swabbing of the cornea. If applied, iodine should not be the sole treatment but used as an adjunctive therapy with other medications.
- Polyene antifungals act by binding to ergosterol in the fungal cell wall, thus altering membrane permeability and causing disruption of the cell.

  - Natamycin (pimaricin) is a polyene antifungal manufactured as a 5% suspension. The drug is effective against filamentous fungi. Therapy is frequent, at least hourly initially, and tapering to every 2–4 hours. Corneal absorption is poor if the epithelium is intact.[148] In addition, only about 2% of natamycin is bioavailable in corneal tissue.[149]
  - Amphotericin B as a topical 0.5%–1% drug has been used and is effective, but unfortunately, it is the most toxic to the cornea of the various agents. Amphotericin B has been recommended subconjunctivally[150] and has been evaluated subconjunctivally as an adjunctive therapy in refractory equine keratomycosis at a dose of 0.2–0.3 mL of a 50 mg/mL solution every 48 hours for an average of three doses.[151] Sixty-one percent of the cases had a positive response to therapy. Amphotericin B is most efficacious against yeasts and *Fusarium* spp.
  - Nystatin is rarely used topically due to toxicity and poor ocular penetration.
- Imidazole antifungals are fungistatic at low concentrations (by inhibiting ergosterol synthesis) and fungicidal at high concentrations (having a direct damaging effect on the cell wall). High concentrations are difficult to obtain or sustain in ocular tissue, so these drugs are essentially clinically fungistatic.[152]

  - Thiabendazole deworming pastes have been used topically to treat fungal keratitis,[153] but with more appropriate products available, their use is no longer recommended. Clotrimazole is available as a dermatologic and vaginal cream that is tolerated by the eye. It is effective against *Aspergillus* spp.
  - Miconazole1% IV solution is used as a topical drop. Vaginal creams are tolerated reasonably well by the eye. However, miconazole does not penetrate the intact corneal epithelium. Miconazole has a broad spectrum of activity against yeasts and filamentous fungi and is a commonly used agent.
  - Ketaconazole is successful as either oral or topical therapy. Topical concentrations of 1%–5% are tolerated.[152]
  - Fluconazole, as topical and oral preparations, may be used as a treatment for fungal keratitis. Oral fluconazole has been used for deep fungal keratitis by giving a loading dose of 2 mg/kg every 12 hours for 1–4 days, followed by a maintenance dose of 1 mg/kg every 12 hours for 2 weeks or more. Based on pharmacokinetic studies, *Latimer* et al. recommend 14 mg/kg every 24 hours as a loading dose and 5 mg/kg every 24 hours as a maintenance dose.[154] Since fluconazole fluctuates in price and at times can be is

very expensive, this regimen can make therapy very expensive. Fluconazole is the least effective of the various imidazoles for *Aspergillus* spp. and *Fusarium* spp. isolates.[155] Fluconazole does have the ability to achieve high tissue levels. Therefore, it has been argued that the *in vitro* sensitivity testing does not reflect the *in vivo* effect.

- Itraconazole 1%/ dimethyl sulfoxide (DMSO) ointment can be formulated, and it achieves good therapeutic corneal concentrations. One study demonstrated the formulation to be effective in 8 of 10 eyes treated. The author has used this preparation extensively and has had only modest success, particularly with *Fusarium* spp.[156,157]
- Voriconazole is the newest of the imidazoles and is commercially available as an oral medication and IV solution. The IV formulation can be used as a 1% topical medication. Based on susceptibility patterns, it is more effective against the usual fungal isolates than natamycin, itraconazole, fluconazole, and ketoconazole. Miconazole is equally as effective *in vitro*.[158,159] Voriconazole has the significant benefit of penetrating the intact cornea and blood aqueous barrier in horses and achieves therapeutic concentrations when administered at a 1% solution every 4 hours and systemically at 4 mg/kg.[160] Intracorneal injection of voriconazole 1% (2 mg) or 5% (22.5 mg) has been used successfully to treat stromal abscesses in horses.[161,162] When injecting intracorneal, the voriconazole is divided into equal volumes and injected around the abscess at 3, 6, 9, and 12 o'clock or at three sites anterior to the abscess. When injecting around the abscess, a 30-gauge needle is angled 30–45° off perpendicular. When injecting anterior to the abscess, the needle is bent at a 30–45° angle near the hub and is inserted nearly parallel to the corneal surface and advanced horizontally across the anterior surface of the abscess. The needle is advanced just beyond the opposite extent of the abscess and is withdrawn slowly as the voriconazole is injected at the site. In the author's experience, repeated intracorneal injections (every 2–3 days) for three treatments and then once a week is beneficial.[163] With practice, the intracorneal injections can be performed with topical anesthetic (proparacaine ophthalmic solution) and standing sedation with intravenous detomidine 0.015 mg/kg and butorphanol 0.01 mg/kg. Prior to injection, the eye is aseptically prepared with 0.5% dilute betadine solution. For best results, adjunctive therapy with topical voriconazole 1%

with or without subconjunctival voriconazole 1% (400–500 µL) is administered.
- Silver sulfadiazine cream has broad antibacterial and antifungal properties. It is available as a 1% cream and is tolerated on the eye.[164] Betbeze et al. report silver sulfadiazine to be fungistatic and fungicidal against all equine fungal isolates tested.[165] In comparison, natamycin was not effective against the same *Fusarium* isolates. Silver sulfadiazine is effective against both yeast and filamentous fungi.

> Antibiotics are also administered in addition to the antifungal agent, as mixed bacterial–fungal infections or secondary bacterial infections are not uncommon. Ocular discomfort is controlled with atropine and NSAIDs. Systemic NSAIDs such as flunixin are used for pain relief and secondary uveitis.

The course of corneal bacterial abscesses and fungal keratitis is typically chronic, and the lesions usually require vascularization to occur before improvement is noted. The vessels may be slow to reach the lesion. Therefore, peripheral corneal lesions usually heal faster. Welch et al. demonstrated *in vitro* antiangiogenic properties of certain isolates from equine fungal keratitis cases.[166] In addition, corneal samples from horses with stromal abscess have abnormally low levels of VEGF-A expression.[120] The production of antiangiogenic properties by fungal organisms and the decreased VEGF-A expression may be responsible for the slow vascularization in cases of fungal keratitis. It is not unusual for the condition to worsen after the initiation of therapy. This has been attributed to the release of exotoxins from the killed fungi. Therapy is usually frequent, and the patient can become uncooperative, necessitating the use of a subpalpebral lavage system. Because of these demands, hospitalization is often necessary. This results in significant expense when treating fungal keratitis.

The prognosis varies with the depth of the lesion. Superficial infections, while expensive to treat, usually carry a good prognosis for vision and function. Andrew et al. report a 95% success in maintaining the eye and a 92% success for visual function with fungal keratitis.[138] Other reports have not been as successful, with 64% retention of a visual eye and 25% enucleation rate with fungal keratitis.[167]

Surgical augmentation of medical therapy with a keratectomy combined with conjunctival grafting enables better sampling for microbiological testing, removal of part of the infectious burden and necrotic tissue, and brings a blood supply to the lesion more rapidly. Smaller deep lesions can be removed entirely by a penetrating keratectomy, posterior lamellar keratoplasty, or deep lamellar endothelial keratoplasties.[168–170] Posterior lamellar keratoplasty (PLK) is performed by dissecting a rectangular, superficial lamellar corneal flap on three sides or by making a semicircular flap, leaving it hinged on the remaining side, and removing the deep abscess by a corneal trephine and placing a preformed corneal graft in the lamellar bed. After placing a donor button in the defect, the superficial lamellar flap is sutured over the deeper graft (**Figure 10.40a,b**).[168,170] A deep lamellar endothelial keratoplasty (DLEK) is performed by making a corneal incision adjacent to the limbus and a stromal pocket is formed over the abscess. The superficial corneal flap is retracted, and the abscess is excised with a corneal trephine. A preformed corneal button is sutured in the defect, and the superficial corneal flap is sutured in place (**Figure 10.41a,b**).[169,170] Alternately, a penetrating keratoplasty can be used to remove the abscess and the defect filled with a porcine submucosal bioscaffold implant and a conjunctival flap (**Figure 10.42**).[171] Despite obtaining deeper tissue surgically, in many cases, an infectious agent is not isolated or observed on histopathology.[112,118–120] Surgical intervention generally has a faster resolution of the disease process than medical therapy alone. In a recent study evaluating outcomes in cases of equine fungal keratitis associated with *Aspergillus* spp. or *Fusarium* spp., 63.6% of the cases required globe sparing surgeries, and 15% required enucleation.[172]

Postoperatively, medical therapy is necessary for an average of 6–12 weeks.[115,169–171] The risks of anesthesia

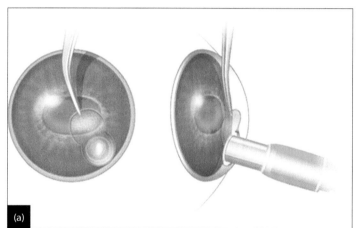
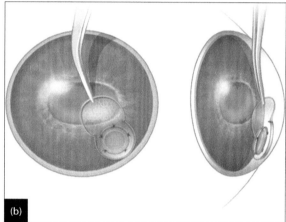

Figure 10.40 (a,b) Illustration of a modified PLK as described by McMullen. (From McMullen, R.J. et al. 2015. *Veterinary Ophthalmology*. 18(5):393–403.)

PLK procedure:

A three-sided rectangular anterior lamellar corneal flap is made two-third the depth of the stroma with a #64 beaver blade over the area of the DSA. The lamellar flap is left hinged on one side. The anterior lamellar flap incision is made 1–2 mm greater than the abscess on each side of the abscess. The anterior corneal flap is dissected and elevated with the use of a corneal dissector. A corneal trephine or biopsy punch (1 mm larger than the abscess) is used to outline the abscess to 75% of the remaining stromal depth. The abscess area is removed using a #65 beaver blade and corneal transplantation scissors. A corneal graft is sutured in the defect with four cardinal sutures. Bisecting sutures are used to secure the graft, and the anterior lamellar flap is secured in position.[168]

Alternatively, a semicircular anterior lamellar corneal flap is made over the DSA. Following formation of the flap, a two-step incision is used to remove the abscess and create a bed for suturing the corneal graft. A corneal trephine or biopsy punch 3 mm larger than the DSA is used to make a midstromal corneal groove. A corneal dissector is used to complete the lamellar keratectomy above the abscess. The abscess is outlined and removed with a trephine or biopsy punch 1–2 mm larger than the abscess, a #65 beaver blade, and corneal transplantation scissors as outlined previously. The corneal graft is sutured in the defect to the out circle of the two-step incision, and the lamellar flap is secured in place.[170]

With both techniques, throughout the procedure, viscoelastic materials are used to maintain the anterior chamber, and 8-0 polyglactin suture is used to suture the corneal graft in place and secure the anterior lamellar flap in place over the graft. In place of a corneal graft, a submucosal bioscaffold implant can be used to fill the defect.

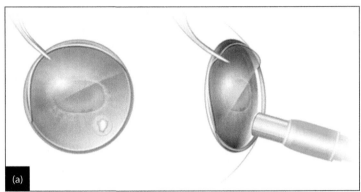
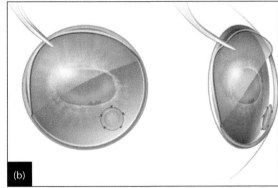

Figure 10.41 (a, b) Illustration of a modified DLEK as described by McMullen. (From McMullen, R.J. et al. 2015. *Veterinary Ophthalmology*. 18(5):393–403.)

DLEK procedure:

A corneal limbal based incision is made two-thirds the depth of the stroma with a #64 beaver blade. A stromal pocket is formed over the DSA with a corneal dissector. The corneal flap is retracted, and the abscess is outlined with a trephine or biopsy punch that is 2 mm larger than the abscess. The abscess is removed with the use of a #65 beaver blade and corneal transplant scissors. The corneal flap is sutured in place with 8-0 polyglactin 910 suture. Prior to complete closer of the corneal flap, a split-thickness corneal graft 1 mm larger in diameter than the defect is placed in the stromal pocket over the old abscess site with Utrata forceps.[169]

Alternatively, following making the corneal flap, a two-step incision is used to remove the abscess and create a bed for suturing the corneal graft. A corneal trephine or biopsy punch 3 mm larger than the DSA is used to make a midstromal corneal groove. A corneal dissector is used to complete the lamellar keratectomy above the abscess. The abscess is outlined and removed with a trephine or biopsy punch 1–2 mm larger than the abscess, a #65 beaver blade, and corneal transplantation scissors as outlined previously. The corneal graft is sutured in the defect to the out circle of the two-step incision, and the corneal flap is secured in place.[170]

With both techniques, throughout the procedure, viscoelastic materials are used to maintain the anterior chamber, and 8-0 polyglactin suture is used to suture the corneal graft in place and secure the corneal flap in place over the graft.

must be weighed against the benefit of surgery. The expense of medical or surgical therapy is roughly equivalent. Despite the difficulty in treating equine mycotic keratitis with early medical and/or surgical intervention, most eyes remain visual.

Viral

Herpesvirus is the main viral agent producing keratitis. The various conditions in different species are discussed under ulcerative keratitis, although nonulcerative syndromes are common.

Lack of tears

Keratoconjunctivitis sicca (KCS) is an important etiology for keratitis in the dog and less so in the cat and other species (see Chapter 9).

Chemical

Chemical injury with a strong alkaline solution is a devastating injury and more damaging to the cornea than a strong acid. Alkaline solutions penetrate deeper into the cornea, whereas acidic solutions precipitate proteins that act as a barrier to deeper penetration. Many of these injuries are of a malicious nature. Immediate therapy is thorough rinsing of the ocular surface and removal of any retained particulate material. Strong soaps for bathing are common causes of superficial ulcerative lesions.

Topical carbonic anhydrase inhibitors (dorzolamide and brinzolamide) can predispose to an immune-mediated keratitis that is nonresponsive to topical corticosteroids.[173] The keratitis is characterized by an ulcerative or nonulcerative keratitis with marked vascularization. Punctate cellular infiltrates are a frequent finding. Histopathological lesions are characterized by infiltrates of plasma cells in the anterior stroma and T-cells and neutrophils in the corneal epithelium. Discontinuation of the carbonic anhydrase inhibitor leads to rapid improvement.

Parasitic

Onchocerca

In the horse, *Onchocerca cervicalis* microfilaria that have died in the cornea may produce a keratitis. It is characterized

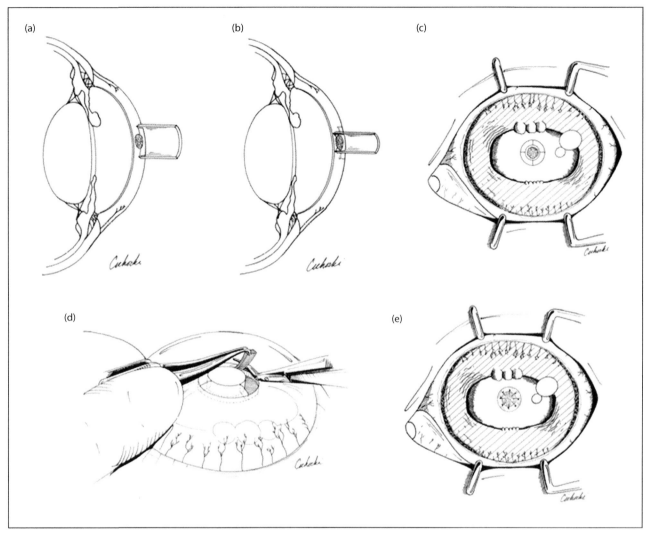

Figure 10.42 Illustration of a modified penetrating keratoplasty with a bioscaffold implant as described by Cichocki. (From Cichocki, B.M. et al. 2016. *Veterinary Ophthalmology.* 20(1):46–52.)

Modified penetrating keratoplasty procedure:

A two-stepped incision is used to remove the abscess. (a) An incision approximately 50% of the stromal depth is made around the abscess with a corneal trephine 3 mm larger in diameter than the abscess. (b) A second incision is made to the level of Descemet's membrane with a corneal trephine 2 mm larger in diameter than the abscess. (c) Four radial incisions are made to 50% of the stromal depth between the two trephinations. (d) A corneal dissector and right and left corneal scissors are used to excise the quadrants. The abscess is removed with a #65 beaver blade and right and left corneal scissors. (e) A bioscaffold implant 2 mm larger in diameter than the abscess is sutured into the central defect. A pedicle conjunctival graft is placed over the bioscaffold implant and sutured to the larger outer trephination.

Throughout the procedure, viscoelastic materials are used to maintain the anterior chamber. The bioscaffold implant is sutured in the defect with 9-0 polyglactin 910 suture, and the conjunctival graft is sutured in place with 8-0 polyglactin suture.[171]

in the acute stages by multifocal opacities and later by vascularization and scarring in the stroma (**Figure 10.43**). Perilimbal follicular formation, anterior uveitis, and conjunctival vitiligo may also be present. The condition is usually bilateral (see **Figure 10.43**). The diagnosis of onchocercal keratitis is often presumptive. Conjunctival snip biopsy containing motile microfilaria is suggestive but not an absolute indicator due to the presence of microfilaria in horses without ocular disease.[174] The role of *Onchocerca* microfilaria in producing ocular lesions has been reduced with the use of routine deworming with broad-spectrum anthelmintics.

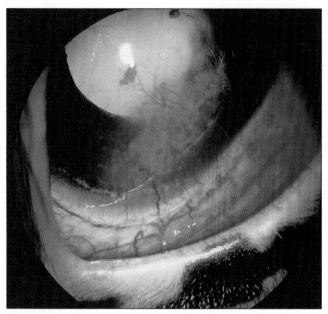

Figure 10.43 Horse with multifocal stromal opacities adjacent to the limbus that were associated with *Onchocerca cervicalis*. Conjunctival perilimbal follicular hyperplasia was also present.

Leishmaniasis

Leishmaniasis may produce a keratoconjunctivitis. Pena et al. report 24% of dogs with leishmaniasis have ocular/periocular lesions, and 34% have some form of keratoconjunctivitis.[175] In addition, 42% of ocular leishmaniasis produced anterior uveitis and/or secondary glaucoma that often resulted in corneal lesions such as corneal edema and neovascularization. The keratitis observed with leishmaniasis varied from focal corneal edema with neovascularization and cellular infiltration adjacent to the limbus, to focal nodular lesions near the limbus.

Diagnosis and therapy

See leishmaniasis involving the eyelid (see Chapter 7, **Figure 7.62**) and anterior uveitis.

Amoeba keratoconjunctivitis

Beckwith-Cohen et al. report a keratoconjunctivitis associated with an unidentified amoeba.[176] Amoeba keratitis is characterized by a fleshy corneal mass that grossly resembles squamous cell carcinoma. Topical long-term immunosuppressive therapy appears to predispose to amoeba keratoconjunctivitis.

Diagnosis and therapy

Diagnosis is by histopathology. Histopathological lesions are consistent with chronic granulomatous superficial keratitis with periodic acid–Schiff (PAS) and Grocott's methenamine silver (GMS) positive microorganisms consistent with amoeba. Treatment consist of a combination of a topical compounded solution of chlorhexidine digluconate (0.02%) and polyhexamethylene biguanide (0.02%) and stopping immune-suppressive therapy.

Immune-mediated

Superficial keratitis due to immune-mediated processes are common but are incompletely understood. The mechanism is often presumed based on bilaterality, lack of infectious or mechanical etiologies, mononuclear cellular infiltrates on histopathologic examination, and response to corticosteroids or other immunosuppressants. Keratitis in many of the infectious diseases also has an immunologic component. Examples of immune-mediated superficial nonulcerative keratitis are described in the following section.

Pannus (chronic superficial keratitis)

Introduction/etiology

Pathologically, pannus is the subepithelial proliferation of vessels and connective tissue. The term pannus is used clinically to signify a bilateral superficial keratitis that is thought to be immune mediated in the German shepherd dog (GSD) and GSD crosses. Similar syndromes have been observed in the greyhound, Shetland sheepdog, Siberian husky, Scotch collie, border collie, Belgian tervuren, Australian shepherd dog, and dachshund.[177,178] The histopathologic changes are characterized by neovascularization and fibroplasia and by plasma cell, lymphocyte, macrophage, and melanocytic cell infiltration. While the epithelium remains intact, it becomes variable in thickness from hyperplastic to thin; surface changes may be observed early in the disease using electron microscopy.[179–181] Petrick and van Rensburg[10] report that GSDs with pannus have very thin corneal epithelial layers compared to other breeds of dogs. In addition, several GSDs in the control group in the same study are reported to have thinned epithelium, loose corneal stroma, and decreased corneal tensile strength. This suggest a predisposing factor for pannus. An increase in eosinophils and mast cells at the limbal regions of GSDs compared to other breeds is reported and may be associated with exposure to light.[182,183] Last, cytoplasmic inclusions are found in corneal fibroblasts, vascular endothelial cells, macrophages, and trabecular cells of GSDs with and without pannus. Viral cultures are negative in dogs with pannus, and the significance of the cytology findings is unknown.[184]

Increase evidence suggest that pannus is immune-mediated disease.[181,185–190] An increase in immunoglobulin IgG is reported in the corneal stroma but not in the epithelium of dogs with pannus[181,185] and is possibly a nonspecific finding associated with stromal inflammation. Anderson et al. report low serum levels of IgG in dogs with pannus.[191] One study suggests that a delayed hypersensitivity reaction is involved in pannus, as leukocytes from dogs with pannus show increased inhibition of migration when exposed to corneal and iridal antigens.[186] However, another study failed to demonstrate lymphocytic stimulation to soluble corneal antigens.[192] Williams reports a predominantly lymphocytic infiltrate in dogs with pannus, with the majority being CD4-expressing lymphocytes and a significant portion of these cells secreting IFN-gamma.[187] These findings support that pannus is associated with an autoimmune disease. The increase expression of MHC II and in particularly the increase expression of DLA class II genes in corneas of dogs with pannus supports it is an immune-mediated disease.[188–190]

Epidemiologic studies relate the occurrence of pannus to geographic areas with an elevation of 4,500 feet or higher in 95% of cases.[177,178] Spontaneous improvement in severe pannus has been achieved by prolonged hospitalization. A genetic predisposition, combined with ultraviolet (UV) exposure at high altitude, altering a corneal antigen so that it is recognized as foreign and resulting in inflammation, has been proposed.[177] Chandler et al. demonstrated an increased expression of MMP2 and MMP9 in dogs with pannus and noted that UV light increases MMP induction in tissue culture.[193] The hypothesis is that UV light increases the expression of MMPs, and these may facilitate the inflammatory reaction. While the breed specificity for the condition and the fact that pannus is more difficult to control in patients from geographic areas of higher altitude suggest a genetic link interacting with environmental factors; the heritability has not been elucidated.

Clinical signs

The age of onset is usually 4–5 years in the GSD, but it may vary with the altitude of the region and the breed of dog. The lesion begins as an area of vascularization and granulation at the temporal limbus, usually in both eyes (**Figure 10.44**). Most dogs have a conjunctivitis, and about 10% may have plasma cell involvement of the third eyelid.[180] The disease progresses over weeks and months with invasion from the medial and ventral areas of the cornea. Eventually, the entire cornea is covered with a gray-to-red, roughened, superficial opacity (**Figure 10.45**). Focal gray spots are often present in the clear cornea adjacent to the infiltrating lesion. Some individuals with pannus develop heavy pigmentation, which obscures the underlying inflammatory reaction. The result is often blindness.

Diagnosis

Diagnosis of pannus is presumptive when bilateral proliferative keratitis is present in a "typical" breed. This is reinforced by the response to anti-inflammatory therapy.

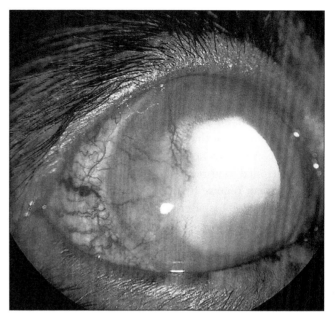

Figure 10.44 Early pannus formation in a Boykin spaniel. The condition was bilateral and responded well to topical corticosteroid therapy.

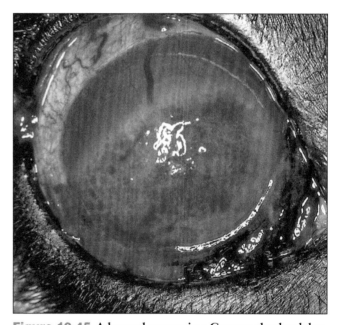

Figure 10.45 Advanced pannus in a German shepherd dog.

Therapy

Glucocorticoids The main therapy for pannus is topical glucocorticoids to suppress corneal inflammation. The route, frequency, and form of glucocorticoid therapy varies with the individual circumstances and preferences. Initial therapy is intensive, but later maintenance therapy is reduced and titrated to the individual response. The duration of therapy is indefinite, perhaps for the life of the animal. Initially, topical prednisolone acetate 1% suspension or dexamethasone 0.1% ophthalmic solution is given every

4 hours for 7–10 days. At this time, a dramatic improvement typically occurs, and the dose can be decreased to every 6 hours for 7–10 days. The frequency is decreased progressively at weekly intervals if improvement is maintained (**Figures 10.46 and 10.47**).

Maintenance therapy of every 12–24 hours is usually achieved but may have to be adjusted periodically. It is extremely important that the owner realizes that the therapy may control but not cure the condition. Many dogs with controlled long-term glucocorticoid medication (for years) may not require further treatment, but the diligent owner at this point is often wary of stopping therapy.

If owner compliance is a problem, topical glucocorticoids can be supplemented with long-acting subconjunctival glucocorticoids such as betamethasone, triamcinolone,

or methylprednisolone. The injections may be repeated if exacerbation occurs, but they do not replace the use of topical glucocorticoids.

Topical cyclosporine, tacrolimus, or primecrolimus

Topical 0.2%–2% cyclosporine, 0.02% tacrolimus solution or ointment, and 1% pimecrolimus have demonstrated efficacy in treating pannus.[194–197] Whether it is best to use these drugs alone or in conjunction with topical corticosteroids for best results is unresolved at this point. They are alternative drugs that can be used in resistant cases and may prevent the necessity for surgery in severe cases. They may also minimize the risk of local (lipid keratopathy) and systemic side effects that corticosteroids may induce. Williams et al. report that topical dexamethasone 0.1% alone and cyclosporine 0.2% alone are equally effective as a treatment for pannus.[197] There is improvement in 95% of the dogs treated with the combination of topical corticosteroids and cyclosporine 2.0%.[198] A topical formulation of tacrolimus 0.02% alone or in combination with DMSO 50% reduces corneal inflammation, neovascularization, and fibrosis in dogs with pannus but does not appear to inhibit the progression of pigment infiltration.[199,200] The author typically initiates therapy with both dexamethasone 0.1% and cyclosporine 2.0% or tacrolimus 0.02%–0.03% and slowly tapers the medications to the lowest frequency that keeps the condition under control.

> The most common error in treating pannus is not to treat intensively for the first 2–3 weeks. It is important for the client to understand that the condition is manageable but not curable and that lifelong therapy is needed to manage the disease.

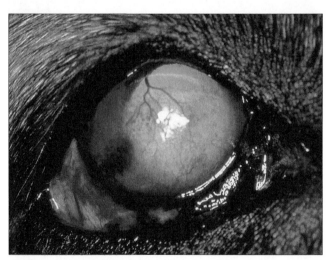

Figure 10.46 Same dog as Figure 10.45 after 2 weeks of topical corticosteroid therapy every 4 hours.

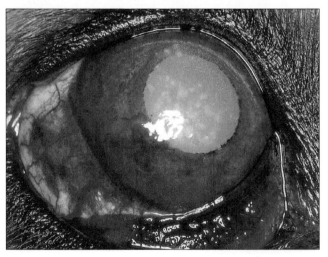

Figure 10.47 Same dog as Figure 10.45 after 10 weeks of topical corticosteroid therapy decreasing in frequency and maintained on every 24-hours of therapy. Note residual corneal pigmentation and focal opacities.

Cryotherapy

Cryotherapy of the corneal surface has been used to slough superficial pigment. When pigmentation is extensive, cryotherapy of the corneal surface for 10–20 seconds at each site using nitrous oxide produces sloughing and clearing of the pigment.[201] Liquid nitrogen spray for 15 seconds and double freezing is also reported to be successful in removing corneal pigment.[202] Liquid nitrogen is more capable of producing permanent corneal edema if performed incorrectly; therefore, nitrous oxide is preferred. Azoulay reports the use of a cryogen consisting of 95% dimethylether, 3% isobutene, and 2% propane to decrease the severity of pigmentary keratitis.[203] Cryotherapy does not take the place of corticosteroids and are continued after healing.

Radiation therapy

β-radiation therapy is an alternative therapy available mainly at teaching institutions. β-radiation may be used to disperse the pigment and suppress inflammation in cases that are difficult to control with topical immuno-suppressive medications. The dose used is quite variable, and bullous keratopathy is a complication from endothelial damage (see section Corneal tumors). Radiotherapy with soft X-rays (15 kv) is reported to be an effective and safe treatment for pannus following a superficial keratectomy. This study suggests that the effect of soft X-rays is superior to Sr-90 irradiation for the treatment of pannus.[204]

Surgery

Superficial keratectomies can produce immediate, but usually temporary, improvement. Keratectomies are used mainly to treat patients with heavy pigmentation and as a last resort (see **Figure 10.120**). The initial improvement from surgery is short-lived as granulation occurs in the healing process. Topical corticosteroids, cyclosporine, and NSAIDs postoperatively are necessary to moderate the inflammatory reaction in the cornea. These drugs must be monitored carefully to avoid complications.

Corneoscleral grafting of the involved area has been reported in four dogs, but this technique has not gained recognition as a legitimate therapy for pannus[205] due to the technical difficulty, expense, questionable results, and difficulty in obtaining donors.

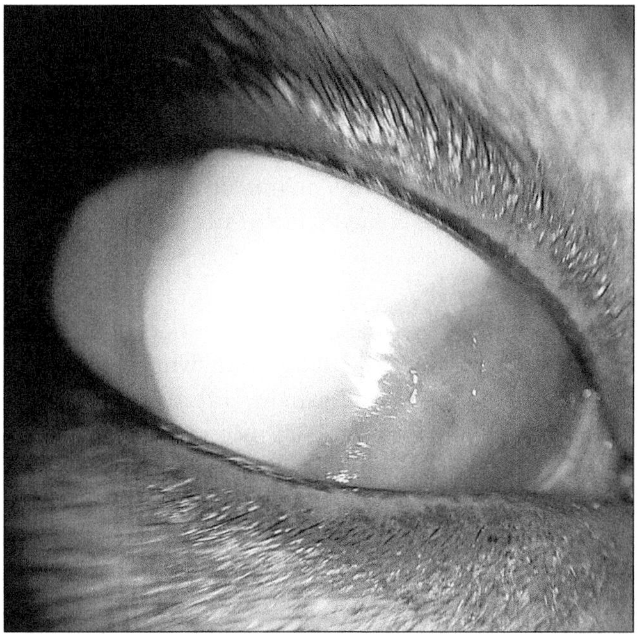

Eosinophilic keratitis

Introduction/etiology

Eosinophilic keratitis is unique to cats and horses. It manifests as a proliferative, progressive, superficial keratitis. The etiology is unknown, but on histopathology, a superficial granulomatous inflammation with numerous eosinophils and mast cells is present. Some cases may have a peripheral eosinophilia, but this and any association with the feline eosinophilic complex is very inconsistent.[206–209] Indirect fluorescent antibody testing for feline herpesvirus-1 (FHV-1) is positive in 33%, and PCR for FHV-1 is positive in 54.5%–76% of cats with eosinophilic keratitis.[209–211] Dean reports that FHV-1 DNA is databale by PCR in 66.7% of the cats with a history and/or presence of a corneal ulceration at the time of initial presentation.[211] Richter et al. reports on four cats with eosinophilic keratitis associated with *Parachlamydia acanthamoebae*.[212]

Clinical signs (cat)

Initially, the keratitis is unilateral, but it may become bilateral. A progressive, red, granulating proliferation usually begins at the superior temporal or inferior nasal limbus and eventually covers the cornea (**Figures 10.48 and 10.49**). Whitish deposits of cheesy consistency that are rich in eosinophils are present in chronic cases. Ulcerative keratitis may be present.

Figure 10.48 Relatively early eosinophilic keratitis at the nasal limbus in a cat. Note the white surface on the proliferative mass. Eosinophils, mast cells, and lymphocytes were readily found on scrapings from the lesion. The patient responded well to topical corticosteroids, but the second eye become involved several months later.

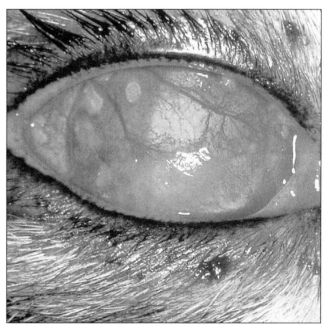

Figure 10.49 Advanced eosinophilic keratitis in a cat. The condition is characterized by superficial white material. The patient was treated with oral megestrol acetate and responded well. (Courtesy of Dr. S. Winston, Atlanta, GA.)

STT values may be decreased but improve with treatment. Blepharospasm is present in about 20% of cases, and the conjunctiva and the third eyelid adjacent to the corneal lesions may be severely affected. Whether this overlaps with eosinophilic conjunctivitis as described in Chapter 8 is unknown. After an initially positive response to therapy, relapse is common (66%) after several months.

Clinical signs (horse)

Two forms have been observed in the horse: An acute multifocal form (**Figure 10.50**) with white plaques in the superficial cornea and a more diffuse limbal based form with white deposits which may be ulcerative.[213,214] Secondary bacterial and fungal infections are not uncommon in cases with ulcerative keratitis.[215] The inflammation stimulates epiphora, blepharospasm, and corneal neovascularization. If corneal ulceration is present, reflex uveitis is a common finding. The white plaques in the multifocal form "shell out" of the cornea with manipulation. Equine eosinophilic keratitis is documented to occur more frequently in the summer months.[216]

Diagnosis

Diagnosis is usually based on the unusual cytology of numerous mast cells and eosinophils. Differential diagnosis includes mast cell neoplasia, which may have similar cytology.

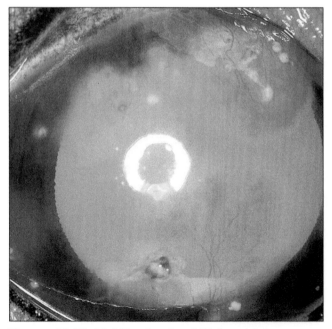

Figure 10.50 Multifocal eosinophilic keratitis in a horse. The white material easily shelled out of the cornea, leaving an ulcer, and it was rich in eosinophils. The patient responded dramatically to topical corticosteroid therapy.

Therapy

Most cases in cats respond to topical immunosuppressive medications (glucocorticoids or cyclosporine). Spiess et al. reports an improvement in 88.6% of cats treated with topical cyclosporine 1.5%.[217] If topical glucocorticoids have not been previously used, they are given as a trial since most cases are responsive. In cats, it is also prudent to treat concurrently with a topical antiviral agent when administering topical immunosuppressives due to the high percentage of FHV-1-positive cats. If relapses or an incomplete response occurs in the cat, megestrol acetate (5 mg every 24 hours for 1 week and 2.5–5 mg/week maintenance) has been recommended. Topical megestrol acetate 0.5% is reported to be effective in 88% of the cats treated for eosinophilic keratitis.[218]

In horses with the multifocal form of eosinophilic keratitis, response to topical glucocorticoid therapy is rapid. Horses treated with systemic oral dexamethasone at 0.04 mg/kg for 1 day, 0.03 mg/kg for 2 days, and 0.02 mg/kg for 3–5 days have a faster resolution of the disease than horses treated with other medication.[215] If infectious ulcerative keratitis is present, treatment with appropriate antibiotics and/or antifungal is warranted prior to treatment with glucocorticoids. The ulcerative and limbal-based forms respond to mast cell stabilizers such as 0.1% Iodoxamide every 6 hours. Alternately, the oral antihistamine, cetirizine at a dose of 0.4 mg/kg can be used to treat equine eosinophilic keratitis and is associated with a decrease risk of recurrence. No matter the treatment used, therapy is often prolonged.

> Eosinophilic keratitis is yet another reason why the clinician should become comfortable in performing cytology of ocular surfaces for diagnostic reasons.

Proliferative keratitis in the cat

Introduction/etiology

This condition is most probably a variant of eosinophilic keratitis.[219] A proliferative chronic superficial keratitis with white, cheesy deposits on the surface is described with clinical signs similar to eosinophilic keratitis. Histopathologically, no eosinophils are present, and the white material is an amorphous eosinophilic deposit.[220,221]

Clinical signs

A superficial proliferative keratitis is present, which usually is bilateral and begins temporally. There are white deposits on the surface of the cornea (**Figure 10.51**). Adjacent conjunctiva may have similar proliferations and deposits. The cats are usually middle aged.

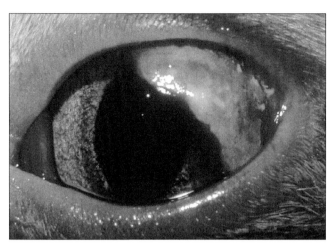

Figure 10.51 **Proliferative keratitis with a white plaque in a cat. This syndrome does not have eosinophils on histopathology. (Courtesy of Dr. V. Pentlarge, Athens, GA.)**

Diagnosis

Biopsy of the lesion and the eosinophilic material near the basal lamina differentiates the condition from eosinophilic keratitis. Corneal scrapings or cytology have not been reported, but presumably eosinophils are absent.

Therapy

The condition is responsive to topical corticosteroids but may relapse or occur in the other eye. If the condition is resistant or relapsing, topical cyclosporine or oral megestrol acetate are considered for treatment. Relapses occur when therapy ceases, so long-term therapy is likely. If topical corticosteroids or cyclosporine are effective, they are preferred to avoid the complications of oral megestrol acetate. To date topical megestrol acetate has not been evaluated for this condition.

Pigmentary keratitis

Introduction/etiology

It is not unusual for clinicians to use this term as a specific diagnosis. However, the condition is not a separate entity but a clinical sign of corneal irritation/inflammation. The term pigmentary keratitis is used for those forms of keratitis in which superficial pigmentation is prominent and is often so dense that the inflammatory response of neovascularization may not be visible. Sources of pigmentation on or in the cornea may be categorized as either endogenous or exogenous in origin. Superficial corneal pigment results from the migration of limbal melanocytes along blood vessels. Corneal neovascularization is thus a prerequisite for superficial stromal pigmentation (melanin).[222] Alternatively, latent or amelanotic melanocytes may be in the cornea and activated by neovascularization, or epithelial pigment may arise from stem cell stimulation

at the limbus. Pigment that is in the epithelial layers may be sloughed with the turnover of epithelium if the cause is corrected or controlled. Stromal pigmentation remains indefinitely. Breeds such as pugs, Shetland sheepdogs, and Dachshunds respond to corneal inflammation with pigmentation more than other breeds.

Deep melanin pigmentation may occur from uveal sources such as persistent pupillary membranes, anterior synechiae, or ruptured iris cysts. Blood staining may occur from hemoglobin breakdown products from some forms of hyphema or from intracorneal hemorrhage (**Figures 10.52 and 10.53**).

Various metals such as iron, copper, gold, and silver may stain the cornea. The most common metallic stain is iron, usually from a retained corneal foreign body. Corneal staining as a complication of silver nitrate stick cauterization of the cornea has been described in a dog.[223]

A variety of topical and systemic medications are documented to produce corneal pigmentation, but most of the drugs are either not often used or are not used long term in veterinary medicine.[224] Long-term topical epinephrine may induce a dark pigmentation in the conjunctiva and the cornea.

Amiodarone is an antiarrhythmic drug that is recognized to produce pigmented fine deposits in the basal cells of the corneal epithelium when used long term in humans. Typically, the deposits are reversible after cessation of therapy. Dogs appear resistant to amiodarone deposits; of six dogs administered amiodarone, only one dog

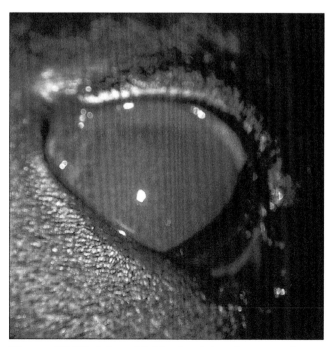

Figure 10.52 **A dog with blood staining the cornea from a chronic hyphema with increased intraocular pressure.**

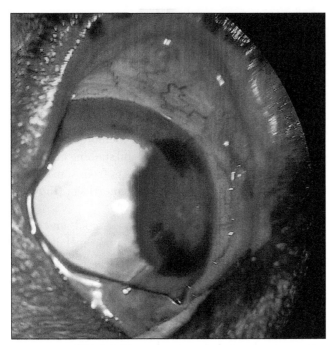

Figure 10.53 Intrastromal hemorrhage in the cornea of a dog that had cobalt radiation therapy and developed a sterile stromal abscess.

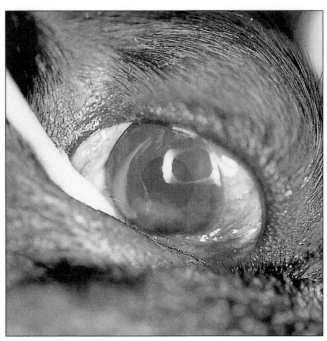

Figure 10.54 Medial corneal pigmentation and granulation in a pug due to irritation from medial entropion. The lesion is still active but will not cover the cornea. Both eyes were treated with a medial canthoplasty.

developed mild deposits after 11 weeks of therapy.[225] On histopathology, the typical cytoplasmic inclusions were found in the basal cells of the affected dog. Nevertheless, periodic ocular examinations are prudent for animals on long-term amiodarone therapy. Lesions, when present, are observed on biomicroscopy as fine dots in the epithelial layer of the cornea.

Pigmentation of the cornea of the cat is common with formation of a corneal sequestrum condition (see section Corneal sequestrum). Dematiaceous fungi can also produce a darkly pigmented cornea.[139–141]

The author categorizes pigmentary keratitis into focal nonprogressive and diffuse progressive forms. The focal form is common in brachycephalic breeds and is usually caused by long-term mechanical irritation such as medial entropion, nasal fold irritation, or a stromal ulcer that has been slow to heal. These often take the shape of a wedge of pigment on the medial cornea that points to the axial cornea (**Figure 10.54**). Often, by the time these areas are recognized by the owner, they are not in the progressive or developing phase.

Diffuse pigmentary keratitis is often insidious and progresses to complete or near complete coverage of the cornea and blindness (**Figure 10.55**). The condition may be unilateral or bilateral. The underlying cause may be KCS, lagophthalmos, or immune-mediated keratitis. Some forms of pannus in the GSD

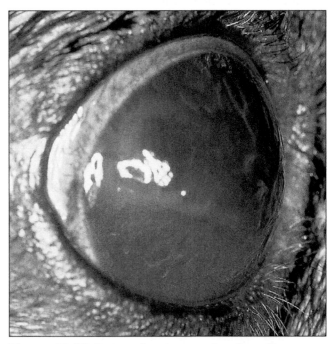

Figure 10.55 Progressive pigmentation that will cover the cornea in this pug if the stromal inflammation is not controlled. Note thickening of the cornea and neovascularization. Vision will improve by controlling the inflammation and thinning the cornea, even if the pigmentation remains.

are characterized more by pigment than by granulation tissue. The underlying inflammation is variably masked by the pigment.

In pugs, pigmentary keratitis is suggested to have a genetic predisposition. Studies have not found a significant correlation with other ocular abnormalities and pigmentary keratitis in the pug.[226,227] For this reason, corneal pigmentation in the pug may be best referred to as pigmentary keratopathy, and it is reported to occur in 82.4% of pugs.[226] It is possible that adnexal disorders and tear film abnormalities may exacerbate the condition. Pugs with severe corneal pigmentation have significantly lower STT values, rapid tear film break-up times, and decreased corneal sensitivity than pugs with milder forms of the disease. It is possible that these decrease values may be secondary to chronic corneal disease and not the cause of the corneal pigmentation.

Clinical signs
Superficial corneal pigmentation is the predominant sign. Focal pigmentation in brachycephalics is usually a limbal based triangle of pigment in the medial cornea (**Figure 10.54**). Diffuse pigmentation may have a vortex appearance with the tip directed to the central cornea. The latter pattern is explained by the pigment following the stem cell migration from the limbus, which occurs in a whorl or vortex pattern.[34]

Depending on the stage of development and cause of the pigment, additional signs of pain, discharge, and neovascularization may be present. Blindness is common when the condition is bilateral and diffuse.

Diagnosis
The underlying cause of pigmentation is determined and treated.

Therapy
Mechanical causes such as medial entropion in brachycephalic breeds are corrected if the keratitis is in the developing stage. However, patients are often presented once the condition is established, and surgery does not change the pigment. As most medial entropions do not cause any visual signs, therapy may be dictated by other signs that are present, such as epiphora.

In the progressive forms, therapy is directed at the cause (e.g., KCS) or the underlying inflammation (e.g., immune-mediated inflammation). If the inflammation is controlled, most animals retain vision despite the presence of diffuse pigmentation. Topical cyclosporine may help decrease the pigmentation, both in cases associated with KCS and with other forms.

> Diffuse pigmentary keratitis is very frustrating to monitor for the owner and the clinician, since the progression is insidious, and the increased pigmentation remains in most cases as a "high water mark" for the inflammation.

Surface cryotherapy and β-radiation therapy have been used to disperse the pigmentation when severe. While the pigment may disperse, residual corneal scarring is often severe. A superficial keratectomy can remove the pigment. However, since the pigment deposition recurs in immune-mediated conditions, keratectomy is not recommended in most patients.[228] Postsurgical complications of infection and melting ulcers are common in brachycephalic breeds if the cornea is not covered or lubricated well.

Equine immune-mediated keratitis
Introduction/etiology
A nonulcerative, noninfectious, immune-mediated keratitis is reported in horses in both the United States and United Kingdom.[229,230] Although there are some differences in the clinical presentation and response to treatment between the disease in the United States and United Kingdom, both are an immune-mediated keratitis. The disease is characterized by a progressive or recurrent corneal opacity with or without minimal ocular discomfort (i.e., mild epiphora, slight blepharospasm). Intraocular inflammation is typically not a presenting sign.

Pate et al., determined that immune-mediated keratitis (IMMK) is secondary to a T-cell-driven process.[231] Immunohistochemical evaluation of corneal samples indicated that both T-helper and T-cytotoxic cells are involved in the disease process. Local humoral involvement is suggested by the presence of immunoglobulins in the corneal samples.

A stromal keratitis that presents clinically similar to IMMK was reported by Rebhun.[232] The potential for aerobic, anaerobic, and equine herpesvirus involvement in the disease process was investigated, but none were proven to be associated with the condition. Cytology demonstrated an acid-fast organism but was not confirmed by culture. However, the lesions resolved in 4–8 weeks with topical aminoglycosides and oral rifampin (4.4 mg/kg b.i.d.).

Whether IMMK is an autoimmune disease or an immune response to an underlying infectious organism has not been determined.

Clinical signs

Clinically, IMMK presents as a nonulcerative, progressive or recurring keratitis (>3 months in duration). It is characterized by corneal opacification, corneal vascularization, mild-to-moderate cellular infiltrate, and corneal edema. A hallmark of IMMK is the absence or presence of mild signs of ocular discomfort. Mild epiphora and/or blepharospasm is a common finding, but there are no clinical signs of uveitis.[229,230,233] IMMK is typically a unilateral disease but can affect both eyes.

There are three distinct clinical presentations for IMMK: Superficial stromal, midstromal, and endothelial. Superficial stromal IMMK is commonly located in the ventral-paracentral cornea, ventral perilimbal cornea, or central cornea. It is characterized by a subepithelial, superficial stromal opacity consisting of diffuse, white-to-yellow cellular infiltrate that is surrounded by superficial corneal neovascularization. The underlying stroma is clear of disease (**Figure 10.56**). Midstromal IMMK clinically appears similar to superficial stromal IMMK. The chief difference is that the cornea appears more opaque, as the cellular infiltrate is denser than with superficial stromal IMMK. In addition, the cellular infiltrate and corneal vascularization is in the central stromal layers. Midstromal IMMK lesions are commonly located in the lateral paracentral, ventral, or central cornea (**Figure 10.57**). Endothelial IMMK (endotheliitis) is commonly located in the ventrolateral or ventral cornea. It is characterized by a chronic, slowly progressive, nonpainful area of deep corneal edema that varies in degree of severity in the areas affected. A dark cellular infiltrate at the level

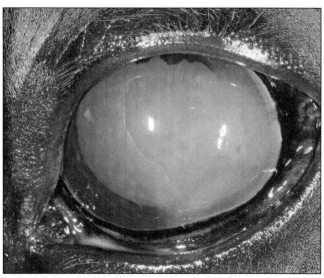

Figure 10.57 Midstromal IMMK. Note the midstromal opacification with corneal neovascularization in the ventrolateral cornea with superficial yellow infiltrate. Corneal edema and neovascularization is present in the lateral cornea. There are multiple stromal opacities of varying depth throughout the cornea. When present, these stromal opacities are more typically limited to the anterior stroma.

of the endothelial cells is present. As with other causes of deep corneal edema, bullous keratopathy, and secondary, focal or multifocal, superficial corneal ulceration may occur (see **Figure 10.65**).

Diagnosis

A presumptive diagnosis is made if there are signs of a chronic (>3 months), progressive or recurring, nonulcerative, noninfectious keratitis consisting of corneal opacification, corneal vascularization, mild-to-moderate cellular infiltration, and corneal edema. The horse is nonpainful or has signs of mild ocular discomfort. The absence of microorganisms is determined by cytology and culture or histopathology. The diagnosis of IMMK can be confirmed by histopathology following a superficial keratectomy/biopsy. Endothelial IMMK can be confirmed by the identification of the dark cellular infiltrate at the edge of the corneal edema by slit lamp biomicroscope. The deep corneal edema associated with endothelial IMMK is similar to that seen with glaucoma or anterior uveitis. The eye is comfortable, the intraocular pressures are normal, and there are no signs of uveitis with endothelial IMMK.[229,233,234]

Histopathology findings of IMMK are consistent with stromal fibrosis, infiltration of lymphocytes and plasma cells, and vascularization.

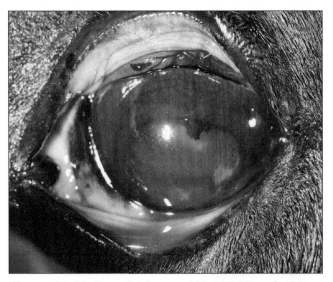

Figure 10.56 Superficial stromal IMMK. Note the faint superficial stromal opacity in the ventrolateral and ventral cornea. Neovascularization is present in the lateral and ventral cornea.

Therapy

Therapy for equine IMMK is topical immunosuppressive medications. Topical dexamethasone 0.1% every 12 hours and cyclosporine A every 12 hours is recommended for the treatment of IMMK.[229,233] The author typically uses topical dexamethasone 0.1% every 6–8 hours and cyclosporine A 2% every 6–8 hours to treat IMMK. The frequency of the topical dexamethasone and cyclosporine are slowly tapered over time. Frequently, the horse must remain on topical cyclosporine to prevent recurrence. Both midstromal and endothelial IMMK are typically less responsive to treatment than superficial IMMK. Gilger et al. have reported the use of episcleral silicone matrix cyclosporine (ESMC) implants for the treatment of IMMK.[235] In this study, the ESMC implants controlled superficial and endothelial IMMK for a mean follow-up period of 176.8 and 207.2 days, respectively. The ESMC implants alone failed to control midstromal IMMK, requiring topical medication and/or surgery. A superficial keratectomy with a conjunctival flap is an effective treatment for refractive cases of superficial and midstromal IMMK. Bromfenac 0.009%, a topical nonsteroidal anti-inflammatory, is reported to be effective in treating endothelial IMMK.[236]

McMullen and Fischer report the use of photothermal therapy following intrastromal injections of indocyanine green as an effective treatment for IMMK.[237] The exact mechanism of this therapy is still under investigation. It may alter corneal antigens and is thought to be cidal to infectious organisms.[238,239] Photothermal therapy appears to hold promise as an effective treatment for refractive cases of IMMK.

> IMMK and fungal keratitis can appear similar. Therefore, it is important to rule out fungal keratitis before initiating treatment with topical immunosuppressive medications.

Intracorneal stromal hemorrhage

Stromal hemorrhage is a rare condition that appears as a focal, bright red to dark red area of blood adjacent to corneal neovascularization (**Figure 10.53**). It typically occurs in older dogs, and the Bichon Frise breed is statistically overrepresented when compared to other patients presented for ophthalmic conditions.[240] Intracorneal hemorrhage may occur in any area of the cornea but is more common in the midperipheral cornea.[241] Concurrent ocular disorders, such as keratoconjunctivitis sicca, cataracts, and corneal ulcers, occur in 91% of the cases, and systemic disorders are present in 59% of the cases. The most common systemic diseases associated with stromal hemorrhages are diabetes mellitus, hyperadrenocorticism, hypothyroidism, and systemic hypertension. Treatment is normally directed toward treating concurrent ophthalmic and systemic disorders. Topical anti-inflammatory medications have no obvious benefit in the resolution of the condition. The blood may reabsorb over time, with or without treatment.

DEEP NONULCERATIVE INFLAMMATORY DISEASE

Stromal or interstitial keratitis

Infectious canine hepatitis (ICH) ocular reaction is described as the typical example of deep keratitis in the dog. Most cases of deep keratitis that are not complications of deep ulcerations accompany an anterior uveitis. Thus, the causes of stromal keratitis are often the same as uveitis.

Neovascularization associated with stromal keratitis is usually characterized by vessels that are relatively straight and, with the slit lamp, can be localized deep in the cornea (**Figure 10.58**). Because the corneal endothelium participates in the process, various degrees of corneal edema and cellular deposits (keratic precipitates) on the endothelium are common (**Figure 10.59**), as are signs relating to an anterior uveitis (synechiae, hypotony, and flare).

An anatomic diagnosis is made by the straight vascular pattern, localization of lesions to the deep cornea, and uveal signs. Therapy is directed at the anterior uveitis and,

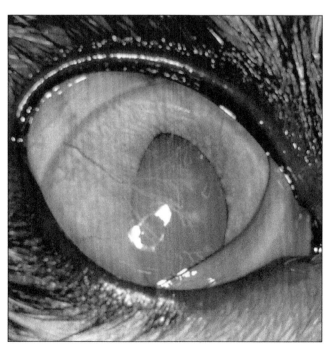

Figure 10.58 Deep stromal vessels with minimal branching in a cat with stromal keratitis.

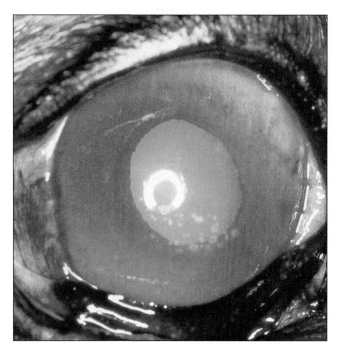

Figure 10.59 Stromal keratitis in a dog with toxoplasmosis-induced episclerokeratouveitis. Note the focal deposits, which are keratic precipitates on Descemet's membrane, and secondary corneal edema from endothelial compromise. An episcleritis was associated with the keratitis dorsally.

if the condition is not thought to be an infectious process, usually consists of corticosteroids. Prednisolone acetate 1% is the best topical steroid for corneal inflammation.

Infectious canine hepatitis

Introduction/etiology

Interstitial keratitis due to infectious canine hepatitis (ICH) is almost an historical disease. The routine use of canine adenovirus-2 (CAV-2) for vaccination has all but eliminated the previous vaccine-related reaction, and since natural ICH is now quite rare, clinicians seldom see the condition. On rare occasions, typical ocular reactions are seen 2 weeks following immunization with CAV-2.

Canine adenovirus-1 (CAV-1), whether virulent or attenuated as a vaccine strain, may produce a condition of acute anterior uveitis and endotheliitis with corneal edema. The ocular signs begin about 10–14 days after vaccination, 6–8 days after IV injection, or in the recovery stage of clinical disease and are the result of an Arthus-type immune reaction.[242,243] The basic lesion is a uveitis, and the corneal edema is due to damage from neutrophilic lysosomal enzymes. Most cases improve spontaneously over 2–3 weeks, but some patients have persistent corneal edema and/or secondary glaucoma. Breeds such

Table 10.3 Possible pathogenesis of infectious canine hepatitis blue eye

Viremia

Viral growth in reticuloendothelial tissue, kidney, liver

▼

± Viral growth in anterior uvea/corneal endothelium (CE)

No growth – No uveitis

Growth – CE, vascular endothelium, trabeculae

▼

Local immune response

Lymphocytes and plasma cells in anterior uvea

Restricted viral growth

▼

Viral growth arrested or viral persistence in restricted sites

No persistence – No clinical signs

Persistence – CE, trabecular meshwork cells

Viral antigen release into aqueous fluid

▼

Immune complex formation (CAV-1 antibody)

Virus/antibody excess: Slight or no pathogenicity

Virus/antibody balance: Complement (C′) binding; pathogenic

▼

C′-mediated release of biologically active components

Leukocyte chemotactic factors

Immune adherence factor

Enhanced phagocytosis of immune complexes

▼

Leukocyte infiltration into anterior chamber

▼

Phagocytosis of immune complexes-C′ by neutrophils and macrophages

▼

Lysosomal enzyme release

Injury (focal) to CE at points of contact with leukocytes?

▼

Infiltration of leukocytes between CE and Descemet's membrane

Aqueous fluid permeates into corneal stroma

Corneal edema

▼

Digestion of immune complexes within phagocytic vacuoles and removal

If lesions in CE focal: Resolution in 1–3 weeks

If lesions extensive: No CE regeneration, persistent or permanent corneal damage. Bullous keratopathy, hydrophthalmos, or extensive corneal pigmentation with complete loss of vision.

Source: Carmichael, L. 1965. *Pathologia Veterinaria* 2(4):344–359.

as the Siberian husky, Afghan hound, and other sight hounds may have an increased incidence of such complications.[244,245] Certain breeds that have goniodysgenesis may be more susceptible to the complication of glaucoma. (See **Table 10.3** for the proposed pathogenesis of ICH ocular lesions.)

Clinical signs

Occasionally, observant owners may present patients with signs only of anterior uveitis such as blepharospasm, miosis, flare, and hypotony. Within 24–36 hours, the familiar sign of corneal edema develops. The deep corneal edema may be focal or diffuse and has the appearance of ground glass (**Figure 10.60**). In 10%–15% of cases, the edema is bilateral. Epithelial bullae may develop and rupture, producing corneal ulceration. If severe hypotony is present, the cornea may develop keratoconus. The conjunctiva is usually hyperemic, and after a lag of 2–3 days, neovascularization of the cornea begins. Most patients improve spontaneously over 2–3 weeks, while others have partial improvement, delayed improvement, or no improvement of the edema with eventual development of pigmentation. Patients whose corneas do not clear in the expected 2–3 weeks may show clearing after a lag of several weeks or months. In these patients, residual pigmentation is usually present in the cornea.

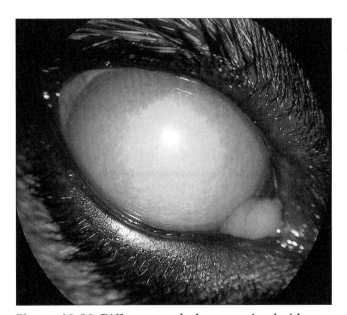

Figure 10.60 Diffuse stromal edema associated with infectious canine hepatitis vaccination with CAV-1, 2 weeks earlier. The uveitis is masked. As most of these reactions occur in puppies, many may spontaneously improve in 2–4 weeks.

Therapy

It is questionable whether therapy alters the course of ICH-induced disease. Most cases improve spontaneously, but if the condition is iatrogenically induced, the clinician may treat using the placebo effect. Topical steroids, nonsteroidals, and atropine are indicated for the uveitis, but the regeneration of the endothelium may not be influenced by these drugs. If the cornea has bullae, steroids are used with caution due to the risk of corneal ulceration. The IOP is monitored since the clinical signs can mask glaucoma until the eye enlarges. Topical carbonic anhydrase inhibitors are indicated for glaucoma.

Herpesvirus stromal keratitis

FHV-1 is a common cause of stromal keratitis in the cat. Herpesvirus stromal keratitis may accompany epithelial erosions with immune suppression (glucocorticoid administration) or develop after the erosions have healed. Stromal keratitis is usually associated with recurrent ocular disease and not with primary ocular disease. Stromal keratitis may be produced by certain strains of herpesvirus that replicate in the stroma, and it is the result of an immune reaction of the host to the virus.[246,247] Townsend et al. and Stiles and Pogranichniy report FHV-1 DNA in approximately half of the cats' corneas without ocular disease, in 41% of the trigeminal ganglia evaluated, and positive viral cultures in six corneas from five normal cats.[248,249] The findings are not conclusive of the cornea being a latent site in the cat, only that viable virus can be present in normal corneas. Volopich S et al. have documented that the presence of FHV-1 DNA in the cat cornea is significantly associated with epithelial keratitis but not stromal keratitis.[250] Experimentally, stromal disease accompanied primary epithelial disease when cats are pretreated with subconjunctival glucocorticoids.[251] Additional ocular lesions in this group consisted of corneal calcification, KCS, and corneal sequestrum. Occasionally, herpesvirus corneal involvement in the cat produces severe edema and bullae, indicating that the endothelium is involved (**Figures 10.58, 10.61, and 10.62**). The iris usually has some color changes, indicating uveitis; the course of the disease is usually weeks to months in duration, with little apparent response to antiviral therapy. Ledbetter et al. described a nonulcerative stromal keratitis in dogs associated with a naturally acquired CVH-1 infection in a colony of laboratory eagles.[252] Clinically, the dogs present with a circumferential ring of peripheral corneal stromal vascularization with limbal, perilimbal, multifocal epithelial, and subepithelial cellular infiltrates.

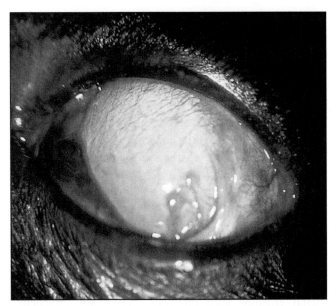

Figure 10.61 Presumed herpes-induced stromal keratitis in a cat. Note also the symblepharon.

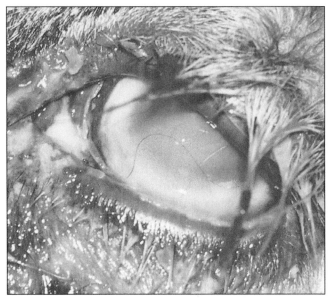

Figure 10.63 Keratouveitis in a young calf due to the (herpesvirus) infectious bovine rhinotracheitis. Intense peripheral leukocytic infiltration is present compared to the central ulcerative lesion found in infectious bovine keratitis. The condition was bilateral, and the calf also had respiratory signs.

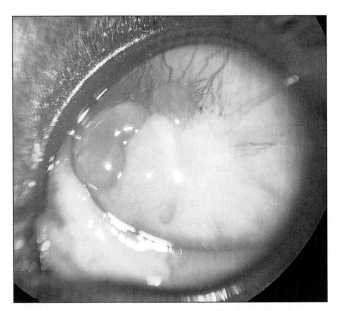

Figure 10.62 Severe herpes-induced keratouveitis in a young Persian cat. The endothelial decompensation produced marked bullae on the corneal surface. The condition was bilateral and took several weeks to abate.

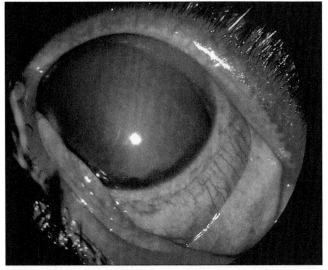

Figure 10.64 Typical corneal edema in a cow with malignant catarrhal fever. The corneal edema from endothelial inflammation is obvious, but a panophthalmitis is produced by the herpesvirus.

Herpesvirus infection in cattle may produce deep stromal keratitis and endothelial damage. The herpesvirus of infectious bovine rhinotracheitis (IBR) may produce a severe nonulcerative keratouveitis (**Figure 10.63**) and needs to be differentiated from "pink eye." The herpesvirus of malignant catarrhal fever (MCF) typically produces a diffusely edematous cornea (**Figure 10.64**) that simulates an ICH eye in the dog. This characteristic of MCF is important in differentiating neurologic diseases of cattle. The edematous cornea masks the preceding uveitis.

Endotheliitis

Acute corneal edema that is not associated with vaccination, systemic disease, increased IOP, or overt anterior

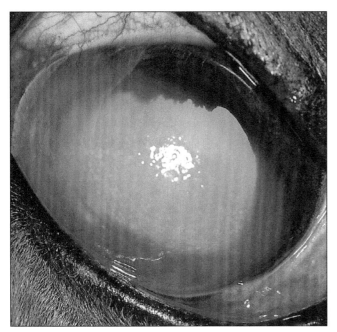

Figure 10.65 Bilateral endotheliitis in a horse without overt anterior uveitis. Cellular deposits are visible at Descemet's membrane, with overlying corneal edema. The patient responded initially to anti-inflammatory therapy, but uveitis occurred with synechia and blindness over a period of 2 years. The cause was unknown but possibly due to herpesvirus.

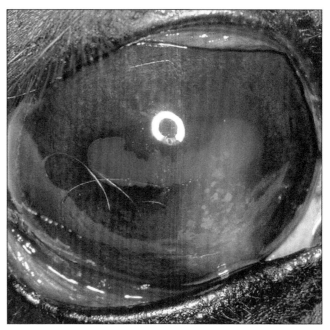

Figure 10.66 Bilateral endotheliitis in a horse without overt anterior uveitis. Cellular deposits are visible at Descemet's membrane, with overlying corneal edema. The patient responded initially to anti-inflammatory therapy, but uveitis occurred with synechia and blindness over a period of 2 years. The cause was unknown but possibly due to herpesvirus.

uveitis may represent focal endotheliitis. Focal opacities at Descemet's membrane, with overlying corneal edema, are typical. In humans, endotheliitis may be associated with autoimmunity and herpesvirus infection.[253–256]

Gratzek et al. described a condition in horses that presents with a focal to multifocal area of corneal edema that is sudden in onset.[234] Overt anterior uveitis is absent, but multifocal opacities at Descemet's membrane are visible (**Figure 10.65**). The condition is responsive to, but not cured by, topical corticosteroids or topical cyclosporine (**Figure 10.66**). The clinical signs and response to immune-suppressive medications is suggestive of endotheliitis of unknown etiology. A similar condition is reported as part of equine IMMK and is referred to as endothelial IMMK[229,230] (see section Equine immune-mediated keratitis). These conditions must be differentiated from the corneal edema of glaucoma, trauma, and anterior uveitis in the horse.

ULCERATIVE INFLAMMATORY DISEASE

Introduction/etiology

Ulcerative corneal disease has the potential to change quickly and subsequently results in disastrous ocular consequences. The signs of ocular pain are often very dramatic, and ulceration must be ruled out whenever ocular pain is present. The basic tenet when evaluating ulcers is to look for, and remove, any underlying cause (especially mechanical). Healing often occurs rapidly after correction but may be delayed for months if the underlying cause is ignored. Many factors are involved as causative agents in the development of corneal ulcers.

Physical

As with nonulcerative keratitis, it is important to look for and remove mechanical causes. Agents such as trauma, trichiasis, distichiasis, insect bites (**Figure 10.67**), and foreign bodies are common causes of ulcers in all species. Thermal burns from house and barn fires may be occasional causes of epithelial ulcerations. In the dog, a single small aberrant cilium that protrudes through the palpebral conjunctiva (see Chapter 7, section Cilia) is a frequently overlooked mechanical cause. High magnification is necessary to identify and locate the hair, but once diagnosed, the ulcer is easily treated. Foreign bodies may lodge under the third eyelid and may not be visible without eversion (see Chapter 8, section Foreign bodies of the third eyelid, **Figure 8.58**). Small foreign bodies embedded in the conjunctiva can be very difficult to detect.

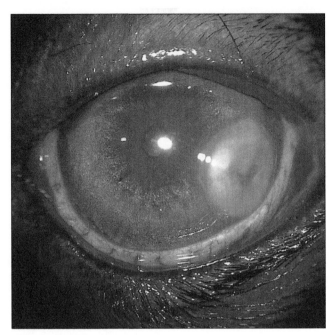

Figure 10.67 A dog with corneal malacia due to a wasp sting. There was evidence of other stings around the head. Note the lack of cellular reaction in the cornea at this time. Compare this appearance to that of a septic ulcer.

Chemical

Chemical agents such as soap and other dermatologic preparations are a common cause of diffuse superficial corneal ulceration in dogs after bathing (**Figure 10.68**). Malicious burns from strong acids or alkalis may occasionally be

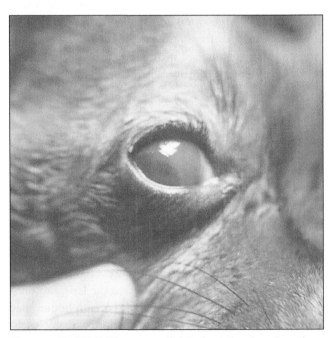

Figure 10.68 Diffuse superficial ulceration in a dog after having been bathed and groomed. Soap or chemical burns are typically diffuse. Note the miosis from corneal pain.

observed. While pet owners frequently blame corneal ulceration on mace and pepper spray, the corneal changes induced by these chemicals are mild.[257]

The defensive spray from walking stick insects (*Anisomorpha* spp.) in the southeastern quadrant of the United States is reported to cause diffuse corneal ulceration in dogs. The venom is capable of causing intense pain, blurred vision, conjunctivitis, keratitis, and corneal ulceration.[258,259]

Infectious

Bacteria, viruses (FHV-1), and fungi are the usual agents involved in ulcerative keratitis. Most surface bacterial infections are not strictly primary; other debilitating conditions often potentiate the pathogenicity of organisms that are indigenous to the ocular surface. Control of the normal ocular flora is maintained by rinsing the ocular surface with tears and blinking that pushes the tears into the nasolacrimal system. Tears also contain IgA and other antibacterial substances such as lactoferrin. Competitive interaction between the indigenous flora helps to keep the organisms low in numbers, whereas disrupting this balance may cause an overgrowth of one species. Debilitating conditions to the ocular surface such as reduced tear secretion, UV radiation, systemic disease with immunosuppression such as diabetes mellitus and Cushing's disease, and trauma which creates breaks in the epithelial barrier may allow indigenous bacteria to adhere to the ocular surface and/or overgrow, thus causing disease.

Bacteria must adhere to replicate and then invade the tissue to become established. Bacteria may differ in their ability to adhere to varying epithelial surfaces, thus explaining why organisms are relatively specific for different tissues. In most cases, adherence does not occur with healthy cells, only with injured cells, frequently associated with prior trauma. The factors involved with adhesion are incompletely understood but require both a bacterial component, such as fimbriae or pilus, and a host cellular receptor. Cellular injury may expose these cellular receptors, or the bacteria may adhere to fibronectin that is bound to the damaged cell. Once adhered, the bacteria are engulfed by the cell and then invade the stroma where inflammation is stimulated.

Inadequate tear film

An absolute lack of tears as in KCS or an inadequate tear film due to excessive exposure from lagophthalmos, facial nerve paralysis, or exophthalmos are common causes of recurrent ulceration. The Pekingese is thought to have an unstable tear film due to retention of mucus on the surface contaminating the lipid layer.[260] The resultant dry spots may result in corneal ulcers. Most nonexophthalmic dogs can tolerate facial nerve paralysis without ulcerative keratitis if the tear production is normal.

Neurotropic

Loss of sensory innervation to the cornea may result in central corneal ulceration that is slow to heal. Corneal epithelial metabolism and mitotic rate may be partially dependent on intact sensory innervation. Neurotropic ulcers may be observed with neurologic patients after laser cyclophotocoagulation[261] and after intraocular surgery.

Immunological

Large corneal epithelial erosions have been observed on occasion in the horse and the dog with autoimmune bullous skin diseases. Immune-mediated ulceration, which is more frequently observed, is indicated by the presence of peripheral ulcers adjacent to the limbus with a small rim of clear cornea (**Figures 10.69 and 10.70**). These ulcers are considered immune mediated if a mechanical cause cannot be found to explain the unusual location and if cytology is negative for infectious agents. These ulcers are typically moderately deep and may develop into a descemetocele. They may be associated with staphylococcal conjunctivitis and are thought to be a result of hypersensitivity to bacteria or toxins. Peripheral furrows that may encircle the cornea have also been observed, similar to Mooren's ulcer in humans (**Figures 10.70 and 10.74**).

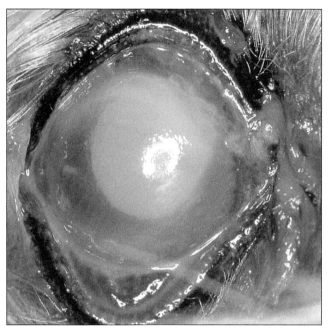

Figure 10.70 **A dog with a marginal furrow paralleling the limbus that was acute in onset. The condition was treated with cyclosporine and responded rapidly. The ulcer healed with granulation. This condition is similar to Mooren's ulcer in humans.**

Peripheral ulcers may be dramatically responsive to topical glucocorticoids or cyclosporine, but therapy must be closely monitored. This condition is one of the few exceptions where glucocorticoids are not contraindicated in treating corneal ulceration.

Macular keratitis or superficial punctate keratitis is observed in the dog and should be differentiated from superficial punctate keratopathy of Shelties. Macular keratitis is characterized by bilateral multifocal, white, superficial stromal infiltrates that are often ulcerative and are accompanied by intense pain and neovascularization (**Figures 10.71 and 10.72**).[262] The condition is typically observed in medium to small breeds of dogs; the longhaired dachshund has a predisposition. Repeated attacks leave a scarred cornea. The condition is very responsive to either topical glucocorticoid or cyclosporine therapy, with improvement noted in 24 hours (**Figure 10.73**). Low-level maintenance therapy is advised to prevent relapse of the disease.

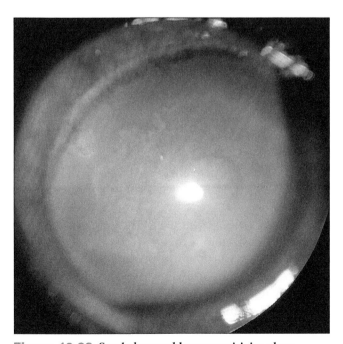

Figure 10.69 **Staphylococcal hypersensitivity ulcer adjacent to the limbus in a dog with staphylococcal keratoconjunctivitis. The central ulcer is almost healed, and this was the initiating problem. The patient responded quickly to topical antibiotic and corticosteroid therapy.**

It is prudent for the clinician to realize that ulceration associated with an immunologic pathogenesis is uncommon. These cases require therapy that is antithetical to dogma for treating most ulcers and, consequently, should be followed closely by the clinician.

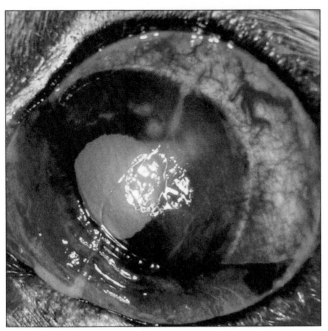

Figure 10.71 Macular keratitis in a cocker spaniel. Multifocal white superficial infiltrates stained with fluorescein are present. The condition was bilateral. Note the intense vascular reaction in the conjunctiva and the cornea. Compare with Figure 10.73 taken after therapy.

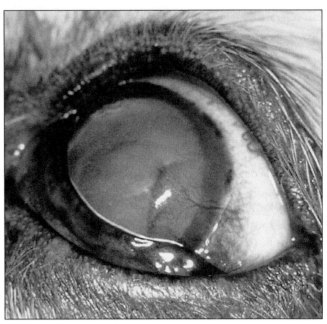

Figure 10.73 Same as patient in Figure 10.71 after only 48 hours of topical cyclosporine and corticosteroid therapy.

Metabolic

Cushing's disease is associated with ulceration characterized by rapid progression and slow healing. It is unknown whether the elevated endogenous steroids induce an ulcer or whether they simply complicate an ulcer from another cause. The elevated steroid levels are thought to activate MMPs (collagenase) and turn an incidental ulcer into a sight-threatening disease. Lassaline-Utter et al. has reported superficial nonhealing ulcerations in horses with pituitary pars intermedia dysfunction (PPID).[263] Horses with PPID have decreased corneal sensitivity, which may be a contributing factor for the slow healing of corneal ulcers in these horses.[20] Increased endogenous cortisol levels in tears following simulated stress in horse has been documented by Monk et al.[264] Whether tear cortisol levels in PPID have a negative effect on corneal healing needs further investigation.

Dystrophic corneal changes

Endothelial dystrophy with severe corneal edema often results in bullae that rupture, producing an ulcer that may heal slowly or allow bacterial contamination. More commonly, spontaneous epithelial erosions that are usually very slow to heal (indolent epithelial ulcers) are thought to result from abnormalities in the basal epithelial cells and consequent basal lamina changes.

A corneal dystrophy that may represent a variant of pellucid marginal degenerations is reported in Friesian horses and is characterized by bilateral symmetric ulcerative corneal lesions that range in depth from superficial

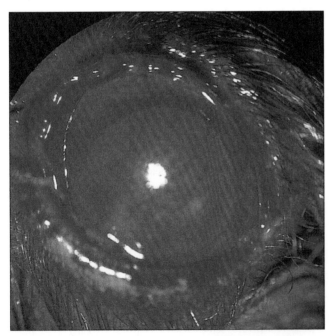

Figure 10.72 Macular keratitis in a miniature poodle. Characteristic multifocal white infiltrates with an intense vascular reaction are present. The condition was bilateral and responded quickly to topical corticosteroids.

facets to perforations.[265] The lesions are typically progressive, located in the inferior cornea, and respond well to surgical treatment. All affected horses share a common ancestor and may represent an inherited corneal dystrophy in the breed.

Clinical signs

Signs of ocular pain such as blepharospasm and epiphora are the most common reason for presentation with a corneal ulcer. Ocular discharge is usually mucopurulent with septic ulcers. Superficial corneal ulcers and erosions often present with more dramatic pain than deep ulcerations. On examination, the normal smooth corneal surface is usually irregular and may have varying degrees of corneal opacification due to focal corneal edema and/or leukocytic infiltration. Corneal neovascularization is stimulated with stromal and septic ulcers, but epithelial erosions may go for weeks without stimulating a vascular response. The duration of the ulcer can often be surmised by the vascular response.

Diagnosis

Fluorescein staining is performed when there is any undiagnosed ocular pain. While fluorescein may not be necessary to diagnose an ulcer, it is valuable in evaluating the healing progress. Descemetoceles have no overlying stroma to retain fluorescein stain (**Figure 10.74**). Stromal ulcers require both fibroplasia and epithelial healing to fill in the defect. Technically, deep ulcers can be "healed" over with epithelium, but they often retain a facet or depression for months and may be mechanically weak. When evaluating facets in the stroma with fluorescein stain, the eye is thoroughly rinsed to remove pooled fluorescein in the tear film and to avoid a false-positive interpretation. Corneal scrapings for cytology are a rapid and inexpensive method to help rule out bacterial and fungal causes of ulcerative keratitis. These methods are routinely used for any progressive or nonhealing ulcer. Cytology results are used to guide therapy until the results of cultures are known.

Therapy

All corneal ulcers have the potential for rapid change and thus must be monitored frequently (every 2–3 days) or the patient hospitalized (for high risk patients such as brachycephalic breeds). Since the epithelial barrier is broken, bacterial infection by resident flora is possible, and topical prophylactic antibiotics are routine therapy. Superficial ulcers are usually more painful than deep ulcers and topical atropine, given every 12–24 hours to reduce reflex ciliary spasms, is the second arm of routine topical therapy. Topical anesthetics are too toxic to use therapeutically. In the horse, systemic prostaglandin (PG) inhibitors are commonly administered for ocular pain. Most uncomplicated ulcers heal in 3–5 days, but indolent or very slow healing superficial ulcers are not uncommon.

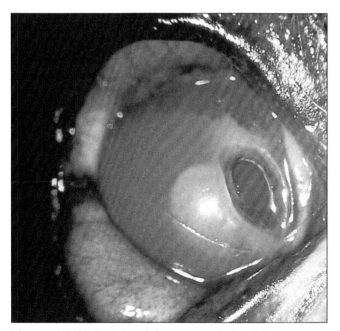

Figure 10.74 **Peripheral descemetocele in a West Highland white terrier. The lesion was sterile and progressed around the circumference, despite performing a hood conjunctival flap. The diagnosis was a probable Mooren's ulcer.**

Indolent epithelial erosion/spontaneous chronic corneal epithelial defects (slow healing ulcer, boxer ulcer, rodent ulcer)

Introduction/etiology

Indolent epithelial ulcers are common and may occur in all species. They may be divided into those with edema and those with little, if any, edema. Those with corneal edema are probably secondary to epithelial and subepithelial bulla formation from endothelial disease, as previously discussed.

Spontaneous ulcers without significant corneal edema are typically epithelial ulcers with little tendency to progress in depth, but they may spread over the surface. It may be months until vascularization is stimulated, and the ulcer heals by granulation.

Indolent epithelial ulcers, originally thought to be specific to boxers,[266] are reported to occur in a variety of breeds.[267–269] Biopsies from superficial keratectomies are characterized by degenerative changes in the basal epithelial cells, loosely adhered epithelium near the ulcer margin, disorganized epithelial maturation, incomplete or absent basal lamina over the ulcer, production of an irregular basal lamina beside the ulcer, and a mild neutrophilic or lymphocytic infiltration.[267,268] Bentley et al. and Murphy et al. have reported similar findings in the epithelium but normal or possibly thicker basal lamina in areas distant to the ulcer.[270, 269] They also report an acellular layer on the ulcer bed that is PAS-positive and covered with fibronectin but irregularly with lamina, collagen IV, and collagen VII. Whether these changes are the cause of the ulcers or the result of chronic epithelial loss is unknown. Murphy et al. reports normal corneal sensation in dogs with chronic epithelial erosions and increased numbers of substance P nerves in the epithelium adjacent to the ulcer.[269]

Occasionally the condition is bilateral, but usually the second eye is affected later. Approximately 50% of patients may have a recurrence in the same or opposite eye. The mean age of onset in the boxer is 6 years, and the right eye is affected most commonly.[267,268,271,272] The relatively recent discovery that the corneal epithelial stem cell is at the limbus may suggest that the problem is at the limbus rather than in the basal cells. In rabbits, loss of limbal epithelium results in recurrent ulceration, delayed healing, and corneal vascularization after a delay of 6 months.[273]

Corneal sensitivity may be altered by disease and surgical procedures at or near the limbus. Diabetic dogs have decreased corneal sensitivity compared to normal dogs, but no correlation exists with either the duration or the control of diabetes.[21] Decreased corneal sensitivity may promote corneal ulceration by reduced blinking and lacrimation, thus exposing the cornea to various traumatic stimuli, or through deficiencies of neurotrophic regulation of epithelial proliferation, migration, and adhesion. The predisposition to epithelial ulcers with altered corneal nerves may also be mediated through substance P nerves.[269]

Indolent epithelial ulcers are observed in the cat and are typically central or paracentral. These ulcers are overrepresented in Persian and Himalayan breeds. La Croix et al. report on 29 cats with 36 indolent ulcers.[274] The mean age of 7.7 years, and no sex predilection is reported in the cats. A history of previous respiratory infection or recurrent conjunctivitis is reported in 72% of the cats, reinforcing the clinical suspicion that many cases are associated with FHV.

Slow to nonhealing epithelial ulcers are described in the horse.[275–279] The clinical signs are like those in the dog with a loose epithelial border. The mean age of horses with superficial nonhealing ulcers is reported to be 12–14 years of age.[277,278] The predominate histological features in horses with superficial nonhealing ulcers are epithelial nonadherence, epithelial dysmaturity, and mild-to-moderate stromal inflammation. The anterior stromal acelluar hyaline zone common in dogs is absent in horses with superficial nonhealing ulcers.[279]

Nonhealing epithelial ulcers in the horse appear refractory to most therapies apart from diamond burr or superficial keratectomy. However, debridement and grid keratotomy have been described as a potential treatment in the horse.[277,278]

Hakanson and Dubielzig have described chronic epithelial ulcers that did not have loose epithelial borders in a subset of horses.[280] These ulcers had a thin, acellular membrane on the anterior stroma. The authors suggest these findings represent a corneal sequestrum. Unlike the cat, the sequestrum remains superficial and does not pigment.

Clinical signs

Superficial epithelial ulcers with loose epithelial borders is the diagnostic criterion for an indolent ulcer (**Figure 10.75**). The ulcer is usually central or paracentral. Unlike a simple abrasion, the ulcer fails to heal within 1 week and may spread around the cornea, healing on one side and extending on the other side. Gross corneal edema is minimal or absent, and neovascularization is not stimulated for an extended period of time. Very chronic lesions heal by granulation. Many dogs exhibit severe pain, but this is quite variable.

Diagnosis

Diagnosis is on the presence of a nonhealing epithelial ulcer with loose, overhanging epithelial borders and with no mechanical cause.

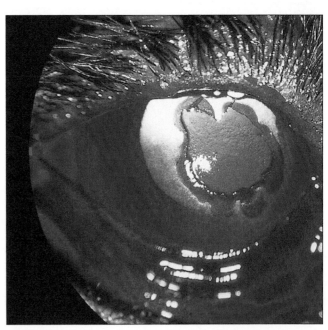

Figure 10.75 A dog with spontaneous epithelial erosion with loose epithelial edges. Note the diffusion of the rose bengal stain under the loose epithelium.

Therapy

Indolent ulcers can be managed in a variety of ways, with no single therapy working consistently. When healing does not occur in the expected time, the condition should be reevaluated to make sure a mechanical cause is not present.

Medical

Routine medical therapy consists of prophylactic topical antibiotics and, if the condition is painful, atropine. Hypertonic topical preparations to dehydrate the cornea are often advised but when compared critically are of no benefit unless the ulcer is accompanied by marked corneal edema. Prominent corneal edema may be seen with granulations tissue or posterior corneal epithelial damage.

Topical fibronectin shows promise in treating persistent epithelial defects; purified fibronectin may be a means of treating the condition in the future.[281] Topical serum is used with success as a source of fibronectin and other growth factors when treating humans with indolent epithelial ulcers from a variety of causes.[282] Topical recombinant epidermal growth factor (100 µg/mL) given every 6 hours healed 8/10 indolent corneal ulcers in dogs.[283] This concentration may be excessive. Studies in the rabbit indicate that >5 µg/mL stimulates healing, and a maximum healing rate is obtained with 20 µg/mL.[284] Epidermal growth factor does not appear to be indicated with erosions from corneal edema or with herpesvirus ulcers.

Topical 5% polysulfonated GAG (PGAG) has been advocated for the treatment of indolent epithelial ulcers, with a healing rate of 82% after corneal debridement.[285] PGAG is an inhibitor of proteolytic enzymes. It may benefit epithelial healing if there is an imbalance in proteolytic activity that promotes epithelial cell migration at the expense of disrupting cellular adhesion. Seventy-seven percent of dogs with epithelial ulcers are reported to have elevated levels of proteolytic activity that were decreased with PGAG therapy and returned to normal levels when healed.[286]

Murphy et al. treated 21 dogs with chronic epithelial defects with topical substance P and achieved 70%–75% healing.[269] While this novel therapy appears highly successful, other procedures are similarly successful. Why additional substance P is beneficial when increased amounts are found in the cornea of dogs with chronic epithelial erosions is not addressed in the study.

Dogs with refractory corneal ulcers treated with topical oxytetracycline (every 8 hours) or oral doxycycline (5 mg/kg, every 12 hours) in conjunction with corneal debridement and grid keratotomy are reported to have a shorter heal time than control dogs.[287] It is speculated that the shorter heal time may be related to the fact that tetracyclines are protease inhibitors and upregulate TGF-β family members and transcription factors. The ability of tetracycline to inhibit MMPs may not be a factor in the increase healing rate, as MMP-2 and MMP-9 are thought not to play a role in the pathogenesis of refractory corneal ulcers in dogs.[288] TGF-β is documented to be decreased in the tears of dogs with refractive corneal ulcers[289] and upregulated by tetracycline in corneal epithelial cells in *in vitro* studies.[290]

In the cat, herpesvirus should be considered when treating a superficial nonhealing ulcer; oral and/or topical antirviral therapy may be indicated.

Soft contact lenses are available for both the dog and the horse and may be used as a pressure bandage to aid healing.[291,292] Depending on the fit and the conformation, the lens may not be retained and, if lost, results in significant financial loss, especially in the horse. In humans, soft contact lenses slow healing and increase the complication rate when used in the treatment of ulcers.[293,294] In cats with intact corneas, extended contact lens wear results in reduced epithelial adhesion due to a reduced concentration of hemidesmosomes.[295] Corneal debridement, grid keratotomy, or diamond burr debridement followed by the placement of a bandage contact lens are shown to decrease the healing time in dogs with indolent ulcers when compared to control groups.[296–299]

An alternative to soft lenses in the dog is to use a commercially available collagen shield. While this tends to be retained better than a soft lens, it dissolves over a period of 3–5 days and may not last long enough to be effective.[300] In a controlled study comparing various therapies for epithelial ulcers, Morgan and Abrams report that debridement alone and collagen shields are the least successful therapies.[301]

Surgical

Debridement

If an epithelial erosion has loose edges or a history of slow healing, the edges are debrided mechanically with a cotton-tip applicator, no matter what other therapy is planned. This is especially important if the margins are loose and nonadherent. Debridement may remove a much larger area of epithelium than the original ulcer, but the epithelium regenerates rapidly and often heals with no further specific therapy (**Figures 10.76 and 10.77**).

Punctate or linear keratotomy

Keratotomy in combination with epithelial debridement is the first choice of many clinicians for surgical therapy in the dog. The technique consists of multiple punctures or crosshatching of the basement membrane with a 25-gauge needle (**Figure 10.78**). This can be performed with topical

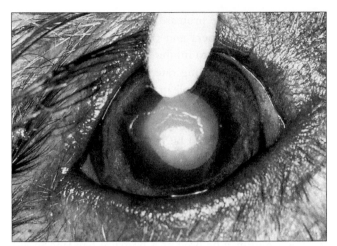

Figure 10.76 A dog with epithelial erosion before debridement with a cotton-tip applicator.

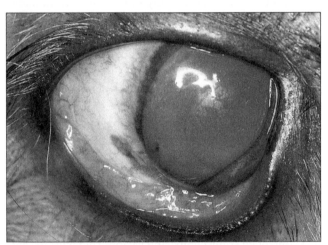

Figure 10.77 Same erosion as Figure 10.76 after debridement of the loose epithelium and application of a soft contact lens. The amount of epithelium removed is often startling for the veterinarian and the owner.

anesthesia alone. Keratotomy exposes the epithelium to the stroma, which promotes a more secure binding of the epithelium. There are many theories to explain the benefit of a keratotomy: Penetrating the basal lamina to expose the epithelial cells to the stroma, thus promoting adhesions; breaching the basal lamina coupled with an abnormal hyaline zone in the superficial cornea may be inhibiting epithelial adhesion;[302] and stimulating extracellular matrix proteins promotes epithelial adhesions.[303] Healing occurs within 1–2 weeks in most instances. The healing rate with a grid keratotomy is variably reported as 72%–85% after one treatment,[301–305] with a mean healing time of 13 days.[302]

Michau et al. treated nonhealing superficial corneal ulcers in horses with either debridement, debridement and grid keratotomy, or superficial keratectomy.[277] The shortest healing time is reported to be 15 days, but only

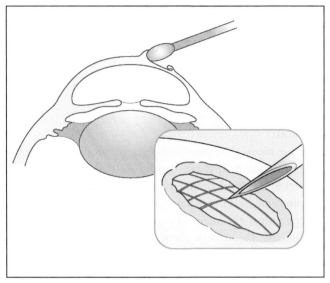

Figure 10.78 Treatment of an indolent epithelial ulcer with debridement of the epithelium and a grid keratotomy with a 25-gauge needle.

63% healed with debridement alone. Seventy-eight percent of the keratotomy group healed with the remainder either undergoing a second keratotomy or a keratectomy. All cases of keratectomies healed. In a study by Brünott et al., eight of nine cases healed with debridement and a grid keratotomy, with a mean healing of 8 days.[278] In the author's experience, most of the slow-healing equine epithelial ulcers have minimal loose epithelium, which can be debrided, and they have not responded to grid keratotomies, even when repeated. Therefore, the author has gone directly to diamond burr or standing superficial keratectomies. The time and type of sedation necessary is the same as a grid keratotomy.

Grid keratotomies are performed as a last resort in the cat. La Croix et al. report that 31% of cats with indolent epithelial ulcers treated by debridement and keratotomies developed a corneal sequestrum, whereas 10% developed a sequestrum when treated by debridement alone.[274] In addition, if the indolent ulcers in the cat is associated with herpesvirus, an additional concern with keratotomies is inoculation of the virus deeper into the stroma to produce a stromal keratitis.

> Keratotomies are utilized only in the treatment of indolent superficial epithelial ulcers and not for the treatment of stromal ulcers.

Diamond burr

Diamond burr debridement is used in refractory indolent ulcers. Corneal debridement with a cotton-tip applicator

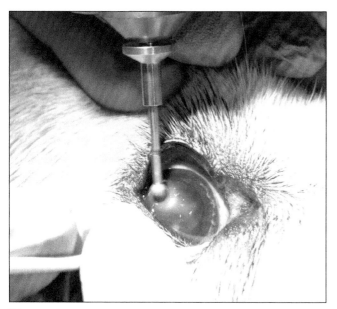

Figure 10.79 Treatment of an indolent ulcer with a diamond burr. Following debridement with a cotton-tip applicator, the loose epithelium and the anterior stroma are debrided with a diamond burr.

is performed just prior to diamond burr debridement to remove loose corneal epithelium. Diamond burr debridement is performed with a handheld, battery-operated diamond burr unit (Algerbrush, Alger Equipment Company) with a 2.5- or 3.5-mm burr in either a fine or medium grit (**Figure 10.79**). With Diamond burr debridement and placement of a bandage contact lens, Gosling et al. report 70% of indolent ulcers in dogs heal in 7 days, and 92.5% heal in 15.5 ± 5.5 days.[298] In a separate study, the healing time with diamond burr debridement and contact lens application is reported to be 9.37 ± 0.42 days.[299] In horses, diamond burr debridement has a 92% heal rate with a healing time of 15.5 days ± 9.32 days.[263] Diamond burr debridement decreases the associated superficial stromal hyaline acellular zone in dogs. The reduction in the hyaline acellular zone is suggested to be a factor in the decreased healing time after diamond burr debridement.[306]

Superficial keratectomy

A superficial keratectomy is successful in 100% of cases, but it is technically more difficult, requires general anesthesia in dogs and cats, and thus is more expensive (see section Dermoid, **Figure 10.120**). The theoretical benefit of a superficial keratectomy is to remove the abnormal basal lamina and underlying hyaline membrane present in the anterior stroma. The author uses superficial keratectomies in dogs only in those patients resistant to other therapies but uses the procedure routinely in cats and horses. In the horse, superficial keratectomies can be performed

standing under heavy sedation combined with topical anesthesia. In cats with refractory ulcers, 85% heal within 4 weeks following a superficial keratectomy.[307]

Temporary tarsorrhaphy/third eyelid flap

Historically, third eyelid flaps have been used in the treatment of indolent ulcers. However, third eyelid flaps are less effective than other procedures in promoting healing of superficial indolent ulcers. The mean healing time following the placement of a third eyelid flap is 17.9 days, with a healing rate of 68%.[308] In the author's opinion, third eyelid flaps are not to be used as the sole treatment. A third eyelid flap does nothing to improve cellular adhesion. Therefore, it is important to at least debride the ulcer before placing a third eyelid flap (see **Figures 10.89 through 10.91**). When treating indolent ulcerations, the author believes that placement of a temporary tarsorraphy is just as effective as or more effective than a third eyelid flap.

Viral ulcers in cats

Introduction/etiology

FHV-1 commonly produces an epithelial ulcer that may be dendritic (linear branching) or geographic (irregular), or when complicated, a stromal ulcer can develop that has the potential to progress into a descemetocele. In severe instances, keratouveitis may develop with marked corneal edema and epithelial bullae formation. One or both eyes may be involved. Affected cats are usually not ill with respiratory disease and typically are young adult cats.[309,310] The epithelial ulceration is usually the primary infection and is self-limiting, being up to 24 days in experimental cats.[251] However, epithelial ulcers may develop in latently infected older cats.

Most cats with herpesvirus become lifelong carriers. The virus resides in a latent form in the sensory ganglia, specifically the trigeminal ganglion for the eye.[311] Recent evidence suggests the corneal stroma may also host the herpesvirus in a latent and an active form in normal feline corneas.[249,312–314]

Clinical signs

The cat usually presents with epiphora and mild blepharospasm. The typical lesion is a superficial, linear or irregular ulcer (**Figures 10.80 through 10.82**), which is usually epithelial if uncomplicated. Lesions begin as small dots that coalesce to form a linear erosion, but they may progress in depth. Due to the small size of the lesions, a blue light and/or magnification may be necessary to detect fluorescein staining. Rose bengal staining may be preferred due to the epithelial necrosis that the virus produces. Stromal keratitis may develop later in one or both

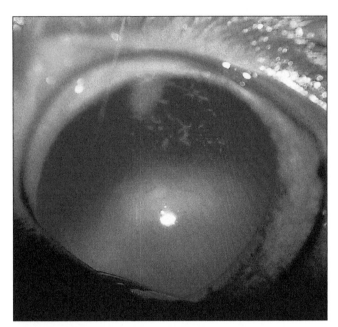

Figure 10.80 Herpesvirus dendritic epithelial ulcer in a cat viewed against the fundus reflection and after staining with fluorescein. Small dots, branching linear lesions, and a geographic erosion are present.

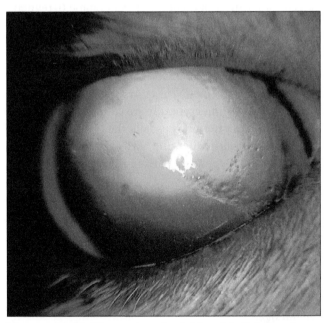

Figure 10.81 Herpesvirus dendritic epithelial ulcer in a cat viewed against the tapetal reflection. Note the linear opacity with small branches and, beyond the linear opacity, small punctate defects.

eyes and appears as diffuse neovascularization with multifocal gray maculae. Epithelial erosions may or may not be present with stromal keratitis (**Figures 10.58, 10.61, and 10.62**). Affected cats may have a history of intermittent sneezing and ocular discharge, indicating a carrier state.

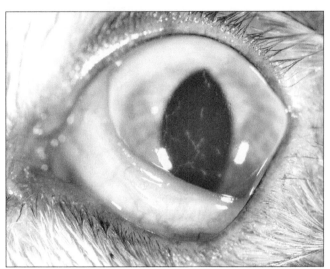

Figure 10.82 A cat with multiple linear dendritic epithelial ulcers noted after fluorescein staining.

Diagnosis

Diagnosis of herpesvirus ocular lesions is often difficult due to the carrier state and the ubiquitous nature of the virus; herpesvirus can be either cultured, or detected with PCR, from 10% of conjunctivae and from 50% of corneas of normal cats.[314] Herpesvirus has been detected in 11% and 28% of normal cats positive for herpesvirus using virus isolation and indirect fluorescent antibody (IFA) testing, respectively.[315]

IFA testing of conjunctiva or corneal scrapings for herpesvirus is the easiest definitive test, but in the author's experience is rarely positive unless performed early in the disease process. Previous fluorescein staining of the cornea has been reported to give a false-positive IFA test. With routine preparation, conjunctival cytology results typically consist of lymphocytes and polymorphonuclear cells, but inclusion bodies are rarely seen.[316] Cytology specimens fixed in Bouin's solution for 1 hour retains the inclusion bodies.[317]

Biopsy via a superficial keratectomy may demonstrate virus particles on electron microscopy or inclusion bodies on light microscopy. Viral cultures have traditionally been considered the gold standard for diagnosing herpesvirus, but PCR testing is more sensitive. The detection of FHV-1 DNA by PCR is dependent on the clinical stage of the disease, collection methods, laboratory methods, and population of cats tested.[250,314,318,319] FHV-1 DNA has been detected in 39% of cats with ocular disease consistent with FHV-1.[250] The percentage of samples positive for FHV-1 DNA depends on whether the cat presents with conjunctivitis, dendritic ulcers, stromal keratitis, or corneal sequestration. FHV-1 DNA can be detected in cats with dendritic ulcers. In samples from cats with cytological identification of intranuclear inclusion bodies consistent with FHV-1, FHV-1 DNA can be detected in 66.6%. FHV-1 DNA has been detected in 54% of conjunctival biopsies and 50% of cytobrush samples from cats with conjunctivitis.[314] As many as 86.6% of cats in a shelter setting with conjunctivitis and respiratory tract disease have tested positive for FHV-1 by PCR.[314] It is pertinent to interpret PRC results for FHV-1 with caution, as false positive and negative results are possible.

When the clinical presentation is a dendritic epithelial ulcer, it is considered pathognomonic for herpesvirus. Sneezing or upper respiratory signs are additional indicative signs of a presumptive diagnosis of herpesvirus infection. Last, the response to specific antiviral therapy may be used retrospectively to diagnose herpesvirus infection.

Therapy
Antiviral
Topical: To be effective, topical antivirals must be given every 4 to 6 hours. Idoxuridine (IDU) was the first specific antiviral agent used to treat herpesvirus ulcerative keratitis. Cidofovir, vidarabine, and trifluorothymidine (TFT) are newer antiherpes medications, with the latter being more effective, less toxic, and having better corneal penetration. The commercially availability of vidarabine is variable and currently must be compounded into a 3% ophthalmic ointment. Vidarabine appears to be well tolerated, but its efficacy is questionable in cats.[320] TFT is the only commercially obtainable antiviral in the United States that is available for use in cats. However, TFT is very expensive, which limits it for routine use. Topical ophthalmic acyclovir (acycloguanosine) is available in Europe, but preliminary tests indicate poor activity against FHV-1.[321,322] Contrary to the *in situ* results, Williams et al. report clinical improvement in feline herpes syndromes with topical 0.5% acyclovir given five times a day.[323] While *in situ* testing indicates limited effectiveness, topical 0.5% cidofovir every 12 hours in experimental herpes significantly decreased the severity of the clinical signs and viral shedding. Cidofovir has the advantage of decreased frequency of dosing because of its long half-life in ocular tissues.[324] Ganciclovir 0.15% ophthalmic gel is approved as a topical ophthalmic preparation for humans. It is effective against FHV-1 *in vitro*,[325,326] but its safety and efficacy *in vivo* has not been evaluated in the cat.

> In the United States, trifluorothymidine 1% ophthalmic solution is the only commercially available topical ophthalmic for use in cats. Acyclovir 5% ophthalmic solution, idoxuridine 0.1%, and cidofovir 0.5% are used off label and must be compounded for topical ophthalmic use.

Oral: Some strains of herpesvirus become resistant to acyclovir because they can replicate with cellular thymidine kinase. Acyclovir is available for systemic use but, unfortunately, is not a good option in the cat because therapeutic levels produce renal, liver, and bone marrow toxicity.[327] Oral famciclovir is effective in treating FHV-1 in cats.[328-330] The published doses for famciclovir are variable. The most commonly recommended dose is 40 mg/kg (every 8 hours).[330,331] However, lower doses at 62.5 mg/kg (every 12–24 hours) and 125 mg/kg (every 8 hours) are reported to be effective.[328] Experimentally, a dose of 90 mg/kg (every 8 hours) is reported to be well tolerated without detectable side effect in cats.[329] This is an off-label use of the drug, so appropriate caution should be exercised.

Interferon Recombinant human leukocyte interferon is synergistic with acyclovir in inhibiting FHV-1 replication in tissue culture.[332] This has prompted either topical or oral use of interferon in conjunction with topical antivirals in patients who have been unresponsive to antivirals alone. Topical interferon is empirically formulated at 0.5–1 IU drop of artificial tear solution and is clinically successful. Vennebusch reports feline omega interferon given five times a day for 20 days produces a 32% improvement in keratitis by day 6 and 70% by day 20.[333] Feline recombinant interferon is not approved in the United States, and human or bovine interferon is usually substituted. In controlled experimental FHV-1 infections in specific pathogen-free (SPF) cats, recombinant feline interferon omega given topically at 10,000 U every 12 hours and orally at 20,000 U every 12 hours for 48 hours before infecting with FHV-1 resulted in no difference from controls in virus load, clinical scores, course of the disease, and virus shedding.[334] The treated group was reported to have more epithelial disease than the control group. In a separate study, Slack et al. reported no improvement in clinical signs or viral shedding in cats with viral keratoconjunctivitis with the topical application of feline recombinant interferon omega and human recombinant interferon α-2b.[335]

L-lysine Oral L-lysine (500 mg every 12 hours) reduces the severity of herpesvirus conjunctivitis in cats[336] and is presumably beneficial in treating corneal manifestations of herpesvirus infection. L-lysine (400 mg every 24 hours) decreases the amount of viral shedding with mild stressors but does not prevent shedding when challenged with glucocorticoid administration.[337] A proposed mechanism of action of L-lysine is by competing with arginine for absorption from the gut and the renal tubule. Arginine is required for *in vitro* replication of herpesvirus, and elevated levels of L-lysine may deprive the virus of arginine.[338]

Oral L-lysine (500 mg every 12 hours) produces elevated plasma levels of lysine but does not affect plasma levels of arginine. This is fortunate for therapy as the cat is very sensitive to a deficiency in arginine.[336,337] There is anecdotal evidence that L-lysine is beneficial in some cats. The current dosage recommendations are to give 500 mg (every 12 hours) to adult cats and 250 mg (every 12 hours) to kittens.[331]

Immunosuppressants The use of immunosuppressants in stromal keratitis may be considered with moderate-to-severe disease, but it is recommended that concurrent antiviral drugs are used. Glucocorticoids are blamed for many of the progressive ulcerative conditions seen in herpesvirus keratitis of humans.[339] Experimental feline herpesvirus infection is made much more severe with glucocorticoid immunosuppression.[311] In addition, glucocorticoid dependence and a rebound effect after cessation of glucocorticoid use may occur.[339,340] Topical cyclosporine may be effective with feline herpesvirus stromal conditions. However, cyclosporine therapy is used with caution and in conjunction with antiviral therapy.[341] Systemic cyclosporine has been documented to prolong and increase the severity of experimental stromal keratitis in rabbits.[342]

Prophylaxis

Prior vaccination against FHV-1 infection may not prevent the development of subsequent ocular manifestations, nor is it of value as therapy. Prior vaccination of animals with an intranasal vaccine failed to alter the latency of FHV-1 or detection of virus shedding in various tissues after experimentally induced relapses.[343] FHV vaccination mainly decreases the severity and the duration of the signs but does not prevent infection or latency.[344] This is of special concern to breeders of cats that develop severe problems. Persian cats seem to have more frequent and more severe ocular symptoms.

Good preventive medicine measures can decrease the incidence of herpesvirus infection in a cattery. Quarantining new cats for several weeks before admission to the cattery, segregation of cats by age group and pregnancy status, good ventilation (10 air exchanges/hour) and sanitation, disposable food, water, and litter trays, and handling the younger cats before the older cats are helpful in decreasing the spread of herpesvirus. Obvious carriers of the virus such as cats with sinusitis and recurrent conjunctivitis are to be removed from the colony. If dealing with a problem cattery, early vaccination with a killed vaccine followed later with a live virus vaccine is recommended.[345]

Screening for FeLV and FIV may be helpful in explaining frequent and severe forms of herpesvirus infection in a cattery. Stressing latent carriers with 5 mg/kg methylprednisolone injections and identifying carriers with viral cultures of saliva 8–10 days later has been useful in a pathogen-free colony to cull carriers and therefore reduce the incidence of upper respiratory disease.[346] This protocol was repeated after an interval of 6 weeks. Nevertheless, 8 months later, another outbreak of herpesvirus upper respiratory tract infection developed after a stressing event.

Viral ulcers in dogs Canine herpesvirus-1 (CHV-1) is present worldwide in the canine population. It is predominately fetal and neonatal infections that result in abortion or death.[347,348] In neonates, ocular disease ranges from extraocular disease (keratitis) to intraocular disease (uveitis, optic neuritis, and retinal dysplasia).[349,350] Recently, studies by Ledbetter et al. identified CHV-1 in adult dogs with ocular disease.[351] Conjunctivitis, ulcerative keratitis (punctate, dendritic, and geographic ulcers), and nonulcerative keratitis (perilimbal superficial corneal neovascularization with leukocyte infiltration) are the most common ocular signs associated with CHV-1 infections in adult dogs.[252] Most dogs that present with CHV-1 ocular disease are systemic and locally immunosuppressed either from disease or medications.[351–355] Treatment consist of topical antibiotics to prevent secondary bacterial infections and topical antiviral medications.[348]

Viral ulcers in horses Equine herpesvirus-1 (EHV-1) has been incriminated as a cause of a multifocal superficial punctate keratitis (**Figure 10.83**). The keratitis may be accompanied by frank corneal ulceration or fine punctate fluorescein staining. The etiology is not proven but is suggested to be herpesvirus-induced based on it is responsive to antiviral therapy.[356] Equine herpesvirus-2 has been isolated from an outbreak of keratoconjunctivitis in foals. The clinical signs of keratoconjunctivitis associated with EHV-2 are characterized by epiphora, mucopurulent discharge, conjunctivitis, and superficial focal macular opacities.[357] Keratoconjunctivitis characterized by epiphora, blepharospasm, and focal crystalline deposits with punctate fluorescein staining has been observed in 12 horses.[358] Equine herpes-2 virus has been isolated from corneal biopsies in two foals with a unilateral keratoconjunctivitis. Two horses with similar lesions responded to antiviral therapy.[359] Topical glucocorticoids results in relapse of the lesions. The significance of herpesvirus in equine keratitis is unknown, but evidence suggests that consideration must be given as an etiology in ulcerative and nonulcerative keratitis. Small subepithelial white foci associated with EHV must be differentiated from superficial fungal keratitis.

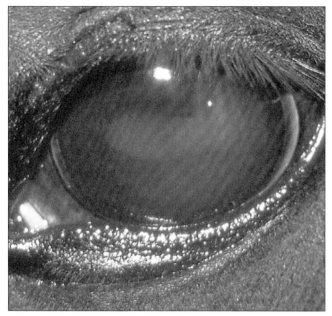

Figure 10.83 Faint subepithelial macular opacities in a horse. Herpesvirus was suspected, but biopsies and culture could not confirm the diagnosis.

Corneal sequestrum (nigrum)

Introduction/etiology

In the Persian, Siamese, and, occasionally, domestic shorthaired (DSH) cats, slow-healing epithelial defects from a variety of causes may result in a corneal nigrum or sequestrum. This is a brown-black plaque or deposit that is usually central or paracentral and stimulates vascularization (**Figure 10.84**). On occasion, the plaque may occupy most of the cornea. The lesion may or may not be painful and occasionally can be bilateral. It may begin as a small superficial spot and progresses quickly (2–3 weeks) in width and depth. The black appearance has been speculated to be iron, catecholamines, and desiccation. A study by Featherstone suggests that melanin may be associated with the sequestrum's color.[360] Souri has suggested that tear film or mucus combined with a small initiating ulcer plays a role in the condition.[361] Although porphyrins have been speculated to be associated with the development of corneal sequestra, Newkirk et al. documented that porphyrins are absent in normal lacrimal glands, cornea, and corneal sequestra of cats, indicating that porphyrins are not the cause of the brown/amber color of corneal sequestra.[362] Cats that develop sequestra usually have a similar colored mucus on the lid margins whenever the eyes are irritated (**Figure 10.85**). This mucus is not from tears (since the mucus is observed in cats with no tears) but apparently from the glands of the conjunctiva or the lids. One study found no difference in tear proteins from normal cats and cats with sequestra.[363] Featherstone has documented

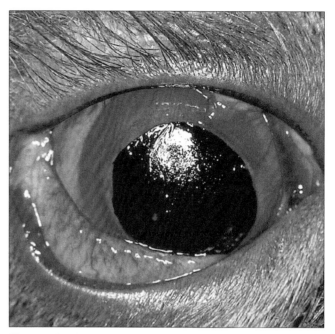

Figure 10.84 Large corneal sequestrum in a Persian cat. Note the conjunctivitis and corneal neovascularization. The patient was treated with a keratectomy and conjunctival pedicle flap.

that cats with cornea sequestra have significantly lower tear lipid than normal-control cats.[360]

The predisposing ulcerative condition may be obvious or occult, such as from small herpesvirus epithelial defects. This is supported by the development of corneal

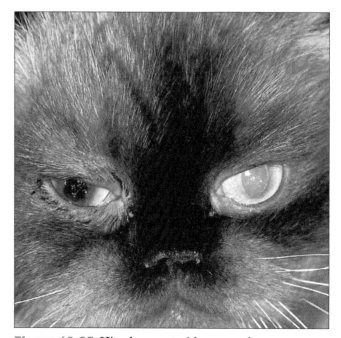

Figure 10.85 Himalayan cat with a corneal sequestrum. Note the blepharospasm and the brown-black discharge caked on the eyelids.

sequestra in 50% of cats with experimental herpesvirus infection and chronic ulcerations secondary to glucocorticoid therapy.[251] Results of PCR testing for herpesvirus in cats with corneal sequestra is variable. The percentage of positive PCR testing for herpesvirus ranges from 18% to 80% depending on the breed.[210,314] In the domestic longhaired (DLH) cat, the rate of recovery of herpesvirus is reported to be 80%, while in the Persian-Himalayan breeds, it is reported to be 50%, suggesting an alternative pathogenesis for the development of corneal sequestrum in these breeds. In cats with sequestra, Cullen et al. report the detection of FHV-1 DNA in 4/9 corneas, toxoplasma gondii DNA in 4/9 corneas, and the detection of both in one cat.[364] The histopathologic lesions of corneal sequestra are desiccated and degenerative stromal necrosis, with an adjacent zone of inflammatory cells.[365–368]

Clinical signs
The appearance of a black plaque on the cat cornea is almost pathognomonic for corneal sequestrum. The surface of the plaque may be smooth or roughened. Normally the plaque is assumed to enlarge slowly; however, progression from a pinpoint spot to a much larger lesion of 6–7 mm in 2–3 weeks can be seen. As the condition progresses, the plaque separates from the adjacent tissue and may eventually slough from the surface. Ocular pain and corneal fluorescein staining is variable.

Diagnosis
Diagnosis is on clinical appearance.

Therapy
Therapy is somewhat controversial, with two camps, the cutters and the observers. If the eye is comfortable, one may wait weeks to months for spontaneous sloughing. The disadvantage of waiting is that the lesion has the tendency to progress in depth and become painful. Therefore, the general recommendation is to surgically remove the sequestrum early by a superficial keratectomy. Often the brown tissue cannot be completely excised due to the depth of the lesion. If the keratectomy site is not covered and the cornea is slow to heal, the nigrum may recur. To help avoid recurrence in the keratectomy bed, most surgeons suggest covering the site with either a corneal graft, a conjunctival graft (**Figure 10.86**), submucosa bioscaffolding implants, amniotic membrane,[369–372] or a third eyelid flap. Featherstone and Sansom report there is no statistical difference in recurrence of the sequestra whether the keratectomy site is covered with a conjunctival graft or not.[373] However, recurrence is possible. Conjunctival grafts have the disadvantage of leaving

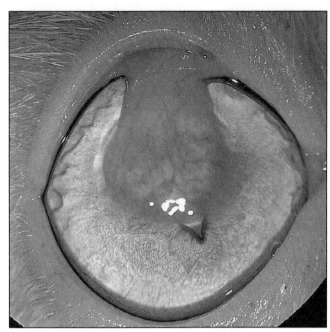

Figure 10.86 Conjunctival pedicle flap in a cat that has healed in place after removal of a sequestrum and is about to be excised or trimmed.

an axial scar. To avoid this problem, a corneoconjunctival transposition is often recommended as the axial corneal scarring with this procedure is typically less than that associated with a conjunctival graft.[374,375] In a large-scale study of 109 eyes with corneal sequestrum treated with a corneoconjunctival transposition, the recurrence rate for the corneal sequestrum is reported to be 10.2%[375] (see **Figures 10.97 and 10.99**). Corneal grafts can be used to treat deep or penetrating corneal sequestrum. Both homologous and heterologous corneal grafts are reported to have a good visual outcome when used to treat corneal sequestrum.[376,377] The recurrence rate for corneal sequestrum following corneal grafts is reported to be 5%, with a mild epithelial pigment formation occurring in 11% of the cases.

Bullous keratopathy (corneal hydrops)
Introduction/etiology
Peracute marked localized swelling of the cornea is observed in both the cat and the horse. The lesions present as ulcerations that have marked focal edema, producing an elevation and a gelatinous stroma with loss of structural integrity (**Figures 10.87 and 10.88**). The surrounding cornea is clear, and infectious organisms are not present unless due to contamination from the surface. The condition usually occurs in young to young adult cats and in foals to young adult horses, and it may sequentially involve the second eye.[378,379] Uveitis may be present but is not a consistent finding, and if present, it is secondary

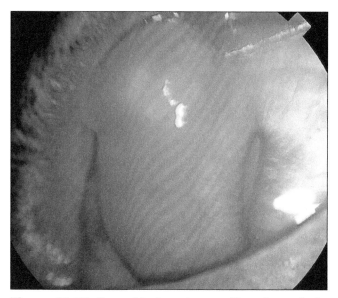

Figure 10.87 **Corneal hydrops in a cat. Note the marked protrusion of the edematous cornea that has been stained with fluorescein. The condition developed peracutely and was treated successfully with a third eyelid flap.**

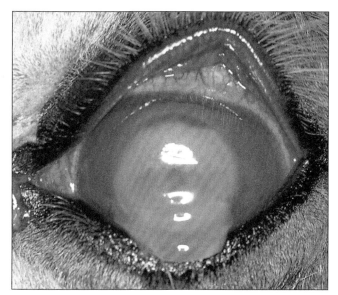

Figure 10.88 **Corneal hydrops in a foal that developed within hours. Culture was negative, and no bacteria were found on histopathology of the tissue. Treatment was by debridement of the malacic cornea and partial tarsorrhaphy, and the lesion healed in 10 days.**

to reflex uveitis. The cornea may become infected, and perforation may occur. The initiating cause is unknown, although the mechanism of progression is probably via MMP digestion. Prior treatment with topical and/or systemic steroids is reported in 78.9% of the cats that develop corneal hydrops/acute bullous keratopathy.[380] Pierce et al.

report an association with the systemic administration of corticosteroids and/or cyclosporine A in the development of acute bullous keratopathy in cats; systemic cyclosporine is a statistically significant risk factor.[381] When observed early, prodromal lesions are small, single, or multifocal ulcerations that may be accompanied by small bullae that rapidly coalesce to form large bullae. In the horse, prior drug therapy has not been associated with the condition. Based on the peracute history, a lack of significant inflammatory cells on cytology and biopsy, sterility on culture, and the tendency for foals and young horses to lie down while sleeping, insect bites are suggested as a possible contributing factor. However, the cause of bullous keratopathy (corneal hydrops) is not known.

Diagnosis

Diagnosis is by appearance of a marked focal edematous lesion of gelatinous stroma, with adjacent normal cornea devoid of edema, leukocytic infiltration, or vascular reaction. Cytology and biopsy of the gelatinous material are typically sterile on culture, lack significant inflammatory cells or bacteria, and consist of disoriented collagen fibrils with marked edema separating the fibrils. Bullous keratopathy must be differentiated from an acute, progressive, melting, septic ulcer that may have organisms and neutrophils on cytology.

Therapy

Therapy entails removing the exposed gelatinous stroma and covering the cornea to "bandage" it. In the cat, a third eyelid flap works well as a pressure bandage

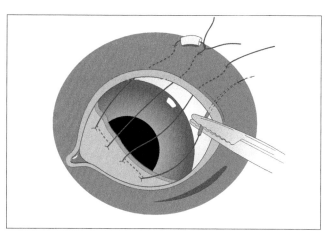

Figure 10.89 **Placement of a third eyelid flap. This is the most common suture pattern used. Note the stints on the skin side, and the suture is placed back from the lid margin to ensure pulling the third eyelid up for pressure, rather than just pulling the upper lid down.**

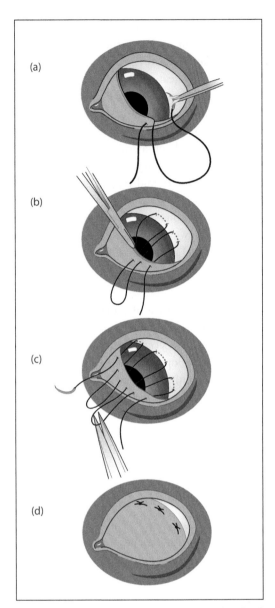

Figure 10.90 (a–d) Technique of suturing the third eyelid to the diametrically opposite episclera. This requires a good ophthalmic cutting needle to pick up the tough episclera, as sutures only in the conjunctiva will pull out. The advantage is that the globe and the third eyelid are a unit rather than independent in their movement.

(**Figures 10.89 through 10.91**). The use of a third eyelid flap is reported to be a successful treatment in 90.5% of the cases.[380] In the horse, the author prefers a partial tarsorrhaphy that provides a pressure bandage, but the lesion remains accessible for treatment and observation (**Figure 7.43**). Topical antimicrobial agents are used but need not be intensive, and systemic analgesics are usually not necessary. Intensive anticollagenases therapy is advised by the author to help stabilize the cornea. In the horse, after two or three debridements of the area, the lesion stabilizes and begins to epithelialize.

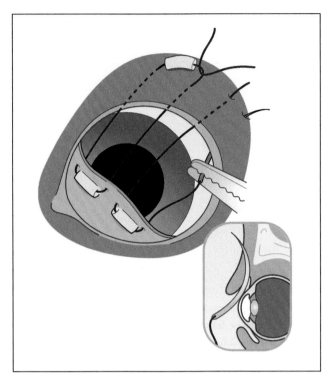

Figure 10.91 Suture pattern used to place a third eyelid flap that allows stints to be used on both sides. This should be considered in dogs or animals that require a lot of tension on the third eyelid to cover the globe. The disadvantage is that often the cartilage of the third eyelid is deformed after removal due to bending over the stint.

Deep corneal ulcers

Introduction/etiology

Progressive and deep corneal ulcers result from tissue damage and stromal loss and are typically secondary to an infectious process. The progressive stromal loss is caused by a combination of toxins liberated by the organism and MMP enzymes liberated by the ocular tissue and neutrophils. MMPs are involved in a variety of normal processes throughout the body, such as tissue remodeling, as well as pathologic conditions such as cancer, wound healing, and angiogenesis.[382] There are >20 MMPs described, based on their substrate specificity, with four endogenous tissue inhibitors of MMPs (TIMPs). Older nomenclature used for these enzymes includes collagenase (MMP-1), gelatinase A (MMP-2), stromelysin-1 (MMP-3), and gelatinase B (MMP-9). Endogenous MMP may be secreted by keratocytes, leukocytes, and, perhaps, corneal epithelium. They normally exist as proenzymes or are latent, but when activated after a lag period, rapid melting of the stroma may occur.

Pseudomonas aeruginosa infection produces progressive, often perforating, ulcers. *P. aeruginosa* has a variety of proteolytic enzymes[383] and has been shown to activate endogenous MMPs of the cornea.[384] Even with organisms such as *Pseudomonas* spp., the host's response is very important in creating the melting ulcers. Specifically, lysosomal enzymes from neutrophils may be more important than direct damage by *P. aeruginosa* exoenzymes.[385] Therapy with agents that inhibit the cyclooxygenase pathway and increase the neutrophilic response will accelerate corneal ulceration.[386] Ulcerations associated with bacteria usually have a more intense leukotactic stimulus, resulting in a dense, creamy white infiltrate, and an intense neovascular response (**Figure 10.92**).

Although *Pseudomonas* spp. produces the classic, progressive, melting corneal ulcer, any organism can activate MMPs, which results in stromal loss. Bacterial isolates from dogs and horses with infectious keratitis are about equally divided between Gram-positive and Gram-negative organisms.[387–390] In the southeastern United States, *Staphylococcus intermedius* (29%), β-hemolytic *Streptococcus* spp., (17%) and *Pseudomonas aeruginosa* (21%) are the most common bacterial isolated from dogs with ulcerative keratitis.[389] Similarly, *Staphylococcus* spp. or β-hemolytic *Streptococcus* (49%) and *Pseudomonas aeruginosa* (31%) are the most common bacteria isolated from dogs with bacterial keratitis in Australia.[390] Historically, *Pseudomonas* spp. and other Gram-negative bacteria organisms are reported to be the most common isolates from ulcerative keratitis in horses.[137] However, more recent studies by the same authors and others show *Streptococcus* spp. and *Staphylococcus* spp. are the most common isolates.[388,391] It is important to note that antibiotic resistance is common for *Streptococcus* spp. and *Staphylococcus* spp. isolated from cases with ulcerative keratitis.[389,390,392] The incidence of Gram-negative isolates and their antibiotic resistance increases with previous therapy.[388] Tolar et al. reports that >80% of β-hemolytic *Streptococcus* spp. isolates are resistant to neomycin, polymyxin B, and tobramycin.[389] In a separate study by LoPinto et al., 23.9% of the *Staphylococcus* spp. isolates are documented to be methicillin-resistant.[392] Although *Staphylococcus* spp., β-hemolytic *Streptococcus* spp., and *Pseudomonas aeruginosa* are the most common bacterial isolates in dogs and horses with bacterial keratitis, other Gram-positive and Gram-negative bacteria are frequently isolated.[387–391] In addition to aerobic bacteria, anaerobic bacteria are isolated in 13% of the cases of domestic animals with ulcerative keratitis[393] (**Figure 10.93**). There are regional variations in bacteria isolated and in their resistance pattern. This underscores the importance of cytology and bacteria cultures and sensitivity when establishing a treatment plan for animals with infectious ulcerative keratitis.

In addition to infectious organisms, melting corneal ulcers can be associated with sterile processes and insect bites such as fire ants, spiders, or bees (**Figure 10.67**).

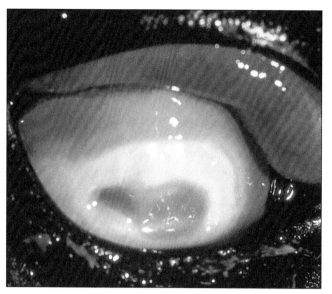

Figure 10.92 *Pseudomonas* **descemetocele in a horse. Note the strong leukotactic response, diffuse corneal edema, and impending vascular response.**

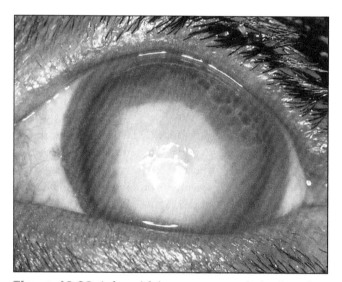

Figure 10.93 **A dog with intense neovascularization of the cornea and a stromal keratitis associated with Listeria monocytogenes. Corneal edema is associated with bullae over the neovascularization. The patient responded well to antibiotics.**

Clinical signs

Crater defects with visible stromal walls indicate that the ulcer has extended into the stroma. Associated corneal edema with thickening of the stroma often exaggerates the depth of the ulcer. If the bottom of the ulcer is clear or dark, it usually indicates that there is no residual stroma, and the ulcer has progressed to Descemet's membrane (**Figure 10.74**).

Varying degrees of white corneal opacity may be present due to combinations of corneal edema and leukocytic infiltration. Marked leukocytic infiltration is indicative of sepsis and is usually more yellow-white than pure stromal edema, which is more gray-white in color (**Figure 10.92**). After a lag time of 48 hours, superficial and deep vascularization starts to develop depending on the chronicity and the stimulus.

Diagnosis

Diagnosis of stromal ulceration is usually based on a defect in the stroma that has sharp sides and deep walls and stains with fluorescein.

Some considerations when interpreting fluorescein staining are:

- If cellular infiltrate is present, the fluorescein staining may appear lime green in color in place of an intense fluorescent green.
- Deep defects may pool fluorescein but may not actually take up stain. These may be healed facets of previous deep ulcers that have not filled in with fibroplasia.
- Descemetoceles do not stain since there is no stromal tissue to take up stain.

The etiologic diagnosis may be made by performing a corneal scraping for cytology and culture, although cultures are often retrospective if the progression is rapid. If tissue necrosis is present, anaerobic bacteria may cause ulceration and may not be diagnosed by the usual culturing techniques.[393–395] Nutritionally variant streptococci require thiol-containing compounds and vitamin B_6 and have been reported to be a significant cause of corneal ulceration.[396] Nutritionally variant streptococci do not grow on most bacteriological media unless a pyridoxal secreting organism such as *Staphylococcus* spp. is also growing, in which case they develop as satellite colonies. Equine ulcers frequently have mixed bacterial and fungal agents, particularly if they have been previously treated.[137] Therefore, both bacterial and fungal cultures are indicated in horses with ulcerative keratitis.

Therapy

Medical   It is recommended to hospitalize most patients with deep corneal ulcers for intensive medical and surgical therapy. Initial medical therapy is best guided by corneal cytology while pending culture and sensitivity results. The antibiotic of choice is constantly changing due to resistance patterns and is based on local and regional sensitivity trends. Since most bacteria isolated

from infectious ulcerative keratitis are *Staphylococcus intermedius*, β-hemolytic *Streptococcus* spp., and/or *Pseudomonas aeruginosa*, a fluoroquinolone such as ciprofloxacin or ofloxacin, or a combination of a first-generation cephalosporin (e.g., cephazolin) and tobramycin are appropriate initial antibiotic therapies.[389,390] The choice between ciprofloxacin and ofloxacin is based on clinician preference and local resistance patterns. The author typically initiates antibiotic therapy with the combination of ofloxacin and cephazolin. If rods are observed on cytology, a fortified ophthalmic gentamicin (10–12 mg/mL) or amikacin solution every hour can be used[397] as initial therapies. Topical fluoroquinolones, such as ciprofloxacin or ofloxacin, may be an appropriate initial therapy for *Pseudomonas aeruginosa*.[390,398] In a study by Ledbetter et al., 88.9%–100% of *Pseudomonas aeruginosa* isolates from dogs with ulcerative keratitis in the Northeast are documented to be susceptible to seven different fluoroquinolones, but regional variations in *Pseudomonas aeruginosa* susceptibility to fluoroquinolones are noted in other studies.[398,389] An alternative to ciprofloxacin or ofloxacin, one of the newer fluoroquinolone antibiotics, such as moxifloxacin, can be used, but these are generally not recommended for initial therapy. Frequent topical antibiotics have been more effective in clearing the cornea of organisms in experimental infections than subconjunctival or parenteral routes.[399,400]

As with dogs, *Streptococcus* spp. and *Staphylococcus* spp. are the most common isolates for horse with bacterial ulcerative keratitis.[387,391] Therefore, as with dogs, an antibiotic with a broad Gram-positive spectrum combined with an antibiotic effective against Gram-negative organisms is appropriate initial therapy in horses. The author typically initiates medical therapy for infected corneal ulcers with the combination of ofloxacin and cephazolin formulated as a 5% solution and a topical antifungal preparation. Aggressive antibiotic therapy of *Pseudomonas* spp. ulcers without surgical intervention resulted in excellent function in 73% of horse cases.[401]

Clinically, EDTA, *N*-acetylcysteine (10%), serum and oral doxycycline are used for their anticollagenase activities. MMP is detectable in the tear film of animals with corneal ulceration[402] and is decreased in activity in the tears 99.4% by EDTA, 96.3% by doxycycline, 98.9% by *N*-acetylcysteine (10%), and 90% by serum.[403] When using anticollagenase inhibitors in the treatment of corneal ulcers, it is often advised to use a combination of the medications as they inhibit different families of proteases. MMP inhibitors (anticollagenase inhibitors) are often administered hourly if the process is in the progressive stages of ulceration. Their effectiveness against *Pseudomonas* spp. has been questioned.[404] Systemic tetracycline may be an alternative. Tetracycline has been shown to be beneficial with *P. aeruginosa* ulcers in an experimental model, and the benefit is thought to be independent of the antibacterial effect.[405] Oral doxycycline at 5 mg/kg and 10 mg/kg in dogs and 20 mg/kg in horses can be detected in the tear film and is suggested to aid in the treatment of corneal ulcerations.[406,407] Vygantas et al. found that bacitracin was more effective *in vitro* in inhibiting MMP-9 from wounded canine corneas than tetracycline, thus adding yet another drug as a possible MMP inhibitor.[408]

Surgical

Unless pinpoint or about 2 mm in diameter, deep ulcers or those involving >75% of the corneal thickness should be considered surgical problems. The procedure of choice depends on the ulcer size, its location, whether it is still in the progressive stage, the clinician's experience, and the instrumentation available.

Tissue glue

Small deep ulcers may have a small amount of tissue glue (cyanoacrylate) applied to reinforce the cornea structurally.[409] The glue must be placed in a very dry ulcer bed and a minimum amount applied, since any excess creates a very irritating surface (**Figure 10.94**). Keeping the cornea dry (often using a hair dryer) and carefully applying a very small drop usually requires general anesthesia. However, with experience, tissue adhesives can be applied under heavy sedation and topical anesthetics. A heal rate of 100% is reported with the application of cyanoacrylate glue to treat indolent ulcers.[410] Any loose corneal epithelium

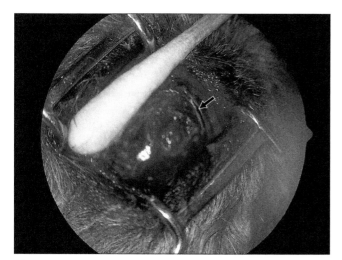

Figure 10.94 **A dog that has had cyanoacrylate glue placed over an ulcer (arrow). It is very difficult to get a small enough drop (even with 25- to 30-gauge needles) that does not extend significantly beyond a small ulcer.**

is removed by corneal debridement prior to application of the tissue glue when treating an indolent ulceration. Watté et al. report an overall heal rate of 89% with the use of cyanoacrylate glue to treat stromal ulcers, descemetoceles, and corneal lacerations.[411] Although tissue glue is a viable alternative to surgery in some circumstances, surgical intervention is generally considered a much better treatment option. The author usually reserves therapy with cyanoacrylate glue to those patients with economic constraints or if general anesthesia is contraindicated.

Corneal sutures

Sutures placed across the ulcer bed to close a lesion may be used in small deep ulcers that are stable. If the condition is still progressive, the sutures may dislodge. The disadvantage is that even a small ulcer produces considerable distortion of the corneal surface when a round defect is closed in a linear pattern. A purse-string pattern is favored over a linear closure. The sutures should not be greater than 7-0 in size and should include a 2- to 3-mm bite on each side to minimize pulling out of the stroma.

Conjunctival flaps

A technique that reinforces or patches the weakened cornea is indicated with deep ulcers of larger size. If the ulcer is acute and in the progressive stage, any procedure that relies on sutures embedded in the adjacent cornea will probably fail if the ulcer is not stabilized medically prior to surgery. A 360° conjunctival flap can be used for large central ulcers that are in a progressive stage (**Figure 10.95**). The hemorrhage that results from conjunctival dissection and the immediate vascularization that the flap brings to the ulcer are beneficial to halting progressive collagenase destruction of the stroma.[412]

Variations of the 360° conjunctival flap are possible, and other than requiring placing fine sutures in the cornea, they are usually easier and faster. Such variations include a hood or 180° flap, a bridge flap (**Figure 10.96**), a conjunctival pedicle flap (**Figure 10.86**), a tarsoconjunctival pedicle flap, and a free conjunctival patch.[413–415] In one study, Dorbandt et al. report an overall success rate of 97% in dogs when a pedicle conjunctival flap is used to treat corneal perforations, descemetoceles, or deep stromal ulcers.[416] Conjunctival flaps are usually a two-step procedure, with the second step (removal of the flap) >3 weeks post surgery. After dissection of excess conjunctival tissue from the adhered region of prior ulceration, topical steroids or NSAIDs are often administered for 2–3 weeks to minimize the scar. The final appearance, with continued shrinkage of the scar, may take several months. A scar may always be present with stromal ulcers due to healing by fibroplasia. Complete 360° conjunctival flaps are easily

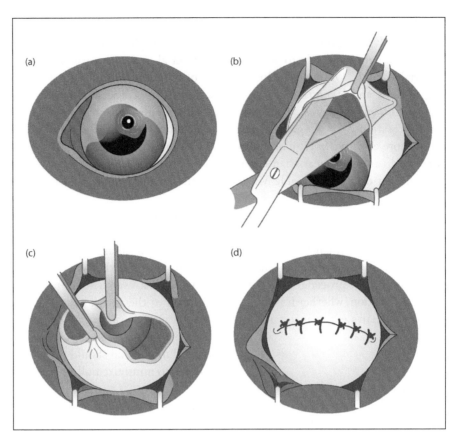

Figure 10.95 Dissection steps for performing a 360° conjunctival flap for a central ulcer. Central corneal ulcer (a). The limbal conjunctiva is excised with scissors for 360° (b). Dissection consists of cutting and then spreading the scissors under the conjunctiva to separate Tenon's fascia. This is thickest dorsally and ventrally adjacent to the rectus muscles. Failure to perform this step correctly results in premature retraction of the conjunctiva. Once the dissection is complete, the conjunctiva should easily pull over the cornea (c) and can be sutured in a variety of patterns (d). The critical time is 5–7 days if retraction is going to occur. The flap is left for approximately 3 weeks and then trimmed, leaving minimal adherence at the ulcer. The conjunctiva does not have to be resutured in place.

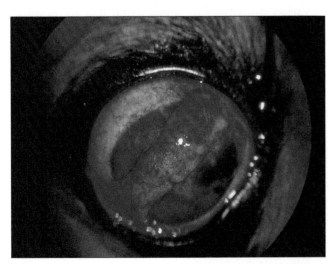

Figure 10.96 A dog with a bridge conjunctival graft in place for a central ulcer. These need to be sutured adjacent to the ulcer to keep them from moving.

dissected in the horse but are more likely to retract prematurely. Pedicle, bridge, or free grafts are more successful than 360° flaps in the horse.

Corneal grafts

Free corneal grafts can be performed to fill defects associated with ulcerations, but a sliding autogenous lamellar graft is more practical and successful if there is enough normal cornea adjacent to the lesion (**Figures 10.97 through 10.99**).[417] In one study, 95% of these grafts are reported to be translucent with reestablishment of the corneal endothelium.[418] This procedure gives better functional results than conjunctival flaps, and while technically more difficult, it is preferred for central ulcers to minimize scarring (**Figure 10.91**). Frozen homologous corneal grafts have been used to patch corneal defects in dogs, cats, and horses. These grafts remain opaque, but they successfully patch

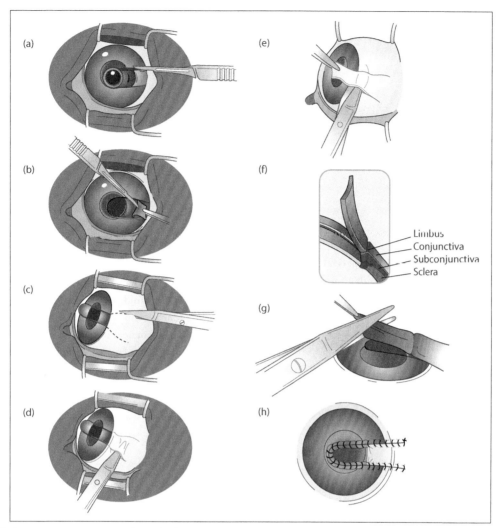

Figure 10.97 Autogenous corneoconjunctival graft. If an ulcer has enough adjacent normal tissue to cover it (a), a half-depth lamellar dissection is performed out to the limbus (b). The width of the dissection should be somewhat wider than the ulcer. The conjunctiva is then excised with scissors, wider than the space to be filled to counteract contraction (c), and the underlying Tenon's capsule is removed (d). The remaining limbal zone is cut, and this allows radial movement of the dissected tissue into the ulcer (e, f). As this procedure is often a source of hemorrhage, it is prudent to do the procedure last. The end of the corneal graft is trimmed to fit the ulcer (g). The entire graft is sutured with 8-0 to 9-0 material (h).

the defect, salvage the eye, and can be used to enlarge the globe for implantation of an intraocular prosthesis.[419] With nonperforating ulcers in the dog and the cat, frozen lamellar grafts provide excellent postoperative results.[420] The grafts become edematous and stimulate intense neovascularization but are clear by 60 days postoperatively.

A variety of materials have been used as "patches" to cover an ulcer, similar to a free-hand conjunctival graft. Porcine small intestinal submucosa,[371,421–423] porcine urinary bladder submucosa,[416,424,425] equine renal capsule,[426] equine and bovine pericardium,[427,428] and xenologous amniotic membrane[429–432] have been used as patches. Covering the ulcer with a patching material when dealing with septic problems has the disadvantage of not bringing a blood supply to the ulcer. The advantage of most of the

nonconjunctival patches is that they leave less scarring but are best utilized in a stable ulcer.

Commercially available bioscaffolding material derived from porcine small intestinal or urinary bladder submucosa are available for use in corneal reconstruction surgeries. These materials can be used alone or in combination with a soft contact lens, temporary tarsorrhaphies, or conjunctival flaps with favorable results.[416,422,424,425] Surgically, a keratectomy is performed to remove the necrotic and infected tissue, and a bioscaffolding material disc is sutured in the wound bed with an 8-0 or 9-0 suture. Following the use of bioscaffolding materials alone or with a soft contact lens to repair complicated corneal ulcers, 86.7% of dogs and cats and 94% of horses are reported to remain visual.[424,425] An 89% success rate is reported when the combination

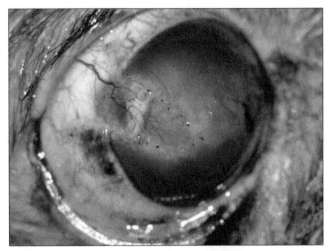

Figure 10.98 Autogenous cornealconjunctival graft to repair a descemetocele in a Shih Tzu 10 days postoperative. Note the corneal edema, neovascularization, and fibrosis in the area of the graft. The corneal vascularization and scarring will decrease over time.

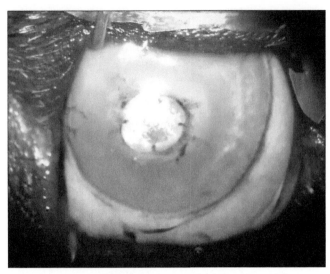

Figure 10.100 Repair of a corneal perforation with the use of a bioscaffolding material composed of porcine urinary bladder submucosa. The bioscaffolding material is sutured in to the corneal defect with four cardinal suture of 8-0 to 9-0 polyglactin suture. A pedicle conjunctival flap is sutured in place over the bioscaffolding material.

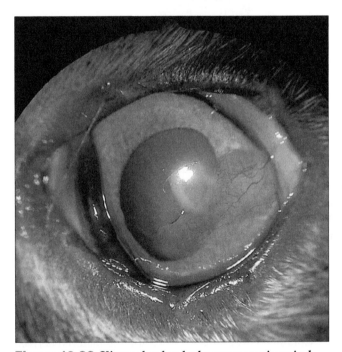

Figure 10.99 Kitten that has had a corneoconjunctival sliding graft for a herpesvirus descemetocele. The vascular portion is the conjunctival part, and the corneal portion is mainly clear. The clinical appearance was clearer than the photograph would indicate.

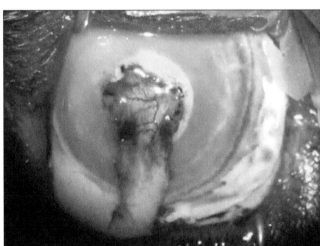

Figure 10.101 Same dog as in Figure 10.100. The pedicle conjunctival flap and the bioscaffolding material are sutured by bisecting sutures with 8-0 to 9-0 polyglactin in to the ulcer margin. Alternatively, a corneal trephine 2 mm larger than the defect can be used with a corneal dissector to make an outer rim for suturing the conjunctival flap similar to Figure 10.42.

of a conjunctival flap and bioscaffolding material is used for repair of corneal perforations, descemetoceles, and deep stromal ulcers.[416] Bioscaffolding materials are typically used for more progressive corneal ulcers in which the structural integrity of the cornea is in question and where a conjunctival flap alone is not appropriate. This accounts for the slight decrease in success rates when bioscaffolding material is used in corneal reconstructive surgery versus the use of a conjunctival flap alone to treat corneal ulceration (**Figures 10.100 and 10.101**).

Amniotic membrane is used in both small animals[430] and horses[431,432] for corneal reconstructive surgery. Amniotic membrane is used for structural support and to promote healing of progressive corneal ulcers. As with bioscaffolding materials, a keratectomy is performed to remove necrotic and infected tissue. The amniotic membrane is sutured in the corneal wound with 8-0 or 9-0 nylon. In a study by Plummer evaluating the use of amniotic membrane in horses to treat progressive corneal ulcers, 91.4% of horses remained visual after surgery.[432]

Corneal collagen cross-linking

Corneal collagen cross-linking (CXL) utilizes UV-A light and riboflavin to improve the biomechanical stability of the cornea. Riboflavin 0.1% is applied to a cornea wound, and the area is exposed to UV-A light, which produces free oxygen radicals that increase the number of intrafibrillar covalent bonds in collagen fibers of the corneal stroma.[433] In addition, the production of free oxygen radicals has antimicrobial activity against bacteria and fungi.[434] An added benefit of CXL is that it prevents proteolytic enzymes from binding to specific cleavage sites.[435] CXL typically has a stabilizing effect on the corneal stroma within 7 days in dogs and cats, with epithelization of the ulcer occurring in approximately 7–14 days.[436-439] Hellander-Edman et al. report an improvement in stromal melting in 4/4 horses within 24 hours and epithelization of the ulcer in 13.5 days following CXL.[440] Currently, there are two commercially available portable CXL systems available for use in veterinary medicine: UV-X Peschke (Meditrade) and KXL™ System (Avedro).

Corneal tattooing

Deep corneal ulcers will invariably have a significant scar. If pigmentation has not accompanied the healing process, a significant cosmetic blemish may compel the owner to seek a solution. Corneal tattooing with platinic chloride offers a cosmetic improvement. After debriding the epithelium, 2% platinic chloride is soaked into the scar and then precipitated with 2% hydrazine.[441] A black precipitate is formed in the scar, which does not improve function but does blend with the usual background of a dark equine iris (**Figures 10.102 and 10.103**).

Infectious bovine keratoconjunctivitis (pink eye)

Introduction/etiology

Infectious bacterial ulcerative keratitis occurs in both cows and sheep. The disease is worldwide and has a significant economic impact from weight loss and cost of treatment. Infectious bovine keratoconjunctivits (IBK) has been documented to occur in one-third of the calves at weaning, with two-thirds of the calves affected unilaterally and one-third affected bilaterally. The average suppression of weight in calves is 11 lb (5 kg) with unilateral involvement and 35 lb (16 kg) in calves with bilateral involvement.[442]

The consensus is that the primary etiology in the cow is *Moraxella bovis*, but multiple factors play a role in

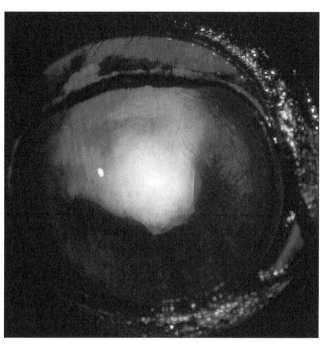

Figure 10.102 Dense corneal leukoma in a horse. The scar was cosmetically objectionable to the owner, who requested corneal tattooing.

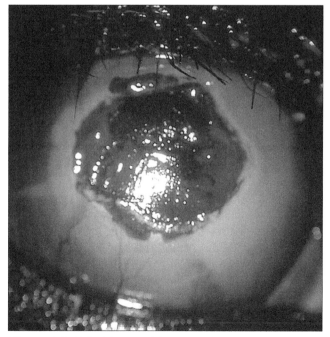

Figure 10.103 A horse with a corneal tattoo immediately after applying platinum chloride. Note the adjacent corneal edema, which detracts from the cosmetic improvement.

both the susceptibility of the animal and the severity of the disease.[443–445]

Enhancing factors

- Strain of *Moraxella bovis*: Piliated hemolytic strains that produce rough cultures are the pathogenic strains. Passage on blood agar quickly reduces the virulence and promotes conversion to smooth cultures that are nonhemolytic.[443,445]
- Age: Young animals have the highest incidence of disease, which suggests that some immunity is acquired from previous exposure.[446]
- Season: Peak incidence of disease is usually in warmer, humid months. Winter outbreaks have been associated with reflected UV light from the snow. In addition, crowded conditions in the winter may lead to outbreaks.
- UV radiation: Outbreaks of IBK can be correlated with peak UV radiation. Experimental infections are created by first irradiating the eyes with UV light. UV radiation produces degeneration and increased sloughing of the epithelial cells and promotes conditions for attachment of *M. bovis*.[447] The most critical wavelength is 270 nm.[448]
- Breed: *Bos indicus* breeds (Brahmam type) are generally resistant.
- Ocular and periocular pigmentation: Breeds and genetic lines of animals with less pigment are more susceptible.[449]
- Flies: *Musca domestica* and *Musca autumnalis* may carry the organisms between animals and may mechanically injure the corneal surface.[443]
- Dust, tall grass, wind: These may produce mechanical irritation to the ocular surface.
- Other infectious agents: Concurrent infection with IBR virus or vaccination with a live IBR virus increases the severity and prevalence of IBK.[450–452] *Mycoplasma* spp. may promote colonization of the conjunctiva by *Moraxella* spp. but does not have a primary role in producing IBK.[453,454.]

Transmission

Direct transmission without the enhancing factors described previously or other enhancing factors is of minimal importance. Only 1 of 20 calves developed clinical IBK from close contact when housed in conditions that minimized other risk factors such as fly control.[455]

Clinical signs
In order of development:

- Epiphora, photophobia, and conjunctivitis are very early signs.

- A focal axial corneal opacity or small abscess develops followed by ulceration in 2–4 days (**Figure 10.104**).
- The central ulcer may heal or progress in depth. Simple ulcerations may heal in 1–2 weeks. Progression of the ulcer in depth often occurs with descemetocele formation or perforation and iris prolapse. Corneal vascularization is stimulated as well as leukocytic infiltration of the cornea (**Figure 10.105**). This produces opacification of the cornea peripheral to the ulcer. Healing of the ulcer bed is frequently by vascular invasion of the ulcer bed, resulting in a raised bed of granulation tissue (**Figure 10.106**). Deep and perforated ulcers heal over in 1–2 months by fibrosis.

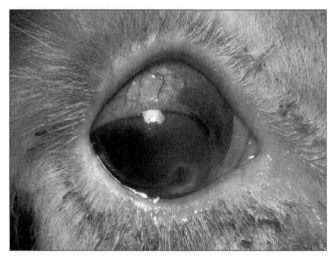

Figure 10.104 Uncomplicated early infectious bovine keratitis lesion in the anterior stroma. The lesion is typically axial.

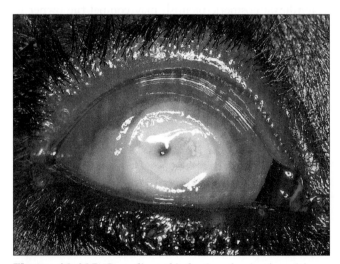

Figure 10.105 Complicated infectious bovine keratitis lesion that has resulted in a descemetocele. The calf was valuable, so it was treated successfully with a pedicle conjunctival graft.

- An endophthalmitis may develop with deep or perforated ulcers.
- A central corneal scar that shrinks in size over several months is present in most recovered animals (**Figure 10.107**).

Therapy

Moraxella bovis is susceptible to a wide variety of antibiotics, but the number of affected animals and difficulty in providing frequent treatments present a challenge. Topical antibiotics are effective, but only if a few animals are affected, and they are confined for treatment. Otherwise, this route is not practical. Subconjunctival injection of an antibiotic is often administered to avoid frequent therapy. Procaine penicillin given either through the upper lid into the dorsal fornix region or subconjunctivally in the bulbar conjunctiva achieves a therapeutic concentration in the conjunctival fluid for 68 and 40 hours, respectively.[456] Parenteral administration of long-acting oxytetracycline, given at 20 mg/kg intramuscularly every 72 hours, is successful both in treating and in eliminating the carrier state.[457] Treatment with long-acting oxytetracycline is approved by the Food and Drug Administration (FDA), except in lactating dairy cows. Florfenicol (a chloramphenicol derivative) is proven to be highly effective in treating IBK; 98% of animals heal with one subcutaneous injection of 40 mg/kg, and 93% heal with two intramuscular injections of 20 mg/kg every 48 hours.[458]

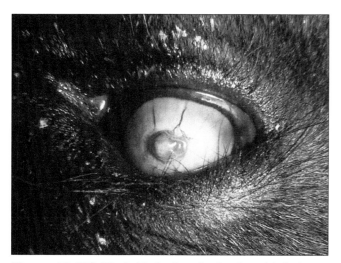

Figure 10.106 Healed infectious bovine keratitis lesion with granulation. The cow develops corneal granulation more readily than other species.

When treating food animals systemically or subconjunctivally, drug withdrawal times prior to slaughter may be an important consideration when choosing the treatment regimen. The current withdrawal times for medications used to treat *Moraxella bovis* are:

- Procaine penicillin: Cattle 14 days, sheep 9 days
- Long-acting oxytetracycline: 28 days; not approved in lactating dairy cows
- Florfenicol: 28 days IM, 38 days subcutaneously

Corticosteroids are often given topically or subconjunctivally with antibiotics for treating IBK; this defies the rule of not using corticosteroids with infection or ulceration. Despite this contradiction, most clinicians feel that it shortens the course of the disease and markedly improves the appearance of the cornea. A frequently used drug combination of penicillin and dexamethasone given subconjunctivally on 3 consecutive days is demonstrated to have no therapeutic benefit when compared to control calves that received no therapy.[459]

Topical atropine ointment may be given for pain, and eye patches may be glued to the skin in severe cases to protect the eye from flies, dust, and sun. Alternatively, a third eyelid flap is frequently used in severe cases. Chromic catgut is used to suture the third eyelid; the gut sutures dissolve spontaneously, which is an advantage when treating animals in large pastures or in great numbers.[460]

Prophylaxis

Because of the significant economic impact of IBK, emphasis should be placed on prevention. Emphasis should be

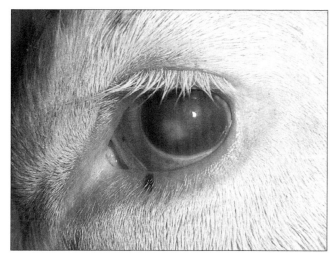

Figure 10.107 Typical axial corneal scar indicative of prior infectious bovine keratitis infection.

placed on good husbandry techniques such as quarantine of all new animals, avoiding purchase of animals from public auction if possible, and/or treating all new animals with long-acting oxytetracycline for two treatments at 3- to 4-day intervals to minimize the risk of carrier animals.

Fly control during the summer with devices such as ear tags or dust bags, and provision of shaded areas, are important to minimize potentiating factors. Live IBR vaccine should be avoided during the IBK season, and subcutaneous vaccination with a bacterin that contains pilus antigens should be considered in problem herds. Vaccination can be as early as 3 weeks of age and should be repeated in 3 weeks and annually thereafter. While experimental evidence suggests that multiple inoculation of a piliated bacterin reduces the incidence of clinical disease, the effectiveness of available vaccines has been questioned.[461,462]

Infectious ovine keratoconjunctivitis

Infectious keratoconjunctivitis is recognized worldwide in sheep. The condition is characterized by conjunctivitis and a peripheral keratitis that is usually not ulcerative. Organisms thought to be responsible are *Mycoplasma conjunctivae* and, less commonly, *Chlamydia psittaci*.[463–466] Ulcerative keratitis may occur in the more severely affected lambs. Animals infected with chlamydial forms of conjunctivitis may also have joint disease. *Mycoplasma*-associated keratoconjunctivitis increases in severity with age. *Branhamella ovis*, *Escherichia coli*, and *Staphylococcus aureus* are commonly cultured from diseased and normal eyes but are not thought to be primary casual agents, although this is controversial.[466] The disease is self-limiting, but the course can be shortened with antibiotics.

Perforated ulcers
Introduction/etiology
Perforated ulcers are managed similarly to deep ulcers but have the additional factors of a protruding iris, alterations of intraocular structures, and an increased risk of intraocular infection. The iris prolapse may appear black, gray, or red, depending on the chronicity and the amount of fibrin layered on the surface (**Figures 10.108 and 10.109**). The fibrin adds to the mass, producing a mushroom shape. The fibrin becomes organized with time, and the condition is often termed a corneal staphyloma at this stage (**Figure 10.110**). The mushroom shape of the protruding iris and layers of fibrin may create a false impression as to the size of the ulcer and consequent assessment of how difficult it may be to repair. Judgment as to the prognosis and means of surgical repair should be made after the iris has been stripped of the fibrin and the extent of the injury determined.

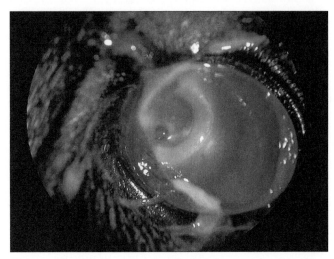

Figure 10.108 Peracute developing descemetocele with small iris prolapse in a Boston terrier. The lesion began as an epithelial ulcer. The iris prolapse is covered with fibrin and thus is not brown or black. Culture was negative. The patient was treated with a 360° conjunctival flap because of the progressive nature of the condition. Vision was retained.

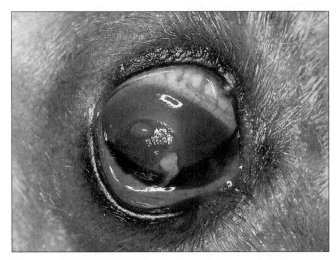

Figure 10.109 Acute iris prolapse from an ulcer in a Yorkshire terrier. Note the lack of adjacent corneal reaction indicating the acute nature. Because of the acute nature, prognosis is good to guarded. The patient was treated successfully with a pedicle flap.

Therapy
The protruding iris is usually excised unless the condition is only a few hours old and/or it is very small. Bleeding may be encountered with iris excision and may be controlled with irrigation, low-temperature cautery, viscoelastic agents, and/or topical epinephrine (1:10,000). Anterior synechiae to the posterior cornea are released by sweeping with a spatula or viscoelastic cannula and the anterior chamber maintained with viscoelastic agents while covering the defect with a surgical patch. The anterior chamber

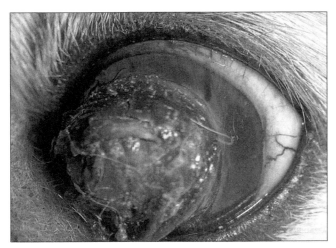

Figure 10.110 Corneal staphyloma in a Pekingese.
This is a chronic problem, and the prognosis for vision is
very poor. Because of the size, either a 360° conjunctival
flap or, preferably, a corneal graft should be used to fill the
defect. The collapsed anterior chamber will be difficult to
reform.

may reform if the perforation is hours or a few days old, but older lesions may resist expansion of the anterior chamber due to posterior pooling of aqueous humor in the vitreal compartment. A surgical patch, usually of conjunctiva or cornea, bioscaffolding material, amniotic membrane, or a combination of these materials is used to repair the corneal defect. Medical treatment consists of intensive topical and systemic antibiotic therapy. Despite the potential gravity of these conditions, the prognosis may be quite good if the anterior chamber can be reformed. Dorbandt et al. report an 89% success rate following surgical repair of corneal perforations in dogs,[416] and Henrisken et al. report 64.9% of horses with iris prolapse maintain vision after surgery.[467] (See **Figures 10.100 and 10.101.**)

> The potential for saving the globe and vision is very good with a perforated cornea and iris prolapse if surgery is performed early.

PENETRATING AND PERFORATING WOUNDS OF THE CORNEA AND GLOBE

A penetrating injury is one that enters but does not pass through the structure, while a perforating injury is one that does pass through the structure. Injuries from missiles, sticks, porcupine quills, and claw wounds may mimic corneal ulcers, but they have a very different prognosis. Pellets and BB shot usually produce multiple injuries at various depths in the globe that can lead to more chronic

complications and blindness. Accurate diagnosis is important so that a precise prognosis can be given.

Injuries to the lens may result in a delayed inflammation (phacoanaphylaxis, phacoclastic uveitis), which usually destroys the eye, and vitreous hemorrhage, often resulting in traction-induced retinal detachment as the hemorrhage organizes. Whenever a peracute iris prolapse occurs without prior ocular signs, a perforating corneal missile injury should be suspected. Many missile injuries are malicious, and thus, an accurate history is often lacking. BB pellets are usually self-sealing, while larger air rifle pellet wounds usually have a small iris prolapse (**Figure 10.111**).

Screening skull radiographs are used to diagnose metallic perforating foreign bodies. With metallic missiles, infection is rarely a problem; therefore, intense steroid therapy is indicated to control the inflammation. Porcupine quills may perforate the eye directly or from the orbital region. Orbital porcupine quills are readily recognized on ultrasound by a double-banded linear hyperechoic lesion.[468] Cat claw injuries are typically in naïve puppies, are often self-sealing, and are recognized by a full-thickness linear lesion. The chance of a corneal cat claw in dogs is calculated to reduce by 1% with each month of age.[469] The lens capsule is often ruptured with claw injuries, and while infection is of concern, surprisingly it often does not materialize.

If the injury is self-sealing, surgical repair of the cornea is not necessary. Paulsen and Kass report a favorable outcome with medical management alone in cats and dogs with corneal lacerations and lens capsular tears.[470] If the lens capsule has suffered a tear >1.5 mm, it recommended

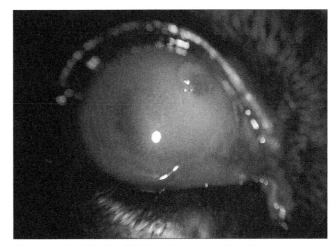

Figure 10.111 Small iris prolapse in a dog that was very
peracute in onset, without a prior history of an ocular
problem. The prolapse was due to a perforating pellet.
X-rays will quickly confirm a metallic foreign body. The
condition should be differentiated from a perforated ulcer
for prognosis and therapeutic reasons.

that the lens be removed to reduce subsequent immune-mediated inflammation.[469,471] All cats and 85.2% of dogs with a corneal laceration and lens laceration >1.5 mm are reported to be visual after surgical repair of the corneal laceration and lens removal by phacoemulsification. Lesions with iris prolapse are managed as a perforated ulcer.

CORNEAL LACERATIONS

Corneal lacerations are relatively easy to manage compared to corneal ulceration, since usually there is no tissue missing (**Figure 10.112**). The prognosis and treatment of lacerations depends on the chronicity and the amount of collateral damage, such as uveal and lens lacerations. The length of the laceration in horses correlates with prognosis, with all lacerations >15 mm resulting in phthisis, blindness, or enucleation.[472] These results indicate that most corneal lesions >15 mm are probably corneal ruptures from blunt trauma. Lavach et al. found that only 12% of horses with corneal perforations involving the cornea and the sclera were managed successfully.[473]

Lacerations require accurate apposition of edges with sutures and treatment for potential infection. Lacerations of the cornea that are not perforating may not require sutures. If the edges of a nonperforating laceration gape, then sutures are indicated. Perforating lacerations require

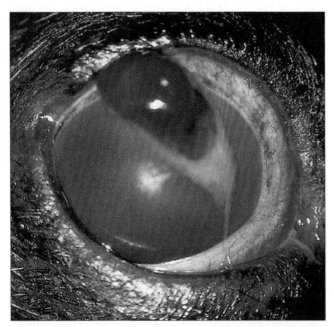

Figure 10.112 Corneal laceration in a dog with iris prolapse. Most acute lacerations have a good prognosis for vision if the lens is not involved. Depending on the extent and the acuteness, the iris may be replaced or excised before suturing.

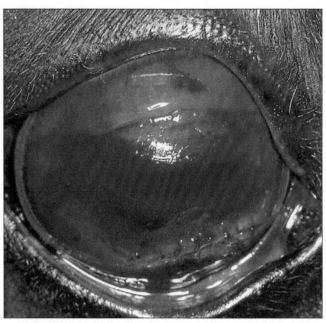

Figure 10.113 Corneal laceration in a horse after suturing. A residual blood clot retracted spontaneously, but tissue plasminogen activator could be injected in a couple of days to hasten the resolution. Lacerations should be differentiated from a corneal rupture.

management of the prolapsed iris by replacement, excision, and freeing any anterior synechiae from the posterior cornea. Whether the iris is replaced into the anterior chamber or excised is dependent on the health of the iris and the length of time it has been prolapsed. The anterior chamber is reformed with viscoelastic agent, and the cornea is accurately sutured. If the anterior chamber has been collapsed for a long time, it may not reform well. Suturing should be with a 7-0 to 9-0 suture material (**Figure 10.113**). Nylon suture can minimize scarring but must be removed at a later time. Lacerations should be differentiated from ruptures of the cornea and the sclera.

RUPTURES OF THE GLOBE

Introduction/etiology

Rupture of the cornea and often the sclera from blunt trauma mimics a laceration, but the prognosis is much worse.[473] The sudden decompressive force associated with a rupture usually results in such severe internal ocular injury that it rarely leaves a functional eye, and the globe frequently becomes phthisical. Horses usually develop ruptures of the cornea and anterior sclera. Ruptures of the cornea frequently extend across the limbus into the sclera. Dogs and cats usually develop posterior ruptures of the sclera, and they are often not visible. Posterior scleral ruptures should be suspected when the globe is very soft (e.g., following an injury such as proptosis of the globe). In small animals, ruptures are usually the result of trauma from automobiles and usually accompany proptosis of the globe; in the horse, ruptures are commonly found as a result of throwing the head or rearing over and hitting the floor, or kicks from other horses. Ruptures of the cornea can be managed similarly to a laceration, but almost invariably, the cornea has severe permanent edema, and the globe becomes phthisical.

Diagnosis

Diagnosis of a rupture as opposed to a laceration is on the history of a blunt injury. Ruptures of the cornea usually extend into the sclera, whereas lacerations are often restricted to the cornea (**Figure 10.114**). Ultrasound of the eye, showing loss of the lens, indicates a ruptured globe.

Therapy

If the diagnosis is certain, enucleation is recommended, because the eye will be blind, with an extensive recovery period that ends in phthisis bulbi. Exploration of the globe during attempts to suture the defects may reveal a ruptured or missing lens. Silicone spheres have been implanted after evisceration of the globe and suture of the rupture, in an attempt to prevent phthisis. A definite risk

of extrusion of the sphere is present when implantation is performed under these conditions.

CORNEAL FOREIGN BODIES

Corneal foreign bodies are usually vegetable matter. A flat, brownish seed hull is the most common foreign body (**Figure 10.115**), and it can usually be removed under topical anesthesia by irrigation or "flicking" it out with a 25-gauge needle or cytobrush. Hydropulsion is an easy method to remove nonpenetrating corneal foreign bodies.[474] A 6-mL syringe is filled with eyewash, and a 25-gauge needle with the needle tip removed is used to dislodge the foreign body (**Figure 10.116**). Splinters in the cornea are more difficult to remove unless one end is protruding from the cornea (**Figure 10.117**). Splinters usually require incising over them so they can be grasped with forceps. A rare complication of vegetable foreign bodies may be fungal keratitis.

MASSES IN THE CORNEA AND SCLERA

Dermoids

Introduction/etiology

A dermoid is a choristoma or a congenital tumor composed of tissues not normally present in that site. Dermoids are observed occasionally in all species but are most common in the dog and the cow. Dermoids are thought to be an

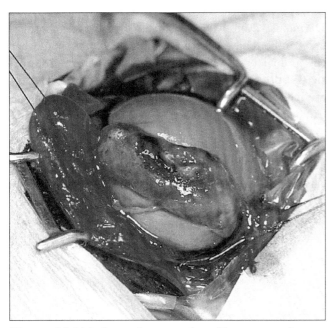

Figure 10.114 Corneal rupture from blunt trauma in a horse. Lesions extend through the limbus on each end, and on exploration, the lens had been expelled. Ultrasound of the eye prior to surgery would reveal loss of the lens and probable retinal detachment. The typical outcome is phthisis bulbi.

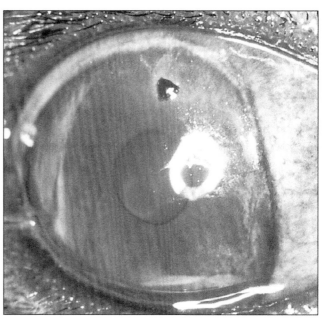

Figure 10.115 Corneal foreign body in a dog. This is a seed hull and a common foreign body in all species. The hull lies in a facet and usually requires mechanical "flicking out" under topical anesthesia.

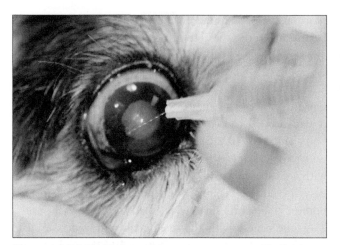

Figure 10.116 Hydropulsion to remove a seed hull in a dog. A 6-mL syringe is filled with eyewash. The needle tip on a 25-gauge needle is removed, and the needle hub is placed on the syringe. A steady stream of fluid is used to dislodge the foreign body.

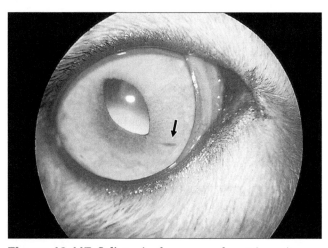

Figure 10.117 Splinter in the cornea of a cat (arrow). These are difficult to remove and require general anesthesia, magnification, cutting down over the splinter, and good forceps to grasp the splinter.

inherited trait in some dog breeds, cattle, horses, and the Burmese cat.[475,476] Dermoids have been observed occurring with coloboma of a hypoplastic third eyelid in the dog (Neapolitan mastiff), the cat, and the horse (**Figure 10.118**). A syndrome of iris hypoplasia, limbal dermoid, and cataract has been observed in the offspring of one quarter horse stallion.[477]

Clinical signs
Owners usually present the patient because of blepharospasm and epiphora resulting from the dermoid hairs. In the dog, most dermoids are unilateral, but they are often bilateral in cattle. The size of the dermoid in the dog and

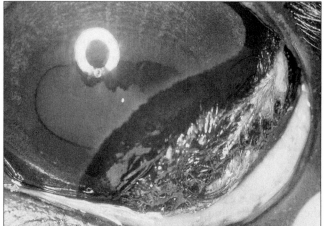

Figure 10.118 Equine dermoid at the lateral limbus accompanied by a coloboma of the third eyelid and of the optic disc.

the cat is usually rather small. The most common site of corneal dermoids in the dog is at the temporal limbus (**Figure 10.119**). In cattle, dermoids often involve the central cornea and may extend onto the third eyelid and conjunctiva (see Chapter 8, **Figure 8.46**).

Diagnosis
Diagnosis of a dermoid is usually obvious because hairs are present on the mass.

Therapy
Dermoids, even when massive, are always superficial and can be removed with a superficial keratectomy when the animal is old enough to undergo general anesthesia (**Figures 10.120 and 10.121**). Until the animal has attained a size to make the surgery practical, ointments can be applied to protect the cornea.

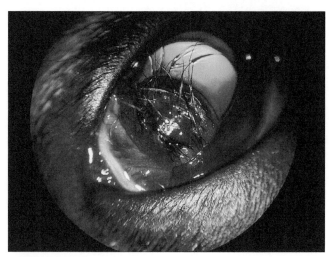

Figure 10.119 German shepherd dog puppy with a corneal dermoid at the lateral limbus.

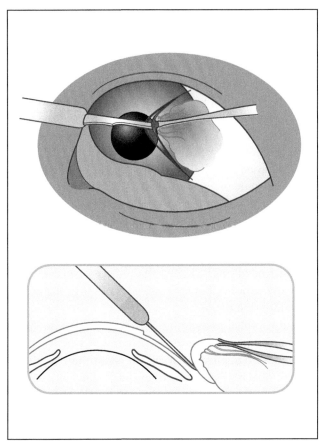

Figure 10.120 Removal of a corneal dermoid with a superficial keratectomy. The dermoid is outlined, and the incision at the tip is extended slightly to make it cruciate, to facilitate picking the tip up. The edges of the incision should have mild gaping to indicate incision into the stroma rather than scratching the epithelium. (Courtesy of Dr. M. Wyman, The Ohio State University.)

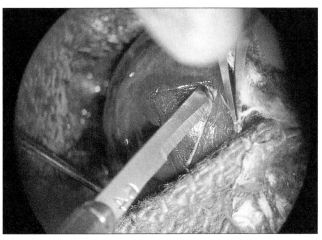

Figure 10.121 Technique for performing a superficial keratectomy. The blade is rotated so it is tangential to the cornea and a blue-white tension line indicates the line of dissection. If the lesion involves the limbus, dissection should start from the corneal side to avoid bleeding during the majority of the dissection. Excess tension on the cornea may leave tufts of torn fibers rather than incised fibers. A variety of specialty blades can be utilized for the dissection.

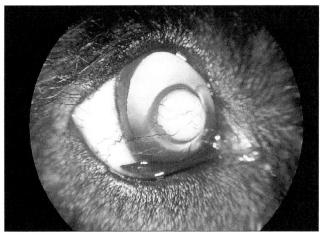

Figure 10.122 Corneal inclusion cyst in a dog. This presents as a raised, smooth mass on the cornea that is pink to creamy in color. Most are superficial and can be dissected with a superficial keratectomy.

Pseudotumors

- Epithelial inclusion cysts are rare, but they may mimic a tumor. They are raised, smooth-surfaced lesions that are filled with a milky fluid (**Figure 10.122**). A central location on the cornea differentiates the cyst from a neoplasia. A history of prior trauma, corneal ulceration, or surgery in the region months previously is helpful but not consistent.[478–480] Diagnosis and therapy is by performing a superficial keratectomy. If incised during surgery, the cystic nature is obvious. Most epithelial inclusion cysts are superficial in the cornea, but depending on their origin, it is possible to have almost full-thickness corneal involvement requiring a surgical patch of conjunctiva or cornea after excision. Choi et al. report the use of equine amniotic membrane to promote healing and to provide structural integrity following the removal of a large cyst in a dog.[481] The author has used bioscaffolding material to aid in healing and structural support following the removal of deep inclusion cysts.
- Nodular granulomatous episclerokeratitis (fibrous histiocytoma) (NGESK) is the most common pseudotumor observed. Collies are predisposed. Fibrous histiocytoma is a misnomer, as this condition is not considered neoplastic in dogs and cats; it is in humans. NGESK manifests as proliferative pink masses, usually at the temporal limbus of one or both eyes (**Figure 10.123**). An arc of lipid is often present

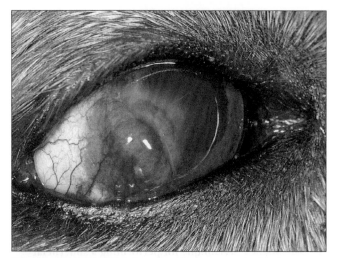

Figure 10.123 Nodular granulomatous episclerokeratitis (NGESK) in a collie. The main differential is a neoplastic process. Both eyes are probably involved in NGESK, and some response may occur with anti-inflammatory therapy.

in the cornea adjacent to the advancing edge of the lesion. Occasionally, the masses are on the lids, third eyelid, and central cornea.[482,483] On histopathologic examination, the masses consist of subepithelial inflammatory cells that range from predominantly lymphocytes and plasma cells to predominantly histiocytes. NGESK is thought to be an immune-mediated disease based on histopathology, breed predisposition, and response to therapy. The masses in NGESK usually respond initially to topical or subconjunctival steroid therapy but often become unresponsive with time. Superficial keratectomy followed by topical steroid therapy may be curative, but systemic azathioprine has supplanted surgery as the therapy of choice.[484] The recommended dose of azathioprine is 2 mg/kg every 24 hours until clinical improvement occurs, reducing to 1 mg/kg every 24 hours, then on alternate days, and finally weekly depending on lesion response and results of weekly hemograms. Therapy may eventually be terminated after long-term maintenance therapy.[485] An alternative to azothioprine is cryotherapy or superficial keratectomy followed by cryotherapy, provided concurrent immunosuppressive therapy is not used.[486] Successful primary treatment of scleritis with oral tetracycline (500 mg every 8 hours) and niacinamide (500 mg every 8 hours) has been reported.[487] The frequency of dose can be reduced to every 12–24 hours based on response. This therapy can also be used when anti-inflammatories have failed.

- Nodular fasciitis: The literature is confusing regarding differentiation of this lesion from NGESK or fibrous histiocytoma. The confusion is compounded by use of the synonym nodular episcleritis.[488,489] Clinically, nodular fasciitis is often a subconjunctival mass attached to the sclera, but it may involve the cornea, the third eyelid, and the lids (**Figure 10.124**). Unlike fibrous histiocytoma, the American Cocker Spaniel and Golden retriever are predisposed to nodular fasciitis.[490] The condition may be static or expand rapidly and behave very aggressively. Histopathologically, the two conditions are similar, with fibroblasts in a lamellar pattern and mononuclear inflammatory cells. The inflammatory cell component is not as severe with nodular fasciitis compared to NGESK.[491-493] Surgical excision is usually curative, but aggressive lesions may require azathioprine therapy.

- Equine limbal pseudotumors: Moore et al. described, in horses, pseudotumors that are raised, smooth, nonulcerated, pink masses in the dorsal limbal or perilimbal region and third eyelid.[494] The horses range in age from 5 to 8 years. On biopsy, the lesions are inflammatory, with a predominant lymphocytic reaction, macrophages, and fibrosis. The lymphocytes are predominantly T cells. In horses, a positive response to surgical excision and/or topical corticosteroid therapy is reported. Relapses may occur, and long-term therapy may be required. The cause is unknown but postulated to be immune mediated.

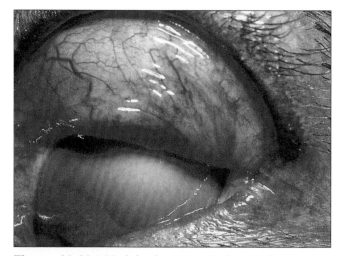

Figure 10.124 Nodular fasciitis (episcleritis) that is invading the peripheral cornea. The lesion was excised for therapeutic and biopsy purposes and controlled with topical corticosteroid therapy.

CORNEAL TUMORS

Introduction/etiology

Tumors of the cornea in the dog and the cat are not common, unlike in the horse and the cow. Most tumors arise near the limbus and extend into the cornea.

Dog and cat

Tumors such as melanomas, melanocytomas, hemangiomas, hemangiosarcomas, papillomas, and squamous cell carcinoma (SCC) have been observed (see also section Conjunctival Neoplasia, Chapter 8) (**Figure 10.125**). While SCC in the dog is rare, chronic KCS or chronic keratitis in general may be a predisposing factor.[495–497]

Epibulbar melanomas are more appropriately termed melanocytomas, considering the predominant plump melanocytes present on histopathologic examination and their benign nature. They are most common in the GSD, Labrador retriever, and Golden retriever.[498–500] In the young dog, the tumor may invade axially into the cornea as well as deeper into the iridocorneal angle and the ciliary body. Some melanocytomas may remain static for long periods of time, and when present in an old dog, they often require only surveillance. The leading edge of the tumor onto the cornea frequently has an arc of lipid in front of the advancing edge (**Figure 10.126**). Epibulbar melanomas should be differentiated from epibulbar extension of an intraocular melanoma. They are relatively benign and rarely metastasize.[498,501,502] Feline epibulbar melanoma appears to be similar to the dog.[503]

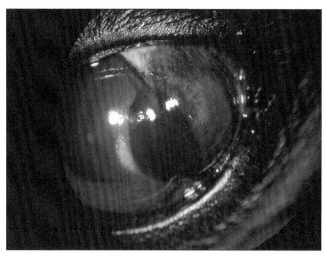

Figure 10.126 Epibulbar melanocytoma in a young German shepherd dog. Note the arc of lipid in advance of the tumor. The patient was treated by excision and corneoscleral graft.

Horse

SCC is the most common tumor of the eye and the adnexa of the horse. It originates from the cornea/limbus in 25%–30% of cases (**Figure 10.127**).[504,505] SCC remains superficial in the cornea until late in the progression of the condition and can be excised even when it covers most of the surface area. About 16% of cases are bilateral. The incidence increases with age, with a mean age ranging

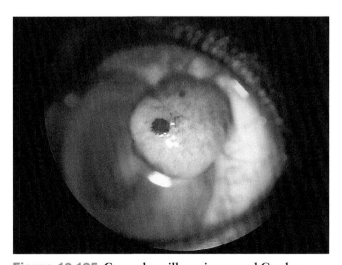

Figure 10.125 Corneal papilloma in an aged Gordon Setter. The papilloma was removed with a superficial keratectomy.

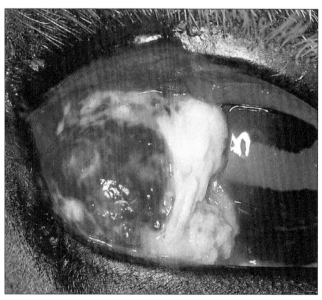

Figure 10.127 Corneal squamous cell carcinoma in a 9-year-old Clydesdale. Despite the extensive invasion, the lesion remains superficial in most instances. The patient was treated with a superficial keratectomy followed by β-radiation therapy.

from 9–12 years. SCC is more common in neutered horses. In intact animals, males are twice as commonly affected as females, and geldings are five times more susceptible than stallions. Draft horses, Appaloosas, and horses with white, cremello, and palomino hair color have a greater risk.[504–508] Haflinger horses appear to have a genetic predisposition for the development of limbal SCC.[509] SCC may occur in any breed or coat collar as exposure to solar radiation for a long duration is a predisposing factor for the development of SCC.[504] Ultraviolet radiation induces mutations in the tumor-suppressor gene p53, and it is overexpressed in equine ocular SCC.[510,511]

SCC has a high recurrence rate (30%–47.7%) but a late and low metastatic rate (6%–15%). Reports vary as to whether the site of origin influences the prognosis: One reports a higher recurrence with eyelid SCC[505] than from the third eyelid or the limbus; another reports a higher recurrence with SCC located at the limbus and the bulbar conjunctiva when compared to other anatomical sites,[512] and another reports no relationship between tumor location and outcome.[508]

Angiosarcomas (hemangiomas, hemangiosarcomas, and lymphangiosarcomas) are relatively rare and may occur on the equine cornea and limbal region. These tumors can usually be identified clinically by their vascular appearance (**Figure 10.128**), but biopsy and histopathology are required to differentiate between the tumors. Angiosarcomas are reported in the horse, the dog, and the cat.[513–517] While they can be excised surgically, they have a high potential for metastasis, and the prognosis for the animal's long-term survival is guarded (18 months).[513–515,517]

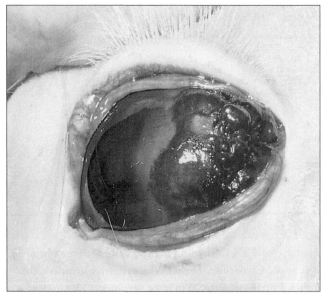

Figure 10.128 Corneal invasion of a limbal hemangiosarcoma. The prognosis is guarded because of the metastatic potential; enucleation is the therapy of choice.

Favorable results are documented with superficial keratectomy or keratectomy and strontium-90 therapy.[518,519]

Other tumors that occur in the cornea of the horse are melanocytomas, basal cell carcinomas, lymphoma, and mast cell tumors.[520–523] Extraocular lymphoma may involve the third eyelid, the corneosclera, the conjunctiva, or the eyelid, with the third eyelid being the most common ocular location.[523] Extraocular lymphoma can be nodular or diffuse. In a recent multicenter study, nodular extraocular lymphoma appears to have a fair to good prognosis with complete surgical excision, where diffuse extraocular lymphoma and eyelid lymphoma have a much worse prognosis.[523] At this time, conclusions cannot be made regarding the use of intralesional steroid injections or systemic chemotherapeutic agents as adjunctive therapies. The potential for ocular manifestation of multicentric lymphoma should be considered, as 27% of the cases of multicentric lymphoma have ocular lesions.[522]

Cow

SCC of the eye and the adnexa is most frequent in Herefords, Hereford crosses, Simmentals, and shorthorns, and it has a significant economic impact. The etiology is multifactorial, with UV light and genetic predisposition being crucial. The amount of circumocular pigmentation has been reported as being associated with neoplasia, but a genetic predisposition exists, independent of pigmentation.[524–526] The horizontal limbal region is the most common site of origin of SCC lesions (70%), which then spread over the cornea. Approximately 10% of cases are bilateral, and 30% have multiple lesions. Precursor lesions to SCC are benign, raised, white, hyperplastic, keratinized plaques and papillomas, and about one-third spontaneously regress, although they may recur.

Metastasis is late, with rates of about 5%–15%. The tumor may invade the globe in advanced cases (20%), but the path of least resistance is across the cornea and outward (**Figures 10.129 and 10.130**).[527]

Diagnosis

The appearance and history of most tumors is usually suggestive of the diagnosis, but excisional biopsy is definitive. Cytology gives numerous spurious results, usually negative ones. Pseudotumors such as fibrous histiocytoma may mimic neoplasia in their appearance by being progressive in nature.

Therapy

If progressive, epibulbar melanocytomas should have either corneoscleral grafting performed (**Figure 10.131**),[498] or keratectomy or superficial keratectomy followed by diode or neodymium:yttrium, aluminum, and garnet (Nd-YAG)

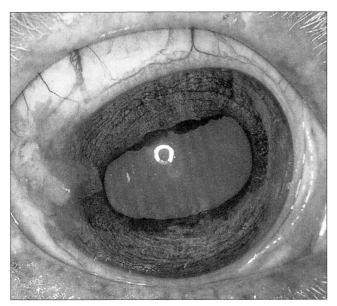

Figure 10.129 Typical location of an early squamous cell carcinoma in a cow. Lesions of this size are easily treated by a variety of modalities, but cryotherapy is probably the most common.

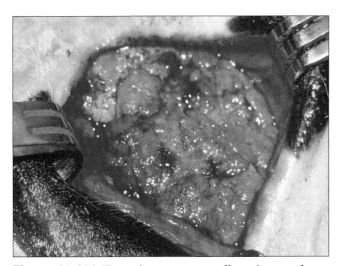

Figure 10.130 Extensive squamous cell carcinoma of the cornea. Range cattle that are not observed at frequent intervals may present at this late stage. The tumor usually prefers to grow outward but later may invade the globe. Enucleation is the most pragmatic therapy at this stage.

laser therapy. Lasering is preferred due to ease.[528,529] The recurrence rate for epibulbar melanocytoma following diode laser photocoagulation and surgical debulking is reported to be 19.05%. Donaldson et al. report excellent results of treating epibulbar melanocytomas with superficial keratectomy and β-radiation.[500] Cryotherapy following surgical resection is a viable alternative if laser or β-radiation are not available.[530] An alternative to a corneal

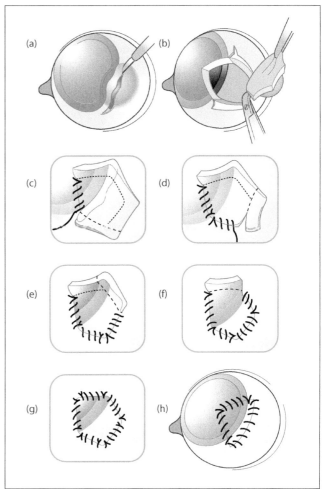

Figure 10.131 Technique of performing a corneoscleral graft for neoplasia of the ocular surface. Removal of a full-thickness piece of cornea and sclera with the neoplasm en bloc (a, b). Placement of a free-hand fresh or frozen graft of sclera and cornea (c–h). The suturing and cutting of the graft are performed one side at a time.

corneoscleral graft is patching the defect with an autogenous cartilage patch from the third eyelid or the pinna, or bioscaffolding material combined with a conjunctival graft.[531–534]

Papillomas and SCCs are removed with a keratectomy. Surgical removal alone of corneal and limbal SCC has the highest rate of recurrence of all treatment modalities and is reported to be as high as 63.6% and 83.3%, respectively.[512] This high recurrence rate is due to the inability to obtain a wide excision in the cornea and limbal region. Therefore, adjunctive therapies of carbon dioxide laser ablation, mitomycin C, or brachytherapy (**Figure 10.132**) are recommended.[535] If these modalities are not available, an alternative is to treat the surgical bed with either cryotherapy, diathermy/hyperthermia, or β-radiation therapy (**Figure 10.132**).[536]

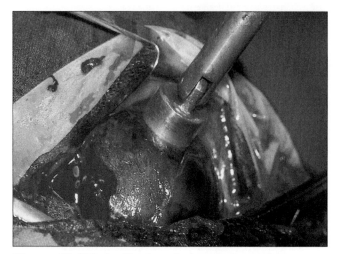

Figure 10.132 Application of a β-radiation probe to a keratectomy site after removal of a squamous cell carcinoma in a horse. This is a soft radiation that does not penetrate more than 2–3 mm.

Surgical debulking combined with cryotherapy is reported to have an overall recurrence rate of 45% for equine ocular SCC.[537] Mosunic et al. report corneal and limbal SCC recurrence rates to be 42.9% and 35%, respectively, following keratectomy and adjunctive cryotherapy.[512] The size of the corneal/limbal neoplasia may correlate with the recurrence rate. Bosch and Klein suggest that keratectomy and adjunctive cryotherapy are an effective treatment for cornea/limbal SCC < 2 cm.[2,537] Success rates as high as 97% are reported with a double-freeze technique for treating bovine SCC[538] and as high as 80%–91% when treated with hyperthermia.[539,540]

Keratectomy combined with adjunctive strontium-90 irradiation is highly effective in treating corneal and limbal SCC.[512,541–543] Mosunic et al. evaluated 157 horses with SCC of the globe and the adnexa treated in a variety of ways; excision with β-radiation therapy has a 12% recurrence rate,[512] corneal SCC treated with adjuvant radiation has a recurrence rate of 35.3%, and limbus and bulbar conjunctival SCC has a 30.8% recurrence rate. A permanent bulbar conjunctival graft or amniotic membrane following keratectomy and strontium-90 irradiation for the treatment of corneal and limbal SCC has been recommended to reduce the potential for postoperative infections and corneal melt.[541,542] Keratectomy combined with strontium-90 irradiation and permanent bulbar conjunctival grafts or amniotic membrane in horses with corneal SCC is reported as having a 17% recurrence success rate[541] and no recurrence at 226 ± 218 days post surgery,[542] respectively. The placement of an amniotic membrane subjectively creates less scarring than a bulbar-conjunctival graft.

Carbon dioxide laser alone, following a superficial keratectomy and/or in association with mitomycin C, is reported to be an effective therapy for corneal and limbal SCC in horses.[544–547] Carbon dioxide laser ablation following a superficial keratectomy and/or conjunctivectomy is reported to have a 12.5%–14.3% recurrence rate following a single treatment and an 8.3% recurrence rate following a second application.[545,546]

The topical application of mitomycin C after surgical debulking of corneal and limbal SCC is reported to be an effective treatment modality. Superficial keratectomy followed by the application of topical mitomycin C intraoperatively and postoperatively is reported to have a recurrence rate of 17.6%,[546] and carbon dioxide ablation followed by a single intraoperatively application of mitomycin C is reported to have a recurrence rate of 20%.[547] Intraoperative mitomycin C (0.04%) solution is applied to the surgical bed via a saturated cellulose sponge for 5 min or by applying a thawed, previously frozen, equine amniotic membrane saturated with 0.4% mitomycin C.[546] Postoperatively, mitomycin C 0.04% is applied after epithelization of the surgical site by a subpalpebral lavage system (0.1–0.2 mL every 8 hours) for a cycle of 7 days on, followed by 7 days off, for one or three cycles. The number of cycles applied is at the discretion of the attending clinician.[546,548] Malalana F et al. report topical mitomycin C alone without surgical debulking to be effective in treating ocular SCC.[548] The study compared two groups: Mitomycin C as the sole treatment and surgical excision combined with topical mitomycin C. The results between the two groups are comparable with a recurrence rate of 25% and 23% for cases treated with mitomycin C alone and with surgery combined with mitomycin C, respectively. The location of the SCC may lower the efficacy of the treatment in particular for those located in the conjunctiva.[548] Topical mitomycin C 0.04% (every 6 hours for 8 weeks) combined with a superficial keratectomy has been used successfully to treat a dog with corneal SCC.[549]

Medical therapy of SCCs with intralesional cisplatin or 5-fluorouracil (5-FU) has become a mode of therapy for lid lesions. Cisplatin injections are repeated at 2-week intervals for 3–4 treatments.[550,551] Intralesional 5-FU should be considered a palliative therapy as it decreases the tumor size and improves comfort levels but does not result in a cure.[552] Two treatment regiments for the use of topical 1% 5-FU are reported to be effective in treating corneal SCC in dogs[553,554]: Topical 1% 5-FU ointment is applied four times a day for 2 weeks, followed by no treatment for 2 weeks, then applied two times a day for 2 weeks,[553] or a pulse-dose regimen of topical 1% 5-FU ointment is applied four times a day for 4 consecutive days once a month, for six treatment cycles.[554] In humans, recurrent corneal and conjunctival SCC has been treated successfully in 6/7 patients with topical α-2b interferon at a concentration of 1 million units/mL every 6 hours.[555]

Suspicious areas for SCC should be biopsied and treated early in the disease process. Small lesions are much more responsive to therapy than larger lesions. Frequent follow-up of cases is important to recognize and treat promptly any early recurrences. The author routinely rechecks 3–4 weeks after initial therapy and at 3-month intervals for the first year. Suspicious areas are biopsied and retreated as needed.

Prophylaxis

Owners are advised to avoid pasturing horses until late afternoon if possible and for the horse to wear a fly mask with UV protection. In cattle, it is important to emphasize the genetic predisposition and cull affected bulls. It is not economically feasible to cull large numbers of grade cows, so early intervention by inspection at 3-month intervals is recommended. Since spontaneous regression occurs in a significant number of cattle (33%), smaller lesions can be observed for growth and, if present, treated with cryotherapy.[526,556]

> Observation of a suspicious area is a poor treatment choice for SCC in horses. Early removal and treatment is the key to decreasing the potential for recurrence of SCC.

DISEASES OF THE SCLERA

Staphyloma

A staphyloma is a thinned outpocketing of the fibrous tunic that is lined by the uveal tunic. It may arise from congenital maldevelopment or may be acquired. Congenital staphylomas may occur with collie eye anomaly and with multiple ocular coloboma abnormalities inherited in the Australian shepherd dog. The term corneal staphyloma is used for a prolapsed iris and associated deposition of multiple layers of fibrin (**Figure 10.110**). As the fibrin organizes and matures, a layer of collagenous tissue covers the protruding iris.

Intercalary staphyloma is located near the limbus and has been described as a late complication of limbal incision with cataract surgery.[557] An additional cause of acquired intercalary staphyloma is chronic glaucoma (**Figure 10.133**) and necrotizing scleritis (see **Figure 10.136**).

Scleritis/episcleritis

Fischer classified canine scleritis/episcleritis based on clinicopathologic changes into:[558]

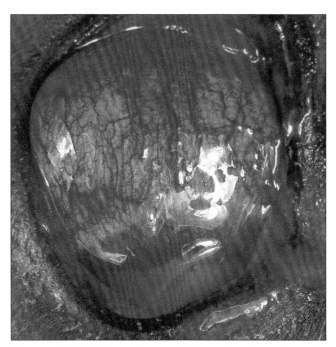

Figure 10.133 Intercalary staphyloma in a Basset hound with chronic glaucoma. Note the blue-black color of the uveal tract bulging under the bulbar conjunctiva.

- Episcleritis
  - Simple
  - Nodular episclerokeratitis
- Scleritis
  - Non-necrotizing
  - Superficial
  - Deep
  - Necrotizing

Simple episcleritis is common and is recognized by engorgement of the superficial episcleral vessels and a diffuse or sector thickening of the episcleral space (**Figures 10.134 and 10.135**). The peripheral cornea usually has a narrow rim of edema and mild neovascularization. The bulbar vascular hyperemia appears similar to intraocular diseases such as glaucoma and anterior uveitis and may be confused with conjunctivitis. Differentiating features are the thickened episclera under the conjunctiva and peripheral corneal edema (**Figure 10.135**) with normal IOP, unless accompanied by anterior uveitis. The condition may be unilateral or bilateral in presentation. An association with positive toxoplasmosis titers has been reported, the significance of which is unknown.[559] An immune panel may have positive antinuclear antibody (ANA) titers, but these are quite variable. The American Cocker Spaniel appears to be predisposed to episcleritis, and in one study, the breed represented 31.5% of the cases.[493] Histopathology of biopsies from dogs with episcleritis reveals that the

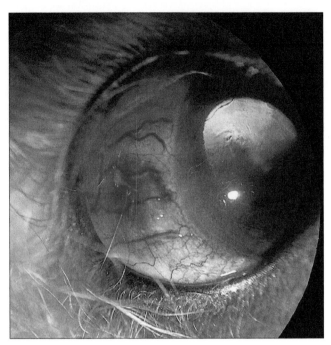

Figure 10.134 Sector episcleritis in an American Cocker Spaniel. Note the selective vascular engorgement and thickening of the episclera. The adjacent cornea may have a mild edema with neovascularization.

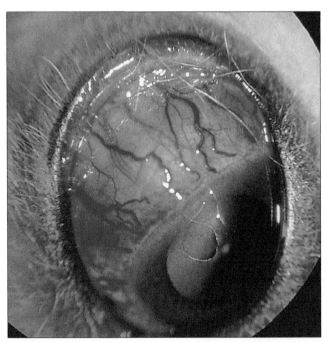

Figure 10.135 Diffuse episcleritis in an American Cocker Spaniel. Note the thickened episclera, selective conjunctival engorgement, and peripheral corneal edema and neovascularization. Because of the breed, these signs might be confused with glaucoma.

predominate inflammatory cells were lymphocytes and histiocytes with the occasional plasma cell.[493] The condition is benign and is responsive to topical or intralesional corticosteroids, although the drugs may have to be given for an indefinite period. Immunohistochemical investigations of the episcleritis biopsies indicated that dogs with a higher percentage of intralesional B lymphocytes required ongoing therapy.[493] Initial topical therapy with prednisolone acetate 1.0% or dexamethasone sodium phosphate 0.1% (every 6 hours) is required to obtain resolution of the condition. After resolution, topical steroids are tapered slowly over weeks to months. Approximately 50% of the cases, whether unilateral or bilateral, require continued medical therapy.[493]

Nodular episclerokeratitis is described earlier (see section Pseudotumors). According to Fischer, fibrous histiocytoma and nodular fasciitis are variations of the same process (**Figures 10.123 and 10.124**). Nodular episcleritis is reported to be significantly different in collies and non-collie breeds on histopathologic examination.[490] Non-collie forms of nodular episcleritis are characterized by degenerate collagen with scattered mononuclear inflammatory cells. Collie nodular episcleritis is characterized by fibroblasts but no degenerative collagen. In collies, the predominate inflammatory cells are lymphocytes and histiocytes with the occasional plasma cells. There is no statistical difference between the percentage of histiocytes, B-cells, and T-cells in collies with nodular episcleritis and non-collie breeds with simple episcleritis.[493]

Williams et al. report two histologically distinctive forms of nodular episcleritis in non-collie breeds: An inflammatory type and a proliferative type.[560,561] The inflammatory form is characterized as inflammatory with the predominant inflammatory cells consisting of epithelioid macrophages that inconsistently form granulomas. An infiltration of neutrophils with fewer plasma cells, eosinophils, and mast cells is a frequent feature of the inflammatory type. Collagen degeneration with a focal inflammatory reaction consisting of neutrophils surrounded by lymphocytes and macrophages is a distinguishing feature. The proliferative form is characterized by the presence of variably sized, spindle-shaped cells that are organized in sheet and whorls. Nodular aggregates of lymphoplasmacytic inflammation with clusters of histiocytic cells is common. In the proliferative form, few neutrophils are seen, and eosinophil, mast cell, and collagen degeneration is not present. The predominate inflammatory cell type in both groups is reported to be T-cells. Although both forms are common, the inflammatory form is more common than the proliferative form. Cocker spaniels and Labrador retrievers are the most common breeds effected with both forms.

Based on the predominate granulomatous inflammatory reaction, nodular episcleritis and nodular episclerokeratitis are often referred to as nodular granulomatous epislceritis. No matter the form or breed, nodular episcleritis typically present as a fleshy, raised, pink mass affecting the temporal limbal region. The lesion may extend into the adjacent cornea and has been reported to extend into the orbit with the dogs presenting with the clinical findings consistent with an orbital mass.[561,562]

Initial treatment for nodular episcleritis and nodular episclerokeratitis consists of topical steroids, either prednisolone acetate 1.0% or dexamethasone 0.1% (every 6 hours). Immunosuppressive doses of corticosteroids, azathioprine, tetracycline, and niacinamide are recommended in refractory cases as described previously (see section Pseudotumors). Surgical excision of an orbital mass associated with orbital extension of nodular episcleritis is reported to be an effective treatment option.[562] The author has successfully treated a Labrador retriever with bilateral orbital extension of nodular episclerokeratitis with an initial combination of oral corticosteroids and azathioprine, and oral doxycycline and niacinamide once in remission.

Non-necrotizing superficial scleritis tends to be bilateral and involves the anterior sclera, the cornea, and the anterior uvea. It manifests as mildly elevated, red lesions in the anterior sclera. The histopathologic changes in the superficial and deep forms are similar, with mononuclear inflammation and a few giant cells. It is responsive to corticosteroid therapy but may relapse.

Deep non-necrotizing scleritis involves the anterior and posterior sclera, the uvea, and the retina. The condition may be bilateral, and loss of ocular function is possible. Fortunately, this is a rare condition. Corticosteroid therapy is frequently unsuccessful, and azathioprine or cyclophosphamide therapy is warranted.

Necrotizing scleritis is uncommon. Histopathologically, necrotizing scleritis is characterized by vasculitis, granulomatous inflammation (macrophages, lymphocytes, and plasma cells), and collagenolysis. Based on immunohistochemical studies, the cellular infiltrate is composed of T-cells, B-cells, MHC class II+ macrophages, and IgG plasma cells. Based on the results of current studies, it is difficult to draw conclusions as to the predominate lymphocyte population.[563,564] Day et al. suggests that the immunopathogenesis of necrotizing scleritis likely involves a primary type IV hypersensitivity with an underlying type III hypersensitivity.[563] In humans, the inflammatory infiltrate predisposes to an imbalance of matrix metalloproteinases and tissue inhibitors of matrix metalloproteinases resulting in collagenolysis.[565] It is likely that a similar process occurs in dogs, as the collagenolysis can progress rapidly, similar to a melting corneal ulcer, resulting in a

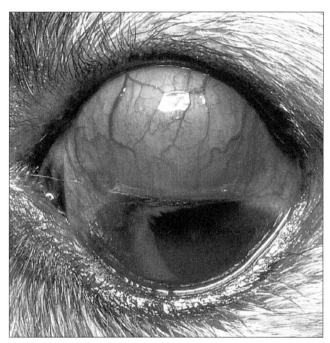

Figure 10.136 Necrotizing scleritis in a dog with *Ehrlichia canis* infection. The condition became bilateral and initially presented because of a uveitis with hemorrhagic overtones.

staphyloma and subconjunctival uveal prolapse (**Figure 10.136**). In addition to extraocular inflammation, intraocular inflammation is a common feature. Anterior uveitis, chorioretinitis (granulomatous and nongranulomatous), and retinal detachments are common with necrotizing sclertitis.[563,564] Necrotizing scleritis can be unilateral or bilateral, and concurrent systemic disease is a possibility. *Ehrlichia canis* infection is reported to be associated with necrotizing scleritis.[559,566]

Parasitic

Parasitic granulomas from *Onchocerca* spp. have been reported in the dog, involving the episcleral/scleral regions adjacent to the limbus.[567–569] In the western United States, an aberrant infection with *O. lienalis* or *O. stilesi*, which normally infect cows, is reported in three dogs. No intraocular involvement is reported in these cases.

Epibulbar involvement with *Onchocerca* spp. appears to be endemic to Greece, and the species involved is postulated to be a unique species that has not been recognized to date and is probably from an unknown wild ungulate.[569] To date, 64 cases have been described in Europe and the United States. Nucleotide sequencing of canine *Onchocerca* indicates that it is a unique species, probably *Onchocerca lupus*, that was originally identified in a wolf.[570] The life cycle is probably indirect, involving biting flies as intermediate hosts. The dog and other canids are probably the definitive host.

Ocular onchocerciasis may be either unilateral or bilateral. In Greece, it is characterized by one or more conjunctival masses on the sclera with associated signs of periorbital swelling, exophthalmos, ocular discharge, ocular pain, conjunctival hyperemia, and protrusion of the third eyelid. Episcleral granulomas are present in most cases, and involvement of the anterior or posterior uvea is a complication in 60%. Peripheral eosinophilia is reported in 34.7% of the cases.

Diagnosis is made by finding the parasite either protruding from the granuloma on clinical examination or in the tissues obtained from surgical excision of the granulomas. Both live and dead parasites of both sexes can be found in the granulomas. Therapy consisted of surgical excision of the granulomas followed by medical therapy with melarsomine (2.5 mg/kg every 24 hours intramuscularly) for 2 days followed by ivermectin (50 μg/kg every 24 hours) for 30 days. Initial therapy results in increased periocular swelling and pruritis that abated within 1 week.

REFERENCES

1. Bayer, J. 1914. *Augenheilkunde.* Wilhelm Braumuller: Leipzig, pp. 1–630.
2. Dice, P. 1981. *Veterinary Ophthalmology.* Lea & Febiger: Philadelphia, PA.
3. Freeman, R. 1980. Corneal radius of curvature of the kitten and the cat. *Investigative Ophthalmology and Visual Science* 19:306–308.
4. Prince, J., Diesem, C., Eglitis, I., and Ruskell, G. 1960. The globe. In: *Anatomy and Histology of the Eye and Orbit of Domestic Animals.* CC Thomas: Springfield, IL.
5. Stapleton, S., and Peiffer, R. 1979. Specular microscopic observations of the clinically normal canine corneal endothelium. *American Journal of Veterinary Research* 42:1803–1804.
6. Peiffer, R., Devanzo, R., and Cohen, K. 1981. Specular microscopic observations of clinically normal feline corneal endothelium. *American Journal of Veterinary Research* 42:854–855.
7. Gilger, B.C., Whitley, R., McLaughlin, S., Wright, J., and Drane, J. 1991. Canine corneal thickness measured by ultrasonic pachymetry. *American Journal of Veterinary Research* 52(10):1570–1572.
8. Moodie, K., Hashizume, N., Houston, D., Hoopes, P., Demidenko, E., Trembly, B. et al. 2001. Postnatal development of corneal curvature and thickness in the cat. *Veterinary Ophthalmology* 4(4):267–272.
9. Chan-Ling, T., Efron, N., and Holden, B. 1985. Diurnal variation of corneal thickness in the cat. *Investigative Ophthalmology and Visual Science* 26:102–105.
10. Petrick, S., and van Rensburg, I. 1989. Corneal anatomical differences in the aetiology of chronic superfical keratitis. *Journal of Small Animal Practice* 30:449–453.
11. Watsky, M., Olsen, T., and Edelhauser, H. 1995. Cornea and sclera. In: *Duane's Foundation of Clinical Ophthalmology.* Tasma, W., Jaeger, E., and Kaufman, P., editors. Lippincott, Williams, & Wilkins: Philadelphia, PA, pp. 1–29.
12. Castoro, J., Bettelheim, A., and Bettellheim, F. 1988. Water gradients across the bovine cornea. *Investigative Ophthalmology and Visual Science* 29:963–968.
13. Barrett, P., Scagliotti, R., Merideth, R., Jackson, P., and Alarcon, F. 1991. Absolute corneal sensitivity and corneal trigeminal nerve anatomy in normal dogs. *Progress in Veterinary and Comparative Ophthalmology* 1:245–254.
14. Chan-Ling, T. 1989. Sensitivity and neural organization of the cat cornea. *Investigative Ophthalmology and Visual Science* 30:1075–1082.
15. Duke-Elder, S., and Gloster, J. 1968. Physiology of the eye and of vision. In: *Systems of Ophthalmology.* CV Mosby: St Louis, MO, pp. 337–363.
16. Wieser, B., Tichy, A., and Nell, B. 2013. Correlation between corneal sensitivity and quantity of reflex tearing in cows, horses, goats, sheep, dogs cats, rabbits and guinea pigs. *Veterinary Ophthalmology* 16(4):251–262.
17. Blocker, T., and Van Der Woerdt, A. 2001. A comparison of corneal sensitivity between brachycephalic and Domestic Short-haired cats. *Veterinary Ophthalmology* 4(2):127–130.
18. Brooks, D., Clark, C., and Lester, G. 2003. Cochet-Bonnet aesthesiometer-determined corneal sensitivity in neonatal foals and adult horses. *Veterinary Ophthalmology* 3:133–137.
19. Rankin, A.J., Hosking, K.G., Roush, J.K. 2012. Corneal sensitivity in healthy, immature, and adult alpacas. *Veterinary Ophthalmology* 15(1):31–35.
20. Miller, C., Utter, M., and Beech, J. 2013. Evaluation of the effects of age and pituritary pars intermedia dysfunction on corneal sensitivity in horses. *American Journal of Veterinary Research* 74(7):1030–1035.
21. Good, K.L., Maggs, D.J., Hollingsworth, S.R., Scagliotti, R.H., and Nelson, R.W. 2003. Corneal sensitivity in dogs with diabetes mellitus. *American Journal of Veterinary Research* 64:7–11.
22. Blocker, T., Hoffman, A., Schaeffer, D.J., and Wallin, J.A. 2007. Corneal sensitivity and aqueous tear production in dogs undergoing evisceration with intraocular prosthesis placement. *Veterinary Ophthalmology* 10(3):147–154.
23. Marfurt, C.F., Murphy, C.J., and Florczak, J.L. 2001. Morphology and neurochemistry of canine corneal innervation. *Investigative Ophthalmology & Visual Science* 42(10):2242–2251.
24. Murphy, C., Reid, T., Mannis, M., and Iwahashi, C. 1990. The role of neuropeptides in corneal wound healing. *Proceedings of the Scientific Meeting of the American College of Veterinary Ophthalmologists* 21:81.
25. Nishida, T., Nakamura, M., Ofuji, K., Reid, T., Mannis, M., and Murphy, C. 1996. Synergistic effects of substance P with insulin-like growth factor-1 on epithelial migration of the cornea. *Journal of Cellular Physiology* 169:159–166.
26. Shamsuddin, A., Nirankari, V., Purnell, D., and Chang, S. 1986. Is the corneal posterior cell layer truly endothelial? *Ophthalmology* 93:1298–1303.
27. Van Horn, D., Sendele, D., Seideman, S., and Buco, P. 1977. Regenerative capacity of the corneal endothelium in rabbits and cats. *Investigative Ophthalmology and Visual Science* 16:597–613.
28. Befanis, P., Peiffer, R., and Brown, D. 1981. Endothelial repair of the canine cornea. *American Journal of Veterinary Research* 42:590–595.
29. Waring, G., Bourne, W., Edelhauser, H., and Kenyon, K. 1982. The corneal endothelium: Normal and pathologic structure and function. *Ophthalmology* 89:531–590.

30. Martin, C., and Anderson, B. 1981. Ocular anatomy. In: Gelatt, K. (editor), *Veterinary Ophthalmology*. Lea & Febiger: Philadelphia, PA, pp. 12–121.

31. Maurice, D. 1957. The structure and transparency of the cornea. *Journal of Physiology* 136:263–286.

32. Goldman, J., Benedek, G., Dohlman, C., and Kravitt, B. 1968. Structural alterations affecting transparency in swollen human corneas. *Investigative Ophthalmology and Visual Science* 7:501–519.

33. Pfister, R. 1975. The healing of corneal epithelial abrasions in the rabbit: A scanning electron microscope study. *Investigative Ophthalmology and Visual Science* 14:648–661.

34. Dua, H., Gomes, J., and Singh, A. 1994. Corneal epithelial wound healing. *British Journal of Ophthalmology* 78:401–408.

35. Kruse, F., Chen, J., Tsai, R., and Tseng, S. 1990. Conjunctival transdifferentiation is due to the incomplete removal of limbal basal epithelium. *Investigative Ophthalmology and Visual Science* 31:1903–1913.

36. Danjo, S., Friend, J., and Thoft, R. 1987. Conjunctival epithelium in healing of corneal epithelial wounds. *Investigative Ophthalmology and Visual Science* 28:1445–1449.

37. Tseng, S., Hirst, L., Farazdaghi, M., and Green, W. 1984. Goblet cell density and vascularization during conjunctival transdifferentiation. *Investigative Ophthalmology and Visual Science* 25:1168–1176.

38. Tseng, S., Hirst, L., Farazdaghi, M., and Green, W. 1987. Inhibition of conjunctival transdifferentiation by topical retinoids. *Investigative Ophthalmology and Visual Science* 28:538–542.

39. Khodadoust, A., Silverstein, A., Kenyon, K., and Dowling, J. 1968. Adhesion of regenerating corneal epithelium: The role of basement membrane. *American Journal of Ophthalmology* 65:339–348.

40. Robb, R., and Kuwabara, T. 1962. Corneal wound healing. I. The movement of polymorphonuclear leukocytes into corneal wounds. *Archives of Ophthalmology* 68:592–642.

41. Weimar, V. 1958. The sources of fibroblasts in corneal wound repair. *Archives of Ophthalmology* 60:93–109.

42. Kitano, S., and Goldman, J. 1966. Cytologic and histochemical changes in corneal wound repair. *Archives of Ophthalmology* 76:345–354.

43. Gasset, A., and Dohlman, C. 1968. The tensile strength of corneal wounds. *Archives of Ophthalmology* 79:595–602.

44. Benezra, D. 1978. Neovasculogenic ability of prostaglandins, growth factors, and synthetic chemoattractants. *American Journal of Ophthalmology* 86:455–461.

45. Glaser, B., D'Amore, P., Michels, R. et al. 1980. The demonstration of angiogenic activity from ocular tissues. *Ophthalmology* 87:440–446.

46. Lutty, G., Liu, S., and Prendergast, R. 1983. Angiogenic lymphokines of activated T-cell origin. *Investigative Ophthalmology and Visual Science* 24:1595–1601.

47. Maurice, D., Zauberman, H., and Michaelson, I. 1966. The stimulus to neovascularization in the cornea. *Experimental Eye Research* 5:168–184.

48. Fromer, C., and Klintworth, G. 1975. An evaluation of the role of leukocytes in the pathogenesis of experimentally induced corneal vascularization. I. Comparison of experimental models of corneal vascularization. *American Journal of Pathology* 79:537–550.

49. Epstein, R., Stulting, R., Hendricks, R., and Harris, D. 1987. Corneal neovascularization: Pathogenesis and inhibition. *Cornea* 6:250–257.

50. Casey, R. 1997. Factors controlling ocular angiogenesis. *American Journal of Ophthalmology* 124:521–529.

51. Roberts, S., Dellaporta, A., and Winter, F. 1966. The Collie ectasia syndrome: Pathology of eyes of young and adult dogs. *American Journal of Ophthalmology* 62:728–752.

52. Molleda, J., Simon, M., Martin, E., Ginel, P., Navales, M., and Lopez, R. 1994. Congenital corneal opacity resembling human sclerocornea concurrent with scleral ectasia syndrome in the dog. *Veterinary and Comparative Ophthalmology* 4:190–192.

53. Roberts, S., and Bistner, S. 1968. Persistent pupillary membrane in Basenji dogs. *Journal of the American Veterinary Medical Association* 153:533–542.

54. Barnett, K., and Knight, G. 1969. Persistent pupillary membrane and associated defects in the Basenji. *Veterinary Record* 85:242–249.

55. Bistner, S., Rubin, L., and Roberts, S. 1971. A review of persistent pupillary membranes in the Basenji dog. *Journal of the American Animal Hospital Association* 7:143–157.

56. Mason, T. 1976. Persistent pupillary membrane in the Basenji. *Australian Veterinary Journal* 52:343–344.

57. Gwin, R., Cunningham, D., and Shaver, R. 1983. Posterior polymorphous dystrophy of the cornea in Cocker Spaniels: Preliminary clinical and specular microscopic findings. *Proceedings of the Scientific Meeting of the American College of Veterinary Ophthalmologists* 14:154–166.

58. Andersson, L.S., Juras, R., Ramsey, D.T., Eason-Butler, J., Ewart, S., Cothran, G. et al. 2008. Equine multiple congenital ocular anomalies maps to a 4.9 megabase interval on horse chromosome 6. *BMC Genetics* 9(1):88.

59. Andersson, L.S., Lyberg, K., Cothran, G., Ramsey, D.T., Juras, R., Mikko, S. et al. 2011. Targeted analysis of four breeds narrows equine multiple congenital ocular anomalies locus to 208 kilobases. *Mammalian Genome* 22(5–6):353.

60. Ramsey, D.T., Ewart, S.L., Render, J.A., Cook, C.S., Latimer, C.A. 1999. Congenital ocular abnormalities of Rocky Mountain horses. *Veterinary Ophthalmology* 2(1):47–59.

61. Ramsey, D., Hauptman, J., and Petersen-Jones, S. 1999. Corneal thickness, intraocular pressure, and optical corneal diameter in Rocky Mountain horses with cornea globosa or clinically normal corneas. *American Journal of Veterinary Research* 60(10):1317–1321.

62. Grahn, B.H., Pinard, C., Archer, S., Bellone, R., Forsyth, G., and Sandmeyer, L.S. 2008. Congenital ocular anomalies in purebred and crossbred Rocky and Kentucky Mountain horses in Canada. *The Canadian Veterinary Journal* 49(7):675.

63. Anderson, L.S., Axelsson, J., Dubielzig, R.R., Lindgren, G., and Ekesten, B. 2011. Multiple congenital ocular anomalies in Icelandic horses. *BMC Veterinary Research* 7(1):21.

64. Plummer, C.E., and Ramsey, D.T. 2011. A survey of ocular abnormalities in miniature horses. *Veterinary Ophthalmology* 14(4):239–243.

65. Depecker, M., Ségard, E., and Cadoré, J.L. 2013. Phenotypic description of multiple congenital ocular anomalies in Comtois horses. *Equine Veterinary Education* 25(10):511–516.

66. Ségard, E.M., Depecker, M.C., Lang, J., Gemperli, A., and Cadoré, J.L. 2013. Ultrasonographic features of PMEL17 (silver) mutant gene–associated multiple congenital ocular anomalies (MCOA) in Comtois and Rocky Mountain horses. *Veterinary Ophthalmology* 16(6):429–435.

67. Komáromy, A.M., Rowlan, J.S., La Croix, N.C., and Mangan, B.G. 2011. Equine multiple congenital ocular anomalies (MCOA) syndrome in PMEL17 (silver) mutant ponies: Five cases. *Veterinary Ophthalmology* 14(5):313–320.

68. Premont, J., Andersson, L., and Grauwels, M. 2013. Multiple congenital ocular anomalies syndrome in a family of Shetland and Deutsches classic ponies in Belgium. *Equine Veterinary Education* 25(11):550–555.

69. Badial, P.R., Cisneros-Àlvarez, L.E., Brandão, C.V.S., Ranzani, J.J.T., Tomaz, M.A., Machado, V.M. et al. 2015. Ocular dimensions, corneal thickness, and corneal curvature in quarter horses with hereditary equine regional dermal asthenia. *Veterinary Ophthalmology* 18(5):385–392.

70. Fischer, C. 1989. Geriatric ophthalmology. *Veterinary Clinics of North America: Small Animal Practice* 19(1):103–123.

71. Sansom, J., and Blunden, T. 2010. Calcareous degeneration of the canine cornea. *Veterinary Ophthalmology* 13(4):238–243.

72. Rebhun, W., Murphy, C., and Hacker, D. 1993. Calcific band keratopathy in horses. *Compendium on Continuing Education for the Practicing Veterinarian* 15:1402–1409.

73. Berryhill, E.H., Thomasy, S.M., Kass, P.H., Reilly, C.M., Good, K.L., Hollingsworth, S.R. et al. 2017. Comparison of corneal degeneration and calcific band keratopathy from 2000 to 2013 in 69 horses. *Veterinary Ophthalmology* 20(1):16–26.

74. Ward, D., Martin, C., and Weiser, I. 1989. Band keratopathy associated with hyperadrenalcorticism. *Journal of the American Animal Hospital Association* 25:583–586.

75. Doughman, D., Olson, G., Nolan, S., and Hajny, R. 1969. Experimental band keratopathy. *Archives of Ophthalmology* 81:264–272.

76. Taravella, M., Stulting, D., Mader, T., and Weisenthal, R. 1994. Calcific band keratopathy associated with the use of topical steroid-phosphate preparations. *Archives of Ophthalmology* 112:608–613.

77. Nevyas, A., Raber, I., Eagle, R., Wallace, I., and Nevyas, H. 1987. Acute band keratopathy following intracameral Visacoat. *Archives of Ophthalmology* 105:958–964.

78. Nevile, J.C., Hurn, S.D., Turner, A.G., and Morton, J. 2016. Diamond burr debridement of 34 canine corneas with presumed corneal calcareous degeneration. *Veterinary Ophthalmology* 19(4):305–312.

79. Dice, P. 1982. Corneal opacities in the Shetland Sheepdog: Preliminary report. *Proceedings of the Annual Meeting of the American Society of Veterinary Ophthalmology and International Society of Veterinary Ophthalmology* 13:58–64.

80. Dice, P. 1984. Corneal dystrophy in the Shetland Sheepdog. *Proceedings of the Scientific Meeting of the American College of Veterinary Ophthalmologists* 15:241.

81. Roth, A., Ekins, M., Waring, G., Gupta, L., and Rosenblatt, L. 1981. Oval corneal opacities in Beagles. III. Histochemical demonstration of stromal lipids without hyperlipidemia. *Investigative Ophthalmology and Visual Science* 21:95–106.

82. Barsotti, G.P.A., Busillo, L. et al. 2008; Corneal crystalline stromal dystrophy and lipidic metabolism in the dog. *Veterinary Research Communications* 32(supplement 1):S227–9.

83. Veenendaal, H. 1937. Dystrophia corneae adiposa bij de hond. *Tijdschr Diergeneesk* 64:913–921.

84. Dice, P. 1974. Corneal dystrophy in the Airedale. *Proceedings of the Scientific Meeting of the American College of Veterinary Ophthalmologists* 5:80–86.

85. Waring, G., Muggli, F., and MacMillan, A. 1977. Oval corneal opacities in Beagles. *Journal of the American Animal Hospital Association* 13:204–208.

86. MacMillan, A., Waring, G., Spangler, W., and Roth, A. 1979. Crystalline corneal opacities in the Siberian Husky. *Journal of the American Veterinary Medical Association* 175:829–832.

87. Waring, G., MacMillian, A., and Reveles, P. 1986. Inheritance of crystalline corneal dystrophy in Siberian Huskies. *Journal of the American Animal Hospital Association* 22:655–658.

88. Crispin, S., and Barnett, K. 1983. Dystrophy, degeneration and infiltration of the canine cornea. *Journal of Small Animal Practice* 24:63–83.

89. Carrington, S. 1983. Lipid keratopathy in a cat. *Journal of Small Animal Practice* 24:495–505.

90. Sandersleben, J. 1986. Lipispeicherkrakheit vom typ der wolmanschen erkrankung des menschen beim Fox Terrier. *Tierärztliche Praxis* 14:253–263.

91. Collins, L., Munnell, J., and Lorenz, M. 1978. The pathology of feline GM_2 gangliosidosis. *American Journal of Pathology* 90:723–730.

92. Cowell, K., Jezyk, P., Haskins, M., and Patterson, D. 1976. Mucopolysaccharidosis in a cat. *Journal of the American Veterinary Medical Association* 169:334–339.

93. Langweiler, M., Haskins, M., and Jezyk, P. 1978. Mucopolysaccharidosis in a litter of cats. *Journal of the American Animal Hospital Association* 14:748–751.

94. Haskins, M., Jezyk, P., Desnick, R., McDonough, S., and Patterson, D. 1979. Mucopolysaccharidosis in a domestic shorthaired cat: A disease distinct from that seen in the Siamese cat. *Journal of the American Veterinary Medical Association* 175:384–387.

95. Breton, L., Guerin, P., and Morin, M. 1983. A case of mucopolysaccharidosis VI in a cat. *Journal of the American Animal Hospital Association* 19:891–896.

96. Shull, R., Munger, R., Spellacy, E., Hall, C., Constantopoulos, G., and Neufeld, E. 1982. Canine alpha-L-iduronidase deficiency: A model of mucopolysaccharidosis I. *American Journal of Pathology* 109:244–248.

97. Haskins, M., Desnick, R., DiFerrant, N., Jezyk, P., and Patterson, D. 1984. ß-glucuronidase deficiency in a dog: A model of human mucopolysaccharidosis VII. *Pediatric Research* 18:980–984.

98. Gwin, R., Polack, F., Warren, J., Samuelson, D., and Gelatt, K. 1982. Primary canine corneal endothelial cell dystrophy: Specular microscopic evaluation, diagnosis, and therapy. *Journal of the American Animal Hospital Association* 18:471–479.

99. Martin, C., and Dice, P. 1982. Corneal endothelial dystrophy in the dog. *Journal of the American Animal Hospital Association* 18:327–336.

100. Bistner, S., Aquirre, G., and Shively, J. 1976. Hereditary corneal dystrophy in the Manx cat: A preliminary report. *Investigative Ophthalmology and Visual Science* 15:15–26.

101. Olin, D., and Tenbroeck, T. 1973. Corneal dystrophy in a cat. *Veterinary Medicine/Small Animal Clinician* 68:1237–1238.

102. Bistner, S., Shaw, D., and Sartori, R. 1981. Ocular manifestations of low-level phenothiazine administration to cattle. *Cornell Veterinarian* 71:136–143.

103. Gratzek, A., Calvert, C., Martin, C., and Kaswan, R. 1993. Corneal edema in dogs treated with tocainide. *Progress in Veterinary and Comparative Ophthalmology* 3:47–51.

104. Murphy, C.J., Burling, T., and Hollingsworth, S. 1993. Thermokeratoplasty for the treatment of chronic bullous keratopathy in the dog. *Proceedings of the Scientific Meeting of the American College of Veterinary Ophthalmology* 24:21.

105. Michau, T.M., Gilger, B.C., Maggio, F., and Davidson, M.G. 2003. Use of thermokeratoplasty for treatment of ulcerative keratitis and bullous keratopathy secondary to corneal endothelial disease in dogs: 13 cases (1994–2001). *Journal of the American Veterinary Medical Association* 222(5):607–612.

106. Gunderssen, T., and Pearlson, H. 1969. Conjunctival flaps for corneal disease: Their usefulness and complications. *Transactions of the American Ophthalmological Society* 67:78–95.

107. Wilkie, D., and Whittaker, C. 1997. Surgery of the cornea. *Veterinary Clinics of North America: Small Animal Practice* 27:1067–1107.

108. Scherrer, N.M., Lassaline, M., and Miller, W.W. 2017. Corneal edema in four horses treated with a superficial keratectomy and Gundersen inlay flap. *Veterinary Ophthalmology* 20(1):65–72.

109. Famose, F. 2016. Evaluation of accelerated corneal collagen cross-linking for the treatment of bullous keratopathy in eight dogs (10 eyes). *Veterinary Ophthalmology* 19(3):250–255.

110. Pot, S.A., Gallhöfer, N.S., Walser-Reinhardt, L., Hafezi, F., and Spiess, B.M. 2015. Treatment of bullous keratopathy with corneal collagen cross-linking in two dogs. *Veterinary Ophthalmology* 18(2):168–173.

111. Walde, I. 1983. Band opacities. *Equine Veterinary Journal* 32(Supplement 2):32.

112. Henriksen, M.D.L., Andersen, P.H., Thomsen, P.D., Plummer, C.E., Mangan, B., Heegaard, S. et al. 2014. Equine deep stromal abscesses (51 cases–2004–2009)–Part 1: The clinical aspects with attention to the duration of the corneal disease, treatment history, clinical appearance, and microbiology results. *Veterinary Ophthalmology* 17(1):6–13.

113. Moore, P., Dietrich, U., Barton, M. et al. 2005. The influence of rainfall and temperature on the frequency of equine fungal keratitis. *Association for Research and Vision and Ophthalmology Abstracts* 46:5067.

114. Voelter-Ratson, K., Pot, S., Florin, M., and Spiess, B. 2013. Equine keratomycosis in Switzerland: A retrospective evaluation of 35 horses (January 2000–August 2011). *Equine Veterinary Journal* 45(5):608–612.

115. Hendrix, D.V., Brooks, D., Smith, P.J., Gelatt, K., Miller, T., Whittaker, C. et al. 1995. Corneal stromal abscesses in the horse: A review of 24 cases. *Equine Veterinary Journal* 27(6):440–447.

116. Proietto, L.R., Plummer, C.E., Maxwell, K.M., Lamb, K.E., and Brooks, D.E. 2016. A retrospective analysis of environmental risk factors for the diagnosis of deep stromal abscess in 390 horses in North Central Florida from 1991 to 2013. *Veterinary Ophthalmology* 19(4):291–296.

117. Rebhun, W. 1982. Corneal stromal abscesses in the horse. *Journal of the American Veterinary Medical Association* 181:677–679.

118. Michau, T., Maggio, F., Pizzirani, S., Davidson, M., and Gilger, B. 2002. Findings from 16 consecutive cases of penetrating keratoplasty for deep stromal abscess in the horse (2001–2002). *Proceedings of the Scientific Meeting of the American College of Veterinary Ophthalmologists* 33:30.

119. Lassaline, M., Andrew, S., Brooks, D., and Detrisac, C. 2002. Histologic analysis of keratectomy specimens from horses undergoing corneal transplantation for stromal abscess. *Proceedings of the Scientific Meeting of the American College of Veterinary Ophthalmologists* 33:32.

120. Henriksen, M.D.L., Andersen, P.H., Mietelka, K., Farina, L., Thomsen, P.D., Plummer, C.E. et al. 2014. Equine deep stromal abscesses (51 cases–2004–2009)–Part 2: The histopathology and immunohistochemical aspect with attention to the histopathologic diagnosis, vascular response, and infectious agents. *Veterinary Ophthalmology* 17(1):14–22.

121. Moore, C.P., Halenda, R., Grevan, V.L., and Collins, B. 1998. Posttraumatic keratouveitis in horses. *Equine Veterinary Journal* 30:366–372.

122. Brooks, D., Millichamp, N., Peterson, M., Laratta, L., Morgan, R., and Dziezyc, J. 1990. Nonulcerative keratouveitis in five horses. *Journal of the American Veterinary Medical Association* 196(12):1985–1991.

123. Dice, P. 1977. Intracorneal acid-fast granuloma. *Proceedings of the Scientific Meeting of the American College of Veterinary Ophthalmologists* 8:91–92.

124. Fyfe, J., McCowan, C., O'Brien, C., Globan, M., Birch, C., Revill, P. et al. 2008. Molecular characterization of a novel fastidious mycobacterium causing lepromatous lesions of the skin, subcutis, cornea, and conjunctiva of cats living in Victoria, Australia. *Journal of Clinical Microbiology* 46(2):618–626.

125. Malaty, R.B.T. 1988. Corneal changes in nine-banded armadillos with leprosy. *Investigative Ophthalmology and Visual Science* 29:140–145.

126. Peiffer, R., and Jackson, W. 1979. Mycotic keratopathy of the dog and cat in the southeastern United States: A preliminary report. *Journal of the American Animal Hospital Association* 15:93–97.

127. Fischer, C., and Peiffer, R. 1987. Acid-fast organisms associated with corneal opacities in a dog. *Proceedings of the Scientific Meeting of the American College of Veterinary Ophthalmologists* 18:241–243.

128. Karpinski, R. 1999. *Veterinary Ophthalmologists*. Listserve.

129. Ford, J., Huang, A., Pflugfelder, S., Alfonso, E., Forster, R., and Miller, D. 1998. Nontuberculous mycobacterial keratitis in south Florida. *Ophthalmology* 105:1652–1658.

130. Scott, E., and Carter, R. 2014. Canine keratomycosis in 11 dogs: A case series (2000–2011). *Journal American Animal Hospital Association* 50:112–118.

131. Ledbetter, E.C., Norman, M.L., and Starr, J.K. 2016. In vivo confocal microscopy for the detection of canine fungal keratitis and monitoring of therapeutic response. *Veterinary Ophthalmology* 19(3):220–229.

132. Nevile, J.C., Hurn, S.D., and Turner, A.G. 2016. Keratomycosis in five dogs. *Veterinary Ophthalmology* 19(5):432–438.

133. Ledbetter, E.C., Montgomery, K.W., Landry, M.P., and Kice, N.C. 2013. Characterization of fungal keratitis in alpacas: 11 cases (2003–2012). *Journal of the American Veterinary Medical Association* 243(11):1616–1622.

134. Labelle, A.L., Hamor, R.E., Barger, A.M., Maddox, C.W., and Breaux, C.B. 2009. Aspergillus flavus keratomycosis in a cat treated with topical 1% voriconazole solution. *Veterinary Ophthalmology* 12(1):48–52.

135. Bourguet, A., Guyonnet, A., Donzel, E., Guillot, J., Pignon, C., and Chahory, S. 2016. Keratomycosis in a pet rabbit (*Oryctolagus cuniculus*) treated with topical 1% terbinafine ointment. *Veterinary Ophthalmology* 19(6):504–509.

136. Voelter-Ratson, K., Monod, M., Braun, U., and Spiess, B.M. 2013. Ulcerative fungal keratitis in a brown Swiss cow. *Veterinary Ophthalmology* 16(6):464–466.

137. Moore, C., Fales, W., Whittington, P., and Bauer, L. 1983. Bacterial and fungal isolates from Equidae with ulcerative keratitis. *Journal of the American Veterinary Medical Association* 182(6):600–603.

138. Andrew, S., Brooks, D., Smith, P., Gelatt, K., Chmielewski, N., and Whittaker, C. 1998. Equine ulcerative keratomycosis: Visual outcome and ocular survival in 39 cases (1987–1996). *Equine Veterinary Journal* 30(2):109–116.

139. Miller, D., Blue, J., and Winston, S. 1983. Keratomycosis caused by *Cladosporium* spp. in a cat. *Journal of the American Veterinary Medical Association* 182:1121–1122.

140. Qualls, C., Chandler, F., Kaplan, W., Bretschwerdt, E., and Cho, D. 1985. Mycotic keratitis in a dog: Concurrent *Aspergillus* spp. and *Curvularia* spp. infections. *Journal of the American Veterinary Medical Association* 186:975–976.

141. Bernays, M., and Peiffer, R. 1998. Ocular infections with dematiaceous fungi in two cats and a dog. *Journal of the American Veterinary Medical Association* 213:507–509.

142. Rheins, M.S., Suie, T., Van Winkle, M.G., and Havener, W. 1966. Potentiation of mycotic ocular infections by drugs. A review. *The British Journal of Ophthalmology* 50(9):533–539.

143. Schmidt, G. 1974. Mycotic keratoconjunctivitis. *Veterinary Medicine, Small Animal Clinician* 69(9):1177–1179.

144. Bistner, S., and Riis, R. 1979. Clinical aspects of mycotic keratitis in the horse. *Cornell Veterinarian* 69:364–374.

145. Moore, P., Dietrich, U., Barton, M., Mosunic, C., Chandler, M., Carmichael, K. et al. 2006. Bacterial isolates cultured in conjunction with equine fungal keratitis. *Proceedings of the 37th Annual Conference of the American College of Veterinary Ophthalmologists* 37:62.

146. Massa, K.L., Murphy, C.J., Hartmann, F.A., Miller, P.E., Korsower, C.S., and Young, K.M. 1999. Usefulness of aerobic microbial culture and cytologic evaluation of corneal specimens in the diagnosis of infectious ulcerative keratitis in animals. *Journal of the American Veterinary Medical Association* 215(11):1671–1674.

147. Zeiss, C., Neaderland, M., Yang, F.C., Terwilliger, G., and Compton, S. 2013. Fungal polymerase chain reaction testing in equine ulcerative keratitis. *Veterinary Ophthalmology* 16(5):341–351.

148. O'day, D., Ray, W., Head, W., and Robinson, R. 1984. Influence of the corneal epithelium on the efficacy of topical antifungal agents. *Investigative Ophthalmology & Visual Science* 25(7):855–859.

149. O'Day, D. 1996. Fungal keratitis. In: Pepose, J., Holland, G.N., and Wilhelmus, K., editors. *Ocular Infection and Immunity*. Mosby: St. Louis, MO, pp. 1048–1061.

150. Beech, J., Sweeney, C.R., and Irby, N. 1983. Keratomycoses in 11 horses. *Equine Veterinary Journal* 15:39–44.

151. Telford, C., and Gilger, B. 2016. Subconjunctival amphotericin B injection adjunctive therapy for refractory equine keratomycosis. *Veterinary Ophthalmology* 19(S2):E21–E43.

152. Johns, K.J., and O'Day, D.M. 1988. Pharmacologic management of keratomycoses. *Survey of Ophthalmology* 33(3):178–188.

153. Joyce, J. 1983. Thiabendazole therapy of mycotic keratitis in horses. *Equine Veterinary Journal* 15:45–47.

154. Latimer, F.G., Colitz, C.M., Campbell, N.B., and Papich, M.G. 2001. Pharmacokinetics of fluconazole following intravenous and oral administration and body fluid concentrations of fluconazole following repeated oral dosing in horses. *American Journal of Veterinary Research* 62(10):1606–1611.

155. Brooks, D., Andrew, S., Dillavou, C., Ellis, G., and Kubilis, P. 1998. Antimicrobial susceptibility patterns of fungi isolated from horses with ulcerative keratomycosis. *American Journal of Veterinary Research* 59(2):138–142.

156. Ball, M., Rebhun, W., Gaarder, J., and Patten, V. 1997. Evaluation of itraconazole-dimethyl sulfoxide ointment for treatment of keratomycosis in nine horses. *Journal of the American Veterinary Medical Association* 211(2):199–203.

157. Ball, M., Rebhun, W., Trepanier, L., Gaarder, J., and Schwark, W. 1997. Corneal concentrations and preliminary toxicological evaluation of an itraconazole/dimethyl sulphoxide ophthalmic ointment. *Journal of Veterinary Pharmacology and Therapeutics* 20(2):100–104.

158. Pearce, J., Giuliano, E., and Moore, C. 2006. Susceptibility patterns of *Aspergillus* and *Fusarium* species isolated from horses with ulcerative keratomycosis. *Proceedings of the 37th Annual Conference of the American College of Veterinary Ophthalmologists* 37:4.

159. Pearce, J.W., Giuliano, E.A., and Moore, C.P. 2009. In vitro susceptibility patterns of Aspergillus and Fusarium species isolated from equine ulcerative keratomycosis cases in the midwestern and southern United States with inclusion of the new antifungal agent voriconazole. *Veterinary Ophthalmology* 12(5):318–324.

160. Clode, A.B., Davis, J.L., Salmon, J., Michau, T.M., and Gilger, B.C. 2006. Evaluation of concentration of voriconazole in aqueous humor after topical and oral administration in horses. *American Journal of Veterinary Research* 67(2):296–301.

161. Tsujita, H., and Plummer, C.E. 2013. Corneal stromal abscessation in two horses treated with intracorneal and subconjunctival injection of 1% voriconazole solution. *Veterinary Ophthalmology* 16(6):451–458.

162. Smith, K.M., Pucket, J.D., and Gilmour, M.A. 2014. Treatment of six cases of equine corneal stromal abscessation with intracorneal injection of 5% voriconazole solution. *Veterinary Ophthalmology* 17(s1):179–185.

163. Beyer, A., Abarca, E., Rodrigues, R., and Moore, P. June 2015. Multiple intrastromal injections of 1% voriconazole for the treatment of a stromal abscess in a horse. *International Equine Opohthalmology Consortium*, Savannah, GA.

164. Mohan, M., Gupta, S., Vajpayee, R., Kalra, V., and Sachdev, M., editors. 1988. *Management of Keratomycosis with 1% Silver Sulfadiazine: A Prospective Controlled Clinical Trial in 110 Cases*. Raven Press: New York.

165. Betbeze, C.M., Wu, C.C., Krohne, S.G., and Stiles, J. 2006. In vitro fungistatic and fungicidal activities of silver sulfadiazine and natamycin on pathogenic fungi isolated from horses with keratomycosis. *American Journal of Veterinary Research* 67(10):1788–1793.

166. Welch, P.M., Gabal, M., Betts, D.M., Whelan, N.C., and Studer, M.E. 2000. In vitro analysis of antiangiogenic activity of fungi isolated from clinical cases of equine keratomycosis. *Veterinary Ophthalmology* 3(2–3):145–51.

167. Gaarder, J., Rebhun, W., Ball, M., Patten, V., Shin, S., and Erb, H. 1998. Clinical appearances, healing patterns, risk factors, and outcomes of horses with fungal keratitis: 53 cases (1978–1996). *Journal of the American Veterinary Medical Association* 213(1):105–112.

168. Andrew, S.E., Brooks, D.E., Biros, D.J., Denis, H.M., Cutler, T.J., and Gelatt, K.N. 2000. Posterior lamellar keratoplasty for treatment of deep stromal abscesses in nine horses. *Veterinary Ophthalmology* 3(2–3):99–103.

169. Plummer, C., Kallberg, M., Ollivier, F., Barrie, K., and Brooks, D. 2008. Deep lamellar endothelial keratoplasty in 10 horses. *Veterinary Ophthalmology* 11(s1):35–43.

170. McMullen, R.J., Gilger, B.C., and Michau, T.M. 2015. Modified lamellar keratoplasties for the treatment of deep stromal abscesses in horses. *Veterinary Ophthalmology* 18(5):393–403.

171. Cichocki, B.M., Myrna, K.E., and Moore, P.A. 2016. Modified penetrating keratoplasty with Acell® bioscaffold implant in seven horses with deep full-thickness corneal stromal abscess. *Veterinary Ophthalmology* 20(1):46–52.

172. Sherman, A.B., Clode, A.B., and Gilger, B.C. 2017. Impact of fungal species cultured on outcome in horses with fungal keratitis. *Veterinary Ophthalmology* 20(2):140–146.

173. Beckwith-Cohen, B.B., Bentley, E., Gasper, D.J., McLellan, G.J., and Dubielzig, R.R. 2015. Keratitis in six dogs after topical treatment with carbonic anhydrase inhibitors for glaucoma. *Journal of American Veterinary Medical Association* 247:1419–1426.

174. Cello, R.M. 1971. Ocular onchocerciasis in the horse. *Equine Veterinary Journal* 3(4):148–154.

175. Pena, M., Roura, X., and Davidson, M. 2000. Ocular and periocular manifestations of leishmaniasis in dogs: 105 cases (1993–1998). *Veterinary Ophthalmology* 3(1):35–41.

176. Beckwith-Cohen, B., Gasper, D.J., Bentley, E., Gittelman, H., Ellis, A.E., Snowden, K.F. et al. 2015. Protozoal infections of the cornea and conjunctiva in dogs associated with chronic ocular surface disease and topical immunosuppression. *Veterinary Ophthalmology* 19(3):206–213.

177. Slatter, D.H., and Lavach, J. 1977. Überreiter's syndrome (chronic superficial keratitis) in dogs in the Rocky Mountain area—A study of 463 cases. *Journal of Small Animal Practice* 18(12):757–772.

178. Chavkin, M., Roberts, S., Salman, M., Severin, G., and Scholten, N. 1994. Risk factors for development of chronic superficial keratitis in dogs. *Journal of the American Veterinary Medical Association* 204(10):1630–1634.

179. Kupper, W. 1975. Oberflachenstruktur der Hornhaut bei der Keratitis superficialis chronica (Uberreiter) des Schaferhundes. *Berl Munch Tierarztl Wochenschr* 88:371–374.

180. Bedford, P., and Longstaffe, J. 1979. Corneal pannus (chronic superficial keratitis) in the German shepherd dog. *Journal of Small Animal Practice* 20(1):41–56.

181. Eichenbaum, J., Lavach, J., Gould, D., Severin, G., Paulsen, M., and Jones, R. 1986. Immunohistochemical staining patterns of canine eyes affected with chronic superficial keratitis. *American Journal of Veterinary Research* 47(9):1952–1955.

182. Peterhans, E. 1978. Histologische untersuchungen zur pathogenese der keratitis superficialis chronica (Ueberreiter des deutschen schaferhundes). *Schweizer Archiv fur Tierheilkunde* 120:41–45.

183. Clerc, B. 1982. Immunological reactions in chronic superficial keratitis (pannus): Attempts to prove the presence of immediate type hypersensitivity in chronic superficial keratitis in the German Shepherd Dog. *Proceedings of the Annual Meeting of the American Society of Veterinary Ophthalmology and International Society of Veterinary Ophthalmology*; Las Vegas, NV, pp. 54–55.

184. Rapp, E., and Kölbl, S. 1995. Ultrastructural study of unidentified inclusions in the cornea and iridocorneal angle of dogs with pannus. *American Journal of Veterinary Research* 56(6):779–785.

185. Tellhelm, E., Reinacher, N., and Tellhelm, B. 1982. Klinische, immunhistologische, und elektronenmikroskopische untersuchungen der keratitis superficials chronica (Uberreiter) des Deutschen schaferhundes. *Kleintierpraxis* 27:131–144.

186. Campbell, L., Okuda, H., Lipton, D., and Reed, C. 1975. Chronic superficial keratitis in dogs: Detection of cellular hypersensitivity. *American Journal of Veterinary Research* 36(5):669.

187. Williams, D. 1999. Histological and immunohistochemical evaluation of canine chronic superficial keratitis. *Research in Veterinary Science* 67(2):191–195.

188. Williams, D. 2005. Major histocompatibility class II expression in the normal canine cornea and in canine chronic superficial keratitis. *Veterinary Ophthalmology* 8(6):395–400.

189. Barrientos, L.S., Zapata, G., Crespi, J.A., Posik, D.M., Díaz, S., Peral-García, P. et al. 2013. A study of the association between chronic superficial keratitis and polymorphisms in the upstream regulatory regions of DLA-DRB1, DLA-DQB1 and DLA-DQA1. *Veterinary Immunology and Immunopathology* 156(3):205–210.

190. Jokinen, P., Rusanen, E.M., Kennedy, L.J., and Lohi, H. 2011. MHC class II risk haplotype associated with canine chronic superficial keratitis in German shepherd dogs. *Veterinary Immunology and Immunopathology* 140(1):37–41.

191. Anderson, L., Keller, W., Blachard, G., and Bull, R. 1974. Serum immunoglobulin changes associated with canine pigmentary keratitis. *Proceedings of the Scientific Meeting of the American College of Veterinary Ophthalmologists* 5:102–118.

192. Peiffer, R. 1978. Chronic superficial keratitis response of lymphocytes from dogs affected with chronic superficial keratitis to soluble homologous corneal antigen. *Proceedings of the Scientific Meeting of the American College of Veterinary Ophthalmologists* 9:51–62.

193. Chandler, H.L., Kusewitt, D.F., and Colitz, C.M. 2008. Modulation of matrix metalloproteinases by ultraviolet radiation in the canine cornea. *Veterinary Ophthalmology* 11(3):135–144.

194. Jackson, P., Kaswan, R., Merideth, R., and Barrett, P. 1991. Chronic superficial keratitis in dogs: A placebo controlled trial of topical cyclosporine treatment. *Progress in Veterinary and Comparative Ophthalmology* 1(4):269–275.

195. Nell, B., Walde, I., Billich, A., Vit, P., and Meingassner, J.G. 2005. The effect of topical pimecrolimus on keratoconjunctivitis sicca and chronic superficial keratitis in dogs: Results from an exploratory study. *Veterinary Ophthalmology* 8(1):39–46.

196. Berdoulay, A., English, R.V., andNadelstein, B. 2005. Effect of topical 0.02% tacrolimus aqueous suspension on tear production in dogs with keratoconjunctivitis sicca. *Veterinary Ophthalmology* 8(4):225–232.

197. Williams, D., Hoey, A., and Smitherman, P. 1995. Comparison of topical cyclosporin and dexamethasone for the treatment of chronic superficial keratitis in dogs. *Veterinary Record* 137(25):635–639.

198. Conceição, D., Luís, S.J., and Delgado, E. 2013. Retrospective study of 53 dogs with chronic superficial keratitis. *Veterinary Ophthalmology* 16(1):E22–5.

199. Balicki, I., and Trbolova, A. 2010. Clinical evaluation of tacrolimus eye drops for chronic superficial keratitis treatment in dogs. *Bulletin of the Veterinary Institute in Pulawy* 54:251–258.

200. Balicki, I. 2012. Clinical study on the application of tacrolimus and DMSO in the treatment of chronic superficial keratitis in dogs. *Polish Journal of Veterinary Sciences* 15(4):667–676.

201. Rickards, D., and Carter, K. 1978. Cryosurgery in canine pannus. *Canine Practice* 5(3):48–50.

202. Holmberg, D., Scheifer, H., and Parent, J. 1986. The cryosurgical treatment of pigmentary keratitis in dogs an experimental and clinical study. *Veterinary Surgery* 15(1):1–4.

203. Azoulay, T. 2014. Adjunctive cryotherapy for pigmentary keratitis in dogs: A study of 16 corneas. *Veterinary Ophthalmology* 17(4):241–249.

204. Allgoewer, I., and Hoecht, S. 2010. Radiotherapy for canine chronic superficial keratitis using soft X-rays (15 kV). *Veterinary Ophthalmology* 13(1):20–25.

205. Kuhns, E., Keller, W., and Blanchard, G. 1973. The treatment of pannus in dogs by use of a corneal-scleral graft. *Journal of the American Veterinary Medical Association* 162(11):950–952.

206. Brightman, A., Vestre, W., Helper, L., and Godshalk, C. 1979. Chronic eosinophilic keratitis in the cat. *Feline Practice (USA)* 9:21–24.

207. Collins, B., Swanson, J., and MacWilliams, P. 1986. Eosinophilic keratitis and keratoconjunctivitis in a cat. *Modern Veterinary Practice (USA)* 67:32–35.

208. Paulsen, M. 1987. Feline eosinophilic keratitis: A review of 15 clinical cases. *Journal of the American Animal Hospital Association* 23:63–69.

209. Morgan, R., Abrams, K., and Kern, T. 1996. Feline eosinophilic keratitis: A retrospective study of 54 cases: (1989–1994). *Veterinary and Comparative Ophthalmology* 6:131–134.

210. Nasisse, M., Glover, T., Moore, C., and Weigler, B. 1998. Detection of feline herpesvirus 1 DNA in corneas of cats with eosinophilic keratitis or corneal sequestration. *American Journal of Veterinary Research* 59(7):856–858.

211. Dean, E., and Meunier, V. 2013. Feline eosinophilic keratoconjunctivitis: A retrospective study of 45 cases (56 eyes). *Journal of Feline Medicine and Surgery* 15(8):661–666.

212. Richter, M., Matheis, F., Gönczi, E., Aeby, S., Spiess, B., and Greub, G. 2010. Parachlamydia acanthamoebae in domestic cats with and without corneal disease. *Veterinary Ophthalmology* 13(4):235–237.

213. Ramsey, D., Whiteley, H., Gerding Jr., P., and Valdez, R. 1994. Eosinophilic keratoconjunctivitis in a horse. *Journal of the American Veterinary Medical Association* 205(9): 1308–1311.

214. Yamagata, M., Wilkie, D., and Gilger, B. 1996. Eosinophilic keratoconjunctivitis in seven horses. *Journal of the American Veterinary Medical Association* 209(7):1283–1286.

215. Lassaline-Utter, M., Miller, C., and Wotman, K.L. 2014. Eosinophilic keratitis in 46 eyes of 27 horses in the Mid-Atlantic United States (2008–2012). *Veterinary Ophthalmology* 17(5):311–320.

216. Edwards, S., Clode, A.B., and Gilger, B.C. 2015. Equine eosinophilic keratitis in horses: 28 cases (2003-2013). *Clinical Case Reports* 3(12):1000–1006.

217. Spiess, A.K., Sapienza, J.S., and Mayordomo, A. 2009. Treatment of proliferative feline eosinophilic keratitis with topical 1.5% cyclosporine: 35 cases. *Veterinary Ophthalmology* 12(2):132–137.

218. Stiles, J., and Coster, M. 2016. Use of an ophthalmic formulation of megestrol acetate for the treatment of eosinophilic keratitis in cats. *Veterinary Ophthalmology* 19(S1):86–90.

219. Prasse, K., and Winston, S. 1996. Cytology and histopathology of feline eosinophlic keratitis. *Veterinary and Comparative Ophthalmology* 6:74–81.

220. Bedford, P., and Cotchin, E. 1983. An unusual chronic keratoconjunctivitis in the cat. *Journal of Small Animal Practice* 24(2):85–102.

221. Pentlarge, V., and Riis, R. 1984. Proliferative keratitis in a cat: A case report. *Journal of the American Animal Hospital Association* 20(3):477–480.

222. Bellhorn, R., and Henkind, P. 1966. Superficial pigmentary keratitis in the dog. *Journal of the American Veterinary Medical Association* 149(2):173–175.

223. Rubin, L., and Koch, S. 1969. Silver nitrate burn of the dog cornea. *Journal of the American Veterinary Medical Association* 155(2):134–135.

224. Pilger, I. 1983. Pigmentation of the cornea: A review and classification. *Annals of Ophthalmology* 15(11):1076–1082.

225. Bicer, S., Fuller, G.A., Wilkie, D.A., Yamaguchi, M., and Hamlin, R.L. 2002. Amiodarone-induced keratopathy in healthy dogs. *Veterinary Ophthalmology* 5(1):35–38.

226. Labelle, A.L., Dresser, C.B., Hamor, R.E., Allender, M.C., and Disney, J.L. 2013. Characteristics of, prevalence of, and risk factors for corneal pigmentation (pigmentary keratopathy) in Pugs. *Journal of the American Veterinary Medical Association* 243(5):667–674.

227. Krecny, M., Tichy, A., Rushton, J., and Nell, B. 2015. A retrospective survey of ocular abnormalities in pugs: 130 cases. *Journal of Small Animal Practice* 56(2):96–102.

228. Stiles, J., Carmichael, P., Kaswan, R., Bounous, D., Moore, A., and Hirsh, S. 1995. Keratectomy for corneal pigmentation in dogs with cyclosporine responsive chronic keratoconjunctivitis sicca. *Veterinary and Comparative Ophthalmology* 56:96–102.

229. Gilger, B.C., Michau, T.M., and Salmon, J.H. 2005. Immune-mediated keratitis in horses: 19 cases (1998–2004). *Veterinary Ophthalmology* 8(4):233–239.

230. Matthews, A. 2000. Nonulcerative keratopathies in the horse. *Equine Veterinary Education* 12(5):271–278.

231. Pate, D.O., Clode, A.B., Olivry, T., Cullen, J.M., Salmon, J.H., and Gilger, B.C. 2012. Immunohistochemical and immunopathologic characterization of superficial stromal immune-mediated keratitis in horses. *American Journal of Veterinary Research* 73(7):1067–1073.

232. Rebhun, W. 1992. Corneal stromal infections in horses. *The Compendium* 14(3):363–370.

233. Matthews, A., and Gilger, B.C. 2009. Equine immune-mediated keratopathies. *Veterinary Ophthalmology* 12(s1):10–6.

234. Gratzek, A.T., Kaswan, R.L., Martin, C., Champagne, E., and White, S.L. 1995. Ophthalmic cyclosporine in equine keratitis and keratouveitis: 11 cases. *Equine Veterinary Journal* 27(5):327–333.

235. Gilger, B.C., Stoppini, R., Wilkie, D.A., Clode, A.B., Pinto, N.H., Hempstead, J. et al. 2014. Treatment of immune-mediated keratitis in horses with episcleral silicone matrix cyclosporine delivery devices. *Veterinary Ophthalmology* 17(s1):23–30.

236. Gilger, B., and Brooks, D. 2009. International Equine Ophthalmology Consortium (IEOC) Symposium;

Havemeyer Workshop Report. *Equine Veterinary Journal* 41(6):606–607.

237. McMullen, R.J., and Fischer, B. 2016. Intrastromal indocyannine green photothermal therapy for the treatment of immune-mediated keratitis in the horse. *International Equine Ophthalmology Consortium*; Malahide, Ireland, p. 44.

238. Omar, G.S., Wilson, M., and Nair, S.P. 2008. Lethal photosensitization of wound-associated microbes using indocyanine green and near-infrared light. *BMC Microbiology* 8(1):111.

239. Topaloglu, N., Yuksel, S., and Gulsoy, M., editors. 2012. Optimization of parameters in photodynamic therapy to kill P. aeruginosa with 809-nm diode laser and indocyanine green. *Proc of SPIE Vol 2012*.

240. Violette, N.P., and Ledbetter, E.C. 2017. Intracorneal stromal hemorrhage in dogs and its associations with ocular and systemic disease: 39 cases. *Veterinary Ophthalmology* 20(1):27–33.

241. Matas, M., Donaldson, D., and Newton, R.J. 2012. Intracorneal hemorrhage in 19 dogs (22 eyes) from 2000 to 2010: A retrospective study. *Veterinary Ophthalmology* 15(2):86–91.

242. Carmichael, L. 1965. The pathogenesis of ocular lesions of infectious canine hepatitis: II. Experimental ocular hypersensitivity produced by the virus. *Pathologia Veterinaria* 2(4):344–359.

243. Carmichael, L.E., Medic, B., Bistner, S.I., and Aguirre, G.D. 1975. Viral-antibody complexes in canine adenovirus type I (CAV-1) ocular lesion: Leukocyte chemotaxis and enzyme release. *Cornell Veterinarian* 65(3):331.

244. Curtis, R., and Barnett, K. 1973. The ocular lesions of infectious canine hepatitis. 1. Clinical features. *The Journal of Small Animal Practice* 14(7):375–389.

245. Curtis, R., and Barnett, K. 1973. The ocular lesions of infectious canine hepatitis 2. FIELD INCIDENCE. *Journal of Small Animal Practice* 14(12):737–745.

246. McNeill, J.I., and Kaufman, H.E. 1979. Local antivirals in a herpes simplex stromal keratitis model. *Archives of Ophthalmology* 97(4):727–729.

247. Wander, A.H., Centifanto, Y.M., and Kaufman, H.E. 1980. Strain specificity of clinical isolates of herpes simplex virus. *Archives of Ophthalmology* 98(8):1458–1461.

248. Townsend, W., Stiles, J., and Krohne, S. 2003. Development of a reverse transcriptase polymerase chain reaction to detect feline herpesvirus 1 latency associated transcripts in the trigeminal ganglia and corneas of clinically asymptomatic cats. *Investigative Ophthalmology & Visual Science* 44(13):4636.

249. Stiles, J., and Pogranichniy, R. 2008. Detection of virulent feline herpesvirus-1 in the corneas of clinically normal cats. *Journal of Feline Medicine and Surgery* 10(2):154–159.

250. Volopich, S., Benetka, V., Schwendenwein, I., Möstl, K., Sommerfeld-Stur, I., and Nell, B. 2005. Cytologic findings, and feline herpesvirus DNA and *Chlamydophila felis* antigen detection rates in normal cats and cats with conjunctival and corneal lesions. *Veterinary Ophthalmology* 8(1):25–32.

251. Nasisse, M., Guy, J., Davidson, M., Sussman, W., and Fairley, N. 1989. Experimental ocular herpesvirus infection in the cat. Sites of virus replication, clinical features and effects of corticosteroid administration. *Investigative Ophthalmology & Visual Science* 30(8):1758–1768.

252. Ledbetter, E.C., Kim, S.G., and Dubovi, E.J. 2009. Outbreak of ocular disease associated with naturally-acquired canine herpesvirus-1 infection in a closed domestic dog colony. *Veterinary Ophthalmology* 12(4):242–247.

253. Green, W.R., and Zimmerman, L.E. 1967. Granulomatous reaction to Descemet's membrane. *American Journal of Ophthalmology* 64(3):555–558.

254. Khodadoust, A.A., and Attarzadeh, A. 1982. Presumed autoimmune corneal endotheliopathy. *American Journal of Ophthalmology* 93(6):718–722.

255. Vannas, A., Ahonen, R., and Mäkitie, J. 1983. Corneal endothelium in herpetic keratouveitis. *Archives of Ophthalmology* 101(6):913–915.

256. Holbach, L.M., Font, R.L., and Naumann, G.O. 1990. Herpes simplex stromal and endothelial keratitis: Granulomatous cell reactions at the level of Descernet's membrane, the stroma, and Bowman's layer. *Ophthalmology* 97(6):722–728.

257. Vesaluoma, M., Müller, L., Gallar, J., Lambiase, A., Moilanen, J., Hack, T. et al. 2000. Effects of oleoresin capsicum pepper spray on human corneal morphology and sensitivity. *Investigative Ophthalmology & Visual Science* 41(8):2138–2147.

258. Dziezyc, J. 1992. Insect defensive spray-induced keratitis in a dog. *Journal of the American Veterinary Medical Association* 200(12):1969.

259. Brutlag, A.G., Hovda, L.R., and Della Ripa, M.A. 2011. Corneal ulceration in a dog following exposure to the defensive spray of a walkingstick insect (*Anisomorpha* spp.). *Journal of Veterinary Emergency and Critical Care* 21(4):382–386.

260. Carrington, S., Bedford, P., Guillon, J., and Woodward, E. 1989. Biomicroscopy of the tear film: The tear film of the pekingese dog. *The Veterinary Record* 124(13):323–328.

261. Johnson, S.M. 1998. Neurotrophic corneal defects after diode laser cycloablation. *American Journal of Ophthalmology* 126(5):725–727.

262. Clerc, B., and Jegou, J. 1996. Superficial punctate keratitis. *Canine Practice* 21:6–11.

263. Lassaline-Utter, M., Cutler, T.J., Michau, T.M., and Nunnery, C.M. 2014. Treatment of nonhealing corneal ulcers in 60 horses with diamond burr debridement (2010–2013). *Veterinary Ophthalmology* 17(s1):76–81.

264. Monk, C.S., Hart, K.A., Berghaus, R.D., Norton, N.A., Moore, P.A., and Myrna, K.E. 2014. Detection of endogenous cortisol in equine tears and blood at rest and after simulated stress. *Veterinary Ophthalmology* 17(s1):53–60.

265. Lassaline-Utter, M., Gemensky-Metzler, A.J., Scherrer, N.M., Stoppini, R., Latimer, C.A., MacLaren, N.E. et al. 2014. Corneal dystrophy in Friesian horses may represent a variant of pellucid marginal degeneration. *Veterinary Ophthalmology* 17(s1):186–194.

266. Roberts, S.R. 1965. Superficial indolent ulcer of the cornea in boxer dogs. *Journal of Small Animal Practice* 6(2):111–115.

267. Gelatt, K., and Samuelson, D. 1982. Recurrent corneal erosions and epithelial dystrophy in the Boxer dog. *Journal American Animal Hospital Association* 18:453–460.

268. Kirschner, S., Niyo, Y., and Betts, D. 1989. Idiopathic persistant corneal erosions: Clinical and pathological findings in 18 dogs. *The Journal of the American Animal Hospital Association (USA)* 25:84–90.

269. Murphy, C.J., Marfurt, C.F., McDermott, A., Bentley, E., Abrams, G.A., Reid, T.W. et al. 2001. Spontaneous chronic corneal epithelial defects (SCCED) in dogs: Clinical features, innervation, and effect of topical SP, with or

without IGF-1. *Investigative Ophthalmology & Visual Science* 42(10):2252–2261.

270. Bentley, E., Abrams, G.A., Covitz, D., Cook, C.S., Fischer, C.A., Hacker, D. et al. 2001. Morphology and immuno-histochemistry of spontaneous chronic corneal epithelial defects (SCCED) in dogs. *Investigative Ophthalmology & Visual Science* 42(10):2262–2269.

271. Křahenmann, A. 1976. Die rezidivierende Hornhaut-Erosion des Boxers (Erosio recidiva corneae). *Schweizer Archiv fur Tierheilkunde* 118:87–97.

272. Scherrer, K. 1983. Histologische untersuchungen zur pathologie der erosio recidiva corneae des Deutschen boxers. *Schweizer Archiv fur Tierheilkunde* 125:337–344.

273. Huang, A., and Tseng, S. 1991. Corneal epithelial wound healing in the absence of limbal epithelium. *Investigative Ophthalmology & Visual Science* 32(1):96–105.

274. La Croix, N.C., Van der Woerdt, A., and Olivero, D.K. 2001. Nonhealing corneal ulcers in cats: 29 cases (1991–1999). *Journal of the American Veterinary Medical Association* 218(5):733–735.

275. Rebhun, W. 1983. Chronic corneal epithelial erosions in horses. *Veterinary Medicine and Small Animal Clinician* 78:1635–1638.

276. Cooley, P., and Wyman, M. 1986. Indolent-like corneal ulcers in 3 horses. *Journal of the American Veterinary Medical Association* 188(3):295–297.

277. Michau, T., Schwabenton, B., Davidson, M., and Gilger, B. 2003. Superficial, nonhealing corneal ulcers in horses: 23 cases (1989–2003). *Veterinary Ophthalmology* 6(4):291–297.

278. Brünott, A., Boevé, M., and Velden, M. 2007. Grid keratotomy as a treatment for superficial nonhealing corneal ulcers in 10 horses. *Veterinary Ophthalmology* 10(3):162–167.

279. Hempstead, J.E., Clode, A.B., Borst, L.B., and Gilger, B.C. 2014. Histopathological features of equine superficial, nonhealing, corneal ulcers. *Veterinary Ophthalmology* 17(s1):46–52.

280. Hakanson, N., and Dubielzig, R. 1995. Chronic superficial corneal erosions with anterior stromal sequestration in three horses. *Veterinary and Comparatice Ophthalmology* 4:179–183.

281. Phan, T.-M.M., Foster, C.S., Boruchoff, S.A., Zagachin, L.M., and Colvin, RB. 1987. Topical fibronectin in the treatment of persistent corneal epithelial defects and trophic ulcers. *American Journal of Ophthalmology* 104(5):494–501.

282. Tsubota, K., Goto, E., Shimmura, S., and Shimazaki, J. 1999. Treatment of persistent corneal epithelial defect by autologous serum application. *Ophthalmology* 106(10):1984–1989.

283. Kirschner, S., Brazzell, R., Stern, M., and Baird, L. 1991. The use of topical epidermal growth factor for treatment of nonhealing corneal erosions in dogs. *The Journal of the American Animal Hospital Association* 27:499–452.

284. Kitazawa, T., Kinoshita, S., Fujita, K., Araki, K., Watanabe, H., Ohashi, Y. et al. 1990. The mechanism of accelerated corneal epithelial healing by human epidermal growth factor. *Investigative Ophthalmology & Visual Science* 31(9):1773–1778.

285. Miller, W. 1996. Using polysulfted glycosaminoglycan to treat persistent corneal erosions in dogs: A pilot clinical study. *Veterinary Medicine* 91:916–922.

286. Willeford, K., Miller, W., Abrams, K., and Vaughn, B. 1998. Modulation of proteolytic activity associated with persistent corneal ulcers in dogs. *Veterinary Ophthalmology* 1(1):5–8.

287. Chandler, H.L., Gemensky-Metzler, A.J., Bras, I.D., Robbin-Webb, T.E., Saville, W.J., and Colitz, C.M. 2010. In vivo effects of adjunctive tetracycline treatment on refractory corneal ulcers in dogs. *Journal of the American Veterinary Medical Association* 237(4):378–386.

288. Carter, R.T., Kambampati, R., Murphy, C.J., and Bentley, E. 2007. Expression of matrix metalloproteinase 2 and 9 in experimentally wounded canine corneas and spontaneous chronic corneal epithelial defects. *Cornea* 26(10):1213–1219.

289. Jurk, I., Gilger, B., Malok, E., Valentine, V., Davidson, M., and Allen, J., editors. 2000. TGF-beta2 levels in tears of normal dogs and dogs with refractory corneal ulcers. *Proceeding American College Veterinary Ophthalmology*.

290. Chandler, H.L., Colitz, C.M., Lu, P., Saville, W.J., and Kusewitt, D.F. 2007. The role of the slug transcription factor in cell migration during corneal re-epithelialization in the dog. *Experimental Eye Research* 84(3):400–411.

291. Schmidt, G., Blanchard, G., and Keller, W. 1977. The use of hydrophilic contact lenses in corneal diseases of the dog and cat: A preliminary report. *Journal of Small Animal Practice* 18(12):773–777.

292. Morgan, R., Bachrach Jr., A., and Ogilvie, G. 1984. An evaluation of soft contact lens usage in the dog and cat. *The Journal of the American Animal Hospital Association* 20:885–888.

293. Williams, R., and Buckley, R.J. 1985. Pathogenesis and treatment of recurrent erosion. *British Journal of Ophthalmology* 69(6):435–437.

294. Ali, Z., and Insler, M. 1986. A comparison of therapeutic bandage lenses, tarsorrhaphy, and antibiotic and hypertonic saline on corneal epithelial wound healing. *Annals of Ophthalmology* 18(1):22–24.

295. Madigan, M.C., and Holden, B. 1992. Reduced epithelial adhesion after extended contact lens wear correlates with reduced hemidesmosome density in cat cornea. *Investigative Ophthalmology & Visual Science* 33(2):314–323.

296. Grinninger, P., Verbruggen, A., Kraijer-Huver, I., Djajadiningrat-Laanen, S., Teske, E., and Boevé, M. 2015. Use of bandage contact lenses for treatment of spontaneous chronic corneal epithelial defects in dogs. *Journal of Small Animal Practice* 56(7):446–449.

297. Wooff, P.J., and Norman, J.C. 2015. Effect of corneal contact lens wear on healing time and comfort post LGK for treatment of SCCEDs in boxers. *Veterinary Ophthalmology* 18(5):364–370.

298. Gosling, A.A., Labelle, A.L., and Breaux, C.B. 2013. Management of spontaneous chronic corneal epithelial defects (SCCEDs) in dogs with diamond burr debridement and placement of a bandage contact lens. *Veterinary Ophthalmology* 16(2):83–88.

299. Dees, D.D., Fritz, K.J., Wagner, L., Paglia, D., Knollinger, A.M., and Madsen, R. 2016. Effect of bandage contact lens wear and postoperative medical therapies on corneal healing rate after diamond burr debridement in dogs. *Veterinary Ophthalmology* 20(5):382–389.

300. Aquavella, J.V., del Cerro, M., Musco, P.S., Ueda, S., and DePaolis, M.D. 1987. The effect of a collagen bandage lens on corneal wound healing: A preliminary report. *Ophthalmic Surgery, Lasers and Imaging Retina* 18(8):570–573.

301. Morgan, R., and Abrams, K. 1994. A comparison of six different therapies for persistent corneal erosions in dogs and cats. *Veterinary and Comparative Ophthalmology* 4:38–43.

302. Stanley, R., Hardman, C., and Johnson, B. 1998. Results of grid keratotomy, superficial keratectomy and debridement

for the management of persistent corneal erosions in 92 dogs. *Veterinary Ophthalmology* 1(4):233–238.

303. Hsu, J.K., Rubinfeld, R.S., Barry, P., and Jester, J.V. 1993. Anterior stromal puncture: Immunohistochemical studies in human corneas. *Archives of Ophthalmology* 111(8):1057–1063.

304. Champagne, E., and Munger, R. 1992. Multiple punctate keratotomy for the treatment of recurrent epithelial erosions in dogs. *The Journal of the American Animal Hospital Association (USA)* 28:213–216.

305. Pickett, J.P. 1995. Treating persistent corneal erosions with a crosshatch keratotomy technique. *Veterinary Medicine* 90:561–572.

306. Dawson, C., Naranjo, C., Sanchez-Maldonado, B., Fricker, G.V., Linn-Pearl, R.N., Escanilla, N. et al. 2017. Immediate effects of diamond burr debridement in patients with spontaneous chronic corneal epithelial defects, light and electron microscopic evaluation. *Veterinary Ophthalmology* 20(1):11–15.

307. Jégou, J.P., and Tromeur, F. 2015. Superficial keratectomy for chronic corneal ulcers refractory to medical treatment in 36 cats. *Veterinary Ophthalmology* 18(4):335–340.

308. Moore, P.A. 2003. Diagnosis and management of chronic corneal epithelial defects (indolent corneal ulcerations). *Clinical Techniques in Small Animal Practice* 18(3):168–177.

309. Bistner, S., Carlson, J., Shively, J., and Scott, F. 1971. Ocular manifestations of feline herpesvirus infection. *Journal of the American Veterinary Medical Association* 159(10):1223–1237.

310. Roberts, S., Dawson, C., Coleman, V., and Togni, B. 1972. Dendritic keratitis in a cat. *Journal of the American Veterinary Medical Association* 161(3):285–289.

311. Nasisse, M.P., Davis, B.J., Guy, J.S., Davidson, M.G., and Sussman, W. 1992. Isolation of feline herpesvirus 1 from the trigeminal ganglia of acutely and chronically infected cats. *Journal of Veterinary Internal Medicine* 6(2):102–103.

312. O'Brien, W.J., and Taylor, J.L. 1989. The isolation of herpes simplex virus from rabbit corneas during latency. *Investigative Ophthalmology & Visual Science* 30(3):357–364.

313. Cook, S.D., Ophth, F., and Hill, J.H. 1991. Herpes simplex virus: Molecular biology and the possibility of corneal latency. *Survey of Ophthalmology* 36(2):140–148.

314. Stiles, J., McDermott, M., Bigsby, D., Willis, M., Martin, C., Roberts, W. et al. 1997. Use of nested polymerase chain reaction to identify feline herpesvirus in ocular tissue from clinically normal cats and cats with corneal sequestra or conjunctivitis. *American Journal of Veterinary Research* 58(4):338–342.

315. Maggs, D.J., Lappin, M.R., Reif, J.S., Collins, J.K., Carman, J., Dawson, D.A. et al. 1999. Evaluation of serologic and viral detection methods for diagnosing feline herpesvirus-1 infection in cats with acute respiratory tract or chronic ocular disease. *Journal of the American Veterinary Medical Association* 214(4):502–507.

316. Cello, R. 1971. Clues to differential diagnosis of feline respiratory infections. *Journal of the American Veterinary Medical Association* 158(6):968–973.

317. Plotkin, J., Reynaud, A., and Okumoto, M. 1971. Cytologic study of herpetic keratitis: Preparation of corneal scrapings. *Archives of Ophthalmology* 85(5):597–599.

318. Stiles, J., McDermott, M., Willis, M., Roberts, W., and Greene, C. 1997. Comparison of nested polymerase chain reaction, virus isolation, and fluorescent antibody testing for identifying feline herpesvirus in cats with

conjunctivitis. *American Journal of Veterinary Research* 58(8):804–807.

319. Sandmeyer, L.S., Waldner, C.L., Bauer, B.S., Wen, X., and Bienzle, D. 2010. Comparison of polymerase chain reaction tests for diagnosis of feline herpesvirus, *Chlamydophila felis*, and *Mycoplasma* spp. infection in cats with ocular disease in Canada. *The Canadian Veterinary Journal* 51(6):629–633.

320. Stiles, J. 1995. Treatment of cats with ocular disease attributable to herpesvirus infection: 17 cases (1983-1993). *Journal of the American Veterinary Medical Association* 207(5):599–603.

321. Nasisse, M., Guy, J., Davidson, M., Sussman, W., and De Clercq, E. 1989. In vitro susceptibility of feline herpesvirus-1 to vidarabine, idoxuridine, trifluridine, acyclovir, or bromovinyldeoxyuridine. *American Journal of Veterinary Research* 50(1):158–160.

322. Owens, J., Nasisse, M., Tadepalli, S., and Dorman, D. 1996. Pharmacokinetics of acyclovir in the cat. *Journal of Veterinary Pharmacology and Therapeutics* 19(6):488–490.

323. Williams, D., Robinson, J., Lay, E., and Field, H. 2005. Efficacy of topical aciclovir for the treatment of feline herpetic keratitis: Results of a prospective clinical trial and data from *in vitro* investigations. *The Veterinary Record* 157(9):254–257.

324. Fontenelle, J.P., Powell, C.C., Veir, J.K., Radecki, S.V., and Lappin, M.R. 2008. Effect of topical ophthalmic application of cidofovir on experimentally induced primary ocular feline herpesvirus-1 infection in cats. *American Journal of Veterinary Research* 69(2):289–293.

325. Maggs, D.J., and Clarke, H.E. 2004. In vitro efficacy of ganciclovir, cidofovir, penciclovir, foscarnet, idoxuridine, and acyclovir against feline herpesvirus type-1. *American Journal of Veterinary Research* 65(4):399–403.

326. van der Meulen, K., Garré, B., Croubels, S., and Nauwynck, H. 2006. In vitro comparison of antiviral drugs against feline herpesvirus 1. *BMC Veterinary Research* 2(1):13.

327. Nasisse, M., Dorman, D., Jamison, K., Weigler, B., Hawkins, E., and Stevens, J. 1997. Effects of valacyclovir in cats infected with feline herpesvirus 1. *American Journal of Veterinary Research* 58(10):1141–1144.

328. Malik, R., Lessels, N.S., Webb, S., Meek, M., Graham, P.G., Vitale, C. et al. 2009. Treatment of feline herpesvirus-1 associated disease in cats with famciclovir and related drugs. *Journal of Feline Medicine and Surgery* 11(1):40–48.

329. Thomasy, S.M., Lim, C.C., Reilly, C.M., Kass, P.H., Lappin, M.R., and Maggs, D.J. 2011. Evaluation of orally administered famciclovir in cats experimentally infected with feline herpesvirus type-1. *American Journal of Veterinary Research* 72(1):85–95.

330. Thomasy, S.M., Covert, J.C., Stanley, S.D., and Maggs, D.J. 2012. Pharmacokinetics of famciclovir and penciclovir in tears following oral administration of famciclovir to cats: A pilot study. *Veterinary Ophthalmology* 15(5):299–306.

331. Stiles, J. 2014. Ocular manifestation of feline viral disease. *The Veterinary Journal* 201:166–173.

332. Weiss, R. 1989. Synergistic antiviral activities of acyclovir and recombinant human leukocyte (alpha) interferon on feline herpesvirus replication. *American Journal of Veterinary Research* 50(10):1672–1677.

333. Vennebusch, T. 2006. Interferon: Topical application in the treatment of the herpes virus keratitis in cats. *Kleintierpraxis* 51(5):274–277.

334. Haid, C., Kaps, S., Gönczi, E., Hässig, M., Metzler, A., Spiess, B.M. et al. 2007. Pretreatment with feline

interferon omega and the course of subsequent infection with feline herpesvirus in cats. *Veterinary Ophthalmology* 10(5):278–284.

335. Slack, J.M., Stiles, J., Leutenegger, C.M., Moore, G.E., and Pogranichniy, R.M. 2013. Effects of topical ocular administration of high doses of human recombinant interferon alpha-2b and feline recombinant interferon omega on naturally occurring viral keratoconjunctivitis in cats. *American Journal of Veterinary Research* 74(2):281–289.

336. Stiles, J., Townsend, W.M., Rogers, Q.R., and Krohne, S.G. 2002. Effect of oral administration of L-lysine on conjunctivitis caused by feline herpesvirus in cats. *American Journal of Veterinary Research* 63(1):99–103.

337. Maggs, D.J., Nasisse, M.P., and Kass, P.H. 2003. Efficacy of oral supplementation with L-lysine in cats latently infected with feline herpesvirus. *American Journal of Veterinary Research* 64:37–42.

338. Maggs, D.J., Collins, B.K., Thorne, J.G., and Nasisse, M.P. 2000. Effects of L-lysine and L-arginine on *in vitro* replication of feline herpesvirus type-1. *American Journal of Veterinary Research* 61(12):1474–1478.

339. Ostler, H.B. 1978. Glucocorticoid therapy in ocular herpes simplex: I. Limitations. *Survey of Ophthalmology* 23(1):35–48.

340. Nasisse, M. 1991. Anti-inflammatory therapy in herpesvirus keratoconjunctivitis. *Progress in Veterinary and Comparative Ophthalmology* 1:63–65.

341. Boisjoly, H.M., Woog, J.J., Pavan-Langston, D., Park, N.-H. 1984. Prophylactic topical cyclosporine in experimental herpetic stromal keratitis. *Archives of Ophthalmology* 102(12):1804–1807.

342. Meyers-Elliott, R., Chitjian, P., and Billups, C. 1987. Effects of cyclosporine A on clinical and immunological parameters in herpes simplex keratitis. *Investigative Ophthalmology & Visual Science* 28(7):1170–1180.

343. Weigler, B., Guy, J., Nasisse, M., Hancock, S., and Sherry, B. 1997. Effect of a live attenuated intranasal vaccine on latency and shedding of feline herpesvirus 1 in domestic cats. *Archives of Virology* 142(12):2389–2400.

344. Tham, K., and Studdert, M. 1987. Clinical and immunological responses of cats to feline herpesvirus type 1 infection. *The Veterinary Record* 120(14):321–326.

345. August, J. 1990. The control and eradication of feline upper respiratory infections in cluster populations. *Veterinary Medicine* 85(9):1002–1006.

346. Hickman, M.A., Reubel, G.H., Hoffman, D.E., Morris, J.G., Rogers, Q.R., and Pedersen, N.C. 1994. An epizootic of feline herpesvirus, type 1 in a large specific pathogen-free cat colony and attempts to eradicate the infection by identification and culling of carriers. *Laboratory Animals* 28(4):320–329.

347. Carmichael, L. 1970. Herpesvirus canis: Aspects of pathogenesis and immune response. *Journal of the American Veterinary Medical Association* 156:1714–1721.

348. Ledbetter, E. 2013. Canine herpesvirus-1 ocular diseases of mature dogs. *New Zealand Veterinary Journal* 61(4):193–201.

349. Percy, D.H., Carmichael, L., Albert, D.M., King, J., and Jonas A. 1971. Lesions in puppies surviving infection with canine herpesvirus. *Veterinary Pathology* 8(1):37–53.

350. Albert, D., Lahav, M., Carmichael, L., and Percy, D. 1976. Canine herpes-induced retinal dysplasia and associated ocular anomalies. *Investigative Ophthalmology & Visual Science* 15(4):267–278.

351. Ledbetter, E.C., Riis, R.C., Kern, T.J., Haley, N.J., and Schatzberg, S.J. 2006. Corneal ulceration associated with naturally occurring canine herpesvirus-1 infection in two adult dogs. *Journal of the American Veterinary Medical Association* 229(3):376–384.

352. Ledbetter, E.C., Kice, N.C., Matusow, R.B., Dubovi, E.J., and Kim, S.G. 2010. The effect of topical ocular corticosteroid administration in dogs with experimentally induced latent canine herpesvirus-1 infection. *Experimental Eye Research* 90(6):711–717.

353. Ledbetter, E.C., da Silva, E.C., Kim, S.G., Dubovi, E.J., and Schwark, W.S. 2012. Frequency of spontaneous canine herpesvirus-1 reactivation and ocular viral shedding in latently infected dogs and canine herpesvirus-1 reactivation and ocular viral shedding induced by topical administration of cyclosporine and systemic administration of corticosteroids. *American Journal of Veterinary Research* 73(7):1079–1084.

354. Ledbetter, E.C., Marfurt, C.F., and Dubielzig, R.R. 2013. Metaherpetic corneal disease in a dog associated with partial limbal stem cell deficiency and neurotrophic keratitis. *Veterinary Ophthalmology* 16(4):282–288.

355. Malone, E., Ledbetter, E., Rassnick, K., Kim, S., and Russell, D. 2010. Disseminated canine herpesvirus-1 infection in an immunocompromised adult dog. *Journal of Veterinary Internal Medicine* 24(4):965–968.

356. Matthews, A., and Handscombe, M. 1983. Superficial keratitis in the horse: Treatment with the antiviral drug idoxuridine. *Equine Veterinary Journal* 15(S2):29–31.

357. Collinson, P., O'Rielly, J., Ficorilli, N., and Studdert, M. 1994. Isolation of equine herpesvirus type 2 (equine gamma herpesvirus 2) from foals with keratoconjunctivitis. *Journal of the American Veterinary Medical Association* 205(2):329–331.

358. Thein, P. and, Böhm, D. 1976. Ätiologie und Klinik einer virusbedingten Keratokonjunktivitis beim Fohlen. *Zoonoses and Public Health* 23(5–6):507–519.

359. Thein, P. 1978. The association of EHV-2 infection with keratitis and research on the occurrence of equine coital exanthema (EHV-3) of horses in Germany. In: Bryans, J., and Gerber, H., editors. *Equine Infectious Diseases IV*. Veterinary Publications: Princeton, NJ, pp. 33–41.

360. Featherstone, H.J., Franklin, V.J., and Sansom, J. 2004. Feline corneal sequestrum: Laboratory analysis of ocular samples from 12 cats. *Veterinary Ophthalmology* 7(4):229–238.

361. Souri, E. 1975. The feline corneal nigrum. *Veterinary Medicine, Small Snimal Clinician* 70(5):531–534.

362. Newkirk, K.M., Hendrix, D.V., and Keller, R.L. 2011. Porphyrins are not present in feline ocular tissues or corneal sequestra. *Veterinary Ophthalmology* 14(s1):2–4.

363. Davidson, H., Gerlach, J., and Bull, R. 1992. Determination of protein concentrations and their molecular weight in tears from cats with normal corneas and cats with corneal sequestrum. *American Journal of Veterinary Research* 53(10):1756–1759.

364. Cullen, C.L., Wadowska, D.W., Singh, A., and Melekhovets, Y. 2005. Ultrastructural findings in feline corneal sequestra. *Veterinary Ophthalmology* 8(5):295–303.

365. Knecht, C., Schiller, A., and Small, E. 1966. Focal degeneration of the cornea with sequestration in a cat. *Journal of the American Veterinary Medical Association* 149(9):1192–1193.

366. Gelatt, K., Peiffer, R., and Stevens, J. 1973. Chronic ulcerative keratitis and sequestrum in the domestic cat. *Journal American Animal Hospital Association* 9:204–213.

367. Formston, C., Bedford, P., Staton, J., and Tripathi, R. 1974. Corneal necrosis in the cat. *Journal of Small Animal Practice* 15(1):19–25.

368. Schmidt, V. 1977. Herdformige Hornhautnekrose der Katze. *Monatshefte fur Veterinarmedizin* 32:493–495.

369. Blogg, J., Dutton, A., and Stanley, R. 1989. Use of third eyelid grafts to repair full-thickness defects in the cornea and sclera. *The Journal of the American Animal Hospital Association (USA)* 25:505–512.

370. Blogg, J., Stanley, R., and Dutton, A. 1989. Use of conjunctival pedicle grafts in the management of feline keratitis nigrum. *Journal of Small Animal Practice* 30(12):678–684.

371. Featherstone, H.J., Sansom, J., and Heinrich, C.L. 2001. The use of porcine small intestinal submucosa in ten cases of feline corneal disease. *Veterinary Ophthalmology* 4(2):147–153.

372. Barachetti, L., Giudice, C., and Mortellaro, C.M. 2010. Amniotic membrane transplantation for the treatment of feline corneal sequestrum: Pilot study. *Veterinary Ophthalmology* 13(5):326–330.

373. Featherstone, H.J., and Sansom, J. 2004. Feline corneal sequestra: A review of 64 cases (80 eyes) from 1993 to 2000. *Veterinary Ophthalmology* 7(4):213–227.

374. Andrew, S.E., Tou, S., and Brooks, D.E. 2001. Corneoconjunctival transposition for the treatment of feline corneal sequestra: A retrospective study of 17 cases (1990–1998). *Veterinary Ophthalmology* 4(2):107–111.

375. Graham, K.L., White, J.D., and Billson, F.M. 2017. Feline corneal sequestra: Outcome of corneoconjunctival transposition in 97 cats (109 eyes). *Journal of Feline Medicine and Surgery* 19(6):710–716.

376. Peña Gimenez, M., and Farina, I.M. 1998. Lamellar keratoplasty for the treatment of feline corneal sequestrum. *Veterinary Ophthalmology* 1(2–3):163–166.

377. Laguna, F., Leiva, M., Costa, D., Lacerda, R., and Peña Gimenez, T. 2015. Corneal grafting for the treatment of feline corneal sequestrum: A retrospective study of 18 eyes (13 cats). *Veterinary Ophthalmology* 18(4):291–296.

378. Glover, T., Nasisse, M., and Davidson, M. 1994. Acute bullous keratopathy in the cat. *Veterinary and Comparative Ophthalmology (USA)* 4:66–70.

379. Dietrich, U., Moore, P., Chandler, M., Mosunic, C., Williams, C., Carmichael, K. et al. 2004. Acute corneal hydrops in horses: 16 cases. *Proceedings of the 35th Annual Confernece of the American College of Veterinary Ophthalmologists* 35:17.

380. Pederson, S.L., Pizzirani, S., Andrew, S.E., Pate, D.O., Stine, J.M., and Michau, T.M. 2016. Use of a nictitating membrane flap for treatment of feline acute corneal hydrops—21 eyes. *Veterinary Ophthalmology* 19:61–68.

381. Pierce, K.E., Wilkie, D.A., Gemensky-Metzler, A.J., Curran, P.G., Townsend, W.M., Petersen-Jones, S.M. et al. 2016. An association between systemic cyclosporine administration and development of acute bullous keratopathy in cats. *Veterinary Ophthalmology* 19:77–85.

382. Clark, A.F. 1998. New discoveries on the roles of matrix metalloproteinases in ocular cell biology and pathology. *Investigative Ophthalmology & Visual Science* 39(13): 2514–2516.

383. Gray, L.D., and Kreger, A.S. 1975. Rabbit corneal damage produced by *Pseudomonas aeruginosa* infection. *Infection and Immunity* 12(2):419–432.

384. Matsumoto, K., Shams, N., Hanninen, L.A., and Kenyon, K.R. 1993. Cleavage and activation of corneal matrix metalloproteases by *Pseudomonas aeruginosa* proteases. *Investigative Ophthalmology & Visual Science* 34(6):1945–1953.

385. Steuhl, K., Döring, G., Henni, A., Thiel, H., and Botzenhart, K. 1987. Relevance of host-derived and bacterial factors in *Pseudomonas aeruginosa* corneal infections. *Investigative Ophthalmology & Visual Science* 28(9):1559–1568.

386. Moreira, H., McDonnell, P.J., Fasano, A.P., Silverman, D.L., Coates, T.D., and Sevanian, A. 1991. Treatment of experimental pseudomonas keratitis with cyclooxygenase and lipoxygenase inhibitors. *Ophthalmology* 98(11):1693–1697.

387. Moore, C., Collins, B., and Fales, W. 1995. Antibacterial susceptibility patterns for microbial isolates associated with infectious keratitis in horses: 63 cases (1986-1994). *Journal of the American Veterinary Medical Association* 207(7):928–933.

388. Moore, C., Collins, B., Fales, W., and Halenda, R. 1995. Antimicrobial agents for treatment of infectious keratitis in horses. *Journal of the American Veterinary Medical Association* 207(7):855–862.

389. Tolar, E.L., Hendrix, D.V., Rohrbach, B.W., Plummer, C.E., Brooks, D.E., and Gelatt, K.N. 2006. Evaluation of clinical characteristics and bacterial isolates in dogs with bacterial keratitis: 97 cases (1993–2003). *Journal of the American Veterinary Medical Association* 228(1):80–85.

390. Hindley, K.E., Groth, A.D., King, M., Graham, K., and Billson, F.M. 2016. Bacterial isolates, antimicrobial susceptibility, and clinical characteristics of bacterial keratitis in dogs presenting to referral practice in Australia. *Veterinary Ophthalmology* 19(5):418–426.

391. McLaughlin, S., Brightman, A., Helper, L., Manning, J., and Tomes J. 1983. Pathogenic bacteria and fungi associated with extraocular disease in the horse. *Journal of the American Veterinary Medical Association* 182(3):241–242.

392. LoPinto, A.J., Mohammed, H.O., and Ledbetter, E.C. 2015. Prevalence and risk factors for isolation of methicillin-resistant Staphylococcus in dogs with keratitis. *Veterinary Ophthalmology* 18(4):297–303.

393. Ledbetter, E.C., and Scarlett, J.M. 2008. Isolation of obligate anaerobic bacteria from ulcerative keratitis in domestic animals. *Veterinary Ophthalmology* 11(2):114–122.

394. Perry, L.D., Brinser, J.H., and Kolodner, H. 1982. Anaerobic corneal ulcers. *Ophthalmology* 89(6):636–642.

395. Rebhun, W., Cho, J., Gaarder, J., Peek, S., and Patten, V. 1999. Presumed clostridial and aerobic bacterial infections of the cornea in two horses. *Journal of the American Veterinary Medical Association* 214(10):1519–1522.

396. da Silva, C.J., Murphy, C., Jang, S., and Bellhorn R. 1990. Nutritionally variant streptococci associated with corneal ulcers in horses: 35 cases (1982-1988). *Journal of the American Veterinary Medical Association* 197(5):624–626.

397. Hyndiuk, R.A., Skorich, D.N., Davis, S.D., Sarff, L.D., Divine, K., and Burd, E. 1988. Fortified antibiotic ointment in bacterial keratitis. *American Journal of Ophthalmology* 105(3):239–243.

398. Ledbetter, E.C., Hendricks, L.M., Riis, R.C., and Scarlett, J.M. 2007. In vitro fluoroquinolone susceptibility of *Pseudomonas aeruginosa* isolates from dogs with ulcerative keratitis. *American Journal of Veterinary Research* 68(6):638–642.

399. Davis, S.D., Sarff, L.D., and Hyndiuk, R.A. 1979. Comparison of therapeutic routes in experimental

Pseudomonas keratitis. *American Journal of Ophthalmology* 87(5):710–716.

400. Leibowitz, H.M., Ryan, W.J., and Kupferman, A. 1981. Route of antibiotic administration in bacterial keratitis. *Archives of Ophthalmology* 99(8):1420–1423.

401. Sweeney, C., and Irby, N. 1996. Topical treatment of *Pseudomonas* sp-infected corneal ulcers in horses: 70 cases (1977–1994). *Journal of the American Veterinary Medical Association* 209(5):954–957.

402. Ollivier, F., Brooks, D., Van Setten, G., Schultz, G., Gelatt, K., Stevens, G. et al. 2004. Profiles of matrix metalloproteinase activity in equine tear fluid during corneal healing in 10 horses with ulcerative keratitis. *Veterinary Ophthalmology* 7(6):397–405.

403. Ollivier, F.J., Brooks, D.E., Kallberg, M.E., Komaromy, A.M., Lassaline, M.E., Andrew, S.E. et al. 2003. Evaluation of various compounds to inhibit activity of matrix metalloproteinases in the tear film of horses with ulcerative keratitis. *American Journal of Veterinary Research* 64(9):1081–1087.

404. Bohigian, G., Valenton, M., Lejeune, C., Okumoto, M., and Caraway, B.L. 1974. Collagenase inhibitors in Pseudomonas keratitis: Adjuncts to antibiotic therapy in rabbits. *Archives of Ophthalmology* 91(1):52–56.

405. Levy, J., and Katz, H. 1990. Effect of systemic tetracycline on progression of *Pseudomonas aeruginosa* keratitis in the rabbit. *Annals of Ophthalmology* 22(5):179–183.

406. Collins, S.P., Labelle, A.L., Dirikolu, L., Li, Z., Mitchell, M.A., and Hamor, R.E. 2016. Tear film concentrations of doxycycline following oral administration in ophthalmologically normal dogs. *Journal of the American Veterinary Medical Association* 249(5):508–514.

407. Baker, A., Plummer, C.E., Szabo, N.J., Barrie, K.P., and Brooks, D.E. 2008. Doxycycline levels in preocular tear film of horses following oral administration. *Veterinary Ophthalmology* 11(6):381–385.

408. Vygantas, K., Janicki, J., Whitley, R., Wright, J., Dillion, A., and Tillson, D. 2001. *In vitro* inhibition of matrix metalloproteinases in experimentally induced corneal ulcers. *Proceedings of scientific meeting of the American College of Veterinary Ophthalmologists* 32:34.

409. Peruccio, C., Bosio, P., and Cornaglia, E. 1984. Indications and limits of cianoacrylate tissue in corneal ulcers and perforations. *Proceedings of Scientific Meeting of the American College of Veterinary Ophthalmologists* 14:135–152.

410. Bromberg, N.M. 2002. Cyanoacrylate tissue adhesive for treatment of refractory corneal ulceration. *Veterinary Ophthalmology* 5(1):55–60.

411. Watté, C.M., Elks, R., Moore, D.L., and McLellan, G.J. 2004. Clinical experience with butyl-2-cyanoacrylate adhesive in the management of canine and feline corneal disease. *Veterinary Ophthalmology* 7(5):319–326.

412. Conn, H., Berman, M., Kenyon, K., Langer, R., and Gage, J. 1980. Stromal vascularization prevents corneal ulceration. *Investigative Ophthalmology & Visual Science* 19(4):362–370.

413. Peiffer Jr., R., Gelatt, K., and Gwin, R. 1977. Tarsoconjunctival pedicle grafts for deep corneal ulceration in the dog and cat. *Journal of the American Animal Hospital Association* 13:387–391.

414. Hakanson, N., and Merideth, R. 1987. Conjunctival pedicle grafting in the treatment of corneal ulcers in the dog and cat. *The Journal of the American Animal Hospital Association* 23:641–648.

415. Scagliotti, R. 1988. Tarsoconjunctival island graft for the treatment of deep corneal ulcers, desmetocoeles, and perforations in 35 dogs and 6 cats. *Seminars in Veterinary Medicine and Surgery (Small Animal)* 3(1):69.

416. Dorbandt, D.M., Moore, P.A., and Myrna, K.E. 2015. Outcome of conjunctival flap repair for corneal defects with and without an acellular submucosa implant in 73 canine eyes. *Veterinary Ophthalmology* 18(2):116–122.

417. Parshall, C. 1973. Lamellar corneal-scleral transposition. *Journal American Animal Hospital Association* 9:270–277.

418. Brightman, A., McLaughlin, S., and Brogdon, J. 1989. Autogenous lamellar corneal grafting in dogs. *Journal of the American Veterinary Medical Association* 195(4):469–475.

419. Hacker, D. 1991. Frozen corneal grafts in dogs and cats: A report on 19 cases. *The Journal of the American Animal Hospital Association* 27:387–398.

420. Hansen, P.A., and Guandalini, A. 1999. A retrospective study of 30 cases of frozen lamellar corneal graft in dogs and cats. *Veterinary Ophthalmology* 2(4):233–241.

421. Lewin, G. 1999. Repair of a full thickness corneoscleral defect in a German shepherd dog using porcine small intestinal submucosa. *Journal of Small Animal Practice* 40(7):340–342.

422. Goulle, F. 2012. Use of porcine small intestinal submucosa for corneal reconstruction in dogs and cats: 106 cases. *Journal of Small Animal Practice* 53(1):34–43.

423. Vanore, M., Chahory, S., Payen, G., and Clerc, B. 2007. Surgical repair of deep melting ulcers with porcine small intestinal submucosa (SIS) graft in dogs and cats. *Veterinary Ophthalmology* 10(2):93–99.

424. Chow, D.W., and Westermeyer, H.D. 2016. Retrospective evaluation of corneal reconstruction using ACell Vet™ alone in dogs and cats: 82 cases. *Veterinary Ophthalmology* 19(5):357–366.

425. Mancuso, L.A., Lassaline, M., and Scherrer, N.M. 2016. Porcine urinary bladder extracellular matrix grafts (ACell Vet® corneal discs) for keratomalacia in 17 equids (2012–2013). *Veterinary Ophthalmology* 19(1):3–10.

426. Andrade, A., Laus, J., Tonanni, R.C., and Paulo, S. 1999. The use of preserved equine renal capsule to repair lamellar corneal lesions in normal dogs. *Veterinary Ophthalmology* 2:79–82.

427. de Moraes Barros, P.S., Safatle, A.D.M.V., Malerba, T.A., Junior, M.B. 1995. The surgical repair of the cornea of the dog using pericardium as a keratoprosthesis. *Brazilian Journal of Veterinary Research and Animal Science* 32:251–255.

428. Dulaurent, T., Azoulay, T., Goulle, F., Dulaurent, A., Mentek, M., Peiffer, R.L. et al. 2014. Use of bovine pericardium (Tutopatch®) graft for surgical repair of deep melting corneal ulcers in dogs and corneal sequestra in cats. *Veterinary Ophthalmology* 17(2):91–99.

429. Barros, P.S., Garcia, J.A., Laus, J., Ferreira, A.L., and Salles Gomes, T. 1998. The use of xenologous amniotic membrane to repair canine corneal perforation created by penetrating keratectomy. *Veterinary Ophthalmology* 1(2–3):119–123.

430. Barros, P.S., Safatle, A., Godoy, C.A., Souza, M.S., Barros, L.F., and Brooks, D.E. 2005. Amniotic membrane transplantation for the reconstruction of the ocular surface in three cases. *Veterinary Ophthalmology* 8(3):189–192.

431. Lassaline, M.E., Brooks, D.E., Ollivier, F.J., Komaromy, A.M., Kallberg, M.E., and Gelatt, K.N. 2005. Equine amniotic membrane transplantation for corneal ulceration

and keratomalacia in three horses. *Veterinary Ophthalmology* 8(5):311–317.

432. Plummer, C.E. 2009. The use of amniotic membrane transplantation for ocular surface reconstruction: A review and series of 58 equine clinical cases (2002–2008). *Veterinary Ophthalmology* 12:17–24.

433. McCall, A.S., Kraft, S., Edelhauser, H.F., Kidder, G.W., Lundquist, R.R., Bradshaw, H.E. et al. 2010. Mechanisms of corneal tissue cross-linking in response to treatment with topical riboflavin and long-wavelength ultraviolet radiation (UVA). *Investigative Ophthalmology & Visual Science* 51(1):129–138.

434. Martins, S.A.R., Combs, J.C., Noguera, G., Camacho, W., Wittmann, P., Walther, R. et al. 2008. Antimicrobial efficacy of riboflavin/UVA combination (365 nm) *in vitro* for bacterial and fungal isolates: A potential new treatment for infectious keratitis. *Investigative Ophthalmology & Visual Science* 49(8):3402–3408.

435. Spoerl, E., Wollensak, G., and Seiler, T. 2004. Increased resistance of crosslinked cornea against enzymatic digestion. *Current Eye Research* 29(1):35–40.

436. Spiess, B.M., Pot, S.A., Florin, M., and Hafezi, F. 2014. Corneal collagen cross-linking (CXL) for the treatment of melting keratitis in cats and dogs: A pilot study. *Veterinary Ophthalmology* 17(1):1–11.

437. Pot, S.A., Gallhöfer, N.S., Matheis, F.L., Voelter-Ratson, K., Hafezi, F., and Spiess, B.M. 2014. Corneal collagen cross-linking as treatment for infectious and noninfectious corneal melting in cats and dogs: Results of a prospective, nonrandomized, controlled trial. *Veterinary Ophthalmology* 17(4):250–260.

438. Famose, F. 2014. Evaluation of accelerated collagen cross-linking for the treatment of melting keratitis in eight dogs. *Veterinary Ophthalmology* 17(5):358–367.

439. Famose, F. 2015. Evaluation of accelerated collagen cross-linking for the treatment of melting keratitis in ten cats. *Veterinary Ophthalmology* 18(2):95–104.

440. Hellander-Edman, A., Makdoumi, K., Mortensen, J., and Ekesten, B. 2013. Corneal cross-linking in 9 horses with ulcerative keratitis. *BMC Veterinary Research* 9(1):128.

441. Pischel, D.K. 1930. Tattooing of the cornea with gold and platinum chloride. *Archives of Ophthalmology* 3(2):176–181.

442. Killinger, A., Valentine, D., Mansfield, M., Ricketts, G., Cmarik, G., Neumann, A. et al. 1977. Economic impact of infectious bovine keratoconjunctivitis in beef calves. *Veterinary Medicine and Small Animal Clinician* 72:618–620.

443. Wilcox, G. 1968. Infectious bovine keratoconjunctivitis: A review. *Vet Bull* 38(6):349–359.

444. Pugh, G., and Hughes, D. 1971. Infectious bovine keratoconjunctivitis induced by different experimental methods. *Cornell Veterinarian* 61:23–45.

445. Nayar, P., and Saunders, J. 1975. Infectious bovine keratoconjunctivitis I. Experimental production. *Canadian Journal of Comparative Medicine* 39(1):20–31.

446. Hughes, D.E., and Pugh, G. 1970. A five-year study of infectious bovine keratoconjunctivitis in a beef herd. *Journal of the American Veterinary Medical Association* 157:433–454.

447. Vogelweid, C., Miller, R., Berg, J., and Kinden, D. 1986. Scanning electron microscopy of bovine corneas irradiated with sun lamps and challenge exposed with *Moraxella bovis*. *American Journal of Veterinary Research* 47(2):378–384.

448. Kopecky, K., Pugh Jr., G., and Hughes, D. 1980. Wavelength of ultraviolet radiation that enhances onset of clinical infectious bovine keratoconjunctivitis. *American Journal of Veterinary Research* 41(9):1412–1415.

449. Pugh Jr., G., McDonald, T., Kopecky, K., and Kvasnicka, W. 1986. Infectious bovine keratoconjunctivitis: Evidence for genetic modulation of resistance in purebred Hereford cattle. *American Journal of Veterinary Research* 47(4):885–889.

450. Pugh Jr., G.W., Hughes, D.E., and Packer, R. 1970. Bovine infectious keratoconjuncti-vitis: Interactions of *Moraxella bovis* and infectious bovine rhinotracheitis virus. *American Journal of Veterinary Research* 31:653–662.

451. Webber, J., and Selby, L. 1981. Risk factors related to the prevalence of infectious bovine keratoconjunctivitis. *Journal of the American Veterinary Medical Association* 179(8):823–826.

452. George, L., Ardans, A., Mihalyi, J., and Guerra, M. 1988. Enhancement of infectious bovine keratoconjunctivitis by modified-live infectious bovine rhinotracheitis virus vaccine. *American Journal of Veterinary Research* 49(11):1800–1806.

453. Pugh, G., Hughes, D., and Schulz, V. 1976. Infectious bovine keratoconjunctivitis: Experimental induction of infection in calves with mycoplasmas and *Moraxella bovis*. *American Journal of Veterinary Research* 37(5):493–495.

454. Rosenbusch, R., and Ostle, A. 1986. Mycoplasma bovoculi infection increases ocular colonization by Moraxella ovis in calves. *American Journal of Veterinary Research* 47(6):1214–1216.

455. Kopecky, K., Pugh Jr., G., and McDonald, T. 1986. Infectious bovine keratoconjunctivitis: Contact transmission. *American Journal of Veterinary Research* 47(3):622–624.

456. Abeynayake, P., and Cooper, B. 1989. The concentration of penicillin in bovine conjunctival sac fluid as it pertains to the treatment of *Moraxella bovis* infection.(I) Subconjunctival injection. *Journal of Veterinary Pharmacology and Therapeutics* 12(1):25–30.

457. Smith, J.A., and George, L. 1985. Treatment of acute ocular *Moraxella bovis* infections in calves with a parenterally administered long-acting oxytetracycline formulation. *American Journal of Veterinary Research* 46(4):804–807.

458. Angelos, J.A., Dueger, E.L., George, L.W., Carrier, T.K., Mihalyi, J.E., Cosgrove, S.B. et al. 2000. Efficacy of florfenicol for treatment of naturally occurring infectious bovine keratoconjunctivitis. *Journal of the American Veterinary Medical Association* 216(1):62–64.

459. Allen, L., George, L., and Willits, N. 1995. Effect of penicillin or penicillin and dexamethasone in cattle with infectious bovine keratoconjunctivitis. *Journal of the American Veterinary Medical Association* 206(8):1200–1203.

460. Anderson, J., Gelatt, K., and Farnsworth, R. 1976. A modified membrana nictitians flap technique for the treatment of ulcerative keratitis in cattle. *Journal of the American Veterinary Medical Association* 168(8):706–708.

461. Lehr, C., Jayappa, H., and Goodnow, R. 1985. Controlling bovine keratoconjunctivitis with a piliated *Moraxella bovis* bacterin. *Veterinary Medicine* 80:96–100.

462. Smith, P., Blankenship, T., Hoover, T., Powe, T., and Wright, J. 1990. Effectiveness of two commercial infectious bovine keratoconjunctivitis vaccines. *American Journal of Veterinary Research* 51(7):1147–1150.

463. Dickinson, L., and Cooper, B. 1959. Contagious conjunctivo-keratitis of sheep. *The Journal of Pathology* 78(1):257–266.

464. Langford, E. 1971. Mycoplasma and associated bacteria isolated from ovine pink-eye. *Canadian Journal of Comparative Medicine* 35(1):18–21.

465. Hopkins, J., Stephenson, E., Storz, J., and Pierson, R. 1973. Conjunctivitis associated with chlamydial polyarthritis in lambs. *Journal of the American Veterinary Medical Association* 163(10):1157–1160.

466. Egwu, G., Faull, W., Bradbury, J., and Clarkson, M. 1989. Ovine infectious keratoconjunctivitis: A microbiological study of clinically unaffected and affected sheep's eyes with special reference to Mycoplasma conjunctivae. *The Veterinary Record* 125(10):253–256.

467. Linde Henriksen, M., Plummer, C., Mangan, B., Ben-Shlomo, G., Tsujita, H., Greenberg, S. et al. 2012. Visual outcome after corneal transplantation for corneal perforation and iris prolapse in 37 horses: 1998–2010. *Equine Veterinary Journal* 44(S43):115–119.

468. Grahn, B.H., Szentimrey, D., Pharr, J.W., Farrow, C.S., and Fowler, D. 1995. Ocular and orbital porcupine quills in the dog: A review and case series. *The Canadian Veterinary Journal* 36(8):488–493.

469. Braus, B.K., Tichy, A., Featherstone, H.J., Renwick, P.W., Rhodes, M., and Heinrich, C.L. 2017. Outcome of phacoemulsification following corneal and lens laceration in cats and dogs (2000–2010). *Veterinary Ophthalmology* 20(1):4–10.

470. Paulsen, M.E., and Kass, P.H. 2012. Traumatic corneal laceration with associated lens capsule disruption: A retrospective study of 77 clinical cases from 1999 to 2009. *Veterinary Ophthalmology* 15(6):355–368.

471. Davidson, M., Nasisse, M., Jamieson, V., English, R., and Olivero, D. 1991. Traumatic anterior lens capsule disruption. *The Journal of the American Animal Hospital Association* 27:410–414.

472. Chmielewski, N., Brooks, D., Smith, P.J., Hendrix, D.V., Whittaker, C., and Gelatt, K. 1997. Visual outcome and ocular survival following iris prolapse in the horse: A review of 32 cases. *Equine Veterinary Journal* 29(1):31–39.

473. Lavach, J., Severin, G., and Roberts, S. 1984. Lacerations of the equine eye: A review of 48 cases. *Journal of the American Veterinary Medical Association* 184(10):1243–1248.

474. Labelle, A.L., Psutka, K., Collins, S.P., and Hamor, R.E. 2014. Use of hydropulsion for the treatment of superficial corneal foreign bodies: 15 cases (1999–2013). *Journal of the American Veterinary Medical Association* 244(4):476–479.

475. Barkyoumb, S.D., and Leipold, H. 1984. Nature and cause of bilateral ocular dermoids in Hereford cattle. *Veterinary Pathology* 21(3):316–324.

476. Christmas, R. 1992. Surgical correction of congenital ocular and nasal dermoids and third eyelid gland prolapse in related Burmese kittens. *The Canadian Veterinary Journal* 33(4):265–266.

477. Joyce, J., Martin, J., Storts, R., and Skow, L. 1990. Iridial hypoplasia (aniridia) accompanied by limbic dermoids and cataracts in a group of related quarterhorses. *Equine Veterinary Journal* 22:26–28.

478. Koch, S., Langloss, J., and Schmidt, G. 1974. Corneal epithelial inclusion cysts in four dogs. *Journal of the American Veterinary Medical Association* 164(12):1190–1191.

479. Schmidt, G., and Prasse, K. 1976. Corneal epithelial inclusion cyst associated with keratectomy in a dog. *Journal of the American Veterinary Medical Association* 168(2):144.

480. Bedford, P., Grierson, I., and McKechnie, N. 1990. Corneal epithelial inclusion cyst in the dog. *Journal of Small Animal Practice* 31(2):64–68.

481. Choi, U.S., Labelle, P., Kim, S., Kim, J., Cha, J., Lee, K.C. et al. 2010. Successful treatment of an unusually large corneal epithelial inclusion cyst using equine amniotic membrane in a dog. *Veterinary Ophthalmology* 13(2):122–125.

482. Smith, J., Bistner, S., and Riis, R. 1976. Infiltrative corneal lesions resembling fibrous histiocytoma: Clinical and pathologic findings in six dogs and one cat. *Journal of the American Veterinary Medical Association* 169(7):722–726.

483. Blogg, J. 1977. Proliferative keratoconjunctivitis in the Collie. *Proceedings of Scientific Meeting of the American College of Veterinary Ophthalmologists* 8:89–90.

484. Paulsen, M., Lavach, J., Snyder, S., Severin, G., and Eichenbaum, J. 1987. Nodular granulomatous episclerokeratitis in dogs: 19 cases (1973-1985). *Journal of the American Veterinary Medical Association* 190(12):1581–1587.

485. Latimer, C., Wyman, M., Szymanski, C., and Winston, S. 1983. Azathioprine in the management of fibrous histiocytoma in two dogs. *The Journal of the American Animal Hospital Association* 19:155–158.

486. Wheeler, C., Blanchard, G., and Davidson, H. 1989. Cryosurgery for treatment of recurrent proliferative keratoconjunctivitis in five dogs. *Journal of the American Veterinary Medical Association* 195(3):354–357.

487. Rothstein, E., Scott, D., and Riis, R. 1997. Tetracycline and niacinamide for the treatment of sterile pyogranuloma/granuloma syndrome in a dog. *Journal of the American Animal Hospital Association* 33(6):540–543.

488. Peiffer Jr., R., Gelatt, K., and Gwin, R. 1976. Use of a corneoscleral homograft to treat proliferative episcleritis in the dog. *Veterinary Medicine/ Small Animal Clinician* 71(9):1273–1278.

489. Schadler, H. 1985. Azathioprine in treatment for ocular nodular episcleritis. *Veterinary Medicine* 80:64–67.

490. Deykin, A., Guandalini, A., and Ratto, A. 1997. A retrospective histopathologic study of primary episcleral and scleral inflammatory disease in dogs. *Veterinary and Comparative Ophthalmology* 7(4):245–248.

491. Bellhorn, R., and Henkind, P. 1967. Ocular nodular fasciitis in a dog. *Journal of the American Veterinary Medical Association* 150(2):212–213.

492. Gwin, R., Gelatt, K., and Peiffer Jr., R. 1977. Ophthalmic nodular fasciitis in the dog. *Journal of the American Veterinary Medical Association* 170(6):611–614.

493. Breaux, C.B., Sandmeyer, L.S., and Grahn, B.H. 2007. Immunohistochemical investigation of canine episcleritis. *Veterinary Ophthalmology* 10(3):168–172.

494. Moore, C.P., Grevan, V.L., Champagne, E.S., Collins, B.K., and Collier, L.L. 2000. Equine conjunctival pseudotumors. *Veterinary Ophthalmology* 3(2–3):57–63.

495. Latimer, K., Kaswan, R., and Sundberg, J. 1987. Corneal squamous cell carcinoma in a dog. *Journal of the American Veterinary Medical Association* 190(11):1430–1432.

496. Ward, D., Latimer, K., and Askren, R. 1992. Squamous cell carcinoma of the corneoscleral limbus in a dog. *Journal of the American Veterinary Medical Association* 200(10):1503–1506.

497. Bernays, M., Flemming, D., and Peiffer Jr., R. 1999. Primary corneal papilloma and squamous cell carcinoma associated with pigmentary keratitis in four dogs. *Journal of the American Veterinary Medical Association* 214(2):215–217.

498. Martin, C. 1981. Canine epibulbar melanomas and their management. *The Journal of the American Animal Hospital Association* 17:83–90.

499. Donaldson, D., Sansom, J., Scase, T., Adams, V., and Mellersh, C. 2006. Canine limbal melanoma: 30 cases

(1992–2004). Part 1. Signalment, clinical and histological features and pedigree analysis. *Veterinary Ophthalmology* 9(2):115–119.

500. Donaldson, D., Sansom, J., and Adams, V. 2006. Canine limbal melanoma: 30 cases (1992–2004). Part 2. Treatment with lamellar resection and adjunctive strontium-90β plesiotherapy–efficacy and morbidity. *Veterinary Ophthalmology* 9(3):179–185.

501. Diters, R.W., Dubelzig, R., Aguirre, G., and Acland, G. 1983. Primary ocular melanoma in dogs. *Veterinary Pathology* 20(4):379–395.

502. Ryan, A.M., and Diters, R. 1984. Clinical and pathologic features of canine ocular melanomas. *Journal of the American Veterinary Medical Association* 184(1):60–67.

503. Harling, D., Peiffer, R., Cook, C., and Belkin, P. 1986. Feline limbal melanoma: Four cases. *Journal of the American Animal Hospital Association* 22(6):795–802.

504. Dugan, S., Curtis, C., Roberts, S., and Severin, G. 1991. Epidemiologic study of ocular/adnexal squamous cell carcinoma in horses. *Journal of the American Veterinary Medical Association* 198(2):251–256.

505. Dugan, S., Roberts, S., Curtis, C., and Severin, G. 1991. Prognostic factors and survival of horses with ocular/adnexal squamous cell carcinoma: 147 cases (1978–1988). *Journal of the American Veterinary Medical Association* 198(2):298–303.

506. Strafuss, A. 1976. Squamous cell carcinoma in horses. *Journal of the American Veterinary Medical Association* 168(1):61–62.

507. Lavach, J., and Severin, G. 1977. Neoplasia of the equine eye, adnexa, and orbit: A review of 68 cases. *Journal of the American Veterinary Medical Association* 170(2):202–203.

508. Schwink, K. 1987. Factors influencing morbidity and outcome of equine ocular squamous cell carcinoma. *Equine Veterinary Journal* 19(3):198–200.

509. Lassaline, M., Cranford, T.L., Latimer, C.A., and Bellone, R.R. 2015. Limbal squamous cell carcinoma in Haflinger horses. *Veterinary Ophthalmology* 18(5):404–408.

510. Teifke, J., and Löhr, C. 1996. Immunohistochemical detection of P53 overexpression in paraffin wax-embedded squamous cell carcinomas of cattle, horses, cats and dogs. *Journal of Comparative Pathology* 114(2):205–210.

511. Pazzi, K.A., Kraegel, S.A., Griffey, S.M., Theon, A.P., and Madewell, B.R. 1996. Analysis of the equine tumor suppressor gene p53 in the normal horse and in eight cutaneous squamous cell carcinomas. *Cancer Letters* 107(1):125–130.

512. Mosunic, C.B., Moore, P.A., Carmichael, K.P., Chandler, M.J., Vidyashankar, A., Zhao, Y. et al. 2004. Effects of treatment with and without adjuvant radiation therapy on recurrence of ocular and adnexal squamous cell carcinoma in horses: 157 cases (1985–2002). *Journal of the American Veterinary Medical Association* 225(11):1733–1738.

513. Hacker, D., Moore, P., and Buyukmihci, N. 1986. Ocular angiosarcoma in four horses. *Journal of the American Veterinary Medical Association* 189(2):200–203.

514. Moore, P., Hacker, D., and Buyukmihci, N. 1986. Ocular angiosarcoma in the horse: Morphological and immunohistochemical studies. *Veterinary Pathology* 23(3):240–244.

515. Bolton, J., Lees, M., Robinson, W., Thomas, J., and Klein, K. 1990. Ocular neoplasms of vascular origin in the horse. *Equine Veterinary Journal* 22(S10):73–75.

516. Chandler, H.L., Newkirk, K.M., Kusewitt, D.F., Dubielzig, R.R., and Colitz, C.M. 2009. Immunohistochemical analysis of ocular hemangiomas and hemangiosarcomas in dogs. *Veterinary Ophthalmology* 12(2):83–90.

517. Gerding, J.C., Gilger, B.C., Montgomery, S.A., and Clode, A.B. 2015. Presumed primary ocular lymphangiosarcoma with metastasis in a miniature horse. *Veterinary Ophthalmology* 18(6):502–509.

518. Pinn, T.L., Cushing, T., Valentino, L.M., and Koch, S.A. 2011. Corneal invasion by hemangiosarcoma in a horse. *Veterinary Ophthalmology* 14(3):200–204.

519. Donaldson, D., Sansom, J., Murphy, S., and Scase, T. 2006. Multiple limbal haemangiosarcomas in a border collie dog: Management by lamellar keratectomy/sclerectomy and strontium-90 beta plesiotherapy. *Journal of Small Animal Practice* 47(9):545–549.

520. Martin, C., and Leipold, H. 1972. Mastocytoma of the globe in a horse. *Journal American Animal Hospital Association* 8:32–34.

521. Hirst, L., Stoskopf, M., Strandberg, J., and Kempski, S. 1983. Benign epibulbar melanocytoma in a horse. *Journal of the American Veterinary Medical Association* 183:333–334.

522. Rebhun, W., and Del Piero, F. 1998. Ocular lesions in horses with lymphosarcoma: 21 cases (1977–1997). *Journal of the American Veterinary Medical Association* 212(6):852–854.

523. Schnoke, A.T., Brooks, D.E., Wilkie, D.A., Dwyer, A.E., Matthews, A.G., Gilger, B.C. et al. 2013. Extraocular lymphoma in the horse. *Veterinary Ophthalmology* 16(1):35–42.

524. Anderson, D.E., Lush, J.L., and Chambers, D. 1957. Studies on bovine ocular squamous carcinoma ("cancer eye"). II. Relationship between eyelid pigmentation and occurrence of cancer eye lesions. *Journal of Animal Science* 16(3):739–746.

525. Nishimura, H., and Frisch, J. 1977. Eye cancer and circumocular pigmentation in Bos taurus, Bos indicus and crossbred cattle. *Australian Journal of Experimental Agriculture* 17(88):709–711.

526. Den Otter, W., Hill, F., Klein, W., Everse, L., Ruitenberg, E., Van der Ven, L. et al. 1995. Ocular squamous cell carcinoma in Simmental cattle in Zimbabwe. *American Journal of Veterinary Research* 56(11):1440–1444.

527. Anderson, W., Davis, C., and Monlux, A. 1957. The diagnosis of squamous cell carcinoma of the eye (cancer eye) in cattle. *American Journal of Veterinary Research* 18(66):5–34.

528. Sullivan, T., Nasisse, M., Davidson, M., and Glover, T. 1996. Photocoagulation of limbal melanoma in dogs and cats: 15 cases (1989–1993). *Journal of the American Veterinary Medical Association* 208(6):891–894.

529. Andreani, V., Guandalini, A., D'Anna, N., Giudice, C., Corvi, R., Di Girolamo, N. et al. 2017. The combined use of surgical debulking and diode laser photocoagulation for limbal melanoma treatment: A retrospective study of 21 dogs. *Veterinary Ophthalmology* 20(2):147–154.

530. Featherstone, H.J., Renwick, P., Heinrich, C.L., and Manning, S. 2009. Efficacy of lamellar resection, cryotherapy, and adjunctive grafting for the treatment of canine limbal melanoma. *Veterinary Ophthalmology* 12(s1): 65–72.

531. Kanai, K., Kanemaki, N., Matsuo, S., Ichikawa, Y., Okujima, H., and Wada, Y. 2006. Excision of a feline limbal melanoma and use of nictitans cartilage to repair the resulting corneoscleral defect. *Veterinary Ophthalmology* 9(4):255–258.

532. Maggio, F., Pizzirani, S., Peña, T., Leiva, M., and Pirie, C.G. 2013. Surgical treatment of epibulbar melanocytomas by complete excision and homologous corneoscleral grafting in dogs: 11 cases. *Veterinary Ophthalmology* 16(1):56–64.

533. Mathes, R.L., Moore, P.A., and Ellis, A.E. 2015. Penetrating sclerokeratoplasty and autologous pinnal cartilage and conjunctival grafting to treat a large limbal melanoma in a dog. *Veterinary Ophthalmology* 18(2):152–159.

534. Plummer, C.E., Kallberg, M.E., Ollivier, F.J., Gelatt, K.N., and Brooks, D.E. 2008. Use of a biosynthetic material to repair the surgical defect following excision of an epibulbar melanoma in a cat. *Veterinary Ophthalmology* 11(4):250–254.

535. Surjan, Y., Donaldson, D., Ostwald, P., Milross, C., and Warren-Forward, H. 2014. A review of current treatment options in the treatment of ocular and/or periocular squamous cell carcinoma in horses: Is there a definitive "best" practice? *Journal of Equine Veterinary Science* 34(9):1037–1050.

536. Rebhun, W. 1990. Treatment of advanced squamous cell carcinomas involving the equine cornea. *Veterinary Surgery* 19(4):297–302.

537. Bosch, G., and Klein, W.R. 2005. Superficial keratectomy and cryosurgery as therapy for limbal neoplasms in 13 horses. *Veterinary Ophthalmology* 8(4):241–246.

538. Farris, H., and Fraunfelder, F. 1976. Cryosurgical treatment of ocular squamous cell carcinoma of cattle. *Journal of the American Veterinary Medical Association* 168(3):213–216.

539. Grier, R., Brewer Jr., W., Paul, S., and Theilen, G. 1980. Treatment of bovine and equine ocular squamous cell carcinoma by radiofrequency hyperthermia. *Journal of the American Veterinary Medical Association* 177(1):55–61.

540. Kainer, R., Stringer, J., and Lueker, D. 1980. Hyperthermia for treatment of ocular squamous cell tumors in cattle. *Journal of the American Veterinary Medical Association* 176(4):356–360.

541. Plummer, C., Smith, S., Andrew, S., Lassaline, M., Gelatt, K., Brooks, D. et al. 2007. Combined keratectomy, strontium-90 irradiation and permanent bulbar conjunctival grafts for corneolimbal squamous cell carcinomas in horses (1990–2002): 38 horses. *Veterinary Ophthalmology* 10(1):37–42.

542. Ollivier, F., Kallberg, M., Plummer, C., Barrie, K., O'Reilly, S., Taylor, D. et al. 2006. Amniotic membrane transplantation for corneal surface reconstruction after excision of corneolimbal squamous cell carcinomas in nine horses. *Veterinary Ophthalmology* 9(6):404–413.

543. Nevile, J.C., Hurn, S.D., Turner, A.G., and McCowan, C. 2015. Management of canine corneal squamous cell carcinoma with lamellar keratectomy and strontium 90 plesiotherapy: 3 cases. *Veterinary Ophthalmology* 18(3):254–260.

544. English, R., Nasisse, M., and Davidson, M. 1990. Carbon dioxide laser ablation for treatment of limbal squamous cell carcinoma in horses. *Journal of the American Veterinary Medical Association* 196(3):439–442.

545. Michau, T.M., Davidson, M.G., and Gilger, BC. 2012. Carbon dioxide laser photoablation adjunctive therapy following superficial lamellar keratectomy and bulbar conjunctivectomy for the treatment of corneolimbal squamous cell carcinoma in horses: A review of 24 cases. *Veterinary Ophthalmology* 15(4):245–253.

546. Clode, A.B., Miller, C., McMullen, R.J., and Gilger, B.C. 2012. A retrospective comparison of surgical removal and subsequent CO2 laser ablation versus topical administration of mitomycin C as therapy for equine corneolimbal squamous cell carcinoma. *Veterinary Ophthalmology* 15(4):254–262.

547. Rayner, S., and Zyl, N.V. 2006. The use of mitomycin C as an adjunctive treatment for equine ocular squamous cell carcinoma. *Australian Veterinary Journal* 84(1–2):43–46.

548. Malalana, F., Knottenbelt, D., and McKane, S. 2010. Mitomycin C, with or without surgery, for the treatment of ocular squamous cell carcinoma in horses. *The Veterinary Record* 167(10):373–376.

549. Karasawa, K., Matsuda, H., and Tanaka, A. 2008. Superficial keratectomy and topical mitomycin C as therapy for a corneal squamous cell carcinoma in a dog. *Journal of Small Animal Practice* 49(4):208–210.

550. Theon, A., Pascoe, J., Carlson, G., and Krag, D. 1993. Intratumoral chemotherapy with cisplatin in oily emulsion in horses. *Journal of the American Veterinary Medical Association* 202(2):261–267.

551. Theon, A., Pascoe, J., and Meagher D. 1994. Perioperative intratumoral administration of cisplatin for treatment of cutaneous tumors in equidae. *Journal of the American Veterinary Medical Association* 205(8):1170–1176.

552. Pucket, J., and Gilmour, M. 2014. Intralesional 5-fluorouracil (5-FU) for the treatment of eyelid squamous cell carcinoma in 5 horses. *Equine Veterinary Education* 26(6):331–335.

553. Dorbandt, D.M., Driskell, E.A., and Hamor, R.E. 2016. Treatment of corneal squamous cell carcinoma using topical 1% 5-fluorouracil as monotherapy. *Veterinary Ophthalmology* 19(3):256–261.

554. Overton, T.L., Allbaugh, R.A., Whitley, D., Ben-Shlomo, G., Griggs, A., Tofflemire, K.L. et al. 2015. A pulse-dose topical 1% 5-fluorouracil treatment regimen in a young dog with corneal squamous cell carcinoma. *Veterinary Ophthalmology* 18(4):350–354.

555. Boehm, M.D., and Huang, A.J. 2004. Treatment of recurrent corneal and conjunctival intraepithelial neoplasia with topical interferon alfa 2b. *Ophthalmology* 111(9):1755–1761.

556. Sloss, V., Smith, T., and Yi, G. 1986. Controlling ocular squamous cell carcinoma in Hereford cattle. *Australian Veterinary Journal* 63(8):248–251.

557. Gelatt, K., and Rubin, L. 1969. Delayed postoperative staphylomas in dogs. *Journal of the American Veterinary Medical Association* 154(3):283–288.

558. Fischer, C. 1982. A clinicopathologic classification of episcleritis and scleritis in the dog. *Proceeding of the Scientific Meeting of the American College of Verterinary Ophthalmogist* 13:1–18.

559. Willis, M., Martin, C., and Stiles, J. 1996. Infectious disease as a possible cause for scleritis and episcleritis in dogs. *Proceedings of the Scientific Meeting of the American College of Veterinary Ophthalmologists* 27:45.

560. Williams, C.O., Dietrich, U.M., Moore, P.A. et al. 2005. The immunopathogenesis of canine nodular ocular episcleritis. *Veterinary Ophthalmology* 8:449.

561. Williams, C., Carmichael, K., Brown, C., and Uhl, E. 2006. The immunopathogeneis of ocular nodular episcleritis. https://getd.libs.uga.edu/pdfs/williams_clara_o_200605_ms.pdf: The University of Georgia.

562. Barnes, L.D., Pearce, J.W., Berent, L.M., Fox, D.B., and Giuliano, E.A. 2010. Surgical management of orbital nodular granulomatous episcleritis in a dog. *Veterinary Ophthalmology* 13(4):251–258.

563. Day, M., Mould, J., and Carter, W. 2008. An immunohistochemical investigation of canine idiopathic granulomatous scleritis. *Veterinary Ophthalmology* 11(1):11–17.

564. Denk, N., Sandmeyer, L.S., Lim, C.C., Bauer, B.S., and Grahn, B.H. 2012. A retrospective study of the clinical, histological, and immunohistochemical manifestations of 5 dogs originally diagnosed histologically as necrotizing scleritis. *Veterinary Ophthalmology* 15(2):102–109.

565. Goetzl, E.J., Banda, M.J., and Leppert, D. 1996. Matrix metalloproteinases in immunity. *The Journal of Immunology* 156(1):1–4.

566. Komnenou, A.A., Mylonakis, M.E., Kouti, V., Tendoma, L., Leontides, L., Skountzou, E. et al. 2007. Ocular manifestations of natural canine monocytic ehrlichiosis (Ehrlichia canis): A retrospective study of 90 cases. *Veterinary Ophthalmology* 10(3):137–142.

567. Orihel, T.C., Ash, L.R., Holshuh, H., and Santenelli, S. 1991. Onchocerciasis in a California dog. *The American Journal of Tropical Medicine and Hygiene* 44(5):513–517.

568. Gardiner, C., Dick Jr., E., Meininger, A., Lozano-Alarcón, F., and Jackson, P. 1993. Onchocerciasis in two dogs. *Journal of the American Veterinary Medical Association* 203(6):828–830.

569. Komnenou, A., Eberhard, M.L., Kaldrymidou, E., Tsalie, E., and Dessiris, A. 2002. Subconjunctival filariasis due to Onchocerca sp. in dogs: Report of 23 cases in Greece. *Veterinary Ophthalmology* 5(2):119–126.

570. Sréter, T., and Széll, Z. 2008. Onchocercosis: A newly recognized disease in dogs. *Veterinary Parasitology* 151(1):1–13.

CHAPTER 11

ANTERIOR UVEA AND ANTERIOR CHAMBER

J. PHILLIP PICKETT

ANATOMY AND PHYSIOLOGY

The uvea is the vascular tunic of the eye and the anterior uvea consists of the iris and ciliary body (**Figures 11.1 and 11.2**). The most striking species differences in the anterior uvea are in pupil shape and reactivity to light. The pupillary light reflexes (PLRs) of ungulates are more sluggish than those of carnivores. Topographically, the iris is divided grossly into a thick peripheral ciliary zone and a thinner central pupillary zone, with the collarette

forming the junctional area (**Figure 11.3**). Remnants of the embryonic pupillary membrane may occasionally be observed arising from the collarette region. The pupillary border has a "ruff" of pigment formed by the central extension of the posterior pigmented epithelial layers. In ungulates, this pigment extension is exaggerated dorsally and ventrally to form the granula iridica or corpora nigra (**Figure 11.4**). In addition to pigmented epithelium, small capillaries are present in the granula iridica.

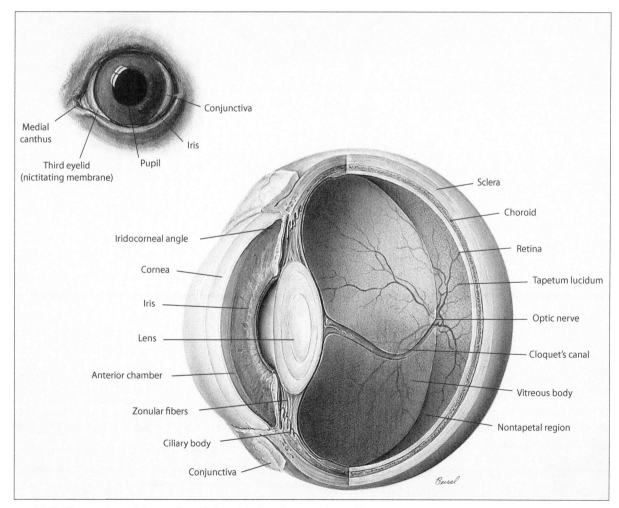

Figure 11.1 Illustration of the canine globe with the three tunics ("fibrous tunic," cornea and sclera; "vascular tunic," iris, ciliary body, choroid; "neural tunic," neuroretina) of the eye.

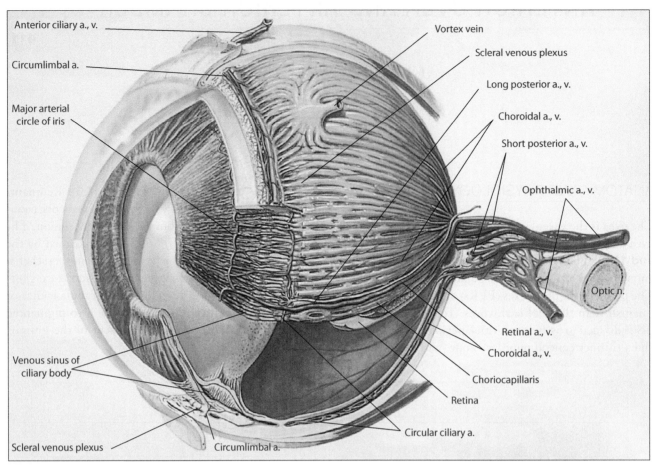

Figure 11.2 Illustration of the canine uveal tract. (a: Artery; v: Vein; n: Nerve.)

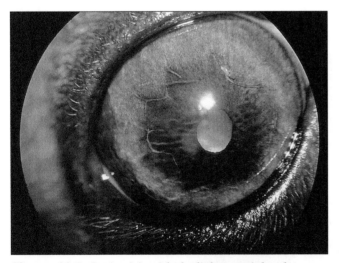

Figure 11.3 Canine iris with the lighter peripheral ciliary zone and the darker pupillary zone. Note the persistent pupillary membranes originating from the collarette region.

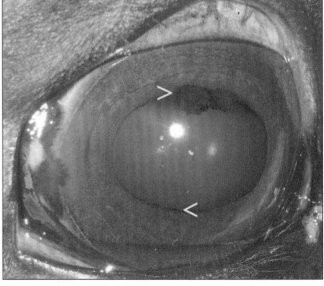

Figure 11.4 Equine corpora nigra or granula iridica on the dorsal pupil margin with subtler granula iridica on ventral pupil margin (arrows). Fine white lines on the cornea are artifactual reflections of the cilia.

The iris rests on the anterior lens surface. When the pupil is midrange or constricted, the iris represents a convex surface. When lens support is lost, iridodonesis or trembling of the iris is noted with movement of the globe. Loss of lens support may occur from a congenitally small lens (microphakia), posterior lens displacement, lens removal, lens resorption, or forward placement of the iris due to peripheral anterior synechiae (congenital or acquired). Normal iris coloration can vary within an eye, between eyes, and between individuals. The darker the iris, the more dense and compact the iris stroma and surface.[1] Crypts or surface defects in the iris, when present, are usually in lighter pigmented irides and in the pupillary zone.

Topographically, the ciliary body is divided into an anterior pars plicata (ciliary processes) and a posterior pars plana. The pars plicata is a ring of 70-plus ciliary processes, and the pars plana is the flat posterior portion between the ciliary processes and the peripheral termination of the retina (ora ciliaris retinae). The width of the pars plana is narrower medially and ventrally due to the more anterior extension of the retina in these quadrants. The usual site for transscleral vitreous centesis is dorsal or dorsolateral, where the pars plana is 7–8 mm posterior to the limbus in a medium-sized dog.[2] The ciliary processes in carnivores are blade-like and are ensheathed with zonular fibers that originate from the pars plana (**Figure 11.5**). The ciliary processes in the horse are capped with a broad band of cells that stops short of the tips of the processes (**Figure 11.6**).

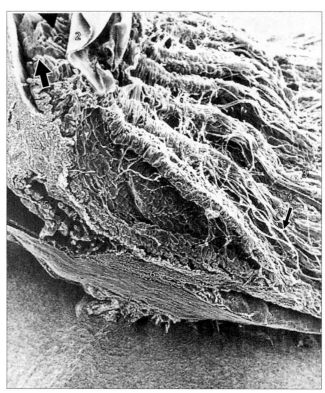

Figure 11.6 Scanning electron microscopy of equine iris and ciliary body. (1: Iris; 2: Lens capsule; 3: Pars plana; 4: Zonules originating from pars plana; 5: Ciliary cleft; 6: Ciliary muscles; 7: Sclera.) Note the convolutions that cap each ciliary process but stop short of the tips (large arrow) (SEM ×18). (From Martin, C., and Anderson, B. 1981. Ocular anatomy. In: Gelatt, K.N., editor. *Veterinary Ophthalmology*. Lea & Febiger: Philadelphia, PA, pp. 12–121.)

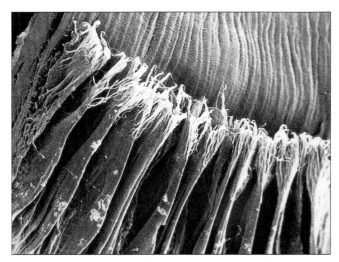

Figure 11.5 Scanning electron microscopy of the canine ciliary body viewed from the vitreous. The blade-like ciliary processes (pars plicata) are ensheathed and capped by the lens zonules. The posterior iris surface is visible dorsal to the zonules (×45).

The anterior chamber is the space demarcated posteriorly by the lens and the iris and anteriorly by the cornea and the iridocorneal angle (**Figure 11.1**). The posterior chamber is delineated anteriorly by the posterior surface of the iris, peripherally by the ciliary body, and posteriorly by the anterior vitreous face/hyaloid membrane.

The iris consists of an anterior border layer, stroma, and posterior epithelium (**Figure 11.7**). The anterior border layer is well developed in the dog and the cat and consists of a layer of fibroblasts and one or more layers of melanocytes; there is not a true endothelial or epithelial layer, as has been previously reported.[1,3,4] Instead of a cellular barrier at the surface of the iris to prevent large molecules and blood products from entering the aqueous humor from the iris vessels (blood–aqueous humor barrier), the iris vasculature endothelial cells form the blood–aqueous humor barrier at the level of the iris. The stroma of the iris contains collagen fibrils, blood vessels, nerves, melanocytes, fibroblasts, and the sphincter and dilator muscles.

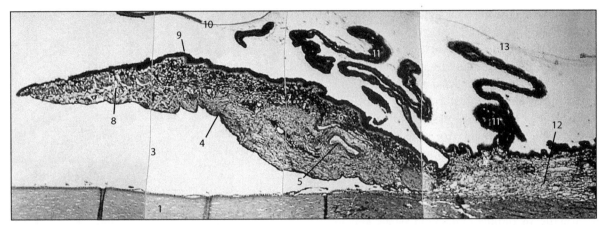

Figure 11.7 Montage of canine iris and ciliary body. (1: Cornea; 2: Limbus; 3: Anterior chamber; 4: Anterior layer of iris; 5: Major arterial circle; 6: Pigment in posterior stroma; 7: Dilator muscle; 8: Sphincter muscle; 9: Posterior pigmented epithelium; 10: Lens capsule; 11: Ciliary processes; 12: Meridional ciliary muscle tendons; 13: Anterior hyaloid membrane; 14: Ciliary stroma [×35]). (From Martin, C., and Anderson, B. 1981. Ocular anatomy. In: Gelatt, K.N., editor. *Veterinary Ophthalmology.* Lea & Febiger: Philadelphia, PA, pp. 12–121.)

The vascular supply to the iris is provided by the long posterior ciliary arteries, which form the major arterial circle of the iris that is visible in the peripheral third of the iris (**Figures 11.2 and 11.7**). The circle is incomplete at 6 and 12 o'clock.[1,5]

> Unless the iris is torn or incised at the 6- or 12-o'clock position, the location of the major arterial circle results in hemorrhage when the peripheral portion of the iris is incised or excised.

The iris muscles of mammals are smooth muscles (in birds and reptiles, iris muscles are striated) with a sphincter muscle located adjacent to the pupil and dilator muscles that run radially from the iris root to near the pupil (**Figure 11.7**). The dilator muscle arises from the anterior epithelial layer of the posterior iris. In species with an elongated pupil, the dilator muscles are poorly developed on the axis of elongation.[6] Each muscle has dual reciprocal autonomic innervation. The sphincter muscle is predominantly under parasympathetic control (cranial nerve [CN] III) with inhibitory adrenergic fibers (mediating relaxation). The sphincter muscle parasympathetic innervation is via the ciliary ganglion to the short ciliary nerves. The short ciliary nerves differ in the dog and the cat. In the dog, multiple branches supply the globe, whereas in the cat, only two branches (malar, laterally, and nasal, medially) are present. The dilator muscles are predominantly under sympathetic control (via the nasociliary nerve of the ophthalmic division of CN V) with inhibitory cholinergic fibers.[8] The two muscles are not equal antagonists, the sphincter muscle being stronger than the dilator muscle. When the pupil dilates, the posterior leaf of the iris initially contracts, and with maximum dilation, the anterior leaf of the iris also contracts. Prostaglandins have been demonstrated to contribute significantly to the muscle tone of the sphincter muscle and, to a lesser extent, the dilator muscle,[9] which is significant when attempting to pharmacologically dilate the pupil with parasympatholytic agents in an eye with anterior uveitis (**Figure 11.8**).

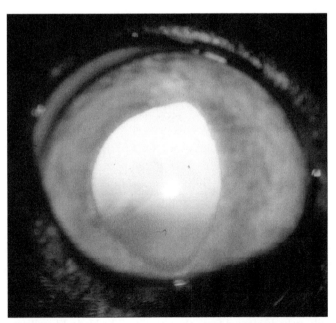

Figure 11.8 Reversed D-shaped pupil in a cat due to hemiparalysis of the malar branch of the short ciliary nerves.

Paralysis of one of the two short ciliary nerves in the cat produces a hemiplegia, resulting in a D-shaped or reversed D-shaped pupil (**Figure 11.8**).

Anisocoria can be classified as a static or dynamic inequality of pupils. Static anisocoria (due to iris hypoplasia, synechia, iris atrophy, unilateral pharmacologic mydriasis, or miosis, etc.) manifests without stimulation of the PLR and is constant, whereas dynamic anisocorias become manifest during or immediately after stimulation of the PLR. For an in-depth explanation of anisocoria due to neurologic deficits, see Chapter 4, Neuro-Ophthalmic Disorders.

Miosis (a constricted pupil) is a common ocular sign and may be from ocular disease, neurologic disease, or pharmacologically induced miosis. Intense miosis is a common manifestation of ocular irritation or pain and is typical of acute anterior uveitis and/or corneal pain (**Figure 11.9**). This miosis is often resistant to dilation with even strong parasympatholytic agents (atropine). Neurologic disease involving the midbrain may produce an intense miosis, whereas the miosis seen with sympathetic denervation (Horner's syndrome) is usually moderate (**Figure 11.10**). The miosis associated with superficial corneal pain may mimic Horner's syndrome by being accompanied by third eyelid protrusion and a narrowed palpebral fissure from blepharospasm. For a more in-depth explanation of neurologic causes of miosis and Horner's syndrome, see Chapter 4, Neuro-Ophthalmic Disorders.

The color of the iris is dependent on the amount of pigment in the stroma and the posterior pigmented

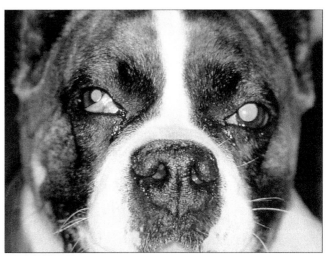

Figure 11.10 Horner's syndrome (right eye and adnexa) in a boxer with chronic otitis. Note the anisocoria, but the miosis is not pinpoint. Classic ptosis, enophthalmos, third eyelid prolapse, and miosis were present.

epithelium. Blue irides have a lack of pigment in the stroma but have pigment in the posterior pigmented epithelium. Albino animals have melanocytes, but due to an enzyme deficiency (usually tyrosinase), they are unable to synthesize pigment granules. White-furred animals may have no melanocytes in the iris stroma due to a neuroectoderm defect and many may also be deaf.[10] A defect in the tapetal and nontapetal pigmentation may also be present in white-furred animals.

The ciliary processes consist of a capillary tuft, stroma, and two layers of epithelium that are a continuation from the retina. The neurosensory retina continues onto the pars plana/plicata as the inner nonpigmented epithelial layer and the retinal pigmented epithelium as the outer pigmented epithelial layer of the ciliary body. The tight epithelial junctions between the epithelial cells are the basis for the blood–aqueous humor barrier (the barrier that prohibits passage of large molecules and blood by-products from the ciliary body vasculature to the normally clear aqueous humor). The capillaries of the ciliary body are fenestrated and do not provide a barrier to large molecules.[11]

The ciliary processes are responsible for aqueous humor formation. The pars plana cells are the origin of the zonules and, in conjunction with the ciliary muscles, have a function in accommodation. The ciliary muscles are not as well developed in domestic animals as in primates, and consequently, the amount of accommodation achieved is very modest. The anterior insertions of the ciliary muscles form the trabecular meshwork in the filtration angle and thus influence aqueous humor outflow (**Figure 11.7**). In birds, the ciliary muscles are striated and very strong, thus

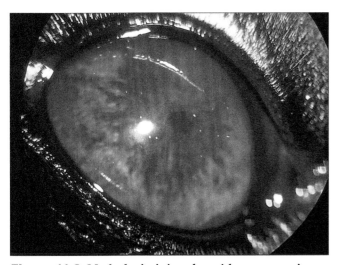

Figure 11.9 Marked miosis in a dog with acute anterior uveitis. Also note the dull iris surface and coloration as well as the subtle cloudiness of the cornea (edema).

allowing for a greater range of accommodation than in most nonprimate mammals.

DISEASES OF THE IRIS AND THE CILIARY BODY

Congenital diseases

Persistent pupillary membrane(s)

Embryologically, the lens is surrounded by a vascular network, the tunica vasculosa lentis (see Chapter 13, Lens), and normally, the anterior remnants of the network disappear by 3–5 weeks of age.[12] When remnants of the embryonic vessels persist, they are visible either on the iris surface or bridging the pupil and are termed persistent pupillary membranes (PPMs). Variable degrees of retained PPMs are frequently observed as a genetic trait in the Basenji, Pembroke Welsh corgi, Golden retriever, Chow Chow, English mastiff, and English Cocker Spaniel. When adherent only to the iris, they present no clinical problem except for genetic counseling (**Figures 11.3 and 11.11**). In the cat, agenesis of the upper lids in kittens is frequently associated with PPMs.[13,14] Peter's anomaly is an embryological maldevelopment of the pupillary membrane, cornea, and lens with corneal opacities, filtration angle anomalies, and anterior cortical cataract formation (**Figure 11.12**). It may be seen in man and in blue-eyed dogs. Aberrant PPMs attached to the cornea (**Figure 11.13**) and

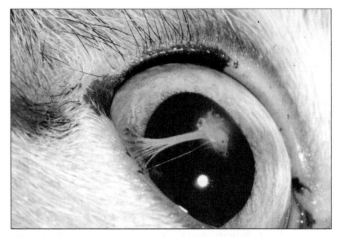

Figure 11.12 Peter's anomaly in a young Great Dane cross. The dog had corneal disease, anterior cortical cataract, and lenticonus, as well as filtration angle malformation. The other eye had a brown iris and no congenital defects. This eye later developed glaucoma and was subsequently enucleated.

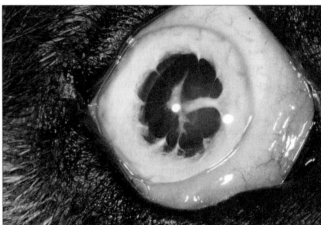

Figure 11.13 Iris to cornea PPM in a cat with resultant corneal opacity (leukoma) due to malformation of corneal endothelium, Descemet's membrane, and posterior corneal stroma.

lens are discussed in Chapter 10, Cornea and Sclera, and Chapter 13, Lens, respectively.

Polycoria

Polycoria is the presence of more than one pupil in the eye, each having a sphincter muscle (**Figure 11.14**). It is rare and is often confused with the more common condition of iris hypoplasia or atrophy that results in holes in the iris near the pupillary border.

Dyscoria

Dyscoria is a congenital or acquired abnormal shape or form of the pupil (**Figure 11.15**). The condition is usually

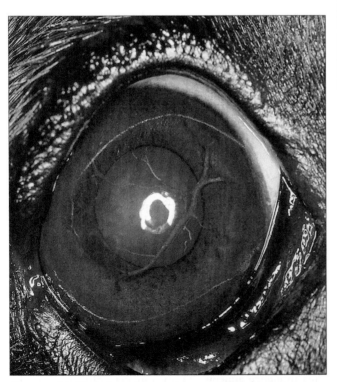

Figure 11.11 A dog with persistent pupillary membranes that are iris to iris. Most originate from the collarette.

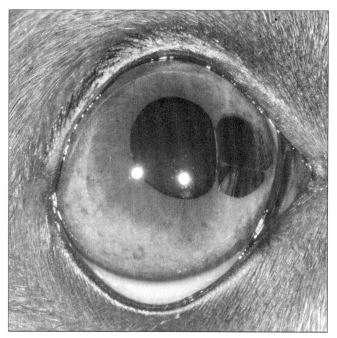

Figure 11.14 Polycoria in a dog. Note the pupillary ruff surrounding all three "pupils." Bright light stimulation resulted in attempted constriction of all three "pupils."

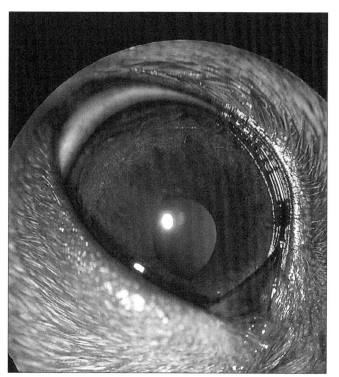

Figure 11.15 Congenital dyscoria in a dog. Note the tented, tilted pupil at the 11-o'clock position.

of no functional importance. It is observed as a congenital finding in the merle ocular dysgenesis syndrome of Australian shepherds, miniature dachshunds, and Great Danes (**Figure 11.16**)[15–17] and is due to an incompletely

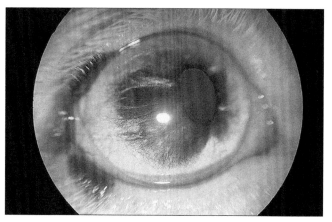

Figure 11.16 Dyscoria and corectopia in an Australian shepherd dog with a hypoplastic iris. Note the transillumination of the iris (10- to 11-o'clock position) from the fundus reflection.

penetrant recessive gene.[18] Dyscoria may be observed with corectopia (nonaxial or displaced pupil). Dyscoria is more commonly observed as an acquired finding secondary to iris degeneration/atrophy, trauma, neoplastic infiltration, and inflammatory synechiae.

Aniridia

Aniridia (absence of the iris) is a misnomer. While an apparent clinical absence of the iris may be present, it is not usually a complete anatomic absence. The condition is more correctly termed iris hypoplasia. The condition is rare and usually manifests as a very dilated pupil. Glaucoma may develop from malformation of the iridocorneal angle. In Belgian horses, it is inherited as an autosomal dominant trait, and thus, genetic influences should be suspected when observed in other species.[19–21] Aniridia and aniridia with limbal dermoids and cataracts have been reported in quarter horses[20,22], the latter thought to be autosomal dominant in nature. Aniridia has been described in Jersey cattle with multiple ocular defects of microphakia, luxated lenses, and cataracts. It was reported as an autosomal recessive trait in the Jersey cow.[23] Two cases of aniridia in related Llanwenog sheep have also been reported.[24] Varying degrees of keratitis have frequently been noted with aniridia, and the cause for this is unknown.

Aniridia presents with bilateral widely dilated pupils that expose the ciliary processes, zonules, and lens equator. Animals usually exhibit photophobia due to the inability of the pupil to constrict with bright light stimulation. Varying degrees of cataract formation are usually present. Superficial keratitis over the dorsal cornea has been observed in many species of animals and in humans with aniridia. The cause is unknown.

Coloboma

Coloboma of the iris is manifested as a notch-like or "keyhole" defect in the iris. A typical coloboma occurs ventrally in the iris due to incomplete closure of the choroidal fissure (**Figure 11.17**), while atypical colobomas occur elsewhere. The condition may be an isolated event or found with other ocular anomalies such as with merle ocular dysgenesis.

Heterochromia

Heterochromia irides is a lack of iris pigmentation within a portion of a pigmented iris (**Figure 11.17a**) or of the

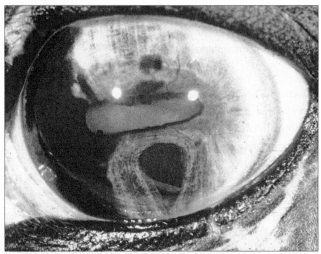

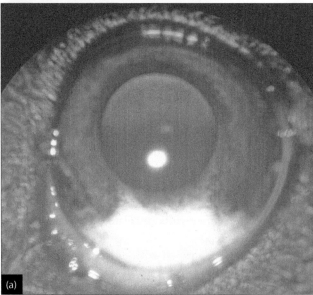

(a)

Figure 11.17 **Typical iris stroma coloboma/hypoplasia in an Appaloosa horse. Note the keyhole-shaped area at 6 o'clock of stromal coloboma with visualization of the deeper posterior pigment epithelium. The young horse also had an immature cortical cataract. (a) Heterochromia irides of the left eye of an Australian shepherd dog. The right iris was a uniform brown color.**

entire iris when the opposite iris is pigmented. In certain breeds of dogs with the merle genome and cats with white haircoats, deafness may be associated with blue eyes.[25–30] In white-furred cats, the eye color may be blue, yellow, or heterochromic; the genes for eye color are independent of white fur, but the blue eye color is expressed only in the presence of the gene for white fur. In white-furred cats, deafness may be unilateral or bilateral; if heterochromia is present, deafness occurs on the side of the blue eye if the deafness is unilateral. Deafness is the result of defective development in the organ of Corti, and degeneration of the inner ear structures begins in the first week of life.[27,28]

The merle coloration gene in the dog is dominant, and in many breeds, homozygous individuals for merling have microphthalmia or severe ocular malformations as well as deafness.[17,26,29] Animals with heterochromia exhibit a mild anisocoria with the blue eye being slightly more dilated.

Siamese cats and Persian cats with Chediak–Higashi syndrome are considered partial albinos; they are not deaf but may have optic chiasmal misrouting of optic nerve fibers.[10,31] Conversely, the white-furred cat has normal routing of optic fibers at the chiasm, with normal retinogeniculate projections. For a further detailed discussion of optic chiasmal misrouting, see discussion in Chapter 4, Neuro-Ophthalmic Disorders.

Ectropion uvea

Ectropion uvea refers to the pupillary margin everting forward to expose the posterior pigmented epithelium. This may occur as a congenital anomaly or, more commonly, is acquired due to contracting membranes on the iris surface (**Figure 11.18**). The contracting membranes (preiridal fibroblastic membranes, PIFMs) are observed with ocular inflammation, neoplasia, or chronic retinal detachment.

Acquired diseases
Altered iris pigmentation
Introduction/etiology

Focal pigment proliferations or densities may be observed on the surface of the iris and should be differentiated from neoplastic pigmentary changes. Iris freckles are clusters of melanocytes on the surface of the iris and are only a few cells thick. This results in a focal, flat, hyperpigmented patch on the surface of the iris. A nevus is a benign accumulation of either the precursors of melanocytes or of atypical melanocytes. It has variable amounts of pigmentation, is more extensively elevated, and extends deeper into the stroma than a freckle.[32,33] Nevi may thicken and may undergo malignant transformation. Most melanomas are thought to originate from nevi. Multiple or diffuse flat, pigmented lesions may be freckles that coalesce

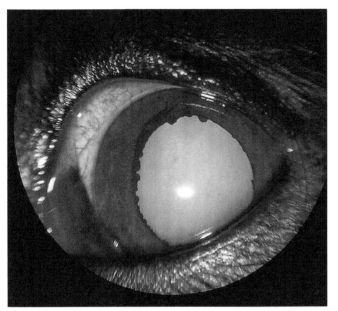

Figure 11.18 Ectropion uvea in a dog. Ectropion of the pupil margin is visible 9 to 1 o'clock. Either preiridal fibrovascular membranes from lens-induced uveitis (note the cataractic lens) or congenital deformity was the suspected cause.

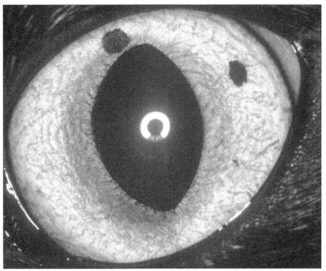

Figure 11.19 Iris nevi in a cat. Pharmacologic mydriasis was even and complete, and the nevi were followed for over 6 years with minimal change.

and may be very difficult to differentiate clinically from malignant progression of a melanoma unless it is bilateral, in which case it is usually a benign lesion. In the cat, these pigmented patches increase with age and pose a special problem for differentiating benign changes from early diffuse melanomas that are seen in this species.

Uniform increases in iridal pigmentation also occur with chronic insidious uveitis in all species. This may be so insidious that the examining clinician does not appreciate it unless it is unilateral.

Clinical signs
A flat, focal, pigmented spot is present on one or both irides. Nevi may be mildly elevated but should have sharp borders (**Figures 11.19 and 11.20**). Nevi and freckles do not distort uniform, complete pharmacologic pupillary dilation, as do stroma masses.

Therapy and prognosis
Pigmented spots of questionable significance should be photographed and observed for change over several months/years. Benign lesions remain static. If the lesion changes in thickness or expands, transcorneal diode or Nd:YAG laser photoablation should be considered.

Iris atrophy
Two forms of iris atrophy are frequently observed and are usually considered senile in origin. A third form of

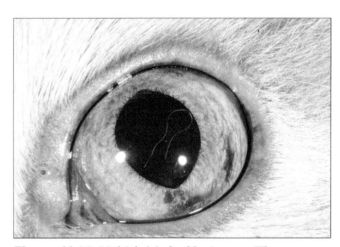

Figure 11.20 Multiple iris freckles in a cat. The contralateral eye had similar findings. The cat was followed for years with minimal change.

iris atrophy is observed secondary to inflammation and/or glaucoma. Iris atrophy is observed most commonly in the dog, although blue-eyed cats frequently manifest both congenital hypoplasia and atrophy with age.

- Sphincter iris atrophy is the most common form of iris atrophy and involves the pupillary portion of the iris. This form is present in many miniature poodles, Chihuahuas, and other toy breeds as they age. Mild sphincter atrophy is characterized by scalloped pupillary margins and loss of the pupillary ruff. As it progresses, asymmetrical or symmetrical loss of the PLR is noted, and depigmented areas of iris at the pupillary margin are visible on transillumination.

Advanced atrophy results in fixed dilated pupils or anisocoria. Pseudopolycoria and/or PPM-like strands are often present at the pupillary margin (**Figure 11.21**).

- Stromal iris atrophy is the second form of iris atrophy and is less frequent. This is usually observed in toy breeds of dogs. It manifests with large defects in the iris stroma and frequently results in almost complete loss of the iris stroma. The pupil may have dyscoria and may be displaced to the opposite side of the atrophy (**Figure 11.22**). This author has seen this with some regularity in "teacup" poodles, and it is many times associated with lens zonular degeneration and lens luxations later in life. A less severe manifestation is seen in blue-eyed cats as simply a thinning of the iris stroma, allowing visualization of the fundic reflection through the irides at the 3- and 9-o'clock positions.

The main clinical significance of iris atrophy is recognition of its presence when interpreting PLRs. When severe iris atrophy is present with cataracts, it becomes difficult to evaluate retinal function without electroretinography, although a strong dazzle reflex is usually indicative of an intact afferent visual pathway, whereas absence of a dazzle reflex is a poor sign concerning retinal function. Glaucoma has not been documented as a complication of iris atrophy in the dog or the cat as it has in humans.

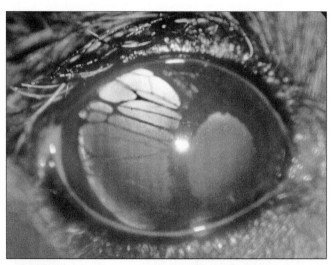

Figure 11.22 Stromal iris atrophy viewed against the fundic reflection in this young "teacup" poodle. Note the dyscoria and corectopia from loss of iris mass. This degeneration was seen in both eyes, and the dog later developed bilateral anterior lens luxations due to lens zonule degeneration.

Uveal (iris and ciliary body) cysts
Clinical signs
Uveal cysts manifest as variably pigmented cystic structures in the anterior or posterior chambers or within the pupillary aperture. The eye may contain one or more cysts, which, in the dog, are often free floating in the anterior chamber. The condition is quite common in the dog, with breeds such as the Boston terrier, Labrador retriever, and Golden retriever predisposed to the formation of cysts. If a cyst is densely pigmented and solitary, it must be differentiated from a pigmented tumor (**Figures 11.23 and 11.24**). Cysts may rupture and become deposited in the angle region, the lens, or on the posterior cornea where they are visible as an irregularly circular pigmented deposit (**Figure 11.25**).

Cysts originate either from the posterior epithelium of the iris or the epithelium of the ciliary body (ciliary body cysts).[34] Uveal cysts are usually of no clinical significance[35,36] except when their axial location impairs vision, or, once collapsed, as minor opacities of the lens or cornea. Ciliary body cysts in the Golden retriever and Great Dane have been associated with glaucoma and uveitis.[37–40] The mechanism of glaucoma production is thought to be through dispersed pigmented cells from the ciliary body and collapsed cysts occluding the filtration angle and the formation of PIFMs that extend across the filtration angle from the anterior surface of the iris. The pathogenesis of PIFMs (preiridal fibrovascular membranes on the iris) with ciliary body cysts is unknown, although inflammatory mediators and debris may be released from ruptured uveal cysts. Marked

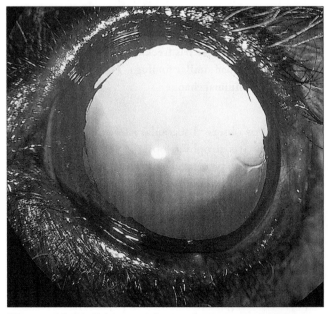

Figure 11.21 Sphincter iris atrophy in an aged miniature poodle. Note the dilated pupil with scalloped borders and isolated strands on the pupil border.

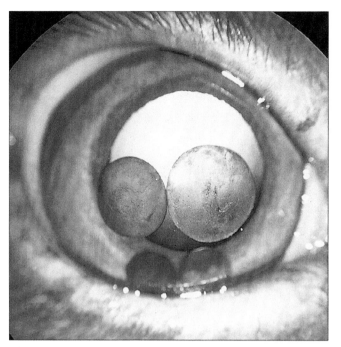

Figure 11.23 Multiple lightly pigmented uveal cysts in the anterior chamber of a basset hound. Note the readily transilluminated largest cyst medially.

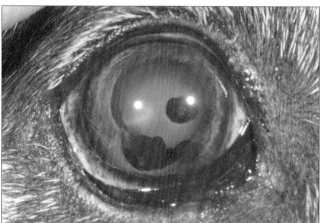

Figure 11.25 Ruptured uveal cyst on the posterior cornea of a dog. The dorsal most irregularly circular black mass is a collapsed cyst on the corneal endothelial surface. Numerous free-floating cysts are noted inferiorly in the anterior chamber. Collapsed iris cysts may be recognized as a round, flat, pigment deposit on the cornea, lens capsule, or in the dependent filtration angle.

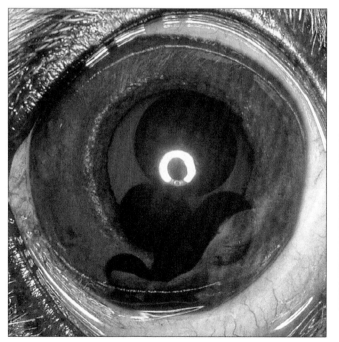

Figure 11.24 Multiple heavily pigmented uveal cysts in the anterior chamber of a basset hound. Due to impairment of the axial visual field, these cysts were aspirated with a 25-gauge needle.

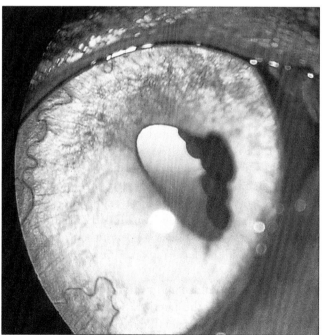

Figure 11.26 Multiple iris cysts in a cluster and attached to the pupil border in a cat.

ciliary body/iris inflammatory cell infiltration is not seen with this syndrome, although other characteristic signs of anterior uveitis (chronic breakdown of the blood–aqueous humor barrier with hyphema, aqueous flare and cells, fibrous membranes across the anterior lens capsule, and posterior synechia) are seen.

Iris cysts in the cat differ in that they typically appear as pigmented clusters still attached to the pupillary margin or protruding from the ciliary body once mydriasis is achieved (**Figures 11.26 and 11.27**). Uveal cysts in cats are rarely free floating as in the dog. Pupillary margin

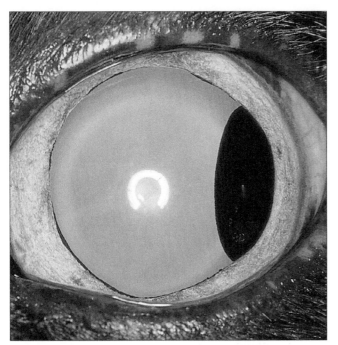

Figure 11.27 An old cat (note nuclear sclerosis) with a large, smooth, uveal cyst that was fixed in place. It was treated with diode laser photocoagulation, which was only partially successful in decreasing the size.

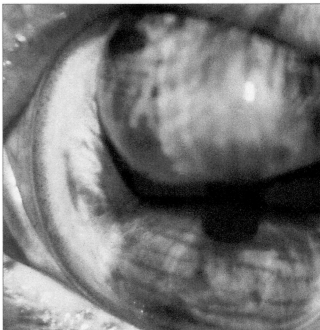

Figure 11.28 Stromal iris cyst in a horse. Note the appearance similar to iris bombe or a mass in the iris. The lesion is most visible on pupil constriction. With pupillary dilation, most cases will "resolve."

cysts may be coincidental with anterior uveitis, but there is usually not a cause-and-effect relationship.

In the horse, stromal iris cysts may manifest as a localized intrastromal swelling.[41] Buyukmihci et al. refuted that they are true cysts and stated that they are hypoplastic areas of the iris, and when the pupil is miotic, the slightly higher pressure in the posterior chamber compared to the anterior chamber pushes the hypoplastic region forward.[42] Clinically, stromal iris cysts most commonly appear as smooth focal swellings that are usually darker than the adjacent iris and are in the basilar aspect of the iris. They are more common in the dorsal region (**Figure 11.28**) but may be found in the ventral iris. The swellings transilluminate when the iris is examined in the miotic state, and they produce a shallowing of the anterior chamber. The condition may be bilateral or unilateral and must be differentiated from iris bombe or a localized intrastromal mass. Equine stromal cysts are more commonly observed in lighter colored irides, and Welsh ponies may have a predisposition.[41]

The most common type of iris cyst in the horse involves the granula iridica, which manifests as large, somewhat spherically shaped swellings attached at the pupillary margin (**Figure 11.29**). Owners frequently feel the cysts are responsible for behavior or performance changes and request cyst removal.

Dziezyc et al. described ciliary body cysts in the inferotemporal quadrant in three ponies of unspecified breed or

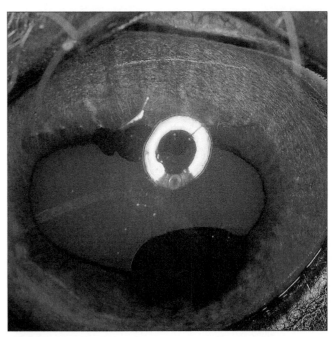

Figure 11.29 Cyst of the lower corpora nigra in a horse. It was treated transcorneally with diode laser photocoagulation, but needle aspiration is as effective, although more invasive.

color, with no other ocular lesions.⁴³ Large cysts of the ciliary body are also observed as the main lesion of anterior segment dysgenesis (ASD) or multiple congenital ocular anomalies (MCOA) syndrome observed in the Rocky Mountain horse and related breeds such as the Kentucky Mountain saddle horse, mountain pleasure horse, various ponies, and Morgan horse.⁴⁴,⁴⁵ ASD/MCOA is a dominant trait with incomplete penetrance that is expressed in color-dilute animals (PMEL17 [silver] genome mutant) with light manes. If the animal is heterozygous, the only lesions are observed by looking obliquely through the dilated pupil are large, thin-walled cysts located temporally behind the iris (**Figure 11.30**). Animals with the full syndrome (homozygotes) may have cornea globosa with myopia (nearsightedness), dyscoria, iris hypoplasia with a smooth nontextured surface appearance and inability to dilate the pupils, cataracts, temporal retinal detachment, retinal dysplasia, PPMs, large palpebral fissures, and persistent hyaloid arteries.⁴⁴

Therapy
Therapy is usually not required for iris cysts, although the cyst(s) can be aspirated through a needle if necessary. Pigmented cysts can be treated noninvasively by diode or Nd:YAG lasering.⁴⁶ In some individuals with numerous cysts, removal may be indicated to clear the visual pathway and to reduce pathology to the cornea and lens. If

there is any difficulty in differentiating cysts from neoplasia because of location or concurrent pathology, ocular ultrasound should be performed. Even when heavily pigmented, cysts are smoother and rounder than most neoplasms. In the color-dilute horses and Golden retriever dogs, the genetic implications should be recognized.

Iridorhexis (iris tears)
Tears in the anterior uvea may occur as the result of blunt or perforating trauma. The tears may be full or partial thickness. Hyphema (blood in the anterior chamber) may result and obscure the uveal pathology. The iris root is the thinnest portion of the iris and is most prone to traumatic tears. Pupillary shape and function may be altered depending on the extent of the tear (**Figure 11.31**). The intraocular pressure (IOP) should be monitored, and therapy is symptomatic for the traumatic uveitis and hyphema or the secondary glaucoma.

Iridoplegia
Introduction/etiology
Iridoplegia (immobile pupils) in a mydriatic state may occur due to end-organ dysfunction (iris sphincter musculature), efferent nerve dysfunction (parasympathetic fibers or nuclei of the oculomotor nerve, CN III), or bilateral afferent limb dysfunction (retina, optic nerve or chiasm, optic tracts) of the PLR. Pharmacologic iridoplegia occurs

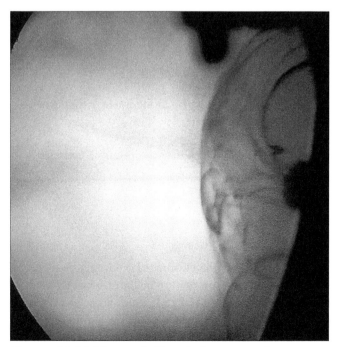

Figure 11.30 Temporal ciliary body cyst in a Tennessee walking horse. This is the typical position for ciliary body cysts in horses heterozygous for the *PMEL 17 (silver)* mutation.

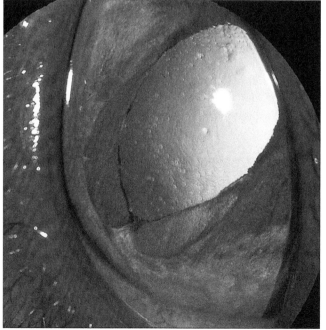

Figure 11.31 Iridodialysis in a dog's iris from blunt trauma. The anterior and posterior leaves of the iris have separated, and the pupil is dyscoric from rupture of the iris sphincter.

from the use of topical mydriatic agents or the ingestion of hyoscyamine, hyoscine, solanine, or belladonna alkaloids from various poisonous plants (black henbane, jimsonweed, nightshades, and ground cherry).

Pharmacologic iridoplegia may last from 4–5 days (dogs and cats) to several weeks (horses) after topical administration of atropine. If the application was accidental, the history may not be helpful, and the cause can only be diagnosed by the lack of synechia or iris atrophy, normal IOP, and the initial lack of response to direct-acting miotic drugs (e.g., pilocarpine). Improvement after several days aids a retrospective diagnosis of drug-induced mydriasis.

Iridoplegia from posterior synechiae and sphincter iris atrophy is a common phenomenon. Anterior uveitis is usually characterized by a tonic pupil in the midpoint to constricted state, and glaucoma by a tonic pupil in the dilated state. Blunt trauma may produce iridoplegia, which may be temporary.

Iridoplegia due to parasympathetic denervation results in a dilated pupil that, depending on the cause, may be unilateral or bilateral. Efferent denervation is characterized by a visual eye (unless multiple nerve injury occurs), lack of a direct or consensual PLR, and positive response to direct-acting cholinergic drugs (e.g., pilocarpine). Peripheral oculomotor nerve injury usually has somatic efferent deficits as well, and depending on the location of injury, multiple nerve deficits may occur. Total ophthalmoplegia from peripheral oculomotor nerve (CN III) lesions results in a dilated, fixed pupil and a ventrolateral deviation of the globe.

Cavernous sinus and orbital fissure syndromes manifest with oculomotor paralysis as well as deficits involving the abducens (CN VI), trochlear (CN IV), ophthalmic (CN V), and maxillary (CN V) nerves. The orbital apex syndrome also involves the optic nerve (CN II). Unless multiple orbital nerve deficits are associated with trauma, such as a proptosed globe, the prognosis is usually guarded for the life of the patient because the cause is often orbital neoplasia, intracranial neoplasia, or intracranial granulomatous inflammation.

Feline dysautonomia (Key–Gaskell syndrome) presents with generalized dysautonomia with dilated pupils. The condition is described mainly in the United Kingdom and sporadically in other regions (Midwestern United States and continental Europe). The etiology is unknown, and the incidence has decreased markedly in the last two decades. It does not appear to be related to feline leukemia virus (FeLV), as does alternating anisocoria (feline spastic pupil syndrome). Cats with dysautonomia may have an initial anisocoria, but subsequently, the pupils are dilated and equal, the eyes are visual, the third eyelid is prolapsed, and the tear secretions are decreased to totally absent. The lesion is characterized as an efferent arm parasympathetic lesion. Additional signs of dysautonomia are megacolon/constipation, megaesophagus/regurgitation, dry mucous membranes, bradycardia, and urinary incontinence.[47–49] It is possible in the cat to have an isolated palsy of one of the two short ciliary nerves (postganglionic parasympathetic fibers). This produces a D-shaped or reversed D-shaped pupil due to the hemidilation (**Figure 11.8**).[8]

Spastic pupils have been observed in FeLV-positive cats that manifest with paradoxical pupillary changes. The animal may have anisocoria that alternates at intervals of hours to days, pupillary hemidilation, or have widely dilated or constricted pupils. The condition is attributed to FeLV involvement of the ciliary ganglia.[50]

> Causes of iridoplegia include:
>
> - Midbrain lesions from trauma, neoplasia, inflammation, or degenerative conditions
> - Cavernous sinus lesions, usually inflammatory or neoplastic
> - Orbital fissure lesions that may be traumatic, neoplastic, or inflammatory
> - Increased IOP, usually >40 mmHg (5.9 kPa)
> - Pharmacologic induction or ingestion of certain toxic plants such as jimsonweed and nightshades
> - Orbital lesions involving the parasympathetic fibers or ciliary ganglion
> - Iris sphincter atrophy
> - Bilateral afferent arm lesions of the PLR, that is, retina, optic nerve, chiasm, or optic tracts
> - Posterior synechia development while the pupil is mydriatic
>
> (For a more thorough description of neurologic disorders causing iridoplegia, see Chapter 4, Neuro-Ophthalmic Disorders.)

Diagnosis

Ocular lesions must be eliminated from the diagnosis by a thorough ocular examination including measurement of IOP. The PLRs are tested and a neurologic examination performed. The response of the pupil to autonomic drugs may be tested (see Chapter 2, Ophthalmic Pharmacology).

Therapy

Therapy is directed at the underlying cause rather than the iridoplegia.

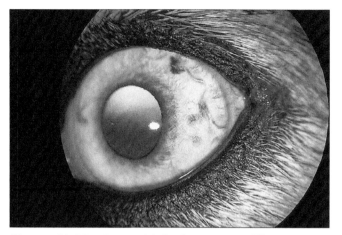

Figure 11.32 Iris petechia/ecchymoses in a Siberian husky with immune-mediated thrombocytopenia.

Iris hemorrhage and hyphema

Introduction/etiology

Petechiae of the iris stroma may be observed in blue irides but are rarely observed in heavily pigmented irides (**Figure 11.32**). Petechiae usually indicate a problem with platelet function or numbers or vasculitis. Tick-borne infectious diseases and thrombocytopenia are the usual causes. Other signs of anterior uveitis may or may not accompany the iris hemorrhage.

Hyphema (blood in the anterior chamber) (**Figure 11.33**) is the result of either blunt or perforating traumatic disruption of the anterior uveal vasculature, a bleeding or clotting defect, systemic hypertension, neoplasia, retinal tear/detachment, or iris neovascularization. The condition is usually unilateral. The blood may

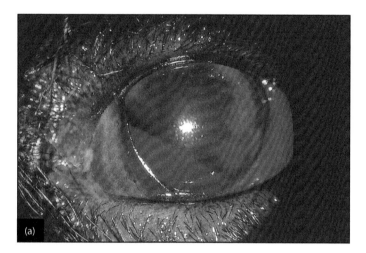

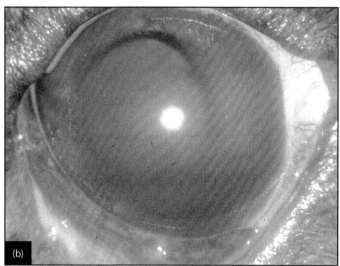

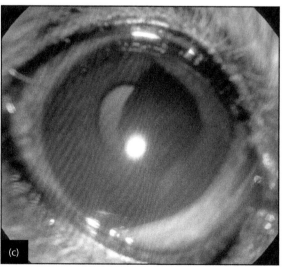

Figure 11.33 (a) Partial hyphema in a dog from blunt trauma. Note the fluid line due to settling of the unclotted blood. Hyphema of this size has a good prognosis if no new bleeding occurs and the cause of the hyphema resolves. (b) Free hyphema that has settled in a dog with lymphosarcoma. Note other signs of anterior uveitis: Posterior synechia with dyscoria, corneal edema, aqueous flare, and vitreous haze obscuring the tapetal reflection. (c) Clotted hyphema partially obscuring pupil in a dog with lymphosarcoma. The clotted blood was adherent to the iris and the lens capsule, thus contributing to posterior synechia formation.

partially or completely fill the anterior chamber and may clot or remain unclotted. The larger the hemorrhage, the more likely it will be clotted. Factors that determine whether the hyphema remains fluid or clots are incompletely understood, but, unlike external hemorrhage, blood in the anterior chamber is immediately diluted with aqueous humor. Blood in the anterior chamber undergoes rapid fibrinolysis due to dilution by aqueous humor and the release of fibrinolytic agents (e.g., tissue plasminogen activator substance or tPA) from the iris. Since coagulation of the blood interferes with removal of hyphema from the anterior chamber, these two factors are beneficial for resorption, but they also favor the possibility of re-bleeding and increased complications. Re-bleeding presents a physiologic dilemma since the intrinsic and extrinsic factors of coagulation are not activated completely.[51]

Hyphema in the acute stages is bright red, but if it is not resorbed and new hemorrhage does not occur, the blood becomes dull and dark; it is designated an "eight-ball hyphema" if the entire anterior chamber is filled with dark blood. Hyphema that is incomplete and fluid settles ventrally if the animal has been quiet (**Figure 11.33b**), whereas clotted blood often remains over the pupil region (**Figure 11.33c**). With fluid hyphema, the amount of blood often appears to change quickly; this is often a function of the animal's activity level. If the animal has been quiet, the blood settles ventrally in the chamber, and the remainder of the anterior chamber begins to clear. Typically, pet owners note that the eye is clearer in the morning after rest but later in the day appears worse due to ocular motion mixing the blood with aqueous humor. Blood pigments may stain the corneal stroma with chronicity, if the endothelium is not functional, or if there is increased IOP.

Blood leaves the anterior chamber through the aqueous humor outflow pathways, with minimal absorption by the iris. The iris is an important source of fibrinolytic products that free erythrocytes from the fibrin, so they may escape the anterior chamber. However, fibrinolytic products may also dislodge blood clots in torn iris or ciliary body vessels, thus causing re-bleeding or secondary hemorrhage.

Etiologies of hyphema include:

- Trauma: Blunt and penetrating/perforating globe injuries are a common source of hyphema. Usually there is history or other ocular/periocular signs consistent with trauma.
- Blood dyscrasias such as hyperviscosity, thrombocytopenia, polycythemia, and leukemia may cause hyphema.
- Bleeding and clotting deficiencies: Dicoumarin poisoning, inherited clotting factor deficiencies, acquired clotting deficiencies with renal and liver failure, and consumption of clotting factors (e.g., disseminated intravascular coagulation or DIC) may cause hyphema.
- Hypertension is a common cause of intraocular bleeding in the cat and may be seen in dogs. Vitreal or retinal/subretinal hemorrhage is more common, but occasionally hyphema is manifested.
- Vascular anomalies such as persistent hyperplastic tunica vasculosa lentis may rarely cause hyphema.
- Neovascularization associated with PIFMs that develop with inflammation, neoplasia, and chronic retinal detachment is a cause of hyphema.[52,53] The conditions that produce PIFMs stimulate diffusible angiogenic factors that stimulate neovascularization of the iris surface. This iris neovascularization is unstable compared to normal vasculature and susceptible to hemorrhage. PIFMs are a common histopathologic finding in the horse, the dog, and the cat but are usually not clinically visible.[52]
- Vasculitis: A variety of diseases such as tick-borne diseases and FIP in cats may cause ocular hemorrhage from vasculitis.
- Erosion of vessels from neoplasia or inflammatory/infectious processes.

Clinical signs

Red-to-black hemorrhage is present to varying degrees in the anterior chamber. If the hemorrhage is unclotted and the animal is quiet, the hemorrhage settles ventrally and has a flat top (**Figure 11.33a and 11.33b**). If the blood appears more diffuse, it is either due to a large amount of blood filling the chamber or due to a partial hyphema that becomes mixed with the aqueous humor after physical activity. Clotted blood is often localized and suspended in the anterior chamber. The pupillary area may retain a clot longer than other areas due to the lack of adjacent iris with fibrinolytic factors (**Figure 11.33c**).

IOP may be increased, decreased, or normal depending on the cause and the extent of the hyphema and accompanying ocular lesions. Concurrent lesions of trauma may include abrasions, punctures, and contusions to the lids, the head, or the body.

The pupil(s), if visible, may be constricted due to anterior uveitis, corneal pain (abrasions or lacerations), or concurrent brainstem hemorrhages causing CN III irritation or stimulation. Pupillary dilation may be due to glaucoma, contusion to the iris with iridoplegia, efferent lesions of the CN III, or from progressive or paralytic brainstem lesions with head trauma.

Diagnosis

The anatomic diagnosis is usually obvious, but the cause often requires an accurate history, good physical examination, ocular ultrasonography, and laboratory testing. The remainder of the ipsilateral globe and orbit and the opposite eye should be examined, and a physical examination should be performed to determine the presence of hemorrhages elsewhere or other lesions of trauma. This is important to provide clinical clues for the origin of the hemorrhage and to give a prognosis.

Therapy

In the past, therapy for hyphema has included a great number of drugs and procedures, most of which, when examined with double-masked studies, have demonstrated little or no benefit. The outcome of hyphema is more dependent on the amount of instantaneous damage done by the trauma than the therapy that is given afterwards.[51,54] If the cause is not trauma, control of the primary processes, such as a blood dyscrasia, bleeding/clotting defect, or hypertension, is essential for resolution of the condition.

The concurrent uveitis is treated with corticosteroids and atropine provided corneal abrasions or ulcerations are not present. If the trauma is a corneal/scleral perforation, glucocorticoids may be contraindicated if sepsis is present. Aspirin and other NSAIDs are usually not given in cases of clotting disorders or thrombocytopenia due to their interference with platelet function, which can promote secondary hemorrhage;[55] however, in cases where uveitis is great (or in a species such as the horse where systemic corticosteroid usage is contraindicated), judicious use of systemic NSAIDs may be tried. Cage rest and tranquilization is probably the most significant therapy for traumatic hyphema but also the most difficult to enforce.

If the IOP is elevated, the patient is treated symptomatically with drugs that decrease production of aqueous humor (topical or systemic carbonic anhydrase inhibitors or topical β-blockers). If traumatic in origin, the presence of glaucoma with complete hyphema of 7–10 days' duration is one of the few indications for invasive surgery or irrigation to remove the blood.[56] While this might seem an obvious choice of therapy, mechanically removing blood from the anterior chamber usually results in more disruption of the blood–aqueous humor barrier with more hemorrhage once the IOP is lowered.

> Surgery is rarely performed to remove hyphema and usually only if associated with trauma.

The use of pilocarpine with hyphema is controversial and is not recommended. Pilocarpine was previously recommended therapy because it constricts the pupil opening the trabecular meshwork pores, allowing erythrocytes easier egress, and it presents a larger iris surface, which is a source for fibrinolytic activity. Pilocarpine also dilates the uveal vasculature, which may increase the chances of re-bleeding, and it causes ciliary muscle spasms that accentuate ocular discomfort if traumatic anterior uveitis is present. Pupillary constriction causes a greater portion of the posterior iris to be in contact with the anterior lens capsule and, thus, may enhance formation of posterior synechia. Vasoconstriction agents such as epinephrine and phenylephrine are often recommended but are of questionable benefit only if continued bleeding occurs.

Fibrinolytic therapy to dissolve blood/fibrin clots and facilitate egress of nonclearing hyphema from the eye has been advocated.[57] Dramatic resolution of fibrin and hemorrhagic clots occurs when 25 μg of tPA is injected into the anterior chamber. Depending on the cause of hyphema, secondary bleeding may be seen.

Experimental clotted hyphema benefited from intravenous mannitol administration. Also, subconjunctival methylprednisolone administered before clotting occurred resulted in poor clot formation and faster resorption.[58] Systemic corticosteroids were thought to be beneficial in humans with traumatic hyphema by decreasing the incidence of secondary hemorrhages, but a double-masked study failed to show any benefit.[59,60]

Uveitis

Introduction/etiology

Iritis is the term used for inflammation of the iris. Cyclitis is the term used for inflammation of the ciliary body. In most cases of inflammation within the anterior segment, both the iris and the ciliary body are involved (and it is difficult to clinically determine if only the iris or the ciliary body is singularly inflamed), and the preferred term is anterior uveitis or iridocyclitis. Posterior uveitis, or choroiditis, indicates inflammation of the choroid, and the term chorioretinitis or posterior uveitis is commonly used descriptively as it is clinically difficult to differentiate choroiditis only from inflammation of the choroid and the adjacent neuroretina. Panuveitis implies inflammation of the iris, ciliary body, and choroid. Endophthalmitis is usually a more severe intraocular inflammatory process involving the ocular cavities (anterior chamber, posterior chamber, and vitreous space) as well. Panophthalmitis has a connotation of extension of the inflammatory process to the fibrous tunic (sclera and cornea) as well as periocular/orbital tissues as well. The causes of uveitis are varied and often elusive in all species. The condition may be unilateral or bilateral and may be chronic or acute in nature.

Unlike many areas of the body, physiologic function in the eye may be impaired by small lesions or scars associated with intraocular inflammation. Consequently, the eye has developed a moderating protective mechanism against the inflammatory reactions of many antigens within the anterior chamber. This is termed anterior chamber-associated immune deviation (ACAID), which downgrades the delayed hypersensitivity inflammatory reaction but preserves the humoral immunity to many antigens that are presented to the anterior chamber.[61] This has the effect of minimizing immune-mediated destruction of sensitive intraocular structures but may allow the antigen (infectious or neoplastic) to progress unchecked. This atypical immune response is not limited to the anterior chamber, as the central cornea, vitreal cavity, and subretinal space also have capacity to generate an ACAID-like immune response.[62,63] This immune privilege is the result of a lack of direct lymphatic drainage from the eye, with antigens bypassing regional lymph nodes and being presented directly to the spleen and the thymus. Suppressor T-cells that downplay cell-mediated responses are produced by the spleen.[64]

Inflammatory damage may be due to cytotoxic effects of an infectious agent, chemical inflammatory mediators produced by the host defense, and proliferative cellular reactions that disrupt normal morphology. Examples of chemical mediators with potentially harmful cellular effects are complement, cell-derived lytic enzymes, cytokines, histamine, and arachidonic acid metabolites. The arachidonic acid metabolites that utilize the cyclooxygenase (prostaglandins, thromboxane, and prostacyclin) and lipoxygenase (leukotrienes, hydroperoxy-tetraenoic, and hydroxyeicosatetraenoic acids) pathways have been studied the most, and they provide the rationale for utilization of NSAIDs in uveitis therapy.[65] Proteolytic enzymes released by neutrophils have previously been assumed to damage intraocular tissues directly, but evidence is accumulating that oxygen metabolites, such as hydrogen peroxide and hydroxyl and superoxide radicals, damage the tissue, potentiate arachidonic acid metabolites, and prolong the life of proteolytic enzymes.[66] Future anti-inflammatory therapy may incorporate antioxidants and hydroxyl radical scavengers.

Species variations exist in the response to ocular injury. Bito argued that species that are grazers or the hunted respond with exaggerated breakdown of the blood–aqueous humor barrier with ocular injury compared to predators.[67] Grazing animals typically have exposed globes that are subject to injury for a wide field of vision. These animals do not typically have sharp vision; therefore, a massive outpouring of protein to seal a corneal perforation or injury salvages the eye and does not greatly hinder function. Animals requiring sharp vision, such as hunters, have more protected eyes and do not respond to injury as dramatically. In the animal kingdom, "blood–aqueous barrier (BAB) integrity" has a definite hierarchy, with primates having more stable BAB than do horses and rabbits. In between these extremes (going from more to less stable BAB) are cattle, cats, and dogs. Interestingly, birds, with their very limited ocular protection but their tremendous dependency on vision for survival, have a very stable BAB, similar to primates.

Causes of uveitis in all species include:

- Infectious agents: Viral, bacterial, protozoan, mycotic, rickettsial, algal.
- Metazoan parasites: Worms, flukes, fly larvae.
- Globe trauma: Perforating and blunt.
- Surface ocular/extraocular disease: Corneal ulceration, corneal stromal abscess/cellulitis, episcleritis, and orbital inflammatory disease.
- Immune mediated: Lens-induced, systemic immune-mediated diseases.
- Neoplastic: Primary intraocular, multicentric, and metastatic.
- Blood dyscrasia: Neoplastic, immune-mediated.
- Idiopathic: Unfortunately, this is a large group in all species.

Clinical signs of anterior uveitis in the dog and the cat

Clinical signs of anterior uveitis typically noted by an owner are a red, cloudy, and painful eye. Other disorders with the same triad of clinical signs include corneal ulcerations, episcleritis, and glaucoma.

- Selective bulbar conjunctival and episcleral vascular injection (**Figures 11.34 and 11.35a**). Conjunctival hyperemia is more of a diffuse red color versus episcleral injection where the deeper episcleral vessels are more individual and distinct. Conjunctival injection alone may be present with surface ocular disease (KCS, surface bacterial or viral infection), and the vessels readily blanch with topical application of 2.5% phenylephrine or 1:10,000 epinephrine. Episcleral injection may be seen in conjunction with primary glaucoma or episcleritis, and the vessels do not readily blanch with topical application of phenylephrine or epinephrine. The canine species usually responds dramatically to anterior uveitis with notable episcleral injection, not always so with the feline species.
- Corneal edema. Poor function of the corneal endothelial cells with subsequent fluid accumulation within the

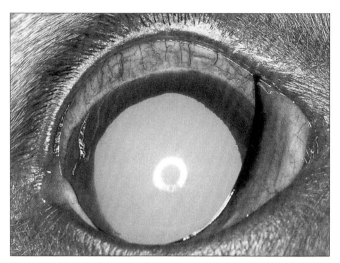

Figure 11.34 Selective injection of the conjunctival and episcleral vessels in a dog with uveitis due to *Brucella canis*. The pupil has been pharmacologically dilated.

corneal stroma (edema, **Figures 11.33b**, **11.35a, and 11.39**) occurs when the abnormal aqueous humor fails to properly nourish the endothelial cells, when the endothelial cells are coated with inflammatory debris (cells, fibrin), or when chronic uveitis results in death of endothelial cells, thereby reducing the critical mass of endothelial cells needed to maintain proper corneal dehydration and clarity. Epithelial defects (ulcers) and primary corneal endothelial cell disease may also cause corneal edema in the absence of anterior uveitis.

- Miosis that does not readily dilate with mydriatics (**Figure 11.9**). In mild and chronic anterior uveitis, the pupils are usually not dramatically constricted but are not as responsive to typical parasympatholytic mydriatic agents (e.g., tropicamide or atropine). Additional causes of pharmacologically unresponsive miosis may include lack of sympathetic innervation (i.e., Horner's syndrome) or posterior synechia.

- Photophobia and blepharospasm, particularly in acute cases. Light stimulation induces pupillociliary spasm (with "brow ache" perceived in humans). These signs can also be seen in animals with iris atrophy and the inability to shade the neuroretina from overstimulation as well as in cases of surface ocular disease (e.g., KCS, corneal ulcers, etc.).

- Plasmoid aqueous humor and possibly fibrin clots in the anterior chamber due to alterations in the BAB. Altered permeability of iris vasculature or tight junctions of the ciliary body epithelium allow blood-borne proteins to leak into the normally protein sparse aqueous humor. The presence of "aqueous flare" from plasmoid aqueous humor is a clinical hallmark of anterior uveitis (**Figure 11.35b** and Chapter 1, **Figure 1.13**). Clotted or unclotted hyphema may be present and the leukotactic stimulation so intense that hypopyon (pooled white blood cells) may develop (**Figures 11.49, 11.50, and 11.54c**).

- Synechiae, both posterior and anterior. With fibrinous exudation from the uveal vasculature, the iris adheres to adjacent structures resulting in variable degrees of synechiae. These may manifest as posterior synechiae (iris adhered to lens), producing immobile

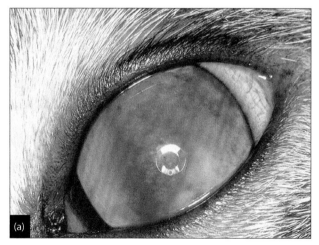

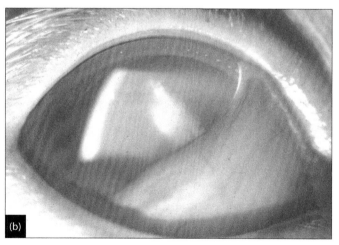

Figure 11.35 (a) Serofibrinohemorrhagic clot in the anterior chamber of a cat with anterior uveitis. Note diffuse corneal edema. Note that despite the apparent intense anterior chamber reaction to inflammation, there is minimal episcleral injection present. This is common in the feline species. (b) Aqueous flare seen via slit lamp biomicroscopy, feline. Note the white beam of light on the corneal surface (to the left) and the trailing white image of the light within the protein rich anterior chamber fluid ("Tyndall effect"). There is also present a large "mutton fat" fibrin clot (keratic precipitate or "KP") on the corneal endothelial surface along with diffuse corneal edema.

or irregular-shaped pupil(s). Uveal pigment disruption and synechiae often result in pigment deposits ("pigment rests") on the anterior lens capsule (**Figure 11.36**). Complete 360-degree posterior synechiae and pupil seclusion result in iris bombe ("ballooning forward") with a shallowing of the anterior chamber (**Figure 11.37**). Peripheral anterior synechiae involving the iridocorneal angle may develop independent of, or secondary to, iris bombe. Synechia may be seen with acute uveitis but may also occur secondary to previous uveitis or injury.

- Change in iris texture and color. The iris becomes thicker, loses its delicate surface mosaic texture, and becomes darker in color with inflammation. Blue and gold irides become brown, which is striking in appearance if it occurs unilaterally (**Figure 11.38**), and brown irides become more black appearing (**Figure 11.36**). This is a sensitive indicator of anterior uveitis, if seen, but can also be due to iridal neoplasia.
- Keratic precipitates (KPs). Cellular and fibrin debris often accumulates on the corneal endothelium, forming KPs. Large deposits ("mutton fat") that can be seen with the unaided eye are formed by macrophages and mononuclear cells, whereas small deposits are usually neutrophils (**Figures 11.35b, 11.39, and 11.40a**). White scars of the endothelial surface may persist long after active inflammation has abated.

- Hypotony is typical of uncomplicated uveitis and is due to decreased active aqueous humor production and potentially increased uveoscleral outflow.[68] Chronic hypotony may persist after the acute inflammation has resolved.
- Synechiae and/or fibrin or cellular debris may block the aqueous humor outflow pathways and produce secondary glaucoma. Secondary glaucoma may persist

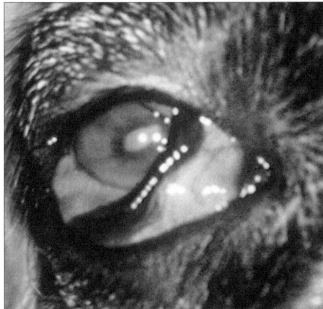

Figure 11.37 Iris bombe in a dog with uveitis associated with *Ehrlichia canis*. Note the dyscoria due to the posterior synechia and the "ballooning forward" with shallowing of the anterior chamber.

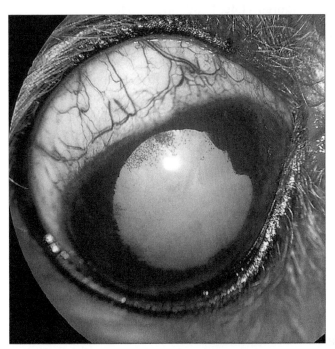

Figure 11.36 Lens-induced uveitis in a miniature poodle. Note the selective episcleral injection and dark iris. The iris is much darker than normal, and the pupil is irregular shaped (dyscoria) from posterior synechiae (1 to 3 o'clock, 5 o'clock, and 7 to 9 o'clock), and the anterior lens capsule is dusted with pigment from the iris ("pigment rests," 9 to 1 o'clock).

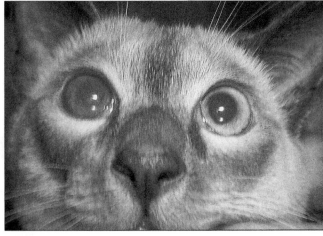

Figure 11.38 Marked darkening of the iris in a Siamese cat with chronic uveitis of undetermined etiology.

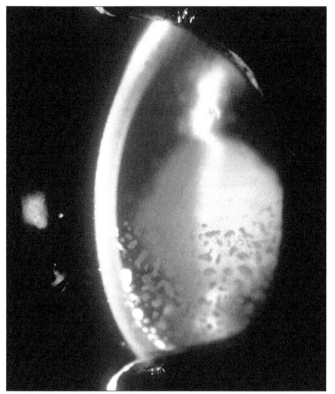

Figure 11.39 Keratic precipitates on the corneal endothelial surface in a dog with diabetes mellitus and lens capsule rupture (phacoclastic uveitis) as seen with slit lamp biomicroscopy. Note the thickened corneal image (corneal edema), debris on endothelial surface, thickened "ballooning forward" iris (iritis and iris bombe), and cataract.

long after active inflammation has resolved due to fibrosis of the filtration angle.
- Deep corneal neovascularization usually accompanies chronic anterior uveitis; conversely, most deep corneal problems (deep septic ulcers or deep stromal infections) also produce anterior uveal inflammation (**Figure 11.54c**).
- Preiridal fibrovascular membranes (PIFM or rubeosis iridis). Neovascularization of the iris surface is present with many cases of chronic uveitis.[52] Rubeosis, while a common histopathologic lesion,[52] is often not clinically visualized due to normal dark iris pigmentation. Rubeosis is most easily detected in lighter pigmented irides (**Figure 11.40a,b**). Rubeosis often extends into the iridocorneal angle and may be responsible for spontaneous hyphema and a very intractable form of glaucoma.
- Cataract. Anterior or posterior cortical or capsular opacities may occur with anterior uveitis and are termed complicated or secondary cataracts. The capsular opacities may be from pigment dispersion, synechiae, "pigment rests," or deposition of inflammatory debris

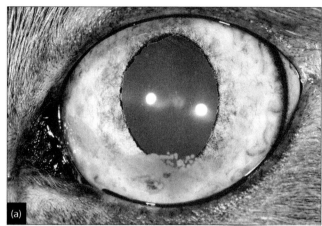

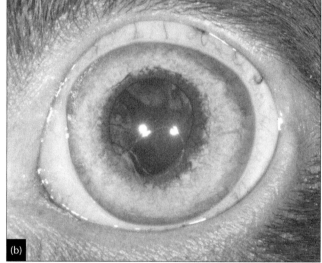

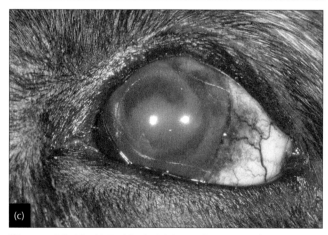

Figure 11.40 (a) Rubiosis irides and "mutton fat" keratic precipitates in a cat with *Bartonella* spp.- associated anterior uveitis. (b) Rubiosis irides/PIFM in a chocolate coated Labrador retriever due to blastomycosis. Note the dyscoria due to posterior synechia and the exudative retinal detachment seen through the pupil due to intense septic chorioretinitis. (c) Anterior uveitis with episcleral injection, corneal edema, aqueous flare, and anterior chamber fibrinohemorrhagic blood clots in a German shepherd dog with ehrlichiosis.

on the capsules. Eventually, impaired nutrition to the lens may result in varying degrees of cortical cataract. Cataracts that are the result of uveitis should be differentiated from cataracts that cause uveitis or cataracts that resulted from a common initiating factor such as trauma or diabetic lens capsule rupture. The most common cause of cataract in adult cats and horses is uveitis induced (see Chapter 13).

• Vision loss. Vision loss may be due to a lack of corneal clarity, lack of aqueous humor clarity, or lack of lens clarity secondary to anterior uveitis. There are other causes of vision loss (glaucoma, retinal disease, optic nerve disease) besides uveitis.

Causes of uveitis in the dog (**Table 11.1**)

Systemic infectious diseases

Infectious canine hepatitis, ehrlichiosis, Rocky Mountain spotted fever (RMSF), systemic mycoses, protothecosis,

toxoplasmosis, leishmaniasis, canine brucellosis, mycobacteria, leptospirosis, and bacterial septicemia are examples of infectious diseases that may cause uveitis. Massa et al. found that in over 100 dogs with uveitis unrelated to the lens or trauma, 18% were related to systemic infectious agents.[69] These authors (based in the southeastern United States) found that the most common agent was *Ehrlichia canis*. Obviously, the infectious agents involved with uveitis varies with what is endemic for the geographical region. Some infectious agents may cause an immune-mediated inflammation, rather than destruction by the infectious agent itself. Anterior uveitis with toxoplasmosis and systemic mycoses may have organisms readily demonstrable in the posterior uvea/subretinal space, but organisms are rarely present in the anterior uvea. This results in speculation that anterior uveitis is more inflammatory mediator induced than due to direct tissue damage by the infecting organism.

Table 11.1 **Causes of canine anterior uveitis.**

ETIOLOGY	DIAGNOSTIC AIDS
Systemic infectious diseases	
Infectious canine hepatitis (ICH)	Recent history of CAV-1 vaccination, age, appearance (corneal edema)
Ehrlichia spp.	Hemorrhagic uveitis, serology, response to tetracycline, low platelet count
Rickettsia rickettsii	Petechiae, serology, response to tetracycline, low platelet count
Brucella canis	Hemorrhagic uveitis, history, serology
Leptospira spp.	Renal and liver disorders, serology
Borrelia burgdorferi	Polyarthritis, renal disease, serology, Western blot
Systemic mycoses	Pulmonary, bone, skin, or CNS signs; thoracic radiography; serology; specific antigen tests; cytology from FNA of lymph nodes/vitreous/subretinal space; breed predisposition (German Shepherd, aspergillosis), geographic location
Toxoplasma gondii	Serology (elevated IgM or rising IgG titers)
Leishmania donovani	History of Mediterranean travel, Fox Hound, cytology of marrow, serology
Prototheca spp.	Hemorrhagic diarrhea; urine, colon mucosa, or subretinal/vitreal cytology
Metazoan parasites	Observation of worm or larva in eye, subretinal tracts in fundus
Trauma	
Blunt or perforating	Physical examination, history, skull radiography or ocular U/S with metallic or nonmetallic foreign body noted
Neoplasia	History, physical examination, ocular U/S, cytology of ocular fluids
Extension from keratitis	Deep ulceration/stromal abscess, history, ocular examination
Immune-mediated processes	
Phacoclastic uveitis	History of penetrating wound, cataract, diabetes mellitus
Lens-induced uveitis	Cataract, associated breed for juvenile cataract
Uveodermatologic syndrome	Bilateral, sterile, cytology nonseptic, typical of syndrome, dermal depigmentation, response to anti-inflammatory drugs
Sclerouveal syndromes	Signs of scleritis/episcleritis
Steroid responsive retinal detachments syndrome	Lack of other systemic signs, large breed dog, bilateral retinal detachments, lack of organisms noted on subretinal FNA and cytology, negative serology for infectious disease

Canine adenovirus-1 (CAV-1, causing infectious canine hepatitis [ICH]) produces a nongranulomatous anterior uveitis with involvement of the corneal endothelium and dramatic corneal edema. The ocular lesions typically manifest 10–14 days after immunization with adenovirus-1 modified live virus (MLV) vaccine or in the convalescing stage of clinical hepatitis. The use of adenovirus-2 MLV vaccines has dramatically decreased but has not eliminated the incidence of vaccine-induced uveitis. Three percent of uveitis cases in a recent report were associated with vaccination.[69] Ocular lesions manifest unilaterally in 85% of cases and occur in young puppies to young adult dogs. Sight hounds and Siberian huskies seem to be at higher risk.[70] The anterior segment reaction is thought to be an immune complex deposition or Arthus-type immune inflammatory reaction.[71,72] Severe instances may result in glaucoma and/or persistent corneal edema, the most serious sequelae. Most cases improve spontaneously over 2–3 weeks (see Chapter 10).

Ehrlichia canis, *E. platys*, and *Rickettsia rickettsii* are tick-borne rickettsial diseases that often produce vasculitis and thrombocytopenia that manifests as unilateral or bilateral anterior uveitis, often with ocular hemorrhage in the anterior or posterior segment (**Figure 11.40c**).[73–79] Approximately one-third of the ehrlichiosis cases in one study[78] had only ocular lesions and no systemic signs. Another study described ocular lesions in 37% of all cases of ehrlichiosis, with 65% of these having ocular lesions as the only sign. In this author's experience, ocular manifestations due to *Ehrlichia* spp. are usually more severe than with RMSF. *Ehrlichia* spp. may also cause posterior uveitis manifested with infiltrates and/or retinal detachment due to exudation. Vasculitis and retinal hemorrhages may be seen with RMSF (see Chapter 14).

Borrelia burgdorferi (Lyme disease) is a tick-borne spirochete that may produce anterior and posterior uveitis and ocular hemorrhage.[80,81] Most reports of disease incidence used antibody testing, which can be unreliable; however, antigen has been demonstrated by PCR within the canine eye.[82] Diagnosis is usually via other systemic signs, paired with serologic data, and response to specific antimicrobial therapy. Contagious bacterial infections such as *Brucella canis*, leptospirosis, and tuberculosis may also manifest with uveitis. *Brucella canis* has been found both experimentally and clinically to produce anterior uveitis, posterior uveitis/retinal detachment, or endophthalmitis, either unilaterally or bilaterally. The uveitis is often accompanied by hemorrhage and, like the systemic disease, becomes a chronic insidious process despite appropriate antimicrobial therapy (**Figure 11.41**). The ocular lesions may be the only clinical signs of brucellosis.[83–88]

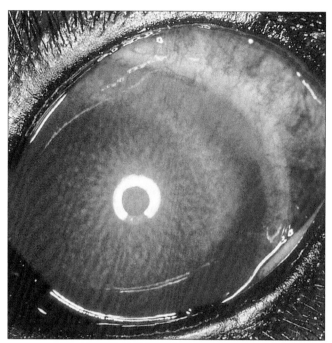

Figure 11.41 A 2-year-old Labrador retriever with anterior uveitis associated with *Brucella canis*. Episcleral injection, corneal edema, and secondary glaucoma were noted. Also note the free blood in the anterior chamber.

As *Brucella canis* is a potential zoonotic agent, if the dog is a housedog, the owners should be educated as to the inherent risk of having a potentially infectious animal in a family environment. Noncontagious bacterial infections from a variety of sources (dental disease, dermatitis, discospondylitis, pyelonephritis) may result in embolization to the eye, with inflammation.

Systemic mycoses often present with anterior uveitis that is usually part of a panuveitis. *Histoplasmosis capsulatum* is the least likely of the systemic mycoses to produce ocular signs in the dog.[89–91] Exposure to a riverine environment is typical for dogs with histoplasmosis. Both histoplasmal and cryptococcal organisms grow well in nitrogen-rich soils and are commonly associated with a history of exposure to bird droppings.[90,92] The incidence of histoplasmosis, blastomycosis, and coccidioidomycosis is often very regional. Cryptococcosis is more sporadic and widespread. Coccidioidomycosis and blastomycosis are common etiologies of uveitis in dogs in their respective endemic regions (coccidioidomycosis, desert southwestern United States; blastomycosis, Midwestern/central southern United States, Ohio and Mississippi River Valleys). The portal of entry is usually the respiratory tract, with hematogenous spread to the eye. Despite the systemic origin of the organism, the ocular complaint is often primary. Blastomycosis and coccidioidomycosis typically produce a granulomatous panuveitis/endophthalmitis (**Figures 11.40b and 11.42**).[92–97]

Cryptococcosis and histoplasmosis usually manifest more as a posterior uveitis. Blastomycosis and cryptococcosis are usually bilateral, while coccidioidomycosis is bilateral in only 20% of patients, and 40% have no systemic signs.[94,95] Blastomycosis involves the eye in >40% of cases with systemic disease.[96,97] Organisms are usually easily demonstrated in the posterior uvea (chorioretinitis with exudative retinal detachment) but are less common in the anterior uvea, suggesting the possibility of an immune-mediated reaction or inflammatory mediators being responsible for the anterior uveitis. Secondary glaucoma from iris bombe is a common complication of anterior uveal involvement (**Figure 11.42**). The complication of blindness with ongoing painful ocular disease, after systemic improvement with therapy, is a common cause for euthanasia request by owners. Disseminated opportunistic fungal diseases associated with saprophytic fungi have a predisposition for the German shepherd dog. Organisms such as *Aspergillus* spp., *Candida* spp., *Penicillium* spp., *Lecythophora canina* sp. nov., *Plectosphaerella cucumerina*, and *Paecilomyces* spp. may disseminate to the eye, causing uveitis.[98,99]

Toxoplasma gondii infection in the dog is worldwide and common, based on serologic and histopathologic surveys; clinical signs and recognition of the disease are relatively rare due to the mildness or ambiguity of the signs.[100,101] Clinical systemic disease is most common in dogs <1 year and in dogs with distemper.[102] The cat is more often affected than the dog. Systemic signs may or may not be present with ocular disease. In the dog, the most common ocular lesions with toxoplasmosis are cyclitis and retinitis (**Figure 11.43**). Organisms are often found in the posterior segment lesions but are usually absent in the anterior uvea.[103,104] Many previously diagnosed cases of toxoplasmosis, based on histopathology, may have been due to *Neospora caninum* due to similarities in morphology of *T. gondii* and *N. caninum*. *N. caninum* is transmitted transplacentally, and thus, most reports are of infection in neonates, where it usually produces an ascending paralysis. Ocular lesions have included retinochoroiditis, anterior uveitis, and extraocular myositis.[105]

Leishmania infantum is transmitted by the sand fly and the dog is a reservoir host. It is endemic in the Mediterranean region, Africa, and Asia. It has been seen sporadically in southern Europe, Germany, and the United Kingdom. The ocular inflammation is usually confined to the anterior uvea, cornea, and lids but may cause endophthalmitis.[106–108] The inflammation is mononuclear, and organisms are present in the histiocytes. Originally, most cases reported in North America had history of travel to the Mediterranean, but *L. donovani* is now endemic in Texas, Oklahoma, and Ohio, although a form of *Leishmania chagasi* is found in South and Central America and in the United States. The fox hound appears uniquely susceptible to *Leishmania chagasi* in the United States.[109] The mode

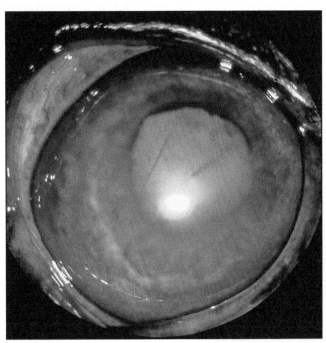

Figure 11.42 Anterior uveitis with exudative retinal detachment in a dog with blastomycosis. The pupil is irregular due to synechia, and the detached retina can be visualized through the pupil.

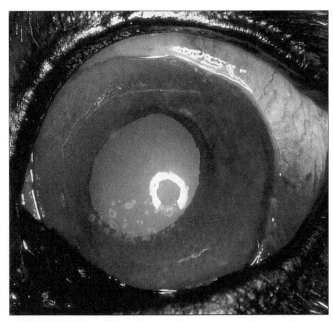

Figure 11.43 A dog with granulomatous uveitis and scleritis associated with toxoplasmosis. Note the keratic precipitates ventrally that are associated with corneal edema; peripheral corneal infiltrates dorsally are associated with scleritis. The iris is darker and thicker than normal.

of transmission in the United States has not been clarified but may involve direct transmission[110] as well as an insect vector.

Prototheca spp. is a ubiquitous algae found in soil and water but is rarely associated with systemic disease in the dog. The portal of entry is thought to be the digestive tract, with hemorrhagic diarrhea being the most common clinical sign. Ocular involvement with a granulomatous posterior uveitis or panuveitis is present in >50% of cases.[111] Ocular lesions have been known to occur without systemic signs.[112]

Aberrant parasites such as fly larvae (ophthalmomyiasis) in the dog and the cat,[113–118] *Elaeophora schneideri* in sheep and elk,[119] *Setaria* spp. in horses and oxen,[120,121] *Halicephalobus deletrix* in a horse,[122] and nemotodes such as *Dirofilaria immitis*,[123–129] *Ancylostoma* spp.,[130] and *Angiostronglus vasorum*[131,132] in dogs may be relatively rare causes of anterior uveitis.

The most common ocular parasites in the dog are immature adult male and female *Dirofilaria immitis* that have been identified as moving between the aqueous humor and the vitreous and are associated with inflammation (**Figure 11.44**). The source of the inflammation may be either mechanical trauma or immune mediated. Removal of the worms results in rapid improvement, although persistent corneal edema may result. Fly larvae may move freely between the anterior and posterior compartments and stimulate anterior uveitis, as well as produce wandering tracks in the subretinal space. A bright light seems to stimulate movement of both types of parasites away from the light.

Trauma

Trauma is a common cause of canine anterior uveitis and may be perforating or blunt. Trauma-induced uveitis is usually unilateral, but it is not infrequent for both eyes to be affected in shotgun pellet injuries. Blunt trauma-induced uveitis may be difficult to diagnose without a complete history or other periocular/head injuries to suggest the cause. Penetrating injuries may mimic perforated corneal ulcers, but the prognosis for penetrating injuries is much worse. Cat claw injuries to puppies and kittens are common, and while intraocular infection is a potential complication (**Figure 11.45**), the most serious complication is usually rupture of the lens capsule during trauma. Tearing of the lens capsule often results in a severe sterile inflammation[133] 2–3 weeks after initial trauma, when the initial traumatic uveitis is subsiding (**Figures 11.46 and 11.47**). Septic implantation syndrome[134] is seen when a penetrating wound seeds the lens cortex with bacteria that leads to septic endophthalmitis 10 days to 4 months (as long as 2 years) after injury. Lens capsule rupture with exposure of large amounts of lens protein to the anterior chamber with secondary intractable uveitis is termed

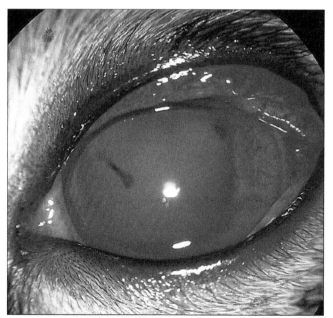

Figure 11.45 Penetrating claw injury that has induced a bacterial uveitis in a young cat. Note the dark linear penetrating corneal injury. Uveitis induced secondary glaucoma is producing mild corneal edema and the dilated pupil. The intraocular infection and the glaucoma responded rapidly to intraocular gentamicin, but vision was not restored.

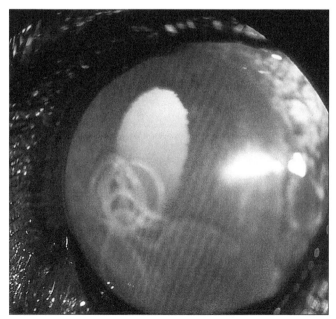

Figure 11.44 Dirofilaria in the anterior chamber of a dog with anterior uveitis. (Courtesy of Dr. M. B. Glaze, Gulf Coast Animal Eye Clinic, Houston, TX.)

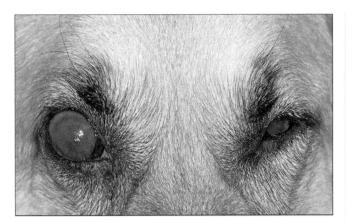

Figure 11.46 Intractable phacoclastic uveitis and secondary glaucoma in a dog. A penetrating scleral injury was responsible. Enucleation was eventually performed.

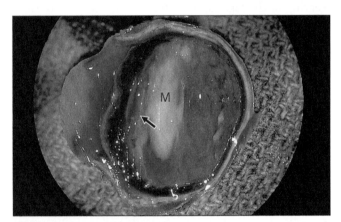

Figure 11.47 Globe from patient in Figure 11.46. Only an empty collapsed capsular bag remains of the lens (arrow). The iris is very thick (to the left of lens capsule), and inflammatory membranes (M) are present behind the lens.

phacoclastic (previously phacoanaphylactic) uveitis and is due to altered tolerance to lens protein.

Neoplasia

Neoplasia mimics simple anterior uveitis by producing tissue necrosis, hemorrhage, and glaucoma. Primary ocular neoplasia is unilateral, but secondary multicentric ocular neoplasia or metastatic neoplasia may be bilateral. The most common secondary ocular tumor in all domestic species is lymphosarcoma.[135] Anterior uveitis, hyphema, iridal masses, secondary glaucoma, vitreal hemorrhage, and retinal detachments are many times seen bilaterally in dogs with ocular manifestations of lymphosarcoma (**Figures 11.33b,c, 11.48, and 11.49**). Krohne et al. found in a prospective study of canine lymphosarcoma cases that 37% of all lymphosarcoma cases had ocular lesions (second only to lymphadenopathy as a presenting sign).[136] Of the ocular signs, 49% of the cases had anterior uveitis, and 14% of the

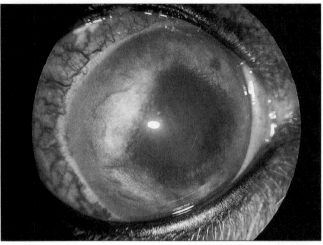

Figure 11.48 An Old English sheepdog with bilateral iris bombe and secondary glaucoma due to lymphosarcoma. The white subconjunctival deposit (11 o'clock) is from a previous injection of methylprednisolone by the referring veterinarian. The dog had advanced lymphadenopathy that was missed because it was not self-evident with the long hair coat. Despite improvement of the uveitis with ocular supportive and systemic chemotherapy, the animal was irreversibly blind from glaucoma.

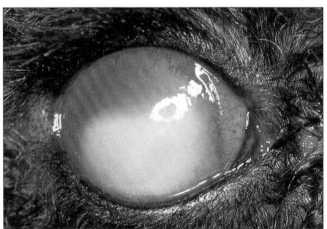

Figure 11.49 Presentation in a dog with bilateral marked hypopyon, uveitis, and secondary glaucoma due to lymphosarcoma. The cornea has perilimbal neovascularization and severe edema. A large mass of neoplastic cells is present in the anterior chamber, and the pupil is dilated from the elevated intraocular pressure.

cases had panuveitis; 100% of cases with anterior uveitis and hyphema were stage V disease. Massa et al. reported that neoplasia accounted for 25% of uveitis cases, and 68% of the neoplasia cases were due to lymphosarcoma.[69] The Rottweiler and the Golden retriever were most commonly affected. All cases of ocular lymphosarcoma had systemic signs of lymphosarcoma. Hemangiosarcoma, transmissible venereal tumor, and adenocarcinoma may metastasize bilaterally to the anterior or posterior uvea.

Secondary to deep corneal ulceration and keratitis

Anterior uveitis secondary to deep corneal inflammation is often sterile even if the corneal ulceration is septic. Bacterial toxins and inflammatory mediators freely diffuse through Descemet's membrane to stimulate anterior uveal inflammation (**Figure 11.50a**). Aqueous humor centesis may be utilized to determine whether sepsis is present in the anterior chamber, but because of aqueous humor turnover, false-negative culture results may occur.

Immune mediated

Many forms of anterior uveitis are sterile and/or cannot be associated with serologic evidence of infection. Such forms are assumed to be immune mediated by exclusion. Massa et al. reported that 58% of uveitis cases in the dog were idiopathic/immune mediated; this figure would have been even higher had they not excluded lens-induced uveitis cases from the series.[69] Circulating immune complexes from elsewhere in the body may localize in the uvea, or humoral and/or cellular immune-mediated processes may be directed against ocular tissue (melanin, retinal S antigen, lens protein), infectious agents, or foreign material in the eye. The ocular inflammation may be part of a systemic immune response or be localized to the eye.

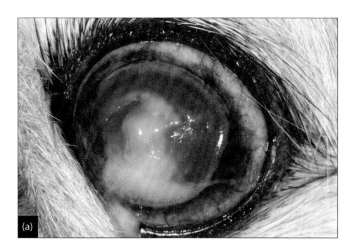

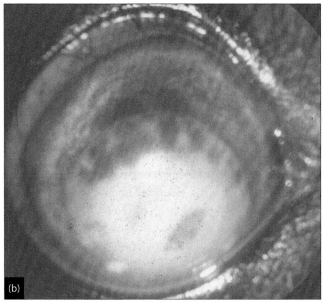

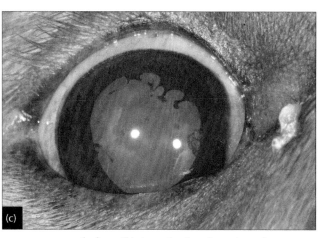

Figure 11.50 (a) Hypopyon in a dog with a septic proteolytic enzyme corneal ulcer. (b) Anterior lens luxation of a hypermature cataractic lens in a poodle. The dog had a hypermature cataract for years, and the lens zonules subsequently degenerated resulting in this anterior lens luxation with secondary glaucoma. (c) "Pigmentary uveitis" (pigmentary and cystic glaucoma in the Golden retriever) in a 9-year-old Golden retriever. The dog presented for vision loss and was noted to have anterior capsular cataract, iris hyperpigmentation, and posterior synechia. Minor aqueous flare was noted. Despite topical corticosteroid and antiglaucoma therapy, blindness due to secondary glaucoma was the final result.

Phacoclastic uveitis and lens-induced uveitis (LIU) are examples of immune-mediated responses against ocular antigens. Phacoclastic uveitis is a chronic severe inflammatory reaction that occurs in some individuals 1–3 weeks after the lens capsule is ruptured. It is a granulomatous reaction in some species, but in the dog, it is characterized by a ruptured lens capsule with neutrophilic invasion within the lens stroma and a lymphocytic–plasmacytic reaction surrounding the lens in the anterior uvea.[137] Perilenticular fibroplasia with iris adhesions frequently results in intractable glaucoma (**Figures 11.46 and 11.47**).[138] The traditional view of phacoclastic uveitis is that the body is reacting to the exposed lens protein because lens protein was sequestered by the lens capsule early in development, and the immune system does not recognize it as "self." This view has been challenged, as normal individuals have circulating antilens antibodies.[139] An alternative theory is that the tolerance to lens protein is altered by the massive exposure to lens antigens, which overrides the effects of intraocular T-suppressor cells.[140] A second type of lens-induced immune-mediated anterior uveitis is more frequent and observed with mature to hypermature cataracts, when the liquefied lens protein passes through an intact lens capsule into the aqueous humor (**Figure 11.36**). This has been called lens induced uveitis (LIU) or phacolytic uveitis.[141–143] LIU is usually mild and easily treated but may result in secondary glaucoma or phthisis bulbi in some animals if untreated.[144] It is characterized by mild lymphocytic–plasmacytic iridocyclitis. With chronicity, the lens zonules may break down due to inflammatory cell enzymes, and the lens may subluxate or luxate (**Figure 11.50b**). While these two forms of uveitis are presented as separate entities, they probably represent opposite ends of a spectrum of inflammatory reactions to lens proteins.

Uveodermatologic syndrome (Vogt–Koyanagi–Harada or VKH-like syndrome) is thought to be an immune-mediated inflammatory response to melanin that results in depigmentation of the skin (vitiligo), hair (poliosis), and uvea (panuveitis).[145,146,149,151–153] Kaya et al. found melanin to lack antigenicity or immunogenic properties; free melanin granules, when injected into the anterior chamber, did not stimulate inflammation, but they did significantly augment intraocular inflammation when incubated with an antigen in sensitized animals.[147] This augmentation was thought to be due to absorption of immunoglobulin or antigen.[147] Two Akitas were immunized with tyrosinase-related protein 1, and a VKH-like syndrome was produced involving the eyes and skin.[145] In humans, VKH syndrome has been associated with meningeal signs in some patients; this is apparently uncommon in the dog, since only one dog has been reported with neurologic signs.[148] VKH syndrome is observed most frequently in the young adult Akita, Irish setter, Siberian husky, and Samoyed. Dogs with heterochromia may have only a unilateral uveitis.[145] The panuveitis is chronic, bilateral, and granulomatous in nature. Depigmentation of the skin and hair often occurs after the initiation of ocular inflammation (see Chapter 7).[145,146,149,151–153] Blindness may occur from secondary glaucoma, retinal detachment, retinal degeneration, and/or complicated cataracts.[145,146,150–153]

Pigmentary uveitis has been described in the Golden retriever and may involve other breeds as well. The condition is chronic, low grade, and progressive, resulting in cataract formation, posterior synechia, secondary glaucoma, and loss of vision in most eyes despite extensive systemic and topical therapy. The condition is characterized by radially oriented pigment deposits on the anterior lens capsule (**Figure 11.50c**), low-grade aqueous flare, fibrin (and occasional hemorrhage) in the anterior chamber, development of PIFM and posterior synechia, filtration angle closure, and iridociliary body cysts.[39,154] The mean age of the patients was 8.6 years,[39] and laboratory testing and histopathology have been negative for systemic disease. Glaucoma led to blindness in 47% of these patients in one study[39] and in all patients in another study.[154] Histopathologically, a very mild lymphocytic infiltration was present in most eyes examined, but in all cases, the patients had received extensive treatment before enucleation, including anti-inflammatory drugs. Pigment infiltration of the ciliary cleft/filtration angle was felt to be the cause of elevated intraocular pressure.[154] The role of iridociliary cysts in uveitis and glaucoma is unclear, but an association has been made by several authors.[37,38] The latest article[154] indicates that the term "uveitis" is a misnomer. Rather, the lack of inflammation noted on histopathology suggests that this disorder should be referred to as "pigmentary and cystic glaucoma in the Golden retriever." A genetic link is also likely since the incidence in the Golden retriever varies with the lineage and thus varies in geographic regions.

A syndrome of bilateral exudative (transudative) retinal detachment, optic neuritis, and anterior uveitis is idiopathic but is thought to be immune mediated, mainly due to a lack of a demonstrable cause and a response to corticosteroids.[155,156] This syndrome is discussed further in Chapter 14.

Causes of uveitis in the cat (see **Table 11.2**)

Many cases of anterior uveitis in the cat are bilateral, and, if granulomatous, they are often indicative of severe systemic disease, with poor prognosis for the cat. Many cats with granulomatous anterior uveitis (especially those with feline infectious peritonitis [FIP], lymphosarcoma, and systemic fungal infections) may die of systemic illness

Table 11.2 **Causes of feline anterior uveitis.**

ETIOLOGY	DIAGNOSTIC AIDS
Systemic infectious diseases	
Feline leukemia virus	FeLV testing (ELISA or/and IFA), +/− systemic signs
Feline immunodeficiency virus	FIV serology (FIV vaccination can cause false positive ELISA, Western blot, and IFA testing), chronic infections, gingivitis
Feline infectious peritonitis	FIP serology, physical examination, elevated globulins
Toxoplasma gondii	Elevated IgM and rising IgG titers on ELISA test
Systemic mycoses	Cytology of ocular centesis, serology for specific fungi
Bartonella henselae	Serology
FHV-1	PCR testing of aqueous, questionable as a cause of uveitis
Trauma	History, physical examination, evidence of ocular perforation/lens rupture
Immune-mediated processes	
Cataract induced	Ocular examination, negative infectious disease serology
Idiopathic	Negative on infectious disease serology, steroid responsive?
Neoplasia	History, ocular ultrasound, ocular cytology, FeLV serology
Idiopathic	Negative on infectious disease titers, older cats

within a few months of diagnosis. Granulomatous uveitis in the cat is usually bilateral with large keratic precipitates (KPs), a chronic course, rubeosis iridis/PIFM formation/posterior synechia, with secondary glaucoma as a sequela. (**Figures 11.35, 11.40a, and 11.51**).

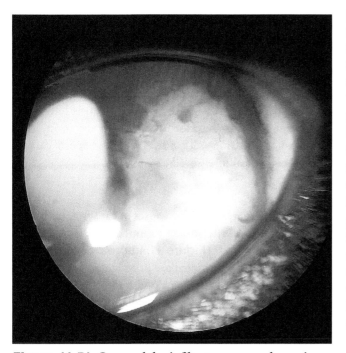

Figure 11.51 Gray nodular infiltrates or granulomas in the iris stroma of a cat. *Cryptococcus* spp. organisms were observed on aqueous humor centesis.

Feline leukemia virus (FeLV) complex

Anterior uveitis has been commonly associated with FeLV, often before systemic signs develop.[157] In one retrospective histopathologic study of feline uveitis, about 20% of cases were due to lymphosarcoma.[158] This was obviously a biased study as it reflected only enucleated eyes. A clinical study of feline uveitis in 53 eyes reported approximately the same percentage of cats had FeLV or lymphosarcoma as the supposed cause of anterior uveitis.[159] Some eyes have obvious mass lesions in the iris with FeLV, but many appear simply as anterior uveitis; aqueous humor aspirates typically have nonmalignant lymphocytes and macrophages (**Figures 11.52 and 11.53**). It is not clear whether the lymphocytic uveitis is always neoplastic. Nonmalignant anterior uveitis has been experimentally produced by subcutaneous injection of feline sarcoma virus and FeLV.[160] Clinically, the frequency of cats presenting with ocular lesions associated with FeLV appears to have dramatically decreased in the last two decades, and the incidence of nonviremic lymphosarcoma has increased.[161] Dubielzig et al. summarized 57 cases of lymphosarcoma submitted for histopathology over a 12-year period and found that 36% of cases with uveitis and lymphosarcoma were positive for FeLV; of eyes with only lymphosarcoma, 16% were positive for FeLV.[162] Extranodal lymphoma or single-tumor masses affecting an organ without systemic illness are usually of B-cell lineage.

Feline infectious peritonitis (FIP)

Anterior uveitis due to FIP occurs either alone or in conjunction with posterior uveitis and optic neuritis

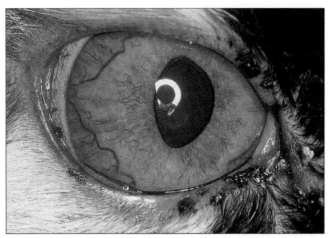

Figure 11.52 Intraocular extranodal lymphosarcoma in a cat that was negative for FeLV on ELISA testing of serum and bone marrow. PCR testing for FeLV was also negative. The FIV serum antibody titer was negative, but FIV antigen was found with PCR. Note the marked iris hyperemia and tan infiltrate of the peripheral iris, producing dyscoria. This resulted in secondary glaucoma and was only mildly responsive to anti-inflammatory therapy. Malignant cells were noted on aqueous humor cytology.

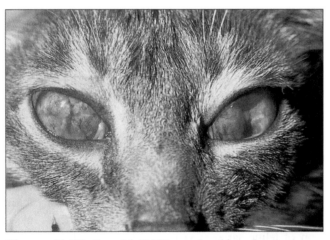

Figure 11.53 Cat with FeLV-associated lymphosarcoma and bilateral iris bombe with secondary glaucoma. The kidneys were also involved.

(**Figure 11.54a**).[163–166] If posterior inflammatory lesions are present, the etiology is more likely to be FIP than FeLV. Typical anterior uveitis symptoms include bilateral corneal edema, granulomatous KPs, large fibrin clots in the anterior chamber, and rubeosis iridis. Ocular lesions are typically associated with the "dry" or noneffusive form of FIP.[165] Cats with the noneffusive form tend to have longer survival times and a more chronic ocular course than do cats with the effusive form of the disease.[164] Ocular lesions were noted in about 50% of

cases with neurologic manifestations, or about 15% of the total cases of FIP, in one study.[166] A histopathologic study of feline uveitis found 20% of the eyes with typical FIP lesions,[158] but in a clinical study of 53 cases of feline uveitis, only one was diagnosed as FIP.[159] The perivascular pyogranulomatous lesions of FIP and the association of a more severe disease in corona virus seropositive cats are compatible with an immune-mediated reaction to mutated virus rather than direct viral toxicity.[163-165]

Systemic mycoses

As in dogs, the incidence of systemic mycoses in cats is often very regional. In endemic riverine areas, histoplasmosis with ocular involvement may be more common in cats than in dogs. Feline histoplasmosis signs may mimic the granulomatous anterior uveitis signs of FeLV and FIP.[168–171] Cryptococcosis is more widespread than other systemic mycoses, and about 20% of reported systemic cases in the cat have ocular lesions. This figure is probably an underestimation, as another series had almost a 50% incidence of ocular lesions when the fundus was examined.[172] In this author's experience, cryptococcosis rarely causes anterior uveitis compared to the incidence of chorioretinitis. Blastomycosis,[173–175] coccidioidomycosis,[176] and candidiasis[177] are rare causes of uveitis in cats. Cats may contract blastomycosis by digging in unsterilized potting soil.[175]

Toxoplasmosis

Toxoplasma gondii has frequently been associated serologically with anterior uveitis, but the organisms are probably not in the anterior uvea.[178–180] The anterior uveitis may or may not be bilateral or granulomatous in nature. Cats with uveitis associated serologically with toxoplasmosis do not usually have concurrent systemic signs. Conversely, 60%–82% of cats with systemic toxoplasmosis have ophthalmic signs, with anterior uveitis being the most common.[181] Co-infection with FIV may predispose cats to acute toxoplasmal disease.[182]

Bartonella henselae

Bartonella henselae, one of the causes of cat scratch disease, has been serologically linked to unilateral chronic anterior uveitis in a cat[183] (**Figure 11.40a**). *Bartonella* spp. are Gram-negative bacteria that are prevalent in cats and may produce disease in cats, dogs, and humans. The importance of *Bartonella* spp. in animals as a cause of uveitis remains to be elucidated.[184–186] Fontenelle et al. compared *Bartonella* titers between normal cats, cats with nonocular disease, and cats with uveitis and found no difference between the incidence and the magnitude of titers between the nonocular group and the uveitis group.[187]

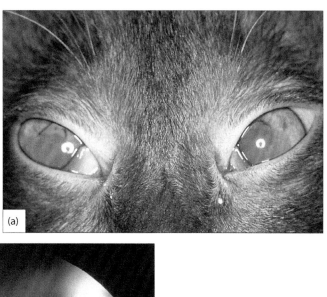

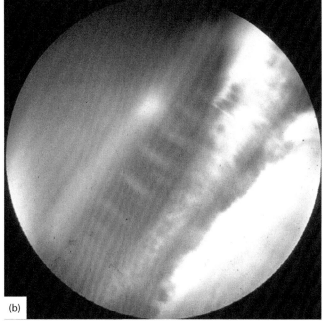

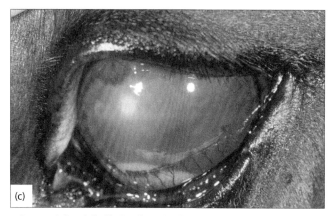

Figure 11.54 (a) Young kitten with FIP-induced bilateral anterior uveitis with fibrin clots in the anterior chambers, KP, and rubiosis irides. Effusions were also present in the chest and abdomen. (b) Pars planitis in an FIV+ older cat. Note the linear gray "snow banking" of inflammatory debris immediately caudal to the ciliary processes. (c) Deep corneal stromal abscess (white intrastromal area dorsomedially) with all the classic clinical signs of anterior uveitis (conjunctival/episcleral injection, increased reflex tearing, corneal edema, aqueous flare, aqueous cells, inferiorly settled hypopyon, deep corneal perilimbal neovascularization). The horse was treated medically for the fungal stromal abscess as well as symptomatically for the uveitis. Once the stroma abscess resolved, the anterior uveitis resolved with no long-term consequences.

The healthy cats had a higher prevalence and higher titers than the cats with uveitis. The mean titer was 1:64 for all groups.

Nongranulomatous anterior uveitis

Nongranulomatous anterior uveitis is common in the cat. Unilateral causes are often due to trauma, neoplasia, or lens injury, with many being idiopathic. Bilateral cases are often presumed to be immune mediated or manifestation of a systemic disease, but often the relationship is tenuous, relying on serologic testing. Viral infections, immune-mediated conditions, bartonellosis, and toxoplasmosis are some etiologies to consider. The division of nongranulomatous from granulomatous anterior uveitis is rather arbitrary based on clinical examination. What appears to be an acute fibrinous anterior uveitis may change with time to a typical granulomatous reaction with mutton fat KPs. In two series, nongranulomatous anterior uveitis/lymphocytic uveitis accounted for 32% and 70% of cases.[158,159]

In a histopathologic study of 158 cat eyes with uveitis,[158] the most common lesion (29%) was diffuse lymphocytic–plasmacytic anterior uveal inflammation. Inflammation was bilateral, with a mean age of 7.4 years with no breed or gender predisposition. No infectious agents were apparent histologically. Two cats were serologically positive for toxoplasmosis, and the remaining cats, when tested, were negative for FeLV and FIP. A nodular form of lymphocytic–plasmacytic uveitis was less frequent (3%), developed in slightly older cats (8.8 years), and was usually unilateral. In the remaining group of eyes in this study, 22% were consistent with FIP lesions, 21% were lymphosarcoma, 10% were traumatic or secondary to keratitis, 8% were LIU, and 5% were secondary to systemic mycotic disease. The study was biased towards the most severe forms of uveitis since the cats either died or had such severe ocular lesions and sequela (glaucoma) that the eyes were enucleated.

A clinical study of 53 cats with nontraumatic uveitis[159] found 70% were considered idiopathic, and 17% were due to FeLV/lymphosarcoma, with one case each of FIP and toxoplasmosis. The idiopathic form was chronic (247 days), free of systemic disease, had a mean age of 9.3 years, was bilateral in 32% of cases, and was more common in the male (4.3:1). Thirty-six percent of the cats had enucleation, and the idiopathic form was characterized by lymphocytic–plasmacytic infiltration of the anterior uvea. Sera from 20 of 53 cats with idiopathic uveitis were retrospectively tested for FIV, and 21% were positive. It is clear from these two cited studies that histopathologic studies are limited in elucidating the etiology of chronic nongranulomatous uveitis.

Serologic testing of feline uveitis cases raises different questions than the histopathologic studies; in one series of 124 cats, 83% had positive serology for at least one disease tested. In this series, *T. gondii* was the most common cause (74%) found on serologic testing (with 54% *Toxoplasma*-positive prevalence in normal healthy cats) followed by FIV (13%), FeLV (12%), and FIP (6%), and 17% were negative.[188] Another series from the same laboratory reported a 90% positive response for infectious agents with serologic testing in feline uveitis patients. In this series, the seroprevalence of infectious disease was 79% for *T. gondii*, 23% for FIV, 6% for FeLV, and 27% for FIP.[189]

The exact role of *T. gondii* in feline anterior uveitis is unknown. The availability of ELISA tests for *Toxoplasma* antigen and feline anti–*T. gondii* IgG and IgM has caused a reassessment of the role of toxoplasmosis in feline uveitis.[190,191] While 74%–79% of cats with anterior uveitis may have serologic evidence of *T. gondii* infection, the histopathology reports from eyes enucleated for secondary glaucoma fail to demonstrate the organism. That *T. gondii* frequently involves the eye in cats that have died from histologically proven systemic toxoplasmosis has been reconfirmed. In this study of 100 cases over a 38-year period, the eyes of 27 of the cats were available for examination, and 82% had intraocular inflammation. *T. gondii* was histologically observed in 45% of these eyes.[181] Multifocal iridocyclochoroiditis was the most common lesion. Fatal toxoplasmosis with histologic confirmation is rare when considering the serologic prevalence.

Davidson and English have summarized the various theories in the literature on the possible link between *T. gondii* and uveitis in humans and other animals.[192] The rarity of finding organisms in the anterior uvea of the cat has led to various hypotheses:

- Anterior uveitis is associated with inflammatory mediators from the posterior segment.
- Organism numbers are so low they are difficult to detect.
- Ocular inflammation is the result of memory immune cells localizing to the eye after exposure to organisms at nonocular sites.
- Molecular mimicry is involved, where peptides of the organism are close to self-antigens that drive the inflammation.
- Circulating immune complexes of *T. gondii* and antibody are deposited in the anterior uvea.
- Nonspecific upregulation of antibody production in uveitis has increased *T. gondii* antibodies.

The response to therapy with clindamycin has been cited as indirect evidence for the role of *T. gondii* in uveitis. Clindamycin (25 mg/kg every 12 hours) alone or with glucocorticoids was more effective in reducing inflammation than glucocorticoids alone.[189] This contrasts to the experimental model where clindamycin therapy increased the morbidity and the mortality of treated animals compared to controls. In a Syrian golden hamster model of retinal toxoplasmosis, of the variety of drugs used to treat toxoplasmosis, none affected the acute clinical course, and only atovaquone reduced the number of tissue cysts and had any affect on the chronic course.[193]

FIV has been associated with anterior uveitis, characterized by anterior uveitis, glaucoma, and pars planitis (**Figure 11.54b**). Inflammation was usually mild to moderate, chronic, and characterized by aqueous flare, peripheral iridal hyperemia, posterior synechia, anterior subcapsular cataracts, and hypotony. Pars planitis is diagnosed by the presence of white cellular infiltrates in the peripheral anterior vitreous that often coalesce posterior to the ciliary plicae.[194]

Feline herpesvirus-1 has also been associated with nongranulomatous uveitis in cats. In a study of idiopathic uveitis cats,[195] 11% (5/44) of uveitis-afflicted cats (that were not determined to be toxoplasmosis-induced uveitis cases) had PCR evidence of viral DNA in their aqueous humor (this compared to 20% [6/29] of toxoplasmosis-induced uveitis cats having viral DNA in the aqueous humor).

Causes of acute uveitis and chronic/intermittent (equine recurrent uveitis or ERU) in the horse

There are multiple etiologies for anterior uveitis in the horse. Blunt trauma to the globe, corneal trauma (superficial, deep, or penetrating), corneal infections (superficial or deep ulcers, superficial or deep stromal abscesses [**Figure 11.54c**]), or primary corneal diseases (immune mediated keratopathy) commonly cause secondary anterior uveitis. The previously mentioned "fragility" of the blood–aqueous barrier in the horse makes for a rather dramatic anterior uveal response to stimulation from corneal disease. Some refer to this as the "corneal-uveal reflex," with the afferent arm of the "reflex" being the ophthalmic branch of CN V, and the efferent arm being iris sphincter/ciliary body smooth muscle spasming due to parasympathetic stimulation from CN III, excessive reflex tearing due to parasympathetic stimulation from CN VII, vasodilation and increased vascular permeability of conjunctival, episcleral, iridal, and ciliary body vasculature due to sympathetic/parasympathetic stimulated vascular changes and effects of intraocular inflammatory mediators (prostaglandins and other inflammatory mediators of the arachidonic acid cascade). Details of these primary corneal diseases are discussed in Chapter 10. Likewise, hematogenous circulating inflammatory mediators stimulated by inflammation from local/nonocular septic processes (e.g., pyometra, mastitis, pneumonia, umbilical abscesses, septicemias, etc.) or sterile systemic inflammatory processes may alter the BAB with resulting signs of anterior uveitis in an animal with no primary ocular disease (**Figure 11.60**). These bouts of anterior uveitis usually resolve with appropriate treatment of the primary disease and supportive care for the eye.

In the horse, however (more than any other species), there is an immune-mediated phenomenon that causes recurrent episodes of nongranulomatous panuveitis and many times subsequent blindness. There are many synonyms for this recurring/chronic uveitis in the equine species: Equine recurrent uveitis (ERU), periodic ophthalmia, and "moon blindness." ERU is seen worldwide, has been known from antiquity (the ancients felt the recurrent nature of the clinical signs had to do with the stages of the lunar calendar, therefore the term "moon blindness"), and is considered the leading cause of blindness in horses and mules. ERU is most commonly manifested clinically as an anterior uveitis but is actually a panuveitis or may be somewhat restricted to the posterior uvea and optic nerve. It is a nongranulomatous uveitis that, if unilateral initially, becomes bilateral, and it is relapsing in nature. Histopathologically, it has been suggested that the findings of infiltration of lymphocytes and plasma cells into the nonpigmented ciliary epithelium, a thick acellular hyaline membrane adherent to the inner aspect of the nonpigmented epithelium, and eosinophilic linear inclusions in the nonpigmented ciliary epithelium are diagnostic of ERU.[196,197]

A wide variety of suggested etiologies have been proposed over the years for recurring uveitis that has a course that varies from acute episodes to chronic and insidious blinding sequela. The acute forms become quiescent with time or therapy but often have relapses or recur at irregular intervals. Early reports discredited genetic influence,[198] hypothyroidism, and nutritional influences (vitamin A and riboflavin[199,200]) on ERU. In humans and mice, the interaction of genetic factors with immunologic reactions has been linked to major histocompatibility antigens. In humans, specific major histocompatibility antigen HLA-B27 has been associated with certain forms of anterior uveitis,[201] and similar associations have been proposed for horses.[202] Newer studies[203,204] have identified genetic risk factors for ERU in Appaloosa horses in the United States and German warmblood horses. Mules are more resistant than horses to recurrent uveitis, and Appaloosas are disproportionately represented (25% of cases).[202,205] Sixty-eight percent of Appaloosas became blind with the disease compared to 36% of non-Appaloosas in one study.[202] Studies at North Carolina State[206] have shown that ERU develops following primary uveitis when the BAB is disrupted, allowing CD4+ T-lymphocytes to enter and remain in the eye. Subsequent episodes of uveitis develop because of new antigenic detection when CD4+ T-lymphocytes are upregulated, resulting in epitope spreading.[207] Subsequent episodes of ERU are associated with an immune response to various ocular autoantigens, such as S-antigen, interphotoreceptor retinoid-binding protein, and cellular retinaldehyde-binding protein.[208]

Several infectious/parasitic agents have been proposed through the years as initiating causes for the cascade of immunological events leading to the immune-mediated disorder ERU. Some of the classic antigens include:

Onchocerca cervicalis microfilaria have long been thought to be a major cause of ERU. *O. cervicalis* microfilaria pass from the lid to the conjunctiva and the cornea and then into the eye with the episcleral blood vessels. Dead larvae are thought to incite the inflammation rather than live larvae. The infection in horses is similar to the onchocerciasis in humans ("river blindness") that is endemic in parts of sub-Saharan Africa. The importance of *O. cervicalis* may vary with geographic region. The incidence of *O. cervicalis* larvae in the United Kingdom is too low to account for ERU, while in the United States, onchocerciasis is found in 50%–87% of horses depending on the region.[209–213] The primary site of microfilaria localization in the eye is at the limbus and adjacent cornea and conjunctiva, which have resulted in attempts to make a diagnosis by snip biopsies at the lateral bulbar conjunctiva.[214] The routine use of broad-spectrum dewormers has markedly decreased *O. cervicalis* as a major cause of equine recurrent uveitis.

Leptospira spp. have been associated with uveitis in the horse experimentally and naturally. *Leptospira* spp. have been isolated from eyes with recurrent uveitis, although the usual method of diagnosis has been high serum or aqueous humor antibody titers. Wollanke et al. were able to culture *Leptospira interrogans* from 52% of vitrectomy samples from horses with chronic ERU, whereas all normal control samples were negative on culture.[215] Finding a higher titer in the aqueous humor than in the serum is presumptive evidence of a causal relationship.[216–220] Experimental infection with *L. interrogans* serovar *pomona* resulted in ocular inflammation after a lag of 1 year or later in 61% of the eyes.[221] While in many geographic areas of the United States, leptospiral titers indicate that *L. interrogans* plays a major role in recurrent uveitis, in the United Kingdom, the prevalence is so low that it is not considered a probable cause.[222] The predominant serovar reported varies with the geographic region. In Germany, it is *L. grippotyphosa* (no *L. pomona* is found).[223] In the United States, *L. pomona* and *L. bratislava* are common serovars associated with equine recurrent uveitis. In a Louisiana study,[224] serology and aqueous humor antibody levels revealed a high incidence of *L. bratislava* and *L. pomona*, but bacterial culture revealed positive growth for only *L. pomona* and *L. grippothyphosa*.

Borrelia burgdorferi has been implicated as causing pan-uveitis in a pony;[225] the organism was isolated from the anterior chamber. Additional cases of borreliosis and uveitis have also been described.[226] This may be an additional cause for recurrent uveitis in endemic areas for Lyme disease.

Brucella abortus in the past has been suggested as a cause of recurrent uveitis, but surveys of normal and affected horses could not find a correlation.[227,228]

Streptococcus equi was suggested as a possible cause of an outbreak of peripapillary chorioretinitis in horses following an earlier outbreak of strangles. Whether the condition resulted from direct intraocular infection or a hypersensitivity to the organism is not known.[229] *Streptococcus* spp. are not thought to play a significant role in ERU.

Strongyle infection (*Strongylus vulgaris*) has been postulated to have a role in ERU. The addition of phenothiazine and riboflavin to the ration prevented outbreaks in a herd, but no controls were used in the feeding trial.[230] Viruses such as adenovirus and influenza virus have been clinically implicated in uveitis.[231]

As stated previously, immune-mediated responses are an important factor potentially in combination with one or more of the other diseases listed above. Delayed hypersensitivity to an antigen (*L. interrogans*) is currently thought to be one of many processes involved with ERU,[232,233] but the inciting antigen might be different in various regions. The histopathology, presence of a predominance of CD4+ T-lymphocytes in the cellular reaction,[206] expression of major histocompatibility complex antigens in ocular cells,[232] and elevated antibody levels against retina S-antigen and other retinal proteins[234,235] are findings compatible with an immune-mediated process. The recurrences may be associated with persistence of antigen, re-exposure to an antigen in the presence of a leaky blood–aqueous humor barrier, or acquired sensitivity to autoantigens through either alteration or suppression of tolerance.[221,231,232]

As with other species, a combination of infectious agent exposure and, more importantly, immunological mechanisms, is the favorite current suspected etiology of ERU. It is probable that the condition has multiple different primary causes in different geographic areas.

Clinical signs of acute episodes of equine recurrent uveitis

- Lids and conjunctiva: Blepharospasm, excessive lacrimation turning to mucopurulent discharge, chemosis, and marked conjunctival hyperemia are typical. The animal may be depressed and anorexic.
- Cornea: The cornea develops varying degrees of edema and may become discolored yellow from neutrophilic infiltration (**Figure 11.55**). Perilimbal deep neovascularization may develop after several days.
- Aqueous humor: Aqueous flare (**Figure 11.35b**) is the hallmark of uveitis, with possible hypopyon and hemorrhage in severe cases (**Figures 11.56 and 11.57**). Aqueous humor formation is decreased, resulting in hypotony.
- Iris: The pupil is miotic, the iris dull, thickened, and hyperpigmented (**Figure 11.54c**). Posterior synechia develops rapidly.
- Lens: Lens changes are a common cause of eventual blindness of the animal. The lens often has pigment deposits or nests of pigment from iris adhesions, a capsular haze develops from deposits of cells and fibrin, and, eventually, cortical cataract develops.

Uveitis is the most common cause of cataract formation in the horse (and the cat).

- Vitreous: The vitreous usually develops inflammatory infiltrates (initially a yellow-green discoloration) which result in a haze and, later, organization into mobile strands within the liquefied vitreous ("floaters").

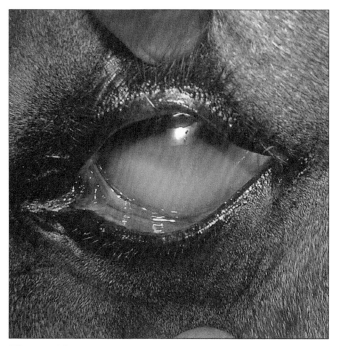

Figure 11.55 **Acute ERU-associated corneal edema masking the intraocular signs of anterior uveitis.**

- Retina and optic nerve: Initially, peripapillary subretinal infiltrate is seen as a gray discoloration with elevation from the surrounding retina. With time, this active inflammation resorbs into peripapillary multifocal to confluent areas of pigment disruption (depigmentation and/or hyperpigmented discrete foci) usually seen in the nontapetum. Vascular alterations of the nerve head and blurring of the nerve margins may be present (see Chapter 14, Vitreous and Ocular Fundus).

Clinical signs of more chronic ERU

Each acute to subacute bout of ERU leaves more scarring in the eye. The pupil is commonly immobile in a constricted position due to posterior synechiae (**Figure 11.57**). While iris adhesions are common, 360-degree posterior synechia with iris bombe and secondary glaucoma (as might be seen in the dog) is not a common complication in horses, and phthisis bulbi is much more likely to develop in the late stages (**Figure 11.58**). Chronicity results in corneal scarring that is usually quite diffuse and is at various levels within the cornea. Band keratopathy or corneal mineralization is a frequent complication (see Chapter 10). The anterior lens capsule becomes fibrosed and covered with pigment rests, and, in the late stages, a dense yellow-white cortical cataract develops. Subluxation of the lens may occur (**Figure 11.59**). The iris is darker

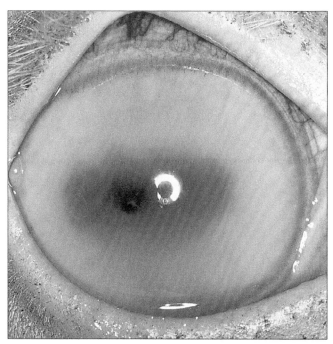

Figure 11.56 **Acute bilateral ERU with miosis and fibrin exudation in the anterior chamber. Note the yellow discoloration of the cornea and the aqueous humor.**

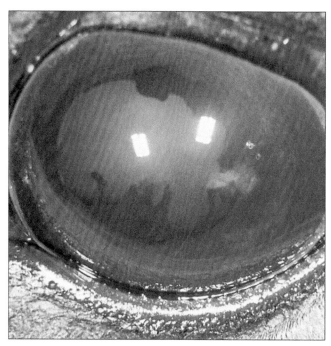

Figure 11.57 **Chronic ERU that is presented with multiple posterior synechiae. Note the anterior capsular cataract and the poor tapetal reflection due to anterior capsular debris and vitreous haze.**

to optic nerve atrophy that is manifest as a pale optic nerve with decreased or no visible retinal vessels (see Chapter 14, Vitreous and Ocular Fundus). While the clinical syndrome usually appears to be primarily an anterior uveitis, Deeg et al., on examining histopathologic specimens of ERU at various stages of clinical disease, found retinal changes in all eyes, and the histopathology was similar whether the eye had clinically active inflammation or was quiescent.[236]

Miscellaneous uveitis syndromes in various species

- Neonatal horses with *Rhodococcus equii* or other bacterial septicemia frequently develop dramatic bilateral uveitis characterized by large fibrin clots and

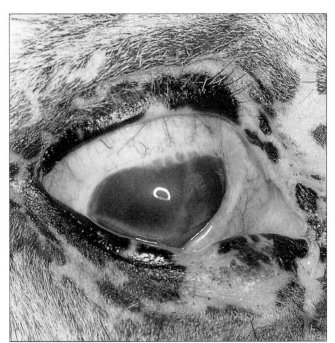

Figure 11.58 Appaloosa with ERU that has resulted in phthisis bulbi. The opposite eye had glaucoma.

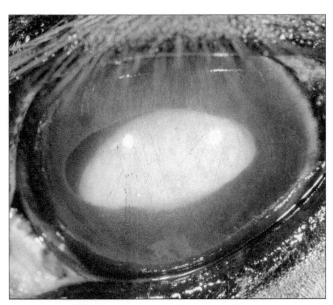

Figure 11.59 Chronic equine recurrent uveitis that has resulted in total cataract and posterior luxation of the lens. Note the diffuse corneal edema, the KPs inferiorly, very dark iris, and total absence of granula iridica.

than normal, dull and thickened, and the granula iridica are often missing.

Vitreal opacities and bands may be visible if the lens is not opaque, and the retina may be detached due to traction bands. Peripapillary scars of varying degrees are the most common fundus lesions. Blindness is frequently due

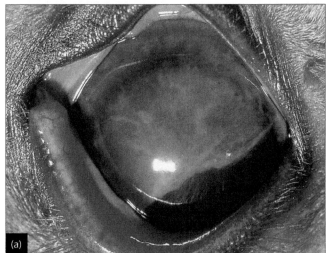

(a)

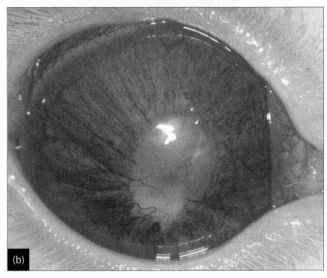

(b)

Figure 11.60 (a) A foal with rhodococcal joint infection that resulted in bilateral uveitis with marked fibrin exudation. (b) Phacoclastic uveitis in a New Zealand white rabbit with *Encephalitozoon cuniculi* infection. Note the severe episcleral injection, rubiosis iridis/PIFM, posterior synechia, lens abscess (5 to 8 o'clock pupil margin), and cataract.

anterior chamber hypopyon (**Figure 11.60**). The foals are systemically ill, and the uveitis usually improves dramatically with systemic antibiotics, topical corticosteroids, and atropine. Intraocular injections of 25–50 µg tissue plasminogen activator (tPA) will rapidly lyse the anterior chamber fibrin clot and synechia.

- As mentioned earlier, anterior uveitis secondary to keratitis is very common in the horse and may be associated with ulcers infected with bacteria or fungi, corneal abscesses from bacteria or fungi (**Figure 11.54c**), and sterile keratouveitis from trauma or unknown causes (see Chapter 10). Topical steroid therapy is not administered with infectious or suspected infectious keratouveitis; rather, the uveitis is treated with appropriate antimicrobials, systemic NSAIDs, and topical atropine. Once the keratitis resolves, the uveitis usually resolves with no long-term ill effects.

- The rabbit has a phacoclastic form of uveitis that is spontaneous and not associated with trauma or swollen mature cataracts. The syndrome is characterized by cataract formation, lens rupture, granuloma in the anterior chamber, and typical signs of anterior uveitis (**Figure 11.60b**). The microsporidium *Encephalitozoon cuniculi* is the causal agent with this syndrome, based on finding organisms in the lens that are morphologically compatible,[237] elevated titers of *E. cuniculi*, and DNA of *E. cuniculi*.[238] The organism may cause lens capsule rupture with secondary intractable phacoclastic uveitis. Therapy is topical glucocorticoids to quiet the eye and lens removal[239] and albendazole 15–30 mg/kg every 24 hours[238] if relapses occur. In the rabbit, *Pasteurella* spp. and *Staphylococcus* spp. septicemias and iridal inflammation can cause a granulomatous anterior uveitis/panuveitis as well.

- Uveitis in cattle is uncommon, but bacterial septicemic diseases such as thromboembolic meningoencephalitis (**Figure 11.61**), listeriosis, neonatal septicemias (**Figure 11.62**), and herpesvirus diseases such as infectious bovine rhinotracheitis (IBR; **Figure 11.63a**) and malignant catarrhal fever (**Figure 11.63b**) may cause anterior uveitis/panuveitis. An idiopathic anterior and posterior uveitis was described in a herd of Holstein cows that affected 65% of the herd. No husbandry problems or infectious disease agents could be identified with extensive testing.[7]

- Equine herpesvirus-1 may cause panuveitis in camelids along with head tilt, nystagmus, and paralysis.[240]

Diagnosis of the cause of uveitis

Anterior uveitis may be unilateral or bilateral, endogenous or exogenous in origin, acute or chronic in course, and

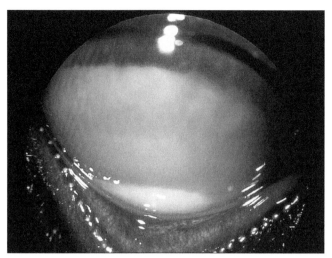

Figure 11.61 A downer cow with infectious thromboembolic meningoencephalitis due to *Hemophilus somnus*. The pupil is constricted, the cornea is diffusely edematous, and hypopyon is present.

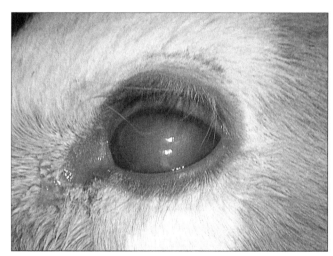

Figure 11.62 A calf with *E. coli* scours and septicemia that developed diffuse corneal edema and anterior uveitis.

granulomatous or nongranulomatous. All these factors may provide diagnostic clues to direct the search for an etiology. A thorough history and general physical examination should be performed to search for a definitive diagnosis. Bilateral uveitis is often a manifestation of systemic disease that may have a guarded prognosis for survival, so as much documentation of underlying cause as possible is desired.

Laterality   Systemic disease should be considered when both eyes are involved, although systemic diseases do not always result in bilateral uveitis, for example, ICH in the dog. With unilateral disease, the clinician should rule out something unique to that eye, such as trauma or neoplasia.

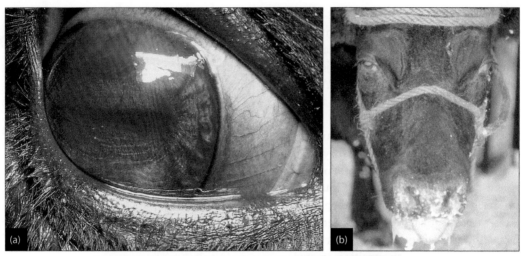

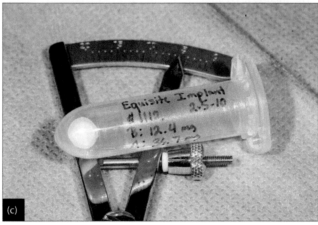

Figure 11.63 (a) Acute bilateral anterior uveitis in a young cow, characterized by corneal edema, miosis, thickening of the iris, and perilimbal corneal neovascularization. Infectious bovine rhinotracheitis was the suspected cause. (b) Malignant catarrhal fever in a cow. Note the bilateral corneal edema from the panuveitis as well as the other signs of a systemic disease. (c) Cyclosporine sustained-release reservoir matrix implant. The implant is 6 mm in diameter and contains 25 mg of cyclosporine.

Bilateral shotgun pellets or multicentric neoplasia such as lymphosarcoma are exceptions of traumatic and neoplastic causes of uveitis that may be bilateral.

Granulomatous versus nongranulomatous

These are pathologic descriptive terms that are subject to error when based on clinical findings, and they change with time. The finding of large or "mutton fat" KPs is the main clinical diagnostic criterion for granulomatous uveitis (**Figures 11.35b and 11.40a**). Focal proliferative lesions may also be present on the iris surface but are not as consistent a finding as large KPs (**Figure 11.51**). An additional limitation of this differentiation is the changing nature of the inflammation over the course of the disease.

Despite these limitations, the terminology persists and, particularly in the cat, may help narrow down the etiology. In the dog, defining the nature of the inflammation is not as helpful in finding the cause, although

a nonviral etiology such as systemic fungal infection should be considered more strongly with granulomatous inflammation.

Ocular centesis with aqueous humor testing

Ocular centesis with cultures and cytology is important in diagnosing sepsis, either bacterial or fungal. Aqueous humor centesis is easily performed but may yield false-negative findings due to the dilution effect of the rapid turnover of aqueous humor. Vitreous aspirates are much more reliable for cultures, but the procedure is also potentially more traumatic to the eye. In general, ocular fluid cytology is not very informative except in sepsis or neoplasia.

PCR testing, looking for minute quantities of DNA, has become a more widespread diagnostic aid and should become even more commonplace in the future. Antibody titers can also be performed on the aqueous humor and, when compared with serum titers, may be higher if local antibody has been produced. The Goldmann–Witmer coefficient or C value theoretically indicates local antibody production if the levels are above 1.[241] The C value for a specific antibody is:

$$\frac{\text{specific IgG in aqueous humor}}{\text{specific IgG in serum}} \times \frac{\text{total IgG in serum}}{\text{total IgG in aqueous humor}}$$

C values have been used extensively to diagnose active toxoplasmosis[180] infections as well as herpes,[195] leptospirosis, bartonella,[185] and others. Even with high C values, caution is recommended in interpreting active toxoplasmosis infection.

Biopsy/fine-needle aspirates

Biopsy of the iris to aid diagnosis (particularly with neoplasia) can be performed by aspiration or excision. Fine-needle vacuuming the surface of a lesion through an ocular paracentesis without iris puncture may yield diagnostic cytology without the risk of hemorrhage. Skin biopsy may also be indicated for uveodermatologic syndrome and lymph node biopsy for lymphoma or lymph node fine-needle aspirate and cytology for systemic fungal infections.

Physical examination

Clinicians are often quick to resort to expensive laboratory testing before obtaining a thorough history and performing a basic physical examination. Physical examination should look for a source of sepsis, other systemic signs, and involvement of other systems. For example, dermal depigmentation may be associated with uveodermatologic syndrome, peripheral lymphadenopathy with lymphoma, petechiae with vasculopathies and blood dyscrasia, and altered kidney size/shape or thyroid size with systemic hypertension in cats.

Blood tests

Serology provides presumptive evidence of infection and should demonstrate either very high or rising titers. *Brucella canis*, toxoplasmosis, leishmaniasis, leptospirosis, systemic mycoses, tick-borne rickettsial diseases, borreliosis, bartonellosis, FIP, and FIV are a few of the etiologies searched for in this manner.

When combined with a sterile ocular centesis, antinuclear antibodies (ANA), rheumatoid factor, and lupus erythematosus cells may occasionally indicate a diagnosis of immune-mediated uveitis. While many causes of uveitis are thought to have an immune component, the diagnosis is usually presumptive based on ruling out all other infectious etiologies and the response to immunosuppressive therapy.

Complete blood count (CBC) and chemistry profile do not usually contribute to the diagnosis in the dog, unless related to a systemic disease such as systemic bacterial infection, blood dyscrasia, lymphosarcoma, or metabolic disease. A CBC, serum biochemistry profile, *Toxoplasma gondii* serology, FIV and FIP serology, and FeLV tests are the initial recommendations for diagnostic workup of most cases of feline uveitis. The immunosuppression produced by FIV and FeLV may make cats susceptible to mixed infections with FIP, bartonella, and *T. gondii*. The testing methodology for *T. gondii* should be noted, as latex agglutination and the indirect hemagglutination tests are not as sensitive and specific as the ELISA technique for detection of *T. gondii*-specific IgG and IgM.[242] An IgM and IgG antibody titer ≥1:64 has been considered positive, but in regions where the titers are ubiquitous, most clinicians require higher titers for diagnosing toxoplasmosis. Elevated IgM or rising IgG titers are considered evidence of active, acute infection.

Additional tests for systemic mycoses in dogs may be performed if initial testing is not diagnostic. ELISA test for cryptococcal capsular antigen in serum has few false-positive results and may be used to monitor therapeutic response. Urine antigen testing for blastomycosis cross-reacts occasionally with histoplasmosis, but it may be used to monitor response to therapy. Urine antigen testing for histoplasmosis is also available.

Imaging

Radiology, ultrasound, CT, and MRI may be useful when both searching for a cause for uveitis and giving a prognosis for vision. Ocular ultrasonography is particularly valuable when the ocular media is so hazy that direct observations cannot be made, and it can help diagnose lens-induced uveitis, trauma, neoplasia, and iris cysts. Imaging is also very important in determining a prognosis for vision based on posterior segment changes such as retinal detachment.

Diagnosis of ERU

A clinical diagnosis of anterior uveitis in the horse is usually not difficult, but whether it is a manifestation of ERU or from an exogenous cause such as trauma or extension from corneal pathology may not always be obvious when the uveitis is unilateral. Bilateral pathology usually indicates ERU (or potential septicemias, especially in foals). The history in chronic cases may indicate recurrent bouts of pain and epiphora. If the condition is acute without evidence of primary corneal pathology, the index of suspicion for ERU is high.

Testing is often restricted to serum and perhaps aqueous humor *Leptospira* spp. titers. Leptospirosis is ideally diagnosed in individual animals by obtaining aqueous humor and serum samples and demonstrating local ocular antibody production.[243] If multiple animals are to be examined, testing is usually limited to sera. Faber et al. were unable to correlate positive aqueous humor cultures of *Leptospira* spp. with serology; however, Wollanke et al. found that of the horses from which *Leptospira* spp. were isolated from the eye, 76% had a fourfold increase in titer from the vitreous compared with the serum.[215,244] Wollanke et al. later contradicted this when they compared vitreal *Leptospira* titers with results of vitreal cultures in ERU eyes in a control group and cultured *L. interrogans* from 52% of the ERU eyes and none of the controls.[245] The mean vitreal titer in ERU eyes was 1:1,332, and the mean serum titer was 1:186. The conclusion was that *Leptospira* persists in ERU eyes, and the ratio between the vitreal and the serum titers may be less than a fourfold difference. In the future, PCR testing for *Leptospira* spp. in aqueous or vitreous humor may be utilized.

> Past dogma was that *Leptospira* spp. organisms were not present in the eye at the time of ERU signs, and the disease was an immune response only. However, there is mounting evidence that *Leptospira* spp. organisms may still be present in the eye at the time of the ERU. A combined therapeutic approach of antimicrobials and immunosuppression may become more commonplace in the treatment of ERU.

Conjunctival snip biopsies can be taken from the lateral bulbar limbal region and examined microscopically for *O. cervicalis* larvae. The tissue is placed in saline, allowed to warm on the microscope slide for a few minutes, and then examined for motile larvae.

> In the author's experience, looking for microfilaria in conjunctival biopsies has a low yield in horses with ERU and is rarely performed today due to the widespread use of avermectin-type parasiticides.

Therapy (all species)

Specific therapy In the horse with a severe, painful, acute uveitis placement, a subpalpebral lavage system to administer topical medications may be indicated. Specific therapy for uveitis may not be feasible. Some of the infectious causes of uveitis may have zoonotic potential, for example, canine brucellosis and canine leptospirosis, and the risk to the owner should be fully explained before recommending

therapy. Even with specific therapy, eliminating the organism from secretions or excretions may be difficult and may require long-term therapy and repeat testing. Systemic and topical antibiotics are indicated if a bacterial cause is suspected (for example, from a perforating injury) or is known to be present (for example, brucellosis, bartonellosis, or tick-borne diseases). Oftentimes systemic antibacterial therapy is used indiscriminately. Despite the potential role of active intraocular *Leptospira* spp. infection in ERU, intraocular antibiotics (except for fluid exchange using dilute gentamicin in mock aqueous humor during vitrectomies) have not been a critical or routine part of therapy, although this may change in the future. Although expensive, systemic (and potentially intravitreal) antibacterial drugs in the treatment of ERU horses with high serum *Leptospira* spp. titers or evidence of *Leptospira* spp. in the eye may prove to be beneficial in conjunction with immunosuppressive therapy.

Topical antiviral agents do not penetrate the intact cornea. Although used systemically to treat herpes viral infections in cats,[246] famciclovir has not been used for therapy of other virally induced causes of uveitis.

Antifungal agents such as systemic amphotericin-B or imidazole therapy are used for systemic mycoses. Intraocular injection of amphotericin-B should be reserved for blind eyes, since it is so toxic it is debatable whether there is a safe dose (see Chapter 2, Ophthalmic Pharmacology). Hendrix et al. could find no difference in the number of *Blastomyces dermatitidis* organisms found on histopathology of the eyes between itraconazole-treated and nontreated affected dogs.[247] This argues for enucleation of blind eyes with blastomycosis to remove a nidus of infection to try to avoid relapse. In the past, systemic glucocorticoid therapy has been considered contraindicated with systemic mycotic infections. Finn et al. reported on 12 dogs with ocular blastomycosis that were treated with topical and systemic prednisolone in addition to systemic antifungal therapy.[248] The duration of the oral prednisolone therapy ranged from 2 weeks to 8.5 months. All eyes with mild-to-moderate lesions and 50% of those with severe ocular lesions were visual at their last examination. The use of systemic glucocorticoids did not adversely affect the systemic outcome. This success rate is significantly better than previous reports on ocular blastomycosis and the visual outcome.[249,250]

Antifilarial treatment for *O. cervicalis* should be administered after the inflammation has subsided, as killing the microfilaria may exacerbate the condition.[214] Ivermectin is very effective in removing dermal microfilaria for about 6 months.[251] On occasion, some ophthalmologists have anecdotally noted uveitis in horses after routine deworming with ivermectin.

In cats with positive *T. gondii* titers and uveitis, clindamycin for 14–21 days may be indicated along with supportive therapy, although this treatment is controversial if there are no systemic signs.

Nonspecific, supportive uveitis therapy

Atropine or mydriatic/cycloplegics. Mydriatic/cycloplegic agents such as atropine are used to treat uveitis to minimize posterior synechiae, relieve the pain from iris sphincter/ciliary spasms, and to help restore the integrity of the BAB.[252,253] Treatment may have to be administered several times a day to effect, and combined therapy with atropine and 10% phenylephrine may give maximum mydriasis. Due to direct effects of prostaglandins on iris sphincter muscles, concurrent use of systemic prostaglandin inhibitors may enhance atropine-induced mydriasis, especially in the horse. In chronic cases with broad posterior synechiae, the pupil cannot usually be mobilized despite using frequent therapy, utilizing concentrations of >1% atropine, or combining with other mydriatics such as phenylephrine and cocaine.

Tissue plasminogen activator (tPA). Intracameral tPA may be used with acute uveitis to dissolve large fibrin/blood clots in the anterior chamber or break down early fibrous synechiae. When dealing with endogenous uveitis as opposed to traumatic uveitis, it may be necessary to give repeated injections, at approximately 5-day intervals, because of an ongoing inflammatory process. In small animals, 25 µg is injected into the anterior chamber, usually using a 30-gauge needle, with or without sedation, after application of a topical anesthetic; in the horse, 50 µg is administered after topical anesthetic application in the standing sedated animal, often with a dramatic resolution of anterior chamber fibrinohemorrhagic clots.

Corticosteroid drugs. Corticosteroids are indicated in sterile uveitis or uveitis in which the immune-mediated response is thought to be a significant factor. Topical, subconjunctival, and systemic routes, either individually or together, may be indicated depending on the severity. Despite the poor prognosis for systemic disease, the granulomatous uveitis of cats with FeLV and FIP is many times responsive to glucocorticoids. If therapy is instituted after extensive synechiae formation, intraocular pressure may become elevated as the inflammation subsides, and antiglaucoma therapy may become necessary.

Topical corticosteroids may be used to treat systemic infection induced anterior uveitis but should not be used in the presence of surface ocular infection, corneal ulceration, or corneal stromal infection/abscessation. In the past, subconjunctival repositol corticosteroids were used to augment topical steroid use, especially in horses with ERU. In theory, this is acceptable therapy, but in practice,

the risk of inappropriate treatment of corneal stromal abscesses and deep corneal infections makes this therapeutic option ill advised.

Nonsteroidal anti-inflammatory drugs (NSAIDs). Systemic nonsteroidal therapy with aspirin (25 mg/kg), phenylbutazone, and flunixin, are important in controlling pain and intraocular inflammation in the horse. In the past, aspirin was advocated for daily use for months to prevent relapse of uveitis that is common with endogenous immune-mediated uveitis such as ERU. With what is currently known about the immunologic cause of ERU, this long-term aspirin therapy cannot be recommended. In the dog, systemic NSAIDs, commonly carprofen and meloxicam, are used.[254] Topical NSAIDs (flurbiprofen and diclofenac) are often used to supplement topical corticosteroids.

Other immunosuppressive agents. Severe ocular inflammation may be unresponsive or incompletely responsive to corticosteroids. Patients with autoimmune uveitis (e.g., uveodermatologic syndrome and others) may not be controlled with corticosteroids, and treatment with systemic alkylating agents, nucleotide analogs, or other antimetabolite/antimitotic drugs (e.g., azathioprine, chlorambucil, cyclophosphamide, or others) may be necessary.[145] The purpose of this class of drugs is to alter the function and numbers of cells responsible for releasing inflammatory mediators. Therapy is initiated with both systemic corticosteroids and azathioprine (2 mg/kg/day for 3–5 days, followed by reduction to 1 mg/kg/day for 10 days, then 0.5 mg/kg/day as needed to maintain disease control[255]); the corticosteroids are tapered off after 3–4 weeks as the inflammation diminishes, the azathioprine blood/tissue levels have plateaued, and the immune competent cells have decreased. Patients treated with these agents should initially have a complete blood count, platelet count, and serum biochemistry performed at biweekly intervals to evaluate bone marrow and liver toxicity. Systemic cyclosporine as well has been used in humans to treat VKH disease[256] and has been recommended for use in dogs.[257]

Intravitreal/suprachoroidal implants containing cyclosporine have been used to control inflammation with ERU and equine experimental immune-mediated uveitis.[258–261] These implants may deliver therapeutic levels of drugs for up to 4 years.[261] Use of these devices reduced the frequency and the severity of uveitis episodes in the population studied[259,261] as well as maintained ocular health and vision. Control of active uveitis prior to implantation is important, as cyclosporine has poor direct anti-inflammatory properties. Horses with secondary cataract formation and glaucoma are also poor candidates for cyclosporine implantation with restoration of vision long-term.[262] These sustained-release implants are not available commercially in North America and are only available to veterinary ophthalmologists from North Carolina State University (**Figure 11.63c**).

Protection from bright light stimulus. Patching the eye and/or keeping the animal in a dark environment are supportive measures for acute uveitis. Most animals with uveitis are sensitive to bright light stimulation in that light stimulation elicits iris sphincter contraction that may lead to further painful anterior uveal muscle spasming. If the eye has been treated with supportive mydriatic/cycloplegic drugs, the dilated pupil may induce further photophobia as well. In small animals, eye patching is rarely performed (and if needed, a temporary tarsorrhaphy or third eyelid flap may be used), especially when frequent therapy is to be administered. In horses, commercially made blinker masks are available to protect the eye from light stimulation, to help avoid self-trauma, and to minimize damage to subpalpebral lavage systems when they are used (**Figure 11.64**).

Surgical therapy. In central Europe and the United States, investigators have performed partial vitrectomies on selected ERU cases. Vitrectomy has produced a significant decrease in recurrence of acute uveitis, although the visual prognosis has not significantly altered, usually because of cataract formation and retinal detachment.[263–266] The goal of vitrectomy is to reduce antigen load in cases

of *Leptospira* spp. induced ERU, to reduce numbers of immunocompetent cells in the vitreous, enhance vision by clearing the vitreous of opaque inflammatory debris, and to provide long-term pain relief.[267] Brooks et al. reported very poor results in horses in Florida, with cataract formation occurring in 46%, and one-third of these becoming complete cataracts.[268] In this study, the incidence of Appaloosa horses may have contributed to the poor outcome.[202]

In all cases of uveitis, secondary glaucoma is not an uncommon occurrence and should be monitored for and controlled with medical and/or surgical therapy to either attempt vision maintenance or minimize pain.

Prevention (all species)

In the not too distant past, an equine vaccine for leptospirosis was not available, but many practitioners in high-risk areas utilized a multivalent bovine vaccine. Anaphylaxis was not uncommon with bovine vaccine use in the equine species, so it was not without some risk. Rohrbach et al. immunized horses with ERU with a bovine vaccine that included six serovars of *Leptospira interrogans* and were unable to demonstrate a statistically significant difference in the number of uveitis episodes after vaccination.[269] No significant adverse effects were noted in the vaccinated horses. Anecdotal recommendations for utilizing bovine vaccines to reduce the incidence of new cases of ERU in predisposed herds had been made. All animals to be immunized were to be examined prior to immunization for signs of ocular inflammation, and serology was to be performed to determine leptospiral antibody titers. Animals with signs of ERU or positive serology for leptospiral antigens were recommended not be immunized.[262] In 2015, Zoetis, Inc. introduced an equine vaccine for *L. pomona* specifically designed to protect the horse from *L. Pomona*-induced uveitis and abortion. In the future, prophylactic immunization of horses against *L. pomona* may reduce the incidence of equine recurrent uveitis. The vaccine should not be useful for treatment of ERU cases; rather, it will hopefully be a preventative for cases of ERU that are instigated by *L. pomona* infection.

In the cat, immunizations for FeLV, corona virus, and FIV may prevent uveitis from these infectious agents. Likewise, in the dog, immunization against canine adenovirus may prevent canine infectious hepatitis and its ocular sequela.

In animals with perforating trauma and lens injury, lens removal in the acute stage to avoid phacoclastic uveitis is indicated if vitreal hemorrhage, retinal detachment, and scleral rupture are not present.[270] Medical management of traumatic corneal laceration and lens capsule rupture has been described,[271] and under certain circumstances,

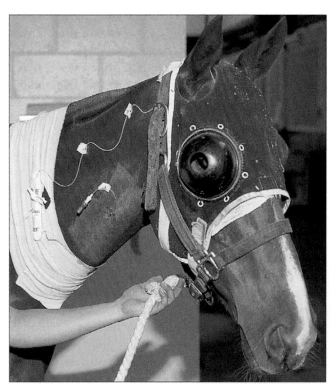

Figure 11.64 Commercial face mask for a horse that provides protection from self-trauma and minimizes photophobia. It is usually used with subpalpebral lavage.

medical management may be superior to surgical management concerning vision and globe maintenance (see Chapter 13, Lens).

Sequelae (all species)

- Interstitial keratitis with corneal scarring and/or endothelial dysfunction with edema.
- Secondary capsular and cortical cataracts.
- Posterior synechiae may result in a fixed/irregular pupil and iris bombe.
- Secondary glaucoma may result from peripheral anterior synechiae/PIFM formation and/or iris bombe.
- Iris color changes (usually hyperpigmentation).
- Prolonged hypotony.
- Phthisis bulbi from cyclitic membrane (a fibrovascular membrane passing from one side of the ciliary body to the other) formation that detaches the ciliary body/ retina and disorganizes ocular anatomy.

Prognosis (all species)

The prognosis for uveitis varies. Chronic or recurrent uveitis, such as ERU and uveodermatologic syndrome in dogs, should always have a guarded to unfavorable prognosis for long-term vision retention. Horses with recurrent uveitis or evidence of prior uveitis episodes should be considered unsound. The Appaloosa has a poorer prognosis than other breeds for maintaining vision.[202,205] Dwyer and Kalsow reported vision loss in one or both eyes in 44%–56% of all horses with uveitis.[205] Blindness occurred in one or both eyes in 36%–46% of non-Appaloosa breeds and in 68%–81% of Appaloosas.[202] Of horses seronegative for leptospirosis, 24%–52% became blind in one or both eyes, while 59% of seropositive horses were blind in one or both eyes. If the horse was seropositive for *L. pomona*, then vision loss in one or both eyes occurred in 100% of Appaloosas and 51% of non-Appaloosas.[205]

Obvious uveitis associated with systemic mycoses also carries an unfavorable prognosis, although focal chorioretinal granulomas may heal with medical therapy. Uveitis associated with penetrating trauma also should be given a guarded prognosis, especially if the cornea is not sealed with continued leakage of aqueous humor, prolapse of uveal contents, and/or the lens capsule is lacerated. Uveitis in cats associated with FIP and FeLV carries a guarded prognosis for sight and an unfavorable prognosis for long-term survival.

ALTERED AQUEOUS HUMOR

As discussed under the signs of anterior uveitis, breakdown of the BAB produces a dramatic increase in the protein content of the aqueous humor. In milder forms of anterior uveitis, this produces murky aqueous humor ("aqueous flare"), but in more severe breaches, a fibrin clot of variable proportions may be formed (**Figures 11.35a and 11.60a**). Variable degrees of cellular exudation are often found with anterior uveitis and, when severe, results in the accumulation of leukocytes in the anterior chamber (hypopyon) (**Figures 11.50a, 11.54c, and 11.61**). These changes may have a degree of hemorrhage associated with them (**Figures 11.33a–c, 11.35a, and 11.40c**). Fibrin clots may be treated by intraocular tPA, as previously discussed, and hypopyon is treated by treating the underlying cause of the uveitis and symptomatic medical therapy (aspiration of hypopyon for other than diagnostic purposes is not warranted).

Lipid leakage into the anterior chamber ("lipemic aqueous") may occur and cause a sudden diffuse gray-white opacity that fills the anterior chamber (**Figure 11.65**). The condition is many times unilateral and occurs in animals that have concurrent hyperlipidemia, either from ingestion of a high-fat meal or from a metabolic problem.[272] It may be confused with a diffuse corneal opacity or a cataract with a dilated pupil. However, with a focal light or slit lamp, the opacity can be localized to the anterior chamber. Lipids are thought to gain access to the anterior chamber from an underlying anterior uveitis with breakdown of the BAB. A rare complication of aqueous laden lipid may be xanthogranuloma. This is an intraocular mass of macrophages, laden with lipids, that results in secondary glaucoma.[273] Miniature Schnauzers are probably predisposed

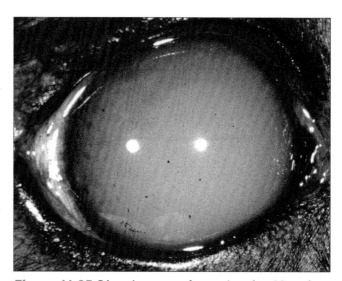

Figure 11.65 Lipemic aqueous humor in a dog. Note the diffuse cloudiness that masks the pupillary outline. The opacity is most dense axially due to the increased depth of the axial anterior chamber versus the peripheral anterior chamber. With slit lamp biomicroscopy, a diffuse white cloudiness of the aqueous humor was readily apparent.

due to their propensity for hyperlipidemia and diabetes mellitus. Therapy is restriction of dietary fats, topical corticosteroids, and/or topical or systemic NSAIDs to treat the anterior uveitis.

NEOPLASIA OF THE IRIS AND THE CILIARY BODY

Primary tumors

Introduction/etiology

The anterior uvea is the most common origin of primary intraocular tumors in all species of domestic animals. Primary intraocular tumors are not common, and as a result, extensive follow-up data to determine epidemiologic statistics has only recently been forthcoming. In the dog, melanoma is about twice as common as all the other primary intraocular tumors combined. Adenocarcinoma and adenoma are the only other primary intraocular tumors occurring with any frequency.[274–277] Other tumors have been reported, including hemangiosarcoma, leiomyosarcoma, fibrosarcoma, ganglioglioma, medulloepithelioma, ganglioneuroblastoma, histiocytic sarcoma, schwannoma, osteosarcoma, retinoblastoma, and hemangioma.[278–285]

Dog

The average age of dogs with ocular melanoma is 9 years (with a wide range from 2 months to 17 years) at the time of diagnosis.[286] Anterior uveal melanomas arise from the anterior surface/stroma of the iris or from the ciliary body and are usually raised, pigmented masses, although amelanotic melanomas occur (**Figures 11.66–11.68**). Melanoma of the iris may be noted earlier as it invades the

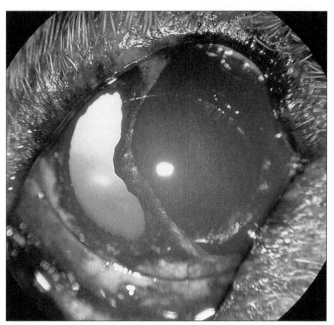

Figure 11.67 Melanoma in a dog that invaded and eroded through the iris but originated in the ciliary body.

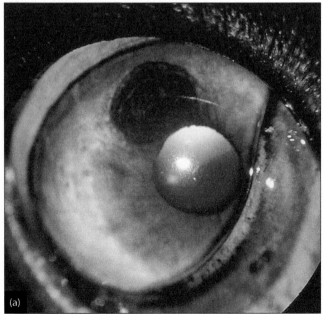

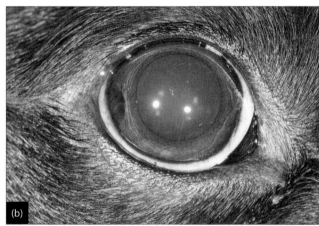

Figure 11.66 (a) Iris melanoma in a dog. The location within the iris, away from the iris base/filtration angle and away from the 9-o'clock position at the base of the greater arterial circle, makes this a favorable candidate for laser photocoagulation/ablation or sector iridectomy to remove the tumor. (b) Iris melanoma over the bifurcation of the greater arterial circle with invasion of the filtration angle makes this a lower potential for successful excision or laser ablation than the mass in Figure 11.66a. Note the "mass effect" (folding of the iris adjacent to the mass) of the tumor upon pupillary dilation.

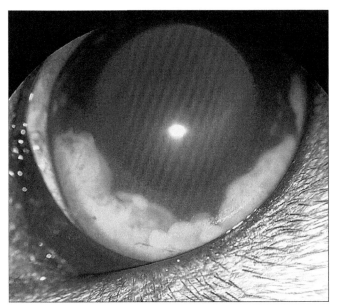

Figure 11.68 Amelanotic melanoma of the ciliary body in a German shepherd dog that extended anteriorly into the iris and the anterior chamber. The type of tumor was difficult to diagnose even with aqueous humor centesis and eventual biopsy.

anterior chamber and distorts the pupil (**Figure 11.66b**). Melanoma of the ciliary body is usually discovered at a later stage after it has invaded into the vitreous, forward into the iris and iridocorneal angle, through the sclera (**Figure 11.69**), or has displaced the lens. Many apparent iris masses have expanded from the ciliary body. Ocular

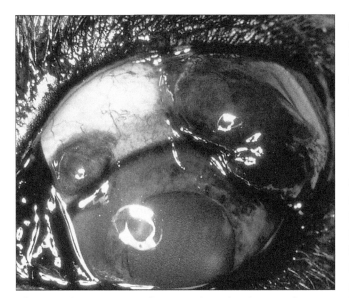

Figure 11.69 Extraocular extension of an intraocular melanoma in a Norwegian elkhound. This should be differentiated from a more benign epibulbar/limbal melanoma.

melanomas may act very aggressively locally with rapid growth and invasion of adjacent structures such as the sclera and into the orbit (**Figure 11.69**).

Efforts to predict the biologic behavior of canine melanomas have resulted in conflicting reports. Bussanich et al. reviewed the literature and found only seven metastases in 190 cases of reported intraocular melanoma.[287] While melanomas frequently cause catastrophic intraocular damage with their growth and invade the sclera and the orbit, <5% metastasize distally. Classification of melanomas by the Callender system (categorizing scheme for human ocular melanomas) to predict biologic behavior in dogs is controversial. This classification grades melanomas by the type of cell in increasing anaplastic characteristics: Spindle A, spindle B, epithelioid, and mixed cell type. Many authors have considered the histopathologic characteristics of Callander's mixed and epithelioid cell types as predictors of malignancy.[288-290] Trucksa et al. considered extrascleral extension and secondary glaucoma the only predictors of metastatic potential, while Wilcock and Peiffer considered the mitotic index to be the only reliable predictor of metastasis.[291, 292] Giuliano et al. studied the survival rate of canine ocular melanoma patients compared to age-matched controls and found no length of survival time correlation to tumor extension, tumor size, or mitotic index, although the malignant melanoma group had a shorter survival time than the benign melanoma (melanocytoma) group.[286] Clinically, it seems prudent to treat those tumors with a history of rapid growth and invasion of adjacent structures more aggressively, that is, with enucleation.

Bilateral melanomas have been described in two reports: One was metastatic to the opposite eye (multiple systemic metastasis),[293] and the other was thought to be primary in both eyes.[294] Breed predisposition for benign melanocytoma and malignant melanoma includes mixed breeds, Labrador retrievers, Golden retrievers, Schnauzers, German shepherds, and cocker spaniels.[286] Inherited melanoma that occurred at a young age (most between 1–2 years) has been described in the Labrador retriever.[295]

Adenocarcinomas and adenomas are typically pink masses arising behind the iris from the ciliary body or invading the iridocorneal angle and peripheral iris (**Figure 11.70**). Many adenomas may contain pigment, and melanomas may be amelanotic (**Figure 11.68**), making it difficult clinically to differentiate epithelial tumors from sarcomas. Labrador and Golden retrievers are susceptible to epithelial tumors[296] as well as melanomas. The biologic behavior of epithelial tumors appears similar to intraocular melanomas in the dog, in that while often locally invasive, even adenocarcinomas appear to metastasize infrequently.[275,277,296–298]

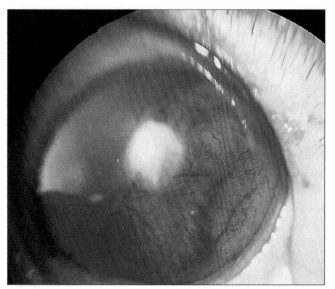

Figure 11.70 Ciliary body adenocarcinoma in a Labrador retriever. Note the pink color and the fact that the tumor is behind the iris (visible most easily from 3 to 5 o'clock and 6 to 9 o'clock).

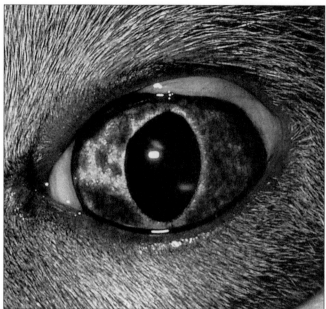

Figure 11.72 Moderately advanced, diffuse iris melanoma in a cat. The apparent invasion of the iris base/filtration angle in this patient bodes poorly for long-term survival.

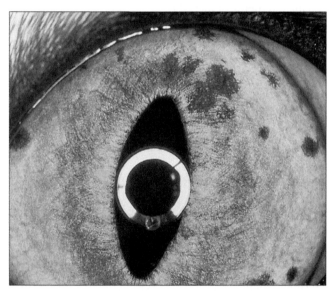

Figure 11.71 Early diffuse iris melanoma in a cat. At this stage, documentation of progression and periodic evaluation are warranted.

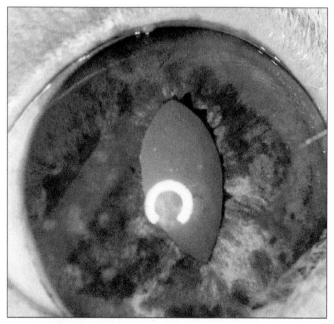

Figure 11.73 Advanced iris melanoma in a cat that has resulted in secondary glaucoma. Statistically, this patient has a much higher potential for eventual distal metastasis than the cat in Figure 11.71.

Cat

In the cat, intraocular melanomas typically arise from the iris as flat, diffuse to multifocal, pigmented lesions, rather than nodular lesions.[299] Initially, feline iris melanoma appears as a focal, flat, dark spot on the iris that is difficult to differentiate from a benign nevus (**Figure 11.19**) or a senile pigment change (**Figure 11.71**). With progression, the lesion not only enlarges, but multifocal pigmented patches develop that eventually coalesce and form a diffuse, thickened, pigmented iris (**Figures 11.72, 11.73, and 11.74a**).

Feline melanomas also differ from canine melanomas in that they metastasize more frequently.[300,301] Melanomas are a disease of older cats (average 11 years), and in one study, 63% of cats with anterior uveal melanomas died from metastatic disease.[302] Duncan and Peiffer reported a 56% mortality rate and found malignancy correlated with the

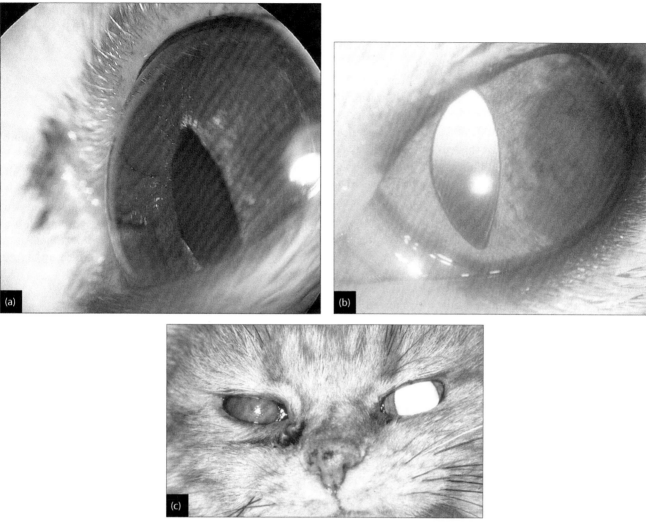

Figure 11.74 (a) Advanced iris melanoma in a cat that is viewed obliquely. The lesion has nodular as well as diffuse characteristics. (b) Posterior iris/ciliary body solitary melanoma in a cat. Despite enucleation, the cat was euthanized within 6 months due to metastasis to the liver. (c) Feline spindle cell sarcoma, right eye. The cat presented for blindness. Note the dilated left pupil. The tumor in the right eye migrated along the optic nerve to the optic chiasm, causing blindness and eventually death. The right eye had been phthisical for 8 years prior to "growing" for 6 months prior to presentation.

mitotic index.[303] In a survival study of feline ocular melanomas, the melanoma group as a whole died earlier than controls, but when stratified according to ocular involvement, the less the invasion of various ocular tissues, the better the survival. Thus, early enucleation when the tumor is confined to the iris improves the survival rate to that of the control population.[304]

Experimentally, feline sarcoma virus (FeSV) injected intraocularly causes disease similar to feline intraocular melanoma.[305] The experimental model has a higher rate of metastasis if the eye is enucleated, as is the case in human melanomas, which raised queries on the advisability of this procedure in the veterinary clinical setting.[306] Kalishman et al. reinforced that early enucleation in the cat improves survival but did not comment on whether late enucleation

hastens metastasis.[304] Stiles et al. found FeLV–FeSV DNA in 3 of 36 melanomas using PCR, the significance of which is unknown, but it tends to bring clinical relevance to the experimental FeSV model of melanomas.[307] A subsequent study, however, failed to confirm an association between FeLV-FeSV and diffuse iris melanomas in cats.[308]

Feline intraocular melanomas arising posterior to the iris have been described and are usually more solitary than diffuse iris melanoma (**Figure 11.74b**). They are characterized by round, pigmented cells that are not typically anaplastic as is found in iridal melanomas.[309] Typically, these tumors are later in their presentation for care than iridal melanomas and may have metastasized.

In the cat, post-traumatic spindle cell sarcoma has been described (**Figure 11.74c**). Trauma usually occurred years earlier resulting in a blind or phthisical eye. The differentiation of the tumor may vary from osteosarcoma to an undifferentiated sarcoma.[310–312] Since tumors often occur in eyes with opaque media, the tumor is usually not discovered until it fills the globe. No instances of distal metastases have been described, but aggressive local invasion of the sclera and the optic nerve may occur.[313] Most cases have rupture of the lens capsule and loss of lens substance, and it has been speculated that the lens epithelium may be the origin of the tumor.[314,315] This is an argument for the enucleation of blind eyes with opaque media or eyes that are phthisical. Cats with spindle cell sarcoma are negative for FeSV and FeLV.[316]

Horse

Anterior uveal melanomas are rare in the horse but are found predominantly in middle-aged gray horses.[317–319] A review of the literature found only 12 reported cases and six possible additional cases.[320] Ten of 12 cases where coat color was known were gray horses, and, thus, other dermal melanomas may coexist with ocular melanomas. Equine ocular melanoma appears to originate from the anterior uvea, and based on the limited data, the cells appear histologically to have a low malignant potential (**Figure 11.75**).

Medulloepithelioma is a rare tumor that has been observed in horses and dogs, arising from the ciliary body or optic nerve region.[281,321–323] The tumor arises from the nonpigmented ciliary epithelium or from undifferentiated cells that form the inner layer of the primitive optic cup.

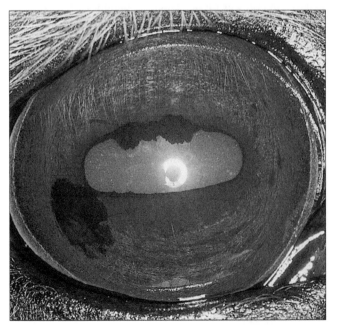

Figure 11.75 Early iris melanoma in a gray horse.

The cells form tubular cords that, when cut on cross section, form rosettes; in the older literature, they were often erroneously called retinoblastomas.[324]

SECONDARY TUMORS

Introduction/etiology

Lymphosarcoma is the most common secondary tumor of the uvea in the dog, the cat, the cow, and the horse.[325,326] In the dog and the horse, advanced systemic signs usually accompany the ocular signs, while in the cat, the ocular signs may be prodromal to the systemic signs. The ocular signs are mainly in the anterior uvea and manifest as bilateral uveitis or hyphema, often with the complication of secondary glaucoma (**Figures 11.33b,c, 11.48, 11.49, 11.52, and 11.53**).[135,327,328]

Metastasis of tumors to the anterior or posterior uveal tract in the dog and the cat is a relatively rare occurrence, but a number of case reports have documented the phenomenon. Adenocarcinomas from a variety of sources have been reported metastasizing to the eye in the dog and the cat.[325,329–333] Several squamous cell carcinomas have been reported in the cat.[334–337] Less frequently, fibrosarcoma, pheochromocytoma, and malignant angioendotheliomatosis have been reported.[328–340] Histiocytic sarcomas have been described in the eye predominantly in Rottweilers, Retrievers, and Bernese Mountain dogs. They were thought to be metastatic to the eye, as most dogs died relatively shortly after enucleation. Without specific stains on histopathology they look like amelanotic melanomas, which carry a good prognosis for survival. In paraffin-embedded tissue, the finding of CD-18-postive cells with no reactivity to melan-A was indicative of histiocytic sarcomas.[283]

Bilateral metastatic lesions have been observed with transmissible venereal tumor, hemangiosarcoma, squamous cell carcinoma, transitional cell carcinoma, seminoma, and pulmonary carcinoma.[336,341–345] Hemangiosarcomas seem to be one of the most common metastatic tumors to the eye (**Figure 11.76**) and usually manifest in the posterior uvea, mimicking hemorrhage (see Chapter 14, Vitreous and Ocular Fundus).

Clinical signs of ocular neoplasia

- A mass on the iris (**Figure 11.66**) or protruding into the pupil region from behind the iris (**Figure 11.70**) is present that may or may not be pigmented.
- Hyphema.
- Secondary glaucoma.
- Progressive iridal color change, usually an increase in pigmentation.

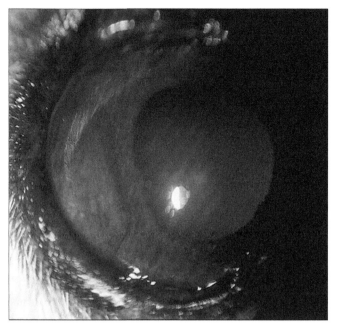

Figure 11.76 Metastatic hemangiosarcoma in the iris of a dog.

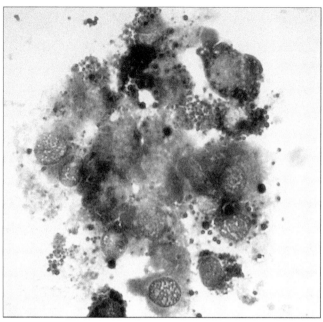

Figure 11.77 Cytology of a feline diffuse iris melanoma obtained by anterior chamber centesis and vacuuming the surface of the lesion.

Diagnosis

Diagnosis of an intraocular neoplasia may be obvious if visualized as a mass protruding from the ciliary body or the iris. However, the lesion may be masked by hemorrhage, aqueous debris, corneal edema, or secondary glaucoma. In the past, the presence of a tumor when the clear media was opaque was usually made after enucleation, but ocular ultrasonography now allows an inexpensive, noninvasive, and rapid method for evaluating these eyes.[346]

The type of tumor cannot be determined with certainty unless cytology, biopsy, or enucleation is performed. FNA of the lesion may be a practical method for making a definitive diagnosis, but only if representative tissue is obtained.[347] "Vacuuming" the surface of iridal lesions with a fine needle can minimize the risk of hemorrhage from mass aspiration (**Figure 11.77**). Hemorrhage and seeding of the tumor along the needle tract are possible complications.[348]

For prognostic reasons, primary intraocular neoplasia should be differentiated from metastatic neoplasia, as the latter disease carries a grave prognosis. Epibulbar neoplasia should be differentiated from extraocular extension of intraocular neoplasia (**Figure 11.69**). Differentiation of primary from metastatic tumor is by history, physical examination, thorax and abdominal imaging, lymph node FNA and cytology, and/or histopathologic examination.

Therapy

Considering the relatively benign nature of most primary intraocular tumors in the dog, consideration should be given to early intervention by excision or laser photocoagulation therapy of focal lesions in an attempt to save the eye. Both Nd:YAG and diode laser photocoagulation/ablation of canine ocular melanoma have been described.[349,350] The best candidate for laser therapy appears to be melanoma of the iris, which is accessible. Melanoma of the ciliary body is usually larger than iridal melanomas by the time it is diagnosed, and it cannot be photocoagulated/ablated with laser energy as effectively due to size and location. Minimal complications occur with smaller iris lesions that do not touch the cornea. Larger tumors of the ciliary body induce significant uveitis, hemorrhage risk, and some degree of cataract formation when treated with laser energy.

Cimetidine has been used successfully to treat or arrest dermal melanoma in three horses, but it has not been tested on intraocular melanoma or in other domestic animals. Cimetidine therapy involves multiple doses each day for months; the optimal response is after 3–4 months of therapy. The action of cimetidine is unknown, but it is described as a "biologic modifier with antitumor properties."[351] It is hypothesized that cimetidine acts by inhibiting histamine activation of suppressor T-cells. Whether intraocular concentrations can be achieved is unknown.

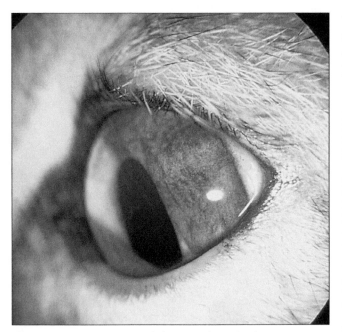

Figure 11.78 A young adult cat with a raised iris mass occupying the dorsolateral quadrant. The cat had a history of a previous mass in the same location that had spontaneously resolved. Aqueous humor centesis and vacuuming of the surface were nondiagnostic. The cat was FeLV negative.

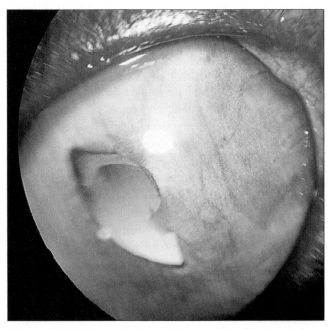

Figure 11.79 Same lesion as Figure 11.78 after 2 months of topical glucocorticoid therapy.

Surgical excision, with or without chemotherapy, has been advocated for ciliary body adenoma and, perhaps, adenocarcinoma.[352,353] Clerc achieved good functional and cosmetic results with surgical excision followed by systemic 5-fluorouracil in five dogs that were diagnosed

with ciliary body adenocarcinoma.[353] Whether the tumors excised were adenocarcinomas rather than adenomas was questioned,[354] and consequently, chemotherapy may not have been necessary.

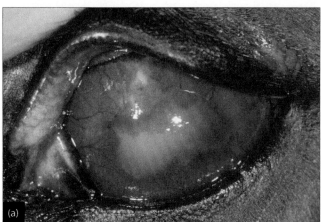

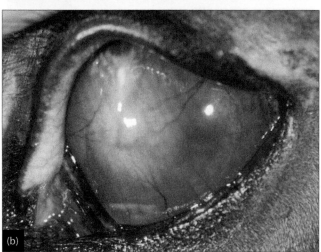

Figure 11.80 (a) Equine patient from Figure 11.54c (and Case 4 in "Sample Cases, Chapter 11," to follow), with presumed corneal stromal abscess/cellulitis. Within 1 week of discontinuing topical corticosteroid therapy and beginning topical antifungal and antibacterial drugs with good corneal penetration capability, the stromal abscess area was infiltrated by deep and superficial corneal neovascularization, and the patient was much more comfortable. (b) At 3 weeks after beginning antifungal/antibiotic therapy, the corneal neovascularization was beginning to consolidate peripherally, the corneal edema was clearing peripherally, the aqueous flare was cleared, and the area of hypopyon was contracting and shrinking in size ("rounding up"). (c) At 6 weeks after beginning appropriate medical therapy, all signs of anterior uveitis were abated, the patient was nonpainful, and the corneal scar was remodeling. Over a 6 month period, all the corneal neovascularization has abated, and the corneal scar had contracted to a 7 mm leukoma in the area of the original cellulitis/abscess. (*Continued*)

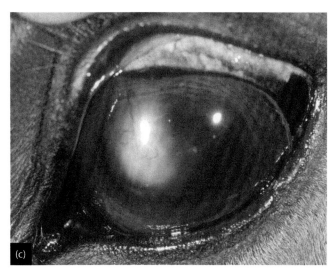

Figure 11.80 (*Continued*) (c) Over a 6-month period, all the corneal neovascularization had abated, and the corneal scar had contracted to a 7-mm leukoma in the area of the original cellulitis/abscess.

The ocular lesions of generalized lymphosarcoma may dramatically regress with successful systemic therapy, but often secondary glaucoma produces permanent blindness/pain necessitating enucleation. Conversely, a worsening of the ocular condition has been noted when medical therapy is given for transmissible venereal tumor. This is presumably due to necrosis of the intraocular metastatic tumor that stimulates severe uveitis.

In the cat, early focal iris melanomas or nevi may be treated with laser ablation, although this therapy is more controversial in cats due to the malignant nature of the tumors; the effectiveness of laser ablation in feline diffuse melanoma has not been evaluated. Many owners refuse permission to enucleate an eye with diffuse iris melanoma that is still visual. It must be remembered, however, that awaiting signs of extensive iris involvement, tumor infiltration into the iridocorneal angle, and glaucoma increases the chance for distal metastasis even after enucleation. Enucleation of eyes with spindle cell sarcoma should include as much of the optic nerve as possible. Histopathologic examination of the nerve should be performed because of the tendency for this tumor to spread up the nerve.

PSEUDOTUMORS (GRANULOMAS OR MANIFESTATION OF LYMPHOCYTIC/PLASMACYTIC IRITIS IN CATS)

Pink to cream-colored iridal masses of 1–2 clock hours or more in FeLV-negative cats was described by Martin in previous editions of this text. Centesis of the eye masses were not described as being diagnostic, and the lesions were said to have regressed with topical steroid therapy. The etiology of these masses was unknown (**Figures 11.78 and 11.79**). This author has seen similar cases, and in some instances, medical therapy was short lived with full resolution of clinical signs.[174]

CLINICAL CASES

CASE 1

A F/S Golden retriever originally presented as a 19-month-old young adult dog with free-floating iris cysts in the anterior chambers of both eyes with one collapsed cyst and pigment on the endothelial surface of the cornea (similar to **Figure 11.25**). Following pupillary dilation, other ciliary body cysts were observed in both eyes. Diode laser coagulation of the cysts in the anterior chambers was performed as the owner felt the free-floating cysts were partially obstructing the dog's vision. Seven years later, at age 9 years, the patient was re-examined for vision loss and change in ocular appearance. The left eye was blind, slightly buphthalmic, with an IOP of 47 mmHg. Both eyes had iris hyperpigmentation, posterior synechia, and radial streaks of pigment deposition on the anterior lens capsules (capsular cataract) as well as incipient/immature cortical cataract

(**Figure 10.50c**). The left eye had optic nerve head degeneration and cupping, and both eyes had subtle strands of anterior vitreal fibrin/old hemorrhage. A diagnosis of Golden retriever pigmentary uveitis/pigmentary and cystic glaucoma in the Golden retriever was made. The left eye was treated with an intravitreal injection of gentamicin, which controlled the glaucoma and eventually led to the left eye becoming phthisical. The right eye was treated with topical corticosteroids and timolol in an attempt to control inflammation and reduce the incidence of glaucoma in that eye. Over a 1-year period, in the right eye, despite additional antiglaucoma therapy, IOP gradually increased, the lens became more opaque, and the patient went blind. This case represents a relatively typical case of pigmentary and cystic glaucoma in the Golden retriever. The age of onset of glaucoma/cataract/synechia and vision loss was typical. Despite traditional therapy for uveitis and glaucoma, the disease progressed, ultimately leading to blindness. Attempt at glaucoma control using cyclodestructive procedures (cyclophotocoagulation and cyclocryotherapy) as would be the case in primary glaucoma has been relatively unrewarding with this disorder.

CASE 2

A 3-year-old intact male chocolate Labrador retriever presented with a painful left eye (**Figure 11.40b**). The left eye had episcleral injection, rubeosis irides, aqueous flare, posterior synechia, and a detached retina. IOP was low (6 mmHg). The right eye was normal. Physical examination revealed a mild fever, a swollen, tender testicle, and numerous swollen peripheral lymph nodes. FNA of lymph nodes and testicle revealed pyogranulomatous inflammation and thick-walled yeast organisms consistent with blastomycosis. Thoracic radiography revealed a diffuse, multifocal pulmonary infiltrate consistent with blastomycosis. Urine antigen for blastomycosis was positive. The patient was initially treated with itraconazole and topical prednisolone, and within one week, the left eye was glaucomatous and buphthalmic. The lymph nodes were shrunken, and the dog was dyspnic/tachypnic. Examination of the right eye revealed two focal granulomas on the nontapetal fundus but no sign of anterior uveitis. Oral prednisolone at an anti-inflammatory dose was added, and within 72 hours, the patient's respiration improved. One week later, the dog was castrated, and the left eye was enucleated. At that time, the fundic lesions of the right eye had not changed. Itraconazole and oral prednisolone were continued for 3 months, at which time the oral prednisolone was discontinued. After a total of 6 months of itraconazole therapy, the dog no longer had lymphadenopathy, was active, had regained lost weight, the lesions in the right eye had resolved to depigmented scars, and the urine blastomycosis antigen was negative. Itraconazole therapy was discontinued, and the dog remained healthy for 2 more years before being lost to follow-up. This case represents a rather typical case of ocular blastomycosis in a young, male, large breed, hunting dog from an area endemic for the disease. The deterioration of the left eye following initiation of antifungal therapy is not uncommon as the dying organisms cause severe intraocular inflammation that can lead to endophthalmitis and secondary glaucoma. The mass die-off of organisms in the pulmonary tissues can also cause respiratory distress, as was seen in this case.

The low-level corticosteroid therapy in this case may have prevented the right eye from deteriorating due to inflammation from dying organisms and antigen stimulation in the anterior uvea. This case is somewhat uncommon in that the dog responded so favorably with an ultimate blastomycosis urinary antigen converting to a negative state and the patient having no signs of disease recurrence after only 6 months of antifungal therapy.

CASE 3

A 6-month-old M/N DSH cat was presented for bilateral blepharospasm. Physical examination was unremarkable, and both eyes had anterior uveitis (as in **Figure 11.54a**) as depicted by mild corneal edema, aqueous flare, fibrinohemorrhagic clots in the anterior chambers, rubeosis irides, ocular hypotension, and cloudy anterior vitreous. Due to the anterior chamber disease, detailed examination of the fundi was not possible. A complete blood count, serum biochemistry panel, urinalysis, FeLV/FIV serology, toxoplasmal serology, and FIP titer were performed. The kitten was found to have polyclonal hyperglobulinemia, hypoalbuminemia, and a FIP/corona virus titer of 1:3200, with all other parameters being normal. A tentative diagnosis of feline infectious peritonitis was made, and medical therapy was begun as topical prednisolone and atropine drops for the anterior uveitis. After 1 week, the ocular signs were greatly improved, and the patient was comfortable. Over the next 3 weeks, the patient became anorexic, dyspneic, and febrile. The kitten developed pulmonary and abdominal effusions. Systemic corticosteroid therapy was administered, but the kitten's general systemic condition deteriorated, and the owner elected humane euthanasia. This case represents a relatively routine case of FIP panuveitis in a young cat. As is typically seen, the kitten presented with bilateral ocular signs with no apparent systemic illness on cursory examination. Despite the ocular disorder responding somewhat favorably to symptomatic therapy, the kitten deteriorated as the disease began to affect other organs/body cavities. Other common infectious diseases causing feline uveitis were tested for and found not to be the culprit in this young cat. Were this cat older, other testing may have included bartonella testing and testing for systemic fungal diseases (depending on if the cat were from an endemic area). As is commonly the case with FIP, ocular signs were seen in this young cat, but ocular signs are not so common in the older cat.

CASE 4

An 8-year-old thoroughbred cross gelding was presented for anterior uveitis of 3 weeks duration that had not responded to symptomatic therapy with topical corticosteroids and atropine and oral NSAIDs. Historically, the patient was evaluated by the referring veterinarian for a painful left eye and was diagnosed with a small fluorescein-positive superficial corneal ulcer. Therapy with topical antibiotic ointment and atropine along with an oral NSAID resulted in epithelialization of the ulceration within 4 days, but the patient remained painful. Topical corticosteroids along with atropine and oral NSAIDs initially reduced pain, but after 2 weeks, the patient became even more painful with worsening of the ocular appearance (worsening corneal edema, beginning of perilimbal corneal neovascularization, and a small, white fluorescein-negative corneal focus in the area where the initial ulceration had been). After 5 more days, the white focus was larger, the neovascularization was more prominent, and the anterior chamber had a ventral fluid line of hypopyon (**Figure 11.54c**). The patient was referred for treatment of suspected equine recurrent uveitis. Slit lamp biomicroscopy revealed that the white corneal focus was an area of infiltrate that was midstromal in depth. A tentative diagnosis of stromal abscess/cellulitis with secondary anterior uveitis was made, and the owner selected conservative medical therapy over surgical intervention. Topical miconazole, chloramphenicol, and atropine were administered on a frequent basis via a subpalpebral lavage system. Systemic NSAIDs were also administered. After one week, the patient was much more comfortable, the corneal stromal focus was infiltrated with blood vessels, and the anterior uveitis signs were improved (**Figure 11.80a**). At 3 weeks after beginning topical antimicrobials and discontinuing topical corticosteroids, the cornea was beginning to clear from the periphery, and the signs of anterior uveitis were abating (**Figure 11.80b**). At 6 weeks, the patient was comfortable, had no signs of anterior uveitis, and the corneal lesion was continuing to resolve (**Figure 11.80c**). Medical therapy at that time was discontinued. At a 6-month recheck, the corneal lesion had shrunk to an avascular leukoma. This case represents an equine patient with an intense anterior uveitis due to corneal disease. The equine species (as well as the rabbit) exhibits rather dramatic anterior uveal inflammation in response to corneal injury/infection. Other therapy for this case could have included surgical excision of the infected corneal stroma and supportive medical therapy (see Chapter 10).

CASE 5

An 8-year-old M/N DSH cat was evaluated for unilateral ocular color change. On initial clinical examination, multifocal areas of iris stromal hyperpigmentation were noted (as in **Figure 11.71**), but there were no signs of anterior uveitis, nor were there any aqueous cells noted on slit lamp biomicroscopic examination. The other eye was normal, as was the physical examination. A tentative diagnosis of diffuse iris melanoma was made, the eye was photographed for future comparative purposes, and observation was recommended on a 6-month frequency. Over the next 3 years, progression of the pigmented focus was slow. The patient showed no signs of ocular irritation, and continued observation was recommended. At 5 years after initial exam, the owner reported dramatic change in the pigmentation, and although the owner had not presented the patient for reexamination in over a year, she presented the cat for reexam. The iris was diffusely pigmented (as in **Figure 11.72**), and pupillary dilation was incomplete with tropicamide application. The surface of the iris was irregular (as in **Figure 11.74**), and there were pigmented aqueous cells seen free floating in the aqueous humor via slit lamp biomicroscopy. Gonioscopy revealed minor accumulation of pigmented cells on the pectinate ligaments inferiorly, but the filtration angle was open. Due to concerns for dispersion of the melanoma to the systemic circulation with distal metastatic disease, enucleation was recommended. CBC, serum biochemistry panel, urinalysis, abdominal ultrasonography, and thoracic radiography were normal. A transpalpebral enucleation was performed, and the patient recovered uneventfully. Histopathological evaluation of the globe and the adnexa revealed no obvious extension of the tumor cells into the aqueous outflow channels that were examined. The patient was healthy for 2 more years before being lost to follow-up. This case describes a typical case of diffuse iris melanoma in a cat. Conservative visual monitoring allowed the patient to maintain a visual eye for over 5 years from initial diagnosis. In this case, despite the rather advanced state when enucleated, there was no systemic dissemination of the tumor, and the cat lived for at least 2 more years without signs of metastatic disease. Had the patient experienced glaucoma or infiltration of the aqueous outflow channels with tumor cells, the potential for distal metastasis to the liver, lungs, or other large organs would have been greater, and the long-term prognosis for survival would have been worse.

GENETIC PREDISPOSITION, ANTERIOR UVEA AND ANTERIOR CHAMBER

PERSISTENT PUPILLARY MEMBRANES (PPM)

Canine—Basenji, Pembroke Welsh corgi, Golden retriever, Chow Chow, English mastiff, English Cocker Spaniel

DYSCORIA

Canine—Australian shepherd, miniature dachshund, Great Dane

ANIRIDIA/IRIS HYPOPLASIA

Canine—Dalmatian

Equine—Belgian, Rocky Mountain horse, Kentucky Mountain saddle horse, Icelandic pony, American quarter horse

Cattle—Jersey

Sheep—Llanwenog

IRIS COLOBOMA

Canine—Australian shepherd

IRIS SPHINCTER ATROPHY

Canine—Miniature poodle, Chihuahua, toy breeds

UVEAL CYSTS

Canine—Golden retriever, Boston terrier, Labrador retriever, Great Dane

Equine—Rocky mountain horse, Kentucky mountain saddle horse, Icelandic pony

ANTERIOR SEGMENT DYSGENESIS/MULTIPLE CONGENITAL OCULAR ANOMALIES

Equine—Rocky mountain horse, Kentucky mountain saddle horse, Icelandic pony, Morgan

UVEODERMATOLOGIC SYNDROME (VKH-LIKE SYNDROME)

Canine—Akita, Irish setter, Siberian husky, Samoyed
Pig—Hormel Sinclair strain pig

ANTERIOR UVEAL MELANOMA

Canine—Labrador retriever, Golden retriever, miniature Schnauzer, German shepherd, American Cocker Spaniel

CILIARY BODY ADENOMA/ADENOCARCINOMA

Canine—Golden retriever, Labrador retriever

REFERENCES

1. Martin, C., and Anderson, B. 1981. Ocular anatomy. In: Gelatt, K.N., editor. *Veterinary Ophthalmology*. Lea & Febiger, Philadelphia, PA, pp. 12–121.
2. Smith, P.J., Pennea, L., MacKay, E.O., and Mames, R.N. 1997. Identification of sclerotomy sites for posterior segment surgery in the dog. *Veterinary and Comparative Ophthalmology* 7:180–189.
3. Shively, J., and Epling, G. 1969. Fine structure of the canine eye: Iris. *American Journal of Veterinary Research* 30:13–25.
4. Donovan, R., Carpenter, R., Schepens, C., and Tolentino, F. 1974. Histology of the normal Collie eye. II. Uvea. *Annals of Ophthalmology* 6:1175–1189.
5. Purtscher, E. 1962. The large arteries of the canine iris. *Berliner und Munchener Tierarztliche Wochenschrift* 74:436–438.
6. Prince, J., Diesem, C., Eglitis, I., and Ruskell, G. 1960. The globe. In: *Anatomy and Histology of the Eye and Orbit in Domestic Animals*. CC Thomas: Springfield, IL, pp. 13–42.
7. Davidson, H.J., Blanchard, G.L., and Coe, P.H. 1990. Idiopathic uveitis in a herd of Holstein cows. *Progress in Veterinary and Comparative Ophthalmology* 2:113–116.
8. Yoshitomi, T., and Ito, Y. 1986. Double reciprocal innervations in dog iris sphincter and dilator muscles. *Investigative Ophthalmology and Visual Science* 27:83–91.
9. Yoshitomi, T., and Ito, Y. 1988. Effects of indomethacin and prostaglandins on the dog iris sphincter and dilator muscles. *Investigative Ophthalmology and Visual Science* 29:127–132.
10. Thibos, L., Levick, W., and Morstyn, R. 1980. Ocular pigmentation in white and Siamese cats. *Investigative Ophthalmology and Visual Science* 19:475–486.
11. Smith, R., and Rudt, L. 1973. Ultrastructural studies of the blood–aqueous barrier. 2. The barrier to horseradish peroxidase in primates. *American Journal of Ophthalmology* 76:937–947.
12. Fox, M. 1963. Postnatal ontogeny of the canine eye. *Journal of the American Veterinary Medical Association* 143:968–974.
13. Bellhorn, R.W., Barnett, K.C., and Henkind, P. 1971. Ocular colobomas in domestic cats. *Journal of the American Veterinary Medical Association* 159:1015–1021.
14. Martin, C.L., Stiles, J., and Willis, M. 1997. Feline colobomatous syndrome. *Veterinary & Comparative Ophthalmology* 7:39–43.
15. Gelatt, K., and Veith, L. 1970. Hereditary multiple ocular anomalies in Australian Shepherd Dogs. *Veterinary Medicine/Small Animal Clinician* 65:39–42.
16. Gelatt, K.N., and McGill, L.D. 1973. Clinical characteristics of microphthalmia with colobomas of the Australian Shepherd Dog. *Journal of the American Veterinary Medical Association* 162:393–396.

17. Gwin, R., Wyman, M., Lim, D., Ketring, K., and Werling, K. 1981. Multiple ocular defects associated with partial albinism and deafness in the dog. *Journal of the American Animal Hospital Association* 17:401–408.

18. Gelatt, K., Powell, G., and Huston, K. 1981. Inheritance of microphthalmia with coloboma in the Australian Shepherd Dog. *American Journal of Veterinary Research* 42:1686–1690.

19. Eriksson, K. 1955. Hereditary aniridia with secondary cataract in horses. *Nordisk Veterinary Medicine* 7:773–793.

20. Joyce, J. 1983. Anridia in a Quarter horse. *Equine Veterinary Journal Supplement* 2:21–22.

21. Irby, N., and Aquirre, G. 1985. Congenital aniridia in a pony. *Journal of the American Veterinary Medical Association* 186:281–283.

22. Joyce, J.R., Martin, J., Storts, R.W., and Skow, L. 1990. Iridal hypoplasia (aniridia) accompanied by limbic dermoids and cataracts in a group of related Quarter horses. *Equine Veterinary Journal Supplement* 10:26–28.

23. Saunders, L., and Fincher, M. 1951. Hereditary multiple eye defects in grade Jersey cows. *Cornell Veterinarian* 41:351–366.

24. Crispin, S.M., Bazeley, K.J., Long, S.E., Gould, D.J., and Watts, J.A. 2000. Two cases of aniridia in Llanwenog sheep. *Veterinary Record* 147:364–365.

25. Bamber, R., and Herdman, E. 1933. Correlation between white coat colour, blue eyes, and deafness in cats. *Journal of Genetics* 27:407–413.

26. Lucas, D. 1954. Ocular associations of dappling in the coat colour of dogs. *Journal of Comparative Pathology* 64:260–266.

27. Bergsma, D., and Brown, K. 1971. White fur, blue eyes, and deafness in the domestic cat. *Journal of Heredity* 62:171–185.

28. Mair, I. 1973. Hereditary deafness in the white cat. *I. Hereditary and clinical aspects. Acta Otolaryngolica Supplement* 314:5–11.

29. Dausch, D., Wegner, W., Michaelis, M., and Reetz, I. 1977. Ophthalmologische befunde in einer merlezucht. *Deutsche Tierärztliche Wochenschrift* 84:453–492.

30. Coulter, D., Martin, C., and Alvarado, T. 1980. A cat with white fur and one blue eye. *California Veterinarian* 9:11–14.

31. Creel, D., Collier, L., Leventhal, A., Conlee, J., and Prieur, D. 1982. Abnormal retinal projections in cats with the Chediak–Higashi syndrome. *Investigative Ophthalmology and Visual Science* 23:798–801.

32. Gelatt, K., Johnson, K., and Peiffer, R. 1979. Primary iridal pigmental masses in three dogs. *Journal of the American Animal Hospital Association* 15:339–344.

33. Peiffer, R. 1981. The differential diagnosis of pigmented ocular lesions in the dog and cat. *California Veterinarian* 5:14–18.

34. Carter, J., and Mausolf, F. 1970. Clinical and histologic features of pigmented ocular cysts. *Journal of the American Animal Hospital Association* 6:194–200.

35. Corcoran, K., and Koch, S. 1993. Uveal cysts in dogs: 28 cases (1989–1991). *Journal of the American Veterinary Medical Association* 203:545–546.

36. Townsend, W.M., and Gornik, K.A. 2013. Prevalence of uveal cysts and pigmentary uveitis in Golden Retrievers in three Midwestern states. *Journal of the American Veterinary Medical Association* 243:1298–1301.

37. Deehr, A., and Dubielzig, R. 1998. A histopathological study of iridociliary cysts and glaucoma in Golden Retrievers. *Veterinary Ophthalmology* 1:153–158.

38. Spiess, B., Bolliger, J., Guscetti, F., Haessig, M., Lackner, P., and Ruehli, M. 1998. Multiple ciliary body cysts and secondary glaucoma in the Great Dane: A report of nine cases. *Veterinary Ophthalmology* 1:41–45.

39. Sapienza, J., Domenech, F., and Prades-Sapienza, A. 2000. Golden Retriever uveitis: 75 cases (1994–1999). *Veterinary Ophthalmology* 3:241–246.

40. Esson, D., Armour, M., Mundy, P. et al. 2009. The histopathological and immunohistochemical characteristics of pigmentary and cystic glaucoma in the Golden Retriever. *Veterinary Ophthalmology* 12:361–368.

41. Rubin, L. 1966. Cysts of the equine iris. *Journal of the American Veterinary Medical Association* 149:151–155.

42. Buyukmihci, N., MacMillan, A., and Scagliotti, R. 1992. Evaluation of zones of iris hypoplasia in horses and ponies. *Journal of the American Veterinary Medical Association* 200:940–942.

43. Dziezyc, J., Samuelson, D.A., and Merideth, S.R. 1990. Ciliary cysts in three ponies. *Equine Veterinary Journal Supplement* 10:22–25.

44. Ramsey, D.T., Ewart, S.L., Render, J.A., Cook, C.S., and Latimer, C.A. 1999. Congenital ocular abnormalities of Rocky Mountain horses. *Veterinary Ophthalmology* 2:47–59.

45. Komaromy, A.M., Rowlan, J.S., LaCroix, N.C., Mangan, B.G. 2011. Equine multiple congenital ocular anomalies (MCOA) syndrome in *PMEL17* (silver) mutant ponies: Five cases. *Veterinary Ophthalmology* 14:313–320.

46. Gemensky, A.J., Wilke, D.A., and Cook, C.S. 2004. The use of semiconductor diode laser for deflation and coagulation of anterior uveal cysts in dogs, cats, and horses: A report of 20 cases. *Veterinary Ophthalmology* 7:360–368.

47. Rochlitz, I. 1984. Feline dysautonomia (the Key–Gaskell or dilated pupil syndrome): A preliminary review. *Journal of Small Animal Practice* 25:587–598.

48. Sharp, N., Nash, A., and Griffiths, I. 1984. Feline dysautonomia (the Key–Gaskell syndrome): A clinical and pathological study of 40 cases. *Journal of Small Animal Practice* 25:599–615.

49. Kidder, A.C., Johannes, C.J., O'Brien, D.P. et al. 2008. Feline dysautonomia in the Midwestern United States: A retrospective study of nine cases. *Journal of Feline Medicine and Surgery* 10:130–136.

50. Scagliotti, R. 1980. Neuro-ophthalmology. In: Kirk, T., editor. *Current Veterinary Therapy VII*, 7th edition. WB Suanders: Philadelphia, PA, pp. 510–517.

51. Pandolfi, M. 1978. Intraocular hemorrhages: A hemostatic therapeutic approach. *Survey of Ophthalmology* 22:322–334.

52. Peiffer, R., Wilcock, B., and Yin, H. 1990. The pathogenesis and significance of pre-iridal fibrovascular membrane in domestic animals. *Veterinary Pathology* 27:41–45.

53. Nelms, S.R., Nasisse, M.P., Davidson, M.G., and Kirschner, S.E. 1993. Hyphema associated with retinal disease in dogs: 17 cases (1986–1991). *Journal of the American Veterinary Medical Association* 202:1289–1292.

54. Havener, W. 1978. *Ocular Pharmacology.* CV Mosby: St Louis, MO, pp. 703–719.

55. Ganley, J., Geiger, J., Clement, J., Rigby, P., and Levy, G. 1983. Aspirin and recurrent hyphema after blunt trauma. *American Journal of Ophthalmology* 96:797–801.

56. Wilson, F. 1980. Traumatic hyphema: Pathogenesis and management. *Ophthalmology* 87:910–919.

57. Lambrou, F., Snyder, R., and Williams, G. 1987. Use of tissue plasminogen activator in experimental hyphema. *Archives of Ophthalmology* 105:995–997.

58. Masket, S., Best, M., Fisher, L., Kronenberg, S., and Galin, M. 1971. Therapy in experimental hyphema. *Archives of Ophthalmology* 85:329–333.

59. Yasuna, E. 1974. Management of traumatic hyphema. *Archives of Ophthalmology* 91:190–191.

60. Spoor, T., Hammer, M., and Belloso, H. 1980. Traumatic hyphema: Failure of steroids to alter its course: A double-blind prospective study. *Archives of Ophthalmology* 98: 116–119.

61. Streilen, J. 1990. Anterior chamber-associated immune deviation: The privilege of immunity in the eye. *Survey of Ophthalmology* 35:67–73.

62. Streilein, J.W., Bradley, D., Sano, Y., and Sonoda, Y. 1996. Immunosuppressive properties of tissues obtained from eyes with experimentally manipulated corneas. *Investigative Ophthalmology and Visual Science* 37:413–424.

63. Zamiri, P., Sugita, S., and Streilein, J.W. 2007. Immunosuppressive properties of the pigmented epithelial cells and the subretinal space. *Chemical Immunology and Allergy* 92:86–93.

64. Streilein, J.W., and Niederkorn, J.Y. 1981. Induction of anterior chamber-associated immune deviation requires an intact, functioning spleen. *The Journal of Experimental Medicine* 153:1058–1067.

65. Wilkie, D.A. 1990. Control of ocular inflammation. *Veterinary Clinics of North America, Small Animal Practice* 20:693–713.

66. Rao, N., Romero, J., Fernandez, M., Sevanian, A., and Marak, G. 1987. Role of free radicals in uveitis. *Survey of Ophthalmology* 32:209–213.

67. Bito, L. 1984. Species differences in the reponse of the eye to irritation and trauma: A hypothesis of divergence in ocular defense mechanism, and the choice of experimental animals for eye research. *Experimental Eye Research* 39:807–829.

68. Toris, C., and Pederson, J. 1987. Aqueous humor dynamics in experimental iridocyclitis. *Investigative Ophthalmology and Visual Science* 28:477–481.

69. Massa, K., Gilger, B., Miller, T., and Davidson, M. 2002. Causes of uveitis in dogs: 102 cases (1989–2000). *Veterinary Ophthalmology* 5:93–98.

70. Curtis, R., and Barnett, K. 1973. The ocular lesions of infectious canine hepatitis. I. Clinical features. *Journal of Small Animal Practice* 14:375–389.

71. Carmichael, L. 1965. The pathogenesis of ocular lesions of infectious canine hepatitis. *Veterinary Pathology* 2:344–359.

72. Bistner, S., and Aguirre, G. 1972. Further studies in the immunopathogenesis of the ocular manifestations of canine hepatitis virus. *Proceedings of the Scientific Meeting of the American College of Veterinary Ophthalmologists*, Dallas, TX, 3:46–68.

73. Keenan, K., Buhles, W., Huxsoll, D., Williams, R., and Hildebrandt, P. 1977. Studies on the pathogenesis of *Rickettsia rickettsii* in the dog: Clinical and clinicopathologic changes of experimental infection. *American Journal of Veterinary Research* 38:851–856.

74. Troy, G., Vulgamott, J., and Turnwald, G. 1980. Canine ehrlichiosis: A retrospective study of 30 naturally occurring cases. *Journal of the American Animal Hospital Association* 16:181–187.

75. Kuehn, N., and Gaunt, S. 1985. Clinical and hematologic findings in canine ehrlichiosis. *Journal of the American Veterinary Medical Association* 186:355–358.

76. Davidson, M., Breitschwerdt, E., Nasisse, M. et al. 1989. Ocular manifestations of Rocky Mountain spotted fever in dogs. *Journal of the American Veterinary Medical Association* 194:777–781.

77. Glaze, M., and Gaunt, S. 1986. Uveitis associated with *Ehrlichia platys* infection in a dog. *Journal of the American Veterinary Medical Association* 188:916–918.

78. Leiva, M., Naranjo, C., and Pena, M.T. 2005. Ocular signs of canine monocytic ehrlichiosis: A retrospective study in dogs from Barcelona, Spain. *Veterinary Ophthalmology* 8:387–393.

79. Komnenou, A.A., Egyed, Z., Sreter, T. et al. 2007. Ocular manifestations of natural canine monocytic ehrlichiosis (*Ehrlichia canis*); a retrospective study of 90 cases. *Veterinary Ophthalmology* 10:137–142.

80. Cohen, N.D., Carter, C.N., Thomas, M.A., Angulo, A.M., and Eugster, A.K. 1990. Clinical and epizootiologic characteristics of dogs seropositive for *Borrelia burgdoreri* in Texas: 110 cases (1998). *Journal of the American Veterinary Medical Association* 197:893–898.

81. Littman, M.P., Goldstein, R.E., Labato, M.A., Lappin, M.R. et al. 2005. Lyme disease in dogs: Diagnosis, treatment, and prevention. *Journal of Veterinary Internal Medicine* 20:422–434.

82. Weigt, A.K., Duncen, R.B., and Pickett, J.P. 2000. A report of Lyme disease (*Borrelia burgdorferi*) with primary ocular involvement in a dog. *Proceedings of the Scientific Meeting of the American College of Veterinary Ophthalmologists*, Montreal, Quebec, Canada, 31:60.

83. Riecke, J., and Rhoades, H. 1975. *Brucella canis* isolated from the eye of the dog. *Journal of the American Veterinary Medical Association* 166:583–584.

84. Saegusa, J., Ueda, K., and Goto, Y. 1977. Ocular lesions in experimental canine brucellosis. *Japanese Journal of Veterinary Science* 39:181–185.

85. Gwin, R., Kolwalski, J., Wyman, M., and Winston, S. 1980. Ocular lesions associated with *Brucella canis* in a dog. *Journal of the American Animal Hospital Association* 16:607–610.

86. Gordon, J., Pue, H., and Rutgers, H. 1985. Canine brucellosis in a household. *Journal of the American Veterinary Medical Association* 186:695–698.

87. Ledbetter, E.C., Landry, M.P., Stokol, T. et al. 2009. *Brucella canis* endophthalmitis in 3 dogs: Clinical features, diagnosis, and treatment. *Veterinary Ophthalmology* 12:183–191.

88. Wanke, M.M. 2004. Canine brucellosis. *Animal Reproduction Science* 82:195–207.

89. Gwin, R., Makley, T., Wyman, M., and Werling, K. 1980. Multifocal ocular histoplasmosis in a dog and cat. *Journal of the American Veterinary Medical Association* 176:638–642.

90. Kerl, M.E. 2003. Update on canine and feline fungal diseases. *The Veterinary Clinics of North America. Small Animal Practice.* 33:721–747.

91. Sano, A., and Miyaji, M. 2003. Canine histoplasmosis in Japan. *Nihon Ishinkin Gakkai Zasshi* 44:239–243.

92. Ajello, J. 1958. Occurrence of *Cryptococcus neoformans* in soils. *American Journal of Hygiene* 67:72–77.

93. Hendrix, D.V., Rohrbach, B.W., Bochsler, P.N. et al. 2004. Comparison of histologic lesions of endophthalmitis induced by *Blastomyces dermatididis* in untreated and treated dogs: 36 cases (1986-2001). *Journal of the American Veterinary Medical Association* 224:1317–1322.

94. Johnson, L.R., Herrgsell, E.J., Davidson, A.P. et al. 2003. Clinical, clinicopathologic, and radiographic findings in dogs with coccidioidomycosis: 24 cases (1995-2000). *Journal of the American Veterinary medical Association* 222: 461–466.

95. Angell, J., Merideth, R., Shively, J., and Sigler, R. 1987. Ocular lesions associated with coccidioidomycosis in dogs: 35 cases (1980–1985). *Journal of the American Veterinary Medical Association* 190:1319–1322.

96. Bloom, J.D., Hamor, R.E., and Gerding, P.A. 1996. Ocular blastomycosis in dogs: 73 cases, 108 eyes (1985-1993). *Journal of the American Veterinary Medical Association* 209:1271–1274.

97. Legendre, A., Walker, M., Buyukmihci, N., and Stevens, R. 1981. Canine blastomycosis: A review of 47 clinical cases. *Journal of the American Veterinary Medical Association* 178:1163–1168.

98. Watt, P.R., Robins, G.M., Galloway, A.M., and O'Boyle, D.A. 1995. Disseminated opportunistic fungal disease in dogs: Ten cases (1982–1990). *Journal of the American Veterinary Medical Association* 207:67–70.

99. Troy, G.C., Panciera, D.L., Pickett, D.P. et al. 2013. Mixed infection caused by *Lecythophora canina* sp. nov. and *Plectosphaerella cucumerina* in a German shepherd dog. *Medical Mycology* 51:455–460.

100. Quinn, P., and McCraw, B. 1972. Current status of *Toxoplasma* and toxoplasmosis: A review. *Canadian Veterinary Journal* 13:247–262.

101. Dubey, J.P. 2004. Toxoplasmosis—A waterborne zoonosis. *Veterinary Parasitology* 126:57–72.

102. Dubey, J. 1985. Toxoplasmosis in dogs: A review. *Canine Practice* 12:7–28.

103. Piper, R., Cole, C., and Shadduck, J. 1970. Natural and experimental ocular toxoplasmosis in animals. *American Journal of Ophthalmology* 69:662–668.

104. Bussanich, M., and Rootman, J. 1985. Implicating toxoplasmosis as the cause of ocular lesions. *Veterinary Medicine* 80:43–51.

105. Dubey, J.P., Koestner, A., and Piper, R.C. 1990. Repeated transplacental transmission of *Neospora caninum* in dogs. *Journal of the American Veterinary Medical Association* 197:857–860.

106. McConnell, E., Chaffee, E., Cashell, I., and Garner, F. 1970. Visceral leishmaniasis with ocular involvement in a dog. *Journal American Veterinary Medicine Association* 156:197–203.

107. Giles, R., Hildebrandt, P., Becker, R., and Montgomery, C. 1975. Visceral leishmaniasis in a dog with bilateral endophthalmitis. *Journal of the American Animal Hospital Association* 11:155–159.

108. Tryphonas, L., Zawidzka, Z., Bernard, M.A., and Janzen, E.A. 1977. Visceral leishmaniasis in a dog: Clinical, hematological, and pathological observations. *Canadian Journal of Comparative Medicine* 41:1–12.

109. Swenson, C.L., Silverman, J., Stromberg, P.C. et al. 1988. Visceral leishmaniasisis in an English Fox Hound from an Ohio research colony. *Journal of the American Veterinary Medical Association* 193:1089–1092.

110. Boggiatto, P.M., Gibson-Corley, K.N., and Metz, K. 2011. Transplacental transmission of *Leishmania infantum* as a means for continued disease incidence in North America. *PLoS Neglected tropical Diseases* 5:e1019.

111. Migaki, G., Font, R., and Sauer, R. 1982. Canine protothecosis: Review of the literature and report of an additional case. *Journal of the American Veterinary Medical Association* 181:794–797.

112. Schultze, A.E., Ring, R.D., Morgan, R.V., and Patton, C.S. 1998. Clinical, cytologic, and histopathologic manifestations of protothecosis in two dogs. *Veterinary Ophthalmology* 1:239–243.

113. Gwin, R., Merideth, R., Martin, C., and Kaswan, R. 1984. Ophthalmomyiasis interna posterior in two cats and a dog. *Journal of the American Animal Hospital Association* 20:481–486.

114. Kaswan, R., and Martin, C. 1984. Ophthalmomyiasis interna in a dog and cat. *Canine Practice* 11:28–34.

115. Johnson, B.W., Helper, L.C., and Szajerski, M.E. 1988. Intraocular *Cuterebra* in a cat. *Journal of the American Veterinary Medical Association* 193:829–830.

116. Harris, B.P., Miller, P.E., Bloss, J.R. et al. 2000. Ophthalmomyiasis interna anterior associated with *Cutereba* spp. In a cat. *Journal of the American Veterinary Medical Association* 216:352–355.

117. Wyman, M., Starkey, R., Weisbrode, S. et al. 2005. Ophthalmomyiasis (interna posterior) or the posterior segment and central nervous system myiasis: *Cuterebra* spp. In a cat. *Veterinary Ophthalmology* 8:77–80.

118. Olliver, F.J., Barrie, K.P., Mames, R.N. et al. 2006. Pars plana vitrectomy for the treatment of ophthalmomyiasis interna posterior in a dog. *Veterinary Ophthalmology* 9:259–264.

119. Abdelbaki, Y., and Davis, R. 1972. Ophthalmoscopic findings in elaeophorosis of domestic sheep. *Veterinary Medicine/Small Animal Clinician* 67:69–74.

120. Shoho, C. 1994. Chronological review of the literature relating to 'the worm in the eye' of the horse and cattle. *Japanese Journal of Veterinary History* 31:19–45.

121. Moore, C.P., Sarazan, R.D., Whitley, R.D. et al. 1983. Equine ocular parasites: A review. *Equine Veterinary Journal, Supplement 2*, November 1983, 76–85.

122. Rames, D.S., Miller, D.K., Barthel, R. et al. 1995. Ocular *Halicephalobus* (syn. *Micronemia*) *deletrix* in a horse. *Veterinary Pathology* 32:540–542.

123. Bellhorn, R. 1973. Removal of intraocular *Dirofilaria immitis* with subsequent corneal scarring. *Journal of the American Animal Hospital Association* 9:262–264.

124. Brightman, A., Helper, L., and Todd, K. 1977. Heartworm in the anterior chamber of a dog's eye. *Veterinary Medicine/Small Animal Clinician* 72:1021–1023.

125. Blanchard, G., and Thayer, G. 1978. Intravitreal *Dirofilaria immitis* in a dog. *Journal of the American Animal Hospital Association* 14:33–35.

126. Forney, M. 1985. *Dirofilaria immitis* in the anterior chamber of a dog's eye. *Veterinary Medicine* 80:49.

127. Miller, W., and Cooper, R. 1987. Identifying and treating intraocular *Dirofilaria immitis* in dogs. *Veterinary Medicine* 82:381–385.

128. Carastro, S.M., Dugan, S.J., and Paul, A.J. 1992. Intraocular dirofilariasis in dogs. *Compendium on Continuing Education for the Practicing Veterinarian* 14:209–217.

129. Dantos-Torres, F., Lia, R.P., Barbuto, M. et al. 2009. Ocular dirofilariasis by *Dirofilaria immitis* in a dog: The first case report from Europe. *The Journal of Small Animal Practice* 50:667–669.

130. Gaunt, P.S., Confer, A.W., Carter, J.D., Trucksa, R.C., Neafie, R.C., and Litchtenfels, J.R. 1982. Intraocular strongylidiasis in a dog. *Journal of the American Animal Hospital Association* 18:120–122.

131. Perry, A.W., Hertling, R., and Kennedy, M.J. 1991. Angiostrongylosis with disseminated larval infection associated with signs of ocular and nervous disease in an imported dog. *Canadian Veterinary Journal* 32:430–431.

132. King, M.C., Grose, R.M., and Startup, G. 1994. *Angiostrongylus vasorum* in the anterior chamber of a dog's eye. *Journal of Small Animal Practice* 35:326–328.

133. Davidson, M.G., Nasisse, M. et al. 1991. Traumatic anterior lens capsule disruption. *Journal of the American Animal Hospital Association* 27:410–414.

134. Bell, C.M., Pot, S.A., and Dubielzig, R.R. 2013. Septic implantation syndrome in dogs and cats: A distinct pattern of endophthalmitis with lenticular abscess. *Veterinary Ophthalmology* 16:180–185.

135. Saunders, L., and Barron, C. 1964. Intraocular tumours in animals. IV. Lymphosarcoma. *British Veterinary Journal* 120:25–35.

136. Krohne, S.G., Henderson, N.M., Richardson, R.C. et al. 1994. Prevalence of ocular involvement in dogs with multicentric lymphoma: Prospective evakluation of 94 cases. *Veterinary & Comparative Ophthalmology* 4:127–135.

137. Wilcock, B., and Peiffer, R. 1987. The pathology of len-induced uveitis in dogs. *Veterinary Pathology* 24:549–553.

138. Fischer, C. 1971. Lens-induced uveitis and secondary glaucoma in a dog. *Journal of the American Veterinary Medical Association* 158:336–341.

139. Denis, H., Brooks, D.E., Alleman, A.R. et al. 2003. Detection of anti-lens crystalline antibody in dogs with and without cataracts. *Veterinary Ophthalmology* 6:321–327.

140. Marak, G. 1992. Phacoanaphylactic endophthalmitis. *Survey of Ophthalmology* 36:325–339.

141. Fischer, C. 1972 Lens-induced uveitis in dogs. *Journal of the American Animal Hospital Association* 8:39–48.

142. van der Woerdt, A., Nasisse, M. et al. 1992. Lens-induced uveitis in dogs: 151 cases (1985-1990). *Journal of the American Veterinary Medical Association* 201:921–926.

143. Van Der Woerdt, A. 2000. Lens-induced uveitis. *Veterinary Ophthalmology* 3:227–234.

144. Lim, C.C., Bakker, S.C., Waldner, C.L. et al. 2011. Cataracts in 44 dogs (77 eyes): A comparison of outcomes for no treatment, topical medical management, or phacoemulsification with intraocular lens implantation. *The Canadian Veterinary Journal* 52: 283–287.

145. Morgan, R.V. 1989. Vogt-Koyanagi-Harada syndrome in humans and dogs. *Compendium on Continuing Education for the Practicing Veterinarian* 11:1211–1218.

146. Kern, T., Walton, D., Riis, R., Manning, T., Laratta, L., and Dziezyc, J. 1985. Uveitis associated with poliosis and vitiligo in six dogs. *Journal of the American Veterinary Medical Association* 187:408–414.

147. Kaya, M., Edward, D., Tessler, H., and Hendricks, R. 1992. Augmentation of intraocular inflammation by melanin. *Investigative Ophthalmology and Visual Science* 33:522–531.

148. Cottrell, B., and Barnett, K. 1987. Harada's disease in the Japanese Akita. *Journal of Small Animal Practice* 28:517–521.

149. Herrera, H.D., and Duchene, A.G. 1998. Uveodermatological syndrome (Vogt–Koyanagi–Harada-like syndrome) with generalized depigmentation in a Dachshund. *Veterinary Ophthalmology* 1(1):47–51.

150. Asakura, I. 1977. Harada's syndrome (uveitis diffusa acuta) in the dog. *Japanese Journal of Veterinary Medicine* 673:445–455.

151. Bussanich, M. 1982. Granulomatous panuveitis and dermal depigmentation in dogs. *Journal of the American Animal Hospital Association* 18:131–138.

152. Romatowski, J. 1985. A uveodermatological syndrome in an Akita dog. *Journal of the American Animal Hospital Association* 21:777–780.

153. Campbell, K., McLaughlin, S., and Reynolds, H. 1986. Generalized leukoderma and poliosis following uveitis in a dog. *Journal of the American Animal Hospital Association* 22:121–124.

154. Esson, D., Armour, M., Mundy, P. et al. 2009. The histopathological and immunohistochemical characteristics of pigmentary and cystic glaucoma in the Golden Retriever. *Veterinary Ophthalmology* 12:361–368.

155. Gwin, R., Wyman, M., Ketring, K., and Winston, S. 1980. Idiopathic uveitis and exudative retinal detachment in the dog. *Journal of the American Animal Hospital Association* 16:163–170.

156. Andrew, S.E., Abrams, K.L., Brooks, D.E., and Kubilis, P.S. 1997. Clinical features of steroid-responsive retinal detachments in 22 dogs. *Veterinary and Comparative Ophthalmology* 7:82–87.

157. Corcoran, K.A., Peiffer, R.L., and Koch, S.A. 1997. Histopathologic features of feline ocular lymphosarcoma. *Veterinary and Comparative Ophthalmology* 5:35–40.

158. Peiffer, R., and Wilcock, B. 1991. Histopathologic study of uveitis in cats: 139 cases (1978–1988). *Journal of the American Veterinary Medical Association* 198:135–138.

159. Davidson, M., Nasisse, M., English, R., Wilcock, B., and Jamieson, V. 1991. Feline anterior uveitis: A study of 53 cases. *Journal of the American Animal Hospital Association* 27:77–83.

160. Lubin, J., Albert, D., Essex, M., Noronha, F., and Riis, R. 1983. Experimental anterior uveitis after subcutaneous injection of feline sarcoma virus. *Investigative Ophthalmology and Visual Science* 24:1055–1062.

161. Miller, P.E., and Dubielzig, R.R. 2007. Ocular tumors. In: *Small Animal Clinical Oncology*, 4th edition. Saunders Elsevier: St. Louis, MO, pp. 686–698.

162. Dubielzig, R., Steinberg, H., Fischer, B., Jackson, M., and Moore, P. 2000 Feline primary ocular lymphosarcoma: Immunophenotyping of leukocytes, FeLV status, and relationship to idiopathic lymphoplasmacytic uveitis. *Proceedings of the Scientific Meeting of the American College of Veterinary Ophthalmologists*, Montreal, Quebec, Canada, 31:46.

163. Andrew, S. 2000. Feline infectious peritonitis. *The Veterinary Clinics of North America. Small Animal Practice* 30:987–1000.

164. Addie, D.D., and Jarrett, O. 1998. Feline coronavirus infection. In: *Infectious Diseases of the Dog and Cat*. WB Saunders: Philadelphia, PA, pp. 58–69.

165. Pederson, N. 1997. An overview of feline enteric coronavirus and feline infectious peritonitis virus infections. *Feline Practice* 23:7–20.

166. Kornegay J. 1978. Feline infectious peritonitis: The central nervous system form. *Journal of the American Animal Hospital Association* 14:580–584.

167. Wiess, R., and Scott, F. 1981. Pathogenesis of feline infectious peritonitis: Pathologic changes and immunofluorescence. *American Journal of Veterinary Research* 42:2036–2048.

168. Mahaffey, E., Gabbert, N., Johnson, D., and Guffy, M. 1977. Disseminated histoplasmosis in three cats. *Journal of the American Animal Hospital Association* 13:46–50.

169. Peiffer, R. 1979. Ocular manifestations of disseminated histoplasmosis in a cat. *Feline Practice* 9:24–29.

170. Wolf, A., and Belden, M. 1984. Feline histoplasmosis: A literature review and retrospective study of 20 new cases. *Journal of the American Animal Hospital Association* 20:995–998.

171. Clinkenbeard, K., Cowell, R., and Tyler, R. 1987. Disseminated histoplasmosis in cats: 12 cases (1981–1986). *Journal of the American Veterinary Medical Association* 190:1445–1448.

172. Blouin, P., and Cello, R. 1980. Experimental ocular cryptococcosis: Preliminary studies in cats and mice. *Investigative Ophthalmology and Visual Science* 19:21–30.

173. Alden, C., and Mohan, R. 1974. Ocular blastomycosis in a cat. *Journal of the American Veterinary Medical Association* 164:527–528.

174. Nasisse, M., van Ee, R., and Wright, B. 1985. Ocular changes in a cat with disseminated blastomycosis. *Journal of the American Veterinary Medical Association* 187:629–631.

175. Miller, P.E., Miller, L.M., and Schoster, J.V. 1990. Feline blastomycosis: A report of three cases and literature review (1961-1988). *Journal of the American Animal Hospital Association* 26:417–424.

176. Angell, J., Shively, J., Meredith, R., Reed, R., and Jamison, K. 1985. Ocular coccidioidomycosis in a cat. *Journal of the American Veterinary Medical Association* 187:167–170.

177. Miller, W.W., and Albert, R.A. 1988. Ocular and systemic candidiasis in a cat. *Journal of the American Animal Hospital Association* 21:521–524.

178. Vainisi, S., and Campbell, H. 1969. Ocular toxoplasmosis in cats. *Journal of the American Veterinary Medical Association* 154:141–152.

179. Lappin, M. 1989. Clinical feline toxoplasmosis: Serologic diagnosis and therapeutic management of 15 cases. *Journal of Veterinary Internal Medicine* 3:139–143.

180. Davidson, M.G. 2000. Toxoplasmosis. The Veterinary Clinics of North America. *Small Animal Practice* 30:1051–1062.

181. Dubey, J., and Carpenter, J. 1993. Histologically confirmed clinical toxoplasmosis in cats: 100 cases (1952–1990). *Journal of the American Veterinary Medical Association* 203:1556–1566.

182. Davidson, M.G., Rottman, J.B., English, R.V. et al. 1993. Feline immunodeficiency virus predisposes cats to acute generalized toxoplasmosis. *The American Journal of Pathology* 143:1486–1497.

183. Lappin, M.R., and Black, J.C. 1999. *Bartonella* spp. infection as a possible cause of uveitis in a cat. *Journal of the American Veterinary Medical Association* 214:1205–1207.

184. Breitschwerdt, E.B., Maggi, R.G., Chomel, B.B. et al. 2010. Bartonellosis: An emerging infectious disease of zoonotic importance to animals and human beings. *Journal of Veterinary Emergency and Critical Care* 20:8–30.

185. Lappin, M.R., Kordick, D.L., and Breitschwerdt, E.B. 2000. *Bartonella* spp. antibodies and DNA in aqueous humor of cats. *Journal of Feline Medicine and Surgery* 2:61–68.

186. Stiles, J. 2011. Bartonellosis in cats: A role in uveitis? *Veterinary Ophthalmology* 14(Supp. 1)9–14.

187. Fontenelle, J.P., Powell, C.C., Hill, A.E. et al. 2008. Prevalence of serum antibodies against *Bartonella* species in the serum of cats with or without uveitis. *Journal of Feline Medicine and Surgery* 10:41–46.

188. Lappin, M., Marks, A., Greene, C. et al. 1992. Serologic prevalence of selected infectious diseases in cats with uveitis. *Journal of the American Veterinary Medical Association* 201:1005–1016.

189. Chavkin, M., Lappin, M., and Powell, C. 1992. Seroepidemiologic and clinical observations of 93 cases of uveitis in cats. *Progress in Veterinary and Comparative Ophthalmology* 2:29–36.

190. Lappin, M., Greene, C., and Prestwood, A. 1989. Enzyme-linked immunosorbent assay for detection of circulating antigens of *Toxoplasma gondii* in the serum of cats. *American Journal of Veterinary Research* 50:1566–1586.

191. Lappin, M., Greene, C., Prestwood, A., Dawe, D., and Tarleton, R. 1989. Diagnosis of recent *Toxoplasmosis gondii* infection in cats by use of an enzynme-linked immunosorbent assay for immunoglobulin M. *American Journal of Veterinary Research* 50:1586–1590.

192. Davidson, M., and English, R. 1998. Feline ocular toxoplasmosis. *Veterinary Ophthalmology* 1:71–80.

193. Gormley, P., Pavesio, C., Minnasian, D., and Lightman, S. 1998. Effects of drug therapy on *Toxoplasma* cysts in an animal model of acute and chronic disease. *Investigative Ophthalmology and Visual Science* 39:1171–1175.

194. English, R., Davidson, M., Nasisse, M., Jamieson, V., and Lappin, M. 1990. Intraocular disease associated with feline immunodeficiency virus infection in cats. *Journal of the American Veterinary Medical Association* 196:1116–1119.

195. Maggs, D.J., Lappin, M.R., and Nasisse, M.P. 1999. Detection of feline herpes-specific antibodies and DNA in aqueous humor from cats with or without uveitis. *American Journal of Veterinary Research* 60:932–936.

196. Cooley, P.L., Wyman, M., and Kindig, O. 1990. Pars plicata in equine recurrent uveitis. *Veterinary Pathology* 27:138–140.

197. Dubielzig, R.R., Render, J.A., and Morreale, R.J. 1997. Distinctive morphologic features of the ciliary body in equine recurrent uveitis. *Veterinary and Comparative Ophthalmology* 7:163–167.

198. Jones, T., and Maurer, F. 1942. Heredity in periodic ophthalmia. *Journal of the American Veterinary Medical Association* 101:248–250.

199. Jones, T., Roby, T., and Maurer, F. 1946. The relation of riboflavin to equine periodic ophthalmia. *American Journal of Veterinary Research* 7:403–416.

200. Jones, T. 1949. Riboflavin and the control of equine periodic ophthalmia. *Journal of the American Veterinary Medical Association* 94:326–329.

201. Saari, K.M., Solja, J., Hakli, J. et al. 1981. Genetic background of acute anterior uveitis. *American Journal of Ophthalmology* 91:711–720.

202. Dwyer, A., Crockett, R., and Kalsow, C. 1995. Association of leptospiral seroreactivity and breed with uveitis and blindness in horses: 372 cases (1986–1993). *Journal of the American Veterinary Medical Association* 207:1327–1331.

203. Fritz, K.L., Kaese, H.J., Valberg, S.J. et al. 2013. Genetic risk factors for insidious equine recurrent uveitis in Appaloosa horses. *International Foundation for Animal Genetics* 45:392–399.

204. Kulbrock, M., Lehner, S., Metzger, J. et al. 2013. A genome-wide association study identifies risk loci to equine recurrent uveitis in German warmblood horses. *PloS One* 8(8):1–6.

205. Dwyer, A., and Kalsow, C. 1998. Visual prognosis in horses with uveitis. *Proceedings of the Annual Meeting of the American Society of Veterinary Ophthalmology*, Seattle, WA, pp. 1–8.

206. Gilger, B.C., Malok, E., Cutter, K.V. et al. 1999. Characterization of T-lymphocytes in the anterior uvea of eyes with chronic equine recurrent uveitis. *Veterinary Immunology and Immunopathology* 71:17–28.

207. Deeg, C.A., Kaspers, B., Gerhards, H. et al. 2001. Inter- and intramolecular epitope spreading in equine recurrent uveitis. *Investigative Ophthalmology and Visual Science* 47:652–656.

208. Deeg, C.A., Hauck, S.M., Amann, B. et al. 2006. Identification and functional validation of novel autoantigens in equine uveitis. *Molecular and Cellular Proteomics* 5:1462–1470.

209. Stannard, A., and Cello, R. 1975. *Onchocerca cervicalis* infection in horses from the western United States. *American Journal of Veterinary Research* 36:1029–1031.

210. Lloyd, S., and Soulsby, E. 1978. Survey for infection with *Onchocerca cervicalis* in horses in the eastern United States. *American Journal of Veterinary Research* 39:1962–1963.

211. Lyons, E., Drudge, J., and Tolliver, S. 1981. Prevalence of microfilariae (*Onchocerca* spp.) in skin of Kentucky horses at necropsy. *Journal of the American Veterinary Medical Association* 179:899–900.

212. Attenburrow, D., Donnelly, J., and Soulsby, E. 1983. Periodic ophthalmic (recurrent) uveitis of horses: An evaluation of the aetiological role of microfilariae of *Onchocerca cervicalis* and the clinical management of the condition. *Equine Veterinary Journal Supplement* 2:48–56.

213. Cummings, E., and James, E. 1985. Prevalence of equine onchocerciasis in the southeastern and Midwestern United States. *Journal of the American Veterinary Medical Association* 186:1202–1203.

214. Cello, R. 1971. Ocular onchocerciasis in the horse. *Equine Veterinary Journal* 3:148–153.

215. Wollanke, B., Rohrbach, B., and Gerhards, H. 2001. Serum and vitreous humor antibody titers in, and isolation of, *Leptospira interrogans* from horses with recurrent uveitis. *Journal of the American Veterinary Medical Association* 219:795–800.

216. Rimpau, W. 1947. Leptospirose being pferde. *Tierarztliche Umschau* 2:177–178.

217. Heusser, H. 1948. Die periodische augenentzundung, eine leptospirose? *Schweizer Archiv fur Tierheilkunde* 90:288–312.

218. Roberts, S. 1958. Sequelae of leptospirosis in horses on a small farm. *Journal of the American Veterinary Medical Association* 133:189–194.

219. Halliwell, R., Brim, T., Hines, M., Wolf, D., and White, F. 1985. Studies on equine recurrent uveitis. II. The role of infection with *Leptospira interrogans* serovar *pomona*. *Current Eye Research* 4:1033–1040.

220. Sillerud, C., Bey, R., Ball, M., and Bistner, S. 1987. Serologic correlation of suspected *Leptospira interrogans* serovar *pomona*-induced uveitis in a group of horses. *Journal of the American Veterinary Medical Association* 191:1576–1578.

221. Williams, R., Morter, R., Freeman, M., and Lavignette, A. 1971. Experimental chronic uveitis. *Investigative Ophthalmology* 10:948–954.

222. Matthews, A., Waitkins, S., and Palmer, M. 1987. Serological study of leptospiral infections and endogenous uveitis among horses and ponies in the United Kingdom. *Equine Veterinary Journal* 19:125–128.

223. Wollanke, B., Gerhards, H., Brem, S., Gothe, R., and Wolf, E. 1999. Studies on vitreous and serum samples from horses with equine recurrent uveitis (ERU): The role of Leptospira, Borrelia burgdorferi, Borna disease virus, and Toxoplasma in the etiology of ERU. *Proceedings of the Scientific Meeting of the American College of Veterinary Ophthalmologists*, Chicago, IL, 29:31.

224. Polle, F., Storey, E., Eades, S. et al. 2014. Role of intra-ocular *Leptospira* infections in the pathogenesis of equine recurrent uveitis in the southern United States. *Journal of Equine Veterinary Science* 34:1300–1306.

225. Burgess, E., Gillette, D., and Pickett, P. 1986. Arthritis and panuveitis as manifestations of *Borrelia burgdorferi* infection in a Wisconsin pony. *Journal of the American Veterinary Medical Association* 189:1340–1342.

226. Knickelbein, K.E., Scherrer, N.M., Engiles, J.B. et al. 2016. Uveitis associated with Borrelia infection in 5 horses. *Proceedings of the Scientific Meeting of the American College of Veterinary Ophthalmologists*, Monterey, CA, 47:84.

227. Jones, T. 1940. The relation of brucellosis to periodic ophthalmia in Equidae. *American Journal of Veterinary Research* 1:54–57.

228. Davis, G., Wood, R., Gadd, J., and Kennedy, R. 1950. The incidence of *Brucella* agglutinins in horses and their relationship to periodic ophthalmia. *Cornell Veterinarian* 40:364–366.

229. Roberts, S. 1971. Chorioretinitis in a band of horses. *Journal of the American Veterinary Medical Association* 158:2043–2046.

230. Quin, A. 1950. The control of equine strongylosis and periodic ophthalmia with a ration additive. *British Veterinary Journal* 106:116–118.

231. Matthews, A., and Handscombe, M. 1983. Uveitis in the horse: A review of the aetiological and immunopathological aspects of the disease. *Equine Veterinary Journal Supplement* 2:61–64.

232. Romeike, A., Brugmann, M., and Drommer, W. 1998. Immunohistochemical studies in equine recurrent uveitis (ERU). *Veterinary Pathology* 35:515–526.

233. Gilger, B.C., Salmon, J.H., Yi, N.Y. et al. 2008. Role of bacteria in the pathogenesis of recurrent uveitis in horses from the southeastern United States. *American Journal of Veterinary Research* 69:1329–1335.

234. Hines, M., and Halliwell, R. 1991. Autoimmunity to retinal S-antigen in horses with equine recurrent uveitis. *Progress in Veterinary and Comparative Ophthalmology* 1:283–290.

235. Maxwell, S., Hurt, D., Brightman, A., and Takemoto, D. 1991. Humoral responses to retinal proteins in horses with recurrent uveitis. *Progress in Veterinary and Comparative Ophthalmology* 1:155–161.

236. Deeg, C.A., Ehrenhofer, M., Thurau, S.R. et al. 2002. Immunopathology of recurrent uveitis in spontaneously diseased horses. *Experimental Eye Research* 75:127–133.

237. Wolfer, J., Wilcock, B., and Percy, D. 1993. Phacoclastic uveitis in the rabbit. *Veterinary and Comparative Ophthalmology* 3:92–97.

238. Stiles, J., Didier, E., Ritchie, B., Greenacre, C., Willis, M., and Martin, C. 1997. *Encephalitozoon cuniculi* in the lens of a rabbit with phacoclastic uveitis: Confirmation and treatment. *Veterinary and Comparative Ophthalmology* 7: 233–238.

239. Wolfer, J., Grahn, B., Taylor, M., and Laperriere, E. 1995. Treatment of phacoclastic uveitis in the rabbit by phacoemulsification. *Proceedings of the Scientific Meeting of the American College of Veterinary Ophthalmologists*, Newport, RI, 26:12.

240. Rebhun, W.C., Jenkins, D.H., Riis, R.C. et al. 1988. An epizootic of blindness and encephalitis associated with herpesvirus indistinguishable from equine herpesvirus 1 in a herd of llamas and alpacas. *Journal of the American Veterinary Medical Association* 192:953–956.

241. Chavkin, M.J., Lappin, M.R., Powell, C.C., Cooper, C.M., Munana, K.R., and Howard, L.H. 1994. *Toxoplasma gondii*-specific antibodies in the aqueous humor of cats with toxoplasmosis. *American Journal of Veterinary Research* 55:1244–1249.

242. Lappin, M., and Powell, C. 1991. Comparison of latex agglutination, indirect hemagglutination, and ELISA techniques for the detection of *Toxoplasma gondii*-specific antibodies in the serum of cats. *Journal of Veterinary Internal Medicine* 5:299–301.

243. Davidson, M., Nasisse, M.P., and Roberts, S.M. 1987. Immunodiagnosis of leptospiral uveitis in two horses. *Equine Veterinary Journal* 19:155–157.

244. Faber, N., Crawford, M., LeFebvre, R. et al. 2000. Detection of *Leptospiral* spp. in the aqueous humor of horses with naturally acquired recurrent uveitis. *Journal of Clinical Microbiology* 38:2731–2733.

245. Wollanke, B.B., Rohrback, B.W., Gerhards, H. 2001. Serum and vitreous humor antbody titers in and isolation of *Leptospira interrogans* from a horse with recurrent uveitis. *Journal of the American Veterinary Medical Association* 219:795–800.

246. Thomasy, S.M., Lim, C.C., Reilly, C.M. et al. 2011. Evaluation of orally administered famciclovir in cats experimentally infected with feline herpesvirus type-1. *American Journal of Veterinary Research* 72:85–95.

247. Hendrix, D., Rohrbach, B., and Bochsler, P. 2004. Comparison of histologic lesions of endophthalmitis induced by *Blastomyces dermatitidis* in treated and untreated dogs:36 cases (1986-2001). *Journal of the American Veterinary Medical Association* 224:1317–1322.

248. Finn, M.J., Stiles, J., and Krohne, S.G. 2007. Visual outcome in a group of dogs with ocular blastomycosis treated with systemic antifungals and systemic corticosteroids. *Veterinary Ophthalmology* 10:299–303.

249. Brooks, D.E., Legendre, A.M., Gum, G.G. et al. 1991. The treatment of canine ocular blastomycosis with systemically administered itraconazole. *Progress in Veterinary and Comparative Ophthalmology* 1:263–268.

250. Bloom, J.D., Hamor, R.E., and Gerding, P.A. 1996. Ocular blastomycosis in dogs: 73 cases, 108 eyes (1985–1993). *Journal of the American Veterinary Medical Association* 209:1271–1274.

251. Herd, R., and Donham, J. 1983. Efficacy of ivermectin against *Onchocerca cervicalis* microfilarial dermatitis in horses. *American Journal of Veterinary Research* 44:1102–1105.

252. van Alphen, G.W., and Macri, F.J. 1966. Entrance of fluorescein into the aqueous humor of cat eye. *Archives of Ophthalmology* 75:247–253.

253. Krohne, S.G., Gionfriddo, J., Morrison, E.A. et al. 1998. Inhibition of pilocarpine-induced aqueous humor flare, hypotony, and miosis by topical administration of antiinflammatory and anesthetic drugs to dogs. *American Journal of Veterinary Research* 59:482–488.

254. Krohne, S.G., Blair, M.J., Bingaman, D., and Gionfriddo, J. 1998. Carprofcn inhibition of flare in the dog measured by laser flare photometry. *Veterinary Ophthalmology* 1:81–84.

255. Moore, C.P. 2001. Ophthalmic pharmacology. In: Adams, H.R., editor. *Veterinary Pharmacology and Therapeutics*, 8th edition. Iowa State University Press: Ames, IA, pp. 1120–1148.

256. Wakefield, D., McCluskey, P., and Reece, G. 1990. Cyclosporine therapy in Vogt–Koyanagi–Harada disease. *Australian New Zealand Journal of Ophthalmology* 18:137–142.

257. Gram, W.D., and Pariser, M. 2011. Uveodermatologic syndrome. In: Tilley, L.P., and Smith, F.W.K., editors. *Blackwell's Five-Minute Veterinary Consult: Canine and Feline*. Wiley-Blackwell: Ames, IA, p. 1283.

258. Gilger, B.C., Malok, E. Stewart, T. et al. 2000. Effect of an intravitreal cyclosporine implant on experimental uveitis in horses. *Veterinary Immunology and Immunopathology* 76:239–255.

259. Gilger, B.C., Salmon, J.H., Wilke, D.A. et al. 2006. A novel bioerodible deep scleral lamellar cyclosporine implant for uveitis. *Investigative Ophthalmology and Visual Science* 47:2596–2605.

260. Gilger, B.C., Wilke, D.A., Davidson, M.G. et al. 2001. Use of an intravitreal sustained-release cyclosporine delivery device for treatment of equine recurrent uveitis. *American Journal of Veterinary Research* 62:1892–1896.

261. Gilger, B.C., Wilke, D.A., Clode, A.B. et al. 2010. Long-term outcome after implantation of a suprachoroidal cyclosporine drug delivery device in horses with recurrent uveitis. *Veterinary Ophthalmology* 13:294–300.

262. Gilger, B.C., and Deeg, C. 2011. Equine recurrent uveitis. In: Gilger, B.C., editor. *Equine Ophthalmology*, 2nd edition. Elsevier-Saunders: Maryland Heights, MO, pp. 317–349.

263. Winterberg, A., and Gerhards, H. 1997. Langzeitergebnisse der pars-plana-vitrektomie bei equiner rezidivierender uveitis. *Pferdeheilkunde* 13:377–383.

264. Fruhauf, B., Ohnesorge, B., Deegen, E., and Boevé, M. 1998. Surgical management of equine recurrent uveitis with single port pars plana vitrectomy. *Veterinary Ophthalmology* 1:137–151.

265. Gilger, B.C., and Spiess, B. 2006. Surgical management of equine recurrent uveitis. In: Stick, J., and Auer, J., editors. *Equine Surgery*. WB Saunders: Philadelphia, PA, Chapter 62, pp. 749–755.

266. Spiess, B. 2011. Pars plana vitrectomy. In: Gilger, B.C., editor. *Equine Recurrent Uveitis. In: Equine Ophthalmology*, 2nd edition. Elsevier-Saunders: Maryland Heights, MO, pp. 344–346.

267. Tomordy, E., Hassig, M., and Spiess, B. 2010. The outcome of pars plana vitrectomy in horses with equine recurrent uveitis with regard to the presence or absence of intravitreal antibodies against various serovars of *Leptospira interrogans*. *Pferdeheikunde* 26:251–254.

268. Brooks, D., Cutler, T., Andrew, S. et al. 2001. Outcome of pars plana vitrectomy in 24 eyes of 18 horses with equine recurrent uveitis. *Proceedings of the Scientific Meeting of the American College of Veterinary Ophthalmologists*, Sarasota, FL, 32:38.

269. Rohrbach, B., Ward, D., Hendrix, D. et al. 2005. Effect of vaccination against leptospirosis on the frequency, days to recurrence, and progression of disease in horses with equine recurrent uveitis. *Veterinary Ophthalmology* 8:171–179.

270. Davidson, M., Nasisse, M., Jamieson, V., English, R., and Olivero, D. 1991. Traumatic anterior lens capsule disruption. *Journal of the American Animal Hospital Association* 27:410–414.

271. Paulson, M.E., and Kass, P.H. 2012 Traumatic corneal laceration with associated lens capsule disruption: A retrospective study of 77 clinical cases from 1999 to 2009. *Veterinary Ophthalmology* 15:355–368.

272. Olin, D., Roger, W., and MacMillan, A. 1976. Lipid-laden aqueous humor associated with anterior uveitis and concurrent hyperlipemia in two dogs. *Journal of the American Veterinary Medical Association* 168:861–864.

273. Zarfoss, M.K., and Dubielzig, R.R. 2007. Solid intraocular xanthogranuloma in three miniature Schnauzer dogs. *Veterinary Ophthalmology* 10:304–307.

274. Bellhorn, R., and Henkind, P. 1968. Adenocarcinoma of the ciliary body: A report of two cases in dogs. *Veterinary Pathology* 5:122–126.

275. Bellhorn, R. 1971. Ciliary body adenocarcinoma in the dog. *Journal of the American Veterinary Medical Association* 159:1124–1128.

276. Peiffer, R., Gwin, R., Gelatt, K., Jackson, W., Williams, L., and Hill, C. 1978. Ciliary body epithelial tumors in four dogs. *Journal of the American Veterinary Medical Association* 172:578–583.

277. Peiffer, R. 1983. Ciliary body epithelial tumors in the dog and cat: A report of thirteen cases. *Journal of Small Animal Practice* 24:347–370.

278. Barron, C., and Saunders, L. 1959. Intraocular tumors in animals. *II. Primary nonpigmented intraocular tumors. Cancer Research* 19:1171–1174.

279. Verwer, M., and Thije, P. 1967. Tumour of the epithelium of the ciliary body in a dog. *Journal of Small Animal Practice* 8:627–630.

280. Saunders, L., Geib, L., and Barron, C. 1969. Intraocular ganglioglioma in a dog. *Veterinary Pathology* 6:525–533.

281. Wilcock, B., and Williams, M. 1980. Malignant intraocular medulloepithelioma in a dog. *Journal of the American Animal Hospital Association* 16:617–619.

282. Brooks, D.E., and Patton, C.S. 1991. An ocular ganglioneuroblastoma in a dog. *Progress in Veterinary and Comparative Ophthalmology* 1:299–302.

283. Naranjo, C., Dubielzig, R.R., and Friedrichs, K.R. 2007. Canine ocular histiocytic sarcoma. *Veterinary Ophthalmology* 10:179–185.

284. Heath, S., Rankin, A.J., and Dubielzig, R.R. 2003. Primary ocular osteosarcoma in a dog. *Veterinary Ophthalmology* 6:85–87.

285. Zarfoss, M.K., Jones, Y., Colitz, C.M., Dubielzig, R.R., Klauss, G. et al. 2007. Uveal spindle cell tumor of blue-eyed dogs: An immunohistochemical study. *Veterinary Pathology* 44:276–284.

286. Giuliano, E., Chappell, R., Fischer, B., Dubielzig, R. et al. 1999. A matched observational study of canine survival with primary intraocular melanocytic neoplasia. *Veterinary Ophthalmology* 2:185–190.

287. Bussanich, N.M., Dolman, P.J., Rootman, J., and Dolman, CL. 1987. Canine uveal melanomas: Series and literature review. *Journal of the American Animal Hospital Association* 23:415–422.

288. Ditter, R., Dubielzig, R., Aguirre, G., and Acland, G. 1983. Primary ocular melanoma in dogs. *Veterinary Pathology* 20:379–395.

289. Ryan, A., and Diter, S.R. 1984. Clinical and pathologic features of canine ocular melanomas. *Journal of the American Veterinary Medical Association* 184:60–67.

290. Schaffer, E., and Funke, K. 1985. Das primar-intraokulare maligne melanom bei hund und katze. *Tierarztliche Praxis* 13:343–359.

291. Trucksa, R., McLean, I., and Quinn, A. 1985. Intraocular canine melanocytic neoplasms. *Journal of the American Animal Hospital Association* 21:85–88.

292. Wilcock, B., and Peiffer, R. 1986. The morphology and behavior of primary ocular melanomas in 91 dogs. *Veterinary Pathology* 23:418–424.

293. Render, J., Ramsey, D., and Ramsey, C. 1997. Contralateral uveal metastasis of malignant anterior uveal melanoma in a dog. *Veterinary and Comparative Ophthalmology* 7:263–266.

294. Roperto, F., Restucci, B., and Crovace, A. 1993. Bilateral ciliary body melanomas in a dog. *Progress in Veterinary and Comparative Ophthalmology* 3:149–151.

295. Cook, C., and Lannon, A. 1997. Inherited iris melanoma in Labrador Retriever dogs. *Proceedings of the Scientific Meeting of the American College of Veterinary Ophthalmologists*, Santa Fe, NM, 28:106.

296. Dubielzig, R., Steinberg, H., Garvin, H., Deehr, A.M., and Fischer, B. 1998. Iridociliary epithelial tumors in 100 dogs and 17 cats: A morphological study. *Veterinary Ophthalmology* 1:223–231.

297. Glickstein, J.M. 1974. Malignant ciliary body adenocarcinoma in a dog. *Journal of the American Veterinary Medical Association* 165:455–456.

298. Zarfoss, M.K., and Dubielzig, R.R. 2007. Metastatic iridociliary adenocarcinoma in a Labrador Retriever. *Veterinary Pathology* 44:672–676.

299. Acland, G., McLean, I., Aguirre, G., and Trucksa, R. 1980. Diffuse iris melanoma in cats. *Journal of the American Veterinary Medical Association* 176:52–56.

300. Bellhorn, R., and Henkind, P. 1970. Intraocular malignant melanoma in domestic cats. *Journal of Small Animal Practice* 10:631–637.

301. Bertoy, R., Brightman, A., and Regan, K. 1988. Intraocular melanoma with multiple metastases in a cat. *Journal of the American Veterinary Medical Association* 192:87–89.

302. Patnaik, A., and Mooney, S. 1988. Feline melanoma: A comparative study of ocular, oral, and dermal neoplasms. *Veterinary Pathology* 25:105–112.

303. Duncan, D., and Peiffer, R. 1991. Morphology and prognostic indicators of anterior uveal melanomas in cats. *Progress in Veterinary and Comparative Ophthalmology* 1:25–32.

304. Kalishman, J., Chappell, R., Flood, L., and Dubielzig, R. 1998. A matched observational study of survival in cats with enucleation due to diffuse iris melanoma. *Veterinary Ophthalmology* 1:25–29.

305. Albert, D., Shadduck, J., Craft, J., and Niederkorn, J. 1981. Feline uveal melanoma model induced with feline sarcoma virus. *Investigative Ophthalmology and Visual Science* 20:606–624.

306. Niederkorn, J., Shadduck, J., and Albert, D. 1982. Enucleation and the appearance of second primary tumors in cats bearing virally-induced intraocular tumors. *Investigative Ophthalmology and Visual Science* 23:719–725.

307. Stiles, J., Bienzle, D., Render, J.A., Buyukmihci, N.C., and Johnson, E.C. 1999. Use of nested polymerase chain reaction (PCR) for detection of retroviruses from formalin-fixed, paraffin-embedded uveal melanomas in cats. *Veterinary Ophthalmology* 2:113–116.

308. Cullen, C.L., Haines, D.M., Jackson, M.L. et al. 2002. Lack of detection of feline leukemia and feline sarcoma viruses in diffuse iris melanomas of cats by immunohistochemistry and polymerase chain reaction. *Journal of Veterinary Diagnostic Investigation* 14:340–343.

309. Harris, B.P., and Dubielzig, R.R. 1999. Atypical primary ocular melanoma in cats. *Veterinary Ophthalmology* 2:121–124.

310. Woog, J., Albert, D., Gonder, J., and Carpenter, J. 1983. Osteosarcoma in a phthisical feline eye. *Veterinary Pathology* 20:209–214.

311. Dubielzig, R. 1984. Ocular sarcoma following trauma in three cats. *Journal of the American Veterinary Medical Association* 184:578–581.

312. Miller, W., and Boosinger, T. 1987. Intraocular osteosarcoma in a cat. *Journal of the American Animal Hospital Association* 23:317–320.

313. Hakanson, N., Shively, J., Reed, R., and Merideth, R. 1990. Intraocular spindle cell sarcoma following ocular trauma in a cat: Case report and literature review. *Journal of the American Animal Hospital Association* 26:63–66.

314. Dubielzig, R.R., Hawkins, K.L., Toy, K.A., Rosebury, W.S., Mazur, M., and Jasper, T.G. 1994. Morphologic features of feline ocular sarcomas in ten cats: Light microscopy, ultrastructure, and immunohistochemistry. *Veterinary and Comparative Ophthalmology* 4:7–12.

315. Zeiss, C.J., Johnson, E.M., and Dubielzig, R.R. 2003. Feline intraocular tumors may arise from transformation of lens epithelium. *Veterinary Pathology* 40:355–362.

316. Cullen, C., Haines, D., Jackson, M., Peiffer, R., and Grahn, B. 1998. The use of immunohistochemistry and the polymerase chain reaction for detection of feline leukemia virus and feline sarcoma virus in six cases of feline ocular sarcoma. *Veterinary Ophthalmology* 1:189–193.

317. Murphy, J., and Young, S. 1979. Intraocular melanoma in a horse. *Veterinary Pathology* 16:539–542.

318. Neumann, S. 1985. Intraocular melanoma in a horse. *Modern Veterinary Practice* 66:559–560.

319. Davidson, H., Blanchard, G., Wheeler, C., and Render, J. 1991. Anterior uveal melanoma with secondary keratitis, cataract, and glaucoma in a horse. *Journal of the American Veterinary Medical Association* 199:1049–1050.

320. Barnett, K.C., and Platt, H. 1990. Intraocular melanoma in the horse. *Equine Veterinary Journal Supplement* 10:76–82.

321. Bistner, S., Campbell, J., Shaw, D., Leininger, J.R., and Ghobrial, H.K. 1983. Neuroepithelial tumor of the optic nerve in a horse. *Cornell Veterinarian* 73:30–40.

322. Riis, R.C., Scherlie, P.H., and Rebhun, W.C. 1990. Intraocular medulloepithelioma in a horse. *Equine Veterinary Journal Supplement* 10:66–69.

323. Ueda, Y., Senba, H., Nishimura, T., Usui, T., Tanaka, K., and Inagaki, S. 1993. Ocular medulloepithelioma in a thoroughbred. *Equine Veterinary Journal* 25:558–561.

324. Bistner, S. 1974. Medulloepithelioma of the iris and ciliary body in a horse. *Cornell Veterinarian* 64:588–595.

325. Barron, C., Saunders, L., and Jubb, K. 1963. Intraocular tumors in animals. III. Secondary intraocular tumors. *American Journal of Veterinary Research* 24:835–853.

326. Rebhun, W., and Piero, F. 1998. Ocular lesions in horses with lymphosarcoma: 21 cases (1977–1997). *Journal of the American Veterinary Medical Association* 212:852–854.

327. Cello, R., and Hutcherson, B. 1963. Ocular changes in malignant lymphoma of dogs. *Cornell Veterinarian* 52:492–523.

328. Lavach, J.D. 1984. Disseminated neoplasia presenting with ocular signs: A report of two cases. *Journal of the American Animal Hospital Association* 20:459–462.

329. Ladds, P., Gelatt, K., Strafuss, A., and Mosier, J. 1970. Canine ocular adenocarcinoma of mammary origin. *Journal of the American Veterinary Medical Association* 156:63–68.

330. Bellhorn, R. 1972. Secondary ocular adenocarcinoma in three dogs and a cat. *Journal of the American Veterinary Medical Association* 160:302–307.

331. Whitley, R., Jensen, H., Andrews, J., and Simpson, S. 1980. Renal adenocarcinoma with ocular metastasis in a dog. *Journal of the American Animal Hospital Association* 16:949–953.

332. Murphy, C.J., Canton, D.C., Bellhorn, R.W., Okihiro, M., Cahoon, B., and Dufort, R. 1989. Disseminated adenocarcinoma with ocular involvement in a cat. *Journal of the American Veterinary Medical Association* 195:488–491.

333. Gionfriddo, J.R., Fix, A.S., Niyo, Y., Miller, L.D., and Betts, D.M. 1990. Ocular manifestations of a metastatic pulmonary adenocarcinoma in a cat. *Journal of the American Veterinary Medical Association* 197:372–374.

334. Hayden, D. 1976. Squamous cell carcinoma in a cat with intraocular and orbital metastases. *Veterinary Pathology* 13:332–336.

335. West, S.C., Wolf, E.D., and Vainisi, S.J. 1979. Intraocular metastasis of mammary adenocarcinoma. *Journal of the American Animal Hospital Association* 15:725–728.

336. Cook, C., Peiffer, R., and Stine, P. 1984. Metastatic ocular squamous cell carcinoma in a cat. *Journal of the American Veterinary Medical Association* 185:1547–1549.

337. Hamilton, H., Severin, G., and Nold, J. 1984. Pulmonary squamous cell carcinoma with intraocular metastasis in a cat. *Journal of the American Veterinary Medical Association* 185:307–309.

338. Fulton, L.M., Bromberg, N.M., and Goldschmidt, M.H. 1991. Soft tissue fibrosarcoma with intraocular metastasis in a cat. *Progress in Veterinary and Comparative Ophthalmology* 1:129–132.

339. Nysk,a A., Hermalin, A., Jakobso,n B. et al. 1992. Intraocular vascular embolization of a malignant canine pheochromocytoma. *Progress in Veterinary and Comparative Ophthalmology* 2:129–132.

340. Kilrain, C.G., Saik, J.E., and Jeglum, K.A. 1994. Malignant angioendotheliomatosis with retinal detachments in a dog. *Journal of the American Veterinary Medical Association* 204:918–921.

341. Barron, C., Saunders, L., Seibold, H., and Heath, M. 1963. Intraocular tumors in animals. V. Transmissible venereal tumor of dogs. *American Journal of Veterinary Research* 24:1263–1269.

342. Szymanski, C. 1972. Bilateral metastatic intraocular hemangiosarcoma in a dog. *Journal of the American Veterinary Medical Association* 161:803–805.

343. Szymanski, C., Boyce, R., and Wyman, M. 1984. Transitional cell carcinoma of the urethra metastatic to the eyes in a dog. *Journal of the American Veterinary Medical Association* 185:1003–1004.

344. Hogenesch, H., Whiteley, H., Vicini, D., and Helper, L. 1987. Seminoma with metastases in the eye and the brain in a dog. *Veterinary Pathology* 24:278–280.

345. Cassotis, N.J., Dubielzig, R.R., Gilger, B.C., and Davidson, M.G. 1999. Angioinvasive pulmonary carcinoma with posterior segment metastasis in four cats. *Veterinary Ophthalmology* 2:125–131.

346. Dziezyc, J., Hager, D., and Millichamp, N. 1987. Two-dimensional real-time ocular ultrasonography in the diagnosis of ocular lesions in dogs. *Journal of the American Animal Hospital Association* 23:501–508.

347. Bussanich, M. 1984. Don't overlook fine-needle aspiration biopsy to differentiate intraocular tumors. *Veterinary Medicine* 79:1055–1060.

348. Karcioglu, Z., Gordon, R.A., and Karcioglu, G. 1985. Tumor seeding in ocular fine needle aspiration biopsy. *Ophthalmology* 92:1763–1765.

349. Cook, C.S., and Wilkie, D.A. 1999. Treatment of presumed iris melanoma in dogs by diode laser photocoagulation: 23 cases. *Veterinary Ophthalmology* 2:217–225.

350. Nasisse, M.P., Davidson, M.G., Olivero, D.K., Brinkmann, M., and Nelms, S. 1993. Neodymium: YAG laser treatment of primary canine intraocular tumors. *Progress in Veterinary and Comparative Ophthalmology* 3:152–157.

351. Goetz, T., Ogilvie, G., Keegan, K., and Johnson, P. 1990. Cimetidine for treatment of melanomas in three horses. *Journal of the American Veterinary Medical Association* 197:449–452.

352. Bellhorn, R.W., and Vainisi, S.J. 1969. Successful removal of ciliary body adenoma. *Modern Veterinary Practice* 50:47–49.

353. Clerc, B. 1996. Surgery and chemotherapy for the treatment of adenocarcinoma of the iris and ciliary body in five dogs. *Veterinary and Comparative Ophthalmology* 6:265–270.

354. Peiffer, R.L. 1997. Letters to the editor: Adenocarcinoma commentary. *Veterinary and Comparative Ophthalmology* 7:3.

CHAPTER 12

GLAUCOMA

J. PHILLIP PICKETT

INTRODUCTION

Glaucoma has been traditionally defined as an elevation of the intraocular pressure (IOP) beyond that which is compatible with the health of the eye. Elevation of IOP may arise from a variety of causes and, thus, is a final common pathway for many disease processes. Therefore, glaucoma should be considered a sign and not the basic disease entity itself, and every effort should be made to understand why the IOP is elevated.

In the last two decades, human glaucoma has been defined as a progressive optic neuropathy, with elevation of the IOP being only one of the causes for optic neuropathy. Glaucoma is now considered a neurodegenerative disease.[1-4] In time, with more sophisticated diagnostic instrumentation, veterinary medicine may also recognize "normal tension glaucoma" as in human ophthalmology, and we may shift our focus in treating glaucoma from controlling IOP to treating neurodegeneration. For the veterinary clinician and the practicing veterinary ophthalmologist, glaucoma for now remains a disease where diagnosis of elevated IOP and therapy to reduce the IOP to a more physiologic state remains the key to prevention of blindness, pain, and disfigurement from this devastating group of disorders.

Glaucoma results in blindness if it is not controlled and thus must be considered one of the main causes of a potentially treatable blindness. In an early survey of 162,000 dogs seen at veterinary teaching hospitals, the diagnosis of glaucoma was made in 1 out of every 204 patients.[5] In one review, glaucoma represented almost 9% of ophthalmologic diagnoses.[6,7] In a later paper,[8] Gelatt and MacKay identified an overall incidence in North America of 0.89% for primary or breed-related glaucomas with some breeds (most notably the American Cocker Spaniel and basset hound) having an incidence of over 5%.

ANATOMY AND PHYSIOLOGY

Aqueous humor is continuously produced by the ciliary processes in the posterior chamber by a process of passive ultrafiltration and active secretion. The emphasis on the importance of secretion versus ultrafiltration has varied over the years, but it is now thought that active secretion is the most important process in aqueous humor formation and takes place in the nonpigmented ciliary epithelium. Hydrostatic and oncotic pressures in the ciliary processes are not great enough to promote ultrafiltration as a major contributor of aqueous humor production. While species variations exist in aqueous humor composition and, perhaps, in formation, Na^+/K^+-activated ATPase is thought to be the major transporter of solutes into the aqueous humor and is found in highest concentration along the lateral cellular membranes of the nonpigmented epithelium.[9] Sodium is thought to be transported into the intercellular channels, creating an osmotic gradient that pulls fluid into the channels and then into the posterior chamber. Oubain, which inhibits Na^+/K^+-activated ATPase, decreases aqueous humor production by up to 70%. Carbonic anhydrase inhibitors (CAIs) have long been known to decrease aqueous humor production, but theories on the mechanism have been somewhat controversial. CAIs decrease both sodium and bicarbonate transport into the aqueous humor, although how this coupling occurs is unknown.[10] The endogenous influences on aqueous humor formation are multiple, complex, and incompletely understood.

Aqueous humor egress

Once secreted into the posterior chamber, aqueous humor passes through the pupil and exits the eye through the iridocorneal angle (angle) (**Figure 12.1**). Fluid in the angle passes through the pectinate ligament to the ciliary cleft or sinus (**Figures 12.2 and 12.3**). The ciliary cleft is filled with a porous uveal trabecular network (**Figures 12.4 and 12.5**). Lying external to the uveal trabecular meshwork is the corneoscleral trabecular meshwork, which separates the small aqueous plexus from the ciliary cleft (**Figure 12.4**). The aqueous plexus vessels are very small and merge into the larger collecting veins and finally into the scleral venous plexus (**Figures 12.1, 12.4, and 12.6**). The scleral veins communicate freely with episcleral veins, anterior ciliary veins, and the vortex venous system (**Figure 12.1**).[11-14] Arteriovenous anastomosis between the anterior ciliary artery and the scleral veins has been

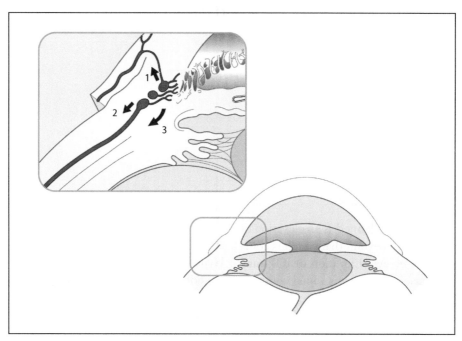

Figure 12.1 Normal canine iridocorneal angle illustrating the alternative routes by which aqueous humor can egress from the angle region. Arrows 1 and 2 indicate the major aqueous humor flow through the vascular pathways. Aqueous humor is collected from the trabecular meshwork into the large scleral venous plexus and may exit anteriorly into the anterior ciliary and conjunctival veins, or posteriorly into the vortex venous system. Arrow 3 indicates the uveoscleral flow through the ciliary muscle interstitium to the suprachoroidal space. (From Martin, C.L. 1983. In: Peiffer, R.L., editor. *Comparative Ophthalmic Pathology*. Charles C Thomas: Springfield, IL, pp. 137–169.)

demonstrated to affect aqueous humor outflow by altering venous pressure.[15] A fine capillary network, that is normally bloodless, runs radially to drain the aqueous humor from the corneoscleral meshwork. These vessels have been variously termed trabecular veins or capillaries, aqueous veins, angular plexus, or aqueous plexus.[14,16–18]

This plexus is oriented radial to the limbus but does have some circumferential anastomosis between channels. The plexus arises within the corneoscleral meshwork (**Figure 12.6**), with outpockets or diverticulae. It drains into larger collecting vessels that join the circumferentially oriented three to four large interwoven channels that form the scleral venous plexus in the midsclera. The scleral venous plexus communicates posteriorly with the vortex venous system, draining the posterior uvea, and anteriorly with

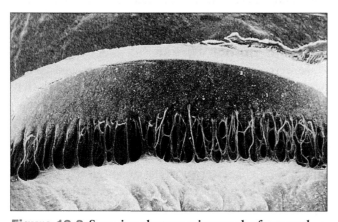

Figure 12.2 Scanning electron micrograph of a normal canine iridocorneal angle showing pectinate ligament morphology as viewed from the anterior chamber or on a gonioscopic view. The iris is pulled down, and the cornea excised and retracted dorsally (×21). (From Martin, C. 1975. *Journal of the American Animal Hospital Association* 11:180–184.)

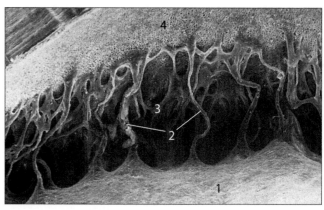

Figure 12.3 Frontal view of the canine iridocorneal angle. (1: Iris; 2: Pectinate ligament; 3: Uveal trabecula; 4: Corneal endothelium) (SEM ×60). (From Martin, C. 1975. *Journal of the American Animal Hospital Association* 11:180–184.)

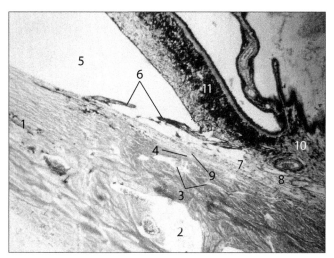

Figure 12.4 Histologic section of the normal canine iridocorneal angle. (1: Limbus; 2: Plexus venosus sclerae; 3: Collecting veins; 4: Aqueous plexus; 5: Anterior chamber; 6: Pectinate ligament (accessory row); 7: Ciliary cleft filled with 8: Uveal trabecula; 9: Corneoscleral trabecula; 10: Ciliary body; 11: Iris.) (From Martin, C.L., and Anderson, B.G. 1981. In: Gelatt, K., editor. *Veterinary Ophthalmology*, 1st edition. Lea & Febiger: Philadelphia, PA, pp. 12–121.)

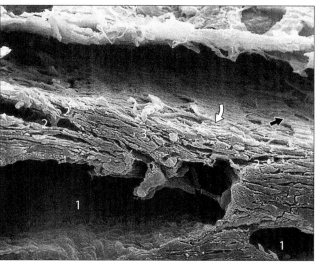

Figure 12.6 Aqueous plexus of a dog viewed on sagittal view. (1: Collecting vein; 2: Trabecular plexus or aqueous plexus; 3: Corneoscleral meshwork.) The inner surface of the trabecular meshwork is covered by a sheet of cells (open arrow). Holes are present in the sheet but may represent artifact in preparation. Dark arrow denotes the direction of the anterior chamber. (SEM ×411.)

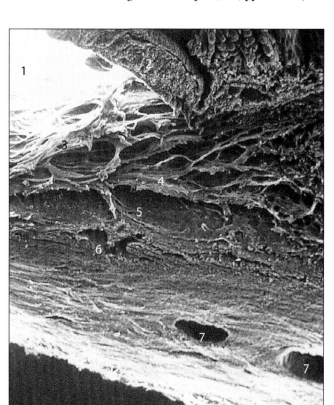

Figure 12.5 Feline iridocorneal angle on sagittal section. (1: Anterior chamber; 2: Iris; 3: Pectinate ligament; 4: Uveal trabecula filling the 5: Ciliary cleft; 6: Aqueous plexus; 7: Scleral venous plexus) (SEM ×43). (From Martin, C.L., and Anderson, B.G. 1981. In: Gelatt, K., editor. *Veterinary Ophthalmology*, 1st edition. Lea & Febiger: Philadelphia, PA, pp. 12–121.)

the episcleral venous plexus (see Chapter 11, **Figure 11.2**).[11,13,14]

The method of entry of aqueous humor into the vascular channels is unknown. Two proposed routes are intracellular/transcellular channels and intercellular channels. Intracellular channels are thought to occur through giant vacuoles or macropinocytosis.[21] These channels are sensitive to IOP changes.[22,23] The significance and, indeed, the existence of intracellular vacuoles has been questioned.[24,25] Demonstrable intercellular channels may be more important for the intravascular transport of aqueous humor.[24,26] Martin, among others, indicated that only infrequently were giant vacuoles identified in the canine endothelium of the aqueous plexus.[19] Direct channels from the trabecular meshwork to the capillaries can be easily demonstrated with injection techniques and scanning electron microscopy (**Figure 12.6**).[16,24,27]

The extracellular matrix (ECM) of the trabecular meshwork has been of interest to investigators because it is thought to be the main source of resistance to aqueous humor outflow from the eye, and alterations within it may be the elusive underlying cause for open-angle glaucoma in man and animal comparative research models. The ECM consists of a variety of macromolecules, of which glycosaminoglycans (GAGs) have been of particular interest because of the observation that perfusion of hyaluronidase in the anterior chamber reduces the outflow resistance.[28,29] GAGs are demonstrable in the trabecular meshwork and trabecular capillaries. Alterations in the composition of GAGs may result in changes in resistance to aqueous humor outflow.[30,31] Chondroitin sulfate is the major GAG present in the normal beagle.[31] Other constituents of the ECM are collagen (types I, III, IV, V, VI, and VIII), elastin, and the adhesive glycoproteins fibronectin, laminin, and vitronectin.[32] A variety of influences such as corticosteroids, growth factors, and matrix metalloproteinases (MMPs) affect the ECM. Weinstein et al. demonstrated MMP-2 and MMP-9 in the normal canine aqueous and iridocorneal angle.[33] Latent MMP-2 was highest in the aqueous and was higher in glaucomatous eyes than in normotensive eyes. Within the trabecular meshwork, latent MMP-9 and active MMP-2 were the relevant MMPs and were higher in glaucomatous eyes than in normotensive eyes.

Myocilin is a glycoprotein that is present in the eyes of dogs and humans and has been studied recently due to the association of a mutant myocilin gene with primary open-angle glaucoma (POAG) in humans. In the normal dog, it can be found in the aqueous and localized to the smooth muscle of the iris and the ciliary body, endothelial cells, cytoplasm of the nonpigmented ciliary epithelium, and the trabecular meshwork extracellular matrix and adjacent sclera. It is elevated in some humans with POAG and in beagles with POAG. The role in the disease is yet to be clarified.[34,35]

In addition to aqueous humor outflow via the aqueous plexus and venous channels, an unconventional or uveoscleral flow of fluid has been demonstrated in various species, including the dog, the cat, and the horse.[36–40] The uveoscleral route passes through the ciliary cleft and into the ciliary muscle interstitium to the suprachoroidal space, to be absorbed by the choroidal veins and transsclerally to the orbital lymphatics (**Figure 12.1**). The relative importance of the two pathways varies with the species. The uveoscleral route accounts for 15% of aqueous humor dispersal in the dog[39] but only 3% in the cat.[36] While not measured in the horse, the uveoscleral flow is thought to be important based on microsphere injection.[40] Additionally, in the horse, a uveovortex flow was demonstrated from the large ciliary sinus at the base of the iris (**Figure 12.7** and Chapter 11, **Figure 11.6**). Spheres from this space progressed into the iris vessels and then to the vortex venous system.[40]

Gonioscopic anatomy

The terminology utilized in describing structures of the iridocorneal angle has varied greatly over time and with investigator. Samuelson summarized the historical comparative anatomy and the terminology of mammalian iridocorneal angles.[18] In carnivores, the predominant structure on frontal or gonioscopic view is the pectinate

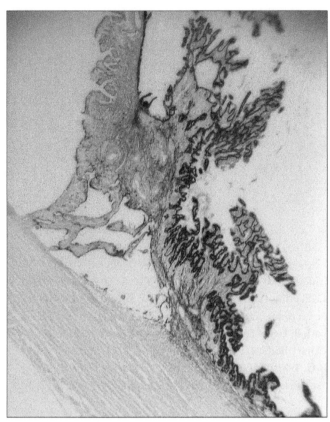

Figure 12.7 Normal equine iridocorneal angle on histology. Note a large ciliary cleft at the base of the iris with a large uveal trabecula and a lack of a significant vascular system in the adjacent sclera compared to the dog (H&E).

ligament structure, which is composed of strands that originate from the base of the iris and insert on the peripheral inner cornea (**Figures 12.2, 12.3, 12.5, 12.8, and 12.9**). Strands of the ligament are usually single but may have branching connections to adjacent ligaments. Thinner strands originate behind the primary row of the pectinate ligaments to form an accessory row.[13,20,41] The primary strands are the same color as the iris and, therefore, are usually pigmented. On histologic section, the pectinate ligament strands are usually incomplete because the section is unlikely to be cut parallel to the full length of the ligament strand (**Figure 12.4**).

The pectinate ligaments insert on the inner peripheral cornea at a uniform level and, in most instances, are associated with deep corneal pigment near the termination of Descemet's membrane. This forms a pigmented zone (deep) that is visible on gonioscopy (**Figure 12.8**). The pigment continues to line the shelf of the limbus or the corneoscleral overlap and is visible on gonioscopy as the superficial pigment zone. This zone is grayer, as it is viewed through the intervening cornea.[13] The presence of the pigmented zones varies between dogs as well as in various quadrants of the same eye.

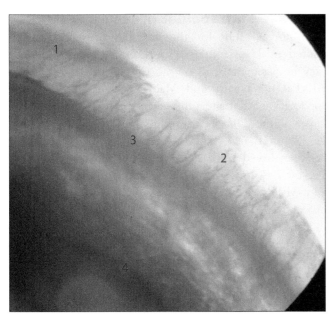

Figure 12.8 Goniophotograph of a canine iridocorneal angle with landmarks. (1: Deep pigmented zone; 2: Pectinate ligaments; 3: Iris base/ciliary zone; 4: Pupil).

The pectinate ligaments are the predominant structures visualized on gonioscopy; if they are not observed, it is because of angle pathology, the angle of observation is incorrect, or the goniolens is not positioned correctly on the corneal apex.

Posterior to the pectinate ligament lies the ciliary cleft that is filled with fine interwoven nonpigmented fibers of the ciliary or uveal trabecular meshwork (**Figures 12.3 through 12.5**). The spaces of the trabecular meshwork are often termed the spaces of Fontana.[42] On gonioscopy, the individual uveal trabecular beams are not recognized, and the region of the uveal trabecular meshwork is seen as a light brown-colored zone behind or through the pectinate ligaments (**Figures 12.8 through 12.10**).[13,20] External (sclerad) to the loose uveal trabecular meshwork are the more compact trabeculae of the corneoscleral trabecular meshwork (cribriform ligament) (**Figure 12.4**).[13,18] The corneoscleral trabeculae are extensions of the longitudinal ciliary muscle that lines the inner sclera and insert at the point of the pectinate ligament insertion. In the horse, a supraciliary space filled with trabeculae lies internal to the ciliary muscle and is the entrance for the uveoscleral flow.[16,43]

The feline iridocorneal angle is similar to the dog, except that the pectinate ligaments tend to be longer and slenderer (**Figures 12.5 and 12.10**). In the horse and other ungulates, the pectinate ligaments are thick cords and are more of a sheet with pores near the iris (**Figures 12.7, 12.11**, and Chapter 11, **Figure 11.6**).[16,18,43] The equine scleral venous plexus is much less developed (**Figure 12.7**), and a large ciliary cleft is present that extends into the base of the iris.[16,18,43,44]

Theoretically, increased IOP may occur from an increased rate of aqueous humor production, obstruction

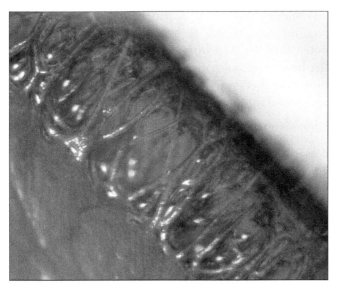

Figure 12.9 High-magnification goniophotograph of a canine iridocorneal angle. To the upper right is the deep pigmented zone and corneal endothelial surface; to the lower left is the iris, with the pectinate ligaments and uveal trabeculae being seen between.

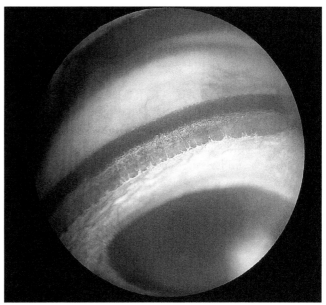

Figure 12.10 Goniophotograph of a feline iridocorneal angle. Note the long, slender pectinate ligaments that do not contrast very much with the uveal trabecula because of the lighter pigmentation.

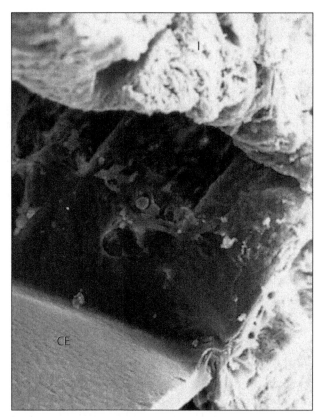

Figure 12.11 Combined sagittal and frontal view of an equine iridocorneal angle. Note the pectinate ligament that is sheet-like with holes near the iris (I) base (SEM ×178). (CE: Corneal endothelium.)

to aqueous humor outflow either at the pupil or angle region, or an increased episcleral and orbital venous hydrostatic pressure. In practice, the obstruction to outflow at the pupil or angle is the usual cause of glaucoma. It may be that the other two possibilities are important but are difficult to assess in clinical veterinary medicine.

CLINICAL SIGNS OF GLAUCOMA

Since glaucoma is a sign rather than the basic disease, it is necessary to study each case as thoroughly as possible to determine the underlying cause(s). Externally, the signs of glaucoma are too nonspecific in most primary glaucoma cases to help differentiate the cause, so special diagnostic procedures must often be pursued.[6,7,45,46]

> The signs of glaucoma vary between species, degree of elevation of IOP, cause of the glaucoma, and chronicity. The dog tends to have the most florid signs; the horse and the cat have more subtle forms.

Increased intraocular pressure

High-normal IOP for the dog has historically been quoted as 25–30 mmHg (3.3–4.0 kPa) and should not vary between the eyes by more than 4–8 mmHg (0.5–1.1 kPa).[45–50] Gelatt and MacKay used four different applanation tonometers in a variety of breeds and found a mean canine IOP of 19 mmHg (2.5 kPa), with a range of 11–29 mmHg (1.5–3.9 kPa).[50] No differences were noted between breeds measured, but IOP did decrease with age by 2–4 mmHg (0.3–0.5 kPa). Utilizing the Tono-Pen, Miller et al. reported a mean IOP of 17 ± 4 mmHg (2.3 ± 0.5 kPa) in the dog, 20 ± 6 mmHg (2.7 ± 0.8 kPa) in the cat, and 23 mmHg (3.1 kPa) in the horse.[51,52,67] In two studies comparing rebound tonometry (TonoVet) with applanation tonometry (Tono-Pen), the rebound tonometer mean IOP in the dog was 9 mmHg versus a mean IOP of 11 mmHg for the applanation tonometer[53] and 11 mmHg versus 13 mmHg, respectively;[53] in the horse, the rebound tonometer mean IOP was 22 mmHg, and the applanation tonometer mean IOP was 21 mmHg.[53] Diurnal IOP variations occur; in the dog, IOP is 2–4 mmHg (0.3–0.5 kPa) higher in the morning, which coincides with variation in endogenous catecholamines.[54] IOP is remarkably similar across a variety of species. Diurnal variations have been recorded in the cat, with IOP about 4 mmHg higher during the dark cycle (9 p.m. to 3 a.m.).[55]

In the horse particularly, the head position while measuring the IOP is critical. In this author's experience, equine IOPs can be quite labile, with marked differences being measured in the same horse depending on restraint, excitement of the patient, and amount of effort required to open lids for measuring. Komaromy et al. noted that the IOP in horses varied significantly with the head position in relation to the heart.[56] The mean difference between head-up and head-down position was 8 mmHg, but in some individuals, it was as much as 28 mmHg.

Elevated IOP is the only specific sign of active glaucoma. The least expensive measuring instrument in small animal ophthalmology is the Schiotz tonometer (see Chapter 1). Two tables calibrating the Schiotz tonometer for use in the dog have been published, and they both yield IOPs several units higher than human tables (1955 Friedenwald chart).[57,58] Glaucoma may erroneously be diagnosed in many normal dogs if these conversion tables are used. Canine and feline IOPs taken with applanation tonometry correlates most closely with 1955 Friedenwald Schiotz conversion tables (that come with the instruments), and while differences exist, they are not clinically significant.[59,60]

Although Schiotz tonometers may frequently be purchased by veterinarians, they are many times infrequently used. Only with practice can consistent, meaningful readings be obtained. Consequently, erroneous readings are common, and confidence in the results is often lacking.

In two early studies, the Tono-Pen overestimated the real IOP in the normal and low range and underestimated the real IOP in the elevated range.[61,62] In the cat, the Tono-Pen XL tonometer uniformly underestimated IOP compared to manometry, while the TonoVet rebound tonometer more accurately estimated IOP.[63] In dogs and cats with ocular pathology, the Tono-Pen applanation tonometer underestimated IOP compared to the TonoVet rebound tonometer.[64] The variations with the two instruments from real IOP are not usually clinically significant and do not cause diagnostic dilemmas; however, if close observation of IOPs is being done to monitor progression of disease, use of the same instrument the same time of day is important.

The Tono-Pen and the TonoVet are the preferred tonometers for veterinary use because of their accuracy, ease of use, and adaptability to various species, but they are relatively expensive (approximately $3000).[51–53,62–67] The TonoVet must be used on the horizontal plane (the Tono-Pen may be used in any position), but the TonoVet can be used through a smaller interpalpebral fissure than the Tono-Pen. These tonometers are accurate, easy to use, and usually quickly pay for themselves if tonometry is routinely performed in general practice.

Pupil and iris changes

Changes in pupil function are common but not specific signs of glaucoma. Elevation in IOP impairs function of the iris sphincter muscle more than the function of the dilator muscle. This results in a defect in the efferent arm of the pupillary light reflex (PLR) that is nonresponsive to pilocarpine constriction.[68] The impairment is associated with, but not entirely due to, iris ischemia that develops when the IOP exceeds the diastolic blood pressure.[69] Because most veterinary patients are presented with IOPs that are very high, that is, >50–60 mmHg (6.7–8.0 kPa), the pupil is usually dilated if there are no iris adhesions (**Figure 12.12**). If the IOP is around 30 mmHg (4.0 kPa), the pupils may be normal in their light reaction or miotic due to uveitis or prostaglandin (PG) release (**Figure 12.13**). With chronicity, the iris sphincter muscles may undergo atrophy, which further interferes with normal pupillary constriction. Iridodonesis (trembling of the iris)

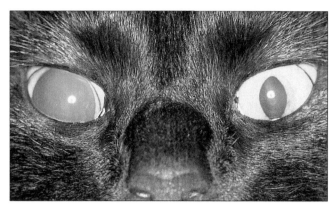

Figure 12.12 A cat with unilateral glaucoma, with the most obvious sign being pupillary dilation, producing anisocoria. Note the lack of obvious corneal edema and conjunctival injection of the limited exposed sclera.

may occur due to a lack of support from a posteriorly displaced lens.

Congestion/engorgement of episcleral vessels and conjunctival veins

Due to the free communication of the ocular venous system, when the posterior intrascleral venous channels are obstructed from scleral distention, the anterior ciliary veins and the episcleral veins become distended. This is typically a selective injection of the episcleral and large conjunctival veins but may, with very acute high pressures

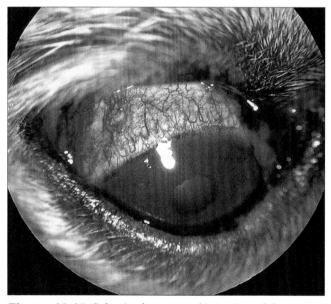

Figure 12.13 Selective large-vessel injection of the episclera/bulbar conjunctiva of a cocker spaniel with an intraocular pressure of 30–40 mmHg (4.0–5.3 kPa). Note the beginnings of deep perilimbal corneal neovascularization ("perilimbal flush"). Also note the lack of pupillary dilation, an uncommon finding with elevated IOP.

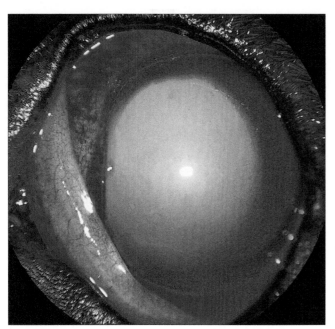

Figure 12.14 A basset hound with acute intraocular pressure of >80 mmHg (10.7 kPa). Intense conjunctival hyperemia, pupil dilation, corneal edema, and a 3+ aqueous flare in the anterior chamber were present. The aqueous humor protein was elevated (4.5 g/dL).

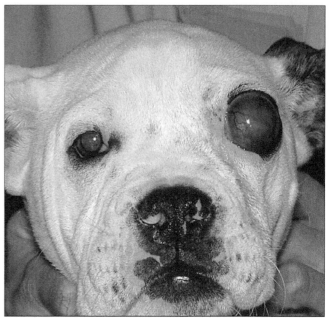

Figure 12.15 Marked buphthalmos in a 4-month-old dog that developed after a perforating cat claw injury. Horizontal corneal diameter was twice that of the normal right eye, and the corneal curvature was very "flat" compared to the normal eye.

or PG release, involve the entire conjunctival vasculature (**Figures 12.13 and 12.14**). Compared to the dog, the horse and the cat have minimal-to-modest congestion of the episcleral and conjunctival veins with glaucoma. In addition, these species have tight lid–globe conformation that makes observation more difficult. In the horse, the lack of congestion may be related to the lack of or rudimentary scleral venous plexus.

Buphthalmos/megaloglobus/ hydrophthalmos

Buphthalmos/megaloglobus/hydrophthalmos (terms used to describe globe enlargement or distension) is frequently noted in the dog, the cat, and the horse due to high IOP and a distensible corneoscleral shell. Buphthalmos occurs most rapidly and dramatically in the young puppy or kitten with glaucoma (**Figure 12.15**). Staphyloma (protrusion of the sclera with visualization of the underlying uvea) may develop from the extreme thinning of the sclera (**Figure 12.16**). Prolonged elevated IOP produces permanent globe enlargement, despite spontaneous or therapeutic lowering of the IOP. Comparison of horizontal corneal diameter can be used to detect questionable enlargements, especially if unilateral. Normal corneal horizontal diameter is 15–17 mm in most dogs and about 17 mm in most adult domestic cats. Corneal curvature with a buphthalmic globe is much flatter than with a normal globe

and may be easier to subjectively evaluate versus corneal diameter measuring. Enlargement of the globe can only be caused by glaucoma, but the presence of buphthalmos does not imply active glaucoma (elevated IOP). Many chronic buphthalmic eyes are soft due to atrophy of the

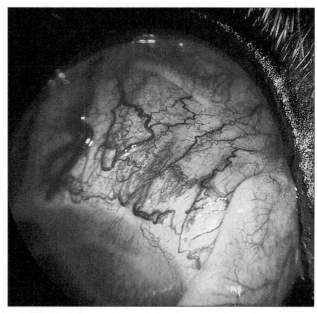

Figure 12.16 Marked episcleral and conjunctival hyperemia and staphyloma from scleral thinning in a basset hound with chronic glaucoma. Also note the deep vascular infiltration of the peripheral cornea ("perilimbal flush").

ciliary body with resultant lack of aqueous humor secretion. Buphthalmos should be differentiated from exophthalmos (see Chapter 6).

Corneal opacification

Corneal opacities may be due to acute disruption of the perfect arrangement of the corneal lamellar layers, true corneal edema, breaks in Descemet's membrane, or corneal neovascularization.

A generalized, diffuse gray discoloration of the cornea may be seen with peracute glaucoma associated with disruption of the perfect lamellar arrangement of the corneal fibers. Magnified examination of the corneal thickness with slit lamp biomicroscopy reveals a normal corneal thickness (versus true corneal edema where the intrastromal fluid causes the cornea to appear thickened). With either medical reduction of IOP or aqueous centesis, this gray discoloration resolves almost instantly. One of this author's favorite student teaching moments is to use a 27-gauge needle and saline-loaded syringe to inflate the anterior chamber of a fresh cadaver specimen via perilimbal centesis. As the IOP is raised, the corneal clarity diminishes only to return to normal clarity once the IOP is lowered. This "instant glaucoma" in a cadaver specimen shows that true corneal edema is not the initial cause of the gray cornea with peracute glaucoma.

True corneal edema is usually due to endothelial damage or compromise and may or may not be rapidly reversed when the IOP is lowered. Edema may be somewhat localized and very dense (**Figure 12.17**) or diffuse and somewhat faint (**Figure 12.14**). Glaucoma associated with an anteriorly displaced lens typically has a circular area of corneal edema where the lens touches the corneal endothelium. Descemet's membrane breaks (Haab's striae) are permanent and manifest as one or more single or branching deep curvilinear double white lines (**Figure 12.18**). They may or may not be associated with more diffuse corneal edema. In the horse, acute breaks in Descemet's membrane with edema (**Figure 12.18a**) are often the presenting sign of glaucoma. Breaks in Descemet's membrane are quite specific for a history of glaucoma, but the process may not be active (i.e., elevated IOP) at the time of examination. Descemet's membrane breaks are one of the most consistent signs with equine glaucoma, but striate keratopathy has also been observed in equine eyes without glaucoma (see Chapter 10, section Striate Keratopathy).

Acute and subacute/chronic cases of glaucoma may have a deep "paintbrush" perilimbal corneal neovascularization pattern ("perilimbal flush," **Figures 12.13 and 12.16**) that differentiates the "red eye" of glaucoma or anterior uveitis from simple conjunctivitis. More superficial aborizing corneal neovascularization and scarring are observed in chronic glaucoma where chronic edema,

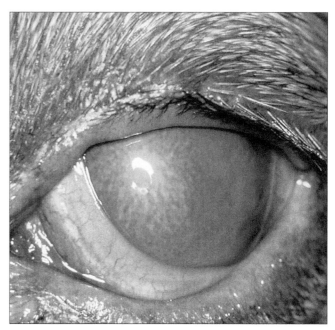

Figure 12.17 True corneal edema associated with glaucoma in a basset hound. Note the "reticulate pattern" of corneal discoloration seen over the dilated pupil background.

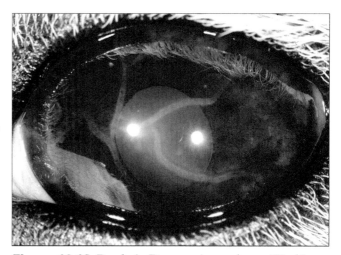

Figure 12.18 Breaks in Descemet's membrane (Haab's striae) producing curvilinear white tracts in a dog with glaucoma. The fine lines dorsally and the white discoloration inferiomedially are corneal surface reflections of lashes and the medial canthus, respectively.

corneal hypoesthesia, and repeated trauma have occurred (**Figure 12.19**). Corneal epithelial erosions and ulcerations may occur associated with the inability to blink over a buphthalmic globe and horizontally oriented axial corneal drying.

Ocular pain

Manifestations of pain or discomfort with uncomplicated glaucoma are often subtle and are related to changes in

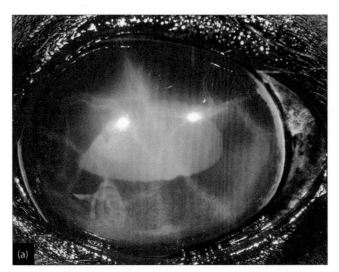

Figure 12.18a Multiple curvilinear breaks in Descemet's membrane (Haab's striae) and diffuse corneal edema in a horse with glaucoma. Note the dyscoria associated with posterior synechia in this case of equine glaucoma associated with equine recurrent uveitis.

temperament, activity, and general well-being rather than obvious ocular discomfort such as blepharospasm (although acute glaucoma is more commonly associated with blepharospasm than are cases of long standing glaucoma). In humans, the pain of acute high IOP is one of a radiating headache. Owners frequently note the temperament changes after the animal improves rather than as it worsens. Glaucoma associated with inflammation often has more acute pain.

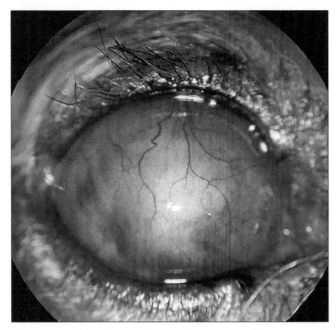

Figure 12.19 Advanced corneal scarring and neovascularization in a Wirehaired fox terrier with absolute or longstanding glaucoma and buphthalmos.

As advocates for the patient, the clinician must assume pain is present with most forms of glaucoma and encourage some form of resolution for ocular pain.

Retinal and optic nerve changes

The observable fundus changes with glaucoma vary from possible papilledema and peripapillary hemorrhage in very acute cases to the more common optic disc atrophy, peripapillary retinal atrophy, optic disc cupping, focal infarcts of the retina, diffuse retinal atrophy/tapetal hyperreflectivity, and attenuation of retinal vessels (**Figures 12.20 through 12.22**). Optic nerve head cupping is the most specific of the fundic changes (**Figure 12.23**) but is difficult to detect early in the dog due to the marked variation in the myelination of the optic disc. With progression, the optic disc becomes atrophied (**Figures 12.20 and 12.22**). The cat normally has a small nonmyelinated optic disc that is slightly cupped and tan to black; consequently, the usual signs of atrophy are difficult to recognize even in advanced feline glaucoma. Because of the size of the globe, optic

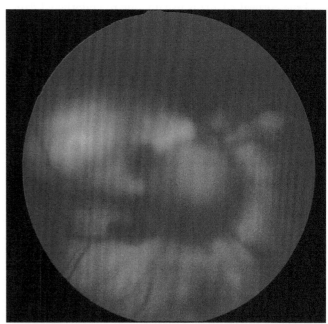

Figure 12.20 Ocular fundus of a Siberian husky with acute closed-angle glaucoma. The optic disc is cupped with retinal vessels stopping at the edge of the disc. Peripapillary hemorrhages (4, 8, and 10 o'clock) and white choroidal infarcts (1–5, 9, and 10–12 o'clock) are present. (From Martin, C., and Vestre, W. 1985. In: Slatter, D., editor. *Textbook of Small Animal Surgery*, vol. 2. WB Saunders: Philadelphia, PA, pp. 1567–1584.)

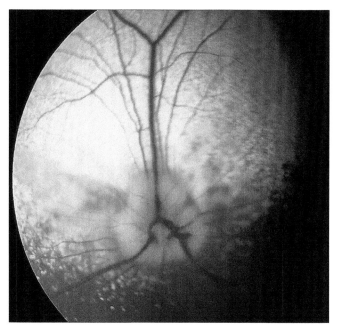

Figure 12.21 Fundus of a dog with acute glaucoma. The gray areas surrounding the optic disc (1–4 and 8–11 o'clock) are acute retinal infarcts/edema. Currently, the vessels, tapetum, and optic nerve appear relatively normal.

nerve head cupping in the horse is difficult to appreciate. A pale disc with loss of peripapillary arterioles and peripapillary depigmented/degenerative changes is most commonly recognized in the longstanding glaucomatous equine eye.

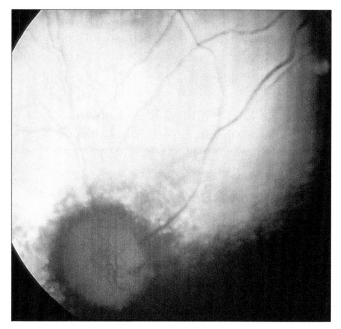

Figure 12.22 Canine fundus with diffuse tapetal hyperreflectivity, retinal vascular attenuation, peripapillary hyperpigmentation, and optic disc contracture/atrophy and cupping from chronic glaucoma.

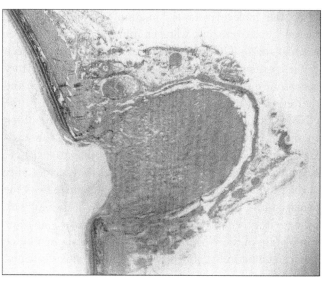

Figure 12.23 Photomicrograph with marked optic nerve cupping from chronic glaucoma in a dog (H&E).

Decreased vision

Vision loss with glaucoma is variable; in some patients, it may become permanent within 1–3 days, while some patients may retain vision despite chronically elevated pressures. The degree and rapidity of elevation of IOP are probably responsible for these variations in tolerance. Grozdanic et al. experimentally elevated the IOP above systolic blood pressure (100–160 mmHg) for one hour and evaluated the eyes for 28 days.[71] One day post elevation, all eyes were blind judged by an absent menace response, although 5/14 had positive PLR, and 10/14 had a positive dazzle reflex. Two weeks after the elevation, all the dogs had a positive menace, PLR, and dazzle reflex despite finding significant thinning of the ventral retina utilizing optical coherence tomography. Damage to the retina and the optic nerve is thought to arise from two mechanisms:

- Ischemic changes to the retina.
- Blockage of axoplasmic flow of the ganglion cells at the lamina cribrosa from a deregistering of the pores. The lamina cribrosa is the weak point of the fibrous tunic, and elevated IOP results in outward bowing, causing the pores within it to deregister. This misalignment pinches the traversing axons.[72–75] Mild-to-modest elevations probably only affect axoplasmic flow, whereas the usual high IOP observed in the dog produces ischemia as well as obstructing axoplasmic flow. Retinal ischemia is presumably responsible for the diffuse full-thickness retinal atrophy observed on histopathology with many forms of high-pressure glaucoma. The retinal ganglion cells are the most sensitive cells in the retina to ischemia, and alpha neurons with large diameter axons are most sensitive to hypoxia and glaucoma.[76]

At the molecular level, ganglion cell death may be caused by excitotoxins, whether initiated by traumatic or vascular injury. Glutamate is one excitotoxin that has been studied extensively. Glutamate is the primary excitatory neurotransmitter in the central nervous system (CNS) and the retina and the most abundant free amino acid in the CNS. Glutamate binds to several receptors that are all ion channels. One important glutamate receptor, *N*-methyl-D-aspartate (NMDA), is highly permeable to calcium. Ischemia or trauma to cells results in increased permeability of the cell membrane and the release of glutamate from the damaged cell. Increased levels of glutamate in the extracellular environment of adjacent normal cells produces an overstimulation of the NMDA receptors on the cell membrane and a resultant influx of toxic levels of intercellular calcium. Toxic levels of intracellular calcium result in activation of a variety of calcium dependent enzymes and apoptosis (cell death).[77,78] This may become a self-perpetuating process and explains how retinal and optic nerve degeneration continues to progress despite normalization of IOP in some patients. Increased glutamate levels have been found in the vitreous of humans, rabbits, and dogs with glaucoma.[79–81]

Aqueous flare

Many of the very congestive cases of glaucoma have high aqueous humor protein content, as well as pigment clumps floating in the anterior chamber. The significance of the breakdown in the blood–aqueous humor barrier is unknown; it may be due to the anterior uveitis that precipitated the glaucoma, or the high pressure may have liberated PGs that broke down the blood–aqueous barrier. On histopathology of 100 dogs with goniodysgenesis-associated glaucoma, pigment dispersion in the anterior segment (evidenced by loss or clumping of posterior iris pigment), pigment in the trabecular meshwork, or pigment cells in the ventral iridocorneal angle was present in 96 of 100 dogs, and neutrophils in the trabecular meshwork in acute cases were present in 86% of the dogs.[82]

Lenticular changes

Subluxation of the lens is often associated with stretching of the globe and rupture of a portion of the ciliary zonules (**Figure 12.24**). Since lens displacement can be an active rather than a passive component in the pathogenesis of glaucoma, it is important to try to determine the cause of the displacement. Primary lens luxation may cause secondary glaucoma (and lens removal may be indicated, especially if the lens is in the anterior chamber, in an attempt to save vision), but chronic glaucoma with secondary lens subluxation may not be improved upon with lens removal. The degree of buphthalmos and close examination of the opposite eye are important in determining the role of the lens in

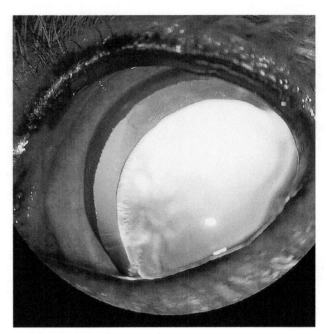

Figure 12.24 Ventrolateral subluxation of the lens secondary to buphthalmos in a dog with glaucoma. Note the aphakic crescent dorsomedially.

glaucoma. Cataract formation is common with chronic glaucoma due to aqueous humor irregularities and lens motility.

DIAGNOSIS OF GLAUCOMA

All signs of glaucoma except elevated IOP are nonspecific for active glaucoma. Despite this, veterinarians still seek to make the diagnosis without this key piece of information because the tonometer is not considered a basic instrument in practice. The diagnosis of glaucoma, per se, is only the first step. The second step is to determine the cause of the glaucoma.

> Early diagnosis of glaucoma can only be accomplished with a tonometer; early therapy has the best chance of preventing blindness.

Provocative testing

Attempts to predict a predisposition to glaucoma by provocative testing have not met with widespread acceptance in veterinary ophthalmology due to the difficulty in reproducibility in untrained animals, expense, difficulties in interpretation, and risk. Testing for glaucoma susceptibility has been performed with the water provocative test, tonography, and mydriasis.

Water loading

The water provocative test forces a water load (1 L), given by stomach tube, onto the vascular system and produces a subsequent increased rate of aqueous humor formation. The normal dog may have an increase in IOP of 3–9 mmHg (0.4–1.2 kPa) at 1 hour.[83,84] If the aqueous humor outflow channels are compromised, the elevation of IOP is beyond the normal range. Acute glaucoma has been produced by this test, so it is not without risk.

Tonography

Tonography is placing the weight of a tonometer (usually a Schiotz indentation tonographer using the 10-g weight or an electronic pneumotonometer) on the cornea for a specific time period (usually 4 minutes) and observing the decay (lowering) of IOP due to the weight of the tonometer. If the aqueous humor outflow channels are compromised, the decay is not as great as in a normal eye. The C value (coefficient of facility of aqueous humor outflow) is 0.24 (SD ± 0.07) (Schiotz tonography instrumentation)[85] or 0.297 (SD ± 0.149) (pneumotonometer instrumentation)[86] µL/mmHg/min in the normal dog with C value of 0.131 (SD ± 0.101) µL/mmHg/min (pneumotonometer instrumentation)[86] in the glaucomatous beagle model, 0.34 µL/mmHg/min in the cat, and 0.24 µL/mmHg/min in humans. While tonography has been used in research colonies of dogs with glaucoma, it has not become a clinical tool despite its advocates.[85,86]

Mydriasis provocative testing

Application of a short acting mydriatic agent (1% tropicamide) may result in significant elevation of IOP (>5 mmHg) within 1–2 hours in dogs with filtration angle closure or narrowing. In the normal dog, IOP increase following mydriasis does not occur. Acute attacks of angle-closure glaucoma may be triggered with the mydriasis provocative test, so short-acting mydriatic agents such as tropicamide should be used instead of longer acting atropine. Reversal of the mydriasis with latanoprost should be performed if the IOP becomes elevated beyond 25 mmHg.

> Because of the expense of instrumentation and the risk of inducing an acute glaucoma event, provocative testing for glaucoma is rarely performed in clinical veterinary ophthalmology.

CLASSIFICATION OF GLAUCOMA

The classification of glaucoma in veterinary medicine (**Table 12.1**) is basically borrowed from terminology in human medicine. This approach is probably valid up to a certain point, but species differences in anatomy and genetic traits have produced marked differences in the prevalence of the different forms of glaucoma.[87] Glaucoma is broadly divided into primary and secondary forms. Primary glaucoma has an implied familial and bilateral tendency. Simplistically, primary glaucoma has no antecedent ocular disease associated with the pressure rise.[46] Secondary glaucoma is associated with concurrent or antecedent intraocular disease. Confusion with these definitions occurs when some of the causes of apparent secondary glaucoma are closely investigated because the obvious secondary cause may have been only a precipitating factor on an already abnormal, but compensated, system.

Congenital glaucoma is associated with congenital anterior segment anomalies and, in humans, may manifest up to the fourth decade in life (translated to approximately 8 years in the dog). As the term congenital glaucoma is a misnomer based on time of onset, and this is the only form of glaucoma where age is considered, it would seem appropriate to place the cause(s) of congenital glaucoma under the appropriate primary or secondary forms of glaucoma and to redefine primary glaucoma. Therefore, primary glaucoma can be defined as a glaucoma that is not associated solely with acquired intraocular lesions or disease.[19] As we learn more about the pathogenesis of glaucoma, these definitions may need modification.

Absolute glaucoma is a clinical term that is frequently used and is simply an end-stage blind eye from any cause of glaucoma and, thus, has no etiologic connotation.

A basic assumption when classifying glaucoma is knowledge of the status of the iridocorneal angle, since both primary and secondary glaucoma are divided into open- and closed-angle glaucoma. This requires gonioscopy, ultrasonic biomicroscopy,[88] or high-resolution ultrasound[89] (see Chapter 1).

Primary open-angle glaucoma

Open-angle glaucoma, as is commonly seen in man, is quite uncommon in animals. The beagle has an autosomal recessive form of primary open-angle glaucoma that has been well documented in a research environment[90] and has been termed by some as the "Florida beagle." Other breeds of dogs, such as the Norwegian elkhound, probably have a form of primary open-angle glaucoma, but it is not as well documented as the Florida beagle.[70,91]

In the Florida beagle, open-angle glaucoma is bilateral, and IOP elevations begin at 6–8 months of age. On gonioscopy, the angles are open in the early and moderately advanced stages (**Figure 12.34**). In the early stages, the clinical signs are subtle, and the IOP is 35–45 mmHg (4.7–6.0 kPa). With chronicity, varying degrees of lens displacement and a secondary closure of the angle usually

Table 12.1 **Proposed classification of veterinary glaucomas.**

Open-angle glaucoma. Glaucoma associated with **a normal iridocorneal angle.**

A. Primary open-angle glaucoma. Glaucoma associated with a normal angle, with no obvious anatomic precipitating factors, bilateral disease potential, and a genetic predisposition.

B. Secondary open-angle glaucoma. Glaucoma associated with an open angle but aqueous contents or vascular hypertension interfere with aqueous egress:
1. Inflammation: Cells, fibrin, or serum products obstruct outflow pathways.
2. Hyphema: Erythrocytes and fibrin obstruct outflow pathways.
3. Obstruction of orbital venous return: Orbital lesion, arteriovenous fistula, or other causes of an elevated episcleral venous pressure that decreases the pressure differential favoring aqueous humor uptake. This is a very rare cause of glaucoma in veterinary species.
4. Pigment deposition or proliferation in the angle that obstructs aqueous humor outflow.
5. Anterior lens luxation: Lens may obstruct access to the angle and aqueous humor outflow (**Figure 12.32**).
6. Vitreous herniation with aphakia or displaced lens (**Figure 12.25**).

Closed-angle glaucoma. Angle is collapsed or covered with peripheral iris or connective tissue.

A. Primary closed-angle glaucoma:
1. Congenitally maldeveloped angle (goniodysgenesis, pectinate ligament dysplasia). Angles are bilaterally involved, often breed predisposition, age of onset of elevated IOP varies (**Figure 12.26**).
2. Acquired closure associated with abnormal anterior segment conformation:
   - Lax lens zonules with forward displacement of the lens that creates a physiologic pupillary block that further aggravates the anterior displacement of the peripheral iris (**Figure 12.27**). In the cat with aqueous humor misdirection, the lens may push forward so far as to almost touch the cornea.
   - Shallow anterior chamber associated with a small/shallow anterior ocular segment. This creates a narrow iridocorneal angle (in degrees) and is more susceptible to pupillary blockade and subsequent forward displacement of the peripheral iris and angle closure (**Figure 12.28**).
   - Plateau iris: The iris plane is flat, but the peripheral iris has a recess adjacent to the iris that is susceptible to closure if pupillary blockage occurs (**Figure 12.29**).

B. Secondary closed-angle glaucoma. Acquired lesions precipitate closure of a normal angle. Also, the angle conformations listed previously (2, bullet points 1–3) have an increased susceptibility to pupillary blockage.
1. Associated with pupil block:
   - Intumescent cataract (**Figure 12.30**).
   - Posterior synechia, iris bombe (**Figure 12.31**).
   - Subluxated lens (**Figure 12.25**).
   - Anterior vitreous herniation with aphakia or displaced lens (**Figure 12.32**).
   - Increased volume in vitreous compartment pushes lens–iris diaphragm forward.
2. No pupil blockage:
   - Neoplasia invasion of angle and iris (**Figure 12.33**).
   - Inflammation with peripheral anterior synechia.
   - Displaced lens pushing iris base forward (see **Figures 12.25 and 12.27**).
   - Fibrovascular membrane proliferation over angle.
   - Corneal epithelial downgrowth into anterior chamber. Seen as a complication of surgery or perforating injury.
   - Pigment proliferation in the angle with obstruction. Cause is unknown.

occurs by 2–3 years of age.[92,93] As the condition progresses, the IOP is often very erratic and high, and the clinical signs are more typical of canine glaucoma (buphthalmos, corneal edema, episcleral injection, pupillary dilation, and lens subluxation).

The cause of the obstruction in aqueous humor outflow is poorly understood, but glycosaminoglycans (GAG) alterations in the angle have been demonstrated.[31,33] The major GAG in normal and glaucomatous beagles is chondroitin sulfate, and the amount of chondroitin sulfate decreases (as does hyaluronic acid) with the duration of the glaucoma, while an enzyme-resistant form of a GAG increases. Myocilin increases in the trabecular meshwork of affected beagles, and one hypothesis is that it increases the resistance to aqueous outflow. It is not known at this time whether myocilin is a cause of the IOP increase or the result, only that it is associated with increased IOP.[34,94,95] Open-angle glaucoma is characterized by its subtlety and its occurrence in both eyes at the same time. While not reported to have anomalous lenses, glaucomatous beagles appear to have small spherical lenses, as judged by the curvature of the lens and the ease of observation of the lens equator (**Figure 12.34**). This author has seen several nonresearch colony, client-owned beagles with open-angle glaucoma and lens instability/anterior lens luxation (sometimes presenting as anterior lens luxation before the onset of glaucoma). Whether these beagles are a nonresearch strain of the Florida beagle or a totally different line of primary open-angle glaucoma in beagles has not been documented. The disease in elkhounds appears similar to

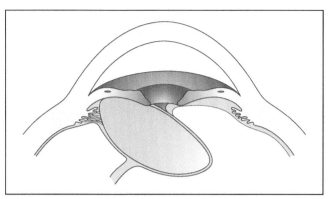

Figure 12.25 Illustration of a tilted subluxated lens pushing forward on the peripheral iris, closing the iridocorneal angle or collapsing the ciliary cleft. Vitreous gel herniation through the pupil may create a pupillary block or obstruct the angle. (From Martin, C.L. 1983. In: Peiffer, R.L., editor. *Comparative Ophthalmic Pathology*. Charles C Thomas: Springfield, IL, pp. 137–169.)

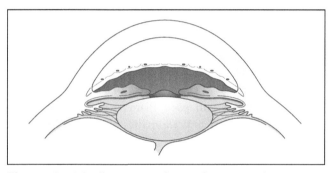

Figure 12.26 Illustration of goniodysgenesis that is characterized by a sheet covering the angle where the pectinate ligaments would normally be visualized. Flow holes are usually present in the sheet on the corneal side. (From Martin, C.L. 1983. In: Peiffer, R.L., editor. *Comparative Ophthalmic Pathology*. Charles C Thomas: Springfield, IL, pp. 137–169.)

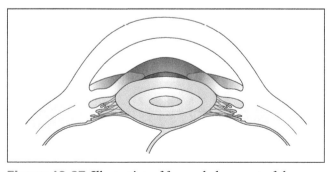

Figure 12.27 Illustration of forward placement of the lens–iris diaphragm that reduces the depth of the anterior chamber and creates a physiologic pupillary block. Note the iris hugs the lens so firmly it outlines the lens. (From Martin, C.L. 1983. In: Peiffer, R.L., editor. *Comparative Ophthalmic Pathology*. Charles C Thomas: Springfield, IL, pp. 137–169.)

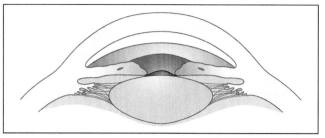

Figure 12.28 Illustration of a shallow anterior chamber that creates a narrow iridocorneal angle. This is more susceptible to closure if pupillary block should occur from lens growth or pathologic conditions. (From Martin, C.L. 1983. In: Peiffer, R.L., editor. *Comparative Ophthalmic Pathology*. Charles C Thomas: Springfield, IL, pp. 137–169.)

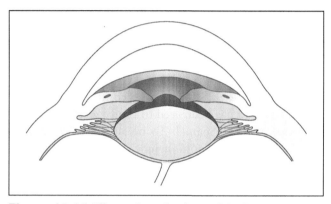

Figure 12.29 Illustration of a plateau iris that is characterized by a recess in the periphery of the iris plane and then a plateau or flat iris plane centrally. On gonioscopy, this may look like a closed angle unless the goniolens is tilted toward the angle under observation. It may lead to peripheral anterior synechiae due to close apposition of adjacent tissues. (From Martin, C.L. 1983. In: Peiffer, R.L., editor. *Comparative Ophthalmic Pathology*. Charles C Thomas: Springfield, IL, pp. 137–169.)

that in the beagle, except the age of onset of clinical signs is somewhat later (6–7 years), and small spherical lenses are not observed.

Primary closed-angle glaucoma

This represents the largest group of primary glaucomas in the dog, but semantics and incomplete knowledge have created a great deal of confusion. The iridocorneal angle may be described as closed as well as narrow. A narrow angle is presumably a potential precursor to a closed angle and is due to a shallowing of the anterior chamber (**Figure 12.35**). In veterinary medicine, the term narrow angle has often been used to describe the apparent narrow or collapsed filtering zone or cleft seen with low-magnification gonioscopy, which is not necessarily related to a shallow anterior chamber as in

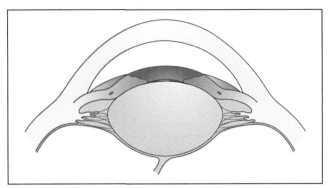

Figure 12.30 Illustration of how an intumescent cataractic lens shallows the anterior chamber, producing a relative pupillary block, which may result in closed angles. Chamber conformations such as those seen in Figures 12.27 through 12.29 may have a higher risk of angle closure with lens intumescence. (From Martin, C.L. 1983. In: Peiffer, R.L., editor. *Comparative Ophthalmic Pathology*. Charles C Thomas: Springfield, IL, pp. 137–169.)

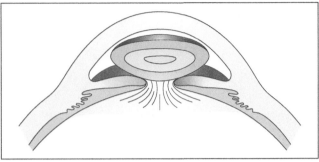

Figure 12.32 Illustration of an anterior lens luxation and how the attached vitreous may produce a pupillary block or the lens may physically block the iridocorneal angle. (From Martin, C.L. 1983. In: Peiffer, R.L., editor. *Comparative Ophthalmic Pathology*. Charles C Thomas: Springfield, IL, pp. 137–169.)

humans (**Figure 12.36**).[96] This definition of narrow-angle glaucoma has been used to typify glaucoma in the American Cocker Spaniel. To be accurate, the gonioscopic description should include descriptions of open, narrow, and collapsed ciliary cleft if possible, as well as open, narrow, and closed iridocorneal angles.[97] It is possible to have a narrowed or closed filtering cleft with a normal open angle (early- to middle-stage open-angle glaucoma) and an open ciliary cleft with a closed or almost closed iridocorneal angle (normotensive eye with goniodysgenesis) (**Figure 12.37**).[98]

A histopathologic study of glaucomatous eyes, in which closed iridocorneal angles were only diagnosed if peripheral anterior synechiae were present,[97] added further confusion to the terminology. In this study, all glaucomatous eyes, whether primary or secondary, (1) had collapsed/closed ciliary clefts, and (2) all primary glaucomas had obstructive tissue in front of the cleft that was interpreted as goniodysgenesis but were still classified as open-angle glaucoma.

For the purposes of this chapter, an angle is closed if it is either covered or collapsed. Primary angle closure may arise from developmental anomalies of the pectinate ligaments (goniodysgenesis, pectinate ligament dysplasia), the result of adhesion of the iris base to the inner sclera from an acquired collapse of the ciliary cleft, or acquired obstruction from the peripheral iris (peripheral anterior synechiae due a narrow angle). The causes of acquired

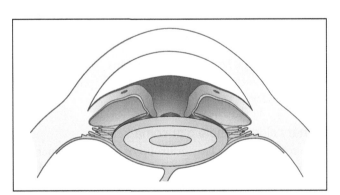

Figure 12.31 Illustration of pupil seclusion from posterior synechiae resulting in iris bombe. The pressure head of the aqueous humor in the posterior chamber balloons the iris forward. Peripheral anterior synechiae and collapse of the ciliary cleft subsequently develop. (From Martin, C.L. 1983. In: Peiffer, R.L., editor. *Comparative Ophthalmic Pathology*. Charles C Thomas: Springfield, IL, pp. 137–169.)

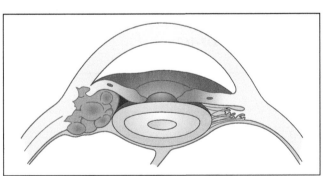

Figure 12.33 Illustration of an intraocular tumor pushing forward on the iris base creating iridocorneal angle closure and infiltrating the angle to obstruct flow directly. Other mechanisms for glaucoma are through stimulation of preiridal fibrovascular membrane formation, hemorrhage, inflammation, and excessive thickening of the iris to close the angles. (From Martin, C.L. 1983. In: Peiffer, R.L., editor. *Comparative Ophthalmic Pathology*. Charles C Thomas: Springfield, IL, pp. 137–169.)

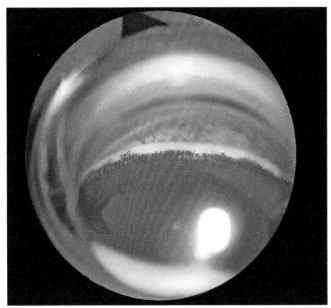

Figure 12.34 Goniophotograph of a beagle with moderately early open-angle glaucoma. Note the relatively normal pectinate ligament and open filtering cleft, but the lens is very round and protruding through the pupil.

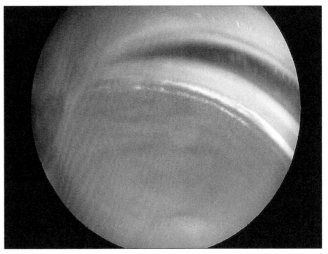

Figure 12.36 Normotensive eye of a 4-year-old cocker spaniel with contralateral glaucoma. Note the apparently narrow filtering cleft that is closed or covered with a sheet that is not pigmented, except for some streaks. This is typical of goniodysgenesis.

closure in primary glaucoma are not known, and while most ophthalmologists believe this phenomenon occurs, progressive closure has not been documented in a systematic way. This author has gonioscopically examined the filtration angle in young American Cocker Spaniels while evaluating the patient for cataract extraction surgery and found the angle to be open/normal. In dogs that were reexamined years later with glaucoma, the gonioscopic impression had changed to one of a closed angle. Unfortunately, the cause of the closure in this subset of patients could not conclusively be determined to be natural progression/closure versus peripheral anterior synechia due to complications from the previous cataract extraction surgery. Acquired collapse of the ciliary cleft is a universal histopathologic finding with most all canine glaucomas (possibly because most glaucoma eyes are enucleated only after they are end stage/blind), but the causes for the collapse in primary glaucoma that does not have obstruction in the angle are not usually understood.

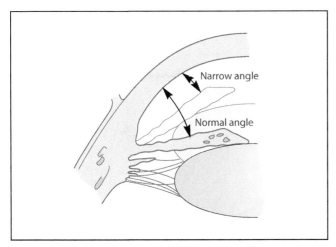

Figure 12.35 Concept of narrow angle in which the anterior chamber depth is reduced, bringing the peripheral iris closer to the cornea and being more susceptible to closure from pupillary block.

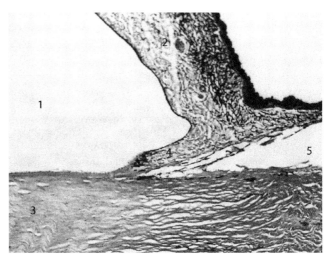

Figure 12.37 Photomicrograph of the normotensive eye from a basset hound with contralateral glaucoma. This micrograph illustrates goniodysgenesis or a closed angle with an open filtering cleft. Note how the base of the iris is pulled forward. (1: Anterior chamber; 2: Iris; 3: Limbus; 4: Pectinate ligament dysplasia; 5: Open ciliary cleft.)

One form of glaucoma that commonly occurs in the American Cocker Spaniel is characterized by collapse of the ciliary cleft, collapse of the pectinate ligaments outward against the cornea, and resultant angle closure. The closure of an angle could also occur due to anatomic predisposition of a shallow anterior chamber that creates a narrow angle (in degrees) between the plane of the iris and the cornea (**Figures 12.28, 12.29, and 12.35**). With a shallow anterior chamber or narrowed iridocorneal angle, occlusion by the adjacent peripheral iris may occur because of various conditions, the most common probably being pupillary block. Increased resistance of fluid flow through the pupil results in posterior chamber aqueous humor pushing the iris base forward, which is more likely to obstruct or close the iridocorneal angle because of the shallow peripheral anterior chamber. This closure may be acute or slow and insidious.[99] A gonioscopic study of Samoyeds found no relationship between goniodysgenesis and glaucoma but did correlate glaucoma with closed angles.[100] This study differentiated between a closed angle from an unspecified cause and severe goniodysgenesis that manifested as a closed angle. No evidence for the presence of peripheral anterior synechiae was given. Further ultrasonography studies in Samoyeds demonstrated that the anterior chamber is not as deep, the lens is thicker and further forward, and the vitreous is longer in eyes with a predisposition to glaucoma versus controls.[100] These findings may be additive or may be eventual decompensating factors on a compromised closed angle from goniodysgenesis. In previous editions of this text, Martin stated that Samoyeds presenting to him with unilateral glaucoma had closed angles from extensive goniodysgenesis in the opposite normotensive eye (**Figure 12.38**).

High magnification is necessary to differentiate a solid (albeit thin) sheet that has linear pigmented streaks that simulate ligaments (as is common with goniodysgenesis) from a collapsed cleft with ligaments that are pushed out and adherent to the inner cornea (closed cleft, as is frequent in the American Cocker Spaniel). High-magnification gonioscopy or scanning electron microscopy indicates that these angles are not narrow, normal angles but closed angles, and they are most compatible histologically with developmental anomalies (**Figures 12.37 through 12.40**).[20,98,101] There is little evidence that these angles are initially normal and then became closed. In support of this point, a study on Flat-coated retrievers with goniodysgenesis found that the severity of the problem was not statistically related to age.[102]

Goniodysgenesis is an arrest in the normal development of the pectinate ligaments that occur as late as 7–14 days postpartum. The pectinate ligaments arise from rarefaction of a sheet of fibrils that arise diffusely from

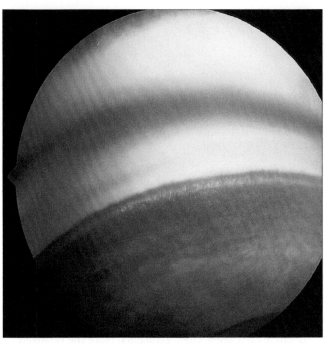

Figure 12.38 Goniophotograph of a normotensive eye of a 2-year-old Samoyed with unilateral glaucoma. The angle is covered or closed by a sheet of tissue that is lighter in pigmentation than the iris and has pigmented streaks. This simulates a narrow cleft but open angle. This is typical of the appearance and degree of goniodysgenesis that is associated with glaucoma.

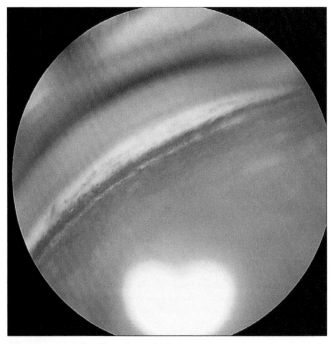

Figure 12.39 Closed angle in a normotensive eye of a basset hound with contralateral glaucoma. Note the narrow white zone that mimics the opening of the ciliary cleft. If the eye is normotensive, microscopic flow holes can be observed around the circumference of the angle.

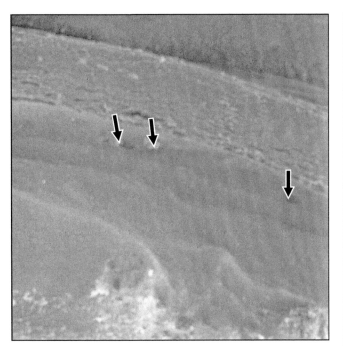

Figure 12.40 Scanning electron micrograph of a normotensive eye of a basset hound with contralateral glaucoma similar to Figure 12.39. Note the solid sheet with microscopic flow holes near the corneal insertion (arrows). (From Martin, C., and Wyman, M. 1978. *Veterinary Clinics of North America* 8:257–286.)

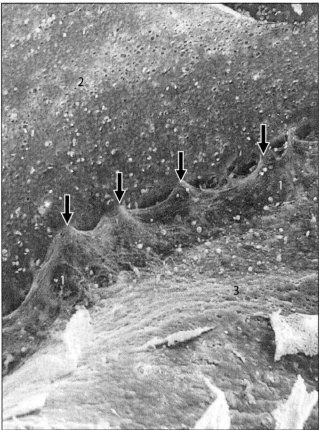

Figure 12.41 Scanning electron micrograph of the iridocorneal angle from a 1-day-old puppy. Note the "hammocking" of a fibrillar sheet (1) across the angle with focal attachments to the corneal side (arrows). The fine pores noted on sheets in the adult (Figures 12.39 and 12.40) correspond to the openings on the corneal side of the embryonic sheet. (2: Corneal endothelium; 3: Iris.) (From Martin, C. 1974. *American Journal of Veterinary Research* 35:1433–1439.)

the peripheral iris and insert by focal attachments to the peripheral cornea (**Figure 12.41**).[103] Various degrees of angle maldevelopment occur where the sheet of fibrils remains as a "web" of tissue versus individual pectinate ligaments or strands, but glaucoma is typically associated with only the very severe forms.[5,20,101,102,104,105] Milder degrees of arrest manifest as an imperfectly developed but recognizable pectinate ligament (**Figures 12.42 and 12.43**); severe degrees of maldevelopment manifest as a solid sheet that pulls the iris forward, creating the appearance of a narrow filtering cleft that is actually a closed angle, with small flow holes visible near the corneal attachment if the eye is normotensive (**Figures 12.36 through 12.40**). If the holes become obstructed, the sheet is forced outward against the cornea, and the ciliary cleft becomes collapsed (**Figure 12.44**). While the predisposition to primary closed-angle glaucoma is bilateral, glaucoma usually manifests sequentially. It is important to examine the normal eye to determine the sequence of events in the affected eye and whether there is a risk to the normotensive eye. The question arises, when examining a diseased organ, whether the lesion is primary or secondary. This can be resolved by looking at the normal twin organ before the secondary effects of increased IOP become apparent. While the sheets of tissue are very obvious, it may be questioned whether deeper angle

structures are also involved with aqueous humor obstruction, or what dynamics within the anterior chamber result in sudden decompensation of a compromised iridocorneal angle. Some authors[102] prefer the term "pectinate ligament dysplasia," as gonioscopically, this is all that can be ascertained. Pectinate ligament dysplasia results in histologic anatomic alterations in the angle, pulling the iris base forward, and an altered relationship between the termination of the corneoscleral trabecula and the ciliary cleft and anomalous ligament (**Figure 12.37**). Thus, the more inclusive term of goniodysgenesis may be correct.

Several interesting and unexplained statistics have arisen repeatedly from studies of closed-angle glaucoma. Several reports have found as high as a 3:1 predominance of females to males for glaucoma.[45,46,104–107] The left eye tends to be affected first in the American cocker and Welsh springer spaniel.[45,46,105] Most cases of closed-angle glaucoma present

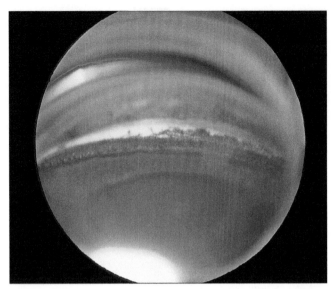

Figure 12.42 Goniophotograph of a normotensive eye of a 6-month-old basset hound. Note that about half of the angle has "webbing" of the proximal pectinate ligament on the iris side due to incomplete rarefaction. This is a mild anomaly without significance for clinical disease.

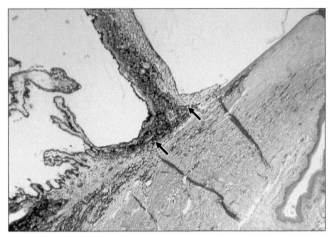

Figure 12.44 Photomicrograph of the iridocorneal angle of a basset hound with goniodysgenesis and a closed ciliary cleft (arrows). The opposite eye had become glaucomatous 1 year previously, and this eye had been normotensive on multiple examinations. The cleft was open in some quadrants and closed in others on histology and scanning electron microscopy. This may represent a preglaucomatous phase with progressive closure of the cleft.

in the winter months.[45–47] The age of onset of glaucoma varies a great deal, with most breeds affected by goniodysgenesis becoming glaucomatous as young adults from 3–6 years old,[104,105,108] but all ages, from the neonate to the aged animal, can be affected. Closed-angle glaucoma in general occurs from 6–8 years of age.[45–47,107]

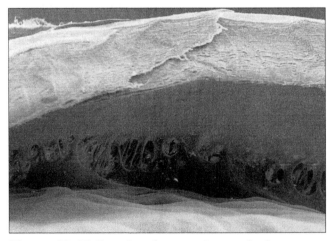

Figure 12.43 Scanning electron micrograph of a basset hound with modest goniodysgenesis, consisting of "webbing" of ligaments, which is on the iridal side of the ligaments. (In the photomicrograph, the cut surface of the cornea appears dorsally and the iris surface appears ventrally.) (From Martin, C. 1975. *Journal of the American Animal Hospital Association* 11:180–184; Martin C. 1975. *Journal of the American Animal Hospital Association* 11:300–306.)

A major unresolved question is the precipitating factor(s) for glaucoma in an eye that has been compensated for years. Anterior uveitis, lipids in the anterior chamber, and decompressing the anterior chamber surgically have been precipitating factors (but not the only ones) for glaucoma in eyes with goniodysgenesis. Owners may relate the onset of glaucoma to a variety of conditions such as weather (barometric changes), diet, and stress. Many basset hounds are initially observed with miosis, flare, and low IOP that rapidly develops into florid glaucoma with dilated pupils. While this might technically be called secondary glaucoma, the plasmoid aqueous humor is much more likely to obstruct an angle with a few flow holes than a normal angle. An analogy would be the decompensation of a chronic nephritis patient into renal failure by stress such as surgery or water restriction. Is the renal failure due to the stress or due to the chronic nephritis? Whether an eye with goniodysgenesis manifests glaucoma, at any age, is a combination of the severity of the abnormality and the presence of the appropriate stress to the eye. The stress may be endogenous or exogenous in origin, and this variability predicts the difficulty in determining the genetics of glaucoma.

A study comparing the number of mast cells in globes enucleated for glaucoma and normal controls found fewer mast cells in the glaucomatous eyes, irrespective of the cause of glaucoma. The significance is unknown, and it is possible that mast cells may not have been identified due to their degranulation.[109] Other factors such as increased thickness of the lens with age, forward placement of the iris and the lens, and enlargement of the vitreous may all contribute to pupillary block and shallowing of the peripheral anterior chamber with eventual closure of the angle[110] (**Figures 12.27 and 12.30**). Much of this configuration could also be produced by severe goniodysgenesis that typically has a sheet of shorter length than the normal pectinate ligaments. Consequently, the iris base is pulled forward (**Figure 12.37**). As previously cited, almost all eyes enucleated for goniodysplasia-related glaucoma had pigment dispersion and inflammatory cells in the angle region.[82] Similarly, retinal pigment damage, breakdown of the blood–retinal barrier, and retinal inflammation were found in dogs with glaucoma with goniodysgenesis.[111] While these findings have been suggested as perhaps being contributory to the glaucoma, some believe that this inflammation represents secondary effects to the acute high IOP elevations resulting in ischemia to most of the intraocular structures.

The conformation of the anterior chamber may vary considerably between individuals, the significance of which is currently unknown. Individual dogs are observed in which the iris "hugs" the lens very tightly, and the outline of the lens is visible through the iris (**Figures 12.27 and 12.45**). These individuals would presumably be more susceptible to pupillary block and subsequent angle closure, but this has not been proven. Also, individuals are observed which have a flat plateau of an iris plane (plateau iris) but a recess at the iris root, which may be more susceptible to angle closure (**Figure 12.29**).

Closed-angle glaucoma is common in the basset hound and American Cocker Spaniel in the United States, but a wide variety of purebred and crossbred dogs have been observed with similar gonioscopic findings.[47,112] The English Cocker Spaniel, Samoyed, Siberian husky, Chow Chow, Shar Pei, Welsh springer spaniel, Bouvier des Flandres, shiba inu, and Flat-coated retriever are also predisposed to closed-angle glaucoma.[41,100,104,105,108,113] Pectinate ligament dysplasia (PLD) in Flat-coated retrievers in the United Kingdom was found in 35% of the examined dogs, and when graded on severity, only those with 63% or more of the angle involved had glaucoma. If the offspring of severely affected dogs were examined, 83% of the offspring had PLD.[102] The heritability was calculated as 0.7 in the Flat-coated retriever.[114] The Bouvier des Flandres has a high incidence of goniodysgenesis (75%) and glaucoma (23% of cases in 155 dogs) in Europe.[104] In the Welsh springer spaniel, goniodysgenesis is possibly a dominant trait.[105] In Norway, English springer spaniels had a prevalence rate of 24% for PLD (goniodysgenesis).[115] Bjerkas et al. found a correlation between PLD and narrow angles and PLD and narrow angles with glaucoma.[115] Glaucoma is considered a familial trait in English

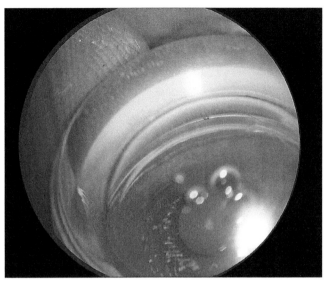

Figure 12.45 Goniophotograph of a normotensive eye of a 2-year-old American Cocker Spaniel with an open angle but a very tight iris–lens contact that outlines the lens through the iris base (see also Figure 12.27). This view is not ideal for showing the angle.

springer spaniels; breedings from normal sires and dams produced 85% of offspring with normal iridocorneal angles, while breedings with either one or both parents having PLD produced abnormal iridocorneal angles in 41%–57% of offspring. A polygenetic trait was postulated for PLD. While goniodysgenesis is probably inherited, and glaucoma has been observed in numerous families of dogs, the genetic mode of transmission of goniodysgenesis or glaucoma in most breeds is unknown. In the shiba inu, myocilin gene mutations were detected, but they did not correlate with glaucoma or goniodysgenesis,[116] illustrating again the differences between open-angle glaucoma and closed-angle glaucoma.

Acquired causes for closed angles in primary glaucoma are not understood, and their progression is rarely documented. Elevation of IOP by itself can cause the ciliary cleft to collapse and the angle to close, as observed in the beagle in the late stages of open-angle glaucoma.[92] In the American Cocker Spaniel, the pectinate ligaments appear to have been forced outward and are collapsed against the inner cornea. This could be explained by a collapse of the ciliary cleft from an unknown cause. PLD has been documented in the American Cocker Spaniel (**Figures 12.46 and 12.47**), but most American Cocker Spaniels with glaucoma appear to have a collapsed and closed ciliary cleft without evidence of PLD.

Diagnosis of closed-angle glaucoma

Diagnosis of closed-angle or closed-cleft glaucoma is based on gonioscopic examination. Often the angle of the

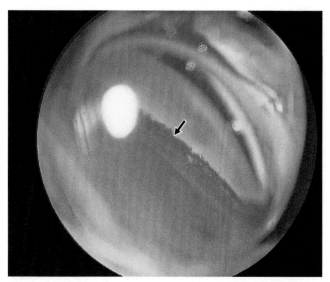

Figure 12.46 Goniophotograph of an American Cocker Spaniel with moderate goniodysgenesis of half of the viewed angle (arrow).

affected eye cannot be examined because of corneal edema or aqueous humor turbidity. It is then necessary to examine the opposite eye to give a prognosis for future glaucoma, as well as to determine the presumed cause of the affected eye. The severe degree of goniodysgenesis on gonioscopic examination typically manifests as a solid sheet with no pectinate ligaments visible (**Figures 12.38 and 12.39**). On low-power gonioscopy, a thin white zone simulates a narrowed filtering cleft with some fine darker radial streaks that may mimic pectinate ligaments. With appropriate high magnification, the angle is covered with solid iridal tissue that is less pigmented as it crosses the angle. A few flow holes can often be detected near the corneal insertion of the sheet of tissue (**Figures 12.39 and 12.40**). The sheet usually occupies 75+% of the circumference when it is associated with glaucoma.[102] The sheet is shorter than the normal pectinate ligaments, which pulls the base of the iris forward and produces a very flat iris plane and, rarely, iridodonesis due to lack of lens support. While clinically the angles with goniodysgenesis look similar whether the IOP is elevated or not, the changes in the deeper angle structures are obvious on histopathologic examination. When flow holes become obstructed, the sheet, which is the pectinate ligament precursor, is pushed outward against the limbal region by the pressure gradient. The ciliary cleft is obliterated, and venous channels in the sclera collapse (**Figures 12.44 and 12.48**). This lesion has erroneously been described as a peripheral anterior synechia.[117] If the eye is normotensive, a sheet is present that pulls the iris root forward, and the ciliary cleft is open, indicating that aqueous humor is passing behind the sheet (**Figures 12.37 and 12.49**).[19]

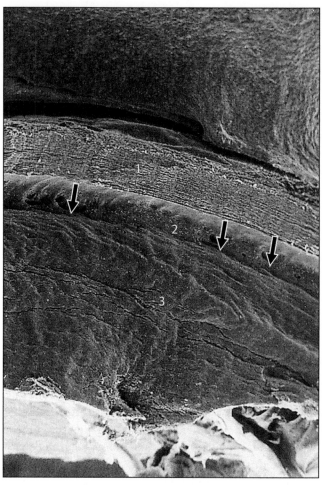

Figure 12.47 Scanning electron micrograph of a 2-year-old American Cocker Spaniel with goniodysgenesis over about half of the angle circumference. The dog was euthanized for nonocular reasons. (1: Cornea; 2: Sheet over filtering cleft; 3: Iris; arrows: Flow holes.) (×56.) (From Martin, C., and Wyman, M. 1978. *Veterinary Clinics of North America* 8:257–286.)

> The role of gonioscopic findings in predicting glaucoma risk is quite controversial within the veterinary ophthalmology community and requires ongoing systematic investigation and statistical analysis. What began as clinical impressions are now being supported by accumulated statistical data in a variety of breeds.

Secondary glaucoma

Secondary glaucomas may be the predominant form of glaucoma in a geographical region due to popularity of certain terrier breeds.[6,7,118] Secondary glaucoma often has rather obvious causes of angle obstruction, but close examination of both eyes may help to explain why some dogs develop ocular hypertension following an insult and others do not. The lens should be looked at critically

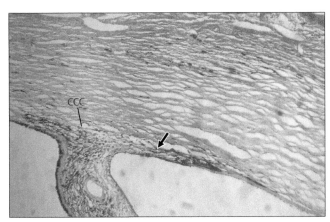

Figure 12.48 Photomicrograph from the eye of a basset hound that has glaucoma (from Figure 12.14). Note the iris-like tissue lining the peripheral cornea (arrow), collapse of the ciliary cleft (CCC), and absence of scleral venous channels.

when assigning it a role in secondary glaucoma. Gelatt and MacKay reviewed a large database (Veterinary Medical Database) and found that 81% of secondary glaucoma cases were associated with cataract formation (lens induced uveitis), with 20% of cataracts developing glaucoma.[119] Lens

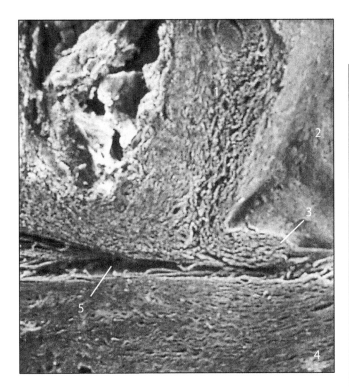

Figure 12.49 Scanning electron micrograph of the normotensive eye of the basset hound depicted in Figures 12.14 and 12.44. Unlike the quadrant viewed in Figure 12.44, this quadrant has an open ciliary cleft. (1: Iris; 2: Anterior chamber; 3: Pectinate ligament dysplasia; 4: Limbus, 5: Ciliary cleft.)

displacement accounted for 12%, postcataract surgery for 5%, uveitis unspecified for 7%, hyphema for 7%, and intraocular neoplasia for 4% of the cases of secondary glaucoma. Johnson et al. reported that secondary glaucomas were diagnosed in 7% of the population of a university-based ophthalmology clinic, and the condition was bilateral in 21% of the patients.[120] Uveitis (not associated with surgery) was the precipitating factor in 45%, surgical uveitis (phacoemulsification) in 15%, and lens displacement in 15% of the cases.

Etiology and mechanisms

Hyphema

Glaucoma associated with acute hyphema usually has an open angle that is occluded with blood and fibrin (**Figure 12.49a,b**). Later, especially with cases of traumatic uveitis/hyphema, posterior synechiae and iris bombe may produce a peripheral anterior synechia and closed-angle glaucoma.

Trauma

Trauma may result in either open- or closed-angle glaucoma. Trauma-induced anterior uveitis may result in anterior (peripheral or central iris to corneal endothelial surface) or posterior (iris to lens) synechiae, with resultant obstruction of aqueous humor outflow (**Figure 12.50**).

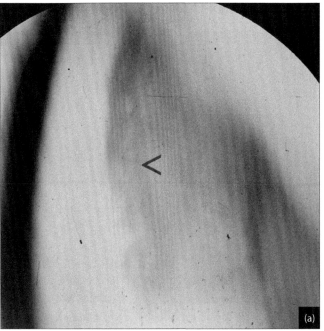

Figure 12.49a Gonioscopic view of a blood/fibrin clot occluded filtration angle (arrow) in a dog with hyphema. The eye had elevated IOP that was controlled with a topical carbonic anhydrase inhibitor diuretic and a topical corticosteroid.

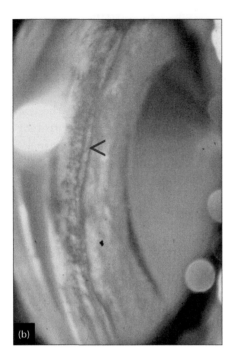

Figure 12.49b Gonioscopic view of same filtration angle as in Figure 12.49a after 2 weeks of therapy with topical corticosteroids and carbonic anhydrase inhibitor diuretics to control IOP. Note the clearance of the blood/fibrin clot and the visualization of pectinate ligaments (arrow).

Trauma may also produce tears in the pectinate ligaments and the ciliary cleft, resulting in recession of the angle. These tears heal by fibrosis, and the resultant loss of

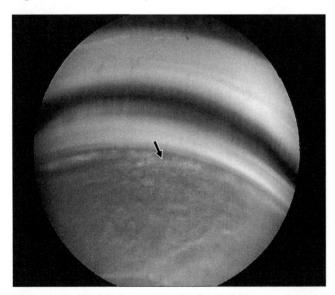

Figure 12.50 Miniature poodle that had blunt trauma from a golf ball hitting the eye 6 months prior to presentation with glaucoma. The eye developed a cataract and a difference in the width of the filtering cleft is present due to peripheral anterior synechiae (arrow). The open portion may represent angle recession as pectinate ligaments are not visible.

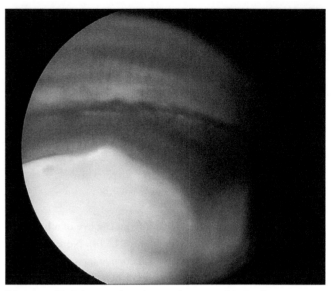

Figure 12.51 Peripheral anterior synechia in the angle of 14-year-old American Cocker Spaniel with a hypermature cataract and lens-induced uveitis. The angle in the contralateral eye was normal. Note the irregular hypermature lens surface. The angle has no visible pectinate ligaments, there is pigment dispersion in the angle, and the width of the angle is irregular.

angle/ciliary cleft function may produce glaucoma months later. Perforating corneal trauma often results in the iris moving forward to plug the defect, and the shallow anterior chamber, combined with inflammation, may result in angle closure. Glaucoma is relatively rare in the horse, and trauma is a significant cause. Four of nine globes in one histopathologic series of equine glaucoma cases showed evidence of perforating or nonperforating trauma.[121]

Inflammation

Intraocular inflammation (uveitis) from a variety of causes is a common cause of secondary glaucoma. Uveitis may produce severe posterior synechiae that results in iris bombe and sufficient shallowing of the anterior chamber to produce secondary closure of the angle with peripheral anterior synechiae (**Figure 12.31**). Alternatively, inflammation may produce peripheral anterior synechiae without posterior synechiae (**Figure 12.51a**) due to vascular endothelial growth factor (VEGF) induced preiridal fibrovascular membrane (PIFM) formation.[122]

Aphakic and pseudophakic glaucoma

Transient ocular hypertension (acute postoperative hypertension, POH) after cataract surgery is common in the dog. The cause is unknown, and it is differentiated from glaucoma because of its transient nature and the lack of optic nerve damage in most cases. The incidence of POH

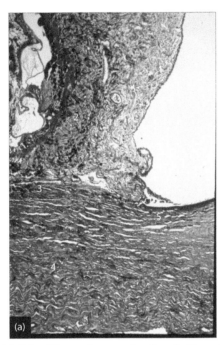

Figure 12.51a Photomicrograph of angle fibrosis and PIFM formation in a dog with longstanding anterior uveitis and secondary glaucoma. Note the totally collapsed ciliary cleft and the lack of scleral drainage channels. (1: PIFM, 2: Iris, 3: Collapsed ciliary cleft, 4: Sclera, 5: Descemet's membrane/posterior cornea).

may approach 50%, and the IOP may exceed 50 mmHg (6.7 kPa). The IOP usually peaks by 3 hours and normalizes by 24 hours.[123] The cause of POH is not totally clear, but the concern is that these patients may be predisposed to glaucoma later. Miller et al., in a nonmasked study in normal dogs undergoing phacoemulsification, demonstrated that the ciliary cleft was narrow 24 hours after surgery despite IOP normalization.[124] The cause and significance of these findings are unknown. Two studies on non-POH glaucoma postcataract surgery found no correlation with transient POH and later development of glaucoma.[125,126]

Glaucoma following cataract surgery may not deserve a separate category and is undoubtedly associated with multiple mechanisms. In one study,[127] the incidence of glaucoma following phacoemulsification for cataract removal was associated with a <10% incidence of postcataract surgery glaucoma. The Boston terrier, American Cocker Spaniel, cocker spaniel-poodle crosses, and Shih Tzus (breeds that are also predisposed to develop primary glaucoma) were at greatest risk for long-term postoperative glaucoma. If routine gonioscopy is performed prior to cataract surgery, varying degrees of acquired closure and goniodysgenesis may often be noted. However, the frequency of non-POH postoperative glaucoma has not yet been correlated with preoperative gonioscopy. Finding gonioscopic lesions does not often abort the cataract

surgery, but it may forewarn the owner and the surgeon of increased postoperative risks.

In another study, Biros et al. retrospectively evaluated the risk factors for glaucoma in a series of cataract surgeries.[125] Of 346 operated eyes, 17% developed glaucoma. More compelling was that 29% of the eyes followed for 12 months developed glaucoma. Median follow-up for all dogs was only 5.8 months, so this figure might significantly underrepresent the true long-term incidence. Risk factors for glaucoma in the study were hypermature cataracts (1 in 4 developed glaucoma), purebreds, aphakia, and male dogs. About 33% of aphakic eyes developed glaucoma compared to 10% for pseudophakic eyes; however, the multiple reasons for not placing an intraocular lens (IOL) at the time of surgery might be the predisposing factor(s), rather than aphakia, per se. Transient POH events after surgery were not found to be predictive of later glaucoma, although half of the eyes that had POH later developed glaucoma.

Neoplasia

Anterior uveal neoplasia may invade the ciliary body and obstruct outflow, shed cells that obstruct the outflow channels, or have necrosis with inflammation and hemorrhage that occludes the outflow channels (**Figure 12.33**). Neoplasia may also stimulate PIFM formation or rubeosis iridis that, when advanced, covers, obstructs, and collapses the iridocorneal angle.[122,128] Lymphosarcoma in the dog and the cat is the most common secondary ocular neoplasia and usually manifests as a bilateral inflammatory secondary glaucoma (see Chapter 11 **Figures 11.48 and 11.53**). Melanoma in the dog and the cat eventually produce glaucoma and may be masked by hyphema or inflammation (see Chapter 11 **Figures 11.67 and 11.73**). When presented with hyphema or cloudiness of the cornea/aqueous humor, ultrasonography is necessary for diagnosis of an intraocular tumor. In a pathologic study of glaucoma in cats, 41% had glaucoma from one of either of these two neoplasms.[129] This study was biased, however, because of the cases evaluated being enucleated specimens only.

Uveal cysts

Cysts in the ciliary body have been associated with glaucoma in the Great Dane[130] and Golden retriever.[131] Normally, most cysts in the anterior chamber are considered benign. In a retrospective pathologic study of canine glaucoma cases, 5% of the glaucomatous globes were from Golden retrievers, and 52% of these Golden retriever globes had iridociliary cysts.[132] Concerning pathophysiology of uveal cyst-associated glaucoma, it was felt that the cysts may mechanically push forward on the lens–iris diaphragm, closing the angle and interfering with aqueous humor flow, or the contents of ruptured cysts may obstruct the trabecular meshwork.[130,132] A more recent study[133] showed that the trabecular meshwork/ciliary cleft was filled with free pigment in Golden retrievers with uveal cysts and glaucoma, peripheral anterior synechia was seen in approximately 30% of cases, posterior synechia was seen in approximately 50% of the cases, and PIFM was seen in about 50% of the cases. These findings may indicate that the contents of the uveal cysts and portions of the ruptured cysts themselves may induce synechia and PIFM formation or may mechanically obstruct aqueous outflow channels leading to secondary glaucoma. In a study by Townsend et al., 164 Golden retrievers underwent clinical evaluation for genetic eye disease with emphasis being placed on identification of uveal cysts.[134] Approximately 24% of eyes (35% of dogs) had the presence of one or more uveal cysts. Subsequent studies (Townsend, personal communication) using high-resolution ultrasonography indicates the incidence of ciliary cysts in the breed is even higher than in the published study. This would indicate that the incidence of glaucoma associated with uveal cysts in the Golden retriever is far less than the incidence of secondary glaucoma.

Pigment proliferation/dispersion

The Cairn terrier, Scottish terrier, boxer, and Labrador retriever have a form of glaucoma associated with increased pigment deposition in the anterior and posterior segments of the eye.[135–139] Clinically, the syndrome is most prevalent

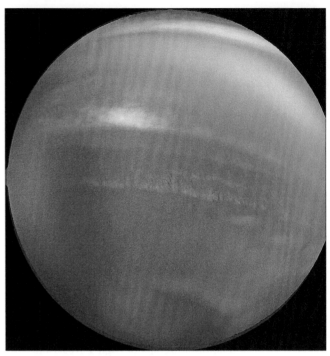

Figure 12.53 Goniophotograph of the normotensive eye of a Scottish terrier with unilateral glaucoma. Note the heavy pigmentation of the angle that has obscured and filled up most of the spaces between the pectinate ligaments.

in the Cairn terrier and manifests initially as a progressive, bilateral, dark peripheral thickening of the iris root followed by scleral/episcleral plaques of pigment adjacent to the limbus (**Figure 12.52**). The latter two signs slowly increase in severity, with pigment clumps in the aqueous and pigmentation in the ventral iridocorneal angle and on the peripheral corneal endothelium (**Figure 12.53**). Glaucoma develops in the latter stages, and the tapetum may have encroachment of pigment beginning peripherally, causing a diminution of the normal tapetal color. The age of onset and the speed of progression of the syndrome is highly variable. The cause of the glaucoma appears to be obstruction of aqueous outflow pathways by the vast amounts of pigment, but the cause for the increased pigment is unknown. van de Sandt et al. found that most of the pigment-containing cells were macrophages.[139] The condition is inherited in the Cairn terrier, possibly as an autosomal dominant trait.[137] Pigment proliferation/dispersion is an insidious disease that has been refractory to therapy.

Lens displacement

Lens displacement is the most significant cause of secondary glaucoma (65%) in terrier breeds,[6,7,118,140–142] but is not restricted to terriers. Anterior lens luxation may physically obstruct aqueous humor flow, or the vitreous adhered to the posterior lens capsule may obstruct the flow at the pupil (**Figures 12.32 and 12.54**). Subluxated lenses are less

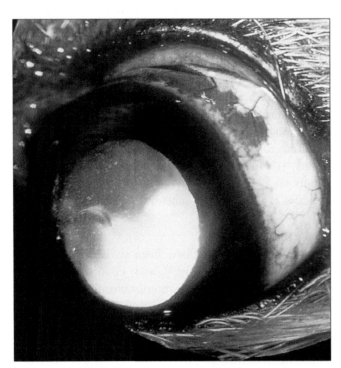

Figure 12.52 Episcleral pigment in a Cairn terrier that may be the precursor to more extensive intraocular pigmentation and glaucoma. The intraocular pressure was high–normal in this patient.

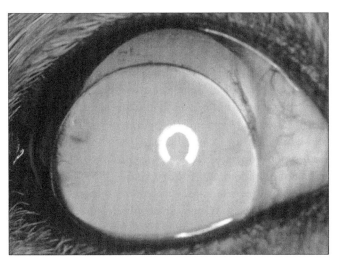

Figure 12.54 Anterior lens luxation in a Jack Russell terrier producing glaucoma. The clear lens may be easily overlooked in the anterior chamber, especially if there is accompanying corneal edema.

likely to produce glaucoma, and it is often less obvious how they interfere with aqueous humor dynamics. Subluxation of the lens to one side may produce a regional shallowing of the chamber and restriction of flow at the ciliary cleft (**Figure 12.25**). Vitreous herniation may produce pupil blockade, or strands of vitreous may obstruct the angle. Posteriorly luxated lenses may produce a low-grade uveitis with progressive peripheral anterior synechiae or changes in the ciliary cleft. (See also Chapter 13.)

Aqueous misdirection glaucoma

In the dog, usually following intracapsular lens extraction but occasionally associated with cataract extraction surgery and disruption of the posterior lens capsule, a rare and frustrating form of aphakic glaucoma occurs associated with anterior vitreous presentation and pupillary block with vitreous and inflammatory membranes or remnants of posterior lens capsule. Termed "malignant glaucoma" in man, the lack of a formed anterior vitreous face following lens removal allows vitreous to displace cranially into the pupillary opening. If aqueous production results in aqueous humor being misguided caudally with a subsequent pressure gradient that pushes more vitreous forward, the continued displacement of vitreous into the pupil and the anterior chamber results in a pupillary block situation, especially if fibrous membranes associated with inflammation and the anterior vitreous or remnants of the posterior capsule span the pupillary opening. Aggressive surgery to remove the fibrous membranes and open the pupil to aqueous flow and to reestablish a new anterior vitreous face caudal to the iris is necessary to try to control IOP and salvage these afflicted eyes. Due to the instability of the vitreous (usually somewhat liquefied due to the movement of the preoperative lens

luxation), continued prolapse of vitreous cranially is common, thereby making control of IOP difficult.

Feline glaucoma

Cats are frequently presented quite late in the course of glaucoma with owner complaint of an enlarged eye or a dilated pupil (**Figure 12.12**). Unlike in the dog, glaucoma in cats is rarely peracute with marked corneal edema, episcleral injection, and blepharospasm, so early diagnosis is uncommon. In cats, most glaucomas are thought to be due to, or associated with, chronic inflammation. Sixty percent and 87%, respectively, of cats in two clinical series[143,144] and 41% of glaucomatous eyes in a pathologic series[129] were associated with inflammation. In the pathologic series, the inflammatory lesion was a lymphocytic–plasmacytic uveitis that could be either diffuse or focal, or both. In most instances, there were obstructive lesions from either the inflammatory cells or collapse of the ciliary cleft and peripheral anterior synechiae (**Figure 12.55**), but in 13% of these eyes, there was no notable inflammatory mechanical cause of glaucoma.[129] In light of the frequent histopathologic finding of mild inflammatory cell presence in the anterior and posterior segments of dogs with primary glaucoma,[82,111] perhaps these histopathologic findings in cats should be reevaluated concerning actual cause of glaucoma. Jacobi and Dubielzig described eight cases of apparent primary open-angle

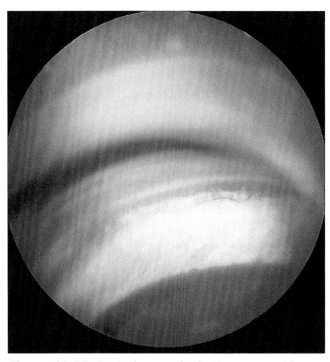

Figure 12.55 Goniophotograph of a Siamese cat with uveitis induced glaucoma in the opposite eye. Note the irregularity of the iris base that is pulled forward because of peripheral anterior synechiae over much of the viewed angle.

glaucoma (six cases were domestic shorthaired or domestic longhaired cats, two were Burmese) from a retrospective histopathology study.[145] The mean age was 9 years, and all had an open ciliary cleft (unlike the case of end-stage open-angle glaucoma in the beagle). Hampson et al. described a form of primary glaucoma in Burmese cats in Australia in which there was no evidence of inflammation, and the angles were open, narrow, or closed.[146] A related group of Siamese cats with multiple anterior segment congenital lesions, including goniodysgenesis, and early-onset glaucoma has been investigated.[147,148] Blocker and van der Woerdt described glaucoma in 82 cats, of which five were thought to be primary glaucomas.[144] Goniodysgenesis does not appear to play a significant role in clinical feline glaucoma, although it has been described.[147–149] There is very little documentation describing the forms of primary glaucoma in the cat, but it may be more prevalent than suspected, based on bilateral involvement in many patients without overt uveitis. As infectious diseases are a leading cause of uveitis, infectious disease serology should be performed on cats with glaucoma. Lens displacement/luxation is frequent with inflammation and may be associated with glaucomatous or normotensive eyes (**Figure 12.56**). Because of the large anterior chamber of the cat, elevated IOP with anterior lens luxation is not as common in the cat, as is the case in the dog.[150]

A unique form of glaucoma occurs in the cat in which the lens–iris diaphragm moves forward and collapses the anterior chamber. The lens is not luxated in that the zonules are still intact, but the pupillary block and collapsed angle result in moderate-to-severe pressure elevations. The condition is usually unilateral and may persist for months. It is thought to represent a form of aqueous humor misdirection glaucoma in which the aqueous humor pools posteriorly in the vitreous, pushing the lens–iris diaphragm forward (**Figure 12.57**). The term aqueous humor misdirection is probably preferable to "malignant glaucoma" as used in man, as neoplasia is not involved in the pathogenesis. Czederpiltz et al. reported a relatively large series of cases with aqueous humor misdirection and found a mean age of 12 years (range of 4–16 years) and females more often affected.[151] The cause of the aqueous humor misdirection is unknown, but it is thought to result in compression of the anterior vitreal elements, resulting in a dense membrane on the anterior vitreal face that blocks the flow of fluid into the anterior chamber. Medical therapy does not relieve the collapsed anterior chamber, although the IOP may moderate. It is obviously prudent not to aggravate the pupillary block by avoiding drugs that are either strong miotics (i.e., latanoprost) or mydriatics. Most clinicians have recommended the use of topical carbonic anhydrase inhibitors to reduce IOP to more normal levels. Phacoemulsification alone or combined with a posterior capsulotomy and/or anterior vitrectomy may help some cases, but in the few cases reported, the results were variable, perhaps due to the chronicity of the condition.[150,151]

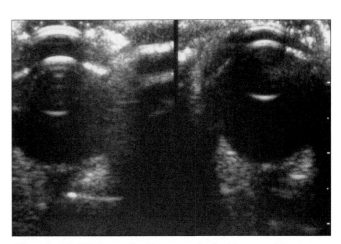

Figure 12.57 B-mode ultrasound of a 15-year-old domestic shorthaired cat with a unilateral shallowing of the anterior chamber and forward displacement of the lens with intact zonules (right frame). Compare the depth of the anterior chamber with the opposite normal eye (left frame). Phacoemulsification of the lens cured the persistent moderately elevated intraocular pressure.

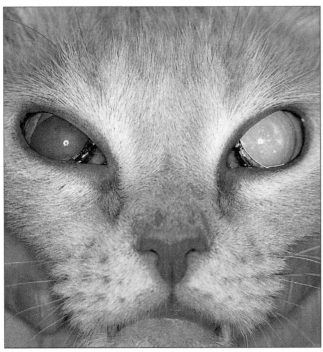

Figure 12.56 Bilateral glaucoma in an aged cat with chronic uveitis. Note one eye with a widely dilated pupil and the other with an anteriorly luxated opaque lens.

Equine glaucoma

As was the case with cats, glaucoma in the horse has in the past been an uncommon clinical diagnosis. The prevalence of glaucoma in horses in one veterinary teaching hospital was 0.11%, and in a national database of teaching hospitals, it was 0.07%.[152] As the use of electronic applanation and rebound tonometry has replaced the crude digital tonometry practiced for years, and as an increased index of suspicion has become more commonplace with primary care equine veterinarians, glaucoma has been increasingly diagnosed in equine patients. As was the case with cats, glaucoma in the horse may rarely be of early onset due to congenital malformations of the internal eye,[152–155] or it may rarely be primary[152,156,157] (glaucoma with no other apparent intraocular or extraocular disease causing a secondary glaucoma) (**Figure 12.58**). Most commonly, glaucoma in the horse is a secondary disorder. Blunt or penetrating trauma,[121] septic or sterile endophthalmitis,[156] anterior lens luxation,[156] and intraocular neoplasia[156,157] are sometimes seen as the initiating event that leads to altered aqueous outflow and secondary glaucoma. The most common cause of glaucoma in the horse, however, is due to sequelae from equine recurrent uveitis (ERU).[152,156–159] Seldom will horses present with acute uveitis with iris bombe and acute-angle closure with IOP elevation as is so commonly seen in the dog with acute uveitis induced glaucoma. Most horses with ERU-induced glaucoma have historically had episodic periods of tearing, blepharospasm, and corneal cloudiness associated with more acute episodes of uveitis. In some cases, ERU has been diagnosed and treated with topical and systemic anti-inflammatory agents and topical mydriatic/cycloplegic drugs with resolution of the more acute signs.

Most horses with ERU-induced glaucoma present with (usually) unilateral corneal cloudiness (**Figure 12.59**) with variable amounts of pain and vision loss that are not responsive to normal drug therapy for ERU. The appearance of curvilinear parallel lines with gray corneal edema between (breaks in Descemet's membrane, Haab's striae, **Figures 12.18a and 12.59**) is considered by some to be almost pathognomonic for equine glaucoma. Elevation of IOP in equine glaucoma is not always present at the time of examination. IOP in the horse is much more variable (and volatile) than in the dog, so repeated measurements of IOP may be needed to definitively diagnose glaucoma. Logistically, there are many variables that need to be reckoned with in obtaining an accurate IOP in the horse. Sedation will invariably reduce IOP,[160,161] and blepharospasm or globe retraction may cause erroneously high IOP readings due to globe compression. For this reason, palpebral nerve blocks are useful in patients with blepharospasm.[160] Head position is another variable to be concerned with when obtaining an accurate IOP in the horse. The head should be at the level of the heart or higher when measuring IOP in the horse in that IOP readings significantly above the true reading are obtained if the head is lower than the heart.[56] Episcleral injection and apparent pain are seldom seen with glaucoma in the horse, unlike in the canine with acute-angle closure glaucoma.[121,152,156–158] A widely dilated pupil is uncommonly seen with equine glaucoma, unless the eye is blind with absolute glaucoma, but the pupil is usually more mydriatic (**Figure 12.59**) than would be expected with a horse with just ERU and no glaucoma. Vision is variable in equine glaucoma. Early on, horses tend to tolerate elevated IOP

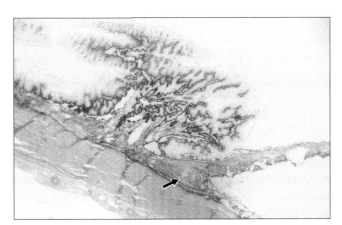

Figure 12.58 Photomicrograph of an equine eye that has glaucoma. This eye is similar to a glaucomatous canine eye because the ciliary cleft and pectinate ligament are collapsed against the inner sclera and the cornea (arrow). Microscopic evidence of uveitis was not apparent, and this may represent a case of primary closed-angle glaucoma.

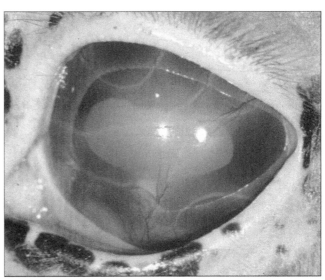

Figure 12.59 Unilateral glaucoma in an Appaloosa that has megaloglobus, pupillary dilation, and multiple breaks in Descemet's membrane with both generalized corneal edema and focal edema within the breaks.

better (less apparent pain and vision loss) than a dog with a similar magnitude of IOP elevation. Chronic glaucoma with hydrophthalmos, lens subluxation, corneal edema, and other signs of absolute glaucoma usually also show optic nerve degeneration/cupping with peripapillary retinal degeneration and subsequent blindness.

The cause of ERU-induced glaucoma in the horse is not completely understood. Some feel that the presence of a PIFM from chronic low-grade inflammation reduces the uveal–scleral outflow facility that is so important in the horse eye.[40,159] Extension of this PIFM across the filtration angle with subsequent scarring and closure of the filtration angle/ciliary cleft also would reduce aqueous humor outflow and cause increased IOP.[159]

As stated earlier, 360 posterior synechia with iris bombe and collapse of the ciliary cleft/filtration angle as an acute event similar to what is commonly seen in the dog does not seem to be problematic in the horse.

Hydrophthalmos with corneal exposure and horizontal linear corneal ulcerations are common with end-stage glaucoma and may lead to corneal rupture or the need to enucleate the eye for pain relief. However, many horses appear comfortable and will with time return to a normotensive state due to ciliary body atrophy associated with the chronic ocular hypertension.[156,158]

The incidence of primary glaucoma in the horse is such that definitive statements concerning breed predisposition are not possible. Because of the rather high incidence of ERU in the Appaloosa breed, this breed should be considered high risk for ERU-induced glaucoma.[152,156,158,159] Glaucoma is usually seen more commonly in older horses,[152,156–159] apart from the aforementioned congenital glaucoma cases.[153–155]

THERAPY OF PRIMARY GLAUCOMA

Glaucoma is a therapeutic challenge, if not an enigma, for the veterinarian. Glaucoma, although theoretically treatable, is a major cause of blindness (and enucleation). Therapy should depend on the type of glaucoma, the functional status of the eye (vision), and the resources and philosophy of the owner. As glaucoma is a final common pathway for a variety of intraocular diseases, specific therapy should vary with the etiologic diagnosis; therefore, diagnosis and therapy should be interdependent.

> Despite the availability of new and more effective topical glaucoma medications and new surgical procedures, it is very difficult to maintain vision in those forms of glaucoma characterized by markedly elevated IOP.

Pragmatically, the prognosis for vision can also modify the intensity and type of therapy. It is difficult to justify costly laser or aqueous diversion surgeries in an eye that is irreversibly blind. In addition, the results of surgery are equivocal; many cases are not controlled (IOP in a normal range) even with long-term medical treatment. Despite newer medications, few cases of primary glaucoma can be controlled indefinitely with medical therapy alone, either due to progressive worsening of the disease state or the eye becoming resistant to the pressure lowering effects of drug therapy over time.

Medical therapy
Emergency therapy for acute glaucoma
All recently visual eyes with glaucoma should have emergency medical therapy to normalize the IOP. The retina may survive for hours only, rather than days, in dogs with glaucoma in which the IOP elevations are commonly 60–90 mmHg (8.0–12.0 kPa).[162] Clines et al. correlated the return of vision with the duration of the initial acute episode, IOP at presentation, and the ability to lower IOP.[163] Forty-two percent of patients that had the IOP medically lowered to <20 mmHg (2.7 kPa) and had signs of <3 days' duration had return of vision. If the IOP was <50 mmHg (6.7 kPa) for <3 days, 52% had return of vision in the short term. Patients with both a history of 3 or more days duration and an IOP >50 mmHg (6.7 kPa) responded less well and only 18% had return of vision. Grozdanic et al. and clinical experience indicate that return of vision may occur as long as 2 weeks after a hypertensive episode if IOP can be returned to a normal state.[71] There should be no hurry to enucleate a blind, acutely glaucomatous globe, provided there are no signs of chronic glaucoma (buphthalmia, lens subluxation, or obvious optic nerve head atrophy/cupping) and the IOP can be returned to a normotensive state. The difficulty is that while the problem may appear "acute" to the owner (painful, red, cloudy, nonvisual eye), frequently the problem is actually chronic.

It is rare that one antiglaucoma medication alone will lower IOP into the normal range. Emergency therapy for the acute-angle closure primary glaucoma canine patient should be a combination of drugs that enhance aqueous humor outflow (miotics and/or prostaglandin analogs), drugs that reduce production of aqueous humor (carbonic anhydrase inhibitor [CAI] diuretics and β-blockers), drugs that dehydrate the vitreous and the anterior segment (osmotic diuretics), and/or surgical removal of aqueous humor from the anterior segment (anterior chamber fine-needle paracentesis).

In the past, one of the most important emergency medical therapies was the use of osmotic diuretics to withdraw fluid from both the aqueous humor and the vitreous.

While several systemically administered hyperosmotic solutions have an ocular effect, only glycerol and mannitol are in widespread use. These drugs remain within the vascular space, setting up a hyperosmotic gradient that draws fluid from the extravascular vitreous and anterior segment spaces into the vessels of the choroid and the retina, and to some extent the iris and the ciliary body. Mannitol must be given intravenously in a slow-push technique over 15–20 minutes. Mannitol (commonly available as a 20% solution) given at 1–2 g/kg produces a reliable and dramatic decrease in IOP within 1–2 hours for 6+ hours and, occasionally, for 2–3 days. Water should be restricted for the first 2–4 hours, or the osmotic effect of the mannitol is decreased. Glycerol (glycerin USP) is given orally at 1–2 mg/kg (approximately 1–2 mL/kg body weight), but, unless diluted with milk or a small amount of soft food, it often results in vomiting. The main advantage of glycerol is low cost and not having to perform venipuncture (glycerin can be dispensed to an owner for outpatient administration). Both preparations can be repeated two to three times at 8- to 12-hour intervals, but it is important to monitor hydration carefully. The response progressively diminishes with multiple doses (i.e., 2–4 days), due presumably to a rebound effect from leakage of the diuretic molecules into the eye. Inflammatory glaucoma may be poorly responsive to mannitol or glycerol or may rarely result in increased IOP due to leakage of the large molecules from the vascular space into the eye pulling fluid into the intraocular chambers. Hyperosmotic agents should be used with extreme caution in animals with heart failure in that acute fluid overload to the vascular space may trigger acute congestive heart failure. Chronic renal insufficiency is not a total contraindication for use of hyperosmotic agents, but clinical dehydration should be avoided to prevent acute renal failure in these patients.

To further reduce IOP by reduction of aqueous humor production, a CAI diuretic may be administered in combination with an osmotic diuretic. Oral acetazolamide is the most commercially available CAI, but it also has the most adverse side effects, so it should be avoided. Acetazolamide is available as an IV preparation but is seldom warranted due to expense and side effects. In years past, dichlorphenamide was a favorite CAI of many ophthalmologists, but it has been withdrawn from the American market and now must be obtained through a compounding pharmacist. A commonly used dose was 2–4 mg/kg every 12 hours. Methazolamide (2–5 mg/kg every 8 to 12 hours) has supplanted dichlorphenamide because of its availability. Skorobohach et al. found the greatest IOP-lowering effect at 3 hours after administration (18%–21%) and an overall 13%–19% decrease in IOP in normal dogs given two different doses (2.5 and 5 mg/kg, respectively) of

methazolamide, but they were unable to demonstrate significant difference in the decrease between dosing at 2.5 mg/kg every 8 hours and 5 mg/kg every 8 hours.[164] This would justify utilizing the lower dose rate to minimize side effects of the drug. Despite administering the drug every 8 hours, the morning IOP returned to baseline, and the evening IOP consistently had a rebound increase compared to baseline.

It is not uncommon to find dogs intolerant to one or all orally administered CAI diuretics at therapeutic doses. Toxicity may manifest initially as panting, gastrointestinal upset (vomiting, diarrhea, anorexia), weakness, depression, and irritability. Weight loss, presumed paresthesia (extremity licking, lameness), and alkaline urine/stone formation may be long-term adverse effects. Long-term use of CAIs has rarely been linked to keratoconjunctivitis sicca (KCS); CAIs are chemically related to sulfonamides. On a short-term emergency basis, some of these signs can be tolerated, but they may be indicators that this form of medical maintenance therapy may not be tolerated and, thus, dictate alternative therapies (surgery). If surgery is anticipated after emergency medical therapy, the dehydration from intensive diuretic therapy, the hypokalemia, and the metabolic acidosis created by CAI diuretics must be considered when assessing the anesthetic risk.[165]

Topical emergency therapy in the form of some combination of miotics (pilocarpine or demecarium bromide), β-blockers (timolol), and CAIs (dorzolamide or brinzolamide) is usually administered, but by themselves, they may not be adequate in the acute, high-pressure, closed-angle glaucoma patient. If a cholinesterase inhibitor miotic (demecarium bromide) is administered frequently for emergency therapy, potent topical or systemic cholinesterase inhibitors (parasite control products) should not be used as significant systemic absorption of topically applied ophthalmic drugs occurs, and toxicity may occur.

With the advent of the prostaglandin analogs (latanoprost, travoprost, and bimatoprost) for the treatment of glaucoma in man, initial emergency therapy with a prostaglandin analog alone has become commonplace with many veterinary ophthalmologists. Topical 0.005% latanoprost is routinely used for emergency therapy in the dog (one drop followed by another drop 15–30 minutes later), as it often reduces IOP within 30–45 minutes in many primary-angle closure glaucoma canine patients. This acute IOP-lowering effect may be due to correction of a "reverse pupillary block" at the level of the iris base/filtration angle[166] or because of decreased production of aqueous humor,[167] or both. Topical latanoprost use often avoids the use of IV mannitol, oral glycerin, and/or systemic CAI diuretics. Latanoprost is not effective in the cat[168,169] or the horse[170] and produces frequent, moderately severe side effects in the horse.[170] Other prostaglandin analogs (travoprost and bimatoprost) may be equally or more effective as latanoprost but have not yet been used as extensively as latanoprost (see Chapter 2).

This author uses a stepwise approach to treat the acute-angle-closure canine glaucoma patient. After topical application of latanoprost, dorzolamide, and timolol, IOP is reevaluated at 1 hour. If the IOP has dropped to a normotensive state, medical therapy is continued as latanoprost every 12 hours and dorzolamide and timolol every 8 hours with reevaluation of IOP and vision at 18–24 hours. If IOP has not returned to a normotensive state by 2 hours after medication, IV mannitol or oral glycerin is administered (or anterior chamber paracentesis is performed, **Figure 12.60**). In the case of hyperosmotic medical therapy, IOP is reevaluated 2 hours following drug administration. The patient is not discharged to the owner's care until the IOP has been returned to a normotensive state.

> Anterior chamber centesis alone is inappropriate therapy for acute glaucoma and should only be undertaken when all other medical options have failed.

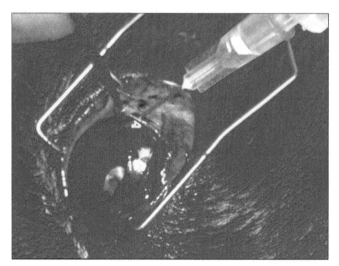

Figure 12.60 Aqueous centesis for emergency treatment of acute glaucoma. A 27-gauge needle is passed through the limbus, parallel to the iris face. Either the aqueous humor is slowly aspirated via syringe to obtain a normotensive state, or a needle alone is passed into the anterior chamber, and the aqueous is allowed to leak out until the needle hub overflows. In the hands of an experienced clinician, the procedure may be accomplished without sedation, but heavy sedation or short-acting injectable anesthetic may be necessary to inhibit accidental injury to intraocular structures (iris and/or lens).

Neuroprotective therapy is a new therapeutic strategy that is being used by many ophthalmologists.[3,78,171,172] A variety of strategies are possible to interrupt the cascade of events that leads to apoptosis of the retinal ganglion cells, but no specific drug that has proven to be of benefit, and approved for this use, is currently available. Consequently, clinicians have resorted to available calcium-channel blockers used in treating systemic hypertension. Amlodipine (0.125 mg/kg every 24 hours) has been used empirically for this purpose in the dog. Neuroprotective therapy is used in addition to pressure lowering medications/techniques. Without reduction of IOP to a normal level, neuroprotective therapy is useless.

Maintenance therapy

Once IOP is normalized with emergency therapy, maintenance medical therapy should aim to maintain a normal and consistent level of IOP. Dogs presented with high IOP and angle-closure glaucoma are usually not controlled well or for very long with traditional medical maintenance therapy. Animals presented with an IOP <50 mmHg (6.7 kPa) or with open-angle glaucoma are more successful candidates for ongoing medical therapy. In the past, maintenance medical therapy comprised an oral CAI diuretic with ancillary topical miotic, miotic-epinephrine, or β-blocker therapy. Epinephrine, dipivalyl epinephrine, pilocarpine, pilocarpine–epinephrine, timolol, and carbachol have been demonstrated to lower the IOP in beagles with open-angle glaucoma more than in normal beagles,[173–176] but the decrease is very modest. Concentrations of 4%–6% timolol are necessary to significantly lower IOP in the dog and the cat.[176] Unfortunately, these concentrations are not available commercially (the highest concentration of commercially available timolol is 0.5%), and these higher concentrations also increase the incidence of systemic side effects (bradycardia, systemic hypotension). Decreases of IOP of 6–10 mmHg (0.8–1.3 kPa) with 4%–6% timolol appear dramatic but must be compared to decreases of 5 mmHg (0.7 kPa) in placebo controls given topical methylcellulose.

It is unusual to control acute-angle-closure glaucoma in the dog with only classic topical glaucoma medication. The newer topical medications (prostaglandin analogs and topical carbonic anhydrase inhibitors) are more likely to control IOP, but many cases that are initially controlled lose IOP control with time. Medical management of visual eyes may only delay surgical intervention, and that may result in more ocular (optic nerve) damage. In dogs, medical control of elevated pressure was reported in an older study to be successful in 10% of cases after 6 months,[177] and only 25% of cases in another older study retained vision.[178] Neither of these studies had the benefit of the newer topical agents such as prostaglandin analogs, CAIs, β-blockers, and α-adrenergic drugs. Clinical experience shows that maintenance of IOP, with or without vision retention, is much more likely today with newer drugs; however, medical therapy alone for angle-closure glaucoma in the dog carries nowhere near the success rate seen in man for medical treatment of chronic open-angle glaucoma.

> Owners may elect medical over surgical therapy for financial reasons, not realizing that it is possible to spend $200–$300 per month on a combination of the newer topical medications and frequent visits for monitoring IOP.

In an older study in cats, only 15% of the cases treated medically were controlled; this low rate of vision retention was attributed to the late stage of presentation to the veterinary specialist.[178] Blocker and van der Woerdt later reported that 72% of feline glaucomatous eyes were blind at the time of initial presentation, but medical management maintained vision in 44% of the visual eyes.[144] As previously mentioned, many cases of glaucoma in the cat are secondary glaucoma due to intraocular inflammation and its chronic effects. Topical corticosteroid administration and topical CAI[179] alone or with a β-blocker (dorzolamide-timolol)[180] administration has been this author's most successful mode of medical therapy in the feline species. Topical prostaglandin analogs do not reduce IOP in cats,[168,181] and their use in an attempt to lower IOP in the cat is not warranted. In the horse, medical therapy of glaucoma may sometimes result in adequate IOP control, but usually only if IOP was not initially greatly elevated. As many cases of equine glaucoma are secondary to inflammation, topical and/or systemic corticosteroids or nonsteroidal anti-inflammatory drugs (NSAIDs) are important in the medical management of glaucoma in the equine species. Adverse side effects of prolonged systemic therapy with NSAIDs should be weighed as well as potential long-term effects of topical corticosteroid use on corneal health. Topical CAIs and β-blockers may be used to lower IOP in the horse.[182–184] Topical atropine has been recommended as a therapy for equine glaucoma because of the presumed importance of the uveoscleral flow.[152] Topical atropine had no effect on IOP in the normal horse in one study[185] but lowered IOP in 10 of 11 horses in another later study.[186] In some normal horses, topical atropine causes IOP elevation, so IOP monitoring is important if topical atropine is to be used in an attempt to lower IOP in a horse. Latanoprost may slightly lower the IOP in the horse, but the frequency of adverse side effects of epiphora, blepharospasm, and blepharoedema was high.[170]

Surgical therapy

If most cases of angle-closure glaucoma in the dog are not controllable with medical therapy, what are the surgical alternatives? Due to the severe obstruction in the outflow pathways, surgical procedures that open the angle (cyclodialysis), remove the obstruction (trabeculectomy), or circumvent the obstruction (filtering procedures, shunts) would be logically indicated; however, all these procedures have failed to give predictable or long-lasting results, although individual cases may be successful.

Filtering

Filtering procedures for the treatment of glaucoma are some of the oldest surgical procedures that have been used to reduce IOP and maintain vision. Most filtering procedures involve making a hole in the sclera (sclerotomy) immediately caudal to the corneoscleral limbus to form a communication with the anterior chamber and either the suprachoroidal space or the subconjunctival space (or both). In addition to the sclerotomy, disinsertion of the base of the ciliary body to enhance aqueous humor flow from the anterior chamber to the suprachoroidal space (cyclodialysis) or splitting of the iris and fixing the resulting pupillary margins of the iris leaflets to the external sclera beneath a conjunctival flap to enhance aqueous humor flow to the subconjunctival space (iridencleisis) is usually performed. Successful results (30%–50%) with filtering surgeries have been reported in the dog[187–189] but are usually relatively short term. The major cause for failure of filtering procedures (return to an elevated IOP state) is fibrosis with closure of the scleral defect. Studies using regional repositol corticosteroid therapy to reduce postop fibrosis and drainage tract failure[189] have been tried, but long-term results did not warrant further work in this area. Long-term complications (cataracts and retinal detachment) often occur in human and veterinary patients alike, despite control of the IOP. In humans, 32% of patients undergoing aqueous humor shunts have serious retinal complications (i.e., retinal detachment), with 67% of these cases requiring retinal surgery.[190] Long-term results with these types of surgical procedures have been poor in the hands of most veterinary ophthalmologists, and with the introduction of anterior chamber shunt devices and selective laser cyclophotocoagulation to reduce intraocular pressure in glaucoma cases, filtering procedures have become antiquated in veterinary ophthalmology.

Cyclocryotherapy

In the past, cyclocryotherapy for acute or chronic glaucoma of visual eyes was the procedure of choice for most veterinary surgeons before it was replaced by laser cyclophotocoagulation. Unlike other surgical procedures that have the objective of enhancing the outflow of aqueous humor, cyclocryotherapy (as well as cyclophotocoagulation) acts to reduce the production of aqueous humor.[191–193] Cyclocryotherapy involves a transconjunctival/transscleral application of a cryogen to noninvasively damage part of the ciliary body. Cryogens evaluated have been either nitrous oxide or liquid nitrogen.[177,191–194] Nitrous oxide is only able to achieve a target tissue temperature of –10°C to –13°C (14–8.6°F), rather than the –20°C (–4°F) necessary for tissue necrosis.[191] The goal of cyclocryotherapy, however, is to impair aqueous humor production versus totally discontinue aqueous humor formation; therefore, the use of nitrous oxide as a cryogen can be successful in maintaining a physiologic IOP postoperatively. In the normal cat, freezing 75% of the ciliary body decreases the aqueous humor production by as much as 50%[193] with subsequent marked reduction of IOP. In the normal dog, the histopathologic changes produced by freezing are reversed 6 months after cryotherapy[191,192] with return of normal preoperative IOP levels.

The following is a brief description of the cyclocryosurgical procedure. If possible, the patient's IOP should be normalized with emergency medical therapy before surgery. Preoperative anti-inflammatory agents (topical/systemic corticosteroids or systemic NSAIDs with topical corticosteroids) are administered. If nitrous oxide is used, the 3 × 6-mm glaucoma probe is centered 5 mm posterior to the limbus, and each site is frozen for 2 minutes (**Figure 12.61**). The probe is applied to the full circumference of the globe (approximately four sites dorsal, four ventral), except at the 3- and 9-o'clock positions, to avoid the long posterior ciliary arteries. After the probe has thawed, freezing is repeated at each site. If liquid nitrogen is used, the 4-mm probe is placed at a similar location posterior to the limbus, but freezing is stopped when the ice ball reaches the corneal limbus. Freezing is repeated after thawing, as was the case with nitrous oxide cryogen. Postoperative antiglaucoma therapy (CAI and β-blockers) and anti-inflammatory therapy (topical and systemic) are continued.

Immediately after freezing, conjunctival chemosis (sometimes intense) is seen that usually abates in 3–5 days with topical corticosteroid therapy. Postoperative IOP may elevate for several hours to several days. If the eye is visual, this temporary elevation should be prevented with aggressive antiglaucoma medication and/or aqueous centesis if necessary. Most eyes have normalized pressure by 3–5 days, and the IOP may continue to decrease for up to 7–14 days. Once the IOP is normal, antiglaucoma therapy may slowly be weaned. In this situation, ocular hypotension (IOP less than 10 mmHg) is preferred. Monitoring of IOP should be weekly for the first month and monthly thereafter to detect the eventual return to the elevated IOP state.

A significant number of dogs (about 30+%) treated with either nitrous oxide or liquid nitrogen cryotherapy have a recurrent increase in IOP within 6–12 months; therefore, visual eyes should be diligently monitored. Liquid nitrogen gives better results than nitrous oxide, particularly if refreezing is necessary.[177,194] Short-term retention of vision (6–12 months) in acute cases was 73% in one series and 25% in another.[178,195]

Chemosis, sometimes very dramatic, is expected for several days post freezing. Transient increases in IOP are common and are the most serious complication that may destroy the remaining vision in a marginally functional eye. A moderate-to-severe degree of anterior uveitis is present with all successful cyclocryotherapy cases. Iris depigmentation may occur with anterior segment necrosis if the anterior ciliary arteries are destroyed. Retinal detachment due to choroidal edema is common and sometimes is self-correcting. Posterior synechia and cataract formation are commonly seen, and phthisis bulbi may occur if aqueous production is decreased too much.

Contraindications for cyclocryotherapy for glaucoma are similar to other antiglaucoma therapies, that is, ocular neoplasia or intraocular infection. Cyclocryotherapy has the inherent disadvantage of a lack of quantitation, that is, a certain amount of freezing cannot be recommended for a given elevation of IOP. Because other more definitive techniques (evisceration and prosthesis, chemical ciliary body ablation with intravitreal gentamicin, or enucleation) are available for treatment of a blind eye, cyclocryotherapy should be reserved for visual eyes when newer

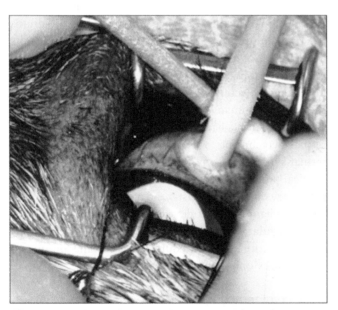

Figure 12.61 Application of a nitrous oxide probe to the globe for cyclocryotherapy. This is usually performed for 360°, avoiding long posterior ciliary arteries at 3 and 9 o'clock.

techniques such as aqueous humor shunt device placement and/or laser cyclophotocoagulation is unavailable.

Cyclophotocoagulation

Transscleral Nd:YAG or diode laser cyclophotocoagulation (CPC) has been successful at controlling IOP in canine, feline, and equine glaucoma.[196–199] Like cyclocryotherapy, the mechanism of action of CPC is ciliary process destruction and a decrease in aqueous humor production.[199–204] The functional changes and morphologic lesions of CPC are not as great in albinotic animals (for this reason some still feel cyclocryosurgery is indicated in these patients), which suggests that melanin absorbs the laser energy, although damage is also present in the ciliary body stroma, pigmented epithelium, and nonpigmented epithelium.[205,206] Due to the expense of the Nd:YAG laser, the diode laser is the more popular alternative in veterinary ophthalmology. Low-energy (2.5-watt) diode lasers are compact and are marketed for the veterinarian (**Figure 12.62**). The wavelengths of the Nd:YAG and diode lasers are similar (1064 and 810 nm, respectively) and are absorbed by pigment and blood. Diode and Nd:YAG lasers produce similar ocular lesions in postmortem eyes: a zone of coagulation necrosis centered at the scleral–ciliary body stroma interface that does not extend to the ciliary epithelium.[203] The diode laser produces lesions at lower energies than the Nd:YAG laser due to better scleral transmittance and better absorption of energy by melanin.[197] The acute lesions produced by the diode laser are hemorrhage and coagulation necrosis of the ciliary epithelium. This is centered in the inner sclera and radiates outward with time to involve the ciliary processes, the peripheral retina, and the trabecular meshwork.[204] Diode laser lesions involve the ciliary epithelium more than the ciliary stroma or sclera[207] compared to Nd:YAG laser

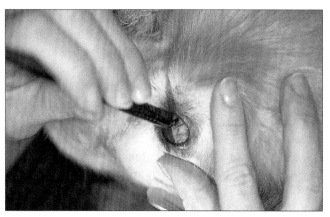

Figure 12.63 Diode laser probe placed to deliver transscleral energy to the ciliary body.

lesions. Because of the lower energy levels utilized with the diode laser, complications of postop uveitis and cataract are less common than with the Nd:YAG laser.

In the dog, lasering 3 mm posterior to the limbus, with the beam aimed at the center of the eye to avoid the lens, will strike the ciliary processes, whereas lasering 5 mm posterior to the limbus with the same angle of application coagulates the pars plana (**Figure 12.63**). In one study, with the Nd:YAG laser, 3–7 J was delivered in 30–40 spots 3 mm posterior to the limbus in either a contact or noncontact mode.[196] When the energy level is held constant, more tissue disruption occurs with the shorter time duration, that is, high watts and short time.[208] This short-time/high-wattage technique, however, has the adverse effect of causing decreased corneal sensitivity and neurotropic keratitis in some animals[209] and should thus be avoided in favor of a longer duration pulse of lower energy. The author's current technique with the diode laser involves a double row of burns, centered 3 and 5 mm posterior to the limbus, approximately 20–25 sites dorsally and 20–25 sites ventrally (avoiding the 3- and 9-o'clock positions) at 5 seconds per site with an energy threshold just below that which elicits an audible "pop" (approximately 500–1000 mW). Postoperatively, the external reaction (conjunctival chemosis) to laser CPC is not near as severe as the usual cyclocryosurgery reaction. The postlaser intraocular inflammation is usually substantially less or occasionally approximates the cryo-induced inflammation.[206] Unfortunately, postlasering IOP spikes occur quite consistently with both Nd:YAG and diode lasers and should be dealt with in the same manner as with cyclocryosurgery. The success rate (IOP in a normal range) in a series of 56 canine eyes using noncontact Nd:YAG laser was 83% during the 3- to 4-month followup. Failures were noted mainly in albinotic eyes of Siberian huskies.[196] The main reported complications were intraocular hemorrhage (16%), cataracts (37%, most were incipient cataracts), and phthisis bulbi in one eye. In one report,

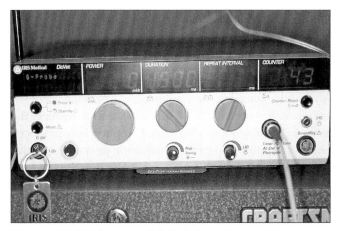

Figure 12.62 Commercial diode laser for veterinary ophthalmology. Attachments for use with the operating microscope, binocular indirect ophthalmoscope, and probes for cyclophotocoagulation and retinopexy are available.

diode laser success rates (IOP in a normal range) in dogs utilizing settings that averaged 1500 mW and 1500 msec were reported as 65% at 6 months (off all medications), and 53% of eyes that were judged to be potentially visual were still visual at 12 months.[197] Combination aqueous humor shunt device placement and cyclophotocoagulation surgeries appear to have a higher long-term success rate than with either procedure alone.[210,211]

Direct visualization and photocoagulation of the ciliary body may be obtained via endoscopic instrumentation. At this writing, endoscopic cyclophotocoagulation paired with phacoemulsification and artificial lens implantation appears to have the greatest potential for IOP control and retention of vision of all techniques listed thus far.[212] Reports of up to 90% of patients having controlled IOP 12 months after surgery, up to 70% of postop patients still having vision, and up to 95% of patients postop being on less antiglaucoma drugs to maintain normal IOP have been made using this modality. Because of the high incidence of post-endolaser cataract formation, phacoemulsification is performed, in conjunction with diode endolaser of 75+% of the ciliary processes using special fiberoptic endolaser delivery systems. Postoperative hypertension necessitating aggressive antiglaucoma medications and possibly aqueous centesis is very commonplace, and the need to hospitalize and monitor patients for up to 1 week postop is common as well. Despite the expensive equipment costs and the learning curve to develop successful technique, this modality is becoming more common with veterinary ophthalmologists in an attempt to save vision and spare suffering at the hands of angle-closure glaucoma.

In the horse, positioning of the laser probe should be 4 mm posterior to the limbus for the ventral quadrant and 4–6 mm posterior to the limbus for the dorsal quadrant to target the ciliary processes. The nasal quadrant should be avoided because the width of the pars plicata and pars plana is very narrow in this region.[213] Current recommended energy/time settings for the horse are 1.2–1.5 W power and 5 seconds duration, 40 laser sites per visual eye and 40–50+ sites per nonvisual eye. Postoperative antiglaucoma medications (with or without aqueous centesis) and anti-inflammatory drugs are necessary to control postop hypertension and inflammation. With this protocol, 59% of lasered eyes were still visual at 49 months postop, although 64% of these horses required some sort of indefinite antiglaucoma medications.[214]

Aqueous humor shunts

Implantation of a tube from the anterior chamber to the subconjunctival or orbital space is a surgical technique that has been attempted repeatedly to control IOP in the canine patient.[215–219] In theory, a tubing passed from the anterior chamber shunts aqueous humor from the anterior chamber into the subconjunctival/orbital space where it is removed by the capillary beds around the exit portal (bleb), thereby bypassing the obstructed normal aqueous outflow channels. In theory, complication such as secondary cataract formation due to decreased aqueous humor production and/or altered aqueous humor quality (uveitis) as occurs with the cyclodestructive procedures would not occur since normal aqueous humor production is not disturbed. These aqueous shunting procedures have been somewhat successful in therapy for glaucoma in man[220] (compared to low success rates in canine cases). In one human study, shunt surgery failures increased with time, and of those failures, 26% failed by 3 months, 63% failed by 12 months, and 80% failed by 24 months.[221] A variety of tube configurations have been devised in conjunction with various medical and surgical protocols, with some techniques offering better long-term success than others,[219,222,223] but to this point, a relatively consistently successful combination for canine glaucoma has not been found; therefore, cyclodestructive techniques remain more the norm for the treatment of canine primary glaucoma. In some investigators' experience, shunt devices function better in normal eyes than in glaucomatous eyes with the reasoning that alteration in aqueous humor in glaucomatous eyes stimulate fibroplasia,[122,224] thereby causing shunt failure due to fibrosis of the bleb. Animals tend to heal with more fibroplasia than humans (adult, Caucasian), which has resulted in veterinary ophthalmology having difficulty in duplicating the success of these shunt devices in humans in our canine patients.

The high rate of failure to reduce IOP with drainage devices is either due to fibrin obstruction of the intraocular portion of the tube (more of an acute complication) or, more commonly, fibrosis of the region adjacent to the external ocular bleb (more of a long-term complication). The latter creates a nonabsorbent bleb with no egress of aqueous from the eye to the subconjunctival/orbital space. The design of the tube does not appear to alter the amount of encapsulation that is produced,[217] but the type of biomaterial is important, with silicone having the least reaction.[220] Various homemade tube designs have been made out of silicone tubing with attached bands and sheets to increase the size of the subsequent filter bleb. Commercially produced shunts are now being marketed with pressure sensitive valves that open at a preset pressure (Ahmed valves). These valved shunt devices inhibit the immediate postoperative hypotension and anterior chamber collapse that was seen with nonvalved shunt devices. These newer valved devices are less extensive than the original encircling Schocket and Joseph implants and, therefore, require less extensive subconjunctival dissection with subsequent less postoperative scarring (**Figures 12.64 and 12.65**).

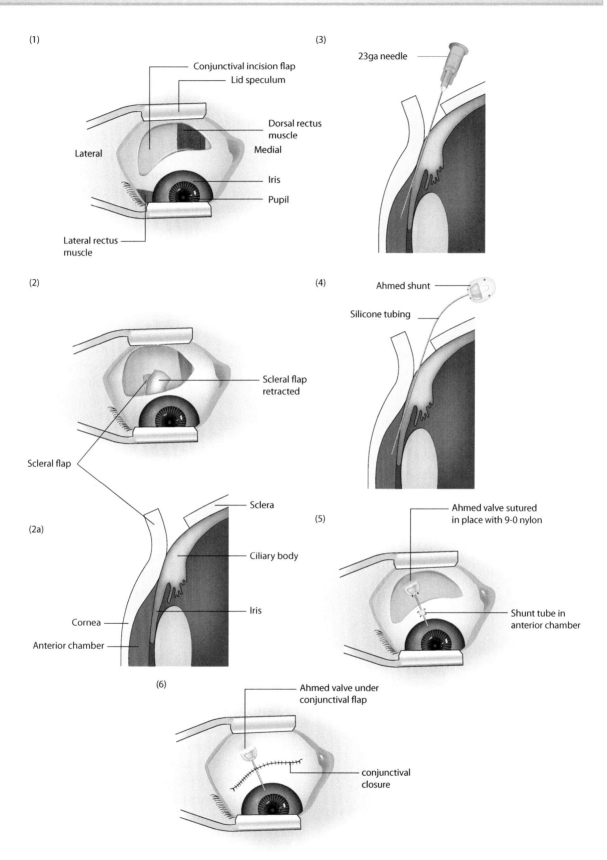

Figure 12.64 **Placement of an aqueous humor shunt.**

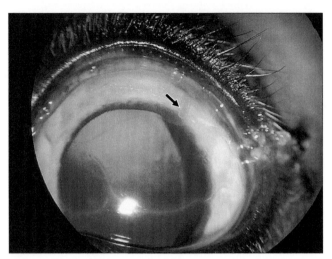

Figure 12.65 A commercial aqueous humor shunt (arrow) in place in a Siberian husky. Note the subluxated lens. The shunt functioned for only 3 weeks when a fibrous walled subconjunctival cyst developed where aqueous humor was accumulating. Attempts to remove the cyst and restore function were unsuccessful. No antifibrotic agents other than glucocorticoids were used.

Additional complications of shunt surgery, in addition to tube occlusion and bleb failure, include extrusion of the tube or implant (**Figure 12.65a**), bacterial infection, cataract formation, collapse of the anterior chamber, hypotony, hyphema, and corneal edema. Despite these

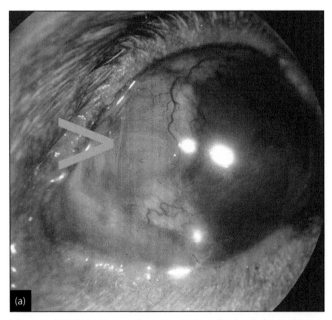

(a)

Figure 12.65a Extrusion of an Ahmed valved shunt device with erosion of device through conjunctiva. This resulted in uncontrolled leakage of aqueous humor from the anterior chamber with anterior chamber collapse, retinal detachment, hyphema, and vision loss.

numerous complications and less than optimal success rates, shunt surgery is a technique that holds promise and deserves much more work on tube design and pharmacologic manipulation of the inflammatory reaction of aqueous humor-stimulated fibrosis. Since shunting of aqueous humor deals with the cause of elevated IOP/glaucoma (inability of aqueous humor to exit the eye), further research is warranted in this direction.

Most research to improve success of controlling IOP with aqueous shunts has centered on the use of topical/locally applied antifibrotic agents to control bleb fibrosis and failure. Antifibrotic agents thus far used are topical 5-fluorouracil and mitomycin C[222,225,226] in addition to topically applied prednisolone acetate.[222] These products have been administered by topical application to the surgical site at the time of surgery, postoperatively, or in some cases have been administered in conjunction with remodeling procedures where the fibrous tissue over the valved device is removed to enhance new outflow pathways.[222] Attempts to alter tissue fibrosis at the distal end have led some investigators to implant the distal end into some very unlikely places such as the nasolacrimal duct, various facial veins, and the frontal sinus.[227–229]

Currently, some clinicians combine laser CPC with aqueous humor shunts. The rationale is that while the shunts may not function long-term, they will probably function long enough to neutralize the post-lasering pressure spike, and either one or both procedures may control the IOP on a long-term basis. Bentley et al. reported that 11 out of 19 cases (58%) were still visual after 1 year with a combined shunt/cycloablation procedure, and 14 out of 19 (74%) had an IOP <25 mmHg (3.3 kPa).[210] Sapienza and van der Woerdt reported that good control of IOP was attained in 76% of treated cases, and 41% of eyes were visual after 12 months.[211]

THERAPY OF SECONDARY GLAUCOMA

Secondary glaucoma due to lens displacement

Lens subluxation and complete luxation are frequently associated with glaucoma. It is often difficult to decide whether lens instability has an active or passive role in producing glaucoma. The objectives of removing an anteriorly luxated lens are: (1) to normalize IOP, (2) to return or retain vision, and (3) to reverse corneal pathology. If the lens is luxated anteriorly, examination of the angle of the contralateral eye (if that eye is normal) is important to determine if there are other associated factors (e.g., angle closure, goniodysgenesis) causing the glaucoma. If the angle in the normotensive eye is pathologic, it is very probable that removal of a luxated lens will not entirely cure glaucoma on a long-term basis. This does not mean that lens removal should not be performed, but it does indicate a more guarded prognosis for cure and the need for long-term medical therapy and postoperative surveillance of IOP.

Acute anterior lens luxation should ultimately be treated by removing the lens, but emergency therapy should be aimed at reduction of IOP (use of drugs that reduce aqueous humor production [topical β-blockers and topical or systemic CAI agents], use of osmotic diuretics but not drugs that cause pupillary constriction), and reduction of intraocular inflammation from the anteriorly luxated lens movement. The clinician should also be aware of the many potential postoperative complications. Persistent postoperative corneal edema, usually focal, is not uncommon due to endothelial damage from the lens, surgery, and postoperative vitreous adhesions. Recurrent IOP elevations may occur from pressure-induced angle pathology, predisposing angle pathology,[230] or pupillary blockage from anterior vitreous herniation or postoperative iridal/vitreous adhesions. Vision is often lost due to the initial high preoperative IOP or, in the long-term postoperative course, from retinal detachments, which are relatively common within the first year. In this author's experience, genetically predisposed anterior lens luxations in young dogs carry a better prognosis than do anterior lens luxations due to hypermature cataracts or senile lens changes in old dogs or any anterior lens luxation in cats or horses. For more detail concerning anterior lens luxation, therapy, and prognosis, see Chapter 13.

Lens removal in an eye with chronic anterior lens luxation is often problematic. The eye may be irreversibly blind, the cornea may have permanent edema and scarring, and the IOP may not be normalized following surgery if, indeed, it is elevated. If the eye is blind with a markedly elevated IOP, ocular evisceration and prosthesis implantation or enucleation should be recommended instead.

Posteriorly luxated lenses are rarely removed. In the case of a total lens luxation to the floor of the vitreous space, chronic miotic therapy to "trap" the lens in the posterior chamber and prevent anterior displacement into the anterior chamber is warranted if the iris sphincter musculature is intact.

Subluxated lenses may be removed if the angles are open, the pressures are not controlled medically, and the clinician can find no other reasons for IOP elevation. An aphakic crescent in a blind buphthalmic patient (**Figures 12.24 and 12.65**) is a sign of end-stage glaucoma, and removal of the lens will not control IOP nor will it restore vision once removed. Topical latanoprost every 12 hours can be used to trap a subluxated lens in place, since it is a very potent miotic as well as a good ocular hypotensive agent. Binder et al. treated primary subluxated or posteriorly luxated lenses with topical 0.25% demecarium bromide every 12 hours and maintained vision in 100% of dogs at 3 months after diagnosis, 80% after 1 year, and 58% after 2 years.[231] The time until anterior luxation was a mean of approximately 3 years if a miotic was used and less than 2 years if no therapy was administered. No difference was noted between when the opposite lens destabilized and when glaucoma developed in the treated and control groups.

Forward displacement of the lens with intact zonules in feline aqueous humor misdirection syndrome may respond well to phacoemulsification with a posterior capsulotomy and partial anterior vitrectomy. Many veterinary ophthalmologists conservatively treat these usually geriatric patients with topical CAI agents with equal long-term success at retaining vision.[148]

Secondary glaucoma due to inflammation

Glaucoma secondary to inflammation is generally not treated surgically, unless posterior synechia is present resulting from previous cataract extraction surgery. Secondary glaucoma associated with active inflammation is often very painful. If vision is still present, and if the process is not due to infection, medical antiglaucoma therapy (drugs that reduce aqueous production, i.e., CAI and β-blockers) and topical/systemic corticosteroid therapy are indicated. Since miotics and prostaglandin analogs may worsen anterior uveitis, their use in the treatment of uveitis-induced glaucoma are usually not indicated. Treating intraocular inflammation with corticosteroids may exacerbate glaucoma due to improvement in ciliary body function and increased aqueous humor formation as the inflammation resolves. If surgery is attempted to break down synechiae, intracameral tissue plasminogen activator (tPA) and viscoelastic agents should be used to maintain tissue separation. If vision is lost and the eye is painful, the patient is treated for absolute glaucoma.

Secondary open-angle glaucoma

Glaucoma associated with hyphema or other substances that clog the angle are treated medically with antiglaucoma drugs that reduce aqueous production. In the case of clotted blood obstructing the filtration angle or pupil, intracameral injection of tPA may liquefy the clot and restore outflow of aqueous humor (Chapter 11). The primary condition is treated if possible.

THERAPY OF ABSOLUTE/END-STAGE GLAUCOMA

Therapy for eyes that are glaucomatous and chronically blind from a variety of etiologies touches on humane and philosophical questions. Most owners are not aware of the pain or suffering of an animal with glaucoma as it often manifests in subtle ways. In man, excessively elevated IOP is perceived as a "sinus headache," and the same may be true in our veterinary patients. Patient comfort should be a consideration for veterinarians when advising clients on chronic glaucoma management.

Enucleation

The most pragmatic treatment for absolute glaucoma is to enucleate the globe, but this may have significant client resistance, especially if the process is bilateral. Enucleation is indicated in secondary glaucoma associated with neoplasia, infection, deep corneal ulceration, and overwhelming inflammation such as phacoclastic uveitis (see Chapter 6 for enucleation techniques). Methyl methacrylate or silicone orbital prosthetic spheres have been used in small animals and horses to minimize the postoperative sunken appearance that most enucleated orbits develop.[232,233] A 40- to 50-mm orbital prosthesis is recommended for the horse and 14- to 25-mm spheres for the dog and the cat, to compensate for postsurgical atrophy of orbital contents. Some feel that cats are not good candidates for sphere implantation as 40% in one study failed due to fluid accumulation in the orbit.[232] This author has found that with meticulous dissection of the lacrimal gland, third eyelid gland, and conjunctival tissue from the orbit, orbital fluid accumulation does not occur. Longhaired dogs may do well without an orbital prosthesis for cosmesis.

Orbital prostheses give an initial cosmetic improvement, but with time and fibrosis, the prosthesis may be pushed forward in the orbit and appear simply as a round subcutaneous object that is sharply outlined, or it may retract caudally within the socket, resulting in questionable long-term cosmetic improvement over a sunken orbit. This author does not place a sphere the size of the enucleated globe; rather, I routinely place a large enough silicone sphere to completely fill the orbit. The sphere has the anterior surface (immediately beneath the closed lids) trimmed flat, so once the postoperative tissue swelling regresses and fibrosis occurs, the surface is flush with the face and the rim of the orbit.

Ocular evisceration with silicone sphere implantation

Pet owners, including horse owners, have an inherent aversion to enucleation and almost always chose an alternative option if presented to them. Ocular evisceration with silicone sphere implantation is an attempt to overcome the aesthetic objections to enucleation (**Figures 12.66 and 12.67**).[234] Ocular evisceration is contraindicated with intraocular neoplasia and infection, and an implant is likely to be extruded when placed in an eye with deep corneal

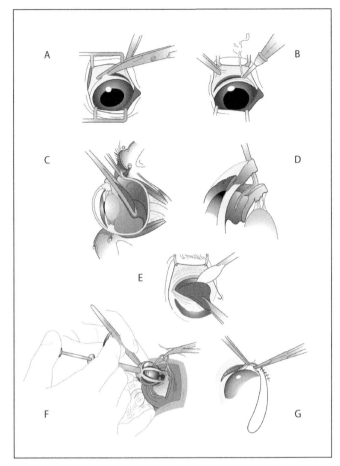

Figure 12.66 Technique for performing ocular evisceration with silicone sphere implantation. **A:** A limbal- or fornix-based flap is dissected to exposure the sclera; **B:** A scleral incision is made with an electroscalpel (or scalpel and scissors) 3–4 mm posterior to the limbus of about 160°; **C, D, E:** The contents of the globe are removed with an evisceration spatula or a lens loop, making sure to include the lens; **F:** The appropriate-sized silicone sphere is introduced with a sphere inserter or by everting the scleral incision edges with forceps; **G:** The sclera is sutured with 6-0 absorbable suture and the conjunctiva with a running 6-0 absorbable suture. (From Martin, C. 1993. Glaucoma. In: *Textbook of Small Animal Surgery*, Vol. 2, D. Slatter (editor), WB Saunders: Philadelphia, pp. 1263–1276.)

ulceration (**Figure 12.67a**). Once the silicone sphere is implanted, the buphthalmic corneoscleral shell contracts around the implant and becomes more normal in size. The sphere diameter implanted should be equal to the normal horizontal corneal diameter, but an additional 2- to 3-mm larger sphere may be implanted in a buphthalmic eye. The intraocular contents should be submitted for histopathologic examination to confirm the clinical diagnosis and avoid missing neoplasia or infectious causes of secondary glaucomas.[235] While it is not to be encouraged, prosthesis

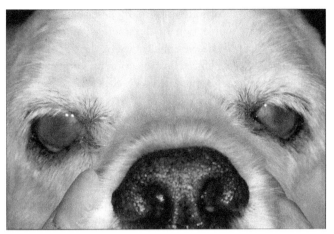

Figure 12.67 An American Cocker Spaniel with bilateral evisceration and prosthesis implantation. While the corneas may not appear normal in many animals, the appearance is cosmetically preferred to bilateral enucleation in the minds of many owners.

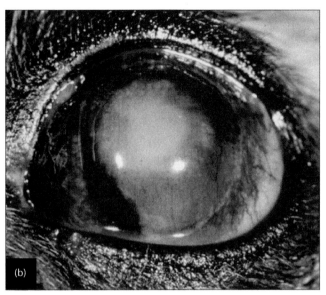

Figure 12.67b Corneal neovascularization 4 weeks following evisceration and prosthesis surgery for end-stage glaucoma. The corneal vasculature eventually met in the axial cornea and then regressed, leaving a diffusely gray, fibrosed cornea and a comfortable globe.

placement with undetected ocular neoplasia may not have regrowth because most canine ocular tumors are benign.[236]

The postoperative recovery time for an evisceration is typically longer than for an enucleation. Immediate postoperative problems are usually limited to lid and orbital swelling and can be reduced by using systemic NSAID therapy preoperatively and postoperatively. A temporary tarsorrhaphy postoperatively is indicated to prevent

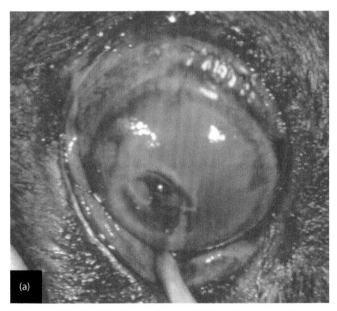

Figure 12.67a Perforated corneal ulcer in an American Cocker Spaniel 2 weeks following evisceration and prosthesis implantation surgery. The case was complicated by the patient having KCS as well as a blind, buphthalmic, glaucomatous globe and an axial corneal ulceration at the time of surgery. The ruptured globe was enucleated.

exposure keratitis while the periocular tissues are swollen; this is especially indicated in the case of an extremely buphthalmic eye or in a brachycephalic breed. Intraocular hemorrhage cannot be avoided, and most eyes undergo various color changes from the remaining blood. Also, some corneas undergo an intense vascular response that subsequently subsides (**Figure 12.67b,c**).

Corneal ulceration may occur due to trauma to a blind buphthalmic eye or may be neurotrophically (total lack of corneal sensation) mediated; the ulcer may perforate and result in extrusion of the implant (**Figure 12.67a**). Anecdotally, many ophthalmologists feel there is an increase in KCS incidence in patients with globes eviscerated for a long time due to lack of corneal sensation and lack of reflex tearing. Last, the occasional globe retracts into the socket up to 2 years after evisceration. This is usually due to orbital content atrophy.

Pena et al. described evisceration of the globe and injection of silicone oil rather than placement of a solid prosthesis.[237] Only five dogs were included in the study, so this technique cannot yet be adequately compared for complications and long-term cosmetic outcome to the more common solid prosthesis.

Chemical ablation of the ciliary body

Chemical destruction of the ciliary body is an inexpensive and relatively reliable means of lowering IOP in blind, painful eyes.[238–240] Bingaman et al. reported a success rate in lowering IOP of 65% in the dog and the cat, with about 9% of

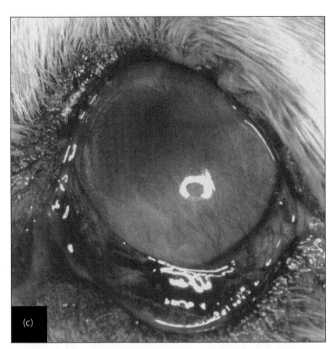

Figure 12.67c Results of evisceration and prosthesis implantation surgery in an American Cocker Spaniel; the patient was 3 months after surgery. Initial corneal neovascularization had regressed leaving a somewhat clear cornea revealing the dark intraocular silicone sphere.

the eyes developing phthisis bulbi.[241] Most clinicians administer gentamicin at a dose of 15–30 mg by injection into the vitreous cavity after removal of an equal volume of vitreous or aqueous. The intraocular dose should not exceed the maximum daily systemic dose of 4.4 mg/kg.[241] Some believe that the higher the IOP, the higher the dose of intravitreal gentamicin necessary to obtain normal IOP. This author is not of that opinion, and I inject 25–30 mg in dogs with the amount dependent more on the volume of the globe than the IOP. Gentamicin at this dose/concentration is toxic to the retina; therefore, the procedure is contraindicated if the eye is visual or potentially visual. Intravitreal gentamicin injection is also contraindicated in secondary glaucoma due to neoplasia or infectious agents nonresponsive to gentamicin (e.g., systemic mycoses or prototheca). This author does not recommend gentamicin injection for treatment of hyphema-induced secondary glaucoma due to the concern of an undiagnosed intraocular tumor. Recent studies have revealed a connection between intravitreal gentamicin injection in cats and undifferentiated sarcoma formation in cats.[242] Therefore, most ophthalmologists do not recommend gentamicin injection for treatment of feline glaucoma. In the horse, a recommended dose of 50 mg gentamicin and 1 mg dexamethasone has been reported.[156] Repeat injection of the canine eye with gentamicin for those eyes failing to respond initially is only 50% successful.[241] It is not uncommon for the equine patient to require a second injection to

normalize IOP.[154] Although originally described by Vainisi et al., concurrent injection of dexamethasone or another corticosteroid into the vitreous cavity of the dog is felt by some to be of no benefit.[238] Postinjection inflammation may usually be adequately controlled with either topical corticosteroids or systemic NSAIDs.

Complications of chemical ablation of the ciliary body are cataract formation, intraocular hemorrhage, and phthisis bulbi (**Figure 12.68**). The eye usually appears normal on a short-term basis, but over several months, a cataract develops, and phthisis bulbi is common, resulting in a poor cosmetic appearance. To decrease the incidence of phthisis bulbi, lower doses may be used, but they are often not successful in softening the eye. A more dependable salvage procedure (uniformity of ocular size and lack of long-term complication) is evisceration and prosthesis implantation or even enucleation, unless the animal's systemic health or the owner's financial limitations are the determining factors.

Cidofovir (Vistide) is a systemic antiviral agent that is used in humans for cytomegalovirus infections, and it was found to produce marked ocular hypotony. This led to it being used intraocularly, where it is supposedly selectively toxic to the ciliary body epithelium, sparing the retina and the lens. The recommended dose in dogs and cats is 100 µg (range from 100 to 500 µg), and it is usually given intravitreally, although sometimes cidofovir is injected into the anterior chamber. At a dose of 100 µg per injection, the success of lowering IOP below 20 mmHg (2.7 kPa) was 40% and 90% at 500 µg per injection. Cats have not been

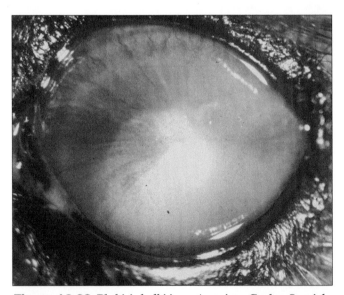

Figure 12.68 Phthisis bulbi in an American Cocker Spaniel several months after intravitreal gentamicin injection. Corneal fibrosis and edema are present as well as secondary cataract formation. Despite aqueous flare and posterior synechia, the patient was comfortable with no medical therapy, and the globe was cosmetically acceptable to the owner.

as responsive, with <30% success.[243] In a later study of canine patients with end-stage glaucoma, 85% of patients receiving 562.5 mcg of intravitreal cidofovir had reduction of IOP to a subnormal/normal level within 2 weeks, with 70% of the patients undergoing phthisis bulbi. With additional injections, 97% of cases were restored to subnormal/normal IOP levels.[244]

PROPHYLAXIS

The use of topical antiglaucoma medications in a prophylactic manner has until recently been empirical.[107,245,246] An early retrospective study found that prophylactic therapy using a variety of drugs (timolol, oral dichlorphenamide, echothiophate) lengthened the time before the onset of glaucoma in the second eye from 5 to 10 months in breeds predisposed to glaucoma.[106] A later prospective study of primary closed-angle glaucoma patients found that either 0.5% betaxolol every 12 hours, or a cholinesterase-inhibiting miotic (0.25% demecarium bromide) plus a corticosteroid (betamethasone) every 24 hours, increased the time interval for the second eye to become glaucomatous to 31 months versus 8 months in the control group.[107] This study performed gonioscopy and used a consistent form of therapy, whereas the former study did not. Two subsequent retrospective studies[245,246] showed that use of various topical prophylactic antiglaucoma drugs

(miotics, prostaglandin analogs, β-blockers, and/or topical CAIs) resulted in prolongation of the time before glaucoma affected the second eye in patients who were presented with unilateral primary glaucoma. A masked prospective study using treated patients versus placebo-treated patients would be definitive as far as the effect of prophylactic therapy, but since studies thus far indicate that there is a dramatic improvement in maintaining vision with prophylactic therapy, the standard of care for veterinary ophthalmologists is to treat the second eye in all cases of primary glaucoma with some sort of medical prophylaxis.

The long-term use of echothiophate should be cautioned due to collapse and proliferative changes in the lamellae of the corneoscleral meshwork, degenerative changes in the ciliary muscle, and inflammation of the ciliary body and the iris in the monkey.[247]

An ounce of prevention is worth a pound of cure! The clinician should remember to treat the normal eye prophylactically in patients with suspected unilateral primary glaucoma. Maintaining the eye for an average of 31 months without glaucoma is far longer than the duration of success when treating glaucoma with any surgical or medical protocol.

CLINICAL CASES

CASE 1

A 3-year-old F/S American Cocker Spaniel was presented for a 2-plus-week history of glaucoma of the left eye unresponsive to medical therapy consisting of topical pilocarpine and antibiotic–corticosteroid drops. Historically, the patient was seen for an acutely painful, cloudy, red left eye with a dilated pupil and elevated IOP. After 2 weeks of medical therapy, the IOP was minimally decreased, and the patient was minimally less painful, as per the owner. Clinically, the left globe was buphthalmic with episcleral injection, corneal cloudiness, a dilated pupil revealing an aphakic crescent dorsomedially due to ventrolateral lens subluxation (as in **Figure 12.24**), and an IOP of 45 mmHg. Funduscopically, the optic nerve was atrophic and cupped, and the peripapillary tapetal fundus was thinned with radiating areas of increased reflectivity (as in **Figure 12.22**). The left eye had no menace, dazzle, or pupillary light reflexes. The right eye was visual with a normal IOP and fundus.

Gonioscopically, the filtration angle in the right eye was abnormal, appearing "closed" or having "goniodysgenesis" (as in **Figure 12.36**). Primary angle-closure glaucoma was diagnosed in the left eye, the left eye was felt to be irreversibly blind, and the right eye was judged to be at risk for acute-angle closure and glaucoma as well. The owner opted for an intravitreal gentamicin injection in the left eye and prophylactic medical therapy (demecarium bromide [DBr] and dexamethasone drops every 24 hours in the evening) for the right eye. The left eye became comfortable but phthisical following the gentamicin injection (as in **Figure 12.68**), requiring no further therapy. The owner (who lived over 4 hours away) dutifully had the patient reexamined on a yearly basis at our referral hospital and every 3 months by her regular veterinarian. Approximately 6 years later, at 9 years of age, the owner called late one night to report that the dog's right eye was red, cloudy, painful like it had been acutely for the other eye, and the patient did not seem visual. The owner was instructed to give the dog oral glycerin and methazolamide (from a "glaucoma emergency kit" that had been sent home with the owner just for this sort of circumstance) and to apply the DBr every 8 hours. The patient was seen 10 hours later and was more comfortable, was visual, and had an IOP of 20 mmHg. The pupil was miotic, which precluded examination of the fundus. Based on the client history and clinical findings, it was assumed that the patient had indeed experienced an acute attack of IOP elevation, and the patient was predisposed to have yet another despite medical therapy. The owner elected cyclophotocoagulation in an attempt to control glaucoma in the right eye and preserve vision. This was performed transsclerally and was without incident. The patient was treated with topical dexamethasone, dorzolamide, timolol, and DBr immediately postop and was weaned to topical dorzolamide and timolol after 2 months when the IOP was stable in the low teens. The DBr was discontinued because the patient was beginning to develop an axial incipient cataract and pupillary miosis-impaired vision. Due to client circumstances, the patient was not seen again until after a year from the date of surgery. The owner indicated that the patient had slowly lost vision and that the right eye seemed red and "bulging," but did not seem painful. Examination revealed the right eye to be slightly buphthalmic with mild episcleral injection and a dilated pupil. The dog had no menace or dazzle response. The fundus was poorly seen due to the immature cataract, but the optic disc was judged to be atrophic and cupped with diffuse tapetal hyperreflectivity. IOP was 35 mmHg. Based on the poor prognosis for vision restoration and the owner's desire to not treat the blind eye, a gentamicin injection was performed in the right eye, and the outcome was similar to the left eye. This case is a good example of angle-closure glaucoma in the American Cocker Spaniel and any other breed predisposed to primary angle-closure glaucoma. The initial eye had an acute episode of IOP elevation that did not respond to nonaggressive medical therapy. By the time the patient presented to the referral center, the eye was blind. Based on gonioscopy, the contralateral eye was felt to be predisposed to a similar scenario. Prophylactic medical therapy in this case was very successful at prolonging the time until the second eye underwent an acute "glaucoma attack." Currently, other medial prophylaxis (dorzolamide, timolol, latanoprost, or other drugs) could be used instead of DBr and dexamethasone. The left and right eyes responded quite well to intravitreal gentamicin injections once the eyes were irreparably blind. Despite phthisis bulbi and cataract formation, both eyes appeared comfortable, did not require medical therapy, and were cosmetically pleasing to the owner. Other salvage procedures (evisceration and prosthesis implantation or enucleation) were offered to the owner, but due to costs and cosmetic concerns, the gentamicin injection was chosen by the owner. When the right eye experienced an "acute attack of glaucoma," aggressive medical therapy resulted in reduction of IOP to a normal level with apparent regaining vision compared to the evening before. Because the IOP was not low (20 mmHg despite aggressive therapy less than 10 hours prior to exam), it was felt that medical management alone would not be enough to control IOP long-term and preserve vision. This patient had a good initial result from the Nd:YAG cyclophotocoagulation, but as is commonly the case, long-term control was poor, even with medical therapy, and the patient ultimately was blinded by glaucoma. Currently, newer drugs (prostaglandin analogs such as latanoprost) may have been able to control the IOP for a longer period and maintained vision longer. Currently, more aggressive surgical therapy (phacoemulsification and cyclophotocoagulation via diode endolaser) may have also maintained a normal IOP longer, dealt with the postlaser complication of cataract formation, and maintained vision in this patient for a longer period of time.

CASE 2

A 12-year-old DLH cat was referred for an anterior lens luxation of the left eye with elevated IOP. Clinically, the left eye had minor episcleral injection, IOP of 35 mmHg, minor ventral keratic precipitates (KP), an anterior lens luxation of an immature cataractic lens, rubeosis irides, and a positive dazzle response. The right eye had minor KP, mild rubeosis irides, and anterior vitreal fibrin and debris. IOP in the right eye was 8 mmHg. A diagnosis of bilateral anterior uveitis was made, with anterior lens luxation and glaucoma in the left eye. CBC, serum biochemistry panel, and urinalysis were within normal limits, FeLV and toxoplasmal serology were negative, but FIV testing was positive as was PCR testing for bartonella. An intracapsular lens extraction was performed, and postoperative medical therapy was oral doxycycline and an anti-inflammatory dose of prednisolone as well as topical antibiotic, prednisolone, and dorzolamide for the left eye and topical prednisolone for the right eye. The left eye's surgical incision healed without mishap, and the patient had a good menace response and pupillary light responses in both eyes for the first 3 months postop. The active intraocular inflammation in both eyes abated, and both eyes were kept on every-24-hour topical prednisolone to control inflammation. Oral antibiotics and prednisolone were discontinued 2 weeks following surgery. IOP in the left eye was initially low postop, so dorzolamide was discontinued after one month. With abatement of intraocular inflammation in the right eye, IOP increased to the high teens. Long-term, IOP in the left eye slowly increased over a 4-month period to the mid-20s, so the patient was started back on topical dorzolamide along with the topical every-24-hour prednisolone. Eventually IOP in the left eye was unresponsive to dorzolamide–timolol, and after one year, the patient was reexamined, and the left eye was found to be buphthalmic, blind, with an IOP of 45 mmHg. IOP in the right eye was in the high-20s. The owner elected enucleation of the blind left eye. The right eye was treated with topical dorzolamide and prednisolone, and for 1-year follow-up from the referring veterinarian, the cat remained visual with IOPs in the mid-to-low teens. This case represents lens luxation-induced glaucoma in the left eye of a cat, complicated by uveitis-induced glaucoma and eventual loss of the left eye to glaucoma. Immediately following removal of the anteriorly luxated lens, IOP in the left eye was easily maintained in a normal range. With time, however, IOP increased (probably due to filtration-angle fibrosis due to smoldering inflammation), and the eye was lost to glaucoma. In the right eye, chronic uveitis was controlled with topical corticosteroids, but secondary IOP elevation was seen, most likely due to filtration-angle scarring from the uveitis. Medical management (topical corticosteroids and dorzolamide) was successful in managing IOP in the right eye for the 1-year follow-up.

CASE 3

A 3-year-old M/N Jack Russell terrier was presented for a red, cloudy, acutely painful left eye. The referring veterinarian had diagnosed glaucoma (IOP greater than 35 mmHg) and an anterior lens luxation. Initial therapy had included topical prednisolone and dorzolamide. When examined 12 hours following initiation of medical therapy, the left eye was visual (positive menace and dazzle response), episcleral injection was less than prior to therapy (as per owner), IOP was 18 mmHg, and the patient was relatively comfortable, only showing mild blepharospasm. The lens was in the anterior chamber (as in **Figure 12.54**), touching the corneal endothelial

surface, resulting in focal corneal edema. The right eye had a deep anterior chamber with strands of pigment-laden vitreous passing through the pupil into the anterior chamber. The right iris had notable iridodonesis, and there was also phacodenesis. Primary lens luxation with secondary glaucoma was diagnosed in the left eye, with the right eye having a posterior lens subluxation as well. Intracapsular lens extraction was performed without mishap in the left eye. Postoperatively, the patient was discharged with topical antibiotic, prednisolone, and dorzolamide drops in the left eye and topical latanoprost in the right eye to constrict the pupil to maintain the right lens in the posterior chamber. Subsequent rechecks of both eyes revealed IOPs less than 10 mmHg, bilaterally, with uneventful healing of the surgical site of the left eye. There was permanent mild corneal edema in the area where the lens had been touching the cornea prior to lens removal. After 6 weeks, topical dorzolamide was discontinued in the left eye, and topical prednisolone was weaned and ultimately discontinued after 12 weeks. The right eye continued to be treated with topical latanoprost, and after 1-year follow-up, the right lens remained in the posterior chamber, and the IOP in the right eye remained less than 10 mmHg. IOP in the left eye stabilized in the mid-teens. This case represents genetic primary lens luxation with secondary glaucoma in a predisposed terrier breed. The immediate medical therapy with a drug to decrease aqueous humor production to lower IOP in the affected eye may have saved the optic nerve from pressure-induced degeneration and may have saved the dog's vision in the left eye. Use of a miotic drug to try to lower IOP (such as pilocarpine or latanoprost), could have further restricted aqueous outflow through the pupil into the anterior chamber and could have resulted in even further increase in IOP instead of lowering IOP. In this case, IOP normalized following lens removal. This is not always the case in that many dogs with primary lens luxation may also have filtration angle anomalies that are also genetic in origin. Many of those dogs may require medical management of glaucoma, even after lens removal. The contralateral eye also had primary lens luxation, but to a lesser extent, at presentation. See Chapter 13, Lens, concerning medical/surgical options for posterior lens luxation in the dog. In this case, the latanoprost-induced miosis helped maintain the lens in the posterior chamber for the 1-year follow-up period. The lower than normal IOP in the right eye was attributed to the enhanced aqueous humor outflow due to latanoprost usage.

CASE 4

A 13-year-old Appaloosa gelding presented for a cloudy left eye. Historically, the horse had experienced occasional episodes of tearing, photophobia, and cloudiness of both eyes, but the owners had not noted any vision impairment (the horse was not ridden regularly). Clinically, the left eye was minimally blepharospastic with mild diffuse corneal edema, Haab's striae, iris hyperpigmentation, foci of posterior synechia, and a midrange, unresponsive to light stimulation pupil (similar to **Figure 12.59**). IOP was 42 mmHg. Menace and dazzle responses were present in both eyes. The right eye had an IOP of 10 mmHg, mild aqueous flare, iris hyperpigmentation, areas of posterior synechia, mild inflammatory debris on the anterior and posterior lens capsules, vitreous syneresis and fibrin strands, and peripapillary areas of chorioretinal scarring, especially ventromedial and ventrolateral to the optic nerve ("butterfly lesion"). A diagnosis of equine recurrent uveitis (ERU) was made with secondary glaucoma in the left eye. Medical (topical corticosteroids, bilaterally, topical dorzolamide-timolol in the left eye, and systemic NSAIDs) and surgical (suprachoroidal cyclosporine implants in both eyes with trans-scleral cyclophotocoagulation in the left eye) options were offered. The owner elected medical therapy initially due to cost/prognosis concerns. Two weeks later, reexamination revealed two visual eyes with no signs of active intraocular inflammation. Diffuse corneal edema was not present, but the Haab's striae were still present in the left cornea. Right eye IOP was 18 mmHg, and the left eye was 20 mmHg. The owner elected surgical therapy bilaterally (cyclosporine implants) for ERU as well as cyclophotocoagulation in the left eye to try to control glaucoma without the need for chronic medical therapy. Surgery in both eyes was uneventful, and postop medical therapy continued as topical corticosteroids, bilaterally, dorzolamide, left eye, and oral NSAIDs. Over a 3-month period, the horse was weaned of all topical and systemic medications with no signs of active uveitis or glaucoma. Eighteen months later, the horse presented with a painful, cloudy right eye. Because the patient was not being treated daily, and the horse was on pasture, the owners were not sure how long the eye had been painful or cloudy. The right eye was enlarged, had moderate diffuse corneal edema and Haab's striae, a mid-dilated unresponsive pupil, and an IOP of 65 mmHg. The lens was subluxated ventromedially and was involved with an immature cortical cataract. There was no menace or dazzle response from the right eye. The left eye was visual and had the previously identified Haab's striae, with an IOP of 15 mmHg. Medical therapy (topical prednisolone, dorzolamide-timolol, oral NSAIDs, and aqueous centesis) failed to control IOP in the right eye. After 5 days of aggressive in-hospital medical therapy, the owner elected to enucleate the blind, painful, glaucomatous right eye. Two-year follow-up revealed a comfortable, nonglaucomatous, visual left eye without any further medical management. This case is typical of glaucoma in the horse. Chronic low-grade uveitis, many times with no overt clinical signs of pain, leads to filtration angle fibrosis, preiridal fibrovascular membrane formation, and other changes that inhibit outflow of aqueous humor. Unlike acute-angle-closure glaucoma in dogs, most horses do not usually appear painful in the early stages of glaucoma. The appearance of Haab's striae indicates ocular distension associated with elevated IOP and is a classic sign of glaucoma in horses. In this author's hospital, Appaloosas are overrepresented for both ERU and glaucoma. The advanced age of this patient was also typical of equine glaucoma. This patient responded quite well to initial medical therapy in the left eye (many do not, as was the case in the right eye) and also responded quite well to the diode laser cyclophotocoagulation for glaucoma in the left eye. Secondary cataract, a common complication from cyclophotocoagulation in all species, was very minor in this patient and could have reflected changes due to the ERU as well as changes associated with the laser procedure.

CASE 5

A 5-year-old M/N German shepherd cross presented for blindness and painful, discolored eyes. Historically, the owner had noticed both eyes being cloudy with blepharospasm for several days prior to vision loss. The referring veterinarian had noted corneal edema, mild hyphema, blindness, and IOPs in the mid-30s in both eyes. Examination revealed no menace but positive dazzle responses bilaterally. Episcleral injection and corneal edema were present bilaterally as well as mild clotted blood and fibrin in both anterior chambers. IOPs were 35 and 38 mmHg. There were mild rubeosis irides, miosis, and subtle retinal detachments seen bilaterally. Gonioscopy revealed blood and fibrin obstructing the filtration angles (**Figure 12.49a**). Physical examination revealed mild fever and lymphadenopathy. Medical workup quickly diagnosed ehrlichiosis as the underlying systemic disease responsible for the uveitis. Initial therapy for the panuveitis of undetermined etiology was topical prednisolone and dorzolamide–timolol, oral doxycycline, and oral NSAIDs. Within 24 hours, IOPs had decreased to less than 10 mmHg, the aqueous humor inflammatory debris and fibrinohemorrhagic clots were resolving, and the dog appeared visual. To prevent posterior synechia and iris bombe, topical tropicamide was used three times daily to "move" the pupils and hopefully inhibit adhesions of the iris to the anterior lens capsule. At a 2-week recheck, the patient was bright and alert, visual, and both eyes were clear of signs of active inflammation. The anterior chamber blood and fibrin clots had cleared, and IOPs were less than 10 mmHg. Gonioscopy revealed clearing of the blood and clots from the filtration angles (**Figure 12.49b**). The pupils were free and dilated due to tropicamide usage. Neither fundus showed signs of the previous retinal detachments. Medical therapy was continued as topical prednisolone and tropicamide (dorzolamide–timolol was discontinued) and oral doxycycline. Over a 2-month period, all drugs were weaned to discontinuance, and the patient was reexamined 1 year later with no signs of glaucoma or uveitis and minimal diffuse tapetal hyperreflectivity being noted

bilaterally. This case of uveitis-induced glaucoma in a dog responded well to symptomatic therapy for the glaucoma (dorzolamide–timolol), uveitis (prednisolone drops and oral NSAIDs), and systemic therapy for the underlying disease (doxycycline for the ehrlichiosis). Had the dog developed posterior synechia with iris bombe and peripheral anterior synechia due to iris/cornea adhesions from debris in the filtration angles, the outcome may not have been as good. In this case, miotic or prostaglandin analog therapy could have exacerbated the anterior uveitis, caused pupillary constriction with posterior synechia and iris bombe, and could have made the glaucoma worse. In this case, diagnosis of the probable underlying disease was quick and accurate, so specific therapy for the infectious disease was begun early, and the patient responded quite well. Lists of potential infectious and neoplastic disorders that may cause anterior uveitis in the dog are to be found in Chapter 11, Anterior Uvea and Anterior Chamber. In the case of some infectious diseases (systemic fungal infections in particular), therapy to kill the infectious organisms many times causes such a massive die-off of organisms with secondary inflammation that leads to worsening of the secondary glaucoma. For this reason, many use systemic anti-inflammatory doses of corticosteroids to reduce inflammation to quell the inflammation and hopefully prevent endophthalmitis and end-stage glaucoma.

GENETIC PREDISPOSITION, GLAUCOMA

PRIMARY OPEN-ANGLE GLAUCOMA

Canine—Beagle ("Florida beagle" and potentially other nonresearch beagles), Norwegian elkhound

CLOSED-ANGLE GLAUCOMA

Canine—American Cocker Spaniel, basset hound, English Cocker Spaniel, Samoyed, Siberian husky, Chow Chow, Shar Pei, Welsh springer spaniel, Bouvier des Flandres, shiba inu, Shih Tzu, Flat-coated retriever

ACUTE POSTOPERATIVE (PHACOEMULSIFICATION) HYPERTENSION

Canine—Labrador retriever, Boston terrier

LONG-TERM POSTCATARACT EXTRACTION SURGERY GLAUCOMA

Canine—Boston terrier, American Cocker Spaniel, Cocker spaniel-poodle mix, Shih Tzu

GLAUCOMA SECONDARY TO UVEAL CYSTS

Canine—Golden retriever, Great Dane

PIGMENT PROLIFERATION/ DISPERSION GLAUCOMA

Canine—Cairn terrier, Scottish terrier, boxer, Labrador retriever

ANTERIOR LENS LUXATION AND GLAUCOMA

Canine—All terrier breeds, Chinese crested, Chihuahua, Shar Pei

REFERENCES

1. Anderson, D. 1980. Glaucoma: The damage caused by pressure. XLVI Edward Jackson Memorial Lecture. *American Journal of Ophthalmology* 108:484–495.

2. Quigley, H.A. 1993. Open-angle glaucoma. *New England Journal of Medicine* 328:1097–1106.

3. Weinreb, R.N., and Levin, L.A. 1999. Is neuroprotection a viable therapy for glaucoma? *Archives of Ophthalmology* 117:1540–1544.

4. Hernandez, M.R., and Pena, J.P.O. 1997. The optic nerve in glaucomatous optic neuropathy. *Archives of Ophthalmology* 115:389–395.

5. Martin, C. 1974. Glaucoma. In: Kirk, R.W., editor. *Current Veterinary Therapy IV*, 4th edition. WB Saunders: Philadelphia, PA, pp. 513–518.

6. Boevé, M., and Stades, F. 1985. Glaucoom bij hond en kat, overzicht en retrospectieve evaluatie van 421 patienten. I. Pathobiologische achtergronden, indeling en raspredisposities. *Tijdschrift Voor Diergeneeskunde* 6:219–227.

7. Boevé, M., and Stades, F. 1985. Glaucoom bij hood en kat. II. Klinische aspecten. *Tijdschrift Voor Diergeneeskunde* 6:228–236.

8. Gelatt, K.N., and MacKay, E.O. 2004. Prevalence of the breed-related glaucomas in purebred dogs in North America. *Veterinary Ophthalmology* 7:97–111.

9. Green, K. 1984. Physiology and pharmacology of aqueous humor inflow. *Survey of Ophthalmology* 29:208–214.

10. Caprioli, J. 1992. The ciliary epithelia and aqueous humor. In: Hart, W., editor. *Adler's Physiology of the Eye*, 9th edition. Mosby Year Book: St Louis, MO, pp. 228–247.

11. Troncoso, M. 1942. The intrascleral vascular plexus and its relations to the aqueous outflow. *American Journal of Ophthalmology* 25:1153–1162.

12. Uberreiter, O. 1959. Die kammerwasservenen reim hunde. *Wiener Tierarztliche Monetsschrift* 46:721–722.

13. Martin, C.L. 1969. Gonioscopy and anatomical correlations of drainage angle of the dog. *Journal of Small Animal Practice* 10:171–184.

14. Van Buskirk, M. 1979. The canine eye: The vessels of aqueous drainage. *Investigative Ophthalmology and Visual Science* 18:223–230.

15. Rohen, J. 1956. Arteriovenose anastomosen im limbusreich des hundes. *Albrecht von Graefes Archiv fur Ophthaalmologie* 157:361–367.

16. Martin, C.L., and Anderson, B.G. 1981. Ocular anatomy. In: Gelatt, K., editor. *Veterinary Ophthalmology*, 1st edition. Lea & Febiger: Philadelphia, PA, pp. 12–121.

17. Bedford, P., and Grierson, I. 1986. Aqueous drainage in the dog. *Research in Veterinary Science* 41:172–186.

18. Samuelson, D. 1996. A re-evaluation of the comparative anatomy of the eutherian iridocorneal angle and associated ciliary body musculature. *Veterinary and Comparative Ophthalmology* 6:153–172.

19. Martin, C.L. 1983. The pathology of glaucoma. In: Peiffer, R.L., editor. *Comparative Ophthalmic Pathology*. Charles C Thomas: Springfield, IL, pp. 137–169.

20. Martin, C. 1975. The normal canine iridocorneal angle as viewed with the scanning electron microscope. *Journal of the American Animal Hospital Association* 11:180–184.

21. Tripathi, R. 1971. Ultrastructure of the exit pathway of the aqueous in lower mammals (a preliminary report on the "angular aqueous plexus'). *Experimental Eye Research* 12:311–314.

22. Lee, W.R., and Grierson, I. 1975. Pressure effects on the endothelium of the trabecular wall of Schlemm's canal: A study by scanning electron microscopy. *Albrecht von Graefes Archives fur Klinische und Experimentelle Ophthalmologie* 196:255–265.

23. Grierson, I., and Lee, W.R. 1997. Light microscopic quantitation of the endothelial vacuoles in Schlemm's canal. *American Journal of Ophthalmology* 84:234–246.

24. Epstein, D., and Rohen, J. 1991. Morphology of the trabecular meshwork and inner-wall endothelium after cationized ferritin perfusion in the monkey eye. *Investigative Ophthalmology and Visual Science* 32:160–171.

25. Sit, A.J., Coloma, F.M., Ethier, C.R., and Johnson, M. 1997. Factors affecting the pores of the inner-wall endothelium of Schlemm's canal. *Investigative Ophthalmology and Visual Science* 38:1517–1525.

26. Ethier, C.R., Coloma, F.M., Sit, A.J., and Johnson, M. 1998. The pore types in the inner-wall endothelium of Schlemm's canal. *Investigative Ophthalmology and Visual Science* 39:2041–2048.

27. Costa-Vila, J., and Ruano-Gil, D. 1988. Scanning electron microscope study of the communications between the anterior chamber and the sinus venosus sclerae in primates. *Acta Anatomica* 131:342–345.

28. Barany, E.H. 1956. The action of different kinds of hyaluronidase on resistance of flow through the angle of the anterior chamber. *Acta Ophthalmologica* 34:397–403.

29. Gum, G.G., Samuelson, D.A., and Gelatt, K. 1992. Effect of hyaluronidase on aqueous outflow resistance in normotensive and glaucomatous eyes of dogs. *American Journal of Veterinary Research* 53:767–770.

30. Richardson, T. 1982. Distribution of glycosaminoglycan in the aqueous outflow system of the cat. *Investigative Ophthalmology and Visual Science* 22:319–329.

31. Gum, G.G., Gelatt, K.N., and Knepper, P.A. 1993. Histochemical localization of glycosaminoglycans in the aqueous outflow pathways in normal Beagles and Beagles with inherited glaucoma. *Progress in Veterinary and Comparative Ophthalmology* 3(2):52–57.

32. Yue, B. 1996. The extracellular matrix and its modulation in the trabecular meshwork. *Survey of Ophthalmology* 40:379–390.

33. Weinstein, W.L., Dietrich, U.M., Sapienza, J.S. et al. 2007. Identification of ocular matrix metalloproteinases present within the aqueous humor and iridocorneal drainage angle tissue of normal and glaucomatous canine eyes. *Veterinary Ophthalmology* 10:108–116.

34. MacKay, E.O., Kallberg, M.E., and Gelatt, K.N. 2008. Aqueous humor Myocilin protein levels in normal, genetic carrier, and glaucomatous Beagles. *Veterinary Ophthalmology* 11:177–185.

35. Hart, H., Samuelson, D.A., Tajwar, J. et al. 2007. Immunolocalization of Myocilin protein in the anterior eye of normal and primary open-angle glaucomatous dogs. *Veterinary Ophthalmology* 10:28–37.

36. McMaster, P., and Macri, F. 1968. Secondary aqueous humor outflow pathways in the rabbit, cat, and monkey. *Archives of Ophthalmology* 79:297–303.

37. Gelatt, K., Glenwood, G., Williams, L., and Barrie, K. 1979. Uveoscleral flow of aqueous humor in the normal dog. *American Journal of Veterinary Research* 40:845–848.

38. Cruise, L., and McClure, R. 1981. Posterior pathway for aqueous humor drainage in the dog. *American Journal of Veterinary Research* 42:992–995.

39. Samuelson, D., Gum, G., Gelatt, K., and Barrie, K. 1985. Aqueous outflow in the Beagle: Unconventional outflow using different-sized microspheres. *American Journal of Veterinary Research* 46:242–248.

40. Smith, P.L., Samuelson, D., Brooks, D., and Whitley, R. 1986. Unconventional aqueous humor outflow of microspheres perfused into the equine eye. *American Journal of Veterinary Research* 47:2445–2453.

41. Bedford, P. 1977. A gonioscopic study of the iridocorneal angle in the English and American breeds of Cocker Spaniel and the Basset Hound. *Journal of Small Animal Practice* 18:631–642.

42. Troncoso, M., and Castroviejo, R. 1936. Microanatomy of the eye with the slit lamp microscope. *American Journal of Ophthalmology* 19:481–492.

43. Samuelson, D., Smith, P., and Brooks, D. 1989. Morphologic features of the aqueous humor drainage pathways in horses. *American Journal of Veterinary Research* 50:720–727.

44. De Geest, J.P., Lauwers, H., and Simoens, P.D.S. 1990. The morphology of the equine iridocorneal angle: A light and scanning electron microscopic study. *Equine Veterinary Journal Veterinary Ophthalmology Supplement* 10:30–35.

45. Magrane, W.G. 1957. Canine glaucoma. I. Methods of diagnosis. *Journal of the American Veterinary Medical Association* 131:311–314.

46. Magrane, W.G. 1957. Canine glaucoma. II. Primary classification. *Journal of the American Veterinary Medical Association* 131:372–374.

47. Lovekin, L.G. 1964. Primary glaucoma in dogs. *Journal of the American Veterinary Medical Association* 145:1081–1091.

48. Bryan, G. 1965. Tonometry in the dog and cat. *Journal of Small Animal Practice* 6:117–120.

49. Heywood, R. 1971. Intraocular pressures in the Beagle dog. *Journal of Small Animal Practice* 12:119–121.

50. Gelatt, K.N., and MacKay, E.O. 1998. Distribution of intraocular pressure in dogs. *Veterinary Ophthalmology* 1:109–114.

51. Miller, P., Pickett, P., Majors, L., and Kurzman, I. 1991. Evaluation of two applanation tonometers in cats. *American Journal of Veterinary Research* 52:1917–1921.

52. Miller, P.E., Pickett, J.P., Majors, L.J., and Kurzman, I.D. 1991. Clinical comparison of the Mackay-Marg and Tono-Pen applanation tonometer in the dog. *Progress in Veterinary and Comparative Ophthalmology* 1:171–176.

53. Leiva, M., Naranjo, C., and Pena, M.T. 2006. Comparison of the rebound tonometer (ICare^R) with the applanation tonometer (Tono-Pen XL) in normotensive dogs. *Veterinary Ophthalmology* 9:17–21.

54. Gelatt, K., Gum, G., Barrie, K., and Williams, W. 1981. Diurnal variations in intraocular pressure in normotensive and glaucomatous Beagles. *Glaucoma* 3:21–24.

55. Del Sole, M.J., Sande, P.H., Bernades, J.M. et al. 2007. Circadian rhythm of intraocular pressures in cats. *Veterinary Ophthalmology* 10:155–161.

56. Kormaromy, A.M., Garg, C.D., Ying, G.S. et al. 2006. Effect of head position on intraocular pressure in horses. *American Journal of Veterinary Research* 67:1233–1235.

57. Peiffer, R.L., Gelatt, K.N., Jessen, C.R., Gum, G.G., Swin, R.M., and Davis, J. 1977. Calibration of the Schiotz tonometer for the normal canine eye. *American Journal of Veterinary Research* 38:1881–1889.

58. Picket, J., Miller, P., and Majors, L. 1988. Calibration of the Schiotz tonometer for the canine and feline eye. *Proceedings of the American College of Veterinary Ophthalmologists*, Las Vegas, NV, 19:45–51.

59. Miller, P., and Pickett, J. 1992. Comparison of the human and canine Schiotz tonometry conversion tables in clinically normal cats. *Journal of the American Veterinary Medical Association* 201(7):1017–1020.

60. Miller, P., and Pickett, J. 1992. Comparison of the human and canine Schiotz tonometry conversion tables in clinically normal dogs. *Journal of the American Veterinary Medical Association* 201(7):1021–1025.

61. Priehs, D., Gum, G., Whitley, D., and Moore, L. 1990. Evaluation of three applanation tonometers in dogs. *American Journal of Veterinary Research* 51:1547–1550.

62. Dziezyc, J., Millichamp, N., and Smith, W. 1992. Comparison of applanation tonometers in dogs and horses. *Journal of the American Veterinary Medical Association* 201:430–433.

63. McLellan, G.J., Kemmerling, J.P., and Miller, P.E. 2013. Validation of the TonoVet^R rebound tonometer in normal and glaucomatous cats. *Veterinary Ophthalmology* 16:111–118.

64. von Spiessman, L., Karck, J., Rohn, K. et al. 2015. Clinical comparison of the TonoVet rebound tonometer and the Tono-Pen Vet applanation tonometer in dogs and cats with ocular disease: Glaucoma or corneal pathology. *Veterinary Ophthalmology* 18:20–27.

65. Knollinger, A.M., La Croix, N.C., Barrett, P.M., and Miller, P.E. 2005. Evaluation of a rebound tonometer for measuring intraocular pressure in dogs and horses. *Journal of the American Veterinary Medical Association* 227:244–248.

66. Gelatt, K. 1977. Evaluation of applanation tonometers for the dog eye. *Investigative Ophthalmology and Visual Science* 16:963–968.

67. Miller, P., Pickett, P., and Majors, L. 1990. Evaluation of two applanation tonometers in horses. *American Journal of Veterinary Research* 51:935–937.

68. Rutkowski, P., and Thompson, S. 1972. Mydriasis and increased intraocular pressure. I. Pupillographic studies. *Archives of Ophthalmology* 87:21–24.

69. Rutkowski, P., and Thompson, S. 1972. Mydriasis and increased intraocular pressure. II. Iris fluorescein studies. *Archives of Ophthalmology* 87:25–29.

70. Martin, C., and Vestre, W. 1985 Glaucoma. In: Slatter, D., editor. *Textbook of Small Animal Surgery*, vol. 2. WB Saunders: Philadelphia, PA, pp. 1567–1584.

71. Grosdanic, S.D., Matic, M., Betts, D.B. et al. 2007. Recovery of canine retina and optic nerve function after acute elevation of intraocular pressure: Implications for canine glaucoma treatment. *Veterinary Ophthalmology* 10:101–107.

72. Minckler, D., and Spaeth, G. 1981. Optic nerve damage in glaucoma. *Survey of Ophthalmology* 26:128–148.

73. Samuelson, D., and Gelatt, K. 1983. Orthograde rapid axoplasmic transport and ultrastructural changes of the optic nerve. Part II. Beagles with primary open-angle glaucoma. *Glaucoma* 5:174–184.

74. Williams, L., Gelatt, K., and Gum, G. 1983. Orthograde rapid axoplasmic transport and ultrastructural changes in the optic nerve. Part I. Normotensive and acute ocular hypertensive Beagles. *Glaucoma* 5:117–128.

75. Brooks, D., Samuelson, D., and Gelatt, K. 1989. Ultrastructural changes in laminar optic nerve capillaries of Beagles with primary open-angle glaucoma. *American Journal of Veterinary Research* 50:929–935.

76. Glovinsky, Y., Quigley, H., and Dunkelberger, G. 1991. Retinal ganglion cell loss is size dependent in experimental glaucoma. *Investigative Ophthalmology and Visual Science* 32:484–491.

77. Schumer, R., and Podos, S. 1994. The nerve of glaucoma! *Archives of Ophthalmology* 112:37–44.

78. Brooks, D.E., Komaromy, A.M., and Kallberg, M.E. 1999. Comparative optic nerve physiology: Implications for glaucoma, neuroprotection, and neuroregeneration. *Veterinary Ophthalmology* 2:13–25.

79. Dreyer, E., Zurakowski, D., Schumer, R., Podos, S., and Lipton, S. 1996. Elevated glutamate levels in the vitreous body of humans and monkeys with glaucoma. *Archives of Ophthalmology* 114:299–305.

80. Brooks, D., Garcia, G., Dreyer, E., Zurakowski, D., and Franco-Bourland, R. 1997. Vitreous body glutamate concentration in dogs with glaucoma. *American Journal of Veterinary Research* 58:864–867.

81. Dreyer, E. 1997. Amino acid abnormalities in the vitreous of the buphthalmic rabbit. *Veterinary and Comparative Ophthalmology* 7:192–195.

82. Keilly, C.M., Morris, R., and Dubielzig, R.R. 2005. Canine goniodysgenesis-related glaucoma: A morphologic review of 100 cases looking at inflammation and pigment dispersion. *Veterinary Ophthalmology* 8:253–258.

83. Lovekin, L. 1971. Water provocative test for glaucoma: Range of normal tonometric responses of the canine eye. *American Journal of Veterinary Research* 32:1179–1183.

84. Gelatt, K., Peiffer, R., Jessen, C., and Gum, G. 1976. Consecutive water provocative tests in normal and glaucomatous Beagles. *American Journal of Veterinary Research* 37:269–273.

85. Gelatt, K.N., Gwin, R.M., Peiffer, R.L., and Gum, G.G. 1977. Tonography in the normal and glaucomatous Beagle. *American Journal of Veterinary Research* 38:515–520.

86. Gelatt, K., Gum, G., and MacKay, E. 1996. Estimations of aqueous humor outflow facility by pneumatonography in normal genetic carrier and glaucomatous Beagles. *Veterinary and Comparative Ophthalmology* 6:148–151.

87. Walde, I. 1984. Klassifikation des glaukomas beim hund. *Tierarztliche Praxis* 12:65–78.

88. Gibson, T., Roberts, S., Severin, S., Steyn, P., and Wrigley, R. 1998. Comparison of gonioscopy and ultrasound biomicroscopy for evaluating the iridocorneal angle in dogs. *Journal of the American Veterinary Medical Association* 213:635–638.

89. Bentley, E., Miller, P.E., and Diehl, K.A. 2003. Use of high-resolution ultrasound as a diagnostic tool in veterinary ophthalmology. *Journal of the American Veterinary Medical Association* 223:1617–1622.

90. Gelatt, K., and Gum, G. 1981. Inheritance of primary glaucoma in the Beagle. *American Journal of Veterinary Research* 42:1691–1693.

91. Ekesten, B., Bjerkas, E., Kongsengen, K., and Narfström, K. 1997. Primary glaucoma in the Norwegian Elkhound. *Veterinary and Comparative Ophthalmology* 7:14–18.

92. Gelatt, K., Peiffer, R., Gwin, R., Gum, G., and Williams, L. 1977. Clinical manifestations of inherited glaucoma in the Beagle. *Investigative Ophthalmology and Visual Science* 16:1135–1142.

93. Peiffer, R., and Gelatt, K. 1980. Aqueous humor outflow in Beagles with inherited glaucoma: Gross and light microscopic observations of the iridocorneal angle. *American Journal of Veterinary Research* 41:861–867.

94. Hart, H., Samuelson, D.A., Tajwar, J., MacKay, E.O. et al. 2007. Immunolocalization of myocilin protein in the anterior chamber of normal and primary open-angle glaucomatous dogs. *Veterinary Ophthalmology* 10:28–37.

95. MacKay, E.O., Kallberg, M.E., Barrie, K.P. et al. 2008. Myocilin protein levels in the aqueous humor of the glaucomas in selected canine breeds. *Veterinary Ophthalmology* 11:234–241.

96. Bedford, P. 1975. The aetiology of primary glaucoma in the dog. *Journal of Small Animal Practice* 16:217–239.

97. Smith, R.I., Peiffer, R.L., and Wilcock, B.P. 1993. Some aspects of the pathology of canine glaucoma. *Progress in Veterinary and Comparative Ophthalmology* 3:16–28.

98. Martin, C., and Wyman, M. 1978. Primary glaucoma in the dog. *Veterinary Clinics of North America* 8:257–286.

99. Yeon, Y., and Jung, H. 1997. Clarifying the nomenclature for primary angle-closure glaucoma. *Survey of Ophthalmology* 42:125–136.

100. Ekesten, B., and Narfström, K. 1991. Correlation of morphologic features of the iridocorneal angle to intraocular pressure in Samoyeds. *American Journal of Veterinary Research* 52:1875–1878.

101. Martin, C. 1975. Scanning electron microscopic examination of selected canine iridocorneal angle abnormalities. *Journal of the American Animal Hospital Association* 11:300–306.

102. Read, R., Wood, J., and Lakhani, K. 1998. Pectinate ligament dysplasia (PLD) and glaucoma in Flat Coated Retrievers. I. Objectives, techniques, and results of a PLD survey. *Veterinary Ophthalmology* 1:85–90.

103. Martin, C. 1974. Development of the pectinate ligament structure of the dog: Study by scanning electron microscopy. *American Journal of Veterinary Research* 35:1433–1439.

104. van der Linde-Sipman, J.S. 1987. Dysplasia of the pectinate ligament and primary glaucoma in the Bouvier des Flandres dog. *Veterinary Pathology* 24:201–206.

105. Cottrell, B., and Barnett, K. 1988. Primary glaucoma in the Welsh Springer Spaniel. *Journal of Small Animal Practice* 29:185–199.

106. Slater, M., and Erb, H. 1986. Effects of risk factors and prophylactic treatment on primary glaucoma in the dog. *Journal of the American Veterinary Medical Association* 188:1028–1030.

107. Miller, P.E., Schmidt, G.M., Vainisi, S.J., Swanson, J.F., and Hermann, M.K. 2000. The efficacy of topical prophylactic antiglaucoma therapy in primary closed-angle glaucoma in dogs: A multicenter clinical trial. *Journal of the American Animal Hospital Association* 36:431–438.

108. Corcoran, K.A., Koch, S.A., and Peiffer, R.L. 1994. Primary glaucoma in the Chow Chow. *Veterinary and Comparative Ophthalmology* 4:193–197.

109. Louden, C., Render, J., and Carlton, W. 1990. Mast cell numbers in normal and glaucomatous canine eyes. *American Journal of Veterinary Research* 51:818–819.

110. Ekesten, B. 1993. Correlation of intraocular distances to the iridocorneal angle in Samoyeds with special reference to angle-closure glaucoma. *Progress in Veterinary and Comparative Ophthalmology* 3:67–73.

111. Mangan, B.G., Al-Yahya, K., Chen, C. et al. 2007. Retinal pigment epithelial damage, breakdown of the blood-retinal barrier, and retinal inflammation in dogs with primary glaucoma. *Veterinary Ophthalmology* 9:117–124.

112. Martin, C., and Wyman, M. 1968. Glaucoma in the Basset Hound. *Journal of the American Veterinary Medical Association* 153:1320–1327.

113. Kato, K., Sasak, N., Matsunaga, S. et al. 2006. Possible association of glaucoma with pectinate ligament dysplasia and narrowing of the iridocorneal angle in Shiba Inu dogs in Japan. *Veterinary Ophthalmology* 9:71–75.

114. Wood, J., Lakhani, K., and Read, R. 1998. Pectinate ligament dysplasia and glaucoma in Flat Coated Retrievers. II. Assessment of prevalence and heritability. *Veterinary Ophthalmology* 1:91–99.

115. Bjerkas, E., Ekesten, B., and Farstad, W. 2002. Pectinate ligament dysplasia and narrowing of the iridocorneal angle associated with glaucoma in the English Springer Spaniel. *Veterinary Ophthalmology* 5:49–54.

116. Kato, K., Sasaki, N., Matsunaga, S., Nishimura, R., and Ogawa, H. 2007. Cloning of canine myocilin cDNA and molecular analysis of the *myocilin* gene in Shiba Inu dogs. *Veterinary Ophthalmology* 10:53–62.

117. Lovekin, L., and Bellhorn, R. 1968. Clinicopathologic changes in primary glaucoma in the Cocker Spaniel. *American Journal of Veterinary Research* 29:379–385.

118. Krahenmann, A. 1978. Sekundar-glaukome beim hund. *Schweizer Archiv fur Tierheilkunde* 120:67–80.

119. Gelatt, K.N., and MacKay, E.O. 2004. Secondary glaucomas in the dog in North America. *Veterinary Ophthalmology* 7:245–259.

120. Johnsen, D.A., Maggs, D.J., and Kass, P.H. 2006. Evaluation of risk factors for development of secondary glaucoma in dogs: 156 cases (1999–2004). *Journal of the American Veterinary Medical Association* 229:1270–1274.

121. Wilcock, B., Brooks, D., and Latimer, C. 1991. Glaucoma in horses. *Veterinary Pathology* 28:74–78.

122. Sandberg, C.A., Herring, I.P., Huckle, W.R., LeRoith, T., Pickett, J.P., and Rossmeisl, J.H. 2012. Aqueous humor vascular endothelial growth factor in dogs: Association with intraocular disease and the development of pre-iridal fibrovascular membrane. *Veterinary Ophthalmolmology* 15(Suppl):21–30.

123. Smith, P., Brooks, D., Lazarus, J., Kubilis, P., and Gelatt, K. 1996. Ocular hypertension following cataract surgery in dogs: 139 cases (1922–1993). *Journal of the American Veterinary Medical Association* 209:105–111.

124. Miller, P.E., Stanz, K.M., Dubielzig, R.R., and Murphy, C.J. 1997. Mechanisms of acute intraocular pressure increases after phakoemulsification lens extraction in dogs. *American Journal of Veterinary Research* 58:1159–1165.

125. Biros, D.J., Gelatt, K.N., Brooks, D.E. et al. 2000. Development of glaucoma after cataract surgery in dogs: 220 cases (1987–1998). *Journal of the American Veterinary Medical Association* 216:1780–1786.

126. Lannek, E., and Miller, P. 2001. Development of glaucoma after phakoemulsification for removal of cataracts in dogs: 22 cases (1987–1997). *Journal of the American Veterinary Medical Association* 218:70–76.

127. Sigle, K.J., and Nasisse, M.P. 2006. Long-term complications after phakoemulsification for cataract removal in dogs: 172 cases (1995–2002). *Journal of the American Veterinary Medical Association* 228:74–79.

128. Peiffer, R., Wilcock, B., and Yin, H. 1990. The pathogenesis and significance of pre-iridal fibrovascular membrane in domestic animals. *Veterinary Pathology* 27:41–45.

129. Wilcock, B., Peiffer, R., and Davidson, M. 1990. The causes of glaucoma in cats. *Veterinary Pathology* 27:35–40.

130. Spiess, B., Bolliger, J., Guscetti, F., Haessig, M., Lackner, P., and Ruehli, M. 1998. Multiple ciliary body cysts and secondary glaucoma in the Great Dane: A report of nine cases. *Veterinary Ophthalmology* 1:41–45.

131. Sapienza, J., Domenech, F., and Prades-Sapienza, A. 2000. Golden Retriever uveitis: 75 cases (1994–1999). *Veterinary Ophthalmology* 3:241–246.

132. Deehr, A., and Dubielzig, R. 1998. A histopathological study of iridociliary cysts and glaucoma in Golden Retrievers. *Veterinary Ophthalmology* 1:153–158.

133. Esson, D., Armour, M., Mundy, P. et al. 2009. The histopathological and immunohistochemical characteristics of pigmentary and cystic glaucoma in the Golden Retriever. *Veterinary Ophthalmology* 12:361–368.

134. Townsend, W.M., and Gornik, K.A. 2013. Prevalence of uveal cysts and pigmentary uveitis in Golden Retrievers in three Midwestern states. *Journal of the American Veterinary Medical Association* 243:1298–1301.

135. Covitz, D., Barthold, S., Diter, R., and Riis, R. 1984. Pigmentary glaucoma in the Cairn Terrier. *Proceedings of the Scientific Meeting of the American College of Veterinary Ophthalmologists*, Atlanta, GA, 15:246–250.

136. Petersen-Jones, S. 1991. Abnormal ocular pigment deposition associated with glaucoma in the Cairn Terrier. *Journal of Small Animal Practice* 32:19–22.

137. Peterson-Jones, S.M., Forcier, J., and Mentzer, A.L. 2007. Ocular melanosis in the Cairn Terrier: Clinical description and investigation of the mode of inheritance. *Veterinary Ophthalmology* 10:63–69.

138. Peterson-Jones, S.M., Mentzer, A.L., and Dubielzig, R.R. 2008. Ocular melanosis in the Cairn Terrier: Histopathological description of the condition, and immunohistological and ultrastructural characterization of the characteristic pigment-laden cells. *Veterinary Ophthalmology* 11:260–268.

139. van de Sandt, R., Boeve, M.H., Stades, F.C. et al. 2003. Abnormal ocular pigment deposition and glaucoma in the dog. *Veterinary Ophthalmology* 6:273–278.

140. Walde, I. 1982. Glaukom beim hunde. IV. Mitteilung. *Klenintier Praxis* 27:387–410.

141. Curtis, R., Barnett, K.C., and Lewis, S.J. 1980. Primary lens luxation in the dog. *The Journal of Small Animal Practice* 21:657–668.

142. Curtis, R., Barnett, K.C., and Lewis, S.J. 1983. Clinical and pathologic observations concerning aetiology of primary lens luxation in the dog. *The Veterinary Record* 112:238–246.

143. Ridgway, M., and Brightman, A. 1989. Feline glaucoma: A retrospective study of 29 clinical cases. *Journal of the American Animal Hospital Association* 25:485–490.

144. Blocker, T., and van der Woerdt, A. 2001. The feline glaucomas: 82 cases (1995–1999). *Veterinary Ophthalmology* 4:81–85.

145. Jacobi, S., and Dubielzig, R.R. 2008. Feline primary open angle glaucoma. *Veterinary Ophthalmology* 11:162–165.

146. Hampson, E., Smith, R., and Bernays, M. 2002. Primary glaucoma in Burmese cats. *Australian Veterinary Journal* 80:672–680.

147. McLellan, G.J., Betts, D., Sigle, K. et al. 2004. Congenital glaucoma in the Siamese cat. *Proceedings of the 35th Annual Conference of the American College of Veterinary Ophthalmologists*, Washington, DC, 35:36.

148. McLellan, G.J., and Miller, P.E. 2011. Feline glaucoma—A comprehensive review. *Veterinary Ophthalmology* 14(Suppl. 1):15–29.

149. Trost, K., Peiffer, R.L., and Nell, B. 2007. Goniodysgenesis associated with primary glaucoma in an adult European Short-haired cat. *Veterinary Ophthalmology* 10:3–7.

150. Sapienza, J.S. 2005. Feline lens disorders. *Clinical Techniques in Small Animal Practice* 20:102–107.

151. Czederpiltz, J.M., La Croix, N.C., van der Woerdt, A. et al. 2005. Putative aqueous humor misdirection syndrome as a cause of glaucoma in cats: 32 cases (1997–2003). *Journal of the American Veterinary Medical Association* 227:1434–1431.

152. Miller, T.R., Brooks, D.E., Gelatt, K.N. et al. 1995. Equine glaucoma: Clinical findings and response to treatment in 14 horses. *Veterinary and Comparative Ophthalmology* 5:170–182.

153. Gelatt, K.N. 1973. Glaucoma and lens luxation in a foal. *Veterinary Medicine/ Small Animal Clinician* 68:261–266.

154. Barnett, K.C., Cottrell, B.D., Paterson, B.W. et al. 1988. Buphthalmos in a Thoroughbred foal. *Equine Veterinary Journal* 20:132–135.

155. Halenda, R.M., Grahn, B.H., Sorden, S.D. et al. 1997. Congenital Equine Glaucoma: Clinical and light microscopic findings in two cases. *Veterinary and Comparative Ophthalmology* 7:105–116.

156. Utter, M.E., and Brooks, D.E. 2011. Glaucoma. In: Gilger, B.C., editor. *Equine Ophthalmology*, 2nd edition. Elsevier Saunders: Maryland Heights, MO, pp. 350–366.

157. Gilger, B.C. 2013. Equine ophthalmology. In: Gelatt, K.N., editor. *Veterinary Ophthalmology*, 5th edition. Wiley-Blackwell: Ames, IA, pp. 1560–1609.

158. Pickett, J.P., and Ryan, J. 1993. Equine glaucoma: A retrospective study of 11 cases from 1988 to 1993. *Veterinary Medicine* 9:756–763.

159. Wilcock, B., and Wolfer, J. 1991. Neovascular glaucoma in five horses. *Proceedings of the Scientific Meeting of the American College of Veterinary Ophthalmologists*, Boston, MA, 22:29–36.

160. van der Woerdt, A., Gilger, B., Wilkie, D., and Strauch, M. 1995. Effect of auriculopalpebral nerve block and intravenous administration of xylazine on intraocular pressure and corneal thickness in horses. *American Journal of Veterinary Research* 56:155–158.

161. McClure, J.R., Gelatt, K.N., Gum, G.G. et al. 1976. The effect of parenteral acepromazine and xylazine on intraocular pressure in the horse. *Veterinary Medicine/Small Animal Clinician* 71:1727–1730.

162. Hayreh, S., and Weingeist, T. 1980. Experimental occlusion of the central artery of the retina. IV. Retinal tolerance time to acute ischaemia. *British Journal of Ophthalmology* 64:818–825.

163. Clines, J., Marrion, R., Ring, R., Stuhr, C.H., Covitz, D., and Roldan, R. 1999. A retrospective study evaluating the prognosis for intraocular pressure reduction and restoration or maintenance of vision following treatment for the acute onset of primary glaucoma in the canine patient. *Proceedings of the Scientific Meeting of the American College of Veterinary Ophthalmologists*, Chicago, IL, 30:58.

164. Skorobohach, B., Ward, D., and Hendrix, D. 2003. Effects of oral administration of methazolamide on intraocular pressure and aqueous humor flow rate in clinically normal dogs. *American Journal of Veterinary Research* 64:183–187.

165. Haskins, S., Munger, R., Helphrey, M. et al. 1981. Effect of acetazolamide on blood acid–base and electrolyte values in dogs. *Journal of the American Veterinary Medical Association* 179:792–796.

166. Miller, P.E., Bentley, E., Diehl, K.A., and Carter, R. 2003. High resolution ultrasound imaging of the anterior segment of dogs with primary glaucoma prior to and following the topical application of 0.005% latanoprost.

Proceedings of the Scientific Meeting of the American College of Veterinary Ophthalmologists, Coeur D' Alene, ID, 34:76.

167. Ward, D.A. 2005. Effects of latanoprost on aqueous humor flow rate in normal dogs. *Proceedings of the Scientific Meeting of the American College of Veterinary Ophthalmologists*, Nashville, TN, 36:15.

168. Studer, M., Martin, C., and Stiles, J. 2000. The effect of latanoprost 0.005% solution on intraocular pressure in healthy dogs and cats. *American Journal of Veterinary Research* 61:1220–1224.

169. McLellan, G.J., and Miller, P.E. 2011. Feline glaucoma—A comprehensive review. *Veterinary Ophthalmology* 14:15–29.

170. Willis, M., Diehl, K., Hoshaw-Woodard, S., Kobayashi, I., Vitucci, M., and Schmall, M. 2001. Effects of topical administration of 0.005% latanoprost solution on eyes of clinically normal horses. *American Journal of Veterinary Research* 62:1945–1951.

171. Ofri, R., and Narfstrom, K. 2007. Light at the end of the tunnel? Advances in understanding and treatment of glaucoma and inherited retinal degeneration. *Veterinary Journal* 174:10–22.

172. Danesch-Meyer, H.V. 2011. Neuroprotection in glaucoma: Recent and future directions. *Current Opinion in Ophthalmology* 22:78–86.

173. Whitley, R., Gelatt, K., and Gum, G. 1980. Dose response to topical pilocarpine in the normotensive and glaucomatous Beagle. *American Journal of Veterinary Research* 41:417–424.

174. Gelatt, K., Gum, G., Brooks, D., Wolf, D., and Bromberg, N. 1983. Dose response of topical pilocarpine–epinephrine combinations in normotensive and glaucomatous Beagles. *American Journal of Veterinary Research* 44:2018–2027.

175. Gelatt, K., Gum, G., Wolf, D., and White, M. 1984. Dose response of topical carbamylcholine chloride (carbachol) in normotensive and early glaucomatous Beagles. *American Journal of Veterinary Research* 45:547–554.

176. Gelatt, K.N., Larocca, R.D., Gelatt, J.K., Strubbe, T., and MacKay, E. 1995. Evaluation of multiple doses of 4% and 6% timolol, and timolol combined with 2% pilocarpine in clinically normal Beagles and Beagles with glaucoma. *American Journal of Veterinary Research* 56:1325–1331.

177. Roberts, S., Severin, G., and Lavach, J. 1984. Cyclocryotherapy. II. Clinical comparison of liquid nitrogen and nitrous oxide cryotherapy on glaucomatous eyes. *Journal of the American Animal Hospital Association* 20:828–833.

178. Stades, F., and Boevé, M. 1986. Methods, techniques, and results of glaucoma therapy in the dog and cat. *Proceedings of the Scientific Meeting of the American College of Veterinary Ophthalmologists and International Society of Veterinary Ophthalmology*, New Orleans, LA, 17:183–194.

179. Rainbow, M.E., and Dziezyc, J. 2003. Effects of twice daily application of 2% dorzolamide on intraocular pressure in normal cats. *Veterinary Ophthalmology* 6:147–150.

180. Dietrich, U.M., Chandler, M.J., Cooper, T. et al. 2007. Effects of topical 2% dorzolamide hydrochloride alone and in combination with 0.5% timolol maleate on intraocular pressure in normal feline eyes. *Veterinary Ophthalmology* 10:95–100.

181. Bartoe, J.T., Davidson, H.J., Horton, M.T. et al. 2005. The effects of bimatoprost and unoprostone isopropyl

on the intraocular pressure of normal cats. *Veterinary Ophthalmology* 8:247–252.

182. van der Woerdt, A., Wilke, D.A., Gilger, B.C. et al. 2000. Effects of single- and multiple-dose 0.5% timolol maleate on intraocular pressure and pupil size in female horses. *Veterinary Ophthalmology* 3:165–168.

183. Willis, A.M., Robbin, T.E., Hoshaw-Woodward, S. et al. 2001. Effect of topical administration of 2% dorzolamide hydrochloride or 2% dorzolamide hydrochloride-0.5% timolol maleate on intraocular pressure in clinically normal horses. *American Journal of Veterinary Research* 62:709–713.

184. Germann, S.E., Matheis, F.L., Rampazzo, A. et al. 2008. Effects of topical administration of 1% brinzolamide on intraocular pressure in clinically normal horses. *Equine Veterinary Journal* 40:662–665.

185. Mughannam, A.J., Buyukmihci, N.C., and Kass, P.H. 1999. Effect of topical atropine on intraocular pressure and pupil diameter in the normal horse eye. *Veterinary Ophthalmology* 2:213–215.

186. Herring, I.P., Pickett, J.P., and Champagne, E.S. 2000. Effect of topical 1% atropine on intraocular pressure in normal horses. *Veterinary Ophthalmology* 3:139–143.

187. Bedford, P. 1977. The surgical treatment of canine glaucoma. *Journal of Small Animal Practice* 18:713–730.

188. Peiffer, R., Gwin, R., Gelatt, K., and Schenk, M. 1977. Combined posterior sclerectomy, cyclodialysis, and trans-scleral iridencleisis in the management of primary glaucoma. *Canadian Practice* 4:54–61.

189. Wheeler, C.A. 1985. A new angle on glaucoma filter procedures: Preoperative subconjunctival injection of triamcinolone. *Transactions of the Sixteenth Annual Scientific Program of the American College of Veterinary Ophthalmologists*, San Francisco, CA, 16:110–116.

190. Law, S., Kalenak, J., Connor, T., Pulido, J., Han, D., and Mieller, W. 1996. Retinal complications after aqueous shunt surgical procedures for glaucoma. *Archives of Ophthalmology* 114:1473–1480.

191. Vestre, W., and Brightman, A. 1983. Ciliary body temperatures during cyclocryotherapy in the clinically normal dog. *American Journal of Veterinary Research* 44:135–143.

192. Vestre, W., and Brightman, A. 1983. Effects of cyclocryosurgery on the clinically normal canine eye. *American Journal of Veterinary Research* 44:187–194.

193. Higginbotham, E., Lee, D., Bartels, S., Richardson, T., and Miller, M. 1988. Effects of cyclocryotherapy on aqueous humor dynamic in cats. *Archives of Ophthalmology* 106:396–403.

194. Roberts, S., Severin, G., and Lavach, J. 1984. Cyclocryotherapy. I. Evaluation of a liquid nitrogen system. *Journal of the American Animal Hospital Association* 20:823–827.

195. Vainisi, S., and Schmidt, G. 1986. Retrospective survey of cyclocryosurgery for the control of canine glaucoma. *Proceedings of the Scientific Meeting of the American College of Veterinary Ophthalmologists and International Society of Veterinary Ophthalmology*, New Orleans, LA, 17:194–201.

196. Nasisse, M., Davidson, M., and English, R. 1990. Treatment of glaucoma by use of trans-scleral neodymium:yttrium aluminum laser cyclocoagulation in dogs. *Journal of the American Veterinary Medical Association* 197:350–354.

197. Cook, C., Davidson, M., Brinkmann, M., Priehs, D., Abrams, K., and Nasisse, M. 1997. Diode laser trans-scleral cyclophotocoagulation for the treatment of glaucoma in dogs: Results of six and twelve month follow up. *Veterinary and Comparative Ophthalmology* 7:148–154.

198. Whicham, H.M., Brooks, D.E., Andrew, S.E., Gelatt, K.N., Strubbe, T., and Biros, D.J. 1999. Treatment of equine glaucoma by trans-scleral neodymium:yttrium aluminum garnet laser cyclophotocoagulation: A retrospective study of 23 eyes of 16 horses. *Veterinary Ophthalmology* 2:243–250.

199. Rosenberg, L.F., Karalekas, D.P., Krupin, T., and Hyderi, A. 1996. Cyclocryotherapy and noncontact Nd:YAG laser cyclophotocoagulation in cats. *Investigative Ophthalmology and Visual Science* 37:2029–2036.

200. Nasisse, M., Davidson, M., and MacLachlan, J. 1988. Neodymium:yttrium, aluminum, and garnet laser energy delivered trans-sclerally to the ciliary body of dogs. *American Journal of Veterinary Research* 49:1972–1978.

201. Schuman, J., and Puliafito, C. 1990. Laser cyclophotocoagulation. *International Ophthalmology Clinics* 30:111–119.

202. Sapienza, J.S., Miller, T.R., Gum, G.G., and Gelatt, K.N. 1992. Contact trans-scleral cyclophotocoagulation using a neodymium:yttrium aluminum garnet laser in normal dogs. *Progress in Veterinary and Comparative Ophthalmology* 2:147–153.

203. Quinn, R., Parkinson, K., Wilcock, B., and Tingey, D. 1996. The effects of continuous wave Nd:YAG and semiconductor diode laser energy on the canine ciliary body: *In vitro* thermographic analysis. *Veterinary and Comparative Ophthalmology* 6:45–50.

204. Nadelstein, B., Wilcock, B., Cook, C., and Davidson, M. 1997. Clinical and histopathologic effects of diode laser trans-scleral cyclophotocoagulation in the normal canine eye. *Veterinary and Comparative Ophthalmology* 7:155–162.

205. Cantor, L., Nichols, D., and Katz, J. 1989. Neodymium-YAG trans-scleral cyclophotocoagulation: The role of pigmentation. *Investigative Ophthalmology and Visual Science* 30:1834–1837.

206. Schubert, H., and Federman, J. 1989. A comparison of CW Nd:YAG contact trans-scleral cyclophotocoagulation with cyclocryopexy. *Investigative Ophthalmology and Visual Science* 30:536–542.

207. Brancato, R., Leoni, G., Trabucchi, G., and Cappellini, A. 1991. Histopathology of continuous wave neodymium:yttrium aluminum garnet and diode laser contact trans-scleral lesions in rabbit ciliary body. *Investigative Ophthalmology and Visual Science* 32:1586–1592.

208. Echelman, D.A., Nasisse, M.P., Shields, B., McGahan, M.C., and Fleisher, L.N. 1994. Influence of exposure time on inflammatory response to Neodymium: YAG cyclophotocoagulation. *Archives of Ophthalmology* 112:977–981.

209. Weigt, A.K., Herring, I.P., Marfurt, C.F., Pickett, J.P. et al. 2002. Effects of cyclophotocoagulation with a Nd:YAG laser on corneal sensitivity, intraocular pressure, aqueous tear production, and corneal nerve morphology in eyes of dogs. *American Journal of Veterinary Research* 63:906–915.

210. Bentley, E., Miller, P.E., Murphy, C.J., and Schoster, J.V. 1999. Combined cycloablation and gonioimplantation for treatment of glaucoma in dogs: 18 cases (1992–1998). *Journal of the American Veterinary Medical Association* 215:1469–1472.

211. Sapiena, J.S., and van der Woerdt, A. 2005. Combined trans-scleral diode laser cyclophotocoagulation and Ahmed gonioimplantation in dogs with primary glaucoma: 51 cases (1996-2004). *Veterinary Ophthalmology* 8:121–127.

212. Bras, I.D., Robbin, T.E., Wyman, M. et al. 2005. Diode endoscopic cyclophotocoagulation in canine and feline glaucoma (abstract). *Proceedings Notes of the 36th Annual Conference of the American college of Veterinary ophthalmologists*, Nashville, TN, 36: 50.

213. Miller, T., Willis, M., Wilkie, D., Hoshaw-Woodard, S., and Stanley, J. 2001. Description of ciliary body anatomy and identification of sites for trans-scleral cyclophotocoagulation in the equine eye. *Veterinary Ophthalmology* 4:183–190.

214. Annear, M.J., Wilkie, D.A., and Gemensky-Metzler, A.J. 2010. Semi-conductor diode laser trans-scleral cyclophotocoagulation for the treatment of glaucoma in horses: A retrospective study of 42 eyes. *Veterinary Ophthalmology* 13:204–209.

215. Pritchard, D., and Hamlet, M. 1970. A silastic-dacron implant for the treatment of glaucoma. *Veterinary Medicine/ Small Animal Clinician* 65:1191–1194.

216. Gelatt, K., Gum, G., Samuelson, D., Mandelkorn, R., Olander, K., and Zimmerman, T. 1987. Evaluation of the Krupin-Denver valve implant in normotensive and glaucomatous Beagles. *Journal of the American Veterinary Medical Association* 11:1404–1409.

217. Peiffer, R., Popovich, K., and Nichols, D. 1990. Long-term comparative study of the Schocket and Joseph glaucoma tube shunts in monkeys. *Ophthalmic Surgery* 21:55–59.

218. Bedford, P. 1989. A clinical evaluation of a one-piece drainage system in the treatment of canine glaucoma. *Journal of Small Animal Practice* 30:68–75.

219. Bentley, E., Nasisse, M., Glover, T., and Nelms, S. 1996. Implantation of filtering devices in dogs with glaucoma: Preliminary results in 13 eyes. *Veterinary and Comparative Ophthalmology* 6:243–246.

220. Lim, K.S., Allan, B.D.S., Lloyd, A.W., Muir, A., and Khaw, P.T. 1998. Glaucoma drainage devices: Past, present and future. *British Journal of Ophthalmology* 82:1083–1089.

221. Lavin, M., Franks, W., Wormald, R., and Hitchings, R. 1992. Clinical risk factors for failure in glaucoma tube surgery. *Archives of Ophthalmology* 110:480–485.

222. Westermeyer, H.D., Hendrix, D.V.H., and Ward, D.A. 2011. Long-term evaluation of the use of Ahmed gonioimplants in dogs with glaucoma: Nine cases (2000–2008). *Journal of the American Veterinary Medical Association* 238:610–617.

223. Garcia, G.A., Brooks, D.E., Gelatt, K.N. et al. 1998. Evaluation of valved and non-valved gonioimplants in 83 eyes of 65 dogs with glaucoma. *Animal Eye Research* 17:9–16.

224. Herschler, J., Claflin, A., and Fiorentino, G. 1980. The effect of aqueous humor on the growth of subconjunctival fibroblasts in tissue culture and its implications for glaucoma surgery. *American Journal of Ophthalmology* 89:245–249.

225. Tinsley, D., Niyo, Y., Tinsley, L., and Betts, D. 1995. *In vitro* evaluation of the effects of 5-fluorouracil and mitomycin-C on canine subconjunctival and subtenon's fibroblasts. *Veterinary and Comparative Ophthalmology* 5:218–230.

226. Tinsley, D., Niyo, Y., Tinsley, L., and Betts, D. 1995. *In vivo* clinical trial of perioperative mitomycin C in combination with a drainage device implantation in normal canine globes. *Veterinary and Comparative Ophthalmology* 5:231–241.

227. Raffan, P.J. 1990. A method of surgical correction of glaucoma in a dog. *Journal of Small Animal Practice* 31:305–308.

228. Hakanson, N.W. 1996. Extraorbital diversion of aqueous in the treatment of glaucoma in the dog. *Veterinary and Comparative Ophthalmology* 6:82–90.

229. Cullen, C.L., Allen, A.L., and Grahn, B.H. 1998. Anterior chamber to frontal sinus shunt for the diversion of aqueous humor: A pilot study in four normal dogs. *Veterinary Ophthalmology* 1:31–39.

230. Lazarus, J.A., Pickett, J.P., and Champagne, E.S. 1998. Primary lens luxation in the Chinese Sharpei: Clinical and hereditary characteristics. *Veterinary Ophthalmology*, 1:101–107.

231. Binder, D.R., Herring, I.P., and Gerhard, T. 2007. Outcomes of nonsurgical management and efficacy of demecarium bromide treatment for primary lens instability in dogs: 34 cases (1990-2004). *Journal of the American Veterinary Medical Association* 231:89–93.

232. Nasisse, M., van Ee, R., Munger, R., and Davidson, M. 1988. Use of methyl methacrylate orbital prosthesis in dogs and cats: 78 cases (1980–1986). *Journal of the American Veterinary Medical Association* 192:539–542.

233. Provost, P., Ortenburger, A., and Caron, J. 1989. Silicone ocular prosthesis in horses: 11 cases (1983–1987). *Journal of the American Veterinary Medical Association* 194:1764–1766.

234. Brightman, A., Magrane, W., Huff, R., and Helper, L. 1977. Intraocular prosthesis in the dog. *Journal of the American Animal Hospital Association* 13:481–485.

235. McLaughlin, S., Render, J., Brightman, A., Whiteley, H., Helper, L., and Shadduck, J. 1987. Intraocular findings in three dogs and one cat with chronic glaucoma. *Journal of the American Veterinary Medical Association* 191:1443–1445.

236. McLaughlin, S., Ramsey, D., Lindley, D., Gilger, B., Gerding, P., and Whitley, R. 1995. Intraocular silicone prosthesis implantation in eyes of dogs and a cat with intraocular neoplasia: Nine cases (1983–1994). *Journal of the American Veterinary Medical Association* 207:1441–1443.

237. Pena, M., Luera, M., and Garcia, F. 1997. A new type of intraocular prosthesis for dogs. *Veterinary Record* 146:67–68.

238. Vainisi, S., and Schmidt, G. 1983. Intraocular gentamicin for the control of endophthalmitis and glaucoma in animals. *Proceedings of the Scientific Meeting of the American College of Veterinary Ophthalmologists*, Chicago, IL, 14:134.

239. Moller, I., Cook, C.S., Peiffer, R.L. Jr., Nasisse, M.P., and Harling, D.E. 1986. Indications for, and complications of, pharmacologic ablation of the ciliary body for the treatment of chronic glaucoma in the dog. *Journal of the American Animal Hospital Association* 22:319–326.

240. Spiess, B. 1986. Erfahrungen mit einer neuen methode zur behandlung des absoluten glaukoms beim hund und bei der katze. *Schweizer Archiv fur Tierheilkunde* 128:469–473.

241. Bingaman, D., Lindley, D., Glickman, N., Krohne, S., and Bryan, G. 1994. Intraocular gentamicin and glaucoma: A retrospective study of 60 dog and cat eyes. *Veterinary and Comparative Ophthalmology* 4:113–119.

242. Duke, F.D., Strong, T.D., Bentley, E., and Dubielzig, R.R. 2013. Feline ocular tumors involving ciliary body ablation with intravitreal gentamicin. *Veterinary Ophthalmology* 16s1:188–190.

243. Peiffer, R., and Harling, D. 1998. Intravitreal cidofovir (Vistide) in the management of glaucoma in the dog and cat. *Proceedings of the Scientific Meeting of the American College of Veterinary Ophthalmologists*, Seattle, WA, 29:29.

244. Low, M.C., Landis, M.L., and Peiffer, R.L. 2014. Intravitreal cidofovir injection for the management of chronic glaucoma in dogs. *Veterinary Ophthalmology* 17:201–206.

245. Strom, A.R., Hassig, M., Iburg, T.M., and Spiess, B.M. 2011. Epidemiology of canine glaucoma presented to University of Zurich from 1995 to 2009. Part 1: Congenital and primary glaucoma (4 and 123 cases). *Veterinary Ophthalmology* 14:121–126.

246. Dees, D.D., Fritz, K.J., MacLaren, N.E. et al. 2013. Efficacy of prophylactic antiglaucoma and antiinflammatory medications in canine primary angle-closure glaucoma: A multicenter retrospective study (2004–2012). *Veterinary Ophthalmology* 17:195–200.

247. Lutjen-Drecoll, E., and Kaufman, P.L. 1979. Echothiophate-induced structural alterations in the anterior chamber angle of the Cynomolgus monkey. *Investigative Ophthalmology and Visual Science* 18:918–929.

LENS

KATE MYRNA

ANATOMY AND PHYSIOLOGY

Introduction

The lens is a biconvex clear structure located behind the iris in the patellar fossa of the anterior vitreous. It is held in place by the zonules or the tertiary vitreous. While the lens is not the major refractive medium of the eye, its ability to vary in refractive power with accommodation makes it unique. The lens is also unique in its transparency, high protein content, high carbonic anhydrase (CA) levels, high glutathione levels, and lack of vascularity and innervation.[1,2] The lens depends on the aqueous humor and the vitreous for nutrition and elimination of waste products. The lens is composed of the lens capsule, lens epithelium, and lens fibers, with very minimal intercellular constituents. In the dog, the lens is about 10.5 mm in diameter and 7.5 mm in axial thickness, in the cat is 9–10.4 mm in diameter and 7.5 mm in axial thickness, and in the horse is 21 mm in diameter and 12.75 mm in axial thickness.[3]

Embryology and anatomy

The lens develops from a plate of surface ectoderm, the lens placode, that is formed by gestational day 15 in the dog. The lens placode invaginates to form a pit and later forms a vesicle (gestational day 19) that migrates into the optic vesicle (gestational day 25). The periphery of the original lens vesicle is lined with epithelium, but the cells from the posterior surface elongate and fill the vesicle (gestational day 30) and are called the primary lens fibers (**Figure 13.1**).[4] The primary lens fibers later lose their nuclei and form the embryonic nucleus in the adult. The original cells that line the vesicle produce the "elastic" basal lamina, or lens capsule, by 35 days of gestation. After the elongation of the primary lens fibers, the epithelium is present only under the anterior half of the lens capsule, as in the adult. The presence of epithelium under the anterior capsule is responsible for the continuing development of the anterior and equatorial capsule, resulting in thicknesses of 40–50 μm at the anterior pole and 3–5 μm at the posterior pole.[5] The anterior capsule is the thickest basal lamina in the body.[2] The cuboidal cells lining the anterior capsular region migrate to the equator, become more columnar, and they form fibers anteriorly and posteriorly that reach toward the opposite equator. Where the fibers from opposite cells abut each other, a suture line or pattern is created that is clinically visible (**Figure 13.2**). Typically, this is an upright "Y" in the anterior lens and an inverted "Y" in the posterior lens, although more complex branching patterns are not uncommon. The lens fibers are hexagonal in cross section and interdigitate snugly. In addition, they attach to adjacent fibers by ball and socket junctions and surface convolutions (**Figure 13.3**).[6,7]

The lens continues to form new fibers throughout most of an animal's life. The region of most recent lens fiber formation is immediately under the capsule and is termed the cortex. Cell nuclei, which have been pushed inward from the equator, form an arc that bends anteriorly, the lens bow (**Figure 13.4**). Older fibers are pushed and compacted toward the middle, and this region is called the nucleus. The nucleus is often subdivided into chronological stages such as embryonal, fetal, and adult (**Figure 13.4**).[8,9]

The various regions of the lens can be seen clinically as "zones of optical discontinuity" with a slit lamp or a focal beam of light as the beam passes through the lens (**Figure 13.5**). The continued growth increases the size of the lens with age, but rather than filling the eye, it becomes more compact, causing a loss of elasticity with age and an increase in light scattering.

The embryonic lens is surrounded by a vascular tunic, the tunica vasculosa lentis, that develops posteriorly from the anterior extension of the hyaloid artery and anteriorly from the vascular network of the pupillary membrane (**Figure 13.6**). The hyaloid artery begins to atrophy by 45 days of gestation, but remains of the tunic are normally seen until 14+ days postpartum in the dog.[4]

The lens is held in place by zonules that attach at and adjacent to the equator (**Figures 13.7 and 13.8**). The zonules are collagenous fibrils that arise from the pars plana of the ciliary body.[10] Helmholtz's theory of accommodation states that the zonules are under tension when the ciliary muscles are in a relaxed state; with contraction of the ciliary muscles, the zonular tension is relaxed, and the lens capsule molds the lens into a more spherical

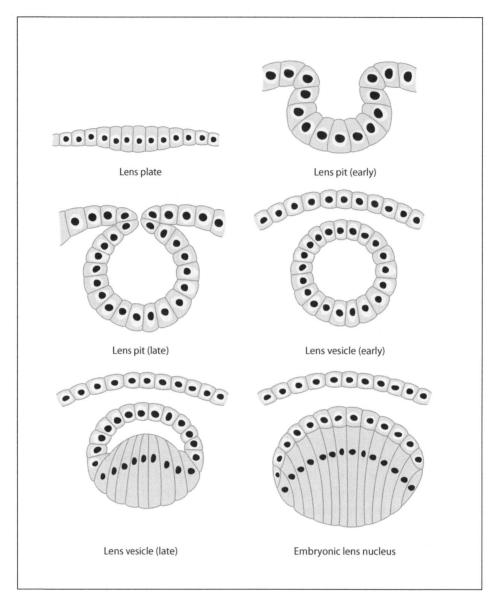

Lens plate

Lens pit (early)

Lens pit (late)

Lens vesicle (early)

Lens vesicle (late)

Embryonic lens nucleus

Figure 13.1 Stages of embryonic lens development. (From Hamming, N.A., and Apple, D. 1980. In: *Principles and Practice of Ophthalmology* Vol. 1. G. Peyman, D. Sanders, M. Goldberg, editors. WB Saunders: Philadelphia, p. 9.)

structure or a stronger converging lens.[11] This process is termed accommodation. It is very limited in domestic animals, being generally about 2–3 D (young humans, 15 D; >40 years, only 2–3 D),[12] and 1 D in the horse.[13,14]

Physiology and biochemistry

The lens is composed of 65% water and 34% protein, the latter concentration being higher than in any other tissue in the body.[1] It also contains a higher concentration of glutathione than any other tissue. Because the lens is walled off by the capsule early in embryonic development, the proteins are sequestered from the body's immunologic surveillance system. This may result in immune-mediated inflammation against the lens proteins if the capsule is ruptured or the proteins "leak out." This traditional

explanation of lens-induced inflammation is being questioned with an alternative hypothesis: Massive exposure of proteins of the lens overwhelms the suppressor T-cells that normally prevent inflammatory reactions to lens proteins.[15]

Metabolism of the lens is mainly by anaerobic glycolysis, of which the first enzyme, hexokinase, is present in limited amounts and is the rate-limiting factor (**Figure 13.9**). Only about 3% of glucose is metabolized aerobically via the Krebs cycle, but it accounts for 25% of the energy produced, and 90% of the energy is used for active transport. While anaerobic metabolism can occur throughout the lens, the TCA cycle is limited to the epithelium. The hexose monophosphate shunt and the sorbitol pathway are also operative in the lens but do not generate significant amounts of energy (**Figure 13.9**).[1]

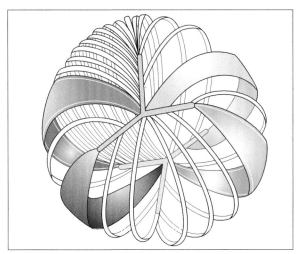

Figure 13.2 Origin of lens sutures from abutment of lens fibers that do not extend across the entire diameter of the lens. (Adapted from Hogan, M., Alvarado, J., and Weddell, J. 1971. *Histology of the Human Eye*. WB Saunders: Philadelphia.)

The lens actively accumulates amino acids, potassium, taurine, and inositol and actively extrudes sodium. A Na/K-ATPase-activated pump results in the lens being low in sodium and high in potassium.[1] Lens clarity is dependent on minimal intercellular water and the tight regular packing of the lens fibers.

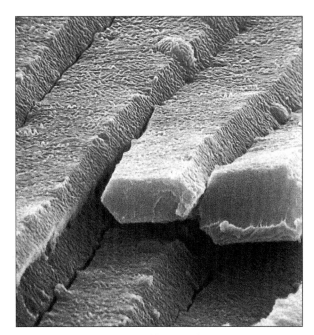

Figure 13.3 Cortical lens fibers of the dog as seen on sagittal section. Note the hexagonal cross section, surface convolutions, and the ball and socket joint along the edges of the fibers (SEM ×4,212). (From Martin, C.L., and Anderson, R.S. 1981. In: Gelatt, K., editor. *Textbook of Veterinary Ophthalmology*. Lea & Febiger: Philadelphia, PA, pp. 12–121.)

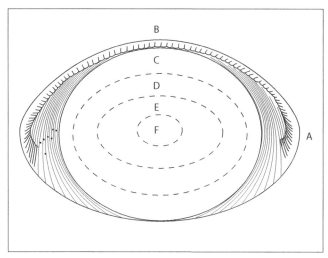

Figure 13.4 Illustration of an adult dog lens with lens bow (A) and various zones. Note the anterior capsule (B) is thicker than the posterior capsule, and the epithelium is only under the anterior capsule. (C: Anterior cortex; D: Anterior adult nucleus; E: Anterior fetal nucleus; F: Embryonal nucleus.) (From Martin, C.L., and Anderson, R.S. 1981. In: Gelatt, K., editor. *Textbook of Veterinary Ophthalmology*. Lea & Febiger: Philadelphia, PA, pp. 12–121.)

Nuclear sclerosis refers to the normal aging changes that occur in the lens and does not result in any appreciable loss of vision, although dogs >10 years old often do not like navigating stairs in reduced light. The continued growth of the lens results in compacting of the lens center and, in combination with biochemical protein changes,

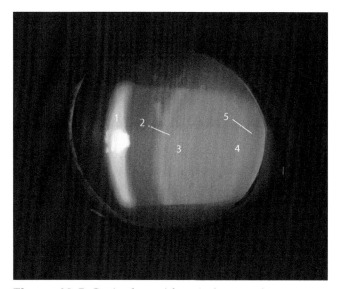

Figure 13.5 Canine lens with optical zones of discontinuity viewed with a slit lamp. The fetal nucleus is not viewed because the beam is off center. (1: Cornea; 2: Anterior cortex; 3: Anterior nucleus; 4: Posterior nucleus; 5: Posterior cortex.)

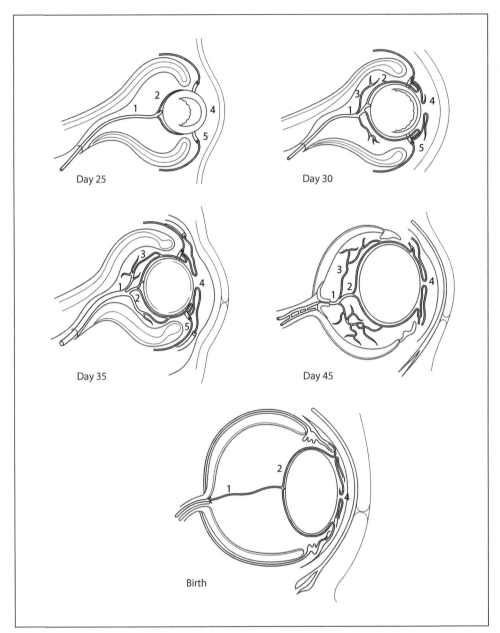

Figure 13.6 The embryonic vascular system of the dog eye at different stages of fetal life. (1: Hyaloid artery; 2: Tunica vasculosa lentis; 3: Vasa hyaloidea propria; 4: Pupillary membrane; 5: Annular vessel.) (From Stades, F. 1983. Utrecht, p. 12.)

produces a noticeable increase in reflection of light. This appears clinically as a very hazy lens or what many owners interpret as a "cataract" in the old animal. While the light is scattered, it is not blocked appreciably, and vision is not lost. On pupil dilation, the central nucleus appears as a lens within the cortex (**Figures 13.10 and 13.11**). Nuclear sclerosis begins to manifest at about 7 years of age in the dog and 15 years in the horse.[16] With experience, the lens density can be used to age an animal as easily and accurately as dental examination. Utilizing a standard for lens transparency and size of specular reflections (Purkinje–Sanson images), a complicated formula was developed to predict the age of dogs and cats.[17]

Nuclear sclerosis is not a senile cataract, does not produce blindness, and is best differentiated from a cataract by examination *after* pupillary dilation.

DISEASES OF THE LENS

Pathological changes in the lens, which are limited in type, are discussed under the following headings: Absence, abnormal size, abnormal shape, opacity, and displacement.

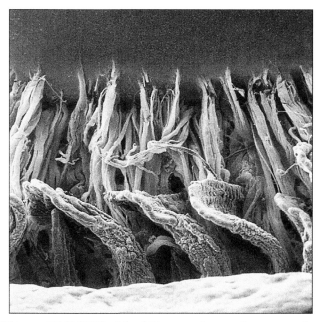

Figure 13.7 SEM of the feline zonular attachments to the lens equator, viewed from the vitreous side. Note how the zonules pass between the ciliary processes and attach both anteriorly and posteriorly to the lens equator (×20).

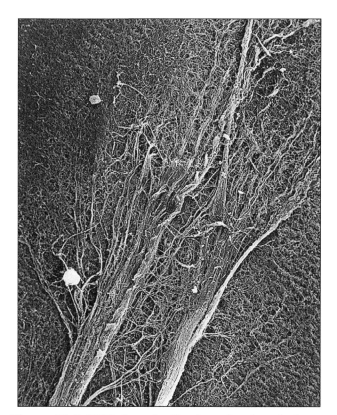

Figure 13.8 SEM of zonular fiber insertions into the lens capsule of a dog. Note how the attachment surface area is increased by the "unraveling" of the larger fibers into the component fibrils (×400). (From Martin, C.L., and Anderson, R.S. 1981. In: Gelatt, K., editor. *Textbook of Veterinary Ophthalmology.* Lea & Febiger: Philadelphia, PA, pp. 12–121.)

Congenital diseases of the lens
Aphakia

Aphakia is a congenital absence of the lens. It is very rare and probably only occurs with multiple ocular anomalies. Primary aphakia is a developmental lack of lens tissue and is associated with severe ocular malformations. The lens plays a critical role in inducing the development of the cornea and the vitreous, and the absence of the lens results in retinal folds and microphthalmos.[18] Secondary aphakia refers to degeneration and resorption or expulsion of the lens from the eye and may not be accompanied by severe ocular anomalies. Microphthalmos, aphakia, acoria, anterior chamber dysgenesis, and retinal dysplasia and detachment have been described in St. Bernards (**Figure 13.12**) and Doberman pinschers and are thought to be inherited.[19–21] Aphakia has also been described with multiple ocular anomalies in a colt, but the genetics are unknown.[22] Primary aphakia may not be diagnosed until histopathologic examination because of ocular anomalies such as absence of the pupil and corneal opacities that obscure examination of the lens region. There is no therapy for aphakia, and owners should be advised about possible inheritance.

Microphakia

Microphakia (a small lens) is not uncommon and may be associated with future dislocation of the lens.[23,24] This abnormality may occur in a normal globe or be associated with a proportional decrease in globe size (microphthalmos); it may also be associated with spherophakia (a round lens). Microphthalmos has been suggested to be a dominant inherited trait in the beagle[25] and is more commonly seen in dogs than in cats. Microphakia may be associated with spherophakia. Most of the reported cases of microphakia in cats have been reported in the Siamese.[26,27]

Microphakia is recognized easily by observing the lens equator when the pupil is dilated. In the cat, elongated ciliary processes that attach to the lens are present. Accompanying lens displacement is common.[23,26] No therapy is necessary unless the lens is luxated or subluxated (**Figures 13.13 and 13.14**) (see section Displaced lens).

Coloboma
Introduction/etiology

A coloboma of the lens is manifested as an equatorial defect or a flattening of the lens and is uncommon. Lens coloboma may be associated with iris coloboma or, if isolated, may be occult due to its peripheral location, or it may be observed incidentally when the pupil is dilated. The lens coloboma may be secondary to a coloboma of the zonules in that area and a resultant lack of tension on the lens equator.[24]

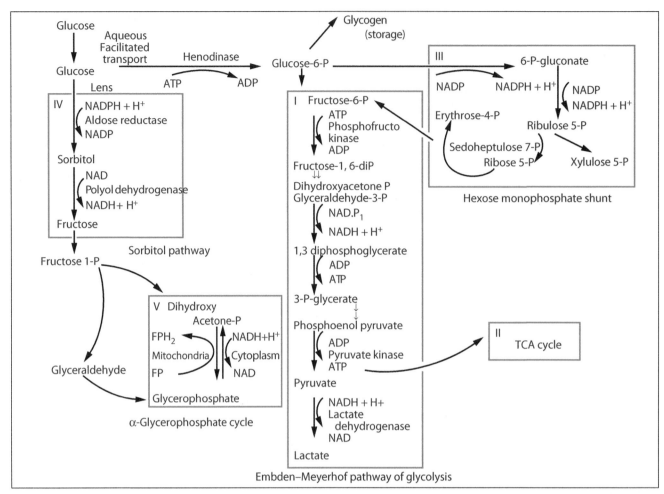

Figure 13.9 Pathways of sugar metabolism in the lens. The Roman numerals indicate the importance of the respective pathways, with I being the most important. (From Jose, J. 1983. In: Anderson, R., editor. *Biochemistry of the Eye*. American Academy of Ophthalmology: San Francisco, CA, pp. 111–144.)

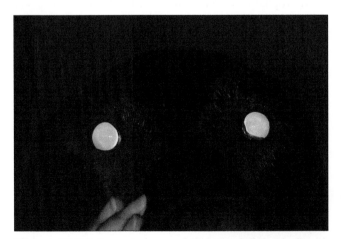

Figure 13.10 Lens structures highlighted through the technique of retroillumination. Both eyes have nuclear sclerosis and bright consistent tapetal reflections.

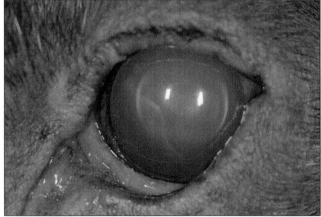

Figure 13.11 Nuclear sclerosis in a dog when viewed against the tapetal reflection and a dilated pupil. Note the "lens within the lens" appearance.

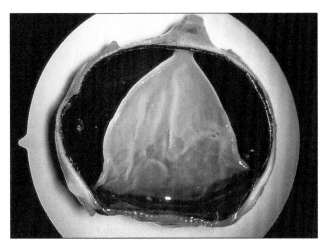

Figure 13.12 Central calotte of a buphthalmic globe from a St. Bernard puppy with bilateral aphakia and acoria. Note the retinal detachment and no lens behind the iris.

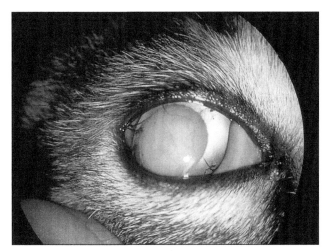

Figure 13.13 Young cat with bilateral microphakia and anterior luxation. Note the few remaining anomalous zonules and the corneal neovascularization from the lens contact.

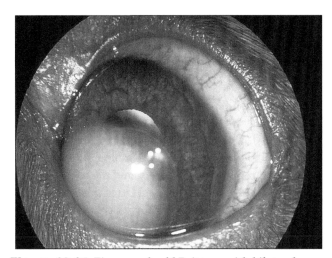

Figure 13.14 Five-month-old Brittany with bilateral anterior luxations associated with microphakia. Note the small clear lens behind the corneal edema.

Clinical signs
- Flattening of the peripheral equatorial lens that is visible on pupillary dilation (**Figure 13.15**).
- Lack of zonules in the area of equatorial flattening (**Figure 13.16**).
- The lens coloboma may or may not be associated with other ocular anomalies or colobomas.

Differential diagnosis
Congenital coloboma may be difficult to differentiate from shrinkage of the lens with a hypermature cataract, or it may be confused with an aphakic crescent with a sub-luxated lens.

Therapy
No therapy is necessary.

Lenticonus and lentiglobus
Introduction/etiology
Lenticonus is a rare lenticular anomaly characterized by a conical protrusion of the lens, usually axially, on either the anterior or posterior surfaces. Lenticonus may be an isolated anomaly or be associated with multiple ocular anomalies in a variety of breeds.[28–36] Lenticonus may not be observed except by ultrasound when accompanied by severe ocular anomalies. The appearance of primary lenticonus may be confusing if it is not observed with a slit lamp.

Lentiglobus is a spherical protrusion of the lens. The protrusion may be clear or opaque and is usually unilateral.

Clinical signs
Protrusion of the anterior or, more commonly, the posterior curvature of the lens is observed. An opacity at the

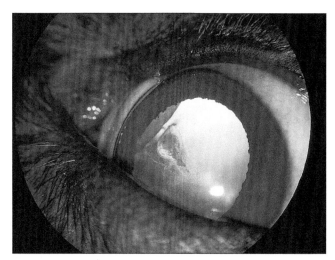

Figure 13.15 Lens coloboma observed in an 8-year-old Old English sheepdog. Note the flattened lens equator and focal cataract in the adjacent lens. Due to the lack of signs, the congenital lesion was not detected in the young dog.

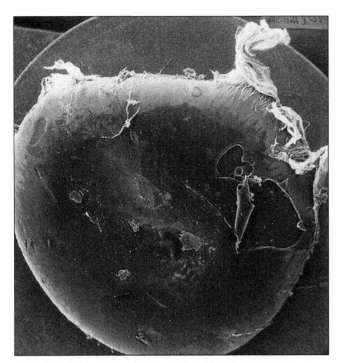

Figure 13.16 SEM of a lens coloboma from a young Australian shepherd dog with an iris coloboma and multiple other ocular anomalies. Note the lack of zonules in the colobomatous region compared to the adjacent equator (×10). (From Martin, C. 1978. *Journal of the American Animal Hospital Association* 14:571–579.)

margin of the protrusion or over the entire protrusion may produce a circular opacity with a clear center or a saucer-shaped opacity, respectively (**Figure 13.17**). Because the posterior capsule is anomalous, rupture of the capsule may occur, risking phacoclastic uveitis.

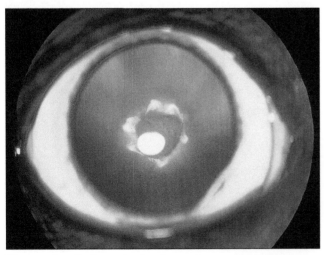

Figure 13.17 Posterior lenticonus in a young Siberian husky. The lenticonus is demarcated by the axial circular lenticular opacity.

Therapy

Therapy is not usually necessary, and lenticonus is not known to be a genetic trait when observed alone.

Prophylaxis

In the Akita, Doberman pinscher, Cavalier King Charles spaniel, Staffordshire bull terrier, bloodhound, and miniature schnauzer, lenticonus is part of a more generalized ocular syndrome that is inherited (see Chapter 15).

Cataracts

A cataract is any opacity of the lens or its capsule. The definition does not specify any particular degree of severity or that blindness is a consequence.

Introduction/etiology

Cataracts can be classified by various schemes and the classifications are often combined.

- *Cataracts classified according to anatomic location*: Anterior capsular, anterior cortical, equatorial, anterior nuclear, fetal nuclear, posterior nuclear, posterior cortical, posterior subcapsular, posterior capsular, axial, and sutural are some of the anatomic descriptors.
- *Cataracts classified according to age*: Congenital, neonatal, juvenile (up to 5–6 years in the dog), and senile are age classifications. Nuclear sclerosis, a normal physiologic process that begins at approximately 7 years of age in the dog, should be differentiated from senile cataracts. All very old animals can develop a significant gray cast to the lens from the light scattering that occurs from nuclear sclerosis, and this is easily confused with a senile cataract.
- *Cataracts classified according to stage or degree of opacification*: This is a common method of describing cataracts and is somewhat arbitrary. The incipient cataract is an early small opacity that owners would not observe (**Figure 13.18**), while the immature cataract is a more diffuse cortical opacity but does not block all light to the fundus, and the animal is still visual if the pupil is dilated. The immature cataract is easily observed (**Figure 13.19**). The mature cataract is a complete opacity that blocks the fundus or tapetal reflection completely, and the eye is blind (**Figure 13.20**). Light still penetrates this opacity but is scattered and does not form a coherent image. The pupillary light reflex (PLR) and dazzle reflex are normal with a bright light, but a menace response is absent with a mature cataract. The mature cataract is often swollen or intumescent from fluid imbibition that produces dark fluid clefts through

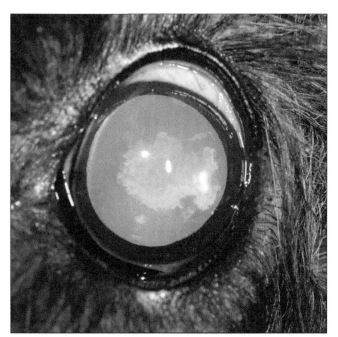

Figure 13.18 Example of an incipient cataract in a dog. This would not be noted by the owner or produce visual symptoms.

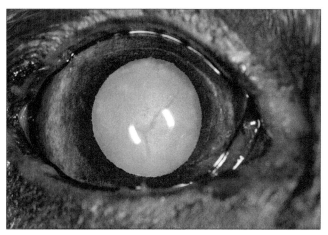

Figure 13.20 Mature cortical cataract in a dog that blocks all tapetal reflection. Note the prominent anterior cortical suture lines and small pigment deposition on the anterior lens capsule.

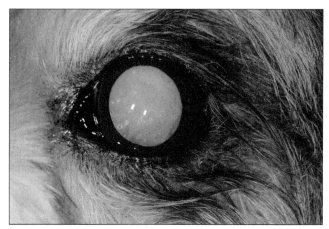

Figure 13.21 A hypermature cortical cataract in a dog that is shrinking in size. Note the refractile plaques and capsular fold in the ventrolateral quadrant.

the anterior cortex and in the suture pattern where fluid can accumulate. The hypermature cataract has undergone a variable degree of resorption of water and, often, protein. This is recognized by the resultant shrinkage of the lens and wrinkling of the lens capsule (**Figure 13.21**). The opacity often has a fine granular texture that may be due to cholesterol crystals from breakdown of cell membranes.[37] Lens resorption can be partial or complete (usually in dogs <2 years of age), resulting in the retention of the capsule with variable amounts of calcific deposits (**Figure 13.22**).

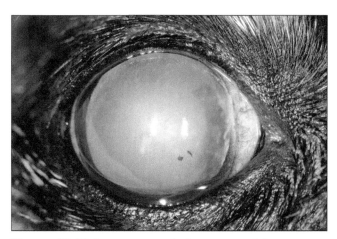

Figure 13.19 Immature cortical cataract and dense nuclear sclerosis. Note the green tapetal reflection around the periphery. Often these dogs are still functional, particularly with pupil dilation.

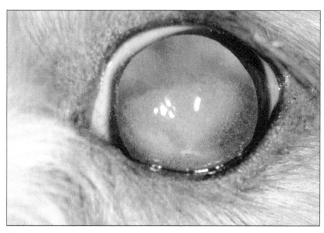

Figure 13.22 Almost complete lens resorption in a dog, leaving a capsular bag filled with crystals.

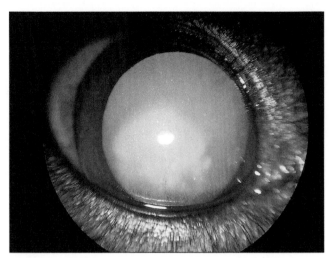

Figure 13.23 Morgagnian cataract in a 2-year-old miniature poodle. Note the denser nucleus settled ventrally in the lens because the cortex is liquified.

The Morgagnian cataract is a hypermature cataract that has a liquefied cortex with the solid nucleus settled within the capsule (**Figure 13.23**). Animals with marked resorption often regain variable amounts of their vision if there is no other ocular pathology such as a retinal detachment or retinal atrophy.

• *Cataracts classified according to the cause*: A variety of etiologies are possible, but in clinical practice, only a few are of significance. Causes include congenital, inherited, and toxic and are discussed individually.

Diagnosis

Good pupil dilation is important to determine the full extent of a cataract and to differentiate it from nuclear sclerosis. A focal slit beam is helpful in localizing the depth of the opacity. The Purkinje–Sanson images from the anterior and posterior capsules are of some aid in depth localization. Nuclear sclerosis after pupil dilation appears as a lens within the cortex or a lens within the lens, but when viewed through a moderate- to small-sized pupil, the light scattering it produces mimics a senile cortical cataract. The importance of differentiating nuclear sclerosis is that it does not produce blindness or clinical signs, whereas a cortical cataract often results in blindness.

Congenital cataracts

Congenital cataracts may be inherited or be due to other *in utero* insults. They may be an isolated anomaly (primary) or one of several ocular anomalies (secondary congenital cataract), such as with microphthalmos. If an isolated event, the cataract is often stationary, with improvement in vision occurring with further growth of normal new fibers. When observed in the older animal, congenital

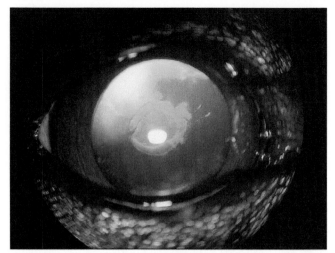

Figure 13.24 Young Scottish terrier with a fetal nuclear cataract. All three dogs in the litter were affected with the same opacity. There was no history of orphan milk supplementation. Opacities in this region are stable and do not progress.

cataracts are typically in the center of the lens or on the anterior or posterior capsule (**Figure 13.24**). The center of the lens represents the embryonal and fetal region, while anterior and posterior capsule opacities are often associated with persistent remnants of the embryonic vascular tunic of the lens, such as persistent pupillary membranes (PPMs) and persistent tunica vasculosa lentis (PTVL) (**Figures 13.25 and 13.26**). When the retention of vascular elements on the posterior capsule is associated with excessive glial or scar tissue, it is termed persistent hyperplastic tunica vasculosa lentis (PHTVL). Congenital cataracts are not synonymous with inherited cataracts. The author has observed entire litters of affected puppies with cataracts from normal parents; repeat breeding from the parents resulted in normal litters.

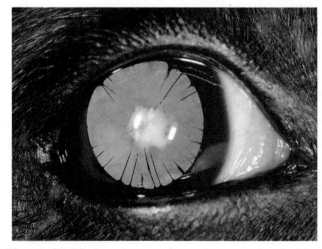

Figure 13.25 Anterior capsular cataract associated with persistent pupillary membranes.

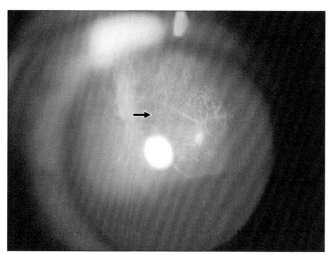

Figure 13.26 Doberman pinscher puppy with posterior capsular markings (arrow) associated with persistent tunica vasculosa lentis and hyaloid artery. While the condition has been studied extensively in the Doberman pinscher, these capsular markings are common in a variety of breeds and are often familial with no documented detrimental effect.

Dog

Congenital cataracts as part of an inherited microphthalmos have been described in the Akita, Cavalier King Charles spaniel, miniature schnauzer, Australian shepherd dog, and Old English sheepdog.[30,32,35,38–40] Cataracts associated with PHTVL are often inherited. Cataracts may be associated with persistent pupillary membranes in the Basenji, beagle, red cocker spaniel, Welsh corgi, and many other breeds. A common appearance is a nest of pigmented dots on the axial anterior capsule that is presumed to be an area of touching or attachment of previous pupillary membranes (Figure 13.27). These are

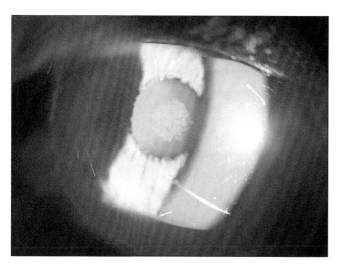

Figure 13.27 Anterior axial capsular pigment deposits, presumably from pupillary membranes. These are common findings in a variety of breeds and are often familial.

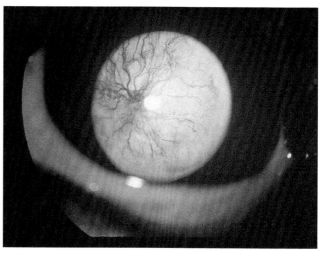

Figure 13.28 Persistent hyperplastic tunica vasculosa lentis in a Bernese Mountain dog puppy. Both puppies in a litter of two were affected. Note the white capsular opacities in addition to the retrolental blood vessels. A subsequent litter from the bitch was normal.

familial and are seen in a wide variety of breeds. Similarly, posterior capsular vascular markings that are white are very common (PTVL). However, persistent hyperplastic primary vitreous (PHPV) and persistent hyperplastic tunica vasculosa lentis (PHTVL) are relatively rare (Figure 13.28) but are inherited in the Doberman pinscher, Staffordshire bull terrier, and Bouvier des Flandres.[34,36,41–44] Lenticular hemorrhage, vitreous hemorrhage, and phacoclastic uveitis may develop from spontaneous rupture of the lens capsule in the severe forms of PHPV/PHTVL. (See Chapter 14, for further discussion of PHPV/PHTVL.)

> Minor anterior and posterior capsular markings produced by the embryonic tunica vasculosa lentis are very common and are of minimal clinical significance as they do not progress.

Congenital cataracts and corneal opacification are part of inherited retinal dysplasia–skeletal dysplasia in the Labrador retriever,[45] skeletal dysplasia–retinal detachment in the Samoyed,[46] and retinal dysplasia in the English springer spaniel.[47]

Cat

Complete congenital cataracts are relatively rare in the cat,[48] although minor lens opacities are not uncommon. Congenital inherited cataracts have been occasionally described in cats, usually in breeds with a Persian background (Figure 13.29).[49]

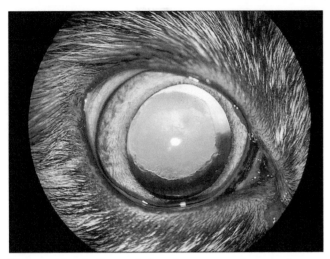

Figure 13.29 Congenital nuclear cataract in a cat about 6 months old. Note the clear peripheral cortex. As new lens fibers are normal, the opacity will not progress in size.

Horse

Congenital cataracts represent 35% of the ocular anomalies in the horse.[50] While they may be associated with microphthalmos, the remainder of the eye is usually normal.[51,52] Congenital cataracts may involve just the suture lines, in which case they are nonprogressive and nonblinding,[53] but they usually involve the entire nucleus and produce visual impairment (**Figure 13.30**). Often the cause of the cataracts is unknown, but they are known or suspected to be inherited in Belgian horses, quarter horses, Morgan horses, and thoroughbreds.[54–56] In the Morgan horse, the opacities are in the fetal nucleus without any visual impairment. While familial, the mode of inheritance has not been determined.[56] In the Belgian horse, cataracts may be observed with aniridia and as a dominant trait.[54] Lens subluxations were noted in one foal with congenital cataracts.[57]

Cow

Inherited congenital cataracts have been reported in the Jersey, Hereford, Holstein, shorthorn, and Holstein–Friesian.[58–60] In the Jersey, lens displacement, microphakia, and buphthalmos may occur as a simple recessive trait.[59] In shorthorns, the cataracts occur with microphthalmos and multiple ocular anomalies as well as hydrocephalus, cerebellar hypoplasia, and myopathy.[60,61]

Clinical signs

- Visual impairment: In dogs and cats, if the lens opacities are complete, or the cataracts are part of severe ocular anomalies, blindness is noted at 4–5 weeks of age when puppies and kittens start to move around. Improvement in vision may be noted after a period of growth if the opacities are stationary and other ocular anomalies do not preclude vision.
- Incidental capsular or nuclear opacities: Congenital opacities may be noted on either the anterior or posterior capsule or the central lens as an incidental finding in the older animal and can usually be traced to their temporal origin by their location and, perhaps, vascular shape (**Figures 13.24, 13.26, and 13.27**).
- Cataracts associated with PHPV/PHTVL may be associated with the unusual occurrence of hemorrhage into the lens (**Figure 13.31**). This may be associated with acute blindness. Vascular remnants varying from pigment or gray markings on the capsule to obvious vascular structures that may or may not have blood in the lumen may be present with PHTVL (**Figures 13.26 and 13.28**).

Diagnosis of congenital origin

- Observation in the first few weeks of life may date the origin of the opacity, but in the dog, neonatal cataracts,

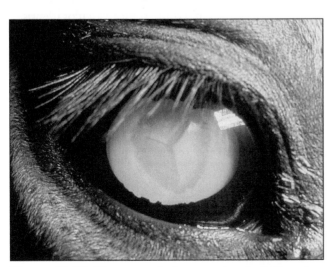

Figure 13.30 Mature cortical cataract in a foal. Note the lens suture which was fractured due to fluid imbibition.

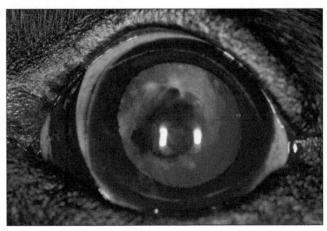

Figure 13.31 Intralenticular hemorrhage from persistent hyperplastic tunica vasculosa lentis.

such as those induced by orphan milk formulas, must be differentiated from congenital cataracts.

- Nuclear opacification of the lens or cataracts located on the capsule with associated embryonic vascular remnants dates the origin of the opacity.
- Lenticular opacities in association with other congenital anomalies.

Acquired cataracts
Inherited cataracts

Inherited genetic defects are the most common cause of cataract in the dog and are relatively uncommon in the cat.[48] The age of onset of inherited cataracts may be congenital, juvenile, or senile. Most have a recessive inheritance, but some are thought to be dominant. (See **Table 13.1** for a list of inherited cataracts.) The most common forms of inherited cataracts are in the juvenile age range (<6 years). While many juvenile cataracts are progressive and result in blindness, a common form found in many retriever breeds, Malamutes, Siberian huskies, and others is a focal axial posterior subcapsular opacity that is either triangular or saucer-shaped. These posterior subcapsular opacities are usually, but not invariably, nonprogressive (**Figure 13.32**).

Inherited cataracts in individual instances are often diagnosed by association rather than by firm genetic evidence. Usually inheritance is presumed, based on the typical appearance and the age in a breed known to be predisposed to cataracts. While more objective evidence such as having afflicted littermates, parents, or relatives is preferred, the individual pet owner often cannot provide this information. Gelatt and Mackay surveyed a large data base of teaching hospital medical records (Veterinary Medical Database) and found the prevalence of dogs presented with cataracts had increased by 255% from 1964 to 2003.[62] Fifty-nine breeds had cataract prevalence above the base line for mixed breeds dogs. Those with the highest prevalence were: Smooth fox terrier (11.7%), Havanese (11.6%), Bichon Frise (11.5%), Boston terrier (11%), miniature poodle (11%), silky terrier, (10%), and toy poodle (10%). Breeds with the greatest number of cataracts were: Boston terrier (11%), miniature poodle (11%), American Cocker Spaniel (9%), standard poodle (7%), and miniature schnauzer (5%). It should be emphasized that many of these cataracts may not have been blinding.

Metabolic cataracts
Hyperglycemia

While a variety of sugars are experimentally capable of inducing cataracts, only glucose and galactose are clinically important, where the pathogenesis has been studied extensively. On initial presentation and without complete ophthalmic examinations, cataracts are noted in almost 60% of cases of canine diabetes mellitus,[63] whereas they were noted in none of a series of 30 cats with diabetes.[64] Williams and Heath screened 50 diabetic patients and found cataracts in 48/50 cats; the mean age was younger (5.6 years) than the normal group of cats that was examined.[65] Roughly half of these cats had the same type of minor opacities found in the normal group, while 26 had more significant, but not blinding, opacities. While this study may contradict other papers, from a clinical standpoint, it appears that feline diabetic cataracts are not usually problematic and require surgery, as is the case in the dog. Bean et al. found that 50% of dogs with diabetes developed cataracts by 6 months, and 75% developed cataracts by 1 year.[66] The importance of galactose in veterinary medicine is uncertain.

The proposed pathogenesis of hyperglycemic cataracts is that the increase in glucose in the aqueous humor is also manifested in the lens, which overloads glycolysis and the hexose monophosphate shunt (**Figure 13.9**). The extra sugar is shunted into the sorbitol pathway where polyols (sorbitol) are formed. Polyols accumulate because they diffuse poorly out of the lens and are not metabolized rapidly.[67] This creates an osmotic gradient that pulls water into the lens, creating vacuoles and, later, protein aggregates (**Figure 13.33**). One of the reasons for species variation in susceptibility to diabetic cataracts may be due to variable aldose reductase activities. Those animals with high levels of aldose reductase, such as the dog, convert more glucose into sorbitol and consequently develop cataracts.[1,68–70] Richter et al. found that lenses from dogs and young cats had high aldose reductase activity when incubated with glucose *in vitro* and developed cataracts.[68] Lenses from older cats (>4 years) *in vitro* had low aldose reductase activity and were resistant to glucose-induced cataracts. As most cats develop diabetes when older, this is probably the reason for the infrequent appearance of cataracts in the diabetic cat.

The younger dog is more susceptible to sugar cataracts; typically, cataracts begin as accentuation of the anterior and posterior sutures and then vacuoles at the equator (**Figure 13.34**), extending into the anterior and posterior cortex. This process often progresses to complete cortical opacification.[69,70] Experimentally, inhibitors of aldose reductase can inhibit the onset and severity of sugar cataracts.[69,71–73] The experimental drug Kinostat is still under investigation but may become commercially available in the future.

Hypocalcemia

Hypocalcemia associated with parathyroid dysfunction, postparturient hypocalcemia, and severe nutritional

Table 13.1 **Inherited or suspected inherited cataracts in the dog.**

BREED	APPROXIMATE AGE OF ONSET	MODE OF INHERITANCE	CHARACTERISTIC EARLY APPEARANCE	COURSE OCULAR LESIONS	ASSOCIATED
Afghan hound	6 months–2 years	AR	Equatorial, cortical	P	–
Akita	C	?	Nuclear	S	Microphthalmos
American Cocker Spaniel	1–2 years; 3–5 years	AR	Posterior, axial, cortical; anterior cortical	P	–
Australian shepherd dog	C	AR with incomplete penetrance 1–2 m AR HSF4 mutation	Nuclear, cortical	S	Microphthalmos
Beagle	C	?	Axial, anterior subcapsular	S	Persistent pupillary membranes +
Beagle	1 year	?	Axial, posterior subcapsular	S	–
Boston terrier	4–6 months; 3–4 years; senile	AR HSF4 mutation	Cortical; nuclear; equatorial	P; P – slow, P – slow	–
Cavalier King Charles spaniel	C; J–	?; –	Nuclear, posterior cortical; Posterior capsular, cortical	P+; P	Lenticonus+; microphthalmos
Chesapeake retriever	6 months– 6 years	Dominant	Axial, posterior subcapsular triangle	S (usually)	–
Doberman pinscher	C	AR?	Posterior capsular	P+	Posterior lenticonus, PHPV/ PHTVL, microphakia
English Cocker Spaniel	C	AR	Nuclear, cortical, sutural	–	Retinal dysplasia
French bulldog	6 months	AR HSF4 mutation			
German shepherd dog	C; 8 weeks	Dominant, AR	Axial, anterior; Posterior sutural	S; P but not blindness	–
Golden retriever	6 months– 6 years	AR	Axial, posterior subcapsular	S (usually)	–
Labrador retriever	C	?	Nuclear, cortical	S	Corneal opacity, retinal dysplasia, retinal detachment
Old English sheepdog	C	?	Nuclear, cortical	P+	Retinal detachment, + microphthalmos
Poodle, miniature/toy	2–10 years	?	Cortical	P	–
Poodle, standard	Several months	AR	Equatorial	P	–
Red cocker spaniel	C	?	Axial, anterior subcapsular	S	PPMs+
Siberian husky	6 months–6 years	AR	Posterior subcapsular	S	–
Schnauzer, miniature	C; J	AR; ?	Nuclear, cortical; cortical	P+; P	Microphthalmos+; –
Staffordshire bull terrier	2–6 months; C	AR; AR	Nuclear; posterior capsular AR HSF4 mutation	P; S (usually)	–; PHPV/PHTVL, microphthalmos
Welsh corgi	J	AR?	Posterior cortical	–	–
Welsh springer spaniel	8 weeks	AR	Posterior cortical vacuoles	P – blind by 2 years	–
West Highland white terrier	C?	AR?	Posterior sutural	P – some	–

AR: Autosomal recessive; C: Congenital; J: Juvenile; P: Progressive; PHPV/PHTVL: Persistent hyperplastic vitreous/persistent tunica vasculosa lentis; S: Stationary. For references, see Chapter 15: Presumed Inherited Ocular Diseases.

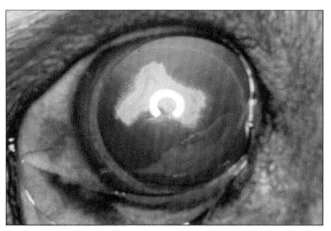

Figure 13.32 Axial posterior subcapsular triangular cataract in a Golden retriever that is typical of juvenile cataracts in retrievers. The opacity has been moved off center to avoid the bright specular reflection.

imbalances in the young animal produces characteristic multifocal anterior and posterior cortical opacities.[74,75] The opacities do not seem to progress and, thus, do not produce signs of blindness (**Figures 13.35 and 13.36**). The mechanism is probably through alterations of lens cell membrane permeability from altered extracellular levels of calcium.[2]

Nutritional deficiencies

Feeding orphan milk replacement diets to wolf puppies produced cataracts, which were attributed to an arginine deficiency in the diet.[76] Cataracts have also been observed clinically in the dog and the cat with commercial orphan diets,[77] home formulated diets, and goat's milk. Nutritional cataracts have been reproduced experimentally in puppies and kittens but were quite mild and improved after weaning.[78,79] In the author's experience, cataracts produced by orphan diets are more severe when the diets are fed to nondomesticated species, such as wolves, raccoons (**Figure 13.37**), coyotes, and, perhaps, large breeds of dogs. Additional arginine and methionine has been added to commercial milk formulas,[80] but this does not appear to have completely eliminated the problem. It is important to dog breeders for the examiner to differentiate nutritional cataracts from inherited forms. Typically, the orphan diet cataract is posterior cortical in the puppy (**Figure 13.38**), posterior sutural in wolf puppies, and becomes nuclear in older animals.

In hatchery-raised fish, cataracts have been produced by a variety of nutritional deficiencies. In trout and Atlantic salmon, diets deficient in methionine, thiamine, zinc, riboflavin, or tryptophan produced cataracts.[81-84]

Trauma

Blunt or perforating trauma is an etiology that must be considered with a unilateral cataract. Perforating trauma that has ruptured the lens capsule is the most obvious cause and may initiate severe intraocular inflammation, termed phacoanaphylaxis or phacoclastic uveitis. The hallmark of a cataract due to a perforating injury is a duplicate opacity of the overlying cornea (**Figure 13.39**). A history of blunt trauma may not be known, and the cataract not be observed until long after the incident. Thus, the appearance of the cataract may be difficult to correlate with the cause (**Figure 13.40**). Braus et al. reported successful cataract extraction in 6/6 cats and 23/27 dogs with traumatic lens rupture.[85] Glaucoma was the most common complication and resulted in loss of the eye.

> No matter the cause of a cataract, most owners can associate its presence with a traumatic incident in the dog's life.

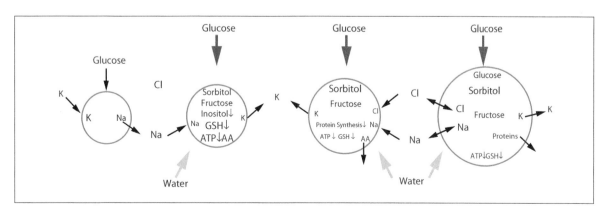

Figure 13.33 Sequence of events leading to a diabetic cataract. As the glucose in the lens increases, it becomes shunted to the sorbitol pathway due to overwhelming of hexokinase in the glycolysis pathway. Sorbitol cannot diffuse out of the capsule, resulting in an osmotic gradient to pull water into the lens. (From Kinoshita, JH. 1986. *American Journal of Ophthalmology* 102:685–692.)

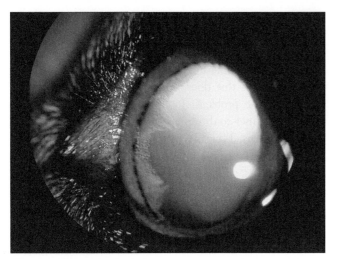

Figure 13.34 Early diabetic cataract in a dog. Note the vacuoles from the lens equator extending axially.

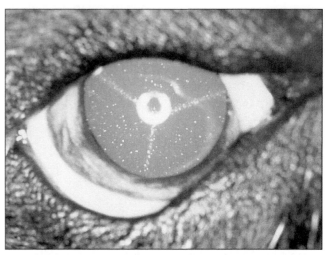

Figure 13.36 Hypocalcemic cataracts in a puppy with severe nutritional calcium/phosphorous imbalance. This puppy had marked osteoporosis.

Intraocular disease

Cataracts secondary to intraocular disease are often termed complicated or secondary cataracts. Three common causes for complicated cataracts are:

- *Inflammation*: Cataracts associated with inflammation may be capsular due to deposition of cells, pigment, and fibrin on the surfaces, or in the lens associated with impaired nutrition. This is the most common type of cataract in the cat and the horse (**Figure 13.41**).
- *Secondary to retinal degenerations*: Certain breeds with progressive retinal atrophy (PRA) almost always develop cataracts, usually late in the disease. Whether the cataracts are associated with a diffusible product that is released by the degenerating retina

or a gene associated with PRA is unknown. The appearance of these cataracts is not unique, so they cannot be distinguished from other forms of inherited cataracts.

- *Secondary to chronic glaucoma*: Animals with chronic glaucoma often develop cataracts, and the cause is unknown, although multiple causes are possible. The stagnation of aqueous humor that occurs with glaucoma probably has a deleterious nutritional effect on the lens. In addition, the prolonged elevated intraocular pressure (IOP) may affect the lens epithelium. These factors, combined with the variety of drugs and surgical insults used to treat glaucoma, are possible contributing factors to cataractogenesis.

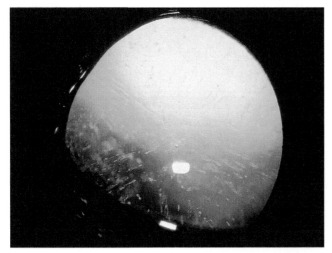

Figure 13.35 Typical hypocalcemic cataracts characterized by dot and linear opacities along a specific level of cortical lens fibers that were forming during the hypocalcemic episode. This dog had hypoparathyroidism.

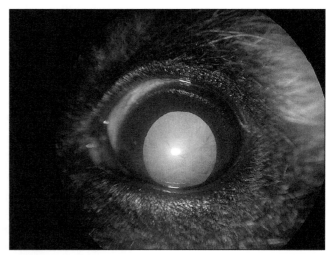

Figure 13.37 Complete cortical cataract in a racoon raised on a commercial canine orphan milk substitute.

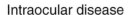

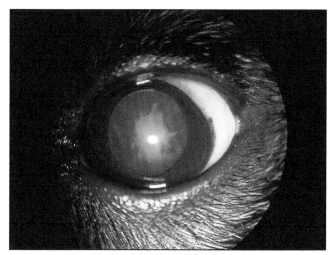

Figure 13.38 Typical nuclear cataract in a collie puppy raised on a commercial orphan milk substitute.

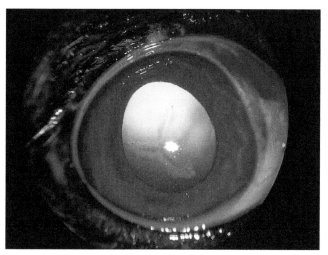

Figure 13.40 Blunt trauma- (proptosed globe) induced cataract in a dog outlining the anterior suture.

Toxic cataracts

Various compounds either ingested or injected parenterally or intraocularly may produce cataracts. The author has observed toxic cataracts most commonly in the cat, often as an incidental finding. While a variety of chemicals may produce cataracts in the laboratory, there are not many examples of involvement of drugs that are routinely used in veterinary medicine. Most animals that develop drug-related cataracts have been given drugs because of systemic signs. Whether stress, systemic disease, or the drug are causal factors, either individually or in combination, is unknown. Antibiotics have usually been the suspected cause of these cataracts, and they are often transient. The vacuolar opacities may resolve rapidly when the drugs are changed, or the animal improves. One example of oral paromomycin, an aminoglycoside that is poorly absorbed

from the gastrointestinal tract, induced acute renal failure and cataracts in four cats treated for enteritis.[86]

The following is a list of toxic agents reported to cause cataract. Except for ketoconazole, these are largely academic as the drugs are not commonly used. Disophenol, an injectable whipworm medication, may produce cataracts in puppies. However, the cataracts are usually transient, and the cataractogenic dose is 2–3 times the clinical dose.[87,88] Diazoxide (an antihypertensive agent) administered intravenously in the dog also produces transient cataracts attributed to drug-induced hyperglycemia consisting of vacuoles at the equator.[89] Dimethyl sulfoxide in the dog, administered orally or applied dermally, may cause an increase in nuclear haze or, conversely, decrease in cortical relucency.[90,91] Hypolipidemic drugs such as

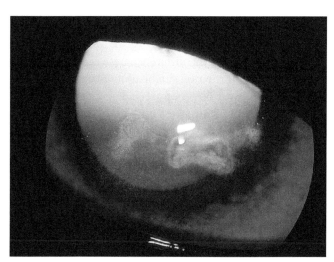

Figure 13.39 A dog with a cataract induced by a perforating cat claw injury. Note the scar in the cornea that is aligned with the lens opacity.

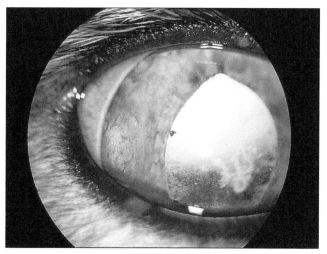

Figure 13.41 Complicated cataract in a cat that had FeLV-associated anterior uveitis and lymphoma that were treated successfully for 1 year. Note the opacity is mainly associated with capsular inflammatory debris.

the hydroxymethylglutaryl-CoA (HMG-CoA) reductase inhibitors can produce posterior or anterior subcapsular cataracts in dogs at doses of 40–60 times the clinical dose. The posterior suture becomes increasingly prominent and may continue to a complete cortical cataract.[92] Oral long-term ketoconazole administration has produced bilateral, rapidly progressive cataracts in dogs. The mean duration of therapy before cataracts were noted was 15 months, with a range of 3.5–37 months of treatment.[93]

Topical glucocorticoids and miotic agents are known to produce cataracts in humans, but animals seem resistant, and the risk is considered minimal. In cats, topical dexamethasone has produced cataracts and mild ocular hypertension. Topical prednisolone and dexamethasone produce subcapsular opacities after 40 days of application, and they continue to progress while the animal is on therapy.[94] Significant cataract development has been documented in groups of experimental cats given systemic dexamethasone to induce diabetes mellitus as well (**Figure 13.42**).

Radiation

Ionizing radiation is cataractogenic and is recognized mainly after cancer teletherapy. Species variations may exist as gamma radiation exposure to cattle, swine, and burros resulted in cataract formation in only 6.7% of cattle.[95] Cataracts were produced in 11% and 28% of canine patients treated with cobalt-60[96] or megavoltage teletherapy, respectively.[97]

Cataracts develop 3–9 months after therapy and are usually bilateral and progressive (**Figure 13.43**). While

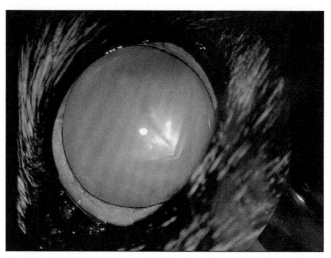

Figure 13.43 Radiation-induced cataracts in a cat 1 year after receiving cobalt therapy to the head region.

microwave radiation can induce anterior and posterior subcapsular cataracts experimentally in dogs, the clinical importance of this form of radiation is unknown.[98] Long-term exposure to ultraviolet (UV) from sunlight is thought to be a major cause of senile cataracts in humans.[2]

Electricity

Animals that have had an electrical shock may develop a typical axial anterior subcapsular cataract months after the shock.[99]

Prognosis

The location of the cataract may be a clue to the potential progression and cause. Most cataracts have no distinguishing features regarding cause or progression, and only repeated examinations can help in giving a prognosis. Capsular and subcapsular opacities are variable but usually stationary in their course. Fetal nuclear opacities do not progress (**Figures 13.24 and 13.29**), but equatorial and cortical opacities may progress (**Figure 13.34**).

In a given patient, the difference between eyes in their stage of cataract formation can be quite marked, and thus, a unilateral cataract does not preclude genetic influences. The speed of cataract progression is highly variable, ranging from days to years. Rapidly developing cataracts are usually accompanied by lenticular osmotic changes that pull water into the cortex, and thus, they are often swollen. These cataracts are characterized by vacuoles and clefts when the opacity is viewed with magnification in the early stages.

While rapid progression with vacuole formation may occur with many forms of cataracts, diabetes mellitus should be considered when the condition is bilateral and symmetrical. Posterior synechiae or aqueous flare does not necessarily indicate that a cataract is secondary to

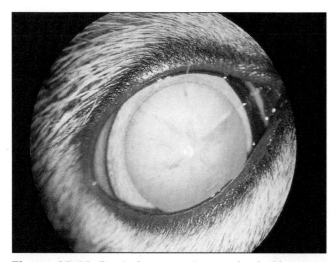

Figure 13.42 Cortical cataracts in a cat that had been given systemic dexamethasone and growth hormone to induce diabetes mellitus. All the cats in the research colony given the protocol developed cataracts, and several developed bullous keratopathy.

inflammation. Phacogenic or lens-induced uveitis is a very common phenomenon and, if an accurate history is not available, may be confusing to the clinician. Lens-induced uveitis usually develops with late immature to hypermature cataracts.

Therapy

Cataracts can either be monitored or surgically removed.

Through the years, a variety of medical therapies have been empirically touted in veterinary medicine for treating nuclear sclerosis or cataracts in general. Oral selenium,[100,101] intraocular superoxide dismutase (orgotein),[102] and topical zinc ascorbate were said to have anticataractogenic benefits, but they have been discounted as effective medical therapy for established cataracts.[103,104] In humans during the last decade, aspirin and oxygen scavengers, including various vitamins, have been variably reported in their effectiveness in preventing cataracts.[105–110] Williams and Munday evaluated an over-the-counter preparation of 2% N-acetyl carnosine, which also contains various other antioxidants, that has been marketed for its anticataractogenic effect in dogs.[111] Therapy was administered every 8 hours over 8 weeks to dogs with varying degrees of cataract formation. Based on comparison of digitized photos at these intervals, they found a small but statistically significant improvement in the group of immature cataracts and those with nuclear sclerosis. Eighty percent of owners thought that their dog's vision had improved while on the medication. Most ophthalmologists are skeptical of these results and point to flaws in the methodology. Ideally, the study should be repeated using a masked study with the drug and a placebo. Therapy or cessation of therapy may arrest the advancement of certain types of cataracts, such as diabetic and toxic cataracts. Aldose reductase inhibitors have been used to prevent experimental diabetic and galactose cataracts.[69,71]

Congenital, neonatal, and early juvenile cataracts can be ignored for a period of time to assess whether they are arrested or may resorb.[112] With the advent of phacoemulsification and an increased success rate of surgery, most surgeons would not wait for resorption in juvenile cataracts since the rate of complications can increase. A concern in congenital cataracts is whether amblyopia may occur if the brain is not subjected to visual images at an early age. Amblyopia is known clinically in humans and can be experimentally reproduced in animals.

Waiting for resorption of cataracts increases the risk of lens-induced uveitis and luxation of the lens. The complication of lens-induced uveitis may result in mild-to-severe intraocular sequelae such as secondary glaucoma or phthisis bulbi. Also, posterior segment changes occur with hypermature cataracts as manifested by a low-amplitude electroretinography (ERG) and an increased incidence of retinal detachment. Lens-induced uveitis is usually responsive to topical glucocorticoids, but in cataract surgery performed in eyes with previous uveitis, the postoperative inflammation is usually more severe.

> Ignoring diffuse cataracts is not an option. Chronic cataracts that do not have lens-induced uveitis (LIU) controlled often become luxated, and the eye may become glaucomatous or eventually phthisical.

Medical therapy

Medical therapy of central lens opacities consists of topical atropine 2–3 times a week to maintain pupil dilation and allow vision around the central opacity. Topical glucocorticoids and/or nonsteroidal anti-inflammatory drugs (NSAIDs) are administered if a lens-induced uveitis develops or to prevent lens-induced uveitis.

Surgical therapy in the dog

Cataract surgery should be performed by a specialist. The investment in instruments, the practice necessary to perform the procedure smoothly, the number of complications, and the fact that it is an elective procedure make it questionable whether the generalist should carry out the surgery. Nevertheless, it is very helpful for any veterinarian referring cataract patients to know some details about the procedure to gain an understanding of the postoperative complications and limitations of the procedure.

Phacoemulsification or using ultrasonic energy to fragment the lens and then aspirate the pieces is the standard technique for cataract surgery in small animals in the last decade. The technique often looks deceptively simple in a soft cataract but requires considerable practice to master and requires the use of an operating microscope. The following text addresses phacoemulsification as the primary mode of cataract extraction.

Patient selection

Patient selection should be based on the understanding that cataract surgery is an elective surgery. With the advent of better surgical results from phacoemulsification, the ease of removing the softer earlier cataracts versus the hard hypermature nucleus, and the documentation of increased complication rates with late cataracts, the philosophy of patient selection has changed significantly. Surgeons prefer to operate on the late immature cataracts while the lens is soft and before lens-induced uveitis has developed. This often translates into operating on a dog that is still visual or has only a unilateral cataract.

Operating when only one eye is blind has the disadvantage that the owner may not note any improvement, but in the author's experience, most owners note an increase in activity level in dogs and cats that have had unilateral cataract surgery. The advantage of operating when one eye is blind is that the animal is never completely blind.

Patients selected for cataract surgery should have cataracts that are not associated with other blinding lesions such as progressive retinal atrophy (PRA), retinal detachment, or optic nerve disease. Most retinal diseases are ruled out by an ERG, but in the absence of an ERG, practitioners must rely on early fundus examination before the cataracts are dense or, less ideally, the pupillary light reflex (PLR) and the dazzle reflex. PLRs are subjective and often erroneously interpreted. PLRs should be normally reactive with dense cataracts, but secondary changes such as uveitis, adhesions, and atrophy of the iris sphincter interfere with iris mobility and interpretation of the PLR. Ocular ultrasound is now routinely performed on all candidates for surgery to detect retinal detachment and vitreous disease. Retinal detachment was found on preoperative ultrasound in 19% of cases with hypermature cataracts, 7% with mature cataracts, and 4% with immature cataracts.[113]

Patients should have their lens-induced uveitis under control. In one study, the success rate in the eyes with uveitis was 78% and 39% at 2 and 6 months, respectively, while in the noninflamed eye, the success rate was 85% and 71%.[114] Secondary cataracts from inflammation are common in the horse and the cat. Patients with secondary cataracts are not good candidates for surgery since the postoperative complications are increased significantly, and posterior segment disease is common.

Cataract surgery patients should have a good temperament because they will be handled frequently, and struggling with patients is often destructive to the eye. Owners must be committed to the postoperative effort, which is often months in duration and is very important. Patients should have good systemic health. Age is not a reason for denying surgery. Diabetes mellitus should be ruled out as a cause of the cataracts. Diabetic patients can be operated upon, but control of diabetes and client education should precede surgery. It is amazing how many owners are preoccupied with the cataracts in their diabetic dogs but do not have the same dedication to the diabetes treatment and control.

Diabetic patients may have different and significant complications. Although Bagley and Lavach found the complication rate was no higher in diabetic dogs than in nondiabetic dogs undergoing phacoemulsification with no intraocular lens (IOL) implants, the author has experienced increased numbers of preoperative and postoperative corneal erosions in diabetic dogs, as have others.[115,116] Corneal erosions complicate the use of anti-inflammatory therapy. An increase in postoperative corneal edema may also be noted in diabetic animals, since the corneal endothelium may be compromised, and surgical trauma hastens decompensation. Additionally diabetic dogs have reduced corneal sensitivity and an increase incidence of keratoconjunctivitis sicca in postoperative patients. One unique and transient postoperative risk to diabetic patients and other patients with lipid metabolic problems (miniature schnauzers) is lipid developing in the anterior chamber associated with lipemia.

Preoperative therapy

Preoperative therapy varies for each individual but usually consists of obtaining maximal pupillary dilation, treating and preventing infection with antibiotics, and treating and minimizing intraocular inflammation with anti-inflammatory drugs. The route of administration, frequency, and duration of preoperative medication vary from surgeon to surgeon.

Anesthesia

Anesthesia with intraocular surgery is greatly facilitated with neuromuscular blockade. The author's preference is for atracurium neuromuscular blockade because of its short duration. One dose of atracurium is adequate for one eye, and if a bilateral procedure is performed, a second dose is administered. When using neuromuscular blockade, the clinician should be aware that a variety of systemic drugs may potentiate the length of paralysis. Drugs known to lengthen neuromuscular blockade include the aminoglycosides, lincomycin, clindamycin, bacitracin, polymyxin B, verapamil, and anesthetics such as enflurane, isoflurane, and halothane.[117,118]

Surgery

Different surgeons use different techniques for extracapsular lens extraction. Variations in technique include position of the animal, fixation of the eye for surgery, method and location of entering the eye, method of opening the anterior lens capsule and removal of the lens, method of irrigation of lens fragments, placement of an intraocular lens, method of suturing and type of suture used to close the eye, method of reforming the anterior chamber, and whether or not the eye is covered.

Patient positioning for phacoemulsification is usually in dorsal recumbency. Phacoemulsification techniques can be carried out using a one-handed technique with one incision or a two-handed technique with two incisions. The phacoemulsification handpiece has the capability of irrigation, irrigation/aspiration, or irrigation/

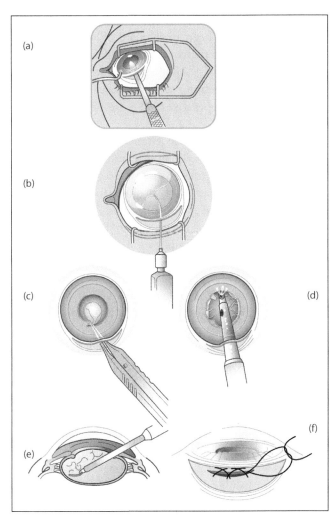

Figure 13.44 Phacoemulsification and placement of an IOL. (a) 3-mm stab incision is made in a groove prepared for enlargement to 8 mm for IOL placement; (b) injection of viscoelastic agent; (c) a circular capsulorrhexis is made with Utrata forceps; (d) phacoemulsification; (e) soft cortex is removed with irrigation-aspiration handpiece; (f) incision is closed if no IOL is placed.

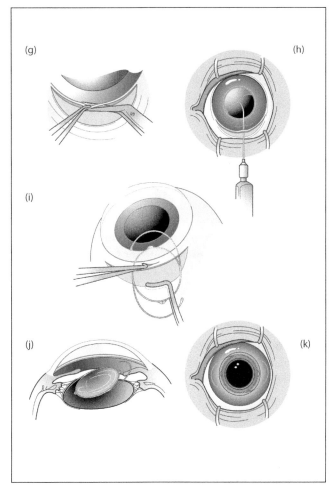

Figure 13.45 Phacoemulsification and placement of an IOL. (g) Enlargement of original 3-mm incision is made with scissors to accommodate the IOL; (h) capsular bag and anterior chamber are filled with viscoelastic; (i) IOL is introduced into the anterior chamber; (j) distal haptic is placed in the capsular bag, and the proximal haptic is then dialed into the bag or placed with forceps; (k) IOL is in the bag, and the eye is sutured after removal of the remaining viscoelastic.

aspiration/ultrasound, depending on the position of the foot pedal. Phacoemulsification is performed through a small incision(s), and fluid infusion maintains the anterior chamber throughout the procedure until an IOL is inserted (**Figures 13.44 and 13.45**).

The actual technique of phacoemulsification varies, but the goal is to preserve the posterior capsule and remove all the lens material. The most common (17% of cases) intraoperative complication is rupture of the posterior capsule, which is only about 5 μm thick.[119] The dorsal nucleus and the cortex are the most difficult parts to reach and visualize.

Placement of an IOL has been practiced for several years and has become routine for many surgeons (**Figures 13.46 and 13.47**). Some surgeons prefer not to place an IOL. The availability of lenses specifically designed for the dog and at a modest price has facilitated their use. The lens power has increased dramatically to the current recommended standard of about 41.5 D.[119–122] While IOLs are not necessary for functional vision postoperatively, the clinical impression is that the animals can see better and are more rapidly visually rehabilitated. Vision in aphakic patients can be quite variable, from clinically normal to markedly disorientated. The author's impression is that older dogs do not adjust well to aphakia. Through objective measurements utilizing visual evoked responses, emmetropic beagles' visual acuity was equivalent to 20/60

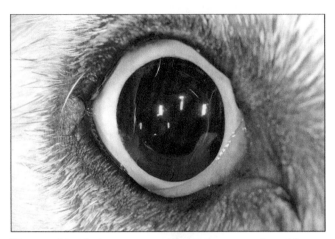

Figure 13.46 Appearance of a dog postoperative with an acrylic foldable IOL in place. Note the haptics (arms) of the IOL.

to 20/80, and aphakic visual acuity (14 D defocus) was 20/850 in one study.[123]

The results of cataract surgery have been frequently reported, but often the results are flawed by the design of the study. Follow-up has often been by owner observation,

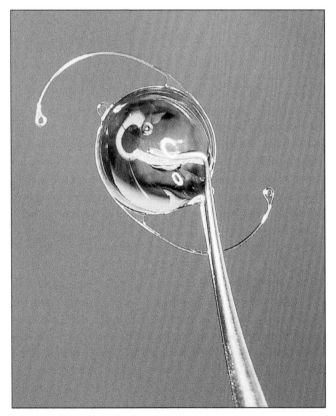

Figure 13.47 Typical appearance of a one-piece polymethylmethacrylate lens for veterinary use. The haptics are the arms that hold the lens in place. The holes at the end of the haptics and on the optics are variably present and are for dialing the lens into position.

the criteria for success are vague, and the duration of follow-up has often been inadequate. The success rates reported based on a return of "functional vision" have varied from 30%–95%.[124–131] The success rate has increased with phacoemulsification, earlier surgical intervention, and improved intraoperative and postoperative medical management.

A success rate with phacoemulsification of >90% is expected on a 3-week to 3-month postoperative evaluation. The reported success rate of extracapsular surgery at around 2 years postoperatively declines to 50%–80% and to about 85% with phacoemulsification.[124,125,128] This figure for phacoemulsification is considered rather optimistic by many surgeons (see Complications).

Complications

The technique and the preoperative and postoperative regimes vary greatly, and yet the results of most experienced surgeons are similar. Whereas complications from corneal trauma and extensive synechiae such as iris bombe are the most common complication of extracapsular extraction,[127,129,132,133] phacoemulsification complications are mainly retinal detachment,[124] posterior capsule opacification, corneal edema, and glaucoma.[128,134] Posterior synechiae are often present with phacoemulsification but are usually very focal and do not disrupt function or create iris bombe, as with extracapsular extraction.

Posterior capsular opacification (PCO) of some degree is common with phacoemulsification, but it is usually not blinding (**Figure 13.48**). Minor or early PCO has been treated in the dog, as in humans, with the Q-switched YAG laser, but severe capsular fibrosis does not respond.[135] PCO is due to the proliferation, migration, and metaplasia of retained lens epithelial cells from the equatorial and anterior capsule regions.[136] The epithelial cells undergo metaplasia to fibrocytes that form plaques and have contractile properties, producing wrinkles in the capsule. The design of the IOL, the IOL material,[137,138] atraumatic surgery, meticulous removal of all cortex,[139] type of capsulorrhexis,[140] and age of the animal all affect the degree of PCO.[136] Several design features of the IOL can decrease PCO, although nothing is known to eliminate it completely. Young animals most consistently produce marked PCO. The use of heparin in the irrigating solution decreases the incidence of PCO by 50% in rabbits and is routinely used by many surgeons for minimizing intraoperative and postoperative fibrin formation.[141]

In the dog, Bras et al. found no differences in PCO after 1 year between diabetic and nondiabetic patients or patients with LIU, or with breed, age, or gender.[142]

Davidson et al. found that the most frequent blinding complication of phacoemulsification was retinal

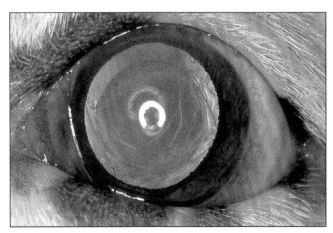

Figure 13.48 Canine patient 4 months after surgery, with mild capsular fibrosis. This would be considered an excellent postoperative result by most surgeons.

detachment, which occurred in 5% or more of cases followed for a mean of 22 weeks.[124] Retinal detachment may be present before surgery, and preoperative ultrasound examination of the eye is used to detect these patients. Since posterior capsular rupture increases the risk for postoperative retinal detachment, focal transscleral cryopexy or laserpexy of the retina at multiple spots is often performed 2 weeks prior to phacoemulsification. Random transscleral retinopexy in Bichon Frise with cataracts, who are genetically predisposed to retinal detachments, decreased the incidence of retinal detachments from 55% to 60% in controls to 12% for those having retinopexy and cataract surgery.[143] However, a retrospective study from Bras et al. demonstrated that Bichon Frise in the United Kingdom are not predisposed to retinal detachment, and Pryor et al. demonstrated that there was no indication for prophylactic retinopexy in a retrospective study of Bichons from the Midwestern United States.[144,145] Johnstone and Ward refuted the association of posterior capsule disruption and retinal detachments.[146] In their analysis of 244 cataract surgeries, the posterior capsule was disrupted in 14%, whether accidental or planned, and they found no difference in the visual outcome or complications.

Glaucoma remains the most significant long-term complication with phacoemulsification, despite the lack of obvious pupillary blockage. Biros et al. reported that 16% of eyes developed glaucoma postoperatively by 6 months, and 29% had glaucoma by 12 months.[134] The mean follow-up was only 5.8 months, so these percentages may be underestimating the risk. Risk factors for glaucoma are hypermature lenses (25% develop glaucoma), purebred breeds, aphakia, and female dogs. No relationship was observed between transient postoperative hypertension

and later development of glaucoma. Aphakia, per se, may not predispose to glaucoma, but the reasons for not placing an IOL may predispose to glaucoma, that is, uveitis and posterior capsule tears. Lannek and Miller evaluated postoperative glaucoma in a select group of patients that had minimal or no preoperative LIU.[147] Sixteen percent of the dogs developed glaucoma. Risk factors for glaucoma were breed, specifically Boston terriers, operative hemorrhage, and concurrent (often minor) ocular disease such as iris atrophy and iris cysts. Transient postoperative hypertension, mild LIU, and posterior capsule rupture with or without vitreous herniation did not increase the risk of postoperative glaucoma. Glaucoma developed from 1 week to 55 months (mean 10 months) after surgery and was often a gradual increase in IOP that was amenable to treatment for a median of 14 months. The potential for glaucoma development to occur months to years after surgery argues for periodic rechecks so that therapy can be initiated before blindness develops. In general, the pathogenesis of postoperative glaucoma and how it is associated with various risk factors is speculative.

Gerardi et al. examined 16 postcataract surgery glaucomatous globes and found a membrane lining various anterior segment structures that was derived from the lens epithelial cells.[148] Thus, like posterior capsular opacities, exuberant proliferation by remaining lens epithelium may produce long-term complications of glaucoma.

Postoperative infection is a relatively rare but devastating complication of intraocular surgery. Most bacterial infections originate from the patient's flora, but infections can originate from improper sterilization of tubing and instruments. Surgeons typically use antibiotics via a variety of routes preoperatively and even intraoperatively and prepare the eye with antiseptics. However, it is disturbing to find that these precautions do not seem to lessen the ability to culture bacteria from the aqueous humor during surgery. Taylor et al. found bacterial contamination of 24% of canine eyes undergoing lens removal, although no patients developed endophthalmitis, nor was the surgical outcome affected.[149] The usual isolates were Gram-positive organisms, but no correlation was found between cultures from the adnexa and the aqueous humor. Phacoemulsification was associated with a lower contamination rate than large incision lens surgery, and this was attributed to the smaller incision. The continuous infusion present with phacoemulsification may also have diluted and washed out any contamination. In humans, similar rates of aqueous humor contamination have been found with similar organisms (24%,[150] 20%–29%,[151] 27%–31%[152]). No statistical differences were found with the technique of lens extraction or use of preoperative antibiotics or intraoperative heparin.

While phacoemulsification and newer drug protocols have increased the short-term success of cataract surgery in veterinary medicine, it is not without serious ocular complications and usually requires long-term follow-up and reassessment. Owner compliance to therapy and rechecks is critical for the long-term success of the procedure.

Postoperative therapy

Postoperative therapy consists of mydriatics, antibiotics, and anti-inflammatory drugs administered in a variety of routes, frequencies, and durations. Mydriatic therapy is not used as vigorously as in the past, with the usual intent only of keeping the pupil mobile by letting it dilate and constrict. Some surgeons prefer the use of tropicamide rather than atropine for this due to its short duration of action. Postoperative topical glucocorticoids and/or nonsteroidal anti-inflammatory drugs (NSAIDs) are often administered for months at a low-frequency maintenance dose.

Cataract surgery in the cat

Cataract surgery in the cat is similar to the dog but is relatively infrequently performed. While series of postoperative results have not been published, the impression is that the cat has less postoperative inflammation than the dog, and consequently, the results are very good. If an IOL is placed, the strength should be 52–53 D and the haptics 18 mm in diameter.[153,154] Obviously, a dog IOL is not a good substitute for use in the cat.

Cataract surgery in the horse

The most common form of cataract operated upon in the horse has been congenital. These traditionally have been removed by an irrigation–aspiration technique but are now easily removed with phacoemulsification. The success rates with the older aspiration techniques for equine cataracts operated on in the first year of life are 77% in foals <6 months and 60% in foals 6–12 months old.[155] Because the cataracts are soft in the young horse, phacoemulsification can be performed even though the available needles for most machines are short. The lens of the horse appears softer than the dog's, allowing short phacoemulsification times. Because the vitreous face pushes forward, even with neuromuscular blockade, tears in the posterior capsule are common. A modified lithotripter, which has a longer needle, has been utilized, but additional equipment, a lack of coordinated fluid infusion, postoperative corneal edema, and corneal ulceration

adjacent to the needle from thermal burns indicate that this technique needs more modifications.[156,157] Most recently, congenital cataracts undergoing phacoemulsification were reported to have an 88% success rate, traumatic cataracts a 100% success rate, and equine recurrent uveitis (ERU)-induced cataracts an 80% success rate.[158] The latter statistic for ERU-associated cataracts is very optimistic, but the numbers in the group were very small. Lassaline et al. reported on 12 eyes from 10 horses with acquired cataracts undergoing phacoemulsification.[159] Six of the 10 horses had ERU, and 5/6 were blind. Two of the five with ERU had sight restored. These statistics are more in line with the traditional estimation of less than 50% success rate in cataracts associated with ERU. Two long-term studies of postsurgical success after phacoemulsification in horses (157 total) had a 95% initial success rate but only 25%–54% in horses greater than 2 years after surgery.[160,161] These studies also support a negative outcome for cataract surgery in horses with ERU.

Rigid and foldable IOL (14–21 D) are now available for the horse, but the aphakic horse performs very well. A common problem with cataract surgery in young horses is the behavior of the horse rather than the surgery. Postoperative problems often result from trauma to the eye and contamination from lying down, despite the routine use of a protective mask. Postoperative infection several days after surgery appears to be more common in the horse than in other species.[157]

DISPLACED LENS

Introduction/etiology

The lens may be displaced completely (luxated) anteriorly into the anterior chamber or posteriorly into the vitreous cavity. Partial displacement (subluxation) may be dorsal, ventral, or sideways. Lens dislocation may or may not produce other ocular complications and may or may not be produced by other ocular conditions. Primary lens luxation (PLL) refers to a condition that occurs without antecedent ocular disease, and it is usually thought to be familial or inherited.

Primary lens displacement

On rare occasions, congenital or early-onset lens displacement may occur. Martin described a case in an 8-week-old Brittany that had bilateral lens luxation accompanied by microphakia and moderately severe corneal edema (**Figure 13.13**).[24] On scanning electron microscopy (SEM), the zonular attachments to the equator were significantly reduced and abnormal in appearance (**Figure 13.49**). Similarly, microphakia with lens luxation has been reported rarely in the young cat.[23,26] Lens luxation in a litter (10 puppies) of soft-coated Wheaten terriers has been described.[162] Most of these puppies also had a wide variety of ocular lesions (PPM, choroidal coloboma, posterior staphyloma, microphthalmos), and three had cardiovascular anomalies.

Primary lens displacement is observed most commonly in adult dogs usually 4–5 years of age. It is common in terrier breeds such as the wirehaired fox terrier, Sealyham terrier, Tibetan terrier, Jack Russell terrier, and terrier crosses.[163–167] Primary lens displacement without intraocular disease is also seen sporadically in a variety of other breeds, including the border collie, Australian blue heeler, German shepherd dog, and Shar Pei.[168–170] These are usually isolated cases presented by pet owners, and thus, the genetic influence is unknown or questionable. In the Tibetan terrier and the Shar Pei, primary lens luxation has been documented as an autosomal recessive trait,[163,164,167–170] and it has been suggested that it is also recessive in other terriers.[164] The ADAMTS17 mutation has been identified as a causal mutation for primary lens luxation in 17 terrier breeds including the Jack Russell terrier, Lancashire heeler, and miniature bull terrier.[171]

A very rare cause of primary lens luxation is complete manifestation of Ehlers–Danlos syndrome. Barnett and Cottrell described a Cavalier King Charles spaniel crossbred that exhibited skin fragility with joint laxity, lens luxation, cataract, lens coloboma, corneal edema, and a thin blue sclera.[172] Most cases of Ehlers–Danlos syndrome manifest lid conformational problems without ocular lesions.

Primary luxation is a bilateral disease, although the onset of displacement varies between eyes. Primary lens displacement is thought to be due to zonular malformations. Curtis found on SEM that the zonules attaching to the posterior capsule in Tibetan and Jack Russell terriers had a fine reticular network over and between the ciliary processes that were not observed in normal dogs.[173] He postulated that these represented weak abnormal zonules that fracture over time. Zonular pathology from primary luxations occurring in 4- to 5-year-old dogs has been reported from a variety of breeds.[24] The lenses had evidence of prior attachment of torn zonules at the equator (**Figure 13.50**), compatible with Curtis' finding that the zonular defect was more proximal near the ciliary processes. Morris and Dubielzig studied the zonular fiber morphology of primary lens luxations with histochemistry and light microscopy.[174] They detected two abnormal staining patterns, which they termed zonular dysplasia and zonular collagenization. Both syndromes appear to be characterized by the presence of an abnormal protein, but only the zonular dysplasia staining was unique and

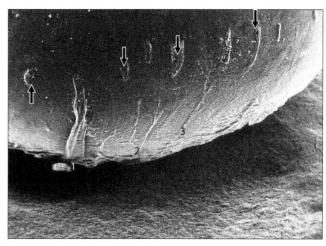

Figure 13.49 SEM of the luxated canine lens seen in Figure 13.14 with microphakia and early luxation. Note the infrequent anomalous areas of zonular attachment (arrows). Only one large anomalous zonule is present in this quadrant (1). Vitreous fibrils (2) and anterior hyaloid (3) face are collapsed onto the posterior lens (SEM ×23). Compare to Figure 13.54. (From Martin, C. 1978. *Journal of the American Animal Hospital Association* 14:571–579.)

mainly in terriers and Shar Peis. The type of staining was not consistent within breeds, and the tissues studied were end-stage glaucoma eyes or eviscerated contents. When bilateral specimens were available, the same pattern of staining was present in both specimens. While the study is not definitive, it does lend support to the hypothesis that not only is the zonular arrangement and morphology

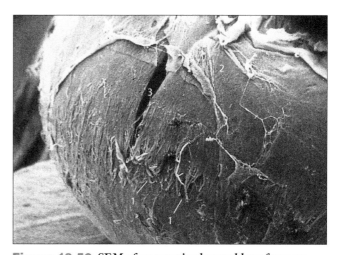

Figure 13.50 SEM of an anterior luxated lens from an Australian blue heeler with primary lens luxation. This area has numerous fractured zonules (1) indicating a mechanical tearing. The anterior vitreous face (2) is collapsed on the lens. (3: Artefact.) (SEM ×24). (From Martin, C. 1978. *Journal of the American Animal Hospital Association* 14:571–579.)

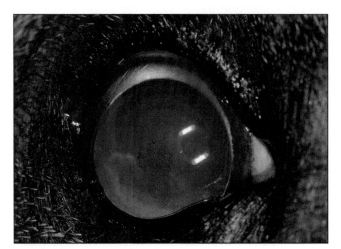

Figure 13.51 Secondary posterior subluxated lens in a Shar Pei with buphthalmos. Note the dorsal aphakic crescent and incident pigment spots on the anterior lens capsule.

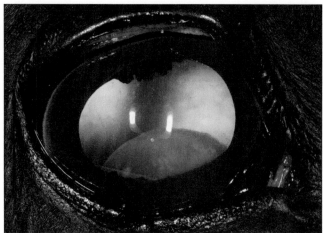

Figure 13.52 Secondary and chronic posterior luxation of the lens in a horse with ERU. Note the hypermature cataractous changes in the lens.

abnormal, but the biochemistry is probably also abnormal. The most likely protein abnormality is in the glycoprotein fibrillin-1.

Secondary lens displacement

An increased circumference of the globe with buphthalmos frequently results in rupture of some of the zonules and a subluxated lens (**Figure 13.51**). Displaced lenses can also precipitate glaucoma, and thus, the history, the examination of the second eye, and the degree of displacement may be clues as to the role of the lens in glaucoma. The triad of glaucoma, uveitis, and displaced lens is common; usually, uveitis is considered the basic underlying disease when all are found together. In the horse, lens subluxation is usually associated with uveitis or buphthalmos (**Figure 13.52**).

In the dog, lens displacement is a common syndrome associated with advanced cataracts. The degenerative process of cataract formation may extend to the zonules and capsular attachment, or lens-induced uveitis with inflammatory cell zonulysis may result in lens displacements with advanced cataracts (**Figure 13.53**).

Lens luxation in aged cats is a distinct condition. A study of 332 cases found Siamese cats and males to be overrepresented, and the most common age was 7–9 years.[175] While usually unilateral, bilateral displacement occurred in 21% of cases. Uveitis was commonly coincident (67%) with lens luxation, which suggested zonulysis by leukocytes. Of 31 tested cats, all were negative for FeLV, but 5/9 cases (55%) were positive for feline immunodeficiency virus (FIV).

Another study of *Toxoplasma gondii* serologic prevalence in cats with uveitis found that all cats with a displaced lens were positive for *T. gondii*, and 13% of the cats studied with

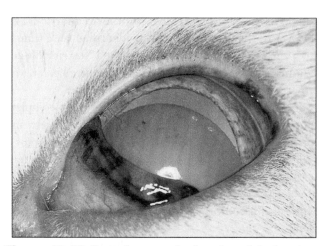

Figure 13.53 Secondary anterior luxation of the lens in a cat with chronic uveitis. In the cat, the IOP is often normal with anterior luxation.

uveitis had displaced lenses.[176] Glaucoma may or may not be present, and frequently animals are blind at the time of presentation despite being normotensive (**Figure 13.54**).

> Trauma is usually overrated as an etiology, and excluding ruptures of the globe, trauma is not an important cause of lens displacement.

> Lens luxations/subluxations and glaucoma represent the classic question of "which came first, the chicken or the egg?" The answer has important implications for therapy and prognosis of the condition.

Clinical signs

Anterior luxation Anterior lens luxation usually manifests with acute epiphora and blepharospasm. Luxation of the lens into the anterior chamber is frequently, but not invariably, associated with increased IOP. Selective vascular injection of the large conjunctival vessels is almost invariable and can occur with or without an elevation of IOP. The lens is usually readily visualized in the anterior chamber if it is opaque or sclerotic (**Figures 13.52 and 13.53**), but it may be overlooked if corneal edema is severe or if the lens is perfectly clear (**Figure 13.54**). Chronic luxation results in cataract formation. Corneal edema may occur where the lens touches the endothelium and is often permanent despite removal of the lens (**Figure 13.54**). The lens may migrate back and forth through the pupil, and the signs can vary depending on the location.

Subluxation Mild or early subluxated lenses may be asymptomatic, with the only sign of ocular disease being vitreous strands in the anterior chamber. Usually, the conjunctiva and episclera are injected, and if the pupil is dilated, an aphakic crescent is visible (**Figure 13.55**). Iridodonesis (iris trembling) and phacodonesis may be present, and the IOP may be elevated. Localized shallowing or deepening of the anterior chamber may occur from the lens pushing the iris anteriorly or posteriorly, depending on the lens position. The mechanism of glaucoma with a subluxated lens is often not clinically obvious, and other predisposing factors for glaucoma should be ruled out in the affected (as well as the normal) eye, since lens removal may not be curative.

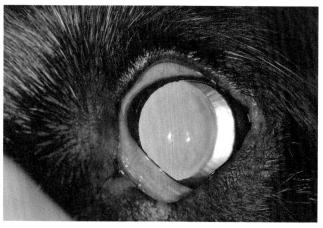

Figure 13.55 Aphakic crescent with subluxation of the lens and visible stretched zonular attachments.

Posterior luxation Posterior lens luxation into the ventral anterior vitreous produces a large aphakic crescent, and, if opaque, the lens is visualized lying in the ventral vitreous (**Figure 13.56**). Often, the only sign of posterior luxation is modest selective conjunctival injection from low-grade uveitis.

Diagnosis

Unless the cornea is opaque, or the pupil is not or cannot be dilated, displaced lenses are easily diagnosed based on the clinical appearance. It may be more difficult to differentiate primary from secondary forms of displacement. Primary displaced lenses are differentiated by breed, lack of other predisposing causes, and findings in the opposite eye.

Therapy

Posterior luxation is treated conservatively with topical glucocorticoids and miotics in most instances. The

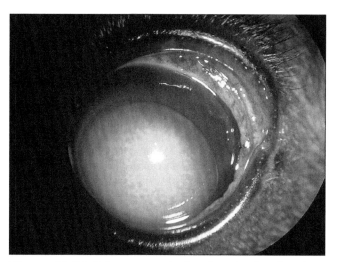

Figure 13.54 Primary anterior lens luxation in a beagle. Note the conjunctival injection and corneal edema. The eye was soft, and the vascular hyperemia was due to irritation rather than glaucoma.

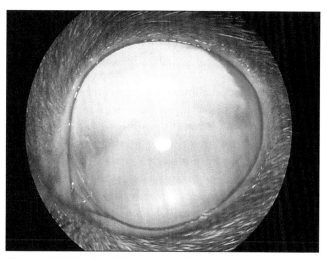

Figure 13.56 Aphakic crescent due to posterior lens luxation in an aged cat. The lens is tilted backwards and is visible because of the widely dilated pupil from glaucoma.

therapy for a subluxated lens is more controversial and is determined by the severity of signs, the surgeon's preference, and the owner's financial resources and concern with surgery. Subluxation may be treated conservatively, if glaucoma is not a problem, by using miotics or latanoprost to try and trap the lens in the posterior chamber. Latanoprost (1 drop every 12 hours) has been more successful in producing sustained miosis than cholinergic drugs. Conservative therapy with topical demecarium bromide for subluxated lenses resulted in 80% of patients being visual at 1 year and a median vision retention time of 1313 days; this was not statistically different to untreated eyes, nor did therapy delay the onset of glaucoma or the second eye from developing signs of lens instability. The median time before anterior luxation occurred was 1131 versus 602 days for nontreated eyes.[177] Topical steroids are indicated if the eye is inflamed. If the IOP is elevated, the lens should probably be removed if the angles appear open in both eyes. Medical therapy often only delays surgery until complete luxation occurs.

Acute anterior luxations require emergency treatment in the dog, as most are associated with glaucoma. Treatment is either transcorneal reduction of the anterior lens luxation or surgical lensectomy. Montgomery et al. describes a technique for repositioning the lens into the posterior segment through an intact cornea.[178] This technique was successful in 85% of eyes, with vision retained in 54.5% of eyes at 1 year. The surgical removal of a luxated lens is intracapsular and carries a high risk of complications from vitreous herniated into the anterior chamber. Vitreous herniation may produce pupillary block glaucoma, may touch the cornea and produce edema, or posterior adhesions may produce retinal holes and tears resulting in retinal detachment.

Glover et al.[169] reported a 14% incidence of retinal detachment 4–6 weeks after intracapsular lens extraction, and this percentage undoubtedly increases over a longer follow-up.[169] Many surgeons now perform prophylactic laser retinopexy after intracapsular extraction to minimize this complication.[143] The use of a cryophake to attach to the lens for removal allows a less traumatic and more controlled means of delivering the lens, while simultaneously wiping the vitreous from the posterior lens.

Closed techniques utilizing phacoemulsification can be performed on an anteriorly luxated lens but, if performed on a hard subluxated lens, may result in the lens falling into the vitreous. Typically, postoperative inflammation is less with intracapsular lens extraction than with extracapsular extraction. Glover et al. reported a success rate of 72% 4 weeks after surgery, but this is too short a follow-up to give a true picture of the complications.[169] Glaucoma persisted in 23% of cases at 4 weeks, but this can be expected to increase over time.

Chronic anterior luxation is sometimes a dilemma. If the eye is blind from glaucoma, it is difficult to rationalize an expensive lensectomy, but the IOP may not be medically controlled. Cyclocryotherapy, cyclophotocoagulation, or evisceration with a silicone ball implantation may be performed in patients with glaucoma and a blind eye. If the eye is soft, no therapy is needed unless uveitis is present.

REFERENCES

1. Jose, J. 1983. The lens. In: Anderson, R., editor. *Biochemistry of the Eye*. American Academy of Ophthalmology: San Francisco, CA, pp. 111–144.
2. Paterson, C., and Delamere, N. 1992. The lens. In: Hart, W., editor. *Adler's Physiology of the Eye*. 9th edition. Mosby Year Book: St Louis, MO, pp. 348–390.
3. Bayer, J. 1914. *Augenheilkunde*. Mosby Year Book: Leipzig, pp. 1–630.
4. Aguirre, G.D., Rubin, L.F., and Bistner, S.I. 1972. Development of the canine eye. *American Journal of Veterinary Research* 33:2399–2414.
5. Donovan, R.H., Carpenter, R.L., Schepens, C.L., and Tolentino, F.I. 1974. Histology of the normal collie eye. III. Lens, retina and optic nerve. *Annals of Ophthalmology* 6:1299–1307.
6. Dickson, D.H., and Crock, G.W. 1972. Interlocking patterns on primate lens fibers. *Investigations in Ophthalmology* 11:809–815.
7. Martin, C.L., and Anderson, R.S. 1981. Ocular anatomy. In: Gelatt, K., editor. *Textbook of Veterinary Ophthalmology*. Lea & Febiger: Philadelphia, PA, pp. 12–121.
8. Berliner, M.L. 1966. *Biomicroscopy of the Eye; Slit Lamp Microscopy of the Living Eye*. Hafner Publishing: New York, p. 152.
9. Martin, C.L. 1969. Slit lamp examination of the normal canine anterior ocular segment. II. Description. *Journal of Small Animal Practice* 10:151–162.
10. Tucker, R. 1973. Comparative and functional studies on the suspensory apparatus of the lens (Mammalia). *Zeitschrift fur Morphologie Tiere* 74:171–191.
11. Helmholtz, H. 1855. Ueber die accommodation des auges. *Albrecht Von Graefes Arch Klin Exp Ophthalmol* 1:1–89.
12. Kuszak, J.R., Mazurkiewicz, M., Jison, L., Madurski, A., Ngando, A., and Zoltoski, R.K. 2006. Quantitative analysis of animal model lens anatomy: Accommodative range is related to fiber structure and organization. *Veterinary Ophthalmology* 9:266–280.
13. Henderson, T. 1926. The anatomy and physiology of accommodation in Mammalia. *Proceedings of the Ophthalmology Society of the United Kingdom* 46:280–308.
14. Knill, L.M., Eagleton, R.D., and Harver, E. 1977. Physical optics of the equine eye. *American Journal of Veterinary Research* 38:735–737.
15. Marak, G.E.J. 1992. Phacoanaphylactic endophthalmitis. *Survey of Ophthalmology* 36:325–339.
16. Lavach, J. 1990. *Lens*. CV Mosby: Philadelphia, PA, pp. 185–208.
17. Tobias, G., Tobias, T.A., Abood, S.K., Hamor, R.E., and Ballam, J.M. 1998. Determination of age in dogs and cats by use of changes in lens reflections and transparency. *American Journal of Veterinary Research* 59:945–950.

18. Coulombre, A.J. 1969. Regulation of ocular morphogenesis. *Investigations in Ophthalmology* 8:25–31.

19. Martin, C.L., and Leipold, H.W. 1974. Aphakia and multiple ocular defects in Saint Bernard puppies. *Veterinary Medicine, Small Animal Clinician* 69:448–453.

20. Peiffer Jr., R.L., and Fischer, C.A. 1983. Microphthalmia, retinal dysplasia, and anterior segment dysgenesis in a litter of Doberman Pinschers. *Journal of the American Veterinary Medical Association* 183:875–878.

21. Bergsjo, T., Arnesen, K., Heim, P., and Nes, N. 1984. Congenital blindness with ocular developmental anomalies, including retinal dysplasia, in Doberman Pinscher dogs. *Journal of the American Veterinary Medical Association* 184:1383–1386.

22. Trapp, C.W. 1957. Congenital maldevelopment of the eyes of a colt. *Cornell Veterinarian* 47:467–468.

23. Aguirre, G.D., and Bistner, S.I. 1973. Microphakia with lenticular luxation and subluxation in cats. *Veterinary Medicine, Small Animal Clinician* 68:498–500.

24. Martin, C. 1978. Zonular defects in the dog: A clinical and scanning electron microscopic study. *Journal of the American Animal Hospital Association* 14:571–579.

25. Rubin, L. 1971. Hereditary microphakia and microphthalmia syndrome in the Beagle. *Proceedings of the Scientific Meeting of the American College of Veterinary Ophthalmologists* 2:50–55.

26. Molleda, J.M., Martin, E., Ginel, P.J., Novales, M., Moreno, P., and Lopez, R. 1995. Microphakia associated with lens luxation in the cat. *Journal of the American Animal Hospital Association* 31:209–212.

27. McLellan, G.J., Betts, D., Sigle, K., and Grozdanic, S. 2004. Congenital glaucoma in the Siamese cat. *Proceedings of the 35th Annual Conference of the American College of Veterinary Ophthalmologists*, 35, p. 36.

28. Aguirre, G., and Bistner, S.I. 1973. Posterior lenticonus in the dog. *Cornell Veterinarian* 63:455–461.

29. Venter, I.J., van der Lugt, J.J., van Rensburg, I.B., and Petrick, S.W. 1996. Multiple congenital eye anomalies in Bloodhound puppies. *Veterinary and Comparative Ophthalmology* 6:9–13.

30. Barrie, K., Peiffer, R., Gelatt, K., and Williams, L. 1979. Posterior lenticonus, microphthalmia, congenital cataracts, and retinal folds in an old English Sheepdog. *Journal of the American Animal Hospital Association* 15:715–717.

31. Gelatt, K.N., Samuelson, D.A., Barrie, K.P. et al. 1983. Biometry and clinical characteristics of congenital cataracts and microphthalmia in the Miniature Schnauzer. *Journal of the American Veterinary Medical Association* 183:99–102.

32. Laratta, L.J., Riis, R.C., Kern, T.J., and Koch, S.A. 1985. Multiple congenital ocular defects in the Akita dog. *Cornell Veterinarian* 75:381–392.

33. Lavach, J., and Severin, G. 1977. Posterior lenticonus and lenticonus internum in a dog. *Journal of the American Animal Hospital Association* 13:685–687.

34. Leon, A., Curtis, R., and Barnett, K. 1986. Hereditary persistent hyperplastic primary vitreous in the Staffordshire Bull Terrier. *Journal of the American Animal Hospital Association* 22:765–774.

35. Narfström, K., and Dubielzig, R. 1984. Posterior lenticonus, cataracts, and microphthalmia; congenital ocular defects in the Cavalier King Charles Spaniel. *Journal of Small Animal Practice* 25:669–677.

36. Stades, F. 1980. Persistent hyperplastic tunica vasculosa lentis and persistent hyperplastic primary vitreous (PHPTVL/

PHPV) in 90 closely related Doberman Pinschers: Clinical aspects. *Journal of the American Animal Hospital Association* 16:739–751.

37. Brooks, A.M., Drewe, R.H., Grant, G.B., Billington, T., and Gillies, W.E. 1994. Crystalline nature of the iridescent particles in hypermature cataracts. *British Journal of Ophthalmology* 78:581–582.

38. Rubin, L.F., Koch, S.A., and Huber, R.J. 1969. Hereditary cataracts in miniature schnauzers. *Journal of the American Veterinary Medical Association* 154:1456–1458.

39. Gelatt, K.N., and Veith, L.A. 1970. Hereditary multiple ocular anomalies in Australian shepherd dogs (preliminary report). *Veterinary Medicine, Small Animal Clinician* 65:39–42.

40. Donovan, R. 1971. Congenital cataracts in the Miniature Schnauzer. *Proceedings of the Scientific Meeting of the American College of Veterinary Ophthalmologists*, vol. 2, pp. 36–43.

41. Barnett, K.C., and Knight, G.C. 1969. Persistent pupillary membrane and associated defects in the Basenji. *The Veterinary Record* 85:242–248.

42. Hirth, R.S., Greenstein, E.T., and Peer, R.L. 1974. Anterior capsular opacities (spurious cataracts) in Beagle dogs. *Veterinary Pathology* 11:181–194.

43. Olesen, H.P., Jensen, O.A., and Norn, M.S. 1974. Congenital hereditary cataract in Cocker Spaniels. *Journal of Small Animal Practice* 15:741–750.

44. van Rensburg, I., Petrick, S., van der Lugt, J., and Smit, M. 1992. Multiple inherited eye anomalies including persistent hyperplastic tunica vasculosa lentis in Bouvier des Flandres. *Progress In Veterinary & Comparative Ophthalmology* 2:133–139.

45. Carrig, C.B., MacMillan, A., Brundage, S., Pool, R.R., and Morgan, J.P. 1977. Retinal dysplasia associated with skeletal abnormalities in Labrador Retrievers. *Journal of the American Veterinary Medical Association* 170:49–57.

46. Meyers, V.N., Jezyk, P.F., Aguirre, G.D., and Patterson, D.F. 1983. Short-limbed dwarfism and ocular defects in the Samoyed dog. *Journal of the American Veterinary Medical Association* 183:975–979.

47. Lavach, R., Murphy, J., and Severin, G. 1978. Retinal dysplasia in the English Springer Spaniel. *Journal of the American Animal Hospital Association* 14:192–199.

48. Peiffer, R.L., and Gelatt, K.N. 1975. Congenital cataracts in a Persian kitten (a case report). *Veterinary Medicine, Small Animal Clinician* 70:1334–1335.

49. Collier, L., Moore, C., and Prieur, D. 1987. Familial congenital cataracts in cats. *Proceedings of the Scientific Meeting of the American College of Veterinary Ophthalmologists*, vol. 18, pp. 22–30.

50. Priester, W.A. 1972. Congenital ocular defects in cattle, horses, cats, and dogs. *Journal of the American Veterinary Medical Association* 160:1504–1511.

51. Garner, A., and Griffiths, P. 1969. Bilateral congenital ocular defects in a foal. *British Journal of Ophthalmology* 53:513–517.

52. Dziezyc, J., Kern, T., and Wolf, D. 1983. Microphthalmia in a foal. *Equine Veterinary Journal Supplement* 2:15–17.

53. Walde, I. 1983. Some observations on congenital cataracts in the horse. *Equine Veterinary Journal Supplement* 2:27–28.

54. Eriksson, K. 1995. Hereditary aniridia with secondary cataract in horses. *Nordisk Veterinaermedicin* 7:773–793.

55. Joyce, J. 1983. Aniridia in a Quarter horse. *Equine Veterinary Journal Supplement* 2:21–22.

56. Beech, J., Aguirre, G., and Gross, S. 1984. Congenital nuclear cataracts in the Morgan horse. *Journal of the American Veterinary Medical Association* 184:1363–1365.

57. Matthews, A., and Handscombe, M. 1983. Bilateral cataract formation and subluxation of the lenses in a foal: A case report. *Equine Veterinary Journal Supplement* 2:23–24.

58. Detlefson, J. 1920. The inheritance of congenital cataract in cattle. *American Naturalist* 54:277–280.

59. Gregory, P., Mead, S., and Regan, W. 1943. A congenital hereditary eye defect of cattle. *Journal of Heredity* 34:125–128.

60. Gelatt, K.N. 1971. Cataracts in cattle. *Journal of the American Veterinary Medical Association* 159:195–200.

61. Leipold, H.W., Gelatt, K.N., and Huston, K. 1971. Multiple ocular anomalies and hydrocephalus in grade beef Shorthorn cattle. *American Journal of Veterinary Research* 32:1019–1026.

62. Gelatt, K.N., and Mackay, E.O. 2005. Prevalence of primary breed-related cataracts in the dog in North America. *Veterinary Ophthalmology* 8:101–111.

63. Ling, G.V., Lowenstine, L.J., Pulley, L.T., and Kaneko, J.J. 1977. Diabetes mellitus in dogs: A review of initial evaluation, immediate and long-term management, and outcome. *Journal of the American Veterinary Medical Association* 170:521–530.

64. Schaer, M. 1977. A clinical survey of thirty cats with diabetes mellitus. *Journal of the American Animal Hospital Association* 13:23–27.

65. Williams, D.L., and Heath, M.F. 2006. Prevalence of feline cataract: Results of a cross-sectional study of 2000 normal animals, 50 cats with diabetes and one hundred cats following dehydrational crises. *Veterinary Ophthalmology* 9:341–349.

66. Beam, S., Correa, M.T., and Davidson, M.G. 1999. A retrospective-cohort study on the development of cataracts in dogs with diabetes mellitus: 200 cases. *Veterinary Ophthalmology* 2:169–172.

67. Kinoshita, J.H. 1974. Mechanisms initiating cataract formation. Proctor lecture. *Investigations in Ophthalmology* 13:713–724.

68. Richter, M., Guscetti, F., and Spiess, B. 2002. Aldose reductase activity and glucose-related opacities in incubated lenses from dogs and cats. *American Journal of Veterinary Research* 63:1591–1597.

69. Sato, S., Takahashi, Y., Wyman, M., and Kador, P.F. 1991. Progression of sugar cataract in the dog. *Investigative Ophthalmology & Visual Science* 32:1925–1931.

70. Wyman, M., Sato, S., Akagi, Y., Terubayashi, H., Datiles, M., and Kador, P.F. 1988. The dog as a model for ocular manifestations of high concentrations of blood sugars. *Journal of the American Veterinary Medical Association* 193:1153–1156.

71. Fukushi, S., Merola, L.O., and Kinoshita, J.H. 1980. Altering the course of cataracts in diabetic rats. *Investigative Ophthalmology & Visual Science* 19:313–315.

72. Kinoshita JH. 1986. Aldose reductase in the diabetic eye. XLIII Edward Jackson memorial lecture. *American Journal of Ophthalmology* 102:685–692.

73. Kador, P.F., Webb, T.R., Bras, D., Ketring, K., and Wyman, M. 2010. Topical KINOSTAT ameliorates the clinical development and progression of cataracts in dogs with diabetes mellitus. *Veterinary Ophthalmology* 13:363–368.

74. Goldman, H. 1929. Experimentelle tetaniekatarakt. *Albrecht von Graefes Archiv für Ophthalmologie* 122:146.

75. Kornegay, J., Greene, C., Martin, C., Gorgacz, E., and Melcon, D. 1980. Idiopathic hypocalcemia in four dogs. *Journal of the American Animal Hospital Association* 16:723–734.

76. Vainisi, S.J., Edelhauser, H.F., Wolf, E.D., Cotlier, E., and Reeser, F. 1981. Nutritional cataracts in timber wolves. *Journal of the American Veterinary Medical Association* 179:1175–1180.

77. Glaze, M., and Blanchard, G. 1983. Nutritional cataracts in a Samoyed litter. *Journal of the American Animal Hospital Association* 19:951–954.

78. Martin, C., and Chambreau, T. 1982. Cataract production in experimentally orphaned puppies fed a commercial replacement for bitch's milk. *Journal of the American Animal Hospital Association* 18:115–119.

79. Remillard, R.L., Pickett, J.P., Thatcher, C.D., and Davenport, D.J. 1993. Comparison of kittens fed queen's milk with those fed milk replacers. *American Journal of Veterinary Research* 54:901–907.

80. Ralston, S., Isherwood, J., Chandler, M., Poffenbarger, E., Severin, G., and Olson, P. 1990. Evaluation of growth rates and cataract formation in orphan puppies fed two milk replacer formulas. *Conference on Veterinary Perinatology in Conjunction with the Neonatal Society*, Cambridge, England, p. 56.

81. Hughes, S.G., Riis, R.C., Nickum, J.G., and Rumsey, G.L. 1981. Biomicroscopic and histologic pathology of the eye in riboflavin deficient rainbow trout (Salmo gairdneri). *Cornell Veterinarian* 71:269–279.

82. Ketola, H.G. 1979. Influence of dietary zinc on cataracts in rainbow trout (Salmo gairdneri). *British Journal of Nutrition* 109:965–969.

83. Poston, H.A., Riis, R.C., Rumsey, G.L., and Ketola, H.G. 1977. The effect of supplemental dietary amino acids, minerals and vitamins on salmonids fed cataractogenic diets. *Cornell Veterinarian* 67:472–509.

84. Poston, H.A., and Rumsey, G.L. 1983. Factors affecting dietary requirements and deficiency signs of L-tryptophan in rainbow trout. *British Journal of Nutrition* 113:2568–2577.

85. Braus, B.K., Tichy, A., Featherstone, H.J., Renwick, P.W., Rhodes, M., and Heinrich, C.L. 2017. Outcome of phacoemulsification following corneal and lens laceration in cats and dogs (2000–2010). *Veterinary Ophthalmology* 20:4–10.

86. Gookin, J.L., Riviere, J.E., Gilger, B.C., and Papich, M.G. 1999. Acute renal failure in four cats treated with paromomycin. *Journal of the American Veterinary Medical Association* 215:1821–1823.

87. Martin, C.L. 1975. The formation of cataracts in dogs with disophenol: Age susceptibility and production with chemical grade, 2,6-diiodo-4-nitrophenol. *The Canadian Veterinary Journal* 16:228–232.

88. Martin, C.L., Christmas, R., and Leipold, H.W. 1972. Formation of temporary cataracts in dogs given a disophenol preparation. *Journal of the American Veterinary Medical Association* 161:294–301.

89. Schiavo, D.M. 1976. Reversible lenticular aberrations in Beagle dogs given diazoxide intravenously. *Veterinary Medicine, Small Animal Clinician* 71:190–195.

90. Rubin, L.F., and Mattis, P.A. 1966. Dimethyl sulfoxide: Lens changes in dogs during oral administration. *Acta Agriculturae Scandinavica Section A Animal Science* 153:83–84.

91. Smith, E.R., Mason, M.M., and Epstein, E. 1969. The ocular effects of repeated dermal applications of dimethyl

sulfoxide to dogs and monkeys. *Journal of Pharmacology and Experimental Therapeutics* 170:364–370.

92. Gerson, R.J., MacDonald, J.S., Alberts, A.W. et al. 1990. On the etiology of subcapsular lenticular opacities produced in dogs receiving HMG-CoA reductase inhibitors. *Experimental Eye Research* 50:65–78.

93. da Costa, P.D., Merideth, R.E., and Sigler, R.L. 1996. Cataracts in dogs after long-term ketoconazole therapy. *Veterinary and Comparative Ophthalmology* 6:176–180.

94. Zhan, G.L., Miranda, O.C., and Bito, L.Z. 1992. Steroid glaucoma: Corticosteroid-induced ocular hypertension in cats. *Experimental Eye Research* 54:211–218.

95. Brown, D.G., Magrane, W.G., Cross, F.H., and Reynolds, R.A. 1972. Clinical observations of eyes of cattle, swine, and burros surviving exposure to gamma and mixed neutron-gamma radiation. *American Journal of Veterinary Research* 33:309–315.

96. Jamieson, V., Davidson, M., Nasisse, M., and English, R. 1991. Ocular complications following cobalt 60 radiotherapy of neoplasms in the canine head region. *Journal of the American Animal Hospital Association* 27:51–55.

97. Roberts, S.M., Lavach, J.D., Severin, G.A., Withrow, S.J., and Gillette, E.L. 1987. Ophthalmic complications following megavoltage irradiation of the nasal and paranasal cavities in dogs. *Journal of the American Veterinary Medical Association* 190:43–47.

98. Lipman, R.M., Tripathi, B.J., and Tripathi, R.C. 1988. Cataracts induced by microwave and ionizing radiation. *Survey of Ophthalmology* 33:200–210.

99. Brightman, A., Brogdon, J., Helper, L., and Everds, N. 1984. Electric cataracts in the canine: A case report. *Journal of the American Animal Hospital Association* 20:895–898.

100. Poulos, Jr., P. 1966. Selenium-tocopherol treatment of senile lenticular sclerosis in dogs (four case reports). *Veterinary Medicine, Small Animal Clinician* 61:986–988.

101. Brooksby, L.O. 1979. A practitioner's experience with selenium-tocopherol in treatment of cataracts and nuclear sclerosis in the dog. *Veterinary Medicine, Small Animal Clinician* 74:301–302.

102. Brainard, J., Hanna, C., and Petursson, G. 1982. Evaluation of superoxide dismutase (orgotein) in medical treatment of canine cataract. *Archives of Ophthalmology* 100:1832–1834.

103. MacMillian, A., Nelson, D., and Munger, R. 1986. A comparison of zinc ascorbate versus saline placebo in the treatment of canine cataracts. *Proceedings of the Scientific Meeting of the American College of Veterinary Ophthalmologists and International Society of Veterinary Ophthalmology* 17:484.

104. Yakely, W.L., and Filby, R.H. 1971. Selenium in the lens of the dog. *Journal of the American Veterinary Medical Association* 158:1561–1565.

105. Cotlier, E. 1983. Aspirin and senile cataract in rheumatoid arthritis. *Lacet* 1:338–339.

106. Gupta, S.K., Joshi, S., Velpandian, T., and Varma, S.D. 1997. Protection against cataract by pyruvate and its ocular kinetics. *Annals of Ophthalmology* 29:243–248.

107. Mares-Perlman, J.A., Lyle, B.J., Klein, R. et al. 2000. Vitamin supplement use and incident cataracts in a population-based study. *Archives of Ophthalmology* 118:1556–1563.

108. Seddon, J., Christen, W., and Manson, J. 1991. Low-dose aspirin and risks of cataracts in a randomized trial of U.S. physicians. *Archives of Ophthalmology* 109:252–255.

109. West, S.K., Munoz, M.S., Newland, H.S., Emmett, E., and Taylor, H.R. 1987. Lack of evidence for aspirin use and prevention of cataracts. *Archives of Ophthalmology* 105:1229–1231.

110. Hankey, G., Richards, S. and Warlow, C. 1992. Does aspirin affect the rate of cataract formation? Cross-sectional results during a randomised double-blind placebo controlled trial to prevent serious vascular events. UK-TIA Study Group. *British Journal of Ophthalmology* 76:259–261.

111. Williams, D.L., and Munday, P. 2006. The effect of a topical antioxidant formulation including *N*-acetyl carnosine on canine cataract: A preliminary study. *Veterinary Ophthalmology* 9:311–316.

112. Rubin, L., and Gelatt, K. 1968. Spontaneous resorption of the cataractous lens in dogs. *Journal of the American Veterinary Medical Association* 152:139–152.

113. van der Woerdt, A., Wilkie, D.A., and Myer, C.W. 1993. Ultrasonographic abnormalities in the eyes of dogs with cataracts: 147 cases (1986–1992). *Journal of the American Veterinary Medical Association* 203:838–841.

114. van der Woerdt, A., Nasisse, M., and Davidson, M. 1990. Phacolytic uveitis in the dog: A retrospective study of 151 cases. *Proceedings of the Scientific Meeting of the American College of Veterinary Ophthalmologists*, vol. 21, p. 161.

115. Bagley II, L.H., and Lavach, J.D. 1994. Comparison of postoperative phacoemulsification results in dogs with and without diabetes mellitus: 153 cases (1991–1992). *Journal of the American Veterinary Medical Association* 205:1165–1169.

116. Good, K.L., Maggs, D.J., Hollingsworth, S.R., Scagliotti, R.H., and Nelson, R.W. 2003. Corneal sensitivity in dogs with diabetes mellitus. *American Journal of Veterinary Research* 64:7–11.

117. Forsyth, S.F., Ilkiw, J.E., and Hildebrand, S.V. 1990. Effect of gentamicin administration on the neuromuscular blockade induced by atracurium in cats. *American Journal of Veterinary Research* 51:1675–1678.

118. Plumb, D. 2002. *Veterinary Drug Handbook.* Iowa State Press: Ames, IA, pp. 77–78.

119. Nasisse, M., Davidson, M., Jamieson, V., English, R., and Olivero, D. 1991. Phacoemulsification and intraocular lens implantation: A study of technique in 182 dogs. *Progress In Veterinary & Comparative Ophthalmology* 1:225–232.

120. Gaiddon, J., Rosolen, S.G., Steru, L., Cook, C.S., Peiffer Jr., R. 1991. Use of biometry and keratometry for determining optimal power for intraocular lens implants in dogs. *American Journal of Veterinary Research* 52:781–783.

121. Murphy, C., Nasisse, M., Olivero, D., Brinkman, M., Campbell, L., and Hellkamp, A. 1991. Refractive state of the pseudophakic canine eye. *Proceedings of the Scientific Meeting of the American College of Veterinary Ophthalmologists*, 22, p. 95.

122. Peiffer, R., and Gaiddon, J. 1991. Posterior chamber intraocular lens implantation in the dog: Results of 65 implants in 61 patients. *Journal of the American Animal Hospital Association* 27:453–462.

123. Murphy, C.J., Mutti, D.O., Zadnik, K., and Ver Hoeve, J. 1997. Effect of optical defocus on visual acuity in dogs. *American Journal of Veterinary Research* 58:414–418.

124. Davidson, M., Nasisse, M., Jamieson, V., English, R., and Oliverso, D. 1991. Phacoemulsification and intraocular lens implantation: A study of surgical results in 182 dogs. *Progress In Veterinary & Comparative Ophthalmology* 1:233–238.

125. Davidson, M.G., Nasisse, M.P., Rusnak, I.M., Corbett, W.T., and English, R.V. 1990. Success rates of unilateral vs. bilateral cataract extraction in dogs. *Indian Journal of Veterinary Surgery* 19:232–236.

126. Knight, G.C. 1957. The extraction of dislocations and the cataractous crystalline lens of the dog with the object

of preserving some useful vision. *The Veterinary Record* 68:318.

127. Magrane, W.G. 1969. Cataract extraction: A follow up study (429 cases). *Journal of Small Animal Practice* 10:545–553.

128. Miller, T.R., Whitley, R.D., Meek, L.A., Garcia, G.A., Wilson, M.C., and Rawls Jr., B.H. 1987. Phacofragmentation and aspiration for cataract extraction in dogs: 56 cases (1980-1984). *Journal of the American Veterinary Medical Association* 190:1577–1580.

129. Rooks, R.L., Brightman, A.H., Musselman, E.E., Helper, L.C., and Magrane, W.G. 1985. Extracapsular cataract extraction: An analysis of 240 operations in dogs. *Journal of the American Veterinary Medical Association* 187:1013–1015.

130. Spreull, J.S., Chawla, H.B., and Crispin, S.M. 1980. Routine lens extraction for the treatment of cataract in the dog. *Journal of Small Animal Practice* 21:535–554.

131. Startup, F.G. 1967. Cataract surgery in the dog. II. Published results. *Journal of Small Animal Practice* 8:671–674.

132. Paulsen, M., Lavach, J., Severin, G., and Eichenbaum, J. 1986. The effect of lens-induced uveitis on the success of extracapsular cataract extraction: A retrospective study of 65 lens removals in the dog. *Journal of the American Animal Hospital Association* 22:49–56.

133. Startup, F.G. 1967. Cataract surgery in the dog. 3. Factors responsible for failure. *Journal of Small Animal Practice* 8:675–679.

134. Biros, D.J., Gelatt, K.N., Brooks, D.E. et al. 2000. Development of glaucoma after cataract surgery in dogs: 220 cases (1987–1998). *Journal of the American Veterinary Medical Association* 216:1780–1786.

135. Nasisse, M., Davidson, M., English, R., Roberts, S., and Newman, H. 1990. Neodymium: YAG laser treatment of lens extraction-induced pupillary opacifications in dogs. *Journal of the American Animal Hospital Association* 26:275–281.

136. Apple, D.J., Solomon, K.D., Tetz, M.R. et al. 1992. Posterior capsule opacification. *Survey of Ophthalmology* 37:73–116.

137. Hollick, E.J., Spalton, D.J., Ursell, P.G. et al. 1999. The effect of polymethylmethacrylate, silicone, and polyacrylic intraocular lenses on posterior capsular opacification 3 years after cataract surgery. *American Journal of Ophthalmology* 106:49–54.

138. Hayashi, H., Hayashi, K., Nakao, F., and Hayashi, F. 1998. Quantitative comparison of posterior capsule opacification after polymethylmethacrylate, silicone, and soft acrylic intraocular lens implantation. *Archives of Ophthalmology* 116:1579–1582.

139. Ram, J., Apple, D.J., Peng, Q. et al. 1999. Update on fixation of rigid and foldable posterior chamber intraocular lenses. Part II: Choosing the correct haptic fixation and intraocular lens design to help eradicate posterior capsule opacification. *American Journal of Ophthalmology* 106:891–900.

140. Hollick, E.J., Spalton, D.J., and Meacock, W.R. 1999. The effect of capsulorrhexis size on posterior capsular opacification: 1-year results of a randomized prospective trial. *American Journal of Ophthalmology* 128:271–279.

141. Zaturinsky, B., Naveh, N., Saks, D., and Solomon, A.S. 1990. Prevention of posterior capsular opacification by cryolysis and the use of heparinized irrigating solution during extracapsular lens extraction in rabbits. *Ophthalmic Surgery* 21:431–434.

142. Bras, I.D., Colitz, C.M., Saville, W.J., Gemensky-Metzler, A.J., and Wilkie, D.A. 2006. Posterior capsular opacification in diabetic and nondiabetic canine patients following cataract surgery. *Veterinary Ophthalmology* 9:317–327.

143. Schmidt, G.M., and Vainisi, S.J. 2004. Retrospective study of prophylactic random transscleral retinopexy in the Bichon Frise with cataract. *Veterinary Ophthalmology* 7:307–310.

144. Braus, B.K., Rhodes, M., Featherstone, H.J., Renwick, P.W., and Heinrich, C.L. 2012. Cataracts are not associated with retinal detachment in the Bichon Frise in the UK–A retrospective study of preoperative findings and outcomes in 40 eyes. *Veterinary Ophthalmology* 15:98–101.

145. Pryor, S.G., Bentley, E., McLellan, G.J. et al. 2016. Retinal detachment postphacoemulsification in Bichon Frises: A retrospective study of 54 dogs. *Veterinary Ophthalmology* 19:373–378.

146. Johnstone, N., and Ward, D.A. 2005. The incidence of posterior capsule disruption during phacoemulsification and associated postoperative complication rates in dogs: 244 eyes (1995–2002). *Veterinary Ophthalmology* 8:47–50.

147. Lannek, E.B., and Miller, P.E. 2001. Development of glaucoma after phacoemulsification for removal of cataracts in dogs: 22 cases (1987–1997). *Journal of the American Veterinary Medical Association* 218:70–76.

148. Gerardi, J.G., Colitz, C.M., Dubielzig, R.R., and Davidson, M.G. 1999. Immunohistochemical analysis of lens epithelial-derived membranes following cataract extraction in the dog. *Veterinary Ophthalmology* 2:163–168.

149. Taylor, M.M., Kern, T.J., Riis, R.C., McDonough, P.L., and Erb, H.N. 1995. Intraocular bacterial contamination during cataract surgery in dogs. *Journal of the American Veterinary Medical Association* 206:1716–1720.

150. Chitkara, D.K., Manners, T., Chapman, F., Stoddart, M.G., Hill, D., and Jenkins, D. 1994. Lack of effect of preoperative norfloxacin on bacterial contamination of anterior chamber aspirates after cataract surgery. *British Journal of Ophthalmology* 78:772–774.

151. Beigi, B., Westlake, W., Mangelschots, E., Chang, B., Rich, W., and Riordan, T. 1997. Peroperative microbial contamination of anterior chamber aspirates during extracapsular cataract extraction and phacoemulsification. *British Journal of Ophthalmology* 81:953–955.

152. Manners, T.D., Turner, D.P., Galloway, P.H., and Glenn, A.M. 1997. Heparinised intraocular infusion and bacterial contamination in cataract surgery. *British Journal of Ophthalmology* 81:949–952.

153. Gilger, B.C., Davidson, M.G., and Colitz, C.M. 1998. Experimental implantation of posterior chamber prototype intraocular lenses for the feline eye. *American Journal of Veterinary Research* 59:1339–1343.

154. Gilger, B.C., Davidson, M.G., and Howard, P.B. 1998. Keratometry, ultrasonic biometry, and prediction of intraocular lens power in the feline eye. *American Journal of Veterinary Research* 59:131–134.

155. Gelatt, K.N., Myers Jr., V.S., and McClure Jr., J.R. 1974. Aspiration of congenital and soft cataracts in foals and young horses. *Journal of the American Veterinary Medical Association* 165:611–616.

156. Dziezyc, J., Millichamp, N., and Keller, C. 1991. Use of phacofragmentation for cataract removal in horses:

12 cases (1985–1989). *Journal of the American Veterinary Medical Association* 198:1774–1778.

157. Millichamp, N.J., and Dziezyc, J. 2000. Cataract phacofragmentation in horses. *Veterinary Ophthalmology* 3:157–164.

158. Gemensky-Metzler, A.J., Bras, I.D., Colitz, C.M., Wilky, D.A., and Klages, D.C. 2004. Clinical features and outcomes of phacoemulsification in 39 horses: A retrospective study (1993–2003). *Proceedings of the 35th Annual Conference of the American College of Veterinary Ophthalmologists*, vol. 35, p. 30.

159. Lassaline, M.E., Plummer, C.E., Brooks, D.E., Kallberg, M.E., and Gelatt, K.N. 2005. Phacofragmentation for acquired cataracts in adult horses. *Proceedings of the 36th Annual Conference of the American College of Veterinary Ophthalmologists*, vol. 36, p. 41.

160. Brooks, D.E., Plummer, C.E., Carastro, S.M., and Utter, M.E. 2014. Visual outcomes of phacoemulsification cataract surgery in horses: 1990–2013. *Veterinary Ophthalmology* 17(Suppl. 1):117–128.

161. Edelmann, M.L., McMullen Jr., R., Stoppini, R., Clode, A., and Gilger, B.C. 2014. Retrospective evaluation of phacoemulsification and aspiration in 41 horses (46 eyes): Visual outcomes vs. age, intraocular lens, and uveitis status. *Veterinary Ophthalmology* 17(Suppl. 1):160–167.

162. van der Woerdt, A., Stades, F.C., van der Linde-Sipman, J.S., and Boevé, M.H. 1995. Multiple ocular anomalies in two related litters of Soft Coated Wheaten Terriers. *Veterinary and Comparative Ophthalmology* 5:78–82.

163. Curtis, R., and Barnett, K.C. 1980. Primary lens luxation in the dog. *Journal of Small Animal Practice* 21:657–668.

164. Curtis, R., Barnett, K.C., and Lewis, S.J. 1983. Clinical and pathological observations concerning the aetiology of primary lens luxation in the dog. *The Veterinary Record* 112:238–246.

165. Formston, C. 1945. Observations on subluxation and luxation of the crystalline lens in the dog. *Journal of Comparative Pathology* 55:168–184.

166. Lawson, D.D. 1969. Luxation of the crystalline lens in the dog. *Journal of Small Animal Practice* 10:461–463.

167. Willis, M.B., Curtis, R., Barnett, K.C., and Tempest, W.M. 1979. Genetic aspects of lens luxation in the Tibetan terrier. *The Veterinary Record* 104:409–412.

168. Foster, S., Curtis, R., and Barnett, K. 1986. Primary lens luxation in the Border Collie. *Journal of Small Animal Practice* 27:1–6.

169. Glover, T.L., Davidson, M.G., Nasisse, M.P., and Olivero, D.K. 1995. The intracapsular extraction of displaced lenses in dogs: A retrospective study of 57 cases (1984–1990). *Journal of the American Animal Hospital Association* 31:77–81.

170. Lazarus, J.A., Pickett, J.P., and Champagne, E.S. 1998. Primary lens luxation in the Chinese Shar Pei: Clinical and hereditary characteristics. *Veterinary Ophthalmology* 1:101–107.

171. Gould, D., Pettitt, L., McLaughlin, B. et al. 2011. ADAMTS17 mutation associated with primary lens luxation is widespread among breeds. *Veterinary Ophthalmology* 14:378–384.

172. Barnett, K.C., and Cottrell, B.D. 1987. Ehlers–Danlos syndrome in a dog: Ocular, cutaneous, and articular abnormalities. *Journal of Small Animal Practice* 28:941–946.

173. Curtis, R. 1983. Aetiopathological aspects of inherited lens dislocation in the Tibetan Terrier. *Journal of Comparative Pathology* 93:151–163.

174. Morris, R.A., and Dubielzig, R.R. 2005. Light-microscopy evaluation of zonular fiber morphology in dogs with glaucoma: Secondary to lens displacement. *Veterinary Ophthalmology* 8:81–84.

175. Olivero, D., Riis, R., Dutton, A., Murphy, C., Nasisse, M., and Davidson, M. 1991. Feline lens displacement: A retrospective analysis of 345 cases. *Progress In Veterinary & Comparative Ophthalmology* 1:239–244.

176. Chavkin, M., Lappin, M., and Powell, C. 1992. Seroepidemiologic and clinical observations of 93 cases of uveitis in cats. *Progress In Veterinary & Comparative Ophthalmology* 2:29–36.

177. Binder, D.R., Herring, I.P., and Gerhard, T. 2007. Outcomes of nonsurgical management and efficacy of demecarium bromide treatment for primary lens instability in dogs: 34 cases (1990–2004). *Journal of the American Veterinary Medical Association* 231:89–93.

178. Montgomery, K.W., Labelle, A.L., and Gemensky-Metzler, A.J. 2014. Trans-corneal reduction of anterior lens luxation in dogs with lens instability: A retrospective study of 19 dogs (2010–2013). *Veterinary Ophthalmology* 17:275–279.

179. Hamming, N.A., and Apple, D. 1980. In: *Principles and Practice of Ophthalmology*. Vol. 1. G. Peyman, D. Sanders, M. Goldberg, editors. WB Saunders, Philadelphia, p. 9.

180. Hogan, M., Alvarado, J., and Weddell, J. 1971. *Histology of the Human Eye*. WB Saunders, Philadelphia.

181. Stades, F. 1983. Development of the vitreous and related (vascular) structures in persistent hyperplastic tunica vasculosa lentis and persistent hyperplastic primary vitreous (PHTVL/PHPV) in the Doberman Pinscher. Utrecht p. 12.

VITREOUS AND OCULAR FUNDUS

EVA ABARCA

VITREOUS

Anatomy and physiology

The vitreous is the largest of the ocular structures, occupying the space bounded anteriorly by the lens and the zonules and peripherally by the ciliary body, the retina, and the optic nerve (**Figure 14.1**). The vitreous is a transparent, elastic hydrogel consisting of 99% water, while approximately 1% of the vitreous consists of a network of collagen fibrils and hyaluronic acid. The vitreous has very few cells, with the normal cellular components being hyalocytes, which originates from blood macrophages and are mainly (hyalocytes) that originate from the blood.[1] Most of the hyalocytes are located in the peripheral vitreous near the ciliary body.[1] Noncross-linked type II collagen fibers make up the framework, and hydrated hyaluronic acid polymers fill the spaces.[2] Hyaluronic acid is responsible for the viscosity of the vitreous, and the relative amounts of collagen and hyaluronic acid determine whether the vitreous is in a gel or a fluid state. These polymers are negatively charged, thus causing expansion of the gel. The addition of positively charged ions causes the vitreous gel to collapse due to the neutralization of the repulsive negative charges.[3] Hyaluronic acid is produced by the hyalocytes and is in highest concentration in the peripheral vitreous.[4]

Embryologically and anatomically, the vitreous is divided into primary, secondary, and tertiary vitreous.

- **Primary vitreous** is the first tissue to develop between the primitive lens and the inner layer of the optic cup. It consists of ectodermal components and the mesodermal origin hyaloid artery system that supplies the fetal lens (see Chapter 13, **Figure 13.6**). The primary vitreous is surrounded (begins about 25 days post fertilization) by the newer secondary vitreous of neuroectoderm origin, which is the majority of the postnatal vitreous.[5,6] The primary vitreous regresses with further development but is still demonstrable in normal animals as a clear narrow central tunnel, which is called Cloquet's canal. In the young animal, the tunnel is straight but sags with growth, developing a sinusoidal curve (**Figure 14.1**).[7]

- **Secondary vitreous** forms as the fetal fissure closes and the primitive hyalocytes produce collagen fibrils. The secondary vitreous is most firmly attached to the peripapillary region, the peripheral retina/ora ciliaris retinae, and the posterior lens capsule. The peripheral attachment is called the vitreous base. The lenticular attachment is the hyaloideocapsular ligament (Wieger's ligament), and this is relatively firm in the dog and the cat, making intracapsular lens extraction difficult without vitreous loss. The major portion of the vitreous face is easily separated from the retina. The secondary vitreous is divided into the peripheral cortical vitreous and the central vitreous. In the dog and the cat, the cortical vitreous is fluid, and the central vitreous is dense.[8,9]

- **Tertiary vitreous** is the zonular system that maintains the lens in place.

The vitreous plays an important role in growth of the eye, ocular metabolism, and mechanical role. The vitreous provides both mechanical and structural support to the lens and the retina, making the vitreous the most important intraocular tissue in the pathogenesis of retinal detachment.[10,11] The vitreous has been demonstrated to have a substance(s) that inhibits angiogenesis.[12] A lack of this antiangiogenic factor may be responsible for the lack of regression and overgrowth of the tunica vasculosa lentis in some breeds of dogs, for example, the Doberman pinscher.[13] Healthy vitreous is a relatively transparent structure. The vitreous cavity should be assessed for the presence of opacities, membranes, or mass-like structures. Diseases of the vitreous cavity include hemorrhage, inflammation (endophthalmitis), membrane formation, vitreal degeneration, and, less frequently, embryologic remnants.

DISEASES OF THE VITREOUS

Developmental disorders

The involution and disappearance of the primary vitreous is somewhat variable in time. In the young pup or the kitten, the course of the hyaloid artery is straight and

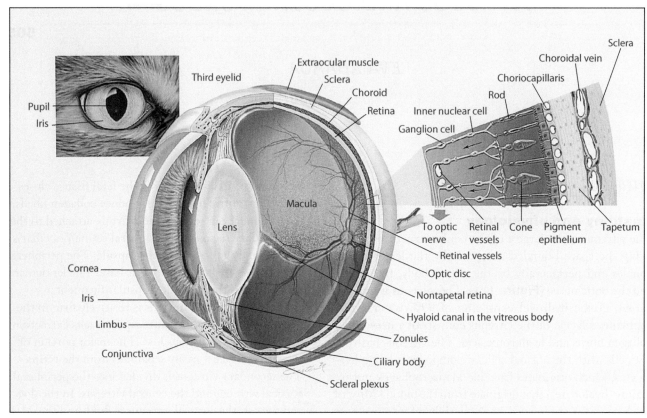

Figure 14.1 Schematic eye of a cat. Note the sinusoidal hyaloid or Cloquet's canal traversing the vitreous from the optic nerve to the back of the lens.

continuous between the optic nerve and the lens, and occasionally it may be patent and contain blood. The closure of the hyaloid artery in Beagle pups usually occurs between 5–17 days postpartum.[14] Munroe found an intact hyaloid artery in the majority of foals up to 4 days of age, and Koch et al. found remnants up to 30 days.[15,16] Blood was often present in the hyaloid artery in the first neonatal day, but only one foal had blood in the artery 2 days after birth.[16,17] A persistent hyaloid artery has been found in 54% of calves aged 6 weeks of age.[18]

With the normal development growth of the eye and involution of the hyaloid artery system, the artery is disrupted, and only the anterior extremity is noted in the sinuous-shaped Cloquet's canal. The anterior extremity is routinely observed as a white dot (Mittendorf's dot) just behind the lens capsule and ventral to the junction of the posterior cortical sutures.[19] Mild glial proliferation on the surface of the disc from incomplete involution of the hyaloid artery is termed Bergmeister's papilla and can be frequently observed as incidental clinical finding in dogs. In ruminants such as the cow (**Figure 14.2**) and sheep, Bergmeister's papilla is routinely visualized as a gray, translucent linear structure protruding from the center of the optic disc into the vitreous cavity.[20]

Persistent hyaloid artery (PAH)

While small remnants of the anterior extremity of the hyaloid artery are a normal finding, some dogs retain a very dense, white, straight hyaloid artery. This trait is

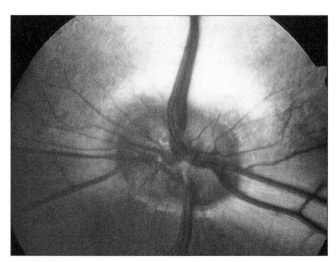

Figure 14.2 Bovine fundus with a dark nonmyelinated oval disc. Note a pinkish white proliferation at the confluence of the retinal vessels that is the remnant of the hyaloid artery (Bergmeister's papilla).

common in Australian shepherd dogs in Australia and has no known clinical significance.[21] Retention of remnants of the tunica vasculosa lentis may be evidenced by small, white, linear or dot opacities or pigmented dots on the posterior capsule, with no opacity in the lens.

Persistent hyperplastic tunica vasculosa lentis/persistent hyperplastic primary vitreous (PHTVL/PHPV)

Persistent hyperplastic primary vitreous (PHPV) is also discussed in Chapter 13.

PHTVL/PHPV may occur secondary to other developmental disorders or may be due to a spontaneous failure of vascular regression associated with proliferative changes that are fibrovascular or fibrous in nature (hyperplastic).[22] These may manifest in the anterior and/or posterior extremity of the hyaloid system. This condition has been described as an inherited trait in the Doberman pinscher, Staffordshire bull terrier, and Bouvier de Flandres. In these breeds, PHTVL/PHPV typically affects the anterior portion of the hyaloid system.[5,6,23,24]

Anterior hyperplastic changes are recognized as axial posterior capsular cataracts with vessels intermixed. Posterior hyperplastic changes are usually recognized by their association with anterior PHPV and manifest with proliferative changes on the optic disc (papillary) or adjacent to the optic disc (peripapillary) (**Figure 14.3**).[22] The condition may be unilateral or bilateral and may be accompanied by persistence of the tunica vasculosa lentis.

PHPV/PHTVL is rare in the cat but has been reported without indication of it being an inherited trait.[25]

Clinical signs
- Mild: Pigmented dots and linear streaks on the posterior lens capsule. The hyaloid artery may be

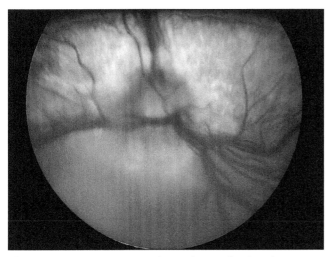

Figure 14.3 Posterior persistent hyperplastic primary vitreous in a poodle.

prominent and may contain blood (see Chapter 13, **Figure 13.26**).
- Moderate: Posterior axial subcapsular cataract, posterior lenticonus, retained hyaloid artery, and possibly vitreal hemorrhage may occur. The ciliary processes may rarely be elongated and visible in the pupil.[26]
- Severe: Extensive cataract, lenticonus, hemorrhage into the lens, lens coloboma, extensive pigment on posterior capsule, and extensive fibrovascular membrane on or adjacent to the optic disc may be present (**Figure 14.3**). Hyphema, uveitis, and secondary glaucoma may be severe complications of PHPV.[27]

Therapy
Therapy is not usually necessary in mild-to-moderate cases, except to advise on the genetic implications. If ultrasound is not routinely performed on all cataract patients, the surgeon may not be aware of PHPV/PHTVL before surgery. If cataract surgery is performed on the severe manifestations of PHPV, a posterior capsulectomy with vitrectomy and coagulation of the hyaloid artery may be necessary.[28] In this situation, the prognosis is less favorable than in routine cataract surgery due to the risk of complications.[27]

Miscellaneous conditions

Several congenital vitreal anomalies of unknown significance have been observed including abnormal vitreal development and vitreous syneresis (a liquefied vitreous) with Collie eye anomaly, in microphthalmic eyes with retinal dysplasia of the Bedlington terrier, and in retinal dysplasia–skeletal dysplasia in Labrador retrievers.[7,29–31] Congenital vitreal syneresis is probably more common than is reported. Pronounced vitreal veils are noted in some individuals, particularly in miniature Schnauzers, Italian greyhounds, and many brachycephalic breeds. The significance of vitreal degeneration is unknown at this time, but ophthalmologists are concerned about an association with lens instability and/or retinal detachments.

Acquired diseases
Vitreal hemorrhage
Introduction/etiology
Vitreous hemorrhage may be produced by or be associated with a number of conditions including systemic hypertension, hyperviscosity syndrome, inflammation, blunt or perforating trauma, neoplasia, clotting disorders, and vascular lesions such as congenital malformations.[32–34] Hemorrhage into formed vitreous results in clots that remain for extended periods of time, whereas if the vitreous is liquefied, the hemorrhage will become diffuse (**Figure 14.4a**). The blood exerts a destructive effect on

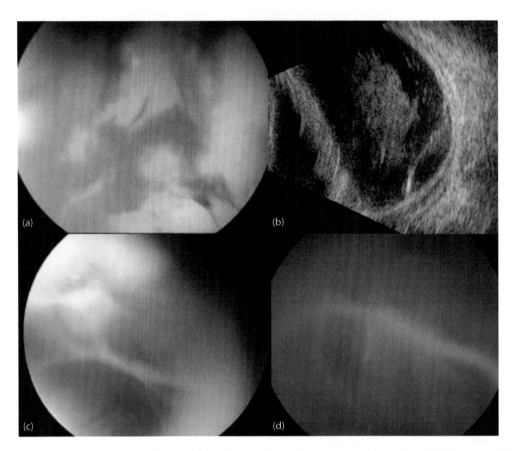

Figure 14.4 (a) funduscopy view; Vitreal hemorrhage (flame shape in appearance) in a dog. (b) Ultrasound image (10 MHz). Vitreous hemorrhage appears in this eye as a well-organized low reflective echogenic area within the posterior vitreous cavity; a partial retinal detachment is noted as a linear hyperechoic line. (c and d) Multifocal areas of chronic vitreal hemorrhage in two canine patients. The vitreous contains old well-organized vitreal hemorrhage forming membranous surfaces within the vitreous cavity. (a and b Courtesy of E. Abarca, Auburn University. c and d Courtesy of GA. Garcia, Oftalvet)

the gel structure, resulting in liquefaction and collapse of vitreal strands around the hemorrhage that can exhibit movement within the vitreous cavity.[32] Hemoglobin and iron stimulate macrophage migration into the vitreous to phagocytize hemosiderin after cellular hemolysis.[35] The low-grade inflammation is an additional stimulation for glial cell migration into the vitreous through small breaks in the inner limiting membrane of the retina. Müller's cells, retinal astroglial cells, and retinal pigment epithelium (RPE) are additional sources of cells that can produce fibrous membranes (**Figure 14.4c,d**).[36] If the membrane is attached to the retina, contraction of the membrane results in traction and subsequent detachment.

> The course and resolution of vitreal hemorrhage is very difficult to predict. The prognosis should be guarded because contractile forces during the resolution of clots may produce retinal detachments.

Clinical signs

Decreased vision may be noted if significant bilateral hemorrhage occurs. As little as 12.5 μL of blood in 5 mL decreases vision in humans to hand motions or worse.[37] The hemorrhage is recognized as red clots suspended in the vitreous (**Figure 14.4**) or diffuse redness if the vitreous is liquefied. Clots gradually shrink and turn to a gray residue in the vitreous. Ultrasonic evaluation of the vitreous cavity for the presence of inflammatory opacities, membranes, retinal detachment, and foreign body is especially important when the inflammatory response precludes visualization of the posterior segment.[38,39] Vitreous hemorrhage appearance on ultrasound depends on its age and its severity. In fresh, mild hemorrhage, dots and short lines of low-reflective mobile vitreous opacities are displayed. The more dense the hemorrhage, the greater the number of opacities and the higher their reflectivity. In more severe older hemorrhages, blood organizes and forms membranous surfaces on B-scan (**Figure 14.4b**).[38,39]

Therapy

Medical therapy depends on the underlying cause; however, the medical treatment is of no known value for vitreal hemorrhage. In humans, vitrectomy or removal of the vitreous is performed for vitreal hemorrhage and membrane formation. However, in veterinary medicine, because of the accompanying ocular lesions or the underlying cause, vitrectomy is rarely performed for vitreal hemorrhage.

Degenerative diseases

Vitreal degeneration

The term "vitreous degeneration" is used to indicate changes that are consistent with breakdown of the vitreous hydrogel.[40] Vitreal degeneration is a vague term used to describe changes in the vitreous, ranging from strands of vitreous appearing in the anterior chamber to increased membranes and disorganized membranes floating in the anterior vitreous that is often liquefied. The variation in the appearance of the anterior vitreous between breeds of dogs and between various age groups can be quite striking. Vitreous herniation into the anterior chamber is thought to indicate zonular defects and to be a risk factor for subsequent lens displacement. While finding vitreal strands in the anterior chamber is obviously not normal, the predictive value for future lens displacement has yet to be proven.

Signs of vitreous degeneration include liquefaction (e.g., syneresis) or opacities (e.g., vitreous "floaters," asteroid hyalosis, and synchysis scintillans).[40] The variation in the appearance of the anterior vitreous between breeds of dogs and between various age groups is noticeable. Vitreous degeneration, especially mild vitreal syneresis (liquefaction), is not uncommon in normal dogs; that has been shown to be an age-related condition.[41] The probability of having vitreous degeneration increased with the age of the dog (odds ratio = 6.7 for dogs of 7+ years compared with 0–6 years) and also increased in females compared with males (odds ratio = 3.6).[41]

Syneresis

Liquefaction of the vitreous can result from a degenerative change that increases with age, inflammation, hemorrhage, or as a part of a congenital syndrome (Collie eye anomaly). A common complication of this progressive liquefaction is the separation of the posterior vitreous (vitreal detachment) in humans. Vitreal diseases are poorly understood in the dog; however, it is known that vitreous liquefaction predisposes to retinal detachment (RD), especially in certain breeds, including the Shih Tzu, Brussels Griffon, Chihuahua, Chinese Crested dog, Havanese, Italian greyhound, Löwchen, Papillon, and Whippet.[40–43]

Vitreal opacities

Asteroid hyalosis Asteroid hyalosis is a degenerative condition in which white spherical particles (asteroid bodies) are suspended in the vitreous of one or both eyes (**Figure 14.5**).[44] With ocular movement, they vibrate, but the bodies do not completely settle out in the ventral vitreous when the eye is motionless. The incidence increases with age, and the condition is bilateral in about 50% of patients. While there was no correlation with specific ocular disease, 33 of 40 dogs (82%) with asteroid hyalosis had lesions of the posterior ocular segment.[45,46] The density of the bodies may cause the fundus to be somewhat hazy, but signs referable to the asteroid hyalosis are unusual. Severe asteroid hyalosis is a common finding when evaluating older and diabetic cataract patients with ultrasound. Poor visual performance has been observed after cataract surgery on animals with asteroid hyalosis; this improved after vitrectomy. Asteroid hyalosis is not responsible for the "fly biting" syndrome in the dog.

Asteroid bodies are liquid crystals composed of calcium and phospholipids.[44,47] Therapy is not necessary in the vast majority of patients.

Synchisis scintillans Synchisis scintillans is a rare condition characterized by multiple cholesterol crystals that gravitate ventrally in a liquefied vitreous and disperse with movement of the eye. The crystals have been associated with vitreal hemorrhage, retinal atrophy, and posterior uveitis.[48] It should be differentiated from the more common condition of asteroid hyalosis.

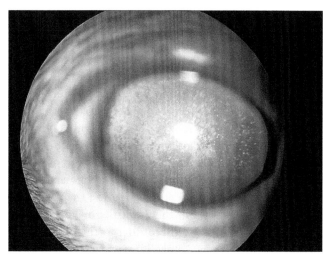

Figure 14.5 Severe asteroid hyalosis in a dog viewed through a dilated pupil. This can be differentiated from cataractous changes by the vibration of the spherical bodies with ocular movement and their position behind the lens.

Other diseases

Inflammation of the vitreous (hyalitis)

Introduction/etiology

Hyalitis or vitritis is part of any endophthalmitis and may be sterile or septic. Primary hyalitis may occur with penetrating injuries or postsurgically, and it can in turn spread to the retina and uvea. Cellular infiltration of the vitreous produces a hazy appearance and results in an inability to focus sharply on the fundus during ophthalmoscopy. Focal hyalitis is common over any active area of retinal or optic nerve head inflammation, particularly if infectious in origin. If septic endophthalmitis is suspected, the vitreous is a more reliable source for culturing than the aqueous humor due to the high turnover rate of fluid in the aqueous humor.

Clinical signs

Loss of vision is common with hyalitis. Episcleral injection is intense. Hyalitis is recognized biomicroscopically by the presence of cells and haze in the anterior vitreous. Cells in the anterior vitreous are differentiated by color and size. Pigmented cells are noted by color and large size, erythrocytes by their color and small uniform size, and leukocytes by their intermediate size and uniformity.

Therapy

Adequate drug levels are very difficult to achieve in the vitreous because of its inert nature. If septic hyalitis is suspected, high levels of antibiotics that penetrate the blood–aqueous humor barrier and intravitreal injection of antibiotics are indicated. Surgical removal of the vitreous combined with intravitreal antibiotics may be employed in veterinary ophthalmology as in human ophthalmology.

Aberrant parasitic migrations

Different parasite migration may affect the vitreous, including *Dirofilaria immitis* (see Chapter 11, **Figure 11.44**), *Angiostrongylus vasorum*,[49] *Echinoccus* sp. *Toxocara canis* larvae,[50] and various fly larvae (ophthalmomyiasis interna posterior),[51] especially *Cuterebra* spp. (order Diptera).

Ophthalmomyiasis can be divided into external and internal infestations, with the internal form subdivided into anterior and posterior types depending on the region of the eye affected. Ocular invasion has been reported in cattle, sheep, horses, deer, cats, dogs, and humans.[52] The host reaction to the larval presence varies; therefore, the ocular signs also vary. The therapy, either medical and/or surgical, should be chosen according to the ocular signs observed in the presence of the intraocular parasite.[52,53]

OCULAR FUNDUS

The ocular fundus is composed of the retina, the choroid, and the optic nerve head (ONH). Direct and indirect

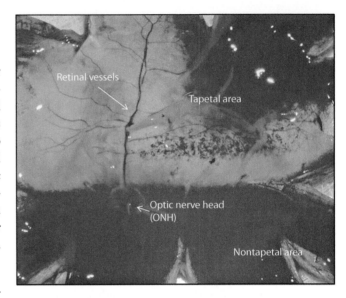

Figure 14.6 Picture of an anatomical specimen of a cow fundus depicting the four major structures that should be evaluated in funduscopy (tapetal area, nontapetal area, optic nerve head, and retinal vessels). (Courtesy of E. Abarca, Auburn University.)

ophthalmoscopy are both used in veterinary ophthalmology to visualize the fundus (**Figure 14.6**). Examination of the fundus is a great clinical tool; however, it is the most challenging aspect of the complete ophthalmic exam for most practitioners. Normal funduscopy appearance can be highly variable and is influenced by the animal's species, breed, age, and coat color. The major fundic structures as viewed from inner to outer are: retina, choroid (which includes the tapetum), and sclera (**Figure 14.7**). The healthy neuroretina is transparent with the exception of the retinal blood vessels and minor reflections off the internal limiting membrane. "Outer" refers to locations

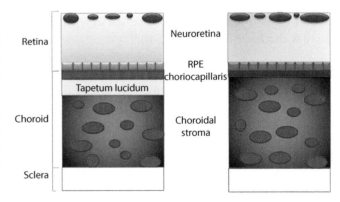

Figure 14.7 Schematic drawing representing the major fundic structures as viewed from inner to outer are: Retina, choroid, and sclera. Note the differences between the tapetal and nontapetal area. (E. Abarca, Auburn University.)

closer to the sclera, and "inner" refers to locations closer to the vitreous body.

Anatomy and physiology

Retina

The retina is composed of the neurosensory retina (neuro-retina) and the retinal pigment epithelium (RPE) (**Figure 14.7**). The RPE is usually pigmented in all areas except where it overlies the tapetum. Normal variations in RPE pigmentation contribute to the ability to visualize underlying choroid in normal variations of the fundic appearance. The retinal histology is classically divided into 10 layers, nine of which are the neurosensory retina and the tenth being the RPE. The original embryonic optic vesicle space is the potential space between the neurosensory retina and the RPE, and it is loosely adherent. Retinal detachment is essentially retinal separation between the neurosensory retina and the RPE. The retina of the puppy or the kitten is immature at birth, reaching maturity histologically and by electroretinography (ERG) 6–9 weeks postnatally.[54-58]

The neurosensory retina is composed of the outer photoreceptor layer (rod and cone inner and outer segments), external limiting membrane, outer nuclear layer (nuclei of rods and cones), outer plexiform layer (synapses between the photoreceptors and inner nuclear layer), inner nuclear layer (contains the nuclei of amacrine cells, horizontal cells, bipolar cells, and Müller's cells), inner plexiform layer (synapses of inner nuclear layer to the ganglion cells), ganglion cell layer, nerve fiber layer (axons of ganglion cells), and the internal limiting membrane (**Figure 14.8**).[54]

Photoreceptors, rods and cones, have different morphology and retinal distribution. Several rods are connected to a single ganglion cell (convergence or summation), which makes them more sensitive to changes in light levels and detection of motion but results in poor visual resolution. Cones have less convergence so that one cone may affect one ganglion cell, which results in more discrimination. Cones are responsible for high-resolution and color vision (**Figure 14.1**, insert). Rods greatly outnumber cones, although the ratio varies with the location in the retina. The *area centralis* is a specialized region in carnivores similar to the *fovea* present in birds and humans. This region is responsible for the highest visual resolution of the animal. In the *area centralis* in carnivores, the cones are at their highest concentration but are still outnumbered by rods (11:1). The periphery of the retina has a ratio of 65:1 to 100:1 of rods to cones, although the absolute number of rods may be less than in the central retina.[60,61] Rods are used in dim light (scotopic vision) and cones for daylight (photopic vision), discrimination, and color vision.

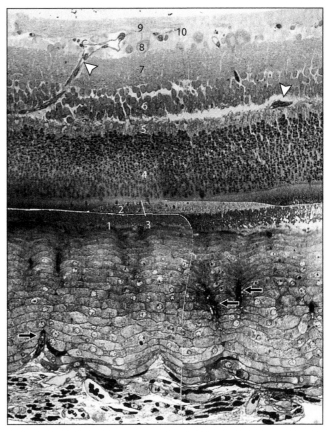

Figure 14.8 **Montage of kitten retina and inner choroid. (C: Choroid with numerous blood vessels and melanocytes; T: Tapetal cells, arrows point to capillaries penetrating tapetum; 1: Retinal pigment epithelium [not pigmented over the tapetum]; 2: Layer of rods and cones; 3: External limiting membrane; 4: External nuclear layer; 5: External plexiform layer; 6: Internal nuclear layer; 7: Internal plexiform layer; 8: Ganglion cell layer; 9: Nerve fiber layer; 10: Internal limiting membrane; arrowheads indicate retinal blood vessels.) (1 μm section ×175.) (From Martin, C., and Anderson, B. 1981. In: Gelatt, K., editor. *Veterinary Ophthalmology*, 1st edition. Lea & Febiger: Philadelphia, PA, pp. 88, 92, 98.)**

The double membrane discs of the outer segments of the rods and the cones contain the photopigments (**Figure 14.9**). Four types of photopigments may be present in species with color vision: three in the cones with peak absorption sensitivity at blue, green, and red wavelengths, and rhodopsin in the rods. Most animals have two cone populations, called dichromatic vision. The photopigment's main function is transduction, or converting light energy into a neurologic electrical signal. Rhodopsin, the most studied form of the photopigments, consists of a vitamin A aldehyde (retinal) and a glycoprotein (opsin). The photoactive form is 11-cis-retinal. Light striking the 11-cis isomer (peak absorption is 500 nm or dark green

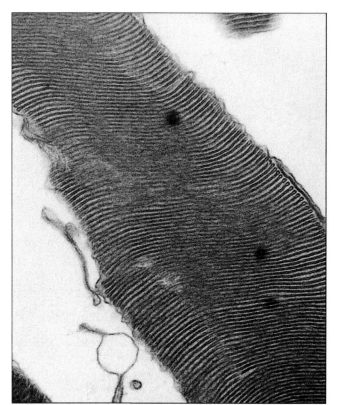

Figure 14.9 Canine rod outer segment composed of disks or lamella that are separated from each other. (From Martin, C., and Anderson, B. 1981. In: Gelatt, K., editor. *Veterinary Ophthalmology*, 1st edition. Lea & Febiger: Philadelphia, PA, pp. 88, 92, 98.)

light) converts it to the all-trans isomer through a series of unstable conformational changes, which are the earliest events in transduction. Light is only necessary for the first step, and energy is not necessary for this transformation. The final step is the separation of the retinal from the opsin and the reduction of retinal to retinol (alcohol) (**Figure 14.10**).[62]

Regeneration of active rhodopsin does require energy and takes place mostly in the RPE, although a small amount of regeneration occurs in the outer segments. Retinol is stored in the RPE as an ester. The photoreceptors in the dark are maintained in a depolarized state by being permeable to sodium and pumping out calcium. Activation of the photopigment alters the calcium pump so that calcium accumulates in the cytoplasm; it in turn alters the channels for sodium leakage, blocking sodium influx, and resulting in hyperpolarization (increased intracellular electronegativity).

RPE cells are hexagonal and are loosely adherent to the photoreceptors. They have occluding junctions between them that act as the blood–retinal barrier for the outer half of the retina against diffusion of substances or drugs from the very leaky underlying choriocapillaris.[63] The

RPE does not contain melanin granules over the tapetum or in individuals with an albinotic fundus. The function of the pigment is not certain but has been postulated to act as a scavenger for free radicals, to minimize light reflection between photoreceptors, and to absorb and convert light energy into heat.[64] One of the functions of the RPE is to phagocytize the shedding discs of the distal rod and cone outer segments. This serves to conserve vitamin A and polyunsaturated lipids. As a by-product of this process, lipofuscin accumulates in the RPE. The discs of the rods and the cones are produced at the base of the outer segment. Older ones are shed and phagocytized at the distal or scleral end, so that every 6 days, there is a turnover of the entire average canine outer rod segment.[65,66] This shedding and production of new discs is cyclic and requires a photoperiod. The period of most intense shedding for the rods is at the beginning of the light cycle (morning), and for the cones, it is at the beginning of the dark cycle (night or sleep).[67] The RPE is important in collecting and storing vitamin A from the blood for future use in the photoreceptors. It also actively takes up taurine and fatty acids from the blood.

There are two sources of blood supply to the mammalian retina: Retinal blood vessels and choroidal blood vessels. Retinal vessels are autoregulated or unaffected by moderate changes in perfusion pressure and have tight cellular vascular junctions, unlike the leaky uveal vasculature. The retinal endothelium is part of the blood–retinal barrier for the inner half of the retina. In general, when they are present, the retinal vessels supply nutrition to the inner half of the retina. The retinal vascular pattern has been categorized into holangiotic, in which the entire retinal surface receives a direct blood supply (cat, dog, cow, sheep); merangiotic, in which the vessels are localized laterally and medially to the peripapillary region (rabbit); paurangiotic, where the vessels are limited to the immediate peripapillary region (horse, guinea pig); and anangiotic, in which retinal blood vessels are absent (certain rodents, bat, armadillo, sloth, birds).[68]

Choroid

The choroid is the posterior portion of the uveal tract (vascular tunic). The main function of the choroid is to provide nutritional support to the retina, and it is composed mainly of pigment and blood vessels disposed in different layers (**Figure 14.1** insert and **Figure 14.7**): The choroidal stroma with large blood vessels, stroma with medium-sized blood vessels, and finally the choriocapillaris. In some species, a tapetum lucidum is present between the choroidal stroma and the choriocapillaris. The vascular beds are supplied mainly by the short and long posterior ciliary arteries that enter around the optic

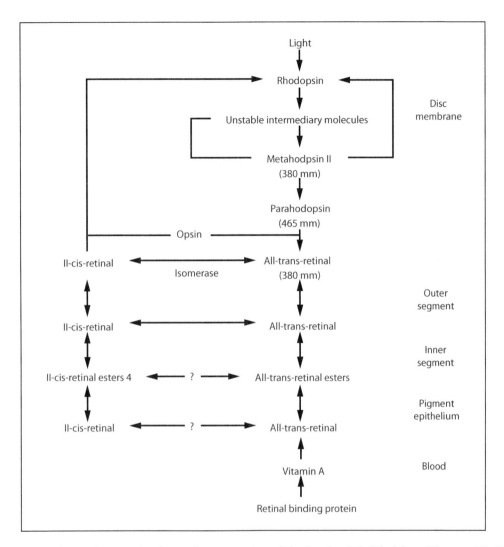

Figure 14.10 Proposed steps in transduction and regeneration of rhodopsin. (Modified from Marmor, M. 1980. In: Peyman, G., Sanders, D., and Goldberg, M., editors. *Principles and Practice of Ophthalmology*. WB Saunders: Philadelphia, PA, pp. 823–856.)

nerve and end in the choriocapillaris that lies just under the RPE. The choriocapillaris supplies nutrition by diffusion to the outer half of the retina. The choroidal capillaries are fenestrated in contrast to the nonfenestrated retinal capillaries; however, the diffusion of substances from the choroid is obstructed by the tight junctions of the RPE. The venous system is freely anastomotic and drains anteriorly via the vortex veins and posteriorly around the optic nerve to the orbital veins (see Chapter 11, **Figure 11.2**). Sensory nerves have been demonstrated in the choroid.[59]

The tapetum lucidum is a reflective structure that is present in most domestic animals except in the pig and birds. It is located in the dorsal one-half to one-third of the choroid and lies just external to the choriocapillaris (**Figure 14.7**). Its function is to reflect light back onto the photoreceptors to amplify light in dim or dark conditions.

Two forms of tapetum exist in domestic animals: A cellular form that is found in carnivores (**Figure 14.8**) and a fibrous form composed of collagenous fibers, that is found in ungulates (**Figure 14.11**). The color varies between individuals, and the pigment in the tapetum varies with the species. The fibrous tapetum is not pigmented; the color is due to the refraction of light. The cat has a high concentration of riboflavin in the tapetum, and the dog has a high concentration of zinc cysteine. Many fish have a tapetum with guanine as the pigment.[69] A more detailed review of the types of tapetum in various species can be found in Ollivier et al.[70]

Normal canine fundus

The first task, once the technique of ophthalmoscopy is mastered, is to understand the layers of the fundus (**Figure 14.7**) and to recognize normal variations in the fundus.

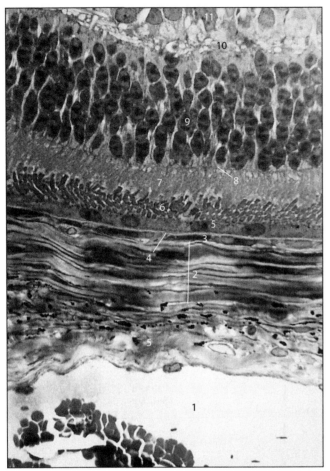

Figure 14.11 Inner choroid and outer retina of a young horse. Large choroidal veins (1) lie under the fibrous tapetum (2) that is separated from the outer retinal pigmented epithelium by the choriocapillaris (3) and Bruch's membrane (4). The pigment epithelium (5) contains very few pigment granules over the tapetum. (6: Photoreceptor outer segments; 7: Photoreceptor inner segments; 8: External limiting membrane; 9: Outer nuclear layer; 10: Outer plexiform layer; 11: Inner nuclear layer.) (×375) (From Martin, C., and Anderson, B. 1981. In: Gelatt, K., editor. *Veterinary Ophthalmology*, 1st edition. Lea & Febiger: Philadelphia, PA, pp. 88, 92, 98.)

This challenge of differentiating normal from abnormal is greatest in the dog, where there is an infinite variability. Even the experienced examiner may have difficulty in differentiating extremes in normal variation from mild pathologic changes.

For discussion purposes, the fundus is divided into tapetal area, optic disc, retinal blood vessels, and nontapetal area (**Figures 14.2 and 14.6**).

Tapetal area

In the adult dog, the tapetum is a brightly colored, right scalene triangle, with the right angle at top and the most

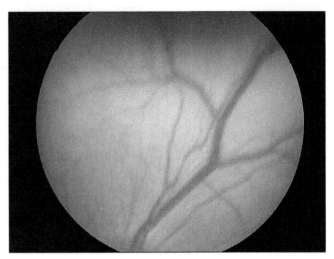

Figure 14.12 Future tapetal region in a 4-week-old puppy.

acute angle positioned nasally.[71] Its function is to stimulate twice the photoreceptors, increasing their light sensitivity.

The tapetum is a choroidal structure (localized between the choriocapillaris and the choroidal stroma) and develops after birth. Thus, adult coloration may not be present until 10–12 weeks of age. In the 4- to 5-week-old puppy, the tapetal region is a brownish to gray color (**Figure 14.12**) that changes to blue and violet colors at about 6–7 weeks (**Figure 14.13**), becoming adult in color by 3 months in most puppies (**Figure 14.14**).

The combination of the tapetum lucidum and the absence of pigment in the RPE are the anatomical basis for the tapetal area in contrast to the nontapetal area where the RPE is typically well pigmented (**Figure 14.7**).

The absence of a visible tapetum can be a normal variation and is most common in animals with blue irides or

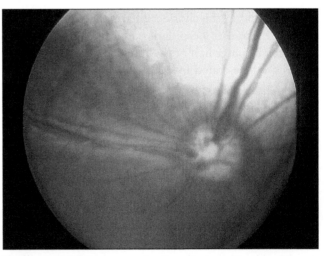

Figure 14.13 Immature fundus of a 6- to 7-week-old puppy with a blue-violet colored tapetum and a small incompletely myelinated optic disc.

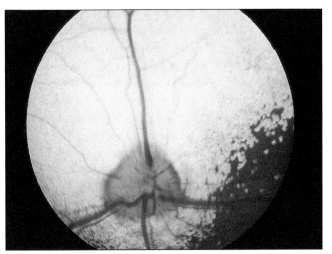

Figure 14.14 Adult canine fundus with a well-developed tapetum. This is a large breed of dog, and the disc is within the tapetum and is well myelinated, imparting a triangular shape and white color. Note the dark spot in the center of the disc. This is the physiologic pit.

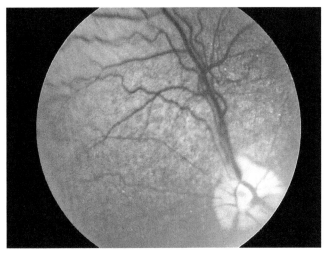

Figure 14.16 Canine fundus with a poorly developed tapetum represented by a few islands of color, but the overall area is gray or pigmented. This is common in breeds such as the Labrador retriever.

subalbinotic eyes. Subalbinotic eyes typically lack retinal and choroidal pigment (**Figure 14.15**). Conversely, pigment in the RPE and/or hypoplasia of the tapetum may obscure the view of the tapetum (**Figure 14.16**).

The tapetal coloration varies a great deal, with no correlation to coat color. The tapetum may have predominant hues of blue, green, yellow, or orange. The mosaic aspect of the tapetum varies from very uniform and homogeneous in texture (**Figure 14.17**) to being composed of individual beads or clumps of beads (**Figure 14.18**). The size of the tapetum varies with the size of the dog; larger dogs have a relatively larger tapetum, with

the optic disc being within the tapetum (**Figure 14.14**), whereas smaller dogs have a small tapetum, usually with the disc outside the tapetum.[68,71] The junction of the tapetal–nontapetal border is sharp in shorthaired dogs (**Figure 14.14**), whereas longhaired dogs have a transitional zone.

Changes in tapetal reflectivity, whether hyporeflective or hyperreflective, generally indicate pathology, although minor variations of normal may be seen. Conus is an area of hyperreflectivity around part or all of the optic disc and is considered normal. Hyperreflectivity of the tapetum is usually attributed to thinning of the overlying retina, the latter acting as a neutral density filter.

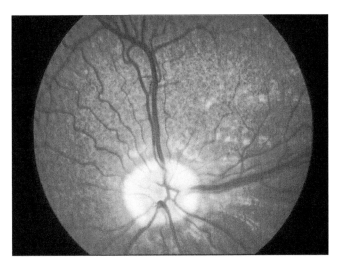

Figure 14.15 Normal canine subalbinotic fundus with an absence of tapetum and pigment. The dense choriocapillaris imparts the diffuse redness, although the white sclera can be observed in small patches. This dog will have blue irides.

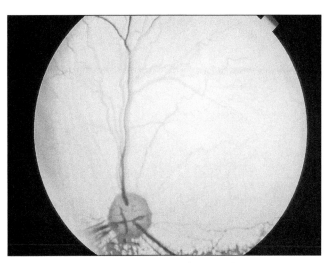

Figure 14.17 Canine fundus with a very homogeneous yellow tapetum. The optic disc has very little myelination and is "cat like."

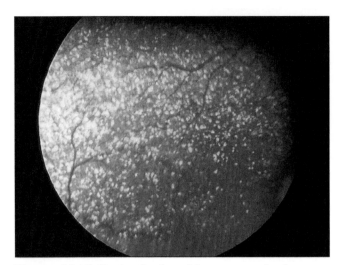

Figure 14.18 Canine fundus with a tapetum that is very granular, composed of individual yellow, green, and orange beads.

Optic nerve head (ONH)

The optic nerve head, disc, or papilla in the dog is routinely myelinated (**Figure 14.19**). The optic disc should be evaluated in color, shape, size, and position. Depending on the size of the tapetal area, the ONH can be located either the tapetal area, nontapetal area, or the junction between both of them (**Figures 14.14 and 14.20**). The disc of the dog has great variations in shape, elevation, and color due to the amount of myelination in individual animals. The color of the disc varies from white to pink. The added myelin may also give the disc an overlying white appearance instead of a pinkish-white color (**Figure 14.19**). The shape may be circular, triangular, or quadrangular. Myelin tends to follow the larger blood vessels on the disc (usually 3–4), and this may impart a triangular shape to the disc. Occasionally, myelin does extend more peripherally into the retina (myelinated nerve fibers). The disc is 1.5–2 mm in diameter and is located ventrotemporally to the anatomic axis. Extreme amounts of myelin may occur in large breed dogs and can produce marked elevation of the entire disc or the rim of the disc. In these individuals, it is difficult to detect mild papilledema.

A small dark spot, the physiologic pit, can be very prominent in the center of some discs, representing the remnant of the embryonic hyaloid artery system (**Figures 14.14 and 14.16**). Conus is an area of hyperreflectivity around part or all of the optic disc and is considered normal.

Retinal blood vessels

Canine retinal vasculature is classified as holangiotic. The retinal vasculature consists of arterioles and venules. The retinal vessels in domestic animals are cilioretinal (originate from short posterior ciliary or choroidal arteries) in origin, and a central retinal artery is absent. Retinal venules are wider and darker in color than the retinal arterioles. The largest vessels are the primary veins (two to five in number). Most dogs have three to four primary veins, and these have an anastomotic arc or a circle in the center of the disc (**Figures 14.15, 14.19, and 14.20**). The arc often appears to pulsate when under observation, but the pulsations do not correlate with the cardiac pulse. The pulsations are caused by the blanching of the vessels when increased pressure is placed on the globe during retraction of the eye into the orbit.

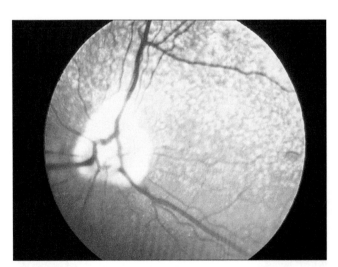

Figure 14.19 Canine ocular fundus with a well-myelinated optic disc. The disc is triangular, elevated around the rim from the myelin, and is more depressed in the center.

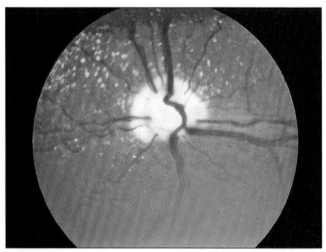

Figure 14.20 Canine ocular fundus. Note the optic disc is in the nontapetum, the presence of two primary veins dorsally, and the dark nontapetum that is lighter in a zone adjacent to the disc.

Secondary veins are the same size as the arterioles but can be differentiated by their origin from the anastomotic arc. The arterioles are up to 20 in number (but are usually 10–12), are small, and originate from the edge of the optic nerve (not the papilla due to the myelin). The arterioles are not paired with a vein as in some species. The tortuosity of the vessels, their size, and number varies greatly with age, breed, and family of dogs. The retinal capillaries extend to the interface of the outer plexiform layer and the inner nuclear layer.[72]

Nontapetal area

The ventral fundus area is called the nontapetal area where the cells in the RPE are well pigmented (**Figure 14.7**). In the ventral fundus, most dogs have fairly dense pigmentation of the RPE that in turn obscures visualization of the choroid and the sclera. Usually, the ophthalmoscope light needs to be brighter to see any detail in this region. The peripapillary region is often lighter and may have pigment disruption and clumping before merging into the more peripheral homogeneous darker nontapetal area (**Figure 14.20**).

Normal feline fundus

The feline fundus has much fewer variables than the canine fundus. The tapetum is usually present (**Figure 14.21**), except in blue-eyed, white-furred cats. The tapetum in the cat is large, with the optic disc always localized within it (**Figure 14.21**). The color of the tapetum can vary from yellow to blue to blue-green and does not have as much beadiness or mosaic appearance as is present in some dogs.

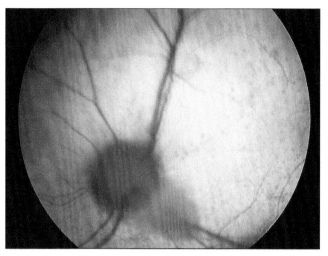

Figure 14.22 Myelination of the nerve fiber layer adjacent to the disc of a cat. This produces a blurred region that may be erroneously interpreted as inflammation.

The ONH IN cats is not myelinated. The myelination of the cat optic nerve stops at the lamina cribrosa, and thus, the optic disc does not have the variability in size, shape, and elevation that is present in dogs. The feline ONH is typically gray, small, and circular in shape.

Occasionally, myelination of the nerve fiber layer adjacent to the disc may be observed (**Figure 14.22**). Fine focusing on the surface often demonstrates a grid-like pattern that is the exposed lamina cribrosa. All blood vessels originate from the periphery of the disc. There are usually three pairs of primary arterioles and veins, with one pair dorsonasally that curves temporally, one pair ventronasally, and one pair ventrotemporally. A relatively avascular area is present 3–4 mm dorsotemporally from the optic disc, which represents the area centralis (**Figure 14.21**). Smaller vessels are present between the major pairs of vessels that supply the peripapillary region.[73,74]

> The variations in the normal dog and cat fundus are quite remarkable and often make it difficult to determine early pathology of the fundus. Despite the extreme variation, owners do not seem to detect any functional change in vision, that is, owners of atapetal dogs do not note nyctalopia in their dogs.

Normal variations in the normal dog and cat fundus

The large variation in normal fundus appearance, especially in the canine species, adds to the complexity in the differentiation between the normal and abnormal appearance. There are three main normal variations that are important to recognize: Tapetal hypoplasia, tigroid fundus, and subalbinotic fundus. The tigroid or subalbinotic

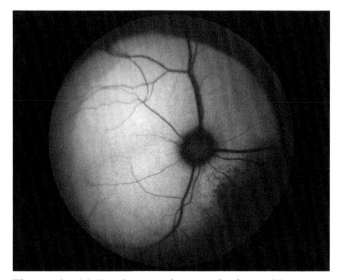

Figure 14.21 Funduscopy photograph of a cat. Note the disc is within the tapetum, the avascular area centralis dorsotemporal to the disc, and the pairing of arteries and veins. (E. Abarca, Auburn University.)

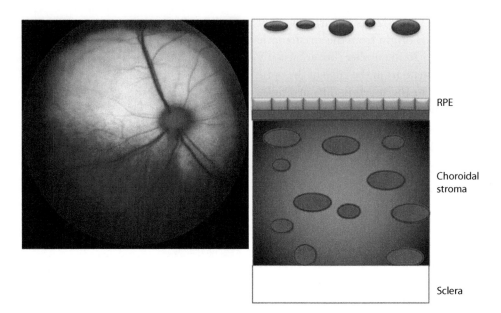

Figure 14.23 Tigroid nontapetal fundus typical for Siamese cats. Schematic drawing representing the lack of pigment in the RPE in the nontapetal area. Note the presence of a well-developed tapetum lucidum. Compare to Figure 14.26 from a white-furred blue-eyed cat. (E. Abarca, Auburn University.)

fundi are frequently misinterpreted as retinal hemorrhage or detachments.

Tapetum hypoplasia: In this variation, there is a partial lack of the tapetum, which can be represented just by a few islands of color (**Figure 14.16**).

Tigroid fundus: In this variation, there is a lack of RPE pigment in the nontapetal area (**Figure 14.23**), and the tapetum may or may not be present. This, combined with the pattern of the underlying choroidal vessels, imparts an orange color to the nontapetal area (**Figure 14.24**). This is a frequent variation in the Siamese cat.

Subalbinotic fundus: The absence of a visible tapetum can be a normal variation and is most common in animals with blue irides or subalbinotic eyes. Subalbinotic eyes typically lack retinal (RPE) and choroidal pigment, which gives a reddish appearance (**Figures 14.25 and 14.26**). This is due to the choroidal blood vessels, which in some cases can be clearly seen with white sclera visible between the vessels. The choroidal vessels are not as dark as the primary retinal veins.

Normal equine fundus

The horse has a paurangiotic fundus, with retinal vessels limited to the peripapillary region. The horse has about 50 vessels radiating in a kidney-shaped pattern 15 mm horizontally and 10 mm vertically (1–2 disc diameters). The arterioles cannot be distinguished from venules, and the vessels traverse only in the nerve fiber layer. The vessels all originate from just within the optic disc border. The optic disc is typically located in the nontapetal region,

ventrolateral to the posterior pole. The disc is pinkish-white in color, oval with the long axis horizontal, and cupped (**Figures 14.27 and 14.28**). The disc dimensions are 5–7 mm horizontally and 3.5–5 mm vertically. Foals have a more circular disc. Often a faint grid can be seen in the center, which is the lamina cribrosa. A narrow non-pigmented zone frequently partly surrounds the optic disc (**Figure 14.28**).

Horses typically have a blue-green tapetum with distinct fine dark spots (stars of Winslow), but the color may be more yellow to red (**Figures 14.27 and 14.28**). The most

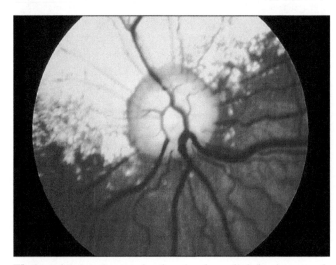

Figure 14.24 Canine fundus that has a lightly pigmented nontapetal area, which is typical for individuals with liver coat colors.

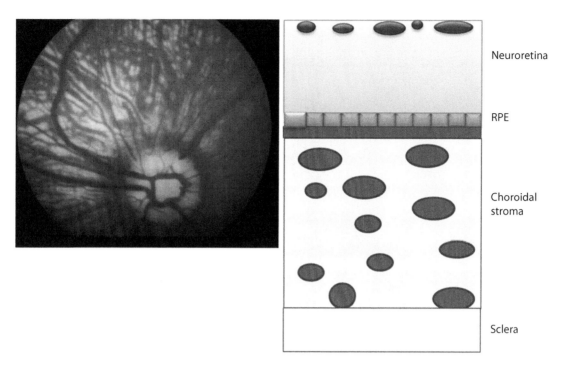

Neuroretina

RPE

Choroidal stroma

Sclera

Figure 14.25 Subalbinotic fundus. Schematic drawing representing the lack of pigment in retina and choroid typical of a subalbinotic fundus; sclera is visible. (E. Abarca, Auburn University.)

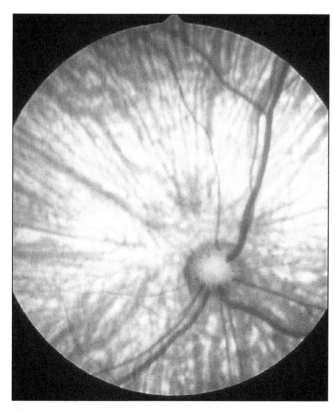

Figure 14.26 Normal subalbinotic fundus of a white-furred, blue-eyed cat. The sclera is visible between the choroidal veins. Note the small circular disc with the retinal blood vessels at the periphery of the disc.

common fundus variable is related to color-dilute animals that may lack part or all of a tapetum and have varying degrees of choroidal vasculature exposed (**Figures 14.29 and 14.30**).[75,76] While the optic nerve is myelinated, myelin does not typically extend to the intraocular portion of the nerve; however, excessive myelination occurs occasionally as a minor anomaly (**Figure 14.31**). A distinct ophthalmoscopically fovea is not present, but a linear horizontal band above the disc that parallels the lower edge of the tapetum is said to represent the area centralis, which

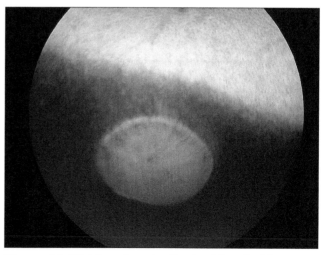

Figure 14.27 Normal equine fundus. Note the blue-green tapetum, which is the most common color, and the oval disc in the nontapetum with fine barely visible blood vessels.

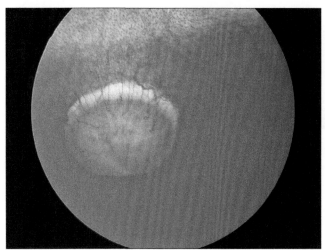

Figure 14.28 Normal equine fundus from a Palomino. Note the yellow tapetum and the retinal blood vessels are more easily visualized because the fundus is not as dark. A narrow white rim is present above the optic disc.

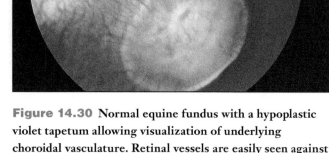

Figure 14.30 Normal equine fundus with a hypoplastic violet tapetum allowing visualization of underlying choroidal vasculature. Retinal vessels are easily seen against this background.

served as the area of maximum visual acuity.[68] The nontapetum is typically homogeneous dark brown, except in color dilute animals. The nontapetal peripapillary region is the frequent location for multifocal depigmented lesions.

Normal bovine and ovine fundus

The bovine eye has a holangiotic fundus. The bovine optic disc is oval with the long axis horizontal, and it is located in the nontapetal region, with the dorsal aspect just touching the tapetum. The average size is 4.2 × 3.5 mm; however, in bulls, the disc may be more circular. The optic disc is typically nonmyelinated, resulting in a dark color (**Figure 14.2**). The disc is cupped, and the veins originate from near the center. Three to four primary veins are present that are accompanied by arterioles. The dorsal pair of arterioles and veins is usually intertwined. The arterioles originate more peripherally on the disc. Fifteen to 20 smaller vessels originate from the disc and disappear 1–2 disc diameters away from the disc. The larger vessels are epiretinal (on the surface) rather than running in the nerve fiber layer. A gray spot in the center of the disc represents the remnant of the hyaloid

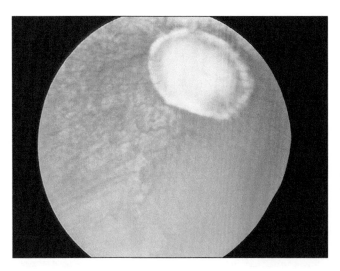

Figure 14.29 Normal equine fundus of a Palomino that has a slash of hypoplastic pigmentation of the retinal pigment epithelium and choroid that exposes the choroidal vasculature.

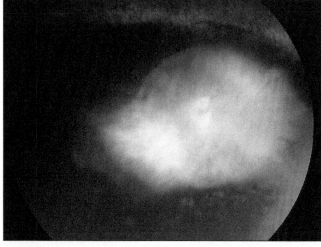

Figure 14.31 Excessive myelination of the optic nerve of a horse. The condition was bilateral, and it was found on a soundness examination where it may have created a question for the examiner.

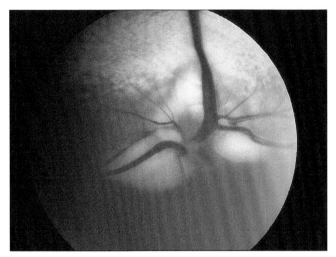

Figure 14.32 Myelination of the optic disc of a cow producing a dramatic departure from the normal dark, cupped disc. Compare to Figure 14.2.

artery or Bergmeister's papilla. In calves, the hyaloid vessel usually has blood present for several months.[20] Partial myelination of the optic disc may occasionally be observed (**Figure 14.32**).[77]

Tapetal colors vary but are usually dark green and stippled, with dark spots or stars of Winslow. Distinct pigment islands are frequently present in the nasal tapetal region and are bilateral. Albino cattle, like other species with subalbinotic eyes, variably have a tapetum, and the nontapetal region is tigroid with the choroidal vasculature visible against the sclera.[78]

The ovine fundus is similar to the cow, but the disc is kidney-shaped (**Figure 14.33**) with a hilus or indentation on the ventral surface. Myelinization of the optic nerve fibers normally stops at the lamina cribrosa.

DISEASES OF THE RETINA AND THE CHOROID

Congenital diseases

Coloboma

Introduction/etiology

A coloboma is a cup or pit-like tissue defect that is congenital and nonprogressive. Classically, colobomatous malformations involve failure of the optic fissure to close (cleft in the optic cup where the hyaloid vasculature gains entry into the fetal eye). Ocular colobomas most frequently involve the vascular tunic of the eye (iris and choroid). Unless extreme, colobomas are not accompanied by an appreciable loss of vision. They are classified as typical if located ventronasally at the 6-o'clock position (**Figure 14.34**) and are considered atypical if located elsewhere. Colobomas frequently involve the optic disc or the immediate region around the disc (peripapillary region) but may be located in the peripheral fundus (**Figure 14.35**).[79]

Coloboma manifests as a sharply circumscribed, usually pale, depigmented area with reduced or anomalous vasculature and is often cupped. Examples of inherited colobomatous defects are found in albino Herefords, Collie eye anomaly, Australian shepherd dogs (**Figure 14.35**), Basenji, and Charolais cattle.[78,80–82]

In the cat, multiple ocular colobomatous syndrome has been described in snow leopards and the domestic cat, and it has been associated with eyelid agenesis.[83,84] Posterior segment lesions include large choroidal colobomas, scleral

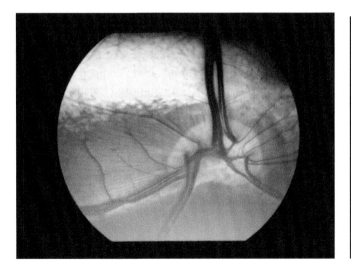

Figure 14.33 Normal ovine fundus with a kidney-shaped disc and Bergmeister's papilla under the venous arch. The striations in the nontapetal region are from the nerve fiber layer. (Picture E. Abarca.)

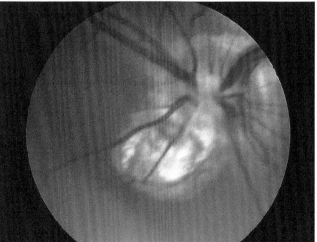

Figure 14.34 Typical coloboma found in a young calf. Note the white hyaloid artery remnant. The coloboma is cupped, as evidenced by the deviation of the vessel passing over the center.

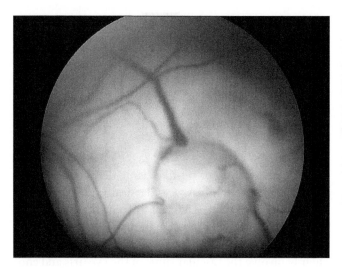

Figure 14.35 Intercalary staphyloma and coloboma in the far periphery of the fundus in an Australian shepherd dog. This is not the optic disc but a cupped lesion in the far periphery. Note the relative lack of choroidal vasculature and cilioretinal vessels emerging from the coloboma.

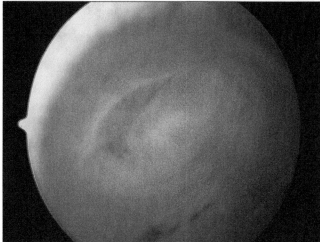

Figure 14.37 A 3-month-old quarter horse that has bilateral coloboma and optic nerve atrophy. The coloboma involves the disc and peridisc region and is cupped and avascular. The animal is blind.

ectasia, retinal dysplasia, and tapetum lucidum hypoplasia (**Figure 14.36**). Entire litters have been reported to be affected, with variable degrees of anomalies, but the cause is unknown.[84]

Colobomas of the choroid are relatively common among cattle. In Charolais cattle, the colobomas are inherited as a dominant trait, with complete penetrance in bulls and incomplete penetrance in cows (**Figure 14.34**).[82] Typical colobomas of the optic disc in Charolais cattle are bilateral, though not symmetrical.[85]

Posterior colobomas involving the optic nerve and the peripapillary region have been observed sporadically in the horse. Colobomas have been observed in the foal

(**Figure 14.37**) with dermoids and malformed third eyelids. No therapy is available except genetic counseling.[86]

Collie eye anomaly
Introduction/etiology
Collie eye anomaly (CEA) is a congenital, bilateral, inherited canine ocular disorder affecting the posterior segment of the eye. CEA is a pleomorphic syndrome, with variability in manifestation and severity of clinical lesions.[80,87,88] The two main ophthalmoscopic changes are regional choroidal hypoplasia and coloboma of the optic disc or adjacent areas. The disease can be complicated by secondary retinal detachment and intraocular hemorrhage.[87] CEA has been widely described in Collie breeds and less frequently in non-Collie breeds including Shetland sheepdog, Australian shepherd dog, Border Collie, Nova Scotia Duck Tolling retriever, Boykin spaniel, Longhaired Whippet, Lancashire Heeler, Hokkaido inu, and even in mixed breeds.[87,89–93]

The incidence in Collies has been reported to be 80% or higher in surveys in the United States,[94,95] 41% in Norway,[96] 13% in Austria,[97] and 32% in Switzerland.[98] The incidence in the Shetland sheepdog is much less in the United States, but it was 48% in one small series in the Netherlands.[91] Many studies have been performed to determine the mode of inheritance for this syndrome. Wallin-Hakanson et al. disputed the recessive mode of inheritance and postulated a polygenetic trait.[99–101] The authors additionally noted that mating of parents with colobomas resulted in smaller litter size. The primary phenotype of choroidal hypoplasia is a simple recessive gene (intronic deletion in NHEJ1) with almost complete penetrance. The responsible gene has been identified for

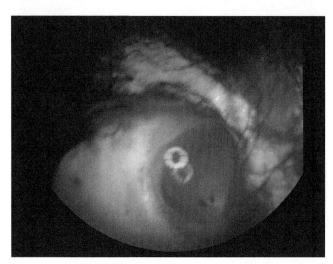

Figure 14.36 Posterior pole coloboma in a kitten with multiple ocular coloboma syndrome.

choroidal hypoplasia, and a DNA test is available for the previously mentioned breeds (http://www.://optigen.com/opt9_test). However, a recent study has shown that the deletion in NHEJ1 is not predictive for choroidal hypoplasia in the Danish Rough Collies.[102] Early studies found no relationship to sex or coat color.

Clinical signs

The two main ophthalmoscopic changes are regional choroidal hypoplasia and coloboma of the optic disc or adjacent areas, with partial or complete retinal detachment and intraocular hemorrhage being less frequently reported. While choroidal hypoplasia is a bilateral finding, colobomatous lesions are often asymmetrical.

Choroidal hypoplasia Choroidal hypoplasia is considered the diagnostic lesion for CEA. Choroidal hypoplasia is a variably sized, pale region located temporal to the disc. The pale area may be separated or confluent with the disc. It is a region of attenuated pigment in the choroid and the retina, with a thinned hypoplastic choroid and tapetum. The choroidal vasculature in this white area is decreased in density (**Figures 14.38 through 14.40**). Choroidal hypoplasia is essentially a static lesion, with the exception of the 4- to 5-week-old puppy. In the very young puppy, very mild degrees of choroidal hypoplasia can be observed as small breaks in the pigmentation temporal to the disc. By 6–8 weeks, these become pigmented and appear normal. These puppies are significant in that they later breed as affected (homozygous) individuals. Breeders refer to this condition as "go normal." In the blue merle Collie with a blue iris,

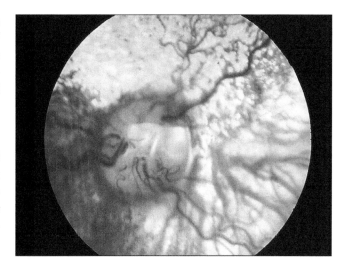

Figure 14.39 Collie eye anomaly with retinal vascular tortuosity, choroidal hypoplasia adjacent to the disc, and an oval pit or coloboma in the disc. The pit is a different color, has no vasculature, and has a vertical ridge.

the fundus is subalbinotic and mild-to-moderate choroidal hypoplasia is difficult or impossible to recognize with confidence. One study found that when examining puppies, all puppies with colobomas had choroidal hypoplasia, but in older dogs, 11 of 66 (17%) had colobomas without choroidal hypoplasia. This was thought to represent individuals who pigmented with age or the "go normal" population.[96]

Dogs that manifest with only choroidal hypoplasia have no visual disturbance and may function well as a pet, but they should not be used for breeding. Affected dogs, no matter how mild, are of course, genetically undesirable,

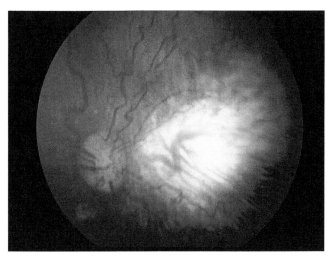

Figure 14.38 Collie eye anomaly in a 6-week-old puppy with moderate choroidal hypoplasia temporal to the disc and a small typical coloboma under the disc. Note the lack of pigment, hypoplastic choroidal vasculature, and tortuous retinal vessels.

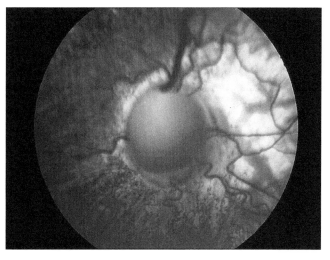

Figure 14.40 Collie eye anomaly with vascular tortuosity, choroidal hypoplasia, and a coloboma that involves the entire nerve head. Note the vessels originating from the edge of the anomalous disc.

but most breeders use mildly affected dogs. Some individuals will always "breed true" with mildly affected offspring, but others will produce litters with the entire range of lesions for CEA. Wallin-Hakanson et al. found that breeding Collies with choroidal hypoplasia increases the incidence of choroidal hypoplasia from 54% to 68%.[100,101] However, the prevalence of dogs with colobomas (8%) is not affected and, thus, is not compatible with a simple recessive gene for the entire CEA.

Posterior polar colobomas The colobomas may affect any portion of the optic nerve head (ONH) or involve the entire peripapillary region, resulting in the disc being positioned at the bottom of a large staphyloma (**Figures 14.41 and 14.42**). Other terms used with severe manifestations of coloboma involvement are posterior scleral ectasia and posterior staphyloma. These colobomas are usually classified as atypical colobomas in that they are not limited to the ventronasal region of the optic disc or peripapillary region.[103] Most colobomas are very evident on examination, but some are masked by glial tissue. Despite the frequent dramatic appearance, little or no visual deficits are noted. The disc is often misshaped and tilted. The vast majority of Collies with these colobomas also have choroidal hypoplasia but not the reverse. In breeds such as the Shetland sheepdog and German shepherd dog, colobomas may be observed without choroidal hypoplasia. About one-third of affected Collies in early surveys had colobomas, but this has decreased due to selective breeding.[94,95,104]

Retinal detachment Retinal detachment occurs in 4%–5% of affected eyes.[95,104] It may start as focal bullous detachment adjacent to a coloboma (**Figure 14.43**),

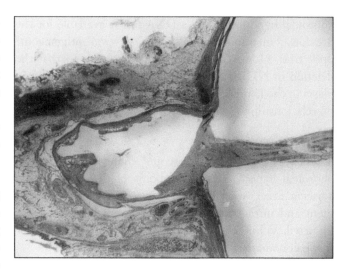

Figure 14.42 Histopathology of a Collie eye with a retinal detachment and a large optic nerve coloboma/posterior scleral ectasia such as in Figure 14.41.

but most are complete detachments with retinal dialysis or giant peripheral retinal tears (**Figure 14.44**). Detachment is present in most cases in the 6-week-old puppy and may represent retinal nonattachment. They are most often unilateral, but bilateral cases occur sporadically. Bullous detachment may progress to complete detachment or actually regress over a matter of months. Rhegmatogenous retinal detachment is associated with holes in the retina that allows fluid vitreous to gain access to the subretinal space.[105] CEA is asymptomatic in most instances, unless retinal detachments are present, and this is undoubtedly why the gene became so disseminated through the Collie population.

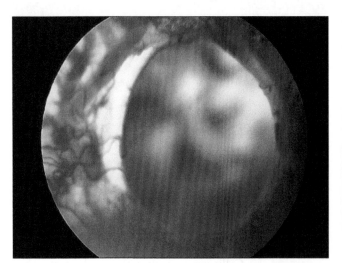

Figure 14.41 Collie eye anomaly with a large posterior scleral ectasia involving not only the optic disc but the peridisc region as well.

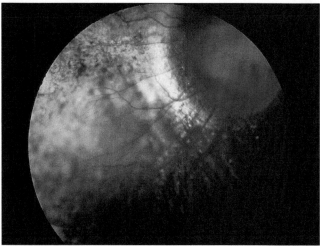

Figure 14.43 Collie eye anomaly with a optic nerve coloboma and a bullous detachment adjacent to the disc. The detachment is recognized by the slightly blurred background from subretinal fluid.

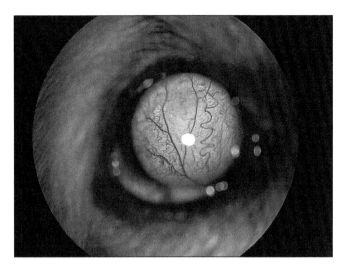

Figure 14.44 Collie puppy with a complete retinal detachment recognized by the presence of retinal blood vessels in focus through the pupil.

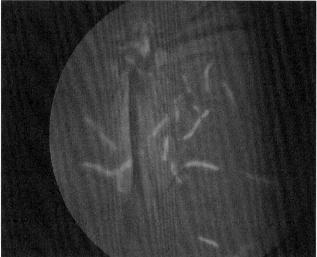

Figure 14.45 Vermiform folds or retinal folds in a Collie puppy.

Vitreal or anterior chamber hemorrhage may occur when the retina detaches. Vascular anomalies may also contribute to intraocular hemorrhage in some families of dogs. Ocular hemorrhage is not considered a basic part of the disease, rather a result of it.

Ancillary findings found in Collie puppies unrelated to CEA are tortuous retinal vasculature, opacities at the tips of the posterior lens sutures, band opacities on the cornea, and vermiform folds in the retina, all of which disappear with age. Vermiform folds (**Figure 14.45**) are curvilinear lines in the puppy retina, which represent folds that subsequently flatten out as the eye grows.

CEA is still very prevalent in the breed due to the continued breeding from dogs with choroidal hypoplasia. However, it is difficult to fault breeding from mildly affected dogs when the vast majority of the gene pool for the breed would be culled for a condition that only produces visual complaints or blindness in about 4%–5% of affected animals.

Diagnosis

Diagnosis is based on the clinical examination of young animals, and the preferred age of examination to detect mild cases of choridal hypoplasia ("go normals") is 5–7 weeks of age. A commercial mutation detection test has been developed, which helps identify the homozygous normal animals.[102]

Therapy

Therapy is not usually necessary. Mildly affected dogs with choroidal hypoplasia are bred by most breeders. Most dogs with mild-to-moderate colobomas will make acceptable pets with little risk of later vision problems.

Focal posterior bullous detachments associated with colobomas have been successfully treated by transpupillary laser retinopexy.[106] Occasional attempts at retinal detachment surgery have been reported[107–109] but are not performed routinely. Most cases presented in the advanced stages of detachment are not ideal candidates for surgery.

Retinal dysplasia

Introduction/etiology

Retinal dysplasia results from an abnormal differentiation of the primitive retinal tissue, which leads to disorganized development. Retinal dysplasia is a congenital or neonatal malformation that is characterized on histopathologic examination by rosettes, formed of tubules of primitive photoreceptors cut on cross section (**Figure 14.46**).[110]

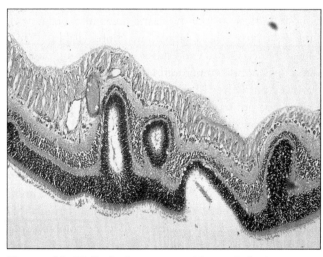

Figure 14.46 Retinal rosettes on histopathologic examination of a retinal detachment (H&E).

Table 14.1 *In utero* insults known to cause retinal dysplasia.

Trauma
Viral infection: Panleukopenia in the cat, BVD in cattle, blue tongue virus in sheep, parvovirus and herpesvirus infection in the dog
Radiation
Nutrition: Vitamin A deficiency
Drug toxicity: Antimitotic drugs
Inherited syndromes

The rosettes may be classified according to the number of cell layers from one to three. Three-layered rosettes are basically the normal retina which is thrown into a fold. The two- and single-layered rosettes represent abnormal differentiation of a more primitive retina. Retinal dysplasia is a pathologic diagnosis, but through correlation with the clinical appearance and known syndromes in certain breeds, it is often used as a clinical diagnosis.

Retinal dysplasia is a manifestation of the retina's limited ability to respond to injury at a critical stage of development and may result from a variety of injuries (see **Table 14.1**). The resulting lesions range in severity from multifocal retinal dysplasia, where histologically there is folding of retinal layers or duplication of one or more retinal neuronal layers, to more severe lesions including larger geographic regions of retinal malformation or even retinal detachment or nonattachment.[110,111]

Defining a clinical syndrome with a pathologic term that has such diverse connotations to the eye has created a great deal of confusion among veterinarians and breeders regarding the prognosis, significance, cause, and amount of overlap between conditions.

Although retinal dysplasia is usually considered a static disease, small focal folds of dysplastic retina may flatten out and become less evident with age or degeneration, and gliosis of the dysplastic areas may occur with time,[112] making them larger and more visible. While considered congenital and thus visible in young puppies, some forms of presumed retinal dysplasia have not been observed until after 10 weeks of age.[112] The nature of the lesions was not documented, but they were characteristic of what most examiners have assumed to be retinal dysplasia.

Retinal dysplasia has been described in miniature horses and in Rocky Mountain horses with anterior segment dysgenesis (ASD)[113,114] (see Chapter 6) and in kittens with feline colobomatous syndrome.[84] The origin of ASD in horses is genetic, but the cause of feline colobomatous syndrome in cats is unknown.

Retinal dysplasia may be due to a variety of *in utero* insults that result in hyperplastic extension of the retina away from the retinal pigment epithelium (RPE), retinal nonattachment, defective RPE, or necrosis of developing retina.[115] RPE is thought to play a critical role in retinal development, and loss of contact or damage to the RPE results in retinal dysplasia. *In utero* insults that have resulted in retinal dysplasia are listed in **Table 14.1**.

Inherited retinal dysplasia in dogs The terminology used in retinal dysplasia is confusing when attempts are made to correlate findings with the prognosis for sight. For purposes of prognosis, retinal dysplasia is discussed in three categories of severity:

- Focal or multifocal, in which there are single or multiple retinal folds
- Geographic, where there are larger areas of defective retinal development
- Generalized, in which there is retinal detachment or nonattachment[111]

However, overlaps occur between categories in the eyes of individuals and between individuals of the same breed (**Table 14.2**). Further evidence that inherited retinal dysplasias have fundamental differences in embryonic origin is illustrated in differences in RPE between diseases. Detailed examination of English springer spaniels has found no morphologic changes in the RPE, whereas RPE morphologic changes are evident in the Australian shepherd dog.[112,116]

Table 14.2 Inherited retinal dysplasia in dogs.

BREED	TYPE OF DYSPLASIA	MODE OF INHERITANCE
Australian shepherd dog	Generalized	Recessive
Akita	Multifocal/microphthalmos	Recessive
American Cocker Spaniel	Multifocal	Recessive
Beagle	Multifocal	?
Bedlington terrier	Generalized	Recessive
Cavalier King Charles spaniel	Circinate and multifocal	?
Doberman pinscher	Generalized	Recessive
Labrador retriever	Multifocal	Incomplete dominant
Old English sheepdog	Multifocal/microphthalmos	Recessive
Rottweiler	Multifocal	?
Saint Bernard	Generalized	?
Sealyham terrier	Generalized	Recessive
English springer spaniel	Focal	Recessive
Yorkshire terrier	Generalized	Recessive

- *Generalized retinal dysplasia:* Associated with retinal nonattachment or detachment, vitreal dysplasia, vitreal liquefaction, and, usually, multiple ocular anomalies including microphthalmos. It is inherited in many breeds of dogs (as the Labrador retriever, Sealyham, Yorkshire and Bedlington terriers) and species.[81,116–127] Animals with this condition are usually unilaterally or bilaterally blind.
- *Geographic retinal dysplasia:* Overlaps with generalized retinal dysplasia in that some individuals develop retinal detachment and have multiple ocular anomalies. Because of the possibility of detachments, the author does not feel it should be grouped with the milder condition of multifocal retinal dysplasia. Geographic retinal dysplasia is most common in field trial strains of the Labrador retriever and the English springer spaniel.

The condition in the Labrador retriever is quite complex genetically and in its manifestations. Mild cases of geographic retina dysplasia in the Labrador retriever have focal hyperreflective perivascular lesions or focal lesions of irregular size, often with pigment clumping (**Figures 14.47 and 14.48**). The lesions are typically above and adjacent to the disc. Dogs with focal lesions may have a loss of central vision that manifests as an inability to see nonmoving objects. Some dogs may develop a retinal detachment up to 1–2 years of age (**Figure 14.49**).

The use of the term retinal dysplasia has perhaps given too much emphasis to the relationship with retinal detachment. Blair et al. found that the detachments are due to

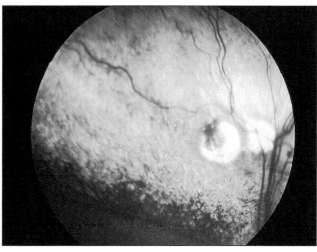

Figure 14.48 Geographic retinal dysplasia in an adult Labrador retriever. The location of the lesion is similar to Figure 14.47, but the lesion is more sharply demarcated and mimics a postinflammatory scar.

giant peripheral circumferential tears or dialysis and are associated with vitreous syneresis and peripheral proliferative vitreous changes that tear the retina.[30,31]

Retinal dysplasia in the English springer spaniel usually manifests similarly to the moderately affected Labrador retriever, that is, focal perivascular or irregularly shaped hyperreflective areas, dorsal and adjacent to the optic disc. The lesions are often asymmetrical in degree of involvement. The 6-week-old puppy has very subtle but observable lesions (**Figure 14.50**). Pigmentary clumping may occur, and retinal detachments may develop. Hyperreflectivity and pigment clumping occur with maturity as secondary atrophy occurs (**Figure 14.51**). Retinal detachments are reported to occur in the first 6 months of life.[110]

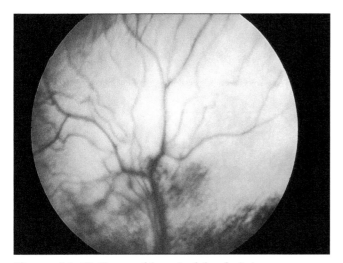

Figure 14.47 Geographic retinal dysplasia in a young Labrador retriever. The lesion is focal and located at 12 o'clock above the disc. A gray lesion with a small orange and pigment spot represents the lesion.

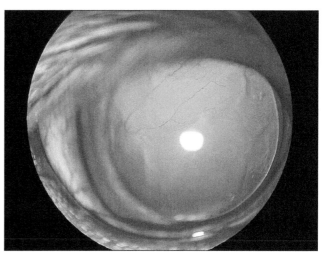

Figure 14.49 Complete retinal detachment in a Labrador retriever with retinal dysplasia. Note the retinal vessels are in focus, indicating forward placement.

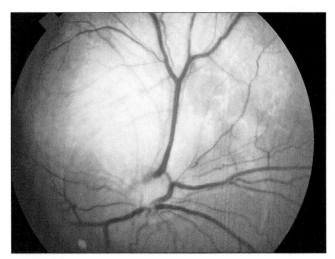

Figure 14.50 Fundus of an English springer spaniel puppy with geographic retinal dysplasia evidenced by aberrant coloration above the disc. Retinal dysplasia is difficult to diagnose at this age but possible.

Congenital cataracts and superficial band keratopathies may be present, the latter resolving with age.[128] The condition is inherited as an autosomal recessive trait.[129]

Oculoskeletal dysplasia. This condition has been described in the Labrador retriever (dwarfism with retinal dysplasia type I, drd1) and in the Samoyed dog (dwarfism with retinal dysplasia type II, drd2) in which there are both ocular lesions and skeletal dysplasia. Homozygous-affected dogs exhibit short-limbed dwarfism and a constellation of ocular changes, which, in the most severe form, are characterized by complete retinal detachment and cataracts. Heterozygous dogs have lesions limited to the retina and consist of unilateral or bilateral focal/multifocal dysplastic changes.[111,130,131] Skeletal dysplasia manifests with bowed short forelimbs with less involvement of the hind limbs, hip dysplasia, ununited

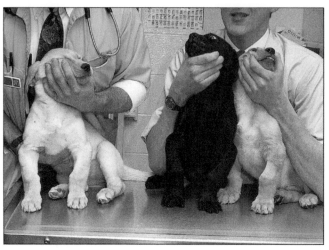

Figure 14.52 Labrador retriever littermates with skeletal dysplasia. Note the bowed forelimbs.

anconeal and coronoid processes, and delayed development of epiphysis (**Figure 14.52**). Animals with skeletal dysplasia are more likely to have retinal detachments, corneal opacities, cataracts, and optic nerve atrophy. A litter may have both mild focal dysplasia and severe ocular anomalies with skeletal dysplasia.[132] The cataracts are congenital, but the retinal detachments occur from 4–6 months of age due to peripheral dialysis or tears. The fundus before detachment has red-brown streaks in the tapetal region, converging to the optic disc in the Samoyed (**Figure 14.53**). In a breeding experiment in the Samoyed dog, two littermates with unilateral detachment and skeletal dysplasia produced offspring with unilateral detachment (at 4 months), focal cataracts, and prominent hyaloid arteries but no clinical or histopathologic

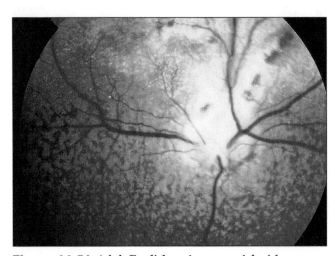

Figure 14.51 Adult English springer spaniel with hyperreflective lesions and pigment clumping in the typical position for retinal dysplasia in this breed.

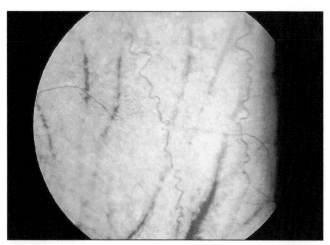

Figure 14.53 Ocular fundus of a young Samoyed with skeletal dysplasia and retinal detachment syndrome. The histopathologic correlation of these breaks in the tapetum are not known, but they were the only lesions before retinal detachment occurred at 4 months of age. No evidence of retinal dysplasia was found on histopathologic examination.

evidence of retinal dysplasia. Conversely, Acland and Aguirre bred from two Samoyeds with multifocal dysplasia and produced a litter with skeletal dysplasia, normal skeletons, and multifocal dysplasia, and a puppy with multifocal cataracts and persistent hyaloid artery.[133] The genetics in the Labrador retriever are more controversial and have been variably reported to be a recessive or dominant gene with incomplete penetrance.[134,135] Carrig et al. more recently postulated that the condition is caused by a single gene that is recessive for skeletal dysplasia and incompletely dominant for ocular lesions.[136] In general, heterozygotes with normal skeletons have mild ocular lesions, and homozygotes with skeletal lesions have severe ocular lesions.

- *Circinate retinal dysplasia:* Is uniquely shaped and is a supposed form of focal retinal dysplasia found in a variety of breeds including the Labrador and Golden retriever, Cavalier King Charles spaniel, and Siberian husky. The shape is circular or U-shaped, with a depressed center and raised periphery (**Figure 14.54**) and may have retinal folds adjacent to it. The condition is usually unilateral and, in retrievers, may not necessarily be congenital, thus raising the question whether it is actually dysplasia.[111] The author has observed circinate lesions of the Cavalier King Charles spaniel in 5- to 6-week-old puppies, and it has also been diagnosed in 4- to 5-year-old adults that have had up to three normal annual examinations by other ophthalmologists. The location may be in either the tapetal or nontapetal region and is often in the midperiphery. To date, retinal detachments have not been associated with the condition, and the histopathology has

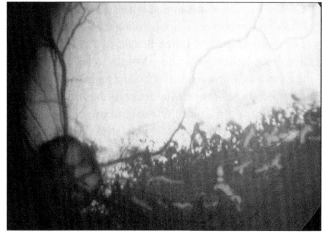

Figure 14.55 Multifocal retina dysplasia or folds in the nontapetum and tapetum of a young adult American cocker spaniel. The lesions in this dog are mainly curvilinear.

not been reported. How it is related to geographic retina dysplasia in the Labrador retriever is unknown.

- *Multifocal retinal dysplasia:* The focal/multifocal form manifests with one or many dots, linear, or linear branching streaks anywhere in the fundus. Tapetal lesions are darker than the tapetum and may have a surrounding hyperreflective border. In the nontapetum, lesions are white (**Figures 14.55 and 14.56**). It has been described as an isolated syndrome in the Beagle, American Cocker Spaniel (**Figure 14.55**), and Rottweiler.[137–139] The condition may be bilateral or, in milder cases, unilateral. In the

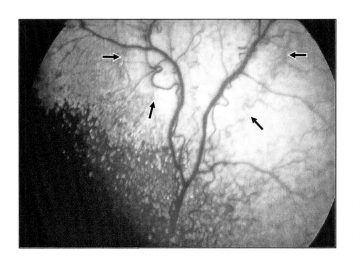

Figure 14.54 Circinate or geographic retinal dysplasia in a Cavalier King Charles spaniel (arrows). The periphery of the lesion is elevated and displaces the retinal blood vessels, while the center is depressed.

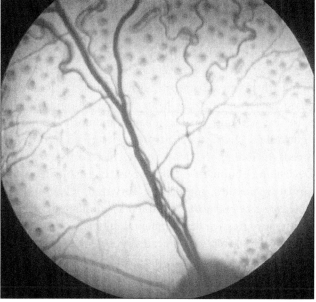

Figure 14.56 Multifocal retinal dysplasia in a dog in which the lesions are mainly dots with a few curvilinear streaks.

Cocker spaniel, it is common with a 12%–20% prevalence reported, and it is thought to be inherited as a recessive trait.[138,140] In the Beagle, 3% of a colony had dysplastic lesions, and while thought to be inherited, the mode is unknown.[137,141,142] Long and Crispin postulated a simple recessive trait for multifocal retinal dysplasia for the Golden retriever in the United Kingdom.[143] Crispin et al. found a prevalence of 3%.[144]

> Retinal dysplasia semantics and the genetic and clinical interplay of the various forms are confusing to the layperson as well as the professional.

Diagnosis

Diagnosis is made on the clinical signs in a known affected breed. Some lesions of focal retinal dysplasia mimic a postinflammatory chorioretinal scar.

Therapy

Genetic counseling is indicated in diffuse and focal forms of retinal dysplasia. It is prudent to advise dog breeders to avoid inbreeding dogs with multifocal dysplasia. In Labradors and Samoyeds dogs with oculoskeletal dysplasia, the identification of the mutation has allowed the development of DNA-based genotyping tests.

Micropapilla, hypoplasia, and aplasia of the optic nerve

Introduction/etiology

The development of the optic nerve (ON) depends on the proper sequence of events during the formation and the closure of the optic fissure and on a complex set of proteins responsible for directing the migration of developing nerve fibers from the retina.[145]

Micropapilla is a clinical syndrome that is observed frequently when screening "normal" dogs. It is characterized by a unilateral or bilateral, small, nonmyelinated optic disc without visual complaints and normal pupillary light reflex. Micropapilla has been described in different breeds including the Irish setter, Flat-coated retriever, Dachshunds, miniature Schnauzers, German shepherds, miniature poodles, and Belgian Tervuren.[146]

Optic nerve hypoplasia is defined as a unilateral or bilateral nonprogressive developmental anomaly of the retina and ON, characterized clinically by a small and gray optic disc(s), dilated pupils, and blindness. In this process, there is a reduction of the centripetal retinal ganglion cells (RGC) axon fibers projecting through the ON.[147,148]

Optic nerve aplasia is a rare, unilateral condition characterized by blindness and no visible optic disc; extremely rare malformation characterized by congenital absence of

the optic nerve, optic disc, retinal ganglion cells and retinal vessels.[149,150]

Optic nerve hypoplasia is the most significant of these syndromes because of the clinical manifestations. Optic nerve hypoplasia is characterized by a reduced number of axons in the nerves and a corresponding decrease in retinal ganglion cells.[147,148] Optic nerve hypoplasia is believed to result from either RGC axon guidance defects, abnormal retinal/optic disc development, or premature RGC death[149,151,152] (**Figure 14.57**).

Normally, many more axons are found in the embryonic optic nerve than in the adult. In the maturation of the optic nerve, there is a normal loss or atrophy of these supernumerary axons to the level of the adult state.[151] In hypoplasia of the optic nerve, it is theorized that this atrophy does not stop but is carried to an extreme.[152] Histopathological features include variable degrees of ON hypoplasia and gliosis.[149]

The condition has been reported in several breeds, including the Beagle and Shih Tzu.[149,153] Optic nerve hypoplasia may be observed as an isolated ocular anomaly but may also occur with more generalized ocular anomalies, such as microphthalmos. It is thought to be inherited in the miniature and toy poodle.[154]

In the cat, hypoplasia of the optic nerve may result from *in utero* or neonatal panleukopenia infection and may be associated with generalized central nervous system (CNS) anomalies.[155] Complete aplasia of the optic nerve has been described in the cat.[156]

A condition termed optic nerve hypoplasia has been reported in the horse; however, is a rare congenital abnormality.[157] Optic nerve hypoplasia has been described in shorthorn cattle with multiple ocular anomalies of retinal

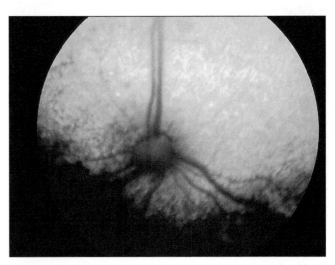

Figure 14.57 Optic nerve hypoplasia in a 3-month-old miniature poodle presented for blindness. The optic nerve is small, gray, circular similar to the feline optic nerve.

dysplasia, cataract, retinal detachment, microphthalmos, and hydrocephalus. The condition is thought to be genetic.[119]

In women, the use of anticonvulsants such as phenytoin during pregnancy has been implicated as causing optic nerve hypoplasia. Veterinarians should, therefore, be on the alert for drug-induced optic nerve hypoplasia in veterinary medicine.[158]

Clinical signs

Optic nerve hypoplasia may be unilateral or bilateral. Blindness with dilated pupils is the presenting sign at 5–8 weeks of age if the condition is bilateral and severe. On ophthalmoscopy, the optic disc(s) is very small and appears "cat like," that is, gray, small, round, cupped, nonmyelinated disc with the vessels at the periphery (**Figure 14.57**). The retinal vasculature may be either normal or tortuous, and either a hyperreflective or dark ring may surround the disc. Unilaterally affected patients are often detected later in life while incidentally looking at the fundus, or if the good eye has suffered a blinding disease or injury. When the condition is unilateral, the unaffected (or less affected) eye can be observed for comparison. Mild-to-moderate degrees of hypoplasia are difficult to diagnose because of the subjectivity and range of normals. If the diameter of the disc is half of normal, the area or volume to hold fibers is a quarter of normal.

The term micropapilla is used for animals with small discs but normal vision.

Therapy

There is obviously no therapy, but owners should be advised to be cautious about breeding because of the potential genetic implications.

Hereditary tapetal dysplasia/degeneration

Introduction/etiology

An inherited trait has been observed in the Beagle, where the tapetum appears to be absent in a pigmented fundus (**Figure 14.58**).[159-161] This is often considered a normal variation but is more likely a pathologic trait. Histologically, the tapetum is present, and the overlying RPE is nonpigmented. The tapetum has irregularly shaped cells, and ultrastructurally, the tapetal rodlets are absent. Abnormally spaced inclusions are present in place of the tapetal rodlets.[71] On chemical analysis, the tapetum is lacking in both zinc and cysteine.[159] Not only are the tapetal rodlets abnormal, but the cells of the RPE of the iris, the ciliary body, and the retina lack pigment granules. In addition, pigment granules are reduced in the stroma of the uvea.[160] Retinal function measured by electroretinography was normal except for a slight elevation of dark-adapted white light thresholds.[161] The condition is thought

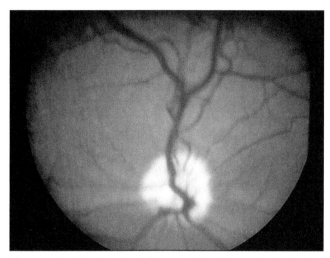

Figure 14.58 Beagle with tapetal dysplasia. The lack of a visible tapetum results in an overall pigmentation to the fundus from choroidal pigment.

to be due to a simple recessive gene.[161] Recently, a case of tapetal dysplasia has been described in a Swedish Vallhund dog.[162] We have also observed pigmented fundi with no apparent tapetum not infrequently in the Labrador retriever.

Clinical signs

Dogs with hereditary tapetal degeneration in the Beagle dog have an absence of tapetum with a pigmented fundus but have no visual complaints.

Acquired diseases

Inherited retinal degenerations/dystrophies

Canine retinal degenerations primarily affect the photoreceptors, RPE, or both. The two main inherited retinal degenerations in the dog include progressive retinal atrophy (PRA) and retinal pigment epithelial dystrophy (RPED), formerly called central PRA (CPRA). This group of retinal diseases may not always belong in the category of "acquired," since detailed studies have shown that while a disease may manifest later in life it starts as dysplasia or maldevelopment.

Progressive retinal atrophy

Introduction/etiology

Progressive retinal atrophy (PRA) is an umbrella name for a variety of familial or hereditary retinal degenerations that have a similar clinical manifestation but a diversity of origins. The condition affects more than 100 dog breeds and is known to be genetically heterogeneous between breeds.[163] By definition, PRA is an inherited, bilateral, progressive degeneration of the retina that eventually results in blindness. Generally, PRA is initially a disease of the photoreceptors that eventually involves all of the retinal layers. If the photoreceptors do not reach their adult maturation before degenerating, the process is termed a photoreceptor dysplasia (not to be confused with retinal dysplasia). If the photoreceptors reach their adult maturation and then begin to degenerate, even at a young age, it is termed an abiotrophy or degeneration. Some conditions initially involve either the rods, the cones, or both the rods and the cones. Therefore, the possibilities exist for a rod dysplasia, cone dysplasia, rod–cone dysplasia, rod degeneration, cone degeneration, or rod–cone degeneration. Additionally, initial dysplasia of one type of photoreceptor may be paired with or initiate subsequent degeneration of the opposite photoreceptor. Without detailed studies, it cannot be anticipated which form of degeneration/dysplasia is occurring in each breed with PRA.

Clinical signs

Despite the dissimilarities in the origin of the PRA, the clinical signs are usually quite similar.

External signs or those noted by the owner

- Night blindness is often the first sign but may not be appreciated or given as the presenting complaint. Night blindness progresses to day blindness over months to years.
- Dilated pupils with increased eyeshine or tapetal reflection.
- Cortical cataracts (appear late in the course). Most dogs in the late stages of PRA develop cortical cataracts, and it is not known whether this is associated with a separate gene or due to the liberation of a substance from the degenerating retina that is toxic to the lens. One such potential substance is docosahexaenoic acid liberated from the photoreceptor outer segments. Docosahexaenoic acid can undergo autoxidation to malondialdehyde and lipid radicals and has been demonstrated to produce cataracts in rabbits.[164] The PRA literature generally avoids discussion of the cause of the associated cataracts.
- Usually a purebred dog.

Ophthalmoscopic signs The lesions of PRA are bilateral and symmetrical. Fundus changes observed in PRA are bilateral and symmetrical and include diffuse tapetal hyperreflectivity in the early stages followed by vascular attenuation, pigmentary changes, and atrophy of the optic nerve head in the later stages of disease.[165]

The hyperreflectivity is generally diffuse and is thought to be due to retinal thinning. Many breeds may develop fan-shaped striations of altered tapetal reflectivity that converge at the disc. Concurrently, retinal blood vessels decrease in number and size. PRA is not, however,

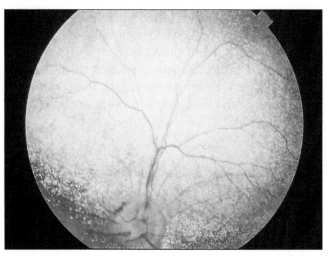

Figure 14.59 Progressive retinal atrophy in an American Cocker Spaniel. The condition is moderately advanced with diffuse tapetal hyperreflectivity and moderate retinal vascular attenuation.

a vascular disease since the photoreceptor degeneration occurs long before the vascular changes are evident (**Figures 14.59 through 14.61**). The retinal vascular attenuation is thought to be associated with thinning of the retina that brings the retinal vasculature in closer apposition to the choroidal vasculature. This increases the oxygen tension in the retina, which is a stimulant to vasoconstriction.[166] Late in the course of PRA, the nontapetal region may develop clumping of pigment or depigmentation (**Figures 14.62 and 14.63**). Generalized depigmentation is more common. Optic atrophy is also a late sign, manifested by a whitish-gray disc, scalloped borders, and disc cupping (**Figure 14.63**).

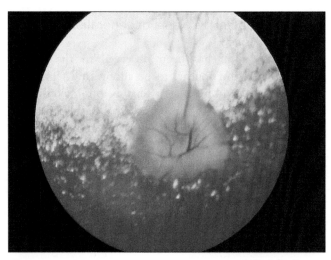

Figure 14.60 Advanced progressive retinal atrophy in a 7-year-old miniature poodle. Note the gray disc, bright tapetum with striations, and loss of almost all retinal vasculature.

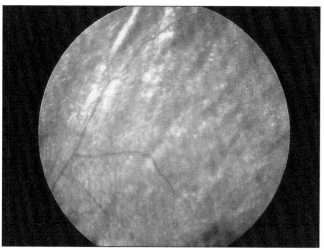

Figure 14.61 Peripheral tapetum of the case in Figure 14.60 with a low strobe light to illustrate the fan-like striations toward the optic nerve.

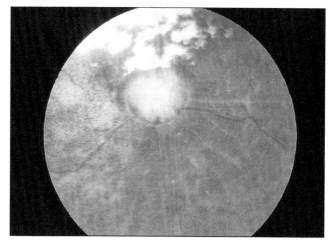

Figure 14.63 Advanced progressive retinal atrophy in an English springer spaniel. The tapetum is hyperreflective, almost all the retinal vessels have disappeared, the nontapetum has lost pigment, and the optic disc is atrophied.

Inheritance

In all breeds studied in detail, PRA has been an autosomal recessive trait except for a form in the Siberian husky and Samoyed, where it is sex-linked,[167] and in the mastiff and Bullmastiff, where it is a dominant trait.[168] Recessive traits pose a dilemma; if only one dog in 1,000 is affected, then one dog in 10 may be a carrier.[169] In the United States, the miniature pinscher, miniature/toy poodle, Irish setter, and Labrador retriever have an increased risk, while the Dachshund, boxer, Beagle, German shepherd dog, and mixed breeds have a low risk. The male Irish setter has 4.5 times the risk as the female.[170] Because PRA is recessive in the vast majority of breeds studied, it can be expected to be found predominantly in purebreds.

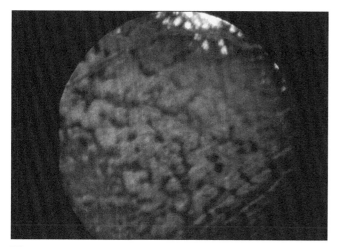

Figure 14.62 Pigment clumping in a "bone corpuscular" pattern in a miniature poodle with progressive retinal atrophy.

When affected (homozygous) dogs of different breeds are bred, the offspring may be normal due to nonallelic genes. This seems to occur with photoreceptor dysplasia (rod–cone dysplasia, rcd)[171] or early-onset PRA. Photoreceptor degeneration (rod–cone degeneration, prcd) is a mid- to late-onset disease and may occur on allelic genes since miniature poodle–American Cocker Spaniel, miniature poodle–English Cocker Spaniel, and American Cocker–English Cocker Spaniel crosses can manifest PRA.[172] In a breeding colony of miniature poodles, when affected females are bred with heterozygous males, the number of affected offspring is 50%. When affected males are bred with heterozygous females, the number of affected pups is fewer than expected (19%), possibly due to gamete selection. The implication of this data is that when test breeding, the results from one litter of seven pups (99% probability of normal subject if all pups are normal) are reliable when testing a male but not when testing a female.[173]

Age of onset

The age of onset of clinical signs varies both with the breed and within the breed. External influences may hasten the course of PRA in individuals. The onset of clinical signs varies from 6 months to 10+ years (**Table 14.3**) and are typically divided between early- and late-onset photoreceptor degeneration.

Early-onset degeneration

Rod–cone dysplasia (rcd, early-onset PRA)

The Irish setter, sloughi, Collie, Welsh corgi, miniature Schnauzer have rcd conditions that have been studied

Table 14.3 **Age of onset of ophthalmic signs of progressive retinal atrophy.**

EARLY ONSET, RAPID PROGRESSION	
Akita	5–18 months
American Cocker Spaniel	2–3 years
Collie	3–6 months
Dachshund	<1 year
English cocker spaniel	2–4 years
Gordon Setter	3–6 months
Irish setter	3–6 months
Longhaired Dachshund	<1 year
Welsh Corgi	3–6 months
LATE ONSET OF CLINICAL SIGNS	
Golden retriever	1–3 years
Miniature poodle	3–5 years
Miniature Schnauzer	2–3 years
Norwegian elkhound	1–2 years
Samoyed	3–5 years
Tibetan terrier	1.5–2.5 years
Toy poodle	3–5 years

in detail. The outer segments of the rods and cones fail to develop normally, and subsequent progressive degeneration of the photoreceptors and the inner retina occurs. Degeneration of the cones is slower than that of the rods. Despite these similarities, the diseases are different biochemically and genetically in being nonallelic genes between breeds.[174] The disease in the Collie, Welsh corgi, Sloughi, and Irish setter, but not in the miniature Schnauzer, is characterized by defects in retinal cyclic nucleotide metabolism that leads to elevations of cyclic guanosine monophosphate (GMP) in the retina. This is the result of a deficiency in the beta subunit of cyclic GMP phosphodiesterase (PDE) in Irish setters and Sloughis (rcd1)[175,176] and the alpha subunit in the Welsh corgi (rcd3).[177] In the defect in the Collie (rcd2), the activity is calmodulin-independent.[178] These biochemical changes can be demonstrated before the subsequent photoreceptor degeneration. In the Irish setter, the Welsh corgi, and the Collie, the photoreceptor and subsequent retinal degeneration progresses rapidly over a few months, while in the miniature Schnauzer, it progresses slowly over a few years.[179–182] PRA in the miniature Schnauzer has been designated a photoreceptors dysplasia, but a PDE deficiency is not present. While abnormal photoreceptor morphology can be observed at 4 weeks of age, and the rod density decreased by 50% by 19 weeks, the process slows down, and clinical signs

are not evident until 1–2 years of age, and blindness is not evident until 4–6 years.[183] Other studies have shown that other genetic defects appear to also be involved in cases of PRA in the miniature Schnauzer.[184]

Rod dysplasia (rd) in the Norwegian elkhound
Rod dysplasia with subsequent cone degeneration has been described in the Norwegian elkhound. This is not a disease of cyclic GMP, as observed in rod–cone dysplasia in the Collie and Irish setter. Despite being dysplasia, the progression of degeneration is relatively slow, manifesting at 1–2 years of age.[185–187] The diagnosis can be made as early as 6 weeks with meticulous ERG techniques utilizing controls. The ERG utilizing a white light is diminished in rod dysplasia but is nonspecific, while the diminished amplitude with red light and dark adaptation is specific.[186,187]

Early retinal degeneration in the Norwegian elkhound
A separate disease, early retinal degeneration (ERD), has been characterized in the Norwegian elkhound. This disease manifests clinically with night blindness at 6 weeks of age and progresses to blindness at 6–12 months of age. The rod and cone outer segments develop abnormally, fail to develop mature synaptic terminals, and subsequently degenerate. The renewal process of the rods is abnormal, appearing cone-like, and may suggest that the disc membranes are contiguous. The condition differs from rod dysplasia in this breed morphologically, electrophysiologically, and in the rate of degeneration. The ERG is characterized by failure of development of the b-wave. In the young dog, the a-wave is normal, but this slowly deteriorates with age. The lack of a b-wave corresponds to the lack of development of the synaptic photoreceptor terminals. This produces a predominantly negative waveform in young animals.[188–190]

Cone–rod dystrophy (crd)
A progressive retinal degeneration is characterized by early degeneration of the rods and cones but with the cones being more severely affected, has been described in the standard wire-haired Dachshund (SWHD) and pit bull terrier.[191–193] In the SWHD, affected animals have abnormal cone ERG responses and may have difficulty navigating in very bright light, but they usually navigate well in ambient light and have very small pupils at 8 weeks of age. The condition slowly progresses, and the fundus is normal until 10 months to 3 years of age, when the typical ophthalmoscopic changes of PRA develop, and the pupils dilate. At this stage, there is advance cone and rod dysfunction.[192,193]

Late-onset degeneration/progressive rod–cone degeneration (prcd)

Rod–cone degeneration is the most common form of PRA and is typically later in onset. The condition affects more than 100 dog breeds and is known to be genetically heterogeneous between breeds. Around 14 mutations have now been identified that are associated with PRA in around 49 breeds, but for the majority of breeds, the mutation(s) responsible has yet to be identified.[165] It has been extensively studied in the miniature poodle, Tibetan terrier, and American and English Cocker Spaniel.

While degeneration can be demonstrated in the miniature and toy poodle electrophysiologically and ultrastructurally as early as 9 weeks of age, the progression is slow, and clinical signs often do not manifest until >3 years of age. The poodle with prcd was initially reported to have an altered ERG at 9 weeks of age, but this is unusual, and 8–12 months is more commonly the age of earliest ERG changes.[194,195] In the poodle, the earliest recognized abnormality is a defect in renewal of photoreceptor outer segment membranes, but the visual pigment in the photoreceptors is normal.[196] The cones degenerate more slowly than the rods, and, consequently, night blindness is an early sign. Most of the prcd conditions investigated to date have an autosomal recessive trait, and many involve allelic genes, as indicated by affected offspring from affected parents of different breeds. No other systemic or local abnormalities (such as deafness) have been associated with prcd.[181,197–200] In the poodle with progressive rod–cone degeneration, plasma levels of docosahexaenoic acid, which is an important constituent of the phospholipids of the outer segments of the photoreceptors, are reduced.[201]

Clinical signs of disease in affected Tibetan terriers manifests rather early compared with those of the prcd-affected dogs. Most recently, it was demonstrated to be a metabolic storage disease, with accumulation of ceroid lipofuscin systemically and in various layers of the retina.[202] This syndrome is distinct from PRA in Tibetan terriers, which is widespread in Europe and is characterized by a reduction of the b-wave by 10 months of age, although patchy disorganization of the outer segments of the rods and the cones has been observed as early as 9 weeks of age. It is thought to be degeneration rather than dysplasia, and the cyclic GMP levels are normal. Night blindness is usually present at 1 year and progresses to blindness by 2–3 years of age.[203]

In the Akita, two ophthalmoscopic patterns of PRA are observed. Night blindness occurs from 1–3 years of age, and at this time, a hyperreflective horizontal band that originates from the area centralis and extends outward is observed in most dogs. This eventually involves the entire tapetum. A second pattern begins as peripheral tapetal reflectivity that progresses to generalized hyperreflectivity.[204,205] Morphologic changes are present in the retina at 11 weeks of age, but ERG changes may not be noted until 15 months of age. The condition is a rod–cone degeneration.

Diagnosis of PRA

- Ophthalmoscopic appearance: PRA is characterized by bilateral, symmetrical, diffuse hyperreflectivity, vascular attenuation, and pale optic nerve. In contrast, nonhereditary forms of retinal atrophy (secondary to chorioretinitis) will usually be asymmetrical in their presentation and show signs of chronic inflammation as focal or multifocal scars with pigment clumping.
- History: Night blindness progressing to day blindness is typical of PRA, but owners seldom volunteer the information unless specifically asked. If the dog is of a breed known to be affected, and there is a history of affected relatives, genetic retinal degeneration may be suspected.
- Electroretinography: Abnormalities in ERG amplitude and latency may occur much earlier than ophthalmoscopic changes. Early detection requires general anesthesia and exacting techniques. Late in the course, the ERG is extinguished or very flat and can be readily detected without anesthesia, utilizing computer averaging techniques. An extinguished ERG is not specific for PRA, since a variety of other severe retinal diseases can extinguish the ERG. Due to the common occurrence of cataracts late in the course, it is important to perform ERGs before undertaking cataract surgery in purebred dogs.
- Genetic testing: Genetic testing is now available to detect a variety of forms of photoreceptor degenerations and dysplasias, with over 35 breeds having DNA tests available. The sample type required may vary between laboratories, but usually either blood samples or cheek swabs are acceptable, with blood samples having less chance for extraneous contamination.

Genetic testing, if widely utilized by breeders, holds the promise of significantly affecting the prevalence of PRA of the prcd (adult type) where screening ophthalmoscopic examinations have not succeeded.

Therapy

No current practical or proven therapy is available to correct or arrest the progression of the inherited retinal degenerations. Experimentally, gene therapy utilizing subretinal injection of a recombinant adenovirus carrying the RPE65 gene for RPE65-deficient Briard dogs was successful in improving ERG and function.[206,207] Neonatal neuroretina has also been transplanted subretinally in Abyssinian cats with inherited rod–cone degeneration, but the functional success was not evaluated.[208] Various vitamin supplements with antioxidants are frequently prescribed and are usually considered placeboes for the owner as well as the dispensing veterinarian.

Other generalized retinopathies

1. *Cone degeneration*: Achromatopsia, day blindness, or cone degeneration (CD) is a congenital and stationary condition that often does not show any fundus abnormalities. It has been described in detail in the Alaskan malamute. In its classical form, the condition is characterized by a profound blindness in daylight conditions but not in dim light. The PLRs and the ocular fundus are normal.[209,210] The condition develops in the young puppy and does not progress to the rods.[209,210] The cones develop normally, but the cone outer segments degenerate, leaving a pure rod retina.[211,212] The condition is inherited as a simple recessive trait.[213]

   More recent reports of cone degeneration in Alaskan malamutes in Australia describe a more complex condition that varies from mild to severe day blindness.[214] The fundus in the Australian dog is normal, similar to other malamutes, and the ERG flicker is fused above 30 Hz. A condition similar to that in malamutes has been observed in the German shorthaired pointer.[215]

   Electroretinography confirms the cone defect by demonstrating a flicker fusion with low-intensity white light at frequencies >25/second (normal is 45–80) and a reduced response to red light in early dark adaptation. White light single flash and blue light ERGs are normal.[215]

2. Congenital stationary night blindness in horses
   Congenital stationary night blindness (CSNB) is a nonprogressive inherited condition reported most commonly in the Appaloosa horse; however, it has also been reported in a Thoroughbred, Quarter Horse, Miniature Horse, and in a Paso Fino horse.[216–218] CSNB is characterized by impaired vision in dark conditions and is present at birth.

Night blindness does not typically progress to day blindness with a normal fundus on ophthalmoscopy. However, more severely affected horses also show signs of visual disturbance in daylight.[216,217] A dramatic difference in the ability to see under dark adaptation or dim light and normal daylight conditions is easily demonstrated. The condition has been demonstrated in a 1-month-old foal and was thought to be congenital, but animals may not be noted to have a deficit until several months of age. In the Appaloosa and miniature horse, CSNB is associated with the leopard complex or spotting patterns that is a dominant trait (LP).[217] CSNB manifested in horses that were homozygous exhibited few dark spots and were mostly white. Diagnosis of CSNB is confirmed by electroretinography (ERG). The characteristic dark-adapted ERG recording consists of an absent b-wave and an a-wave that increases in amplitude as dark adaptation continues. This a-wave dominated ERG is referred to as a "negative ERG."[217] A reduction of the scotopic ERG b-wave may indicate a carrier state, although Sandmeyer et al. were unable to detect ERG changes in heterozygous and normal horses with the leopard complex.[217]

Histologically, the retina in the horse was normal, and thus, combined with the ERG, it has been suggested that the site of the lesion was in the transmission of the neural impulse from the photoreceptors to the bipolar cells.[219,220] There is no treatment; affected animals should not be used for breeding.

3. Hereditary retinal dystrophy in Briard dogs/lipid retinopathy/Leber's congenital amaurosis (LCA)/congenital stationary night blindness in dogs
   The Briard dog is affected with a recessively inherited retinal disorder characterized by congenital night blindness with various degrees of visual impairment under photopic illumination.[221,222] Affected dogs varied from having only night blindness, having night blindness with reduced day vision, or animals that were completely blind. The fundus was normal in affected dogs until the dogs were 2–3 years old, although the resting pupil diameters were increased over controls. Differences in the ERG and ultrastructure indicate that the condition may be related to rcd or a lipid metabolic defect. The ERG is characterized by a decreased b-wave as well as reduced flicker fusion, which indicates cone dysfunction.[221] Ultrastructurally, large lipid inclusions are found in

the retinal RPE at 5 weeks of age that progress to photoreceptor degeneration with time.[223] Plasma lipid abnormalities may also be noted in the Briard.[224,225] The disease in Briards has been extensively studied. It is an animal model for Leber's amaurosis in humans and is due to a deletion of four base pairs in the RPE65 gene.[222] Experimentally, gene therapy utilizing subretinal injection of a recombinant adenovirus carrying the RPE65 gene for RPE65-deficient Briard dogs was successful in improving ERG and function.[206,207] A DNA test is available for the disease in Briards.

4. Retinal pigment epithelial dystrophy (formerly called central progressive retinal atrophy [CPRA]).

Introduction/etiology

Retinal pigment epithelial dystrophy (RPED) is a rare disease in the United States today. Unlike PRA, which is a disease of the photoreceptors, RPED is a disease of the RPE. It is a disease described in the Briard, Labrador retriever, Shetland sheepdog, English Cocker Spaniel, Border Collie, and Collie. It is slowly progressive, causing central vision to be lost so that stationary objects are not recognized. The condition progresses so slowly that the animal may never become completely blind. The RPE cells become abnormal and accumulate a light-brown pigment in the cytoplasm. The pigment from the RPE migrates into the neurosensory retina, resulting in secondary retinal degeneration.[226] It is postulated that the lipofuscin pigment in the neurosensory retina reflects a failure of the RPE to phagocytize adequately the photoreceptor outer segments.[227] In contrast to PRA, cataracts are rarely associated with RPED/CPRA.[228]

In the Briard, a survey in England indicated that about 30% of the population was affected, and it was postulated to be a simple recessive trait.[229] In other breeds, the genetics are still not known, but it has been suggested to be a dominant trait with incomplete penetrance.[230,231] The clinical signs of RPED are very similar to those of experimental and clinical vitamin E deficiency on the canine retina (see section Nutritional retinopathies). The disease seems to have decreased markedly both in the United States and in Europe, perhaps indicating an environmental or nutritional influence.[232] Lower plasma vitamin E levels have been found in affected Briards and in affected Cocker Spaniels and Nizzinis.[232] The latter two breeds show the greatest decrease in vitamin E levels and commonly also have accompanying neurologic signs of proprioceptive deficits, ataxia, and altered spinal reflexes.[232] The biokinetics of vitamin E appear to be abnormal in that vitamin E absorption from an oral dose is near normal, but the plasma levels decline much faster after peaking.[232,233]

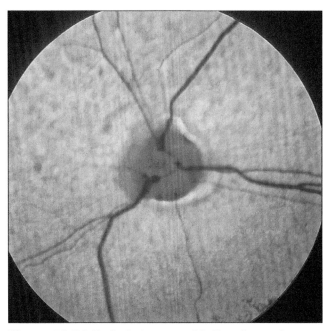

Figure 14.64 Retinal pigment epithelium dystrophy (RPED) or CPRA in a Labrador retriever. Note the multiple light brown accumulations in the tapetal region. Mild vascular attenuation may be present.

Clinical signs

Signs are usually bilateral and symmetrical, but one eye may be more advanced. Early changes are brown clumps of pigment in the central tapetal region. The area of pigmentation increases with time, coalesces, and then may fade late in the course of the disease (**Figure 14.64**). The nontapetal region is usually normal.

The tapetum lucidum develops mild increases in sheen between the pigment clumps, and the retinal vascular caliber decreases but not to the extremes found in PRA. Visual loss is slow and variable, and vision may appear normal for moving and distant objects but impaired for stationary and nearby objects. The earlier the onset, the more rapid the loss of vision. Dilated pupils may occur late in the course of the disease.

RPED/CPRA is rare today in North America and has almost become an historical disease.

Therapy

In light of the link to vitamin E deficiency, supplementation would be prudent.[233]

5. *Multifocal retinopathy*: Canine multifocal retinopathy (CMR) is an inherited condition characterized by multifocal serous retinal detachments that has been associated with various mutations in the bestrophin-1

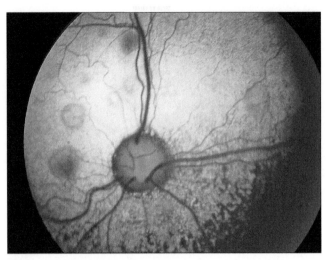

Figure 14.65 Multifocal retinopathy in a Coton de Tulear, noted on screening examination. Some lesions are tan while others are clear. The condition improved spontaneously over a year.

(BEST1) gene.[234] Canine multifocal retinopathy has been described in several breeds including the Great Pyrenees, Coton de Tulear, English and French mastiff, Bullmastiff dogs, and Boerboel.[234–236] The condition does not produce visual complaints and develops in the Great Pyrenees at approximately 13 weeks of age and then slowly regresses. The lesions consist of focal detachment of the RPE with overlying serous detachment of the neurosensory retina. The focal bullae vary in color from gray to tan/orange and are predominantly in the tapetal region (**Figure 14.65**). Secondary focal retinal degeneration occurs with hypertrophy of the RPE. The ERG has shown a lack of progression of the retinal degeneration and the condition is inherited, probably as a simple recessive trait in the Great Pyrenees dog.[234] The condition is thought to be a focal defect in the RPE.[234] A DNA test is now available for the condition.

Inherited PRA in the cat
Introduction/etiology
Inherited retinal degeneration in the cat appears to be rather uncommon, except in the Persian, Abyssinian, Somali, and Siamese cats.[237,238] The Persian cat suffers an autosomal recessive, early-onset retinal degenerative disease.[237] In the Abyssinian breed, both an autosomal-dominant cone–rod dysplasia and recessively inherited rod–cone degeneration have been described.[238–241] Clinical signs are similar to the dog, that is, bilateral tapetal hyperreflectivity and vascular attenuation. The process affects the peripheral fundus first and progresses to the central retina when advanced. The disease in the older cat is primary photoreceptor degeneration with initially severe disorganization of the outer segments of the rods and, later, of the cones.[241] The course in the Abyssinian cats is rapid, and cone–rod dysplasia blindness occurs by 1 year of age, while with rod–cone degeneration blindness is present by 2–4 years of age.[238–242]

Instances of suspected inherited retinal atrophies have been reported occasionally in other breeds.[243–245]

Clinical signs
The ophthalmoscopic signs of inherited retinal degeneration in the cat are detected in an advanced stage with bilateral, symmetrical, diffuse tapetal hyperreflectivity and with an almost complete loss of retinal vasculature (**Figure 14.66**). In the Siamese and DSH, the early lesions of PRA have not been described. In the Abyssinian, gray mottling of the peripapillary region of the fundus on one or both sides of the optic disc is an early sign.[238–242] The gray discoloration progresses and mixes with hyperreflectivity of the tapetum. Retinal vascular attenuation begins in the periphery and progresses to complete loss of vessels. Late in the course, the nontapetum develops pigment clumping and depigmentation.

Diagnosis
The diagnosis of PRA in the cat is based on the clinical signs of bilateral, diffuse, retinal degeneration, supplementing a history that is often incomplete. Inherited atrophies should be differentiated from other causes such as nutritional, toxic, and glaucoma-induced retinal degeneration.

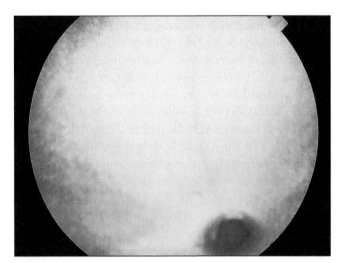

Figure 14.66 Advanced bilateral retinal degeneration in an aged Siamese that had normal taurine blood levels. Since dietary corrections may have occurred, the normal blood levels are of unknown significance.

Retinal degeneration associated with systemic metabolic disease

A variety of metabolic storage diseases have associated histopathologic lesions in the retina, but the animal may not manifest ophthalmoscopic signs. The neurologic signs are often so severe that they overshadow the ophthalmic lesions.

Disorders of amino acid metabolism

Ornithinuria associated with a deficiency of ornithine aminotransferase has been described in the cat. The significant findings are limited to the eye and result in a diffuse retinal atrophy when observed late in the course. The histopathologic changes are extensive neuroretinal and pigment epithelial damage, with a variable decrease in the size of the choriocapillaris.[246] Progressive gyrate atrophy of the choriocapillaris is the typical ophthalmoscopic finding in humans with ornithinuria. This manifests as scalloped white areas of sclera that are visible when the choroid atrophies. The clinical manifestations have been observed occasionally by the author, but whether they represent ornithinurea or choroidal vascular atrophy from other causes is unknown (**Figure 14.67**). The diagnosis is made by finding marked elevations of ornithine in the urine or plasma.

Disorders of lysosomal enzymes

- *GM1 and GM2 gangliosidosis:* GM1 and GM2 gangliosidoses are progressive neurodegenerative lysosomal storage diseases resulting mainly from the excessive accumulation of GM1 and GM2 gangliosides in the lysosomes, respectively.[247] Naturally occurring

GM1 gangliosidosis has been reported in dogs, cats, ruminants, and in wild species such as American black bears and emus.[247] Naturally occurring GM2 gangliosidosis has been reported in dogs, cats, Yorkshire pigs, Jacob sheep, and rabbit.[247] Ocular signs consist of a diffuse haze to the cornea and focal gray spots in the retina. Clear vacuoles are present in fibroblasts, corneal endothelium, and lens epithelium, and lamellated bodies are present in the ganglion cells of the retina.[247,248] Cats with GM gangliosidosis also have neurologic lesions that develop near weaning. The neurologic signs are ataxia and tremors with hypermetria that progress in severity. Abdominal distention and an enlarged liver may be present. A genetic test is now commercially available for the detection of GM1 gangliosidosis in specific breeds as Alaskan husky, shiba inu, Korat and Siamese cats, and for GM2 gangliosidosis in Burmese and Korat cats[249] (https://www.vgl.ucdavis.edu/services/cat/).

- The *mucopolysaccaridoses* are a group of recessively inherited diseases that result from the defective degradation of glycosamino glycans (GAGs). Three different forms have been described in the cat and the dog, based on the specific lysosomal enzyme deficiency. Mucopolysaccharidosis types I, VI, and VII have been described in the cat. All forms have skeletal deformities and facial dysmorphia (shortening), ocular lesions consisting of a diffuse hazy cornea and retinal degeneration, and neurologic deficits. Metachromatic granules are present in leukocytes in types VI and VII.[250–253] Rapid screening for a general diagnosis of mucopolysaccharidosis is by a toluidine blue spot test on the urine.

- Mucopolysaccharidosis types I and VII have been described in the dog. Both forms have corneal clouding and histopathologic accumulation of inclusions in the RPE, but only type VII has retinal degeneration.[254]

- *Mannosidosis* is a recessively inherited condition of defective breakdown of mannose-rich glycoproteins. The defect has been recorded in Persians, DSHs, and domestic longhair cats. The cats exhibit retarded growth, tremors, ataxia, corneal haze, lenticular vacuoles, and resting nystagmus; however, clinical presentation and progression is different in the different breeds.[255]

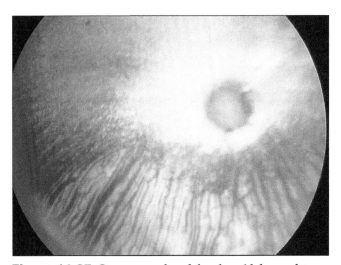

Figure 14.67 Gyrate atrophy of the choroidal vasculature and diffuse retinal atrophy in a Siamese. The cat was hyperthyroid and was noted to be blind after multiple bouts of ketamine anesthesia for diagnosis and treatment of the hyperthyroidism.

Neuronal ceroid lipofuscinosis

Neuronal ceroid lipofuscinosis (NCL) is a group of inherited metabolic diseases characterized by the accumulation of lipopigments (predominantly ceroid) in neurons and other tissues, including the retina. They are not considered lysosomal storage diseases, and the defects are thought to be associated with lipid peroxidation, but the biochemical defect has not been definitively demonstrated.[256,257] NCL has been described in a wide variety of species, including humans, and in a variety of breeds. It is usually a simple recessive trait, but the mutation varies between species and breeds of dogs. Multiple forms or mutations may even affect a single breed. The disease has been studied in most detail in the English setter. While reduced ERG amplitudes in rod- and cone-mediated a- and b-waves and inclusions were present in all the retinal layers, no ophthalmoscopic lesions were reported.[257]

Other affected breeds are the Australian blue heeler, Chihuahua, Border Collie, Saluki, Dachshund, Tibetan terrier, miniature Schnauzer, Polish Owczarek Nizinny, American bulldog, and Cocker Spaniel.[258–261] The Tibetan terrier, Polish Owczarek Nizinny, and miniature Schnauzer manifest clinical fundus changes that are similar to vitamin E deficiency and central progressive retinal atrophy.[259,261] DNA tests are now available for the American bulldog, Border Collie, and English setter (see http://www.caninegeneticdiseases.net).

Nutritional retinopathies
Taurine deficiency in the cat
Introduction/etiology

Taurine is a sulfur-containing amino acid that, in species other than the cat, is not essential, being manufactured in the liver from methionine and cystine. The cat, however, requires taurine in the diet, and the known results of a deficiency include degeneration of the photoreceptors and tapetum, lack of development of the olfactory bulb, cardiomyopathy, reproductive failure, growth retardation, platelet hyperaggregation, and altered immune function.[262–267] This concept of a nutritionally induced diffuse retinal degeneration is reinforced by the production of a similar condition induced by feeding a diet high in casein.[268]

The ophthalmoscopic appearance of early taurine deficiency retinopathy is characteristic of the disease.[269–272] The lesions are usually round to oval, hyperreflective lesions in the area centralis that may extend as a hyperreflective band above the optic disc, and in very severe cases, generalized diffuse retina atrophy can be seen. The focal lesions are asymptomatic and are picked up on routine examination.[262–267]

Although taurine is present in the brain as a neurotransmitter, neurologic signs have not been attributed to a deficiency. Due to the variable levels stored in the liver and the degree of deficiency of the diet, clinical signs may occur from 10–45 weeks after initiating a deficient diet in kittens.[262,263,273–275] The age of onset of the deficiency may affect the rapidity of the lesion's development. Young

animals are thought to be more susceptible; cats 6 months of age took only 11 months to develop focal lesions.[275,276]

Most animal products are high in taurine but heat treatment can destroy taurine.[277,278] Heat-processed can formulations require twice as much added taurine as dry, extruded foods to maintain similar levels of taurine due to bacterial degradation of intestinal taurine.[279] Focal and diffuse retinal degeneration has been described in households with multiple cats fed dog food that is low in taurine.[280]

Clinical signs

Ocular lesions of taurine deficiency initially manifest with bilateral focal mottling or hyperreflective lesions in the area centralis (**Figures 14.68 and 14.69**). The typical lesions progress to a hyperreflective band across the top of the optic disc (**Figure 14.70**). The lesion initially follows the area of highest cone concentration, and at this stage, the condition can be arrested by supplementation. If the diet remains deficient, a diffuse tapetal hyperreflectivity with concurrent decrease in retinal vessel numbers and size occurs (**Figure 14.71**). Blindness is present with diffuse retinal atrophy. Advanced lesions are nonreversible.

Diagnosis

Presumptive taurine deficiency may be suspected by the typical bilateral ophthalmoscopic signs in the area centralis or diffuse retinal degeneration. Plasma amino acid analysis can be performed, but dietary alterations can negate the value of current plasma levels correlating with past disease. Normal cat taurine values are 60–120 μmol/L.

Therapy

Early cases of taurine deficiency with degeneration in the area centralis can be arrested by correcting the nutrition. A dietary taurine level of 500–700 ppm has been suggested

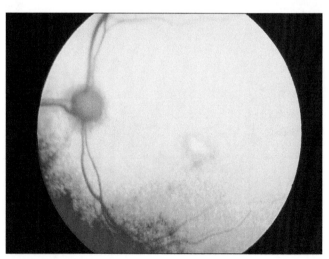

Figure 14.68 Early taurine deficiency in a cat with mild alterations in the area centralis.

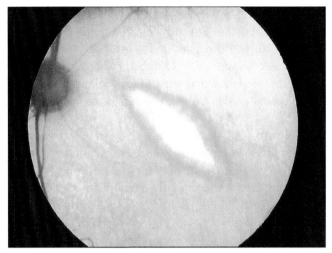

Figure 14.69 More advanced degeneration localized in the area centralis in a cat attributable to taurine deficiency.

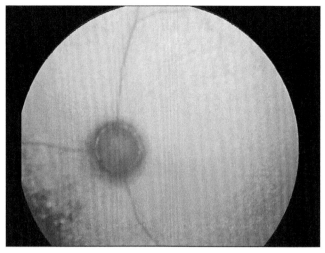

Figure 14.71 A cat with advanced taurine-induced retinal degeneration evidenced by diffuse hyperreflectivity and marked attenuation and loss of retinal vasculature.

as being necessary to prevent retinal disease. If treating for cardiomyopathy, the recommended therapy is 500 mg of taurine every 12 hours.[281] There is no therapy for diffuse retinal atrophy.

Thiamin deficiency in the cat

Thiamin deficiency in the cat is characterized by anorexia and neurologic signs of tremors, ataxia, ventroflexion of the head (**Figure 14.72**), and convulsions. Ocular signs usually consist only of bilateral mydriasis due to midbrain hemorrhages. Rarely, retinal neovascularization, vascular tortuosity, and peripapillary edema are present (**Figure 14.73**).[282,283]

Vitamin E deficiency in the dog

Puppies fed a diet deficient in vitamin E develop retinopathy 3 months after weaning. The lesions develop by

3 months of age as a fine mottling in the posterior tapetal region. By 4 months of age, the puppies are night blind, and the mottling has spread peripherally. At 6 months of age, the mottled areas are surrounded by hyperreflectivity of the tapetum, and vascular attenuation is noted. At 8–12 months of age, the tapetum has discrete multifocal yellow-brown areas and is hyperreflective (**Figure 14.74**). The vasculature is attenuated and has focal constrictions. On histopathology, the focal pigment is lipofuscin, and photoreceptor degeneration is present in the central retina.[284,285] These lesions are very similar to the presumed inherited retinal pigment epitheliopathy (RPED), to Briard RPE65 SNB, and in those breeds with NCL that manifest fundus lesions.[222,261] Lower plasma vitamin E levels have been

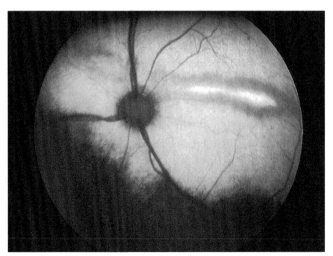

Figure 14.70 A cat with a band of retinal atrophy progressing from the area centralis across the top of the optic disc from taurine deficiency.

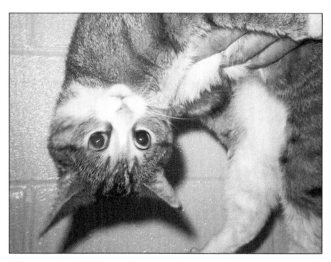

Figure 14.72 Ventroflexion of the head when suspended in a cat with thiamin deficiency. Deficiency was induced by feeding commercial cat food that had the thiamin content destroyed by heat treatment.

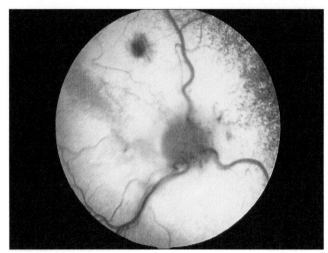

Figure 14.73 Fundus of a cat presented with neurologic signs and responsive to thiamin injections. Retinal hemorrhages, neovascularization, vascular tortuosity, and retinal edema are present. Most cats with thiamin deficiency have a normal fundus.

found in RPED-affected Briards and in RPED-affected Cocker Spaniels and Nizzinis.[232] The latter two breeds show the greatest decrease in vitamin E levels and commonly also have accompanying neurologic signs of proprioceptive deficits, ataxia, and altered spinal reflexes.[232] The biokinetics of vitamin E appear to be abnormal in that vitamin E absorption from an oral dose is near normal, but the plasma levels decline much faster after peaking.[232,233]

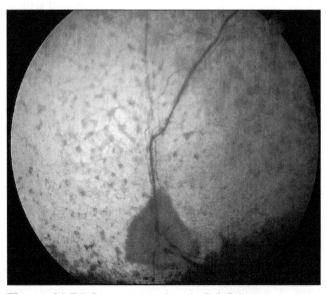

Figure 14.74 Spontaneous vitamin E deficiency retinopathy in a hunting dog with a bizarre homemade diet. Note the multifocal brown accumulations in the tapetal fundus. Compare to Figure 14.64, a case of central retinal atrophy. (Courtesy of Dr. M. Davidson, North Carolina State University, Raleigh, NC.)

Davidson et al. described a cluster of spontaneous vitamin E deficiency in hunting dogs fed food scraps, cattle offal, and turkey carcasses and is associated with slowly progressive blindness.[286] Ophthalmoscopic signs were identical to experimental vitamin E deficiency, consisting of multifocal golden brown accumulations in the central tapetal fundus that gradually increased in severity with age (**Figure 14.74**). Mild tapetal hyperreflectivity and vascular attenuation were also present. Optic nerve atrophy, a decrease in pigment clumping, asteroid hyalosis, and minor cataracts eventually developed with end-stage disease. Serum level of vitamin E was <3 µg/mL (normal range 6–10 µg/mL).[286]

Equine motor neuron disease (EMND)

Equine motor neuron disease (EMND) is a neurodegenerative disease characterized by diffuse neuromuscular disease, weight loss with good appetite, generalized weakness, excessive lying down, sweating, and muscle tremors.[287] Ophthalmoscopic lesions are similar to vitamin E deficiency in the dog, specifically multifocal brown spots in the tapetum and, in addition, a brown band at the junction of the tapetum and nontapetum in a characteristic honeycomb mosaic pattern. Visual deficits are not usually appreciated by the owner. Autofluorescent ceroid lipofuscin accumulates in the RPE and retina with photoreceptor degeneration.[287] Ophthalmoscopy is an excellent field test for diagnosing equine motor neuron disease.

Vitamin A deficiency in the dog

Vitamin A deficiency is a rare disease in carnivores but, when experimentally produced, results in similar neurologic and ophthalmologic signs as in cattle. Neurologic signs of circling, ataxia, agitation, and convulsions are noted. Despite normal cerebrospinal fluid (CSF) pressures, ophthalmic signs of blindness and papilledema develop.[288]

Vitamin A deficiency in cattle
Introduction/etiology

Vitamin A deficiency is a significant disease in cattle. The clinical signs vary with the age of the animal. Vitamin A is provided in cattle feed as retinoids or as a provitamin β-carotene that is found in leafy green plants. Vitamin A is essential for rhodopsin regeneration. Cereal grains are deficient in β-carotene, except for corn. Deficiency can produce signs in 4–8 months, with younger animals developing signs more rapidly. The lag period depends on the residual liver stores and the degree of deficiency in the diet. The conditions under which it is observed are usually in young growing animals on drought-stricken pastures, in animals fed poorly cured and stored forage, or feedlot cattle being fed diets high in grain. Sexual dimorphism in susceptibility probably exists, with males being more susceptible.[289]

The dura mater becomes thickened in response to vitamin A deficiency, and this results in decreased absorption of CSF by the arachnoid villi. This results in increased CSF pressure, which is thought to be the earliest detectable change with vitamin A deficiency and is the cause of seizures. In young animals <6 months of age that have normal remodeling of the skull during growth, the sphenoid bone with the optic canal has a predominant production of bone without resorption. This overproduction of bone and thickened dura mater produces direct compressive forces on the optic nerve, as well as vascular ischemic changes. The compression produces demyelination and malacia of the optic nerve. This does not occur experimentally in older (2-year-old) animals.[290–293]

Clinical signs

In yearling and younger cattle, night blindness is often the first sign, but it is frequently not noted because of husbandry conditions.[294,295] This progresses to total blindness, which is often the first sign noted. This is accompanied by pupillary dilation. The blindness is irreversible.

Bilateral papilledema is the first useful objective sign (**Figure 14.76**). It is reversible in the early stages and is present before blindness occurs. Papilledema precedes optic nerve constriction and is due to increased CSF pressure. Papilledema is not as consistent in adults as it is in growing animals.[296] It manifests in the loss of distinct

borders, enlargement, and elevation of the disc. The disc color changes to pink-white with obscuration of the vessels by the edema.[295,297] Small hemorrhages are common on or adjacent to the disc (**Figure 14.75**). If the condition is chronic, the optic disc becomes atrophic with a gray color and loss of elevation. Retinal degeneration occurs. This is most obvious in the nontapetal peripapillary region as pigment disruption (**Figure 14.76**). Vitamin A is necessary for production of rhodopsin, and deficiency results in disruption of the photoreceptors as well as damage to the RPE.[295]

Miscellaneous ophthalmic signs consist of bilateral exophthalmos and a decrease in corneal sensitivity. Nonophthalmic signs consist of tonic-clonic seizures of short duration, ataxia, gaunt and unthrifty animals, poor growth, decreased mental status, diarrhea, anasarca, and pneumonia.

Vitamin A deficiency in older animals results in less dramatic signs of night blindness that may not progress, papilledema without constriction of the optic nerve, and mottling of the tapetal colors and the nontapetal pigment.[296] Nonophthalmic signs are incoordination, seizures, diarrhea, anasarca, and pneumonia.

Diagnosis

Clinical signs of papilledema, blindness, retinal degeneration, and seizures are highly suggestive when combined with supportive historical data regarding feed. Plasma vitamin A levels <200 µg/L (<20 µg/dL) and liver vitamin A levels <2 µg/g are diagnostic. Liver levels are more reliable than plasma levels in diagnosis as they are not as variable.

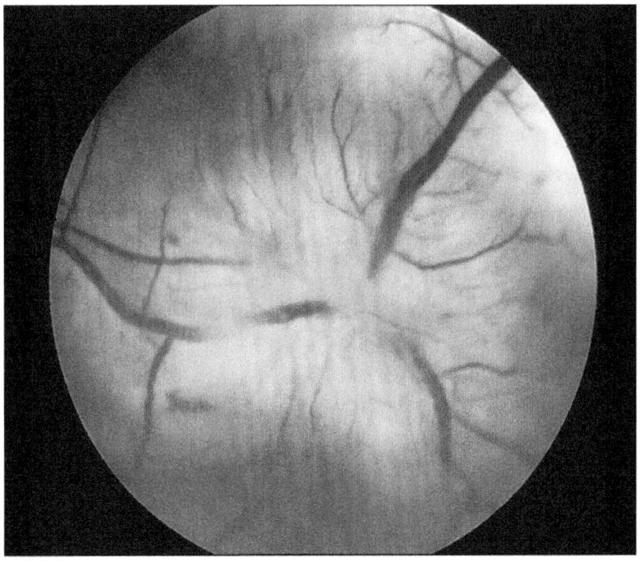

Figure 14.75 Severe papilledema in a steer with vitamin A deficiency. Note the change in color, elevation, hyperemia, and splinter hemorrhages in the disc. Compare to the normal bovine fundus in 14.2.

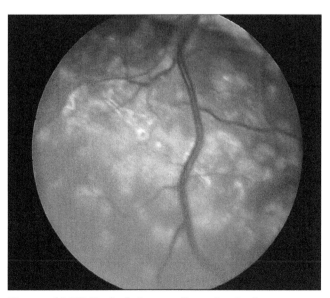

Figure 14.76 Retinal pigment disruption in the nontapetal region in a steer with vitamin A deficiency.

Therapy

Cattle with papilledema but which are not blind may respond to 440 IU/kg vitamin A injection intramuscularly or orally. Dietary supplementation should be up to 80 IU/kg if on a high-energy diet.[297,298]

Prognosis

Adult animals may show improvement of night blindness or vision loss, but young animals, if blind, will not have reversal of blindness due to optic nerve changes. Night blindness and papilledema are reversible if treated before complete blindness occurs.

Drug- and toxin-induced retinal/uveal degeneration

Methylnitrosourea and ketamine hydrochloride

A dramatic, rapid, diffuse retinal degeneration with blindness develops when ketamine is administered to cats also given methylnitrosourea. Either drug alone does not produce the retinal lesion. Twenty-four hours after the combination of ketamine and methylnitrosourea is given, diffuse retinal edema is detected, but PLRs are normal. Retinal degeneration develops 5 days after drug administration and is characterized by vascular attenuation and a hyperreflectivity of the tapetum that is most severe at the tapetal–nontapetal junction. The appearance in chronic cases is similar to advanced retinal atrophy from taurine deficiency. Pathologically, acute lesions are a diffuse and severe loss of photoreceptors and the outer nuclear layer.[299]

A variety of drugs have been demonstrated to have toxicity to the retina or choroid; however, most are not drugs that are used for therapeutic purposes in veterinary medicine, or they are not used in doses sufficient to produce lesions. Examples of such drugs are chloroquine, iodoacetate, phenothiazine derivatives, diphenylalkane derivatives, diethyldithiocarbamate, and hydroxypyridinethione.[299]

Fluoroquinolone-induced retinal degeneration in cats

Fluoroquinolones, specifically enrofloxacin, are known to produce an acute blindness with pupillary dilation and reduced ERG amplitudes in cats.[300] Typical ophthalmoscopic signs in symptomatic cats are usually a diffuse tapetal hyperreflectivity and mild-to-severe retinal vascular attenuation (**Figure 14.77**). Earlier lesions, which are less likely to be observed unless screening patients on therapy, are granular to gray discoloration of the area centralis and visual streak and focal tapetal hyperreflectivity. Generalized tapetal reflectivity is present by day 5–7 post administration of high doses of enrofloxacin at 50 mg/kg by mouth.[301] Additional neurologic signs, weight loss, and

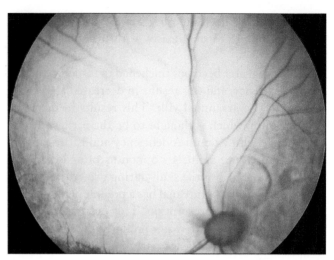

Figure 14.77 Siamese cat presented with acute blindness after receiving enrofloxacin orally. The tapetum is mildly hyperreflective, and the retinal vasculature is attenuated.

decreased food consumption were also noted at experimentally high doses.[301]

The toxic effects of enrofloxacin appear to be dose related and not idiosyncratic. The clinical report suggested that increasing age, IV administration of the drug, the dose, and other systemic factors (as renal and hepatic dysfunction) that may interfere with drug metabolism may be contributing factors to retinal toxicity.[300] Very high doses of orbifloxacin may also induce retinal changes of focal hyperreflectivity.[302] If enrofloxacin is used in cats, it is recommended that the dose does not exceed 5 mg/kg every 24 hours.[300–302] Recently, it has been shown that cats have four specific amino acid sequence differences in the P-glycoprotein ABCG2. Distribution of fluoroquinolones to the retina is normally restricted by the ABCG2 at the blood–retinal barrier.[303] Feline-specific amino acid changes in ABCG2 cause a functional defect of the transport protein in cats. This functional defect may be owing, in part, to defective cellular localization of feline ABCG2.[303]

Ethylene glycol intoxication

Retinal hemorrhages, focal transudative retinal detachment, and a mosaic or gyrate pattern of retinal folds from edema have been described in a cat that survived ethylene glycol poisoning (**Figure 14.78**). The cause of the retinal lesions was postulated to be due to obstruction of choroidal capillaries with transudation of fluid from the choroid to the subretinal space.[304] The author has also observed retinal detachment and retinal vitreal hemorrhage in the dog associated with experimental ethylene glycol intoxication.

Ivermectin toxicity

Massive overdosage of ivermectin to dogs and cats has resulted in blindness, obtundation, tremors, ataxia, emesis,

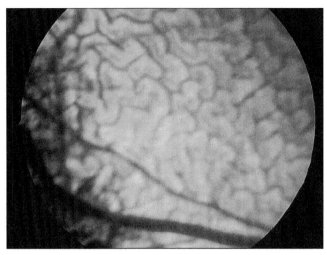

Figure 14.78 Retinopathy observed with ethylene glycol toxicity in a cat. The retina is thrown into gyrate folds due to subretinal fluid transudation from the choroid. The condition resolved following recovery of the cat from the intoxication. (Courtesy of Dr. R. Riis, Ithaca, NY.)

and salivation.[305-307] The overdosage usually occurs when large animal ivermectin preparations are used carelessly in dogs and cats. A genetic defect in MDR-1 has been found as the cause of ivermectin sensitivity.[307] Acute blindness is noted, with poor PLRs. Ophthalmoscopic findings may be papilledema and retinal edema producing retinal folds,[305-309] but in the author's experience, most patients have a normal fundus, dilated pupils, and blindness that improves within 48 hours. Improvement in vision has been observed even when animals have been comatose for days.[305-309] Atrophy of the RPE has been noted with chronic ivermectin therapy (**Figure 14.79**). Diagnosis is

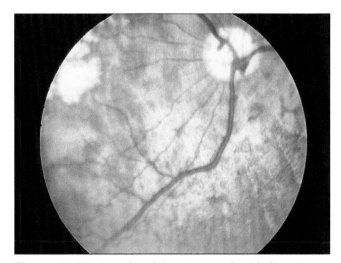

Figure 14.79 Atrophy of the pigmented epithelium in a dog with decreased vision that had been treated with ivermectin for mange.

based on clinical signs, history, toxicological assay results for serum sample, and electroretinogram (ERG).[306,307,309]

Therapy for ivermectin toxicosis is based on supportive care. Use of intravenous lipid emulsion has been described in dogs and cats.[309,310]

Locoweed poisoning

Cattle, sheep, and horses with locoweed (*Astragalus mollissimus*) poisoning are blind, with a dull corneal surface. While the dull appearance is due to tear film problems from lacrimal gland lesions, blindness is probably due to lesions observed in the ganglion and bipolar cells of the retina. Ophthalmoscopic lesions have not been described.[311]

Bracken poisoning

Bracken (*Pteris aquilina*) ingestion by sheep has produced retinal degeneration. The long-term ingestion of bracken produces blindness in sheep usually older than 2 years of age. Ophthalmoscopic signs are a diffuse hyperreflective tapetum, optic disc atrophy, and attenuated retinal vessels. The histologic lesions are initially photoreceptor degeneration and, later, inner retinal cell loss.[312]

Male fern poisoning

Cattle ingesting male fern (*Dryopteris felix mas*) may develop acute blindness, weakness, and constipation. In the acute stages, the ophthalmoscopic signs are dilated pupils, papilledema, and papillary and peripapillary hemorrhage. Some animals may recover vision, but with chronicity, the acute signs develop into optic nerve atrophy, retinal vascular attenuation, and disruption of the pigment in the peripapillary nontapetal region. Histopathologically, the primary lesion is a noninflammatory destruction of the axons and the medullary nerve sheaths of the retrobulbar nerve.[313]

Glaucoma-induced retinal degeneration
Introduction/etiology

Glaucoma is a common cause of retinal and optic nerve degeneration. Depending on the cause of the glaucoma, the fundus changes may be unilateral or bilateral, and sequential or simultaneous in occurrence. The rapidity of the process, degree of intraocular pressure (IOP) elevation, and individual variation in IOP tolerance can produce variable fundus lesions. The pathogenesis of glaucomatous retinal and optic nerve changes may be two-fold: (1) Interference in axoplasmic flow, which damages axons and neurons, and (2) ischemia to the nerve and retina. Acute high-tension glaucoma probably has both mechanisms at work because a full-thickness retinal atrophy usually develops. Lower tension glaucoma may be characterized only by atrophy of the optic nerve, nerve fiber layer, and ganglion cells, which may occur from a mechanical restriction at the disc, interfering with axoplasmic flow of the nerves. This may create retrograde degeneration of the ganglion cells.[314–316] (See Chapter 12, for a more detailed discussion and figures.) Whiteman et al. found evidence of a progressive retinal degeneration from cellular apoptosis in glaucomatous eyes\that began in the ganglion cell layer and progressed to full-thickness retinal cell death.[317]

> Knowledge of the progressive nature of glaucomatous retinal degeneration after the IOP has been normalized adds to the frustration and pessimism associated with treating glaucoma.

Clinical signs

The most typical fundus lesion with glaucoma is a variable degree of optic disc cupping and atrophy. Unless the optic nerve changes are unilateral or observed sequentially, they may be difficult to recognize in the early stages due to the great variability in the canine fundus. The evidence for optic nerve cupping and atrophy is loss of myelin, often with a pigmented ring around the disc visible after receding of the myelin, a gray color to the disc, and posterior deviation of vessels on the disc surface (**Figure 14.80**). These changes are not recognized in the cat unless extreme. In very acute elevations of IOP, papilledema and peripapillary hemorrhages and triangular patches of retinal edema, which may represent infarcts adjacent to the disc, may be present (see Chapter 12, **Figures 12.20 and 12.21**). Vascular attenuation is common but variable, and retinal atrophy is usually observed as tapetal hyperreflectivity.

The pattern of hyperreflectivity may be quite diffuse, patchy, or peripapillary. Choroidal atrophy may be visible in the albinoid fundus as a loss of vasculature and may follow an arcuate pattern. On histopathology, the retina over the tapetal region typically manifests less pathology from glaucoma than the nontapetal area, but this difference is not appreciated on ophthalmoscopy.

Diagnosis

Diagnosis of optic nerve glaucomatous neuropathy is based on clinical signs and history of glaucoma. Usually the specific cause of the retinal atrophy is identified by accompanying ocular signs.

Peripheral cystoid retinal degeneration

Peripheral retinal cysts (Blessig–Iwanoffs cysts in humans) are very common degenerative changes adjacent to the ora ciliaris retinae (**Figures 14.81 and 14.82**). They are usually multiple and are most easily observed with the indirect ophthalmoscope at the temporal and ventral ora ciliaris retinae. In a series of 86 Beagles 8 years of age, 85% had peripheral retinal cysts.[318] They are usually present without evidence of retinal detachment, although idiopathic retinal detachment associated with giant tears of the peripheral retina is not uncommon in the dog. They vary in size, number, and degree of elevation and are considered a normal senile aging change.[319] In one study of senile retinal breaks, 5 out of 100 eyes had ruptured cysts that produced retinal holes.[320] The same study demonstrated that 24% of the eyes had complete retinal breaks, although none of the eyes had retinal detachments, and an additional 38% of the eyes had incomplete breaks. Thus, a total of 62% of the senile eyes had lesions predisposing them to retinal detachment.[320]

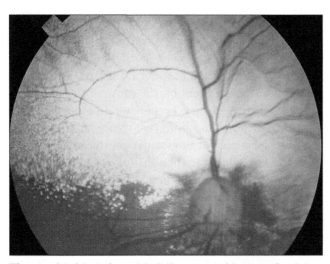

Figure 14.80 A dog with diffuse tapetal hyperreflectivity and optic nerve atrophy and cupping, associated with glaucoma.

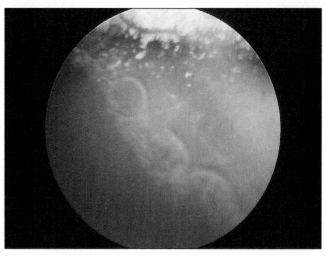

Figure 14.81 Peripheral retinal cysts adjacent to the ora ciliaris retinae in a dog.

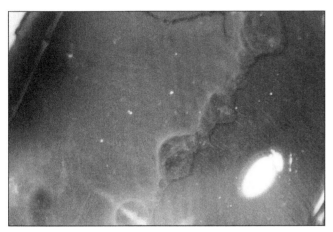

Figure 14.82 Pathologic specimen from a Cocker Spaniel opened to reveal the posterior globe. Note the multiple cysts at the ora ciliaris retinae. The retina is gray from fixation, and the pars plana of the ciliary body is the heavily pigmented side.

Retinal degenerations of unknown cause
Sudden acquired retinal degeneration syndrome (SARDS)

Introduction/etiology

Sudden acquired retinal degeneration syndrome (SARDS) is a syndrome of sudden blindness in dogs that has been recognized with increased frequency in the United States and the rest of the world. SARDS has become a leading cause of currently incurable vision loss in dogs.[321,322] Typically, dogs affected with SARDS present for assessment of rapid vision loss that develops over a period of days to weeks.[322]

SARDS frequently affects middle-aged to elderly and often moderately overweight dogs. The reported mean or median ages of affected dogs range from 7 to 10 years.[322] No breed or genetic predisposition was initially reported, but more contemporary reports indicate that the Dachshund, miniature Schnauzer, Brittany, and Beagle may be at increased risk.[321,323,324] There is sexual dimorphism with 60%–90% of cases occurring in females; the vast majority are in neutered animals.[322,324]

Approximately 50% of the patients have systemic complaints of polyphagia, weight gain, polyuria, and polydipsia.[322]

A variety of exotic and routine laboratory examinations have found no consistent abnormality, nor have epidemiologic questionnaires. Elevation of liver enzymes, white blood cell counts consistent with a stress leukogram, and an abnormal adrenocorticotropic hormone (ACTH) stimulation test or low-dose dexamethasone suppression test are found in many, but not all, animals with SARDS, and 12% to 17% of the cases have laboratory profiles compatible with Cushing's disease, but not all of the series were evaluated critically for Cushing's.[321] Holt et al. found 21% of 38 dogs had a positive screening test for Cushing's disease.[323] Carter et al. in studying 10 neutered dogs with SARDS found nine had systemic signs of glucocorticoid excess, and eight of these had systemic elevations of sex hormone levels, while only five had elevations of cortisol levels post-ACTH stimulation.[325] The investigators interpreted this as evidence of increased adrenal activity. Preliminary results have demonstrated an antiretinal compliment-fixing antibody in the serum of dogs (5/5) affected with SARDS.[326] Keller et al. could not duplicate the finding of serum autoantibodies against retinal proteins when screening 13 dogs with SARDS, nor could Gilmore et al., who compared SARDS with normal dogs and dogs with cancer.[327,328] Gilmore et al. also could find no evidence of either adrenal or pituitary neoplasia in dogs with SARDS using ultrasound and CT imaging.[328] There does not appear to be a comparable syndrome in humans, although paraneoplastic syndromes associated with pulmonary carcinomas and melanomas may have some similarities. These cancer retinopathies are thought to induce an autoimmune reaction to retinal proteins such as recoverin and enolase.

Abnormal melanin synthesis and metabolism in the RPE has been postulated to affect the phagocytosis of the photoreceptor outer segments, which leads to a degenerative process of the photoreceptors. ACTH and melanocyte-stimulating hormone (MSH) may have a hormonal influence on the RPE that leads to this degenerative process.[321]

SARDS may be a syndrome rather than a specific disease. Anecdotal reports of partial blindness, slowly progressive blindness, and unilateral involvement only serve to confuse the issue by adding more variables. A corollary would be our understanding of PRA 30 years ago, when it was considered one disease, but we now know it to be an umbrella term for multiple specific diseases.

An extinguished ERG which, when seen in conjunction with a clinically normal appearing fundus, is considered the hallmark of SARDS and allows differentiation from other neurologic causes of acute vision loss, such as optic neuritis and intracranial neoplasia, where the ERG is generally not affected.[322] In the early stages of the disease, the histopathologic lesions are mainly a total loss of photoreceptor outer segments[325] that die by apoptosis.[322,329]

> An extinguished ERG which, when seen in conjunction with a clinically normal appearing fundus, is considered the hallmark of SARDS.

Clinical signs

Acute SARDS patients are presented as blind and confused, with dilated pupils and a normal fundus. The retinal vessels may have vascular sacculations (inconsistent) or be mildly attenuated in size. This contrasts with most retinal diseases where, if the process is severe enough to produce blindness, obvious retinal changes are usually present.

Chronic SARDS cases develop mild-to-modest tapetal hyperreflectivity and vascular attenuation (**Figure 14.83**). While the pupils are dilated at rest, they react sluggishly to light. This disconnect between having an animal that is blind with a photoreceptor disease yet still having quite robust PLRs with a strong white light is thought to be associated with special ganglion cells that contain the photopigment melanopsin. Retinal ganglion cells containing melanopsin are thought to be responsible for regulating nonvisual photoreceptions such as circadian rhythms and the PLR. These ganglion cells project to the nuclei in the midbrain but not the superior colliculus or lateral geniculate. The ganglion cells also interplay with the rod and cone photoreceptors.[330,331] Grozdanic et al. were able to demonstrate PLRs to a very bright white light in dogs with SARDS, but the PLR response was more sensitive to a blue light, which matches more closely the absorption spectra of melanopsin.[332] The rod and cone-driven PLR was more sensitive to white light than the ganglion cells and was more reactive to the red light than the ganglion cell component. Thus, through the sensitivity both to light intensity and to color spectrum, it is possible to determine which part of the retina has the pathology. On electroretinography of SARDS dogs, the tracing is extinguished or flat. The ERG differentiates retinal blindness from optic nerve blindness, where the ERG is normal.

Therapy

It is generally believed that vision loss with SARDS is permanent, and there is no treatment that can prevent or reverse SARDS-related blindness.[322]

Retinal detachment
Introduction/etiology

As mentioned previously, retinal detachments (RD) are a separation of the neurosensory retina from the underlying RPE (**Figure 14.84**).

There are three main mechanisms that can lead to retinal detachment:

- Serous or exudative RD (subretinal effusion or exudation of fluid).
- Tractional RD (presence of vitreal bands or membranes that produce traction forces on the retina).
- Rhegmatogenous retinal detachment (RRD), or those due to holes and tears in the retina allowing the passage of vitreous into the subretinal space.

Retinal detachment can be related to various pathologic conditions including congenital ocular anomalies such as

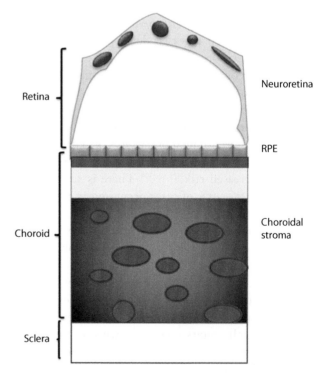

Figure 14.84 Serous retinal detachment. Schematic drawing representing the separation between the neuroretina and the RPE. (E. Abarca, Auburn University.)

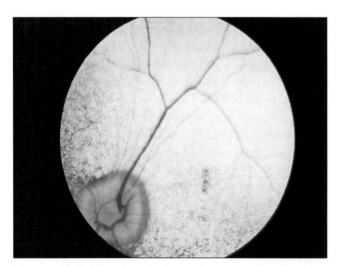

Figure 14.83 Fundus of a dog with acute sudden acquired retinal degeneration syndrome, with mild vascular attenuation and a near normal fundus except for a small linear scar.

retinal dysplasia and CEA, glaucoma, trauma, inflammation, lens-induced uveitis, cataracts, intraocular surgery, vitreal liquefaction and degeneration, and systemic vascular diseases.[333-338]

Serous retinal detachments are often associated with infectious, neoplastic, immune-mediated, and systemic hypertensive etiologies.[333] Detachments of this nature are mostly treated medically, with reattachment of the retina and visual outcome dependent on etiology, chronicity, and patient response to treatment.[333] Tractional retinal detachments are often the result of intraocular inflammation and/or hemorrhage, with resultant inflammatory membrane formation.

RRD is the result of retinal breaks that allow vitreous access to the potential space between the neurosensory retina and RPE. The result is often a progressive retinal tear that leads to retinal dialysis and blindness.[42,333] The basic cause is often unknown, although trauma, microtrauma, and vascular and zonular tension on the peripheral retina may play a role. Posterior capsular rupture with cataract surgery or intracapsular lens extraction is a risk factor for retinal detachment. Johnston and Ward discounted the increased risk of retinal detachment after posterior capsular rupture in the dog.[339] Degenerative changes in the peripheral retina may create holes or circumferential tears and result in retinal detachment. On routine screening, 62% of senile dog eyes have been shown to have partial or complete retinal breaks, but no retinal detachments were found in this series. The lack of either posterior vitreous detachment or liquefied vitreous may have prevented the retina from detaching with these degenerative changes.[320] RRD and pathogenesis of vitreoretinopathy has been extensively studied in Shih Tzu dogs. Affected dogs were middle-aged to older, consistent with previous descriptions of vitreous degeneration in Shih Tzu dogs, which is referred to as an age-related condition.[40,42] This observation suggests a similarity with retinal tear associated with vitreous degeneration in humans, where loss of vitreous gel and the separation of the vitreous body from the retina increase the risk of retinal tear, RD, and age-related nuclear cataract.[40,42]

In horses, equine recurrent uveitis (68%) and trauma (25%) are the major causes of retinal detachment. In one study, bullous detachments were the only form observed, although they also had varying degrees of peripheral giant retinal tears and holes.[340] Despite this, the authors did not think the detachments were rhegmatogenous in origin.

In the cat, although no series of detachments have been reported, the author's experience is that most are classified as serous or exudative and secondary to systemic disease as vascular (hypertension) or inflammatory (chorioretinitis) in nature.

Clinical signs

Unilateral complete retinal detachment may present with a Marcus Gunn (MG) pupil when testing the PLR with the swinging light test. The MG response manifests as a very limited direct reflex in the involved eye, but the pupil constricts with the consensual reflex when the light is swung to the good eye. When the light is then swung back to the involved eye for a repeat of the direct response, the pupil dilates rather than remains constricted.

If the media is clear, variable degrees of retinal detachment may be directly observed with a simple light because the torn retina has moved forward behind the lens (**Figure 14.85**). The retina looks like a grayish veil visible as a vascularized bullae located either directly behind the lens or deeper in the vitreous body. Low partial detachments or complete peripheral dialysis can often only be visualized with an ophthalmoscope (**Figures 14.86 and 14.87**). Traction membranes may occasionally be visible on the retina (**Figure 14.88**). Tearing of retinal vessels when detaching may create vitreal clots or diffuse hemorrhage into both the vitreous and anterior chamber. Chronic retinal detachments are often associated with preiridal fibrovascular membranes and neovascularization of the anterior segment of the eye, which often results in hyphema and/or glaucoma.[336,337] Another mechanism for glaucoma with rhegmatogenous retinal detachment may be obstruction of the outflow channels by photoreceptor

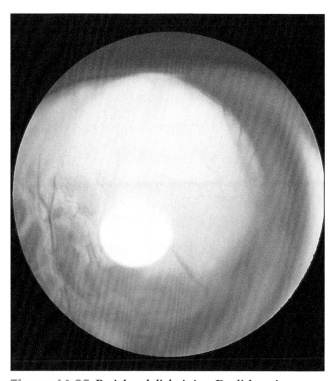

Figure 14.85 Peripheral dialysis in a English springer spaniel associated with retinal dysplasia. The folded retina is visible behind the lens, without an ophthalmoscope.

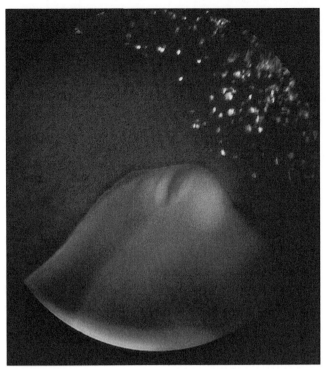

Figure 14.86 A dog with complete peripheral dialysis of the retina that is visible hanging limply from the optic disc.

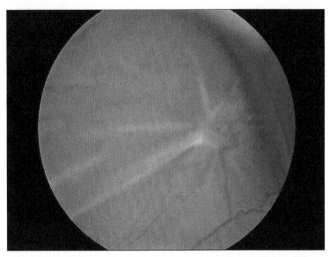

Figure 14.88 Preretinal membrane on the retina causing a focal traction detachment. The detachment was observed originally on a screening genetic eye examination in a Siberian husky and did not change over several years.

outer segments. This mechanism has been implicated in producing glaucoma in humans,[338] and while outer segments have been detected in the aqueous humor of dogs with rhegmatogenous detachments, they have not been associated with glaucoma.[341] Effusive retinal detachments (including steroid-responsive retinal detachment) are discussed with chorioretinitis and hypertension.

Diagnosis

The diagnosis of retinal detachment is made on ophthalmoscopic examination if the media is clear, or by ocular B-mode ultrasound if opacities are present. One of the most important roles of echography is to evaluate the status of the retina in the presence of opaque media.[39] The echographic features of RD are typically quite characteristic: RD generally appears as a bright, continuous echogenic membrane of B-scan (usually linear or curvilinear).[342,343] A complete retinal detachment has been referred to as a V-shaped curvilinear membrane or classic seagull-shaped lesion (with the wings representing the retina, billowing from the remaining anchor points at the ora ciliaris retinae and the optic disc).[342,344]

Therapy

Detachments associated with tears or holes are candidates for retinal detachment surgery, whereas serous/exudative detachments are treated by treating the underlying cause (e.g., inflammation, systemic hypertension). Retinal detachment surgery in veterinary medicine is becoming more available each year. With the newer techniques utilizing intraocular perfluorocarbon gases and silicone oil to tamponade and laser retinopexies, retinal detachment surgery is quite successful. Unilateral retinal detachments are

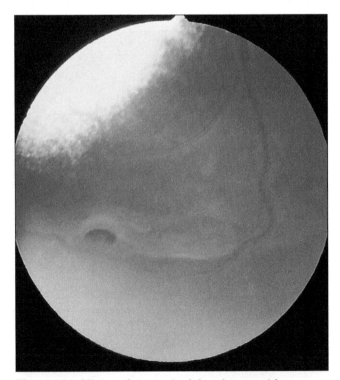

Figure 14.87 Low-lying retinal detachment with a visible hole in the retina. The dog had aplastic anemia, and the lesion was picked up on a screening consultation examination.

often diagnosed late, but surprisingly, even with chronic detachments (i.e., up to 4 weeks or greater duration), visual function may return with successful reattachment.[108,109,345] Success varies with complicating circumstances for the detachment and duration of detachment and may be measured in terms of retinal reattachment and/or return of functional vision rates. Overall, Vainisi and Wolfer reported a 90% reattachment rate and 76% had vision.[345]

Prophylaxis

High-risk patients (e.g., animals with partial detachments or marked vitreal degeneration, the opposite eye previously having a retinal detachment, breed susceptibility to retinal detachments, or even performing surgery on hypermature cataracts) may benefit from prophylactic retinopexy. Laser surgery is best performed in a transpupillary fashion when direct observation of the retina is possible.[43,346]

Inflammation of the retina and choroid

Introduction/etiology

When evaluating a suspected inflammatory fundus lesion, four questions should arise:

- Is this an inflammatory lesion or some other process?
- Is the inflammation active or inactive?
- Is the inflammation granulomatous or nongranulomatous?
- What are the possible causes of the inflammation?

Inflammation of the posterior segment is usually referred to as chorioretinitis or posterior uveitis. If the primary focus is in the retina, it is termed retinochoroiditis; if the primary focus is in the choroid, it is termed chorioretinitis.

Clinical signs

The signs of inflammation of the structures of the fundus are often not specific or dramatic enough to make it obvious whether a lesion is inflammatory, degenerative, vascular, or neoplastic. Furthermore, once a lesion is recognized as inflammatory, there is little evidence morphologically that can determine the cause of the inflammation.

Active inflammation (tapetal versus nontapetal area) (**Figure 14.89**)

Active inflammation in the tapetal area is characterized by edema that may manifest as an opacification or hazy appearance of the retina, hyporeflective lesions (decreased tapetal reflectivity), loss of tapetal mosaic detail, and, perhaps, elevation of the retina with changes in the direction of the retinal vessels (**Figure 14.90**).

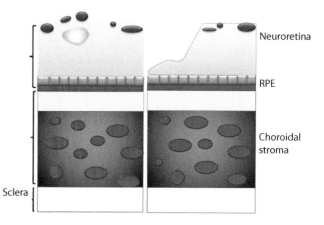

Figure 14.89 **Chorioretinitis (tapetal area) active versus inactive lesions. Schematic drawing representing the difference between active chorioretinitis (left) and inactive chorioretinitis (right) in the tapetal area. (E. Abarca, Auburn University.)**

Changes in the retinal vascular bed (congestive blood vessels and increases in tortuosity) are often difficult to recognize because of the subjectivity of vascular size and tortuosity. Damage to vascular walls may result in hemorrhages at various levels in the fundus (see Chapter 1, section Ophthalmoscopy).

Cellular exudation may be recognized by a haze in the vitreous and "exudates" in the retina. Acute cellular exudation produces soft exudates (**Figure 14.91**). Occasionally, cellular exudation may be perivascular in distribution. Depending on the intensity, perivascular cuffing variably manifests as a white sheath, a perivascular altered reflective zone, or perivascularly aligned focal exudates.

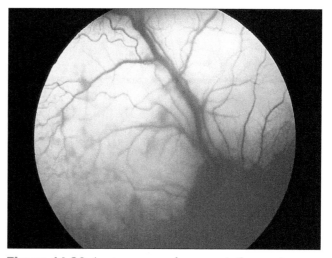

Figure 14.90 **Acute nongranulomatous inflammation over the tapetum in a dog. The lesions are gray with indistinct borders. The lesions were associated with acute distemper infection.**

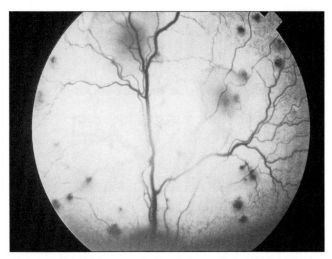

Figure 14.91 Acute and chronic granulomatous lesions in a dog with cryptococcosis. The acute lesions have a halo of edema, whereas the chronic dark lesions are sharply circumscribed.

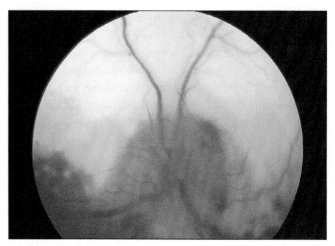

Figure 14.93 Acute inflammation of the optic nerve (papillitis, optic neuritis), evidenced by a hyperemic, swollen blurred disc, and hemorrhages. The dog was also blind, which differentiates this from papilledema.

Acute and active inflammation in the nontapetal region in the acute stages often obscures the pigment with white (depigmented areas) exudation or edema (**Figure 14.92**). Pigment clumping and disruption occurs in the acute stages if the RPE reacts and in the chronic stages as macrophages scavenge.

Inflammation of the optic nerve papilla or disc is manifested by hyperemia of the disc, hemorrhages on and around the disc, elevation of the disc from edema, retinal vessel deviation, haze over the disc from cellular exudation, and peripapillary edema (**Figure 14.93**). Post inflammation, the optic nerve usually manifests varying degrees of atrophy. Atrophy of the optic nerve is recognized by a gray-white coloration, loss of myelin that may convert an elevated disc to a flat or cupped disc, a decrease

in size and number of retinal vessels and, sometimes, peripapillary pigmentary changes (**Figure 14.96**).

Inactive inflammation (tapetal versus nontapetal area)

Presumptive confirmation of active inflammation is often made by watching the dynamic course, that is, it either progresses in severity or improves with or without therapy. Fluorescein angiography can demonstrate active inflammation by vascular leakage. When evaluating lesions, one should attempt to determine whether they are quiescent or active (**Figure 14.89**). Active lesions usually have blurred borders, haziness or dullness, or lack of tapetal detail over the lesion (**Figures 14.90 and 14.91**). Postinflammatory scars are hyperreflective over the tapetal region, have sharp borders, and may have pigment clumping in the center or at the periphery of the lesion. In the nontapetal area, postinflammatory scars are sharply defined and depigmented lesions typically associated with hyperpigmented lesions. (**Figures 14.94 and 14.95**). When inflammation of the fundus has been diffuse, the postinflammatory appearance may be very similar to PRA (**Figure 14.96**). However, inflammatory retinal atrophies are usually asymmetrical in severity between the two eyes, whereas PRA is almost always symmetrical. When possible, it is pertinent to define the inflammation clinically into granulomatous or nongranulomatous lesions, although this is essentially a pathologic diagnosis. Granulomatous lesions usually have an easier definable infectious etiology than nongranulomatous lesions. Granulomatous lesions typically have size or mass to them, resulting in deviated retinal blood vessels and elevation of the retina (**Figure 14.91**, see Blastomycosis). The causes of chorioretinitis are the same as for anterior uveitis (see Chapter 11, **Table 11.3**) plus a few additional agents.

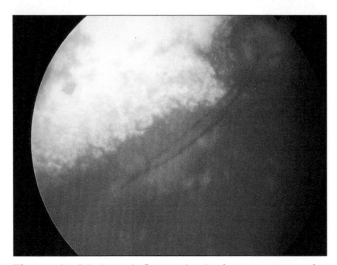

Figure 14.92 Acute inflammation in the nontapetum of an Akita dog with Vogt–Koyanagi–Harada syndrome.

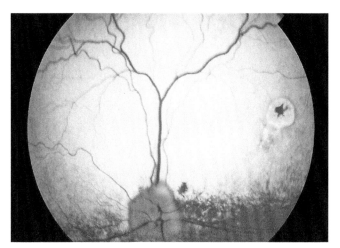

Figure 14.94 Focal chorioretinal scar in a dog, evidenced by hyperreflectivity with sharp borders and pigment clumping within the lesion. The cause was, and is often, unknown at this stage.

Etiology of chorioretinitis

For didactic purposes, chorioretinitis are typically divided in:

Infectious (viral, bacterial, algae, fungal, parasitic and rickettsial)

Noninfectious (immune-mediated, trauma, neoplasia, vascular diseases)

This section reviews the most common causes of chorioretintitis in the different species.

Dog

• *Infectious*: Distemper virus, parvovirus, and herpesvirus (in the neonate), bacterial embolism from focal sepsis, *Brucella canis*, tuberculosis, systemic

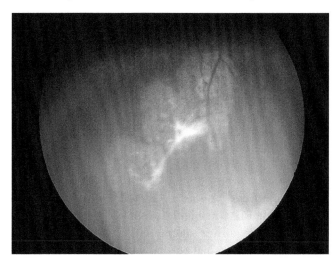

Figure 14.95 A dog with focal, sharply circumscribed, depigmented scars with an overlying glial reaction on the retinal surface.

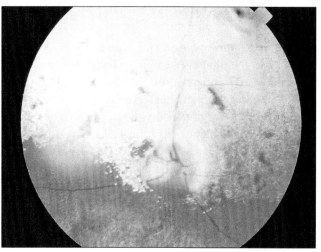

Figure 14.96 Unilateral diffuse retinal degeneration with focal scars in a 6-year-old Chesapeake Bay retriever. The tapetum is diffusely hyperreflective, with marked retinal vascular attenuation and optic nerve atrophy. Superimposed on the diffuse changes are typical focal postinflammatory scars, with pigment clumping and hyperreflective regions. The cause is unknown.

mycoses (as *Aspergillus fumigatus* and blastomycosis), prototothecosis, *Ehrlichia canis* and *E. platys*, *Rickettsia rickettsii*, *Toxoplasma gondii*, *Hepatozoon americanum*, and migrating metazoan parasites.
• *Immune-mediated*: VKH syndrome, steroid-responsive retinal detachments.
• *Trauma*: Blunt or perforating injuries.
• Neoplasia.

Cat

• *Infectious*: FIP, FeLV, panleukopenia (*in utero* and neonate only), FIV, systemic mycoses, *Toxoplasma gondii*, bacterial embolism from focal sepsis, tuberculosis, and migrating metazoan parasites.
• Immune-mediated.
• *Trauma*: Blunt or perforating.
• Neoplasia.

Horse

• *Infectious*: Leptospirosis, *Streptococcus equi*, toxoplasmosis, neonatal and adult septicemia, and metazoan parasites such as *Onchocerca cervicalis*.
• *Immune-mediated*: Equine recurrent uveitis (ERU).

Cow

• *Infectious*: Bovine virus diarrhea (BVD), rabies, malignant catarrhal fever (MCF), infectious thromboembolic meningoencephalitis, listeriosis, septicemia particularly in calves with scours and umbilical infections, tuberculosis, and toxoplasmosis.

Specific diseases

Viral

Canine distemper virus The canine distemper virus (CDV) is a common etiology for nongranulomatous chorioretinitis and optic neuritis in the dog. CDV ocular lesions are most commonly observed in animals during the encephalitic phase, but they may be found during the typical acute catarrhal phase or in animals that have no systemic signs. Typically, distemper produces multifocal retinitis that is characterized by ill-defined, altered reflective areas in the tapetal area (**Figure 14.90**) and focal white hazy lesions in the nontapetal area (**Figure 14.97**). The lesions are usually bilateral, although asymmetrical. The lesions have been reported to be more common in the ventral nontapetal region, but this has not been the author's experience. Lesions may coalesce to become large and fewer in number. Occasionally, perivascular cuffing is recognized.

Optic neuritis may be completely retrobulbar without changes on the optic disc, or it may extend to the nerve head (**Figure 14.98**). If the inflammation extends to the papilla, it is hyperemic, elevated, and hazy, and the animal is blind in the involved eye(s). Distemper fundus lesions are usually asymptomatic, unless the optic nerve or the chiasm is involved. Blindness with dilated pupils associated with distemper is usually due to bilateral optic nerve lesions, chiasm, or bilateral optic tract lesions.

The histopathologic lesions with distemper are more degenerative than inflammatory. Although perivascular cuffing with mononuclear cells may be observed in the retina, more typical changes are neuronal degeneration, edema, atrophy of the photoreceptors, and swelling and proliferation of the RPE. Cytoplasmic inclusion bodies may be observed in the glial cells of the retina and the optic nerve.[347–349]

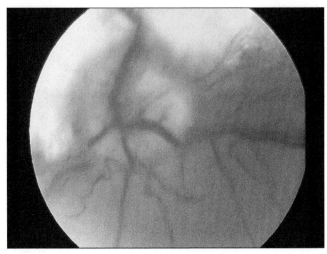

Figure 14.98 **Optic neuritis in a dog that was acutely blind and had distemper. The optic disc is elevated and hazy, and the retinal vessels are hyperemic.**

Canine parvovirus and feline panleukopenia virus In both the puppy and the kitten, parvoviruses, with their affinity for rapidly dividing cells, may affect the developing retina *in utero* or in the early neonatal period. Active inflammation is not present when examined later in life, and the changes are usually noted as an incidental finding. Inflammation in the developing retina results in retinal dysplasia and retinal atrophy. These lesions are noted as multifocal or solitary, sharply demarcated lesions of altered reflectivity in the tapetal region and depigmentation with sharp borders in the nontapetum.[350–352]

Canine herpesvirus (CHV-1) and feline herpesvirus (FHV-1) Herpesvirus in the canine neonate produces a marked panuveitis with keratitis, cataracts, retinal necrosis and disorganization, retinal atrophy and dysplasia, and optic neuritis and atrophy.[353] Since the infection is fatal in most puppies, it is not a recognized clinical syndrome. Surviving puppies would probably demonstrate retinal dysplasia and retinal scars. Feline herpesvirus (FHV-1) has not been proven to produce posterior segment lesions; however, a recent paper in experimental infection in cats describe intraocular and neural FHV-1 involvement during the acute phase of the infection of tissues, including posterior uvea and retina.[354]

Feline infectious peritonitis virus Posterior segment lesions with FIP are highly variable. Ophthalmoscopic lesions include diffuse alterations in tapetal coloration from choroiditis, retinal edema, focal and total exudative retinal detachment, retinal vasculitis, and optic neuritis (**Figures 14.99 and 14.100**). The severe form of the disease causes panophthalmitis, which often precludes

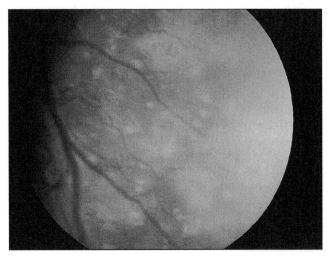

Figure 14.97 **A dog with acute distemper lesions in the nontapetum. Note the hazy borders.**

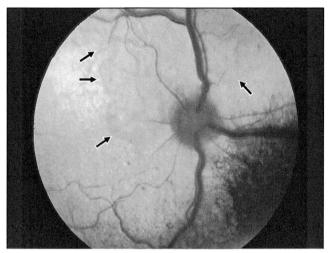

Figure 14.99 Focal bullous detachment dorsal to the disc (arrows) in a cat with FIP and FeLV. The detachment is recognized by the change in texture compared to the adjacent tapetum. Note the vascular hyperemia.

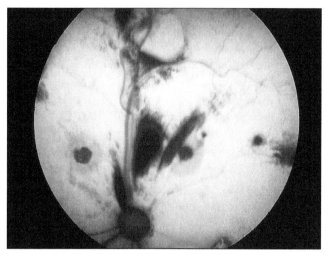

Figure 14.101 Multifocal retinal and preretinal hemorrhages in a cat with pancytopenia associated with FeLV. Note how pale the retinal vessels are from the anemia.

detailed fundus examination. Ocular disease is most common with the noneffusive form of FIP (see Chapter 11).[355]

Feline leukemia virus In the adult, lesions of the posterior segment associated with FeLV are usually due to blood dyscrasias. The most common lesions are various types of hemorrhages associated with severe anemia or thrombocytopenia (**Figure 14.101**). Occasional multifocal, small dark infiltrates are noted in the retina, representing neoplastic infiltration. Chorioretinitis and retinal detachment may also be observed. Feline leukemia virus has been associated with the induction of dysplasia.[356]

Bovine virus diarrhea (BVD) BVD, which is caused by a member of the genus Pestivirus, produces ocular and cerebellar lesions in the fetus if infected during 76–150 days of gestation. The neonate has neurologic signs of ataxia, intention tremors, and may not be able to stand. Ocular lesions include microphthalmos, cataracts, tapetal color changes and loss of texture, attenuated retinal vessels, and focal depigmentation of the nontapetal region (**Figure 14.102**).[357,358] The acute lesions are characterized by a mild-to-moderate retinitis that results in various degrees of destruction of the different layers, mononuclear

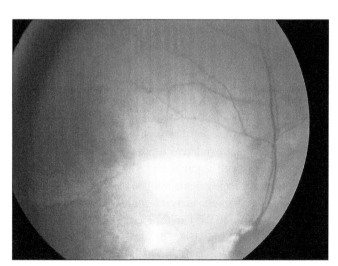

Figure 14.100 More advanced FIP choroiditis in a cat with exudative detachment in the dorsal fundus. Note the altered tapetal coloration from the inflammatory infiltration of the choroid.

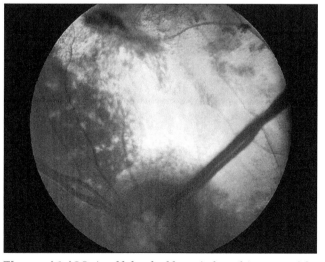

Figure 14.102 A calf that had been infected *in utero* with bovine virus diarrhea and was born with cerebellar ataxia. The tapetum has multifocal patches of pigmentation and altered color, and the nontapetum has numerous sharply demarcated depigmented lesions.

cuffing of inner retinal vessels, proliferation of pigment epithelium, and choroiditis. Residually, there is an absence of cellular elements in the atrophied areas of the retina, frequently a loss of layering, and various numbers of pigment-containing cells.[359]

Bovine malignant catarrhal fever (BMCF) BMCF, which has two forms caused by herpesviruses, produces vasculitis of the entire eye, but anterior uveitis and corneal edema preclude fundus examination in most cases.[360,361]

Bacterial

Bacterial embolism to the eye from a focal source of infection is not very common in small animals. However, it is common in large animals with neonatal septicemia. Many cases are undoubtedly missed if the eyes are not examined. If lesions are limited to the ocular fundus, they are usually "silent" with only focal hemorrhages and retinal/subretinal exudates noted.[362] Lesions have been noted in dogs with bacterial meningitis, endocarditis, and dental infections (**Figure 14.103**).

Endocarditis in a horse has been reported to result in a unilateral optic neuritis and blindness.[363] Calves with scours and infections centered around the joints and umbilicus often develop signs of anterior uveitis, with miosis and a large fibrin clot in the anterior chamber. Embolic lesions may also be visualized in the retina and include hemorrhages, soft exudates, retinal detachment, and papilledema (**Figure 14.104**). Agents include *Streptococcus* spp., *Corynebacterium*, *E. coli*, *Rhodococcus equi*, *Listeria monocytogenes*, and *Pasteurella* spp.

In the dog, contagious bacterial infections characterized by septicemia, such as *Brucella canis* infections, are more

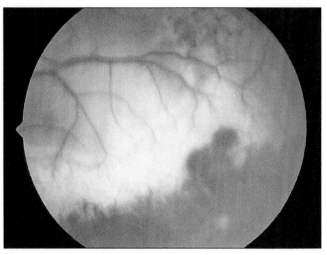

Figure 14.104 Bullous retinal detachment from exudate with multiple hemorrhages and exudates in a calf with vestibular signs. The condition was responsive to antibiotics.

likely to produce ocular lesions. Unilateral or bilateral uveitis has been frequently noted with canine brucellosis (see Chapter 11). In countries with adequate controls, tuberculosis has been rarely reported as a cause of granulomatous chorioretinitis in the cat.[364] *Bartonella vinsonii* (*berkhoffi*) has been reported as producing a mild multifocal chorioretinitis in a dog.[365] As *Bartonella* infections in man may produce a variety of posterior segment inflammatory lesions and are suspected of producing uveitis in cats, perhaps it will be recognized as a significant cause in the dog.

Infectious thromboembolic meningoencephalitis is produced in cattle by *Hemophilus somnus* and is characterized by peracute to acute death in young feedlot cattle. If the animals do not die peracutely, ocular lesions may be found in about 50% of cases and help to make a rapid diagnosis. Externally visible lesions may include strabismus, nystagmus, keratitis, and anterior uveitis with miosis and hypopyon. The most common lesions are in the posterior segment. Ophthalmoscopic lesions are relatively specific and consist of multifocal retinal hemorrhages and exudates that are often seen at the end of retinal vessels (**Figures 14.105 and 14.106**). The exudative lesions consist of inflammatory exudates as well as ganglion cell necrosis. Focal retinal detachment and papilledema may be present.[366]

Leptospirosis is considered a major etiology of equine recurrent uveitis (ERU) in horses. Histopathologically, chorioretinal inflammatory lesions were observed in all cases of ERU.[367] Although clinically visible, these are not observed with this frequency in the author's experience. The fundus lesions are typically located in the peripapillary region, as multifocal alterations in the nontapetal pigment. The lesions are often described as butterfly lesions

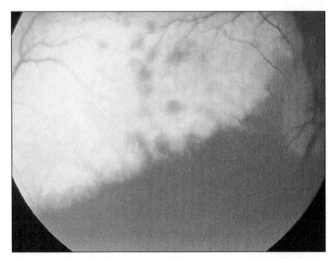

Figure 14.103 Multiple small hemorrhagic lesions near the termination of end arterioles in a dog with bacterial endocarditis.

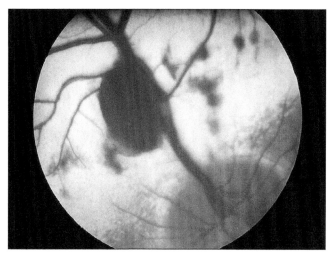

Figure 14.105 Multiple retinal hemorrhages in a yearling feedlot steer with acute neurologic signs associated with thromboembolic meningoencephalitis. Note how many of the hemorrhages are associated with end arterioles.

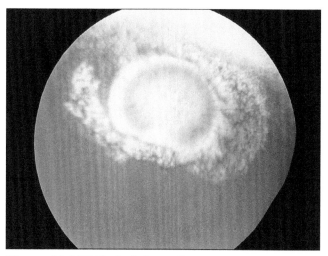

Figure 14.107 Typical "butterfly" scar adjacent to the disc associated with recurrent uveitis in a horse. The lesions are sharply demarcated indicating that they are scars, and while the disc looks pale, the retinal vessels are visible so optic nerve atrophy is not observed.

because of their distribution (**Figure 14.107**). The optic nerve, in the acute stages, is hyperemic with haze from cellular effusion (**Figure 14.108**) in the vitreous. Later the nerve atrophies with loss of retinal vessels and a pale color (see Uveitis, Chapter 11).[368] Retinal detachments are seen in the late stages of the disease (**Figure 14.109**) and may be difficult to recognize because of the paurangiotic vascular pattern of the horse retina.[340] Leptospirosis in a dog was reported with bilateral exudative retinal detachments and chorioretinitis scars.[369]

Systemic mycoses
The systemic mycoses are a significant etiology for chorioretinitis/endophthalmitis in the dog on a regional

basis, although cryptococcosis occurs worldwide[370] (see Chapter 11).

Systemic mycoses (blastomycosis, coccidiodomycosis, histoplamosis, aspergillosis, cryptococcosis) usually enter the body through the respiratory system and reach the eye hematogenously, although CNS cyptococcosis may extend down the optic nerve to the eye.

Canine blastomycosis is a systemic mycotic infection caused by *Blastomyces dermatitidis*, a dimorphic, saprophytic fungus that in the United States is endemic to the Mississippi, Missouri, and Ohio River valleys and the

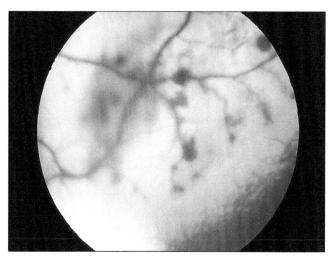

Figure 14.106 Subretinal exudate and hemorrhages associated with end arterioles in a steer with thromboembolic meningoencephalitis.

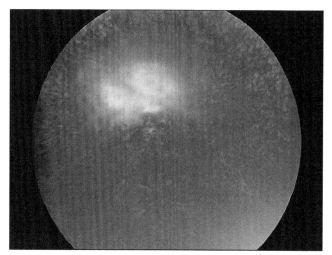

Figure 14.108 A very hyperemic optic disc with overlying cellular reaction in a horse with recurrent uveitis. The hyperemia indicates active inflammation, but the marked pigment disruption around the disc appears chronic and sharply demarcated.

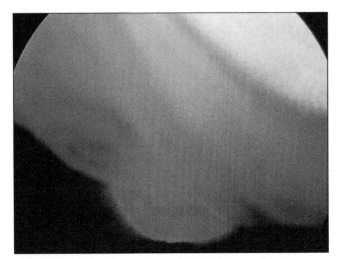

Figure 14.109 Complete retinal detachment in a horse with advanced recurrent uveitis. Detachment may be confused with vitreal membranes as there are no retinal blood vessels visible to allow differentiation.

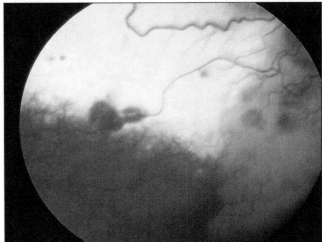

Figure 14.110 Focal subretinal granuloma and retinal hemorrhages in a Labrador retriever with blastomycosis.

mid-Atlantic states.[371] Ocular lesions have been reported to occur in 20% to 52% of dogs with systemic blastomycosis, and approximately 50% of dogs with ocular lesions are affected bilaterally.[372,373]

Histoplasmosis is caused by *Histoplasma capsulatum*, and endemic areas are in the Ohio, Missouri, and Mississippi River Valleys. Both dogs and cats can be affected by histoplamosis.[374]

Systemic aspergillosis with panuveitis is found in German shepherd dogs. Immunosuppression is considered a predisposing factor for such an ubiquitous organism to become disseminated, but the underlying cause in this breed has not been determined.[375]

Ocular lesions related to systemic mycoses involve the posterior segment (choroid) preferentially, where they are readily demonstrable on histopathologic examination. The lesions are characteristically bilateral, focal to multifocal granulomatous lesions that elevate the retina (**Figures 14.91, 14.110, and 14.111**), or, alternatively, a complete exudative retinal detachment is produced (**Figure 14.112**). Optic nerve involvement is common. Vitreous centesis is a rapid means of confirming the etiology.

Algal diseases—Protothecosis
Prototheca spp. is a ubiquitous algae, but infections are relatively rare. When present, the posterior ocular segment is involved in about 50% of cases.[376] The vast majority of dogs are systemically affected with hemorrhagic diarrhea, one of the most frequently seen systemic clinical signs.[376,377] However, systemic signs may be occult, and the animal is presented for blindness.[376,377] Lesions vary from bilateral, multifocal, dark chorioretinal granulomas to large areas of massive, white subretinal accumulations

(**Figure 14.113**). Exudative retinal detachment is the end stage of the process. Inflammatory cell reaction is minimal. Diagnosis is usually made on the basis of finding the organisms in tissue, urine, or ocular aspirates, especially into the subretinal space or vitreal centesis. An overrepresentation of female boxer has been suggested.[378] Prognosis is grave, and recent treatment protocols include the use of a combination of amphotericin B and itraconazole.[378]

Rickettsial infection
Canine ehrlichiosis is a tick-borne disease produced by *Ehrlichia canis*, *E. platys*, and *E. equii*.[379] *E. canis* is the most important agent and is transmitted by the brown dog

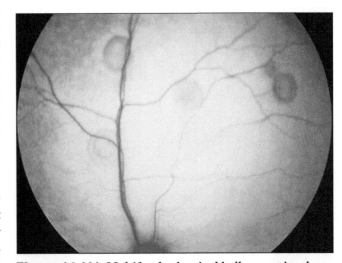

Figure 14.111 Multifocal subretinal bullae associated with cryptococcosis in a cat. The lesions changed minimally over months of treatment. The cat was initially blind, but vision returned rapidly with therapy, and no other CNS signs developed.

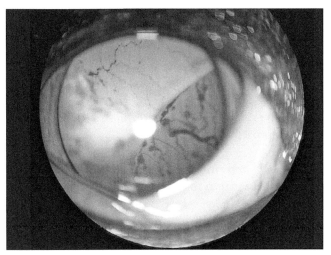

Figure 14.112 Complete exudative retinal detachments in a Beagle with blastomycosis. Note the multiple retinal hemorrhages. The condition was bilateral, and the dog was presented for blindness, not for systemic disease.

tick, *Rhipicephalus sanguineus*. The disease is divided into the acute (1–3 weeks), subclinical (average 11 weeks), and chronic stages. While ocular signs may be present in all stages, animals are not usually presented for diagnosis until the chronic stage. Experimentally, 50% of inoculated dogs developed ocular lesions, and ocular lesions were present in the acute state.[380] The prevalence of ocular lesions has been given as 10%–37% of the cases and, when present, can produce devastating functional results, with uveitis the most common ocular diagnosis.[381,382] Leiva et al. reported that 37% of dogs diagnosed with ehrlichiosis had ocular lesions, and 65% of those with ocular lesions had no apparent systemic signs.[381]

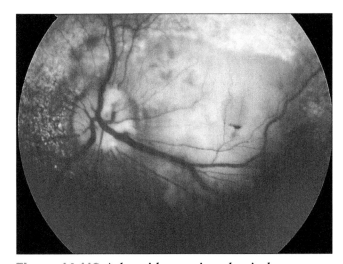

Figure 14.113 A dog with extensive subretinal exudate associated with *Prototheca*. The lesions began as small multifocal dark lesions and progressed to retinal detachment. Diagnosed by vitreal centesis.

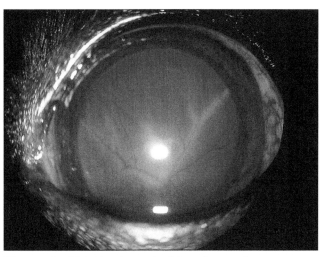

Figure 14.114 Massive retinal detachment due to subretinal hemorrhage in a dog with ehrlichiosis.

The ocular lesions are the result of either platelet deficiency and/or, more commonly, vasculitis. Massive orbital and ocular hemorrhage has been observed. Retinal hemorrhage is common, and retinal detachment may be observed either from massive subretinal hemorrhage or exudates (**Figure 14.114**).[383] Optic neuritis with engorged retinal vessels and papillary hemorrhage may occur. Experimentally, discrete perivascular infiltrates have been described in the subacute stage but have not been described in clinical cases.[384]

Rickettsia rickettsii, the agent of RMSF, produces ocular lesions that are similar but milder than *E. canis*. The vector and reservoir are the ticks *Dermacentor andersoni*, *D. variabilis*, and *Amblyomma americanum*. Retinal petechiae, retinal vasculitis, and mild anterior uveitis are common occurring in 9 out of 11 dogs (82%) in one series (**Figure 14.115**).[385] The ophthalmic lesions generally were mild, and most resolved without complication after systemic administration of appropriate antibiotics.[385] Development of retinal vasculitic foci has been associated with thrombocytopenia, increased concentrations of circulating fibrinogen, and slight prolongation of activated partial thromboplastin.[386]

Protozoa

Toxoplasmosis Toxoplasmosis is caused by the protozoan *T. gondii* and is a well-publicized disease due to its zoonotic potential. While exposure is widespread based on serologic surveys, toxoplasmosis as a systemic clinical disease is not very common. Ocular lesions have been described for both the dog and the cat, and posterior segment lesions are described as retinochoroiditis due to the organism's predilection for the retina. Ophthalmoscopic lesions range from small multifocal infiltrates (**Figure 14.116**) with a ring of edema to focal retinal detachments. Granulomatous anterior uveitis may develop, but organisms are often not

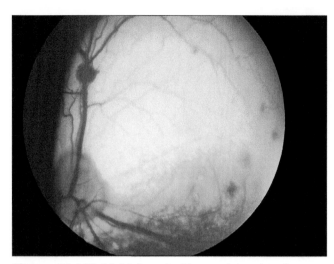

Figure 14.115 Multiple retinal hemorrhages in a dog with Rocky Mountain spotted fever. Note how many hemorrhages are associated with end arterioles.

present with anterior uveal involvement.[387,388] In the dog, toxoplasmosis is frequently associated with distemper, and both agents may produce ocular lesions (see Chapter 11). Many of the previously diagnosed cases of toxoplasmosis may have been caused by *Neosporum caninum*.

Leishmania spp. Leishmaniasis caused by *Leishmania infantum* is a vector-borne zoonotic disease endemic in southern Europe, which is spreading worldwide.[389] Feline cases have been reported from endemic areas in Italy, France, Spain, and Portugal.[389]

Ocular lesions are characterized by granulomatous inflammatory infiltrate in 26.6% of cases. The parasite has been identified immunohistochemically within the globe. Ocular tissues affected, in order of frequency, are

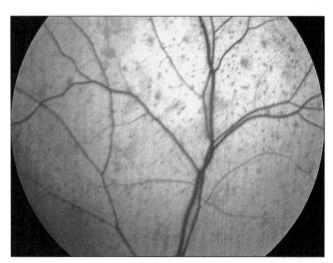

Figure 14.116 Cat with multifocal chorioretinitis associated with toxoplasmosis. Note the larger lesions have fuzzy edges.

conjunctiva and limbus, ciliary body, iris, cornea, sclera and iridocorneal angle, choroid, and optic nerve sheath.[390]

Clinical response to treatment of sick dogs is variable. Clinical cure is often obtained, but clinical recurrence can occur and post-therapy follow-up should be maintained lifelong. In Europe, vaccination can be combined with individual protection with pyrethroids as part of an integrated approach to prevention.[390]

Hepatozoon americanum *Hepatozoon americanum* is a protozoan parasite transmitted by the ticks *Amblyomma maculatum* and *Rhipicephalus sanguineus*; reported cases in the United States have been limited to the Gulf Coast states. It produces a chronic wasting disease with myalgia and lymphadenopathy. Ocular signs consist of ocular discharge, uveitis, and chorioretinal scars. Radiographs of affected dogs in the United States reveal periostitis. Diagnosis is usually made on muscle biopsy. In other parts of the world, hepatozoonosis is often asymptomatic, the organism is found in large numbers in the blood, and bone lesions are rare.[391] Death usually occurs within 24 months of the initial signs. Despite initial improvement in signs with various anticoccidial therapies, relapses occur unless long-term therapy is administered.

Metazoan parasites

Metazoan parasites are an uncommon but interesting etiology for posterior uveitis. Migrating *Toxocara* larvae were initially reported to produce small focal retinal and choroidal granulomas that were of little clinical consequence.[392] Aberrant *Toxocara* larvae have been found associated with severe posterior chorioretinitis and endophthalmitis that often results in blindness.[50,393] Usually, the dogs are of rural origin. Lesions observed are multifocal areas of tapetal hyperreflectivity and hyperpigmentation. When histopathologic examination is performed on young dogs, and the inflammation is active, *Toxocara* larvae are found, and the dogs are still visual. Older dogs are often blind and have more diffuse lesions of retinal and choroidal atrophy, perivascular plasma cell infiltration, hyalitis, and characteristic peripapillary necrosis of the nontapetal retina. The feeding of raw mutton has been postulated to be responsible for the difference between the incidence in urban and rural dogs. *Angiostrongylus vasorum* larvae may be observed in the anterior chamber or the vitreous. Additional ocular lesions may be hemorrhage and inflammation.[49,394,395]

Intraocular migrating *Diptera* (fly) larvae (ophthalmomyiasis interna) have been observed in both the dog and the cat fundus, and they leave characteristic curvilinear wandering paths in the subretinal space. The lesions can be observed as chronic scars without evidence of an active larva, or acute with the larva present (**Figures 14.117 and**

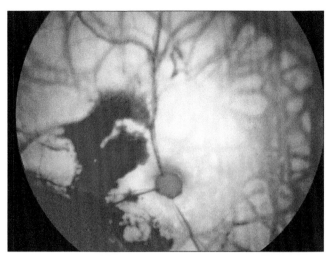

Figure 14.117 Cat with extensive wandering curvilinear retinopathy and retinal hemorrhages, typical of ophthalmomyiasis.

14.118). The larvae can be very motile and seem to be photophobic. The tracts have characteristic dark clumps, and hemorrhages may be present if the tracts are recent.[51,396] The larva in most cases of ophthalmomyiasis interna is usually not identified, but the cattle bot fly (*Hypoderma bovis*) and reindeer warble fly (*Oedemagena tarandi*) have been identified in association with the condition. *Cuterebra* larva have been removed or found in the anterior chamber and the vitreous of both the dog and the cat.[52,53]

Onchocerca cervicalis has been considered to be one of the main known etiologies of uveitis, and migrating larvae have been demonstrated in the posterior uvea on histopathology.[368,397] The peripapillary "butterfly" lesion is characteristic (**Figure 14.107**). The optic nerve in the acute stages may be hyperemic, but it is more often found with

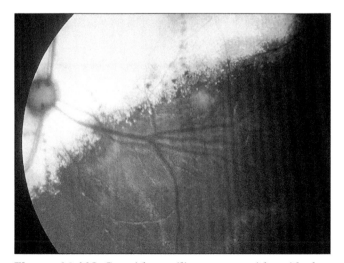

Figure 14.118 Cat with curvilinear tracts with residual debris in the tracts, typical of ophthalmomyiasis. The lesions are not as obvious in the tapetum but are visible.

a loss of retinal blood vessels and a pale color later in the atrophic stage.

In sheep, goats, and wild ruminants, *Elaeophora schneideri*, which inhabits the common carotid and other arteries, may produce ocular lesions in addition to the typical cutaneous lesions of the head. Ocular lesions consist of keratitis, cataract, anterior uveitis, retinal edema, chorioretinal atrophy, retinal vessel attenuation, and optic nerve atrophy.

Immune-mediated chorioretinitis
Most instances of nongranulomatous chorioretinitis are not definitively diagnosed. Immune-mediated disease is often suspected based on associated systemic signs or lack thereof, histopathologic examination in which no infectious agents are found or cultured, and inflammation that is mononuclear or the result of vascular insult.

A transient, multifocal, serous chorioretinitis has been described as an incidental finding in Beagles. On histopathologic examination, only focal serous accumulations of fluid without inflammatory cells between the neurosensory retina and the RPE are observed. The cause is unknown.[398] Similar multifocal retinal lesions were described in a series of Doberman pinschers 10–30 days after receiving sulfadiazine for the first time. The condition was characterized by nonseptic polyarthritis, glomerulonephropathy, polymyositis, skin rash, fever, anemia, leukopenia, and thrombocytopenia, in addition to retinal lesions. The fundus lesions were one-quarter to one-half disc diameter in size and resolved 2 weeks after cessation of therapy. This was hypothesized to be an immune complex disease or a type III hypersensitivity.[399]

Rapidly developing bilateral retinal detachment due to subretinal exudates has been observed in predominantly large breeds of dogs. Associated focal, dark choroidal lesions are often present, and the condition is thought to represent choroiditis and choroidal vasculitis (**Figures 14.119 and 14.120**). Optic neuritis is observed with choroiditis. A lack of systemic signs, negative cultures from the subretinal fluid, histopathologic findings, and improvement with systemic glucocorticoids are suggestive of an immune-mediated choroiditis and retinal detachment.[400,401] The affected dogs present with a history of an acute vision loss. Vitreal hemorrhage has been associated with an increased time to reattachment.[401]

Many dogs in the late stages of Vogt–Koyanagi–Harada (VKH) syndrome develop exudative retinal detachment. The choroid typically has a marked infiltrate of mononuclear cells. The RPE is destroyed, and the neurosensory retina undergoes milder perivascular inflammatory changes and degenerates (**Figure 14.92**). The pigmented portions of the fundus develop patchy depigmentation, which later becomes confluent (**Figure 14.121**).

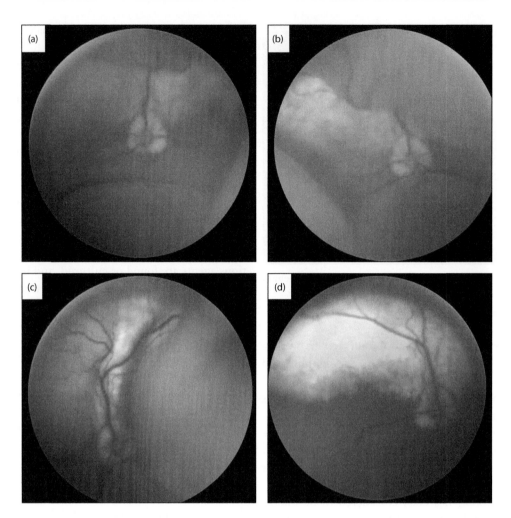

Figure 14.119 A dog with steroid-responsive retinal detachment presented with acute blindness (a) Partial serous retinal detachment at presentation. (b and c) 12 and 24 hours later, the clinical pictures show worsening of the clinical signs (serous retinal detachment) while bloodwork was pending (differential diagnosis infectious chorioretinitis). (d) Positive response to systemic immunosuppressive doses of prednisone.

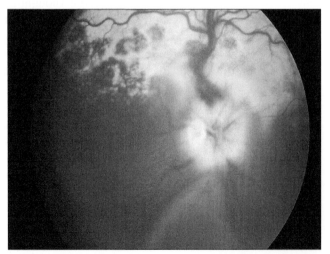

Figure 14.120 A dog with steroid-responsive retinal detachment and focal choroidal infiltrates. Note the vascular hyperemia, swollen disc, and detachment ventrally.

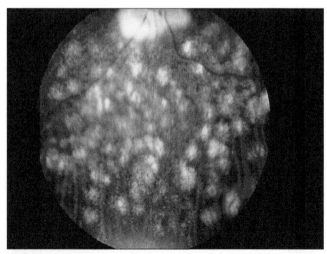

Figure 14.121 An Akita with Vogt–Koyanagi–Harada syndrome and depigmented lesions in the nontapetum. The uveitis was being treated aggressively at this time and was quiescent. Compare to Figure 14.93.

The lesions are presumably due to an immune reaction against melanin (see Chapter 7).

Phacoanaphylaxis or phacoclastic uveitis that is induced by lens capsule rupture predominantly produces a severe anterior uveitis, but the majority of patients also have a lymphocytic–plasmacytic retinal perivascular reaction.[402] The latter lesions are rarely noted clinically due to the severe anterior uveal reaction.

Diagnosis of chorioretinitis

• Like anterior uveitis, nongranulomatous chorioretinitis is often not definitively diagnosed despite exhaustive testing. Appearances are not absolute.

• Lesions should be categorized into granulomatous or nongranulomatous to limit the etiologies.

• Lesions should be correlated with systemic signs and history, that is, environment, exposure. Laboratory tests such as CBC, chemistry profile, immune profile, radiographs of the chest, and serology for various infectious diseases such as brucellosis, systemic mycoses, ehrlichiosis, RMSF, and toxoplasmosis are often indicated in the acute stages. Culture and cytology of vitreous or subretinal fluid are usually reserved for cases with severe active lesions. Patients should be screened for antigens such as FeLV, *Toxoplasma*, and *Cryptococcus*. Enucleation for histopathologic examination is a valid procedure if the eye is nonfunctional and painful.

Chorioretinal lesions with systemic disease are frequently of diagnostic, therapeutic, and prognostic importance. The goal in treating these potentially blinding conditions is to eliminate the inflammation, find the definitive diagnosis, and minimize the potential risk of therapy to the patient.

Therapy

Therapy is directed at the underlying disease, if associated with systemic disease. Because of the difficulty of obtaining therapeutic drug levels in the posterior globe, systemic antibiotics are often administered, if infection is suspected, or immune suppressors administered for immune-mediated or traumatic problems. If acute bacterial infection is known or anticipated, intravitreal antibiotics may be injected (see Chapter 2).

Diseases of the optic nerve
Optic neuritis
Introduction/etiology

The term "optic neuritis" compromises all diseases of the optic nerve that cause primary demyelination and usually manifest themselves as a sudden visual field defect or total loss of vision in one or both eyes.[403–405] Optic neuritis may be part of a condition with generalized fundus lesions (neuroretinitis), or it may be isolated to the optic nerve(s). Optic neuritis may be unilateral or bilateral, and it may involve the optic disc or be confined to the retrobulbar nerve. The cause of optic neuritis is often difficult to determine in the living animal, as neurologic examination, cerebrospinal fluid analysis, and laboratory tests can be normal.[405] The etiology of unilateral optic neuritis can usually be defined, whereas bilateral optic neuritis in systemically healthy animals is often idiopathic.[403–405]

In the dog, distemper should be considered as a cause in all bilateral cases of optic neuritis, even if the animal is vaccinated, and there are no systemic complaints (**Figure 14.98**).[406] The virus of tick-borne encephalitis has been reported to produce an optic neuritis syndrome in the dog in endemic areas of Europe.[407]

Systemic mycoses, toxoplasmosis, ehrlichiosis, orbital neoplasia, orbital cellulitis, orbital trauma such as proptosis, and granulomatous meningoencephalomyelitis (GME, inflammatory reticulosis) are all possible causes of optic neuritis in the dog. GME may extend down both optic nerves from the brain to produce blindness, papilledema, retinal hemorrhage, and retinal detachment (**Figures 14.122 and 14.123**). The condition is usually responsive to systemic glucocorticoids on a short-term basis and should be considered with multifocal neurologic lesions and optic nerve lesions.[408–410] The miniature poodle and other small breeds have an increased incidence of GME.

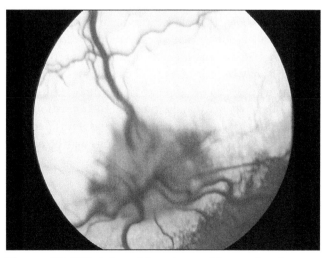

Figure 14.122 A dog with optic neuritis associated with granulomatous meningoencephalomyelitis. Note the peripapillary hemorrhages, elevated disc deviating the retinal vessels, haze over the disc, and vascular hyperemia. The condition was bilateral.

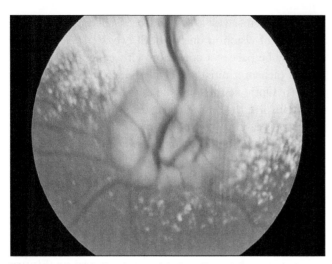

Figure 14.123 Optic neuritis in a dog with granulomatous meningoencephalomyelitis. Blindness was the first sign; later, multifocall neurologic signs developed.

Optic neuritis can be produced by FIP and cryptococcosis in the cat, male fern ingestion in cattle, and guttural pouch infection with *Aspergillus* spp. in the horse. In many instances, the cause of optic neuritis is idiopathic, and these cases are typically systemically normal, acute in onset, and bilateral.

Clinical signs

Optic neuritis may present either unilaterally or bilaterally. If presented with bilateral involvement, the patient is blind with dilated pupils that typically respond very sluggishly and incompletely to light. Affected dogs, even though they are blind, often act photophobic in that they resist the examination light.[405]

The fundus may be normal if the condition is completely retrobulbar, but the typical appearance of optic neuritis is of a swollen optic disc with deviation of retinal blood vessels and loss of the physiologic cup. The retinal vessels are usually congested, as are the capillaries of the disc. Hemorrhages are common on and adjacent to the disc, and peripapillary edema may be present. Inflammation may create a mild haze over the optic disc, and if it is part of a more diffuse disease, chorioretinal lesions may be present (**Figures 14.93, 14.122, and 14.123**).

Diagnosis

Sudden blindness can be caused either by intraocular lesions (optic neuritis or retinopathy as SARDS), postretinal lesions (retrobulbar optic nerve, chiasm, and tracts), or lesions within the cerebrum or the brainstem.[406]

A presumptive clinical diagnosis of optic neuritis is made when a patient is presented with a sudden-onset bilateral blindness and a swollen optic disc. If the condition is retrobulbar neuritis, the main differential diagnosis

is SARDS. The ERG of optic neuritis patients is normal but is extinguished with SARDS.

Optic neuritis is often responsive to glucocorticoid therapy, but such therapy is contraindicated with many of the infectious causes. To avoid inappropriate therapy, a good history, physical and neurologic examination, screening laboratory tests of CBC and serum chemistry profile, and a cerebrospinal tap are indicated. A CT or MRI scan may also provide diagnostic information.

Definitive diagnosis of GME may be difficult, but increased protein and pleocytosis of plasma–lymphocytic cells and, rarely, reticulum cells in the CSF, multifocal neurologic disease, and a temporary response to systemic glucocorticoids are suggestive of the diagnosis.[411]

Differential diagnosis

Differential diagnosis should include any of the diffuse retinal diseases since they produce similar signs of dilated pupils and blindness. Most diffuse retinal diseases that are severe enough to produce blindness are advanced and dramatic, with the major exception of SARDS or retinal toxicity as ivermectin exposure.[309,310]

Cortical blindness is accompanied by brisk PLRs. Papilledema appears similar to optic neuritis ophthalmoscopically, but pure papilledema does not cause blindness. However, the causes of papilledema, such as CNS neoplasia, may produce blindness. In general, the pupils should be reactive if the animal is blind from cortical lesions. Since cortical lesions can also be accompanied by midbrain lesions with pupillary abnormalities, differentiation may be more complex.[412]

Therapy

If an infectious disease is diagnosed, this should be treated specifically. Idiopathic cases, or those thought to be due to GME, should be treated with immunosuppressive doses of systemic prednisone. If GME is diagnosed, the therapy should be prolonged. Alternative therapies to immunosuppressive doses with glucocorticoids have been strong immunosuppressive drugs such as cyclosporine and cytosine arabinoside. Remissions with these drugs have been more complete and with fewer side effects.[413,414] Treatment with cytosine arabinoside requires infrequent dosing compared with glucocorticoids or cyclosporine and is administered at 50 mg/m² subcutaneously every 12 hours for 2 days every 3 weeks. Therapy should be initiated as soon as possible, and if the patient is going to respond, improvement is generally seen in the first 5–7 days. Many of the idiopathic cases, if treated early, have a partial response with a return of some vision and an improvement in PLRs. The optic disc swelling is slower to regress, and over a period of several weeks, variable degrees of optic nerve atrophy become evident.

The treatment of distemper optic neuritis is a dilemma for the clinician. Due to the severity of the signs, that is, blindness, the psychological pressure to treat is great. The risk of immunosuppressive drugs creating a fulminating disease is possible, but there is also rationale for anti-inflammatory therapy of distemper demyelinating lesions.

Papilledema

Introduction/etiology

Papilledema is a passive swelling of the optic disc or papilla, as opposed to the active swelling and hyperemia with optic neuritis. It is usually associated with increased CSF pressure and does not result in blindness, although the basic cause of the increased CSF pressure may produce blindness. The pathogenesis of papilledema is disputed, but it is probably not simply a restriction of venous drainage from the disc. Interference with axoplasmic flow results in swollen axons and is common to most of the etiologies of papilledema. An increase in interstitial fluid in the nerve head from the peripapillary choroid and local blood vessels also occurs but is not as important as the interference in axoplasmic flow in producing swelling.[415] The condition may be unilateral or bilateral. If bilateral, marked asymmetry may still be present. Early papilledema is difficult to recognize in the dog because of the variable amounts of myelin in the nerve head. Serial examinations and comparisons to the opposite eye, if it is normal, allow more critical evaluation. Papilledema is rarely manifest in the cat and horse optic disc, unless very severe.

Any space-occupying mass of the CNS may cause papilledema, but the usual cause is a brain tumor. In one study of brain tumors, 48% of the patients had papilledema.[412] Space-occupying lesions of the orbit such as neoplasia, hemorrhage, and inflammation may impinge on the optic nerve, producing papilledema.

Hydrocephalus is a rare cause of papilledema, with most cases having normal optic discs. Hyperviscosity syndromes such as polycythemia or gammopathy are relatively rare causes of papilledema. Severe systemic hypertension may produce papilledema in the dog, and an association with pancreatitis has been made.

Acute severe hypotony or acute glaucoma are potential causes of papilledema but are rarely recognized. Vitamin A deficiency in young cattle produces dramatic papilledema; papilledema is an early sign in this condition that is present before blindness that is due to bony overgrowth (**Figure 14.75**).[313]

Clinical signs

The optic disc with papilledema becomes elevated and enlarged, causing the retinal vessels to bend upward onto the surface. The disc is typically congested and may have

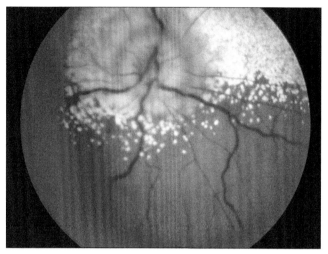

Figure 14.124 Papilledema in a dog with a brain tumor. Note the swollen disc that deviates the retinal blood vessels and the peripapillary edema.

small hemorrhages on or adjacent to the disc. A halo of peripapillary edema may be present in the subretinal space (**Figure 14.124**); however, papilledema is not associated with visual deficits.

Differential diagnosis

In the dog, the normal heavily myelinated optic disc typical of many large breeds of dogs can be difficult to differentiate from mild-to-moderate papilledema. In all species, excessive myelination of the retinal fiber layer may simulate papilledema. Papillitis or optic neuritis may be similar in appearance to papilledema but is accompanied by blindness.

A fundus examination with critical evaluation of the optic disc (color, shape, size) should be part of the physical examination of patients with neurologic signs.

Proliferative optic neuropathy in horses

Proliferative optic neuropathy is an asymptomatic condition that is usually found as an incidental finding on the nerve head of older horses. The condition is unilateral and consists of an elevated grayish, cauliflower-like proliferation on the optic nerve (**Figure 14.125**).[416–418]

The lesion consists of plump cells filled with an eosinophilic foamy cytoplasm. The cytoplasm is partially positive for PAS stain and oil-red-O but negative for luxol-fast blue. The lesion was originally described as neoplastic and termed an astrocytoma.[416]

The neoplastic origin is not accepted today, and the lesion has been compared to xanthelasma in humans.[418]

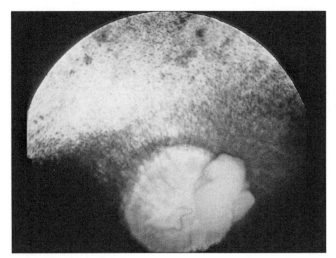

Figure 14.125 Proliferative optic neuropathy found as an incidental finding in one eye of an aged horse. This probably represents extruded myelin.

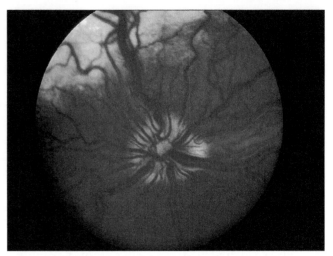

Figure 14.126 A 4-month-old English bulldog with cyanotic congenital heart disease and secondary polycythemia. Note the dark ruddy color and distension of the vessels.

Prognosis for vision with benign proliferative optic neuropathy is excellent, as these lesions are incidental findings. Proliferative optic neuropathy should be differentiated from exudative and ischemic optic neuropathy, which produce vision deficits.

Ischemic optic neuropathy
Proliferative optic neuropathy should be differentiated from ischemic optic neuropathy that is associated with vision loss. Platt et al. reviewed the equine literature on degenerative optic nerve lesions and found proliferative reactions described on the optic nerve in many cases.[419] Common to many was a history of acute blood loss or suspected trauma. Similar lesions are reported in two horses that had undergone occlusion of the internal and external carotid arteries and the greater palatine artery for treatment of guttural pouch mycosis. The horses were blind upon recovery from anesthesia, but the optic disc lesions were not observed until the third postoperative day.[420] There is no treatment for ischemic optic neuropathy, and prognosis for vision is grave. Common clinical signs are a pale optic nerve and severe retinal vascular attenuation.

Blood–vascular diseases of the fundus

A variety of blood dyscrasias and vascular diseases are manifest in the ocular fundus since it is a convenient window to the body's microvasculature. Most of these are systemic diseases, and the fundus lesions may be either a diagnostic clue or the presenting sign.

Polycythemia

Polycythemia, an absolute increase in erythrocytes, must become quite extreme before manifesting in the retinal vasculature. The usual causes are cyanotic congenital heart disease and polycythemia rubra vera. When the packed cell volume (PCV) reaches approximately 66%–69%, the retinal vasculature must accommodate to the increased volume by dilating and increasing in length (tortuous vessels). The blood is also darker in color (**Figures 14.126 and 14.127**). Serous retinal detachment may develop, perhaps associated with hyperviscosity. If the condition is chronic and extreme, retinal and vitreal hemorrhage may eventually occur.[421,422]

Serum hyperviscosity syndrome

Monoclonal gammopathies are the usual etiologies for most hyperviscosity syndromes; the underlying cause is

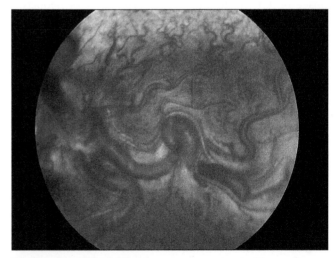

Figure 14.127 Calf with cyanotic congenital heart disease that resulted in severe secondary polycythemia. The vessels have lengthened, resulting in tortuosity, and have dilated to accommodate the additional vascular volume. The blood is also darker than normal.

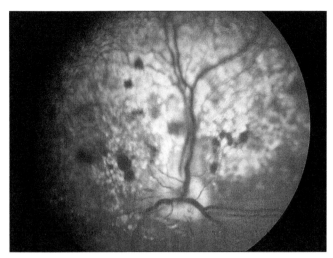

Figure 14.128 A dog with a hypergammopathy with multiple retinal hemorrhages, peripapillary edema, papilledema, and vascular engorgement.

usually a malignancy such as multiple myeloma or lymphoma, but infectious disease may also produce hyperviscosity syndrome.[423] The increased colloidal pressure results in an increased blood volume and dilated, kinked retinal vessels, and may produce sausage-like sacculation. Hemorrhagic diathesis results in retinal hemorrhage, which is the most common lesion, but its cause is not fully understood (**Figure 14.128**).[423–425] Retinal detachment may occur and multiple focal intraretinal cysts under the internal limiting membrane have been observed (**Figure 14.129**). These cysts were initially thought to be focal retinal detachments but their relationship to the retinal blood vessels and biomicroscopy of the retina indicate they are intraretinal. The retinal cysts persist, despite improvement in the systemic disease. In humans, ciliary

body cysts are common with multiple myeloma. Anterior segment lesions of glaucoma and anterior uveitis may also be present.[426]

Severe anemia
Acute anemia with PCVs <7% regularly manifest with pale retinal vessels and varying degrees of retinal hemorrhage, irrespective of the thrombocyte count (**Figures 14.101 and 14.130**). When the condition is combined with thrombocytopenia, the hemorrhage is more extensive. In cats, anemic retinopathy occurs in a high percentage of cats with hemoglobin levels of less than 5 g/dL.[427] Chronic profound anemia has been associated with retinal detachment in the dog.[365] In the horse, acute blood loss may rarely result in blindness associated with retinopathy and optic nerve atrophy (see ischemic optic neuropathy section). The retinal lesions are multifocal with marked pigment disruption.[428]

Thrombocytopenia
The level of platelets that is necessary to prevent hemorrhage appears to have individual variation. In general, platelet counts below 50,000/µl usually result in petechiation. The fundus is a good microvasculature bed to detect petechiation (**Figure 14.131**). Common causes of thrombocytopenia are immune-mediated diseases, rickettsial diseases, and neoplasia.

Clotting disorders
Inherited or acquired clotting disorders may occasionally manifest as retinal hemorrhages.

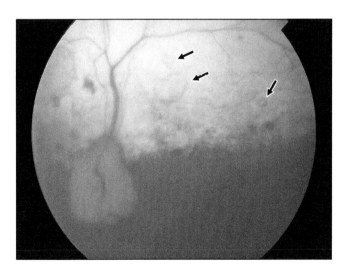

Figure 14.129 Multiple faint intraretinal cysts (arrows) and retinal hemorrhages in a dog with multiple myeloma and a hypergammopathy.

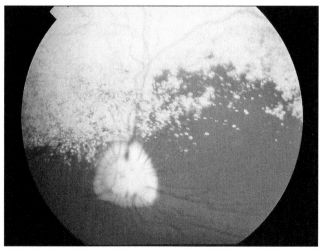

Figure 14.130 Canine fundus manifesting severe anemia with almost no visible blood in the vessels, a pale disc, and some increased tapetal reflectivity. This mimics progressive retinal atrophy, but the dog is visual, and the retinal signs may correct with systemic improvement.

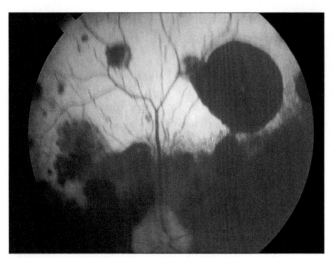

Figure 14.131 Dog with immune-mediated thrombocytopenia and multiple retinal hemorrhages.

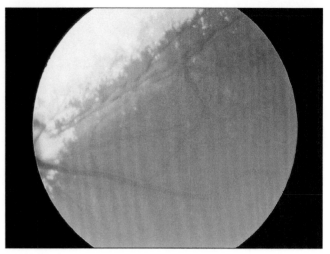

Figure 14.132 Lipemia retinalis in a dog with acute pancreatitis. The pink hue to the vessels is most easily observed against the nontapetal background.

Leukemia

Fundus lesions from various types of leukemias usually manifest as hemorrhages but neoplastic infiltrates may develop.[429] Patients with myelogenous leukemia seem especially prone to retinal hemorrhage. Hemorrhagic diathesis with neoplasia may develop despite normal platelets, and this is thought to represent vasculitis.

Lipemia

Hyperlipemia has been associated with lipids in the anterior chamber, secondary glaucoma, anterior uveitis, corneal lipidosis, and lipemia retinalis.[430] Increases in serum triglycerides above 2500 mg/100 mL may manifest with a pinkish color of the retinal vessels (lipemia retinalis). In animals with a tapetum lucidum, it is easier to detect the color change in the vessels over the nontapetum (**Figure 14.132**).[431] Elevations in cholesterol do not result in a lipemic fundus.

Lipemia is usually associated with diabetes mellitus, hypothyroidism, pancreatitis, liver disease, and familial hyperlipidemia.[432] White retinal deposits with hemorrhage and optic disc hyperemia have been described in a dog with diabetes mellitus that was lipemic but did not manifest lipemia retinalis. The white deposits were thought to be lipids as they resolved with dietary restriction of fat. The hemorrhages and papilledema may have resulted from systemic hypertension.[433]

Systemic hypertension

Introduction/etiology

Examination of the ocular fundus is an excellent method of observing a vascular bed. Hypertension in the dog and cat is being diagnosed with increasing frequency, often because of sudden blindness associated with retinal detachment, retinal hemorrhage, or hyphema. The systemic signs of hypertension are minimal or vague and it is often the fundus lesions that are symptomatic and suggestive of the diagnosis.[434,435] Retinal lesions, caused predominantly by choroidal injury, are common in cats with hypertension. Primary hypertension in cats may be more common than currently recognized.[434,435] Hypertension should be considered in older cats with acute onset of blindness; retinal edema, hemorrhage, or detachment; cardiac disease; or neurologic abnormalities. Cats with hypertension-induced ocular disease should be evaluated for renal failure, hyperthyroidism, diabetes mellitus, and cardiac abnormalities. Blood pressure measurements and funduscopic evaluations should be performed routinely in cats at risk for hypertension (preexisting renal disease, hyperthyroidism, and age >10 years).[435]

Systemic hypertension can be divided in:

Primary
Secondary

- Hypothyroidism is an uncommon cause of systemic hypertension in dogs.[434,436]
- Renal disease: Hypertension has been recognized up to 93% of dogs with chronic kidney disease and 87% of dogs with acute kidney disease.[437] Sixty-one percent of cats with chronic renal failure were found to have hypertension.[437,438]
- Pheochromocytoma (catecholamine secreting tumor of the adrenal medulla) induces hypertension in 43% to 86% of the cases in dogs and up to 100% in cats.[437,439]
- Hyperthyroidism: While untreated hyperthyroidism has been variably reported to cause hypertension in cats (87%[438]; 23%[440]), the link between

hyperthyroidism, hypertension, and hypertensive retinopathy is more tenuous. Stiles et al.[440] found only one of the hypertensive cats in their study with hypertensive retinopathy and van der Woerdt and Peterson[441] examined 100 hyperthyroid cats without a single case of hypertensive retinopathy. Sansom et al.[442] found one cat out of 16 presented for lesions of ocular hypertension had hyperthyroidism.

- High salt diet.[443]
- Hyperaldosteronism in 50% to 100% of the cases in cats.[439,444-446]
- A primary form or essential hypertension has been described as a familial trait in dogs.[437,447,448] Primary hypertension may also be a very significant cause of hypertension in the cat. About 50% of 69 cases of hypertension in the cat had no underlying cause diagnosed.[435]
- Hyperadrenocorticism: 86% of dogs with untreated pituitary dependent hyperadrenocorticism and 100% of dogs with adrenocortical tumors were documented as having systemic hypertension.[449]

Clinical signs

Ocular signs are usually the presenting signs of hypertension but cardiac and neurologic signs may also be associated with hypertension.[435] The underlying cause of hypertension, such as renal failure or hyperthyroidism, also often contributes to the patient's signs. The cat appears to manifest ocular lesions with systemic hypertension more readily than the dog. The mean age of cats presented with signs was 15 years.[435,450]

The lesions observed with hypertension in the dog and cat are typically advanced unless observed on a screening examination. The most common ocular lesions noted in the cat when presented for signs of hypertension are: varying degrees of retinal detachment (62%) and 52% had bilateral detachments; retinal vessel tortuosity; and pre-retinal, vitreal, retinal, or subretinal hemorrhages in 56% of eyes.[435] Multifocal bullae of the retina may be noted early in the course.

Hypertension is manifested in the ocular fundus as dilated tortuous vessels, retinal edema, retinal hemorrhages, vitreous hemorrhages, perivasculitis, papilledema, and focal or generalized transudative retinal detachment (**Figures 14.133 through 14.136**). Sustained increases in blood pressure result in vasoconstriction of autoregulated (as in the retina) peripheral arterioles. This results in hypertrophy and hyperplasia of the tunica media, loss of the internal elastic membrane and, eventually, fibrinoid necrosis.[451] Hayreh et al.[452,453] divided the fundus lesions in primates into hypertensive retinopathy, choroidopathy, and optic neuropathy. The retinal changes occur

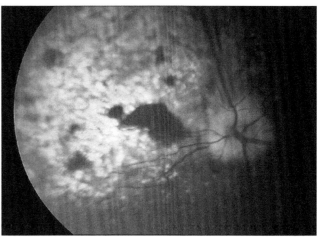

Figure 14.133 Multiple retinal hemorrhages, papilledema, and vascular congestion in a dog with systemic hypertension.

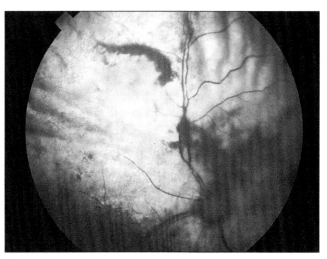

Figure 14.134 Hypertensive retinopathy in an older cat. Multiple retinal and subretinal hemorrhages, a low-lying retinal detachment, and choroidal streaks are visible.

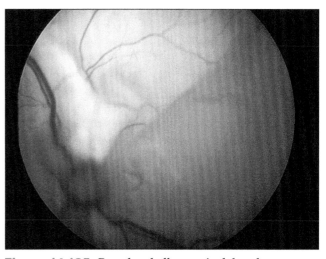

Figure 14.135 Complete bullous retinal detachment associated with systemic hypertension in a cat.

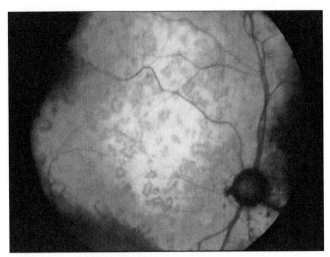

Figure 14.136 Fundus of a cat that has controlled systemic hypertension. Multiple lesions are presumed to be previous bullae that had formed during the hypertensive crisis. In most cases, evidence of previous bullous detachments are folds in the retina from stretching (see Figure 14.140).

significantly earlier than the choroidal and optic nerve changes but the choroidal changes may predominate in the dog and cat.[435,440] The earliest retinal lesions in primates are intraretinal, focal, periarteriolar white transudates that are pinhead size and round and last 2–3 weeks. They are distinguishable from "cotton wool spots" which are ischemic lesions of the terminal arterioles that appear later.[454] The transudates arise from loss of autoregulation of the retinal arterioles, which dilate and, due to damage to the endothelium, become permeable to plasma proteins.[452,453]

Hypertensive choroidopathy is associated with choroidal vascular bed abnormalities, RPE lesions, and serous retinal detachment.[454] If retinal detachment is present, resolution of the hypertension will be accompanied by resolution of the retinal detachment. However, secondary retinal atrophy often precludes a complete return of vision.[455] Secondary glaucoma and hyphema may be noted.

Diagnosis
The measurement of blood pressure (BP) is easily performed by indirect techniques but the interpretation of modest elevations in untrained animals in unfamiliar circumstances is open to dispute. Multiple, consistent readings in relaxed animals of at least moderate elevations in blood pressure are necessary in order to be confident of the results. BP may be affected by stress or anxiety associated with the measurement process and these changes may result in a false diagnosis of hypertension. This anxiety-induced, artifactual increase in BP is often referred to as white-coat hypertension, a reference to the white coat of the medical professional measuring the BP.[437]

A common source of error when performing indirect blood pressure measurements is not using the appropriate size cuff. The cuff width should be 40% and the length 150% of the circumference of the limb. Small cuffs will give erroneously high readings and large cuffs will give low readings.[437] The range of reported normal canine diastolic pressure is 60–110 mmHg and the systolic pressure is 110–190 mmHg. Blood pressures >160 mmHg systolic and 95 mmHg diastolic are considered hypertensive.[456] Feline hypertension is usually established as systolic blood pressure in excess of 165–170 mmHg in a relaxed cat.

> Evaluation of the retinal vascular system is often an inexpensive diagnostic test when a patient has any systemic disease that involves the vascular system or blood elements.

Therapy
When acute blindness is the presenting sign of hypertension, emergency therapy to reduce the blood pressure is indicated. Delay in reducing retinal detachment may result in permanent blindness. Therapy consists of treating any underlying conditions, as well as the lowering systemic blood pressure with anti-hypertensive medication.[437,456] Angiotensin-converting enzyme inhibitor (ACEI) and calcium channel blockers (CCB) are the most widely used antihypertensive agents in veterinary medicine. In dogs, ACEI are usually recommended as the initial agent of choice.[437] In cats, amlodipine (0.625 mg q12–24h) has proven very reliable in producing a rapid (within a few days) drop in blood pressure. Large cats or those not responding to 0.625 mg may have the dose increased to 1.25 mg q12–24h.[435,450] Maggio et al.[435] reported that amlodipine was successful in lowering blood pressure in 31 of 32 cats with systemic hypertension. If detected early in the course of retinal damage, lowering of systemic blood pressure may result in return of visual function.[437]

Solute fluid overload
Patients with renal failure frequently receive very aggressive fluid therapy. The author has noted on several occasions that multiple retinal bullae which progress to complete serous retinal detachment may occur bilaterally in these patients (**Figures 14.137 through 14.139**). Initially, it was thought this was due to hypertension related to renal disease, although the typical retinal hemorrhages of hypertension are not present. The blood pressures are normal, and it is suggested that the detachments

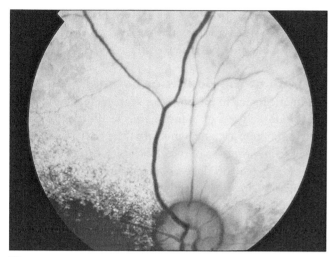

Figure 14.137 A dog in acute renal failure and on fluid therapy that is developing bullous retinal detachments in each eye. The systemic blood pressure was normal.

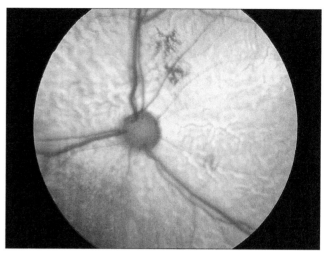

Figure 14.139 Residual retinal folds in a cat that previously had bullous detachment from overhydration. The condition can both manifest and resolve rapidly.

are due to solutes diffusing out of the leaky choriocapillaris into the subretinal space, pulling water with them. Discontinuing the fluids or improvement of renal function may correct the bullous detachments.

Diabetic retinopathy

Retinal vascular lesions are infrequently observed in the diabetic dog.[457] The basic vascular lesion with diabetes mellitus is the microaneurysm (**Figure 14.140**). Experimentally, retinal microaneurysm requires 4 years to develop, but most dogs have developed cataracts by this stage that obscure retinal examination.[458] Most of the reports of diabetic retinopathy have been pathologic, utilizing flat retinal preparations with trypsin digestion to isolate the vasculature. The pathologic vascular lesions

are degeneration and a decrease in numbers of intramural pericytes, resulting in acellular or hypocellular retinal capillaries and a few microaneurysms in the posterior pole.[458–462] Proliferative diabetic retinopathy (hemorrhage, glial membrane proliferation, retinal detachment) has not been reproducible, and the dog is thought to be spared from this disabling change. This has been questioned by the finding of microaneurysm, hemorrhage, irregularity in vascular width, retinal atrophy, and vitreous degeneration in a dog with a 7-year history of diabetes.[463] Monti et al. reported on the ophthalmoscopic findings in 13 spontaneous canine diabetics.[464] They reported clinical findings of dilatation of retinal veins, localized venous sacculations, venous tortuosity, microaneurysm, retinal hemorrhage,

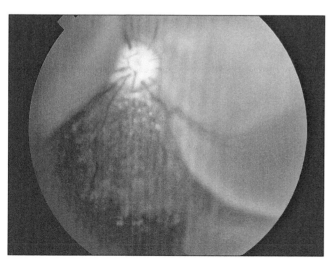

Figure 14.138 Severe bullous detachment as the result of overhydrating a dog in renal failure. The systemic blood pressure was normal.

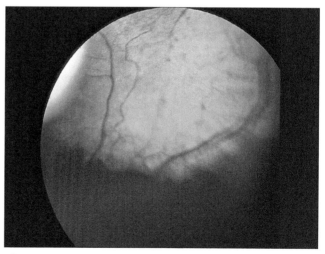

Figure 14.140 Presumed microaneurysms in a diabetic dog. These appear as minute red dots in the fundus. Fluorescein angiography would be needed to confirm that they are microaneurysms.

focal hyperreflectivity of the tapetum, depigmentation of the nontapetal fundus, and retinal exudate. However, the documentation of exudates and microaneurysms in this study is not convincing, and the alterations in venous caliber are subjective and not dramatic. The focal retinal atrophy or scars are nonspecific and may not be related to diabetes. The use of an age-matched control population would help determine whether focal retinal atrophy is found with increased frequency with diabetes. Herring et al. studied the longitudinal prevalence of hypertension, proteinuria, and retinopathy with spontaneous diabetes mellitus.[457] Diabetic vascular complications, including hypertension, proteinuria, and retinopathy, were documented in this longitudinal study, but there were no significant associations between these conditions and time since diabetes mellitus diagnosis or degree of glycemic control.[457] Detectable retinopathy ranged from 9.1% to 20.0% over the 2-year course of the study. The lesions detected in this study were similar to the previously reported.[457]

Diabetes is usually diagnosed in the aged dog, and it may be that most animals do not live long enough to manifest the more serious retinal changes unless the diabetes is juvenile in onset. Long-term administration of megestrol acetate in two cats was thought to be responsible for diabetes mellitus and associated bilateral retinal hemorrhage and exudative retinal detachment. The ocular changes were thought to be due to diabetes, but complications such as hypertension were not eliminated as factors in producing retinal detachment.[465]

Galactose-fed dogs develop microaneurysmal vascular changes similar to diabetic dogs but at an accelerated rate. Microaneurysms developed by 24 months in this model, and proliferative retinopathy developed by 48–60 months of feeding.[466] Lens removal is necessary to observe the retinal changes. Aldose reductase inhibitors prevent the microangiopathy in dogs[467,468] and cats.[469]

Retinal arteriolar aneurysm, independent of diabetes mellitus, has been documented in the dog, possibly due to a congenital defect, and this may result in vitreous hemorrhage.[470]

Oxygen-induced retinopathy

Increased arterial oxygen tension as the result of pure oxygen administration in the early neonatal kitten and puppy (first 2–3 weeks of life) is toxic to the developing retinal vasculature. The developing retinal blood vessels in the peripheral retina undergo vasoconstriction and vaso-obliteration in response to increases in pO_2. Later, a secondary vasoproliferative phase develops at the terminal ends of the developing vascular bed when the patient is returned to normal atmospheric oxygen tension. The vasoproliferation invades the vitreous, hemorrhage from fragile vessels may occur, and contraction of vitreal and vascular membranes may detach the retina.[471–474]

Trauma of the posterior segment

Traumatic injury to the posterior segment and optic nerve may be in the form of blunt injuries to the eye, perforating missile injuries, and avulsion of the retinal–choroidal vessels from proptosis of the globe (see Chapter 6, p. 156). Blunt injury may produce a contrecoup injury that results in fundus hemorrhage and bullous retinal detachment (**Figure 14.141**). Severe blunt injury may rupture the globe, and the sudden decompression may create retinal and choroidal detachments and expulsion of the lens.

Perforating injuries such as BB shot or pellet injuries may be obscured by anterior segment pathology or vitreous hemorrhage. Posterior exit wounds may be observed in the acute or chronic stages. Wounds with vitreous hemorrhage that have a tract that extends to the retina are in danger of producing traction retinal detachment as the hemorrhage organizes.

In the horse, a distinct syndrome of blunt trauma to the back of the head or poll may result in unilateral or bilateral blindness. Injuries to the poll are usually associated with rearing and hitting the head on a beam, or falling over and hitting the poll on the ground. Mild epistaxis is often present, but the amount of blood loss and the resultant pathology are not consistent with neuroretinopathy. On examination of the eyes, they are usually normal within days of the trauma, except for dilated, fixed pupils. The ERG with a diffuse light source is normal. After a period of 4–6 weeks, the ophthalmoscopic examination reveals loss of the retinal vessels and a pale optic

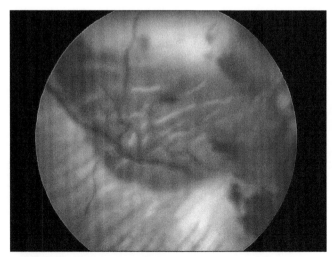

Figure 14.141 Choroidal hemorrhage with overlying retinal folds and retinal and preretinal hemorrhages in a Siamese kitten after head trauma.

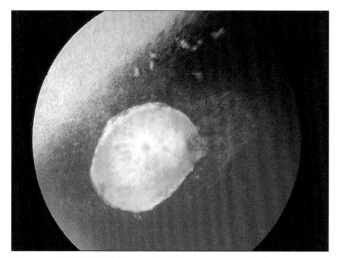

Figure 14.142 Unilateral optic nerve atrophy in a 3-month-old foal after head trauma. Note the lack of retinal blood vessels and the white color of the disc.

disc. Peripapillary pigment disruption may be present but is not consistent (**Figure 14.142**). On pathologic examination of the nerves, the intracanalicular portion of the optic nerve(s) has marked constriction associated with malacia of the nervous tissue (**Figure 14.143**). The pathogenesis of the lesion is thought to be due to stretching of the nerve and associated vessels by the backward momentum of the brain against the fixed intracanalicular portion of the optic nerve.[475]

Clinical signs of posterior segment trauma

Clinical signs associated with blunt or penetrating ocular trauma include marked hemorrhagic chemosis, exophthalmia, and elevation of the nictitans membrane. Ocular hemorrhage at any or multiple levels of the eye is common with trauma. Contrecoup lesions may appear as retinal edema and bullous detachment, and perforating missile injuries may appear as exit wounds in the fundus. Chronic changes are pigment disruption in the fundus and, potentially, complete retinal atrophy or optic nerve atrophy (**Figure 14.144**).

Diagnosis

Diagnosing traumatic fundus lesions is based on the history and evidence from physical examination of concurrent trauma to the head. Penetrating ocular injuries can cause marked disruption and distortion of normal anatomical structures. Ultrasound can demonstrate many of these lesions and is ideal for determining the status of anterior chamber, iris, lens, vitreous, and retina.[476] When the penetrating injury is caused by a sharp object, a hemorrhagic track through the vitreous cavity is usually present, and thickening or detachment of the retina and/or choroid is typically present. CT has particular utility in

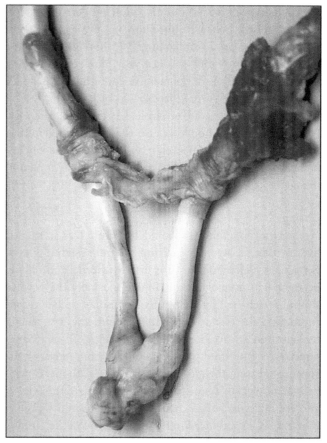

Figure 14.143 Optic nerves and chiasm of a horse that had bilateral blindness secondary to trauma to the poll 6 weeks earlier. Note the marked constriction of the nerves anterior to the chiasm that corresponds to the region of the optic foramen.

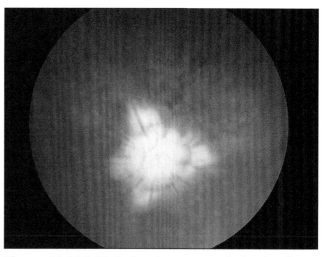

Figure 14.144 Marked optic nerve atrophy in a herding dog that had been previously kicked in the head by a horse. There was no history of a proptosed globe.

the evaluation of orbital trauma, allowing detailed assessment of bony lesions with simultaneous evaluation of soft tissues, globe, orbit, and brain.[344,476] Foreign body and metallic foreign bodies produce very high reflectivity on A-scan, and on B-scan, the metallic foreign body produce a very echo-dense signal that persists at low gain.[344,477,478] MRI is contraindicated in clinical cases with suspicion of metallic foreign body because the magnetic field may induce movement of the foreign body and cause secondary hemorrhage. In these cases, plain radiographs are recommended to screen for metallic foreign bodies.[344]

Therapy

Nonperforating injuries should be treated as nonseptic uveitis, that is, atropine and topical and systemic glucocorticoids. Pellet injuries are usually sterile and should be treated as nonperforating injuries; usually the corneal wound is self-sealing. If the lens capsule has been ruptured, and the tear is larger than 2 mm, the lens should be removed to avoid phacoclastic uveitis or phacoanaphylaxis.[479] Ruptured globes should be enucleated, or the rupture sutured, the globe eviscerated, and an intrascleral prosthesis placed. These globes will undergo phthisis bulbi and are not worth the expense and long-term discomfort that may be experienced to retain the globe in the animal.

There are a lot of controversies surrounding the optimal management of acute cases of traumatic nerve damage/traumatic optic neuropathy (TON). Despite these persisting uncertainties, the main treatment options in current use for TON are as follows: (1) Systemic steroids of varying doses, duration, and mode of administration; (2) surgical decompression of the optic canal; (3) a combination of steroids and surgery; and (4) observation alone (i.e., conservative management).[480–482]

Neoplasia of the fundus

Neoplasias of the ocular fundus (affecting retina, choroid, and optic nerve) are rare in domestic animals. Neoplasms may be classified as primary or secondary (metastatic or systemic/multicentric). When sudden hemorrhage or retinal detachment interferes with a thorough fundus examination, ultrasonography of the eye should be considered to rule out neoplasia.

Primary tumors

Melanoma is the most common primary intraocular tumor; however, intraocular localizations of melanocytic tumors other than extension from the anterior uvea melanoma are uncommon.[483–490] Choroidal melanomas are generally described as a flat, sharply circumscribed, slow-growing pigmented lesion. As the lesion grows, the retina may detach, and extension through the sclera and into the optic nerve may develop.[483] Preiridal fibrovascular membranes may result in hyphema or secondary glaucoma, obscuring visualization of the posterior tumor.[483] On histopathologic examination, the cell type is usually either a plump, pigment-filled cell without evidence of mitosis or a spindle cell.[483,484] Choroidal melanoma have been generally considered benign because of the lack of mitotic figures, cell type, and behavior with similarities to melanocytoma, which is a benign tumor rather than melanoma.[491–494] Extension of the tumor into the optic nerve, the orbit and distant metastasis, however, has been reported.[483,484,486,488]

Primitive neuroectodermal tumors (PNET)

Medulloepithelioma/retinoblastoma are rare congenital tumors of the embryonic neuroepithelium. Although both originate from the primitive neuroepithelial cells of the optic cup, retinoblastomas are malignant tumors arising from the primitive neuroepithelium of the immature retina, while medulloepitheliomas arise from the primitive medullary epithelium of the ciliary body.[495–498] Contemporary literature has reclassified older case reports of retinoblastoma in animals as being medulloepitheliomas.[495] In a recent retrospective study in eight dogs with PNET, Regan et al. showed that four of the eight evaluated tumors displayed histopathological criteria suggestive of retinoblastoma. Interestingly, all retinoblastoma-like tumors occurred in dogs <2 years of age, while all cases of medulloepithelioma occurred in dogs >7.4 years of age, paralleling the clinical presentation of these tumors in humans.[496]

Secondary tumors

Metastatic ocular neoplasia rarely develops in the fundus; however, metastatic tumors can spread to the choroid due to its highly vascular nature. Tumors that metastasize to the anterior uvea may also extend to involve the retina and the choroid. Metastatic lesions are more aggressive and nonpigmented in most instances, which helps to differentiate them from primary neoplasia. Bilateral metastatic lesions rarely occur. Several tumors have been reported including fibrosarcoma[499] hemangiosarcoma, which may mimic fundus hemorrhage (**Figure 14.145**),[500] mammary adenocarcinoma, thyroid adenocarcinoma, renal adenocarcinoma,[501] and myxoid leiomyosarcoma.[502]

Lymphoma

Malignant lymphoma is the most common secondary intraocular tumor affecting dogs and cats. Involvement of the posterior segment has been reported less frequently; however, both the retina and the choroid can be affected.[501,503] An ophthalmological examination may be considered as an important part of staging in lymphoma

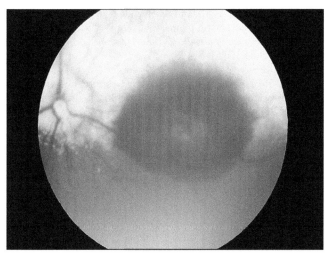

Figure 14.145 A dog with metastatic hemangiosarcoma in the fundus. The condition was bilateral. The ocular lesions must be differentiated from ocular hemorrhages. Lesions may be very small or large. Pulmonary metastasis was also present.

as well as follow-up examination in affected animals.[503] Ophthalmic signs on the posterior segment include posterior uveitis in 3% of the cases, panuveitis in 5%, and retinal hemorrhages in 9%.[504]

Angioinvasive pulmonary carcinoma

In the cat, a unique angioinvasive pulmonary carcinoma has been observed in the choroidal and the retinal vasculature, which results in large infarcts in the retina and the

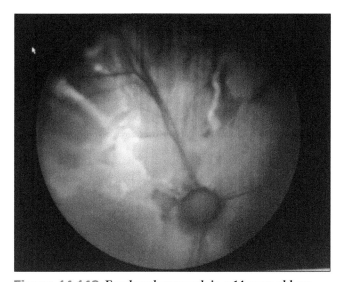

Figure 14.146 Fundus photograph in a 14-year-old cat with presumptive bronchogenic carcinoma. Large, wedge-shaped foci of chorioretinal necrosis are seen as tan-to-black discolored areas associated with profound retinal vascular attenuation. (E. Abarca,Vetsuisse, University of Bern, Switzerland.)

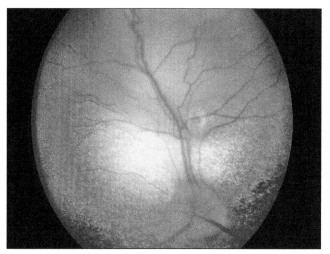

Figure 14.147 Gordon Setter with an orbital osteosarcoma that deformed the globe and produced scleral depression.

choroid[505] (**Figure 14.146**). The condition may be unilateral or bilateral and manifests with retinal detachment, retinal hemorrhage, and retinal vascular attenuation. Unlike other metastatic lesions, this disease does not have mass lesions but rather thrombi or emboli in the retinal and choroidal vasculature.

Orbital neoplasia

Orbital neoplasia or any space-occupying lesion may put compressive forces on the globe and deform it. Ophthalmoscopically, manifestations may vary from pressure striae to indentations of the globe that appear similar to (but are not) bullous detachments (**Figure 14.147**).

Primary neoplasia of the fundus is rare in all of our domestic animals. Lymphoma is the most common secondary intraocular tumor.

REFERENCES

1. Gloor, B. 1973. Zur entwicklung des glaskorpes und der zonula. III. Herkunft, lebenszeit und ersatz der glaskorperzellen beim kaninchen. *Albrecht von Graefes Archiv fur Klinische und experimentelle Ophthalmologie* 187:21–44.
2. Snowden, J., and Swann, D. 1980. Vitreous structure. V. The morphology and thermal stability of vitreous collagen fibers and comparison to articular cartilage (type II) collagen. *Investigative Ophthalmology and Visual Science* 19:610–618.
3. Balazs, E., editor. 1961. Molecular morphology of the vitreous. In: *The Structure of the Eye*. Academic Press: New York, pp. 293–310.
4. Osterlin, S., and Jacobson, B. 1968. The synthesis of hyaluronic acid in vitreous. II. The presence of soluble

transferase and nucleotide sugar in the acellular vitreous gel. *Experimental Eye Research* 7:511–523.

5. Stades, F. 1983. Persistent hyperplastic tunica vasculosa lentis and persistent hyperplastic primary vitreous in Doberman Pinschers: Genetic aspects. *Journal of the American Animal Hospital Association* 19:957–964.

6. Stades, F. 1983. The development of the vitreous and related (vascular) structures in persistent hyperplastic tunica vasculasa lentis and persistent hyperplastic primary vitreous (PHTVL/PHPV) in the Doberman Pinscher. Thesis, Utrecht, pp. 11–21.

7. Tolentino, F., Donovan, R., and Freeman, H. 1965. Biomicroscopy of the vitreous in Collie dogs with fundus abnormalities. *Archives of Ophthalmology* 73:700–706.

8. Eisner, G., and Bachmann, E. 1974. Vergleichend morphologische spaltlampenuntersuchung des glaskorpers bei der katze. *Albrecht von Graefes Archiv fur Klinische und Experimentelle Ophthalmologie* 191:343–350.

9. Eisner, G., and Bachmann, E. 1974. Vergleichend morphologische spaltlampenuntersuchung des glaskorpers von schaf, schwein, hund, affen, und kaninchen. *Albrecht von Graefes Archiv fur Klinische und Experimentelle Ophthalmologie* 192:9–17.

10. Gao, Q.Y., Fu, Y., and Hui, Y.N. 2015. Vitreous substitutes: Challenges and directions. *International Journal for Ophthalmology* 8(3):437–440.

11. Skeie, J.M., Roybal, C.N., and Mahajan, V.B. 2015. Proteomic insight into the molecular function of the vitreous. *PLoS One* 10(5):e0127567.

12. Lutty, G., Thompson, D., Gallup, J., Mello, R., Patz, A., and Fenselau, A. 1983. Vitreous: An inhibitor of retinal extract-induced neovascularization. *Investigative Ophthalmology and Visual Science* 23:52–56.

13. Boevé, M., Linde-Sipman, T., and Stades, F. 1988. Early morphogenesis of persistent hyperplastic tunica vasculosa lentis and primary vitreous. *Investigative Ophthalmology and Visual Science* 29:1076–1086.

14. Duddy, J., Powzaniuk, W., and Rubin, L. 1983. Hyaloid artery patency in neonatal Beagles. *American Journal of Veterinary Research* 44:2344–2346.

15. Munroe, G. 2000. Study of the hyaloid apparatus in the neonatal thoroughbred foal. *Veterinary Record* 146:579–584.

16. Koch, S.A., Cowles, R.R., Schmidt, G.R., Mayo, J.A., and Bowman, R.W. 1978. Ocular disease in the newborn horse: A preliminary report. *Journal of Equine Medicine and Surgery* 2:167–170.

17. Munroe, G. 1999. Subconjunctival haemorrhages in neonatal thoroughbred foals. *Veterinary Record* 144:279–282.

18. Odorfer, G. 1995. Occurrence and frequency of eye disesase among cattle in Austria. *Wien Tierarzlitche Monatsschr* 82:170–178.

19. Martin, C. 1969. Slit lamp examination of the normal canine anterior ocular segment. II. Description. *Journal of Small Animal Practice* 10:151–162.

20. McCormack, J.E. 1974. Variations of the ocular fundus of the bovine species. *Veterinary Scope* 18:21–28.

21. Munyard, K.A., Sherry, C.R., and Sherry, L. 2007. A retrospective evaluation of congenital ocular defects in Australian Shepherd dogs in Australia. *Veterinary Ophthalmology* 10:19–22.

22. Kern, T. 1981. Persistent hyperplastic primary vitreous and microphthalmia in a dog. *Journal of the American Veterinary Medical Association* 178:1169–1171.

23. Leon, A., Curtis, R., and Barnett, K. 1986. Hereditary persistent hyperplastic primary vitreous in the Staffordshire Bull Terrier. *Journal of the American Animal Hospital Association* 22:765–774.

24. van Rensburg, I., Petrick, S., van der Lugt, J., and Smit, M. 1992. Multiple inherited eye anomalies including persistent hyperplastic tunica vasculosa lentis in Bouvier des Flandres. *Progress in Veterinary and Comparative Ophthalmology* 2:133–139.

25. Allgoewer, I., and Pfefferkorn, B. 2001. Persistent hyperplastic tunica vasculosa lentis and persistent hyperplastic primary vitreous (PHTVL/PHPV) in two cats. *Veterinary Ophthalmology* 4:161–164.

26. Rebhun, W. 1976. Persistent hyperplastic primary vitreous in a dog. *Journal of the American Veterinary Medical Association* 169:620–622.

27. Bayon, A., Tovar, M., Fernandez del Palacio, M., and Agut, A. 2001. Ocular complications of persistent hyperplastic primary vitreous in three dogs. *Veterinary Ophthalmology* 4:35–40.

28. Gemensky-Metzler, A.J., and Wilkie, D.A. 2004. Surgical management and histologic and immunohistochemical features of a cataract and retrolental plaque secondary to persistent hyperplastic tunica vasculosa lentis/persistent hyperplastic primary vitreous (PHTVL/PHPV) in a Bloodhound puppy. *Veterinary Ophthalmology* 7(5):369–375.

29. Rubin, L. 1963. Hereditary retinal detachment in Bedlington Terriers. *Veterinary Medicine/Small Animal Clinician* 3:387–389.

30. Blair, N., Dodge, J., and Schmidt, G. 1985. Rhegmatogenous retinal detachment in Labrador Retrievers. I. Development of retinal tears and detachment. *Archives of Ophthalmology* 103:842–847.

31. Blair, N., Dodge, J., and Schmidt, G. 1985. Rhegmatogenous retinal detachment in Labrador Retrievers. II. Proliferative vitreoretinopathy. *Archives of Ophthalmology* 103:848–854.

32. Forrester, J., Lee, W., and Williamson, J. 1978. The pathology of vitreous hemorrhage. I. Gross and histological appearances. *Archives of Ophthalmology* 96:703–710.

33. Stiles, J. 2013. Special ophthalmology: Feline ophthalmology. In: Gelatt, K.N., Gilger, B.C., and Kern, T.J., editors, *Veterinary Ophthalmology* 5th edition: John Wiley & Sons, Inc: Hoboken, NJ, pp. 1477–1559

34. Hendrix, D.V.H. 2013. Disease and surgery of the canine anterior uvea. In: Gelatt, K.N., Gilger, B.C., and Kern, T.J., editors. *Veterinary Ophthalmology* 5th edition. John Wiley & Sons, Inc: Hoboken, NJ, pp. 1146–1198.

35. Burke, J., and Smith, J. 1981. Retinal proliferation in response to vitreous hemoglobin or iron. *Investigative Ophthalmology and Visual Science* 20:582–592.

36. Miller, B., Miller, H., and Ryan, S. 1986. Experimental epiretinal proliferation induced by intravitreal red blood cells. *American Journal of Ophthalmology* 102:188–19.

37. Thompson, J., and Stoessel, K. 1987. An analysis of the effect of intravitreal blood on visual acuity. *American Journal of Ophthalmology* 104:353–357.

38. Gonzalez, E.M., Rodriguez, A., and Garcia, I. Review of ocular ultrasonography. *Veterinary Radiology & Ultrasound* 2001; 42: 485–495.

39. Byrne, S.F., and Green, R.L. 2010. Vitreoretinal disease. In: Byrne, S.D., and Green, R.L., editors. *Ultrasound of the Eye and Orbit* 2nd edition: Jaypee Brothers Medical Publishers (P) Ltd.: New Dheli, pp. 45–86.

40. Papaioannou, N.G., and Dubielzig, R.R. 2013. Histopathological and immunohistochemical features of vitreoretinopathy in Shih Tzu dogs. *Journal of Comparative Pathology* 148(2–3):230–235.

41. Labruyere, J.J., Hartley, C., Rogers, K., Wetherill, G., McConnell, J.F., and Dennis, R. 2008. Ultrasonographic evaluation of vitreous degeneration in normal dogs. *Veterinary Radiology & Ultrasound* 49(2):165–171.

42. Itoh, Y., Maehara, S., Yamasaki, A., Tsuzuki, K., and Izumisawa, Y. 2010. Investigation of fellow eye of unilateral retinal detachment in Shih-Tzu. *Veterinary Ophthalmology* 13(5):289–29.

43. Pizzirani, S., Davidson, M.G., and Gilger, B.C. 2003. Transpupillary diode laser retinopexy in dogs: Ophthalmoscopic, fluorescein angiographic and histopathologic study. *Veterinary Ophthalmology* 6(3):227–235.

44. Wang, M., Kador, P.F., and Wyman, M. 2006. Structure of asteroid bodies in the vitreous of galactose-fed dogs. *Molecular Vision* 12:283–289.

45. Rubin, L. 1963. Asteroid hyalosis in the dog. *American Journal of Veterinary Research* 24:1256–1262.

46. Schaffer, E. 1985. Asteroide hyalose beim hund. *Tierarztliche Praxis* 13:71–75.

47. Miller, H., Miller, B., Rabinowitz, H., Zonis, S., and Nir, I. 1983. Asteroid bodies: An ultrastructural study. *Investigative Ophthalmology and Visual Science* 24:133–136.

48. Leon, A. 1988. Diseases of vitreous in the dog and cat. *The Journal of Small Animal Practice* 29:448–461.

49. Manning, S.P. 2007. Ocular examination in the diagnosis of angiostrongylosis in dogs. *Veterinary Records* 160:625–627.

50. Johnson, B., Kirkpatrick, C., Whiteley, H., Morton, D., and Helper, L. 1989. Retinitis and intraocular larval migration in a group of Border Collies. *Journal of the American Animal Hospital Association* 25:623–629.

51. Kaswan, R., and Martin, C. 1984. Ophthalmomyiasis interna in a dog and cat. *Canine Practice* 11:28–34.

52. Ollivier, F.J., Barrie, K.P., Mames, R.N., Kallberg, M.E., Greiner, E.C., Plummer, C.E., Gelatt, K.N., Strubbe, D.T., and Brooks, D.E. 2006. Pars plana vitrectomy for the treatment of ophthalmomyiasis interna posterior in a dog. *Veterinary Ophthalmology* 9(4):259–264.

53. Wyman, M., Starkey, R., Weisbrode, S., Filko, D., Grandstaff, R., and Ferrebee, E. 2005. Ophthalmomyiasis (interna posterior) of the posterior segment and central nervous system myiasis: *Cuterebra* spp. in a cat. *Veterinary Ophthalmology* 8(2):77–80.

54. Parry, H.G. 1953. Degenerations of the dog retina. I. Structure and development of the retina of the normal dog. *British Journal of Ophthalmology* 37:385–404.

55. Donovan, A. 1966. The postnatal development of the cat retina. *Experimental Eye Research* 5:249–254.

56. Gum, G., Gelatt, K., and Samuelson, D. 1984. Maturation of the retina of the canine neonate as determined by electroretinography and histology. *American Journal of Veterinary Research* 45:1166–1171.

57. Acland, G.M., and Aguirre, G.D. 1987. Retinal degenerations in the dog: IV. Early retinal degeneration (erd) in the Norwegian elkhound. *Experimental Eye Research* 44:491–521.

58. Aguirre, G.D., Rubin, L.F., and Bistner, S.I. 1972. The development of the canine eye. *American Journal of Veterinary Research* 33:2399–2414.

59. Martin, C., and Anderson, B. 1981. Ocular anatomy. In: Gelatt, K., editor. *Veterinary Ophthalmology* 1st edition: Lea & Febiger: Philadelphia, PA, pp. 88, 92, 98.

60. Koch, S., and Rubin, L. 1972. Distribution of cones in the retina of the normal dog. *American Journal of Veterinary Research* 33:361–363.

61. Steinberg, R., Reid, M., and Lacy, P. 1973. The distribution of rods and cones in the retina of the cat (*Felis domesticus*). *Journal of Comparative Neurology* 148:229–248.

62. Marmor, M. 1980. Clinical physiology of the retina. In: Peyman, G., Saunders, D., and Goldberg, M., editors. *Principles and Practice of Ophthalmology*. WB Saunders: Philadelphia, PA, pp. 823–856.

63. Hudspeth, A., and Yee, A. 1973. The intercellular junctional complexes of retinal epithelium. *Investigative Ophthalmology* 12:354–365.

64. Records, R. 1986. Retina: Metabolism and photochemistry. In: Duane, T., and Jaeger, E., editors. *Biochemical Foundations of Ophthalmology*, vol 2., Harper & Row: Philadelphia, PA, pp. 1–23.

65. Buyukmihci, N., and Aguirre, G. 1976. Rod disk turnover in the dog. *Investigative Ophthalmology* 15:579–584.

66. Anderson, D., Fisher, S., and Steinberg, R. 1978. Mammalian cones: Disk shedding, phagocytosis, and renewal. *Investigative Ophthalmology and Visual Science* 17:117–133.

67. Hollyfield, J., and Basinger, S. 1978. Cyclic metabolism of photoreceptor cells. *Investigative Ophthalmology and Visual Science* 17:87–89.

68. Prince, J., Diesem, C., Eglitis, I., and Ruskell, G. (editors) 1960. The globe. In: *Anatomy and Histology of the Eye and Orbit in Domestic Animals*. CC Thomas: Springfield, IL, pp. 13–42.

69. Pirie, A. 1965. The chemistry and structure of the tapetum lucidum in animals. In: Graham-Jones, O., editor. *Aspects of Comparative Ophthalmology*. Pergammon Press: London, pp. 57–75.

70. Ollivier, F.J., Samuelson, D.A., Brooks, D.E., Lewis, P.A., Kallberg, M.R., and Komaromy, A.M. 2004. Comparative morphology of the tapetum lucidum (among selected species). *Veterinary Ophthalmology* 7:11–22.

71. Wyman, M., and Donovan, E. 1965. The ocular fundus of the normal dog. *Journal of the American Veterinary Medical Association* 147:17–26.

72. Engerman, R., Molitor, D., and Bloodworth, J. 1966. Vascular system of the dog retina: Light and electron microscopic studies. *Experimental Eye Research* 5:296–301.

73. Henkind, P. 1966. The retinal vascular system of the domestic cat. *Experimental Eye Research* 5:10–20.

74. De Schaepdrijver, L., Simoens, P., and Lauwers, H. 1997. Morphologic and fluorangiographic study of the feline retina. *Veterinary and Comparative Ophthalmology* 7:216–225.

75. Gelatt, K., and Finocchio, E. 1970. Variations in the normal equine eye. *Veterinary Medicine/Small Animal Clinician* 63:569–574.

76. Barnett, K. 1972. The ocular fundus of the horse. *Equine Veterinary Journal* 4:17–20.

77. McCormack, J. 1977. Appearance of the normal optic disk in cattle. *Veterinary Medicine/Small Animal Clinician* 72:1494–1496.

78. Gelatt, K., Huston, K., and Leiopold, H. 1969. Ocular anomalies of incomplete albino cattle: Ophthalmoscopic examination. *American Journal of Veterinary Research* 30:1313–1316.

79. Briziarelli, G., and Abrutyn, D. 1975. Atypical coloboma in the optic disc of a Beagle. *Journal of Comparative Pathology* 85(2):237–240.

80. Roberts, S. 1969. Collie eye anomaly. *Journal of the American Veterinary Medical Association* 155:859–865.

81. Gelatt, K.; and Veith, L. 1970. Hereditary multiple ocular anomalies in Australian Shepherd Dogs. *Veterinary Medicine/Small Animal Clinician* 65:39–42.

82. Barnett, K., and Ogden, A. 1972. Ocular colobomata in Charolais cattle. *Veterinary Record* 91:592.

83. Gripenberg, U., Blomqvist, L., and Pamilo, P. 1985. Multiple ocular coloboma (MOC) in snow leopards (*Pather uncia*): Clinical report, pedigree analysis, chromosome investigations, and serum protein studies. *Hereditas* 102:221–229.

84. Martin, C., Stiles, J., and Willis, M. 1997. Feline colobomatous syndrome. *Veterinary and Comparative Ophthalmology* 7:39–43.

85. Wijeratne, W.V., and Curnow, R.N. 1978. Inheritance of ocular coloboma in Charolais. *Veterinary Record* 102(23):513.

86. Schuh, J.C. 1989. Bilateral colobomas in a horse. *Journal of Comparative Pathology* 100:331–335.

87. Rampazzo, A., D'Angelo, A., Capucchio, M.T., Sereno, S., and Peruccio, C. 2005. Collie eye anomaly in a mixed-breed dog. *Veterinary Ophthalmology* 8(5):357–360.

88. Roberts, S., and Dellaporta, A. 1965. Congenital posterior ectasia of the sclera in Collie dogs. I. Clinical features. *American Journal of Ophthalmology* 59:180–186.

89. Mizukami, K., Chang, H.S., Ota, M., Yabuki, A., Hossain, M.A., Rahman, M.M., Uddin, M.M., and Yamato, O. 2012. Collie eye anomaly in Hokkaido dogs: Case study. *Veterinary Ophthalmology* 15(2):128–132.

90. Brahm, V., Brahm, E., and Saers, K. 1978. Collie-augen-anomalie (CEA). *Kleinter Praxis* 23:221–224.

91. Barnett, K., and Stades, F. 1979. Collie eye anomaly in the Shetland Sheepdog in the Netherlands. *Journal of Small Animal Practice* 20:321–329.

92. Rubin, L., Nelson, E., and Sharp, C. 1991. Collie eye anomaly in Australian Shepherd Dogs. *Progress of Veterinary and Comparative Ophthalmology* 1:105–108.

93. Lowe, J.K., Kukekova, A.V., Kirkness, E.F., Langlois, M.C. et al. 2003. Linkage mapping of the primary disease focus for collie eye anomaly. *Genomics* 82:86–95.

94. Donovan, E., and Wyman, M. 1965. Ocular fundus anomaly in the Collie. *Journal of the American Veterinary Medical Association* 147:1465–1469.

95. Yakely, W. 1972. Collie eye anomaly: Decreased prevalence through selective breeding. *Journal of the American Veterinary Medical Association* 161:1103–1107.

96. Bjerkas, E. 1991. Collie eye anomaly in the Rough Collie in Norway. *Journal of Small Animal Practice* 32:89–92.

97. Holzhacker, W. 1988. Uber die verbreitung der Collie-augen-anomalie (CEA) in ostosterreich. *Doctor medicinae veterinariae thesis*, Veterinarmedizinischen, University of Wien, pp. 1–102.

98. Kellner, S., and Leon, A. 1985. Augenanomalie bei Collies in der Schweiz. *Kleintierpraxis* 31:63–65.

99. Yakely, W., Wyman, M., Donovan, E., and Fechheimer, N. 1968. Genetic transmission of an ocular fundus anomaly in Collies. *Journal of the American Veterinary Medical Association* 152:457–461.

100. Wallin-Hakanson, B., Wallin-Hakanson, N., and Hedhammar, A. 2000. Influence of selective breeding on prevalence of chorioretinal dysplasia and coloboma in the Rough Collie in Sweden. *Journal of Small Animal Practice* 41:56–59.

101. Wallin-Hakanson, B., Wallin-Hakanson, N., and Hedhammar, A. 2000. Collie eye anomaly in the Rough Collie in Sweden: Genetic transmission and influence on offspring vitality. *Journal of Small Animal Practice* 41:254–258.

102. Fredholm, M., Larsen, R.C., Jönsson, M. et al. 2016. Discrepancy in compliance between the clinical and genetic diagnosis of choroidal hypoplasia in Danish Rough Collies and Shetland Sheepdogs. *Animal Genetics* 47(2):250–2.

103. Latshaw, W., Wyman, M., and Venzke, W. 1969. Embryologic development of an anomaly of the ocular fundus in the Collie dog. *American Journal of Veterinary Research* 30:211–217.

104. Donovan, R., Freeman, H., and Schepens, C. 1969. Anomaly of the Collie eye. *Journal of the American Veterinary Medical Association* 155:872–875.

105. Brown, G., Shields, J., Patty, B., and Goldberg, R. 1979. Congenital pits of the optic nerve head. I. Experimental studies in Collie dogs. *Archives of Ophthalmology* 97:1341–1344.

106. Vainisi, S., Peyman, G., Wolf, D., and West, C. 1989. Treatment of serous retinal detachments associated with optic disk pits in dogs. *Journal of the American Veterinary Medical Association* 195:1233–1236.

107. Rubin, L. 1970. Correction of retinal detachment in a dog. *Journal of the American Veterinary Medical Association* 157:461–466.

108. Dziezyc, J., Wolf, D., and Barrie, K. 1986. Surgical repair of rhematogenous retinal detachments in dogs. *Journal of the American Veterinary Medical Association* 188:902–904.

109. Vainisi, S.J., and Packo, K.H. 1995. Management of giant retinal tears in dogs. *Journal of the American Veterinary Medical Association* 206:491–495.

110. Wilcock, B. 1983. Ocular anomalies. In: Peiffer, R., editor. *Comparative Ophthalmic Pathology*. CC Thomas: Springfield, IL, pp. 3–46.

111. Holle, D., Stankovics, M., Sarna, C., and Aguirre, G. 1999. The geographic form of retinal dysplasia in dogs is not always a congenital abnormality. *Veterinary Ophthalmology* 2:61–66.

112. O'Toole, D., Severin, G., and Neumann, S. 1983. Retinal dysplasia of English Springer Spaniel dogs: Light microscopy of the postnatal lesions. *Veterinary Pathology* 20:298–311.

113. Plummer, C.E., and Ramsey, D.T. 2011. A survey of ocular abnormalities in miniature horses. *Veterinary Ophthalmology* 14(4):239–243.

114. Ramsey, D.T., Ewart, S.L., Render, J.A., Cook, C.S., and Latimer, C.A. 1999. Congenital ocular abnormalities of Rocky Mountain horses. *Veterinary Ophthalmology* 2:47–59.

115. Silverstein, A., Osburn, M., Bennie, I., and Prendergast, R. 1971. The pathogenesis of retinal dysplasia. *American Journal of Ophthalmology* 72:13–21.

116. Cook, C., Burling, K., and Nelson, E. 1991. Embryogenesis of posterior segment colobomas in the Australian Shepherd Dog. *Progress in Veterinary and Comparative Ophthalmology* 1:163–170.

117. Ashton, N., Barnett, K., and Sachs, D. 1968. Retinal dysplasia in the Sealyham Terrier. *Journal of Pathology and Bacteriology* 96:269–272.

118. Rubin, L. 1968. Hereditary of retinal dysplasia in Bedlington Terriers. *Journal of the American Veterinary Medical Association* 152:260–262.

119. Leipold, H., Gelatt, K., and Huston, K. 1971. Multiple ocular anomalies and hydrocephalus in gradebeef Shorthorn cattle. *American Journal of Veterinary Research* 32:1019–1026.

120. Martin, C., and Leipold, H. 1974. Aphakia and multiple ocular defects in Saint Bernard puppies. *Veterinary Medicine/Small Animal Clinician* 69:448–453.

121. Stades, F. 1978. Hereditary retinal dysplasia (RD) in a family of Yorkshire Terriers. *Tijdschrift Voor Diergeneeskunde* 103:1087–1090.

122. Arnbjerg, J., and Jensen, O. 1982. Spontaneous microphthalmia in two Dobermann puppies with anterior chamber cleavage syndrome. *Journal of the American Animal Hospital Association* 18:481–484.

123. Peiffer, R., and Fischer, C. 1983. Microphthalmia, retinal dysplasia, and anterior segment dysgenesis in a litter of Doberman Pinschers. *Journal of the American Veterinary Medical Association* 183:875–878.

124. Bergsjo, T., Arnesen, K., Heim, P., and Nes, N. 1984. Congenital blindness with ocular developmental anomalies, including retinal dysplasia, in Doberman Pinscher dogs. *Journal of the American Veterinary Medical Association* 184:1383–1386.

125. Laratta, L., Riis, R., Kern, T., and Koch, S. 1985. Multiple congenital ocular defects in the Akita dog. *Cornell Veterinarian* 75:381–392.

126. Lewis, D., Kelly, D., and Sansom, J. 1986. Congential microphthalmia and other developmental ocular anomalies in the Doberman. *Journal of Small Animal Practice* 27:559–566.

127. Kaswan, R., Collins, L., Blue, J., and Martin, C. 1987. Multiple hereditary ocular anomalies in a herd of cattle. *Journal of the American Veterinary Medical Association* 191:97–99.

128. Lavach, R., Murphy, J., and Severin, G. 1978. Retinal dysplasia in the English Springer Spaniel. *Journal of the American Animal Hospital Association* 14:192–199.

129. Schmidt, G., Ellersieck, M., Wheeler, C., Blanchard, G., and Keller, W. 1979. Inheritance of retinal dysplasia in the English Springer Spaniel. *Journal of the American Veterinary Medical Association* 174:1089–1090.

130. Pellegrini, B., Acland, G.M., and Ray, J. 2002. Cloning and characterization of opticin cDNA: Evaluation as a candidate for canine oculoskeletal dysplasia. *Genetics* 282(1–2):121–131.

131. Du, F., Acland, G.M., and Ray, J. 2000. Cloning and expression of type II collagen mRNA: Evaluation as a candidate for canine oculoskeletal dysplasia. *Genetics* 255(2):307–316.

132. Meyers, V., Jezyk, P., Aguirre, G., and Patterson, D. 1983. Short-limbed dwarfism and ocular defects in the Samoyed dog. *Journal of the American Veterinary Medical Association* 183:975–979.

133. Acland, G., and Aguirre, G. 1991. Retinal dysplasia in the Samoyed dog is the heterozygous phenotype of the gene (drds) for short-limbed dwarfism and ocular defects. *Proceedings of the Scientific Meeting of the American College of Veterinary Ophthalmologists* 91, p. 44.

134. Barnett, K., Bjorck, G., and Kock, E. 1970. Hereditary retinal dysplasia in the Labrador Retriever in England and Sweden. *Journal of Small Animal Practice* 10:755–759.

135. Carrig, C., MacMillan, A., Brundage, S., Pool, R., and Morgan, J. 1977. Retinal dysplasia associated with skeletal abnormalities in Labrador Retrievers. *Journal of the American Veterinary Medical Association* 170:49–57.

136. Carrig, C., Sponenberg, D., Schmidt, G., and Tvedten, H. 1988. Inheritance of associated ocular and skeletal dysplasia in Labrador Retrievers. *Journal of the American Veterinary Medical Association* 193:1269–1277.

137. Heywood, R., and Wells, G. 1970. A retinal dysplasia in the Beagle dog. *Veterinary Record* 87:178–180.

138. MacMillian, A., and Lipton, D. 1978. Heritability of multifocal retinal dysplasia in American Cocker Spaniels. *Journal of the American Veterinary Medical Association* 172:568–572.

139. Bedford, P. 1982. Multifocal retinal dysplasia in the Rottweiler. *Veterinary Record* 111:304–305.

140. Williams, L., Peiffer, R., Gelatt, K., and Gum, G. 1979. A survey of ocular findings in the American Cocker Spaniel. *Journal of the American Animal Hospital Association* 15:603–607.

141. Weisse, I., Stotzer, H., and Seitz, R. 1973. Die neuroepitheliale invagination, eine form der netzhaut-dysplasie beim Beagle-hund. *Zentralblatt der Veterinärmedizin* 20:89–99.

142. Schiavo, D., and Field, W. 1974. Unilateral focal retinal dysplasia in Beagle dogs. *Veterinary Medicine/Small Animal Clinician* 69:33–34.

143. Long, S.E., and Crispin, S.M. 1999. Inheritance of multifocal retinal dysplasia in the Golden Retriever in the UK. *Veterinary Record* 145:702–704.

144. Crispin, S.M., Long, S.E., and Wheeler, C.A. 1999. Incidence and ocular manifestations of multifocal retinal dysplasia in the Golden Retriever in the UK. *Veterinary Record* 145:669–672.

145. Oster, S.F., Deiner, M., Birgbauer, E., and Sretavan, D.W. 2004. Ganglion cell axon pathfinding in the retina and optic nerve. *Seminars in Cell and Developmental Biology* 15:125–136.

146. Rubin, L.F. 1989. *Inherited Eye Diseases in Purebred Dogs.* Williams & Wilkins: Baltimore, MD.

147. Gelatt, K., and Leipold, H. 1971. Bilateral optic nerve hypoplasia in two dogs. *Canadian Veterinary Journal* 12:91–96.

148. Ernest, J. 1976. Bilateral optic nerve hypoplasia in a pup. *Journal of the American Veterinary Medical Association* 168:125–128.

149. da Silva, E.G., Dubielzig, R., Zarfoss, M.K., and Anibal, A. 2008. Distinctive histopathologic features of canine optic nerve hypoplasia and aplasia: A retrospective review of 13 cases. *Veterinary Ophthalmology* 11(1):23–29.

150. Brodsky, M.C. 2005. Congenital optic disk anomalies. In: Taylor, D., and Hoyt, G., editors. *Pediatric Ophthalmology and Strabismus*, 3rd edition. Elsevier-Saunders: Baltimore, MD, pp. 637–638.

151. Sengelaub, D., and Finlay, B. 1982. Cell death in the mammalian visual system during normal development. I. Retinal ganglion cells. *Journal of Comparative Neurology* 204:311–319.

152. Lambert, S., Hoyt, C., and Narahara, M. 1987. Optic nerve hypoplasia. *Survey of Ophthalmology* 32:1–8.

153. Weisse, V., and Stotzer, H. 1973. Hypoplasie des nervus opticus und kolobom der papille bei einem jungen Beagle. *Berliner und Munchener Tierarztliche Wochenschrift* 86:1–2.

154. Kern, T., and Riis, R. 1981. Optic nerve hypoplasia in three Miniature Poodles. *Journal of the American Veterinary Medical Association* 78:49–54.

155. Greene, C., Gorgacz, E., and Martin, C. 1982. Hydranencephaly associated with feline panleukopenia. *Journal of the American Veterinary Medical Association* 180:767–768.

156. Barnett, K., and Grimes, T. 1974. Bilateral aplasia of the optic nerve in a cat. *British Journal of Ophthalmology* 57:663–667.

157. Roberts, S.M. 1992. Congenital ocular anomalies. *The Veterinary Clinics of North America. Equine Practice* 8:459–478.

158. Hoyt, C., and Billson, F. 1978. Maternal anticonvulsants and optic nerve hypoplasia. *British Journal of Ophthalmology* 62:3–6.

159. Wen, G., Sturman, J., Wisniewski, H., MacDonald, A., and Niemann, W. 1982. Chemical and ultrastructural changes in the tapetum of Beagles with a hereditary abnormality. *Investigative Ophthalmology and Visual Science* 23:733–742.

160. Burns, M.S., Tyler, N.K., and Bellhorn, R.W. 1988. Melanosome abnormalities of ocular pigmented epithelial cells in Beagle dogs with hereditary tapetal degeneration. *Current Eye Research* 7:115–123.

161. Burns, M.S., Bellhorn, R.W., Impellizzeri, C.W., Aguirre, G.D., and Laties, A.M. 1988. Development of hereditary tapetal degeneration in the beagle dog. *Curr Eye Res* 7(2):103–114.

162. Scott, E.M., Teixeira, L.B., Dubielzig, R.R., Komaromy, A.M. 2013. Tapetal dysplasia in a Swedish Vallhund dog. *Veterinary Ophthalmology* 16(Suppl. 1):145–150.

163. Downs, L.M., Bell, J.S., Freeman, J., Hartley, C., Hayward, L.J., and Mellersh, C.S. 2013. Late-onset progressive retinal atrophy in the Gordon and Irish Setter breeds is associated with a frameshift mutation in C2orf71. *Anim Genet* 44(2):169–177.

164. Goosey, J., Tuan, W., and Garcia, C. 1984. A lipid peroxidative mechanism for posterior subcapsular cataract formation in the rabbit: A possible model for cataract formation in tapetoretinal diseases. *Investigative Ophthalmology and Visual Science* 25:608–612.

165. Downs, L.M., Hitti, R., Pregnolato, S., and Mellersh, C.S. 2014. Genetic screening for PRA-associated mutations in multiple dog breeds shows that PRA is heterogeneous within and between breeds. *Veterinary Ophthalmology* 17(2):126–130.

166. Gerstein, D., and Dantzker, D. 1969. Retinal vascular changes in hereditary visual cell degeneration. *Archives of Ophthalmology* 18:99–105.

167. Acland, G., Blanton, S., Hershfield, B., and Aguirre, G. 1994. XLPRA: A canine retinal degeneration inherited as an X-linked trait. *American Journal of Medical Genetics* 52:27–33.

168. Kijas, J., Cideciyan, A., Aleman, T. et al. 2002. Naturally occurring rhodopsin mutation in the dog causes retinal dysfunction and degeneration mimicking human dominant retinitis pigmentosa. *Proceedings of the National Academy of Science* 99:6328–6333.

169. Black, L. 1972. Progressive retinal atrophy: A review of the genetics and an appraisal of the eradication scheme. *Journal of Small Animal Practice* 13:295–314.

170. Priester, W. 1974. Canine progressive retinal atrophy: Occurrence by age, breed, and sex. *American Journal of Veterinary Research* 35:571–574.

171. Aguirre, G. 1976. Inherited retinal degeneration in the dog. *Transactions of the American Academy of Ophthalmology and Otolaryngology* 81:667–676.

172. Aguirre, G., and Acland, G. 1988. Variations in retinal degeneration phenotype inherited at the prcd locus. *Experimental Eye Research* 46:663–687.

173. Acland, G., Boughman, J. and, Aguirre, G. 1981. Inheritance of progressive rod-cone degeneration: A case of gamete selection? *Proceedings of the Scientific Meeting of the American College of Veterinary Ophthalmologists* 12, pp. 115–128.

174. Acland, G., Fletcher, R., Chader, G., and Aguirre, G. 1989. Nonallelism of three genes (rcd1, rcd2, and erd) for early-onset hereditary retinal degeneration. *Experimental Eye Research* 49:983–998.

175. Aguirre, G., Farber, D., Lolley, R., Fletcher, R., and Chader, G. 1978. Rod–cone dysplasia in Irish Setters: A defect in cyclic GMP metabolism in visual cells. *Science* 201:1133–1134.

176. Ray, K., Baldwin, V.J., Ackland, G.M., Blanton, S.H., and Aguirre, G.D. 1994. Cosegregation of codon 807 mutation of the canine rod cGMP phosphodiesterase B gene and rcd1. *Investigative Ophthalmology and Visual Science* 35:4291–4299.

177. Petersen-Jones, S.M., Entz, D.D., and Sargan, D.R. 1999. cGMP phosphodiesterase-α mutation causes progressive retinal atrophy in the Cardigan Welsh Corgi dog. *Investigative Ophthalmology and Visual Science* 40:1637–1644.

178. Woodford, B.J., Liu, Y., Fletcher, R.T., Chader, G.J., Farber, D.B., Santos-Anderson, R., and Tso, M.O. 1982. Cyclic nucleotide metabolism in inherited retinopathy in collies: A biochemical and histochemical study. *Experimental Eye Research* 34:703–714.

179. Aguirre, G., and Rubin, L. 1975. The electroretinogram in dogs with inherited cone degeneration. *Investigative Ophthalmology* 14:840–847.

180. Wolf, E., Vainisi, S., and Santos-Anderson, R. 1978. Rod–cone dysplasia in the Collie. *Journal of the American Veterinary Medical Association* 173:1331–1333.

181. Aguirre, G., Farber, D., Lolley, R. et al. 1982. Retinal degenerations in the dog. III. Abnormal cyclic nucleotide metabolism in rod–cone dysplasia. *Experimental Eye Research* 35:625–642.

182. Chader, G. 1991. Animal mutants of hereditary retinal degeneration: General considerations and studies on defects in cyclic nucleotide metabolism. *Progess in Veterinary and Comparative Ophthalmology* 1:109–126.

183. Parshall, C.J., Wyman, M., Nitroy, S., Acland, G., and Aguirre, G. 1991. Photoreceptor dysplasia: An inherited progressive retinal atrophy of Miniature Schnauzer dogs. *Progress in Veterinary and Comparative Ophthalmology* 1:187–203.

184. Jeong, M.B., Han, C.H., Narfstrom, K., Awano, T., Johnson, G.S., Min, M.S., Seong, J.K., and Seo, K.M. 2008. A phosducin (PDC) gene mutation does not cause progressive retinal atrophy in Korean miniature schnauzers. *Anim Genet* 39(4):455–456.

185. Cogan, D., and Kuwabara, T. 1965. Photoreceptive abiotrophy of the retina in the Elkhound. *Veterinary Pathology* 2:101–128.

186. Aguirre, G., and Rubin, L. 1971. The early diagnosis of rod dysplasia in the Norwegian Elkhound. *Journal of the American Veterinary Medical Association* 159:429–433.

187. Aguirre, G., and Rubin, L. 1971. Progressive retinal atrophy (rod dysplasia) in the Norwegian Elkhound. *Journal of the American Veterinary Medical Association* 158:208–218.

188. Acland, G., Gustavo, A., Parkes, J., and Liebman, P. 1983. A new early-onset inherited retinal degeneration in the

Norwegian Elkhound. *Proceedings of the Scientific Meeting of the American College of Veterinary Ophthalmologists* 14, pp. 98–103.

189. Acland, G., and Aguirre, G. 1987. Retinal degenerations in the dog. IV. Early retinal degeneration (ERD) in Norwegian Elkhounds. *Experimental Eye Research* 44:491–521.

190. Acland, G., O'Brian, P., and Aguirre, G. 1989. Rod renewal is cone-like in early retinal degeneration (erd). *Proceedings of the Scientific Meeting of the American College of Veterinary Ophthalmologists* 20, p. 152.

191. Ropstad, E.O., Bjerkas, E., and Narfstrom, K. 2007. Clinical findings in early onset cone-rod dystrophy in the Standard Wire-haired Dachshund. *Veterinary Ophthalmology* 10(2):69–75.

192. Ropstad, E.O., Bjerkas, E., and Narfstrom, K. 2007. Electroretinographic findings in the Standard Wire Haired Dachshund with inherited early onset cone-rod dystrophy. *Documenta Ophthalmologica* 114(1):27–36.

193. Ropstad, E.O., Narfstrom, K., Lingaas, F., Wiik, C., Bruun, A., and Bjerkas, E. 2008. Functional and structural changes in the retina of wire-haired dachshunds with early-onset cone-rod dystrophy. *Investigative Ophthalmology and Visual Science* 49(3):1106–1115.

194. Aguirre, G., and Rubin, L. 1972. Progressive retinal atrophy in the Minature Poodle: An electrophysiologic study. *Journal of American Veterinary Medical Association* 160:191–201.

195. Sandberg, M., Pawlyk, B., and Berson, E. 1986. Full-field electroretinograms in Miniature Poodles with progressive rod–cone degeneration. *Investigative Ophthalmology and Visual Science* 27:1179–1184.

196. Parkes, J., Aguirre, G., Rockey, J., and Liebman, P. 1982. Progressive rod–cone degeneration in the dog: Characterization of the visual pigment. *Investigative Ophthalmology and Visual Science* 23:674–678.

197. Barnett, K. 1965. Canine retinopathies. II. The Miniature and Toy Poodle. *Journal of Small Animal Practice* 6:93–109.

198. Aguirre, G., Alligood, J., O'Brien, P., and Buyukmihci, N. 1982. Pathogenesis of progressive rod–cone degeneration in Minature Poodles. *Investigative Ophthalmology and Visual Science* 23:610–630.

199. Acland, G., Marsh, R., and Northington, J. 1985. Auditory testing of dogs with inherited retinal degeneration. *Investigative Ophthalmology and Visual Science* 26:785–788.

200. Aguirre, G., and O'Brien, P. 1986. Morphological and biochemical studies of canine progressive rod–cone degeneration. *Investigative Ophthalmology and Visual Science* 27:635–655.

201. Anderson, R., Maude, M., Alvarez, R., Acland, G., and Aguirre, G. 1991. Plasma lipid abnormalities in the Miniature Poodle with progressive rod-cone degeneration. *Experimental Eye Research* 52:349–355.

202. Katz, M.L., Narfstrom, K., Johnson, G.S., and O'Brien, D.P. 2005. Assessment of retinal function and characterization of lysosomal storage body accumulation in the retinas and brains of Tibetan Terriers with ceroid-lipofuscinosis. *American Journal of Veterinary Research* 66(1):67–76.

203. Millichamp, N., Curtis, R., and Barnett, K. 1988. Progressive retinal atrophy in the Tibetan Terrier. *Journal of the American Veterinary Medical Association* 192:769–776.

204. O'Toole, D., and Roberts, S. 1984. Generalized progressive retinal atrophy in two Akita dogs. *Veterinary Pathology* 21:457–462.

205. Paulsen, M., Severin, G., Young, S. et al. 1988. Progressive retinal atrophy in a colony of Akita dogs. *Proceedings of the Scientific Meeting of the American College of Veterinary Ophthalmologists* 19, pp. 1–3.

206. Acland, G.M., Aguirre, G.D., Ray, J., Zhang, Q., Aleman, T.S., Cideciyan, A.V., Pearce-Kelling, S.E. et al. 2001. Gene therapy restores vision in a canine model of childhood blindness. *Nature Genetics* 28(1):92–95.

207. Narfstrom, K., Vaegan Katz, M., Bragadottir, R., Rakoczy, E.P., and Seeliger, M. 2005. Assessment of structure and function over a 3-year period after gene transfer in RPE65-/- dogs. *Documenta Ophthalmologica* 111(1):39–48.

208. Bragadottir, R., and Narfstrom, K. 2003. Lens sparing pars plana vitrectomy and retinal transplantation in cats. *Veterinary Ophthalmology* 6(2):135–139.

209. Rubin, L. 1971. Clinical features of hemeralopia in the adult Alaskan Malamute. *Journal of the American Veterinary Medical Association* 158:1696–1698.

210. Rubin, L. 1971. Hemeralopic in Alaskan Malamute pups. *Journal of the American Veterinary Medical Association* 158:1699–1701.

211. Koch, S., and Rubin, L. 1971. Distribution of cones in the hemeralopic dog. *Journal of the American Veterinary Medical Association* 159:1257–1259.

212. Aguirre, G., and Rubin, L. 1974. Pathology of hemeralopia in the Alaskan Malamute dog. *Investigative Ophthalmology* 13:231–235.

213. Rubin, L., Bourns, T., and Lord, L. 1967. Hemeralopia in dogs: Hereditary of hemeralopia in Alaskan Malamutes. *American Journal of Veterinary Research* 28:355–358.

214. Seddon, J.M., Hampson, E.C., Smith, R.I., and Hughes, I.P. 2006. Genetic heterogeneity of day blindness in Alaskan Malamutes. *Anim Genet* 37(4):407–410.

215. Acland, G. 1998. Day blindness in German Shorthaired Pointers in the United States: Clinical and electroretinographic findings. *Proceedings of the Scientific Meeting of the American College of Veterinary Ophthalmologists* 29, p. 33.

216. Witzel, D., Riis, R., Rebhun, W., and Hillman, R. 1977. Night blindness in the Appaloosa: Sibling occurrence. *Journal of Equine Medicine and Surgery* 1:383–386.

217. Sandmeyer, L.S., Bellone, R.R., Archer, S., Bauer, B.S., Nelson, J., Forsyth, G., and Grahn, B.H. 2012. Congenital stationary night blindness is associated with the leopard complex in the Miniature Horse. *Veterinary Ophthalmology* 15(1):18–22.

218. Nunnery, C., Pickett, J.P., and Zimmerman, K.L. 2005. Congenital stationary night blindness in a Thoroughbred and a Paso Fino. *Veterinary Ophthalmology* 8(6):415–419.

219. Witzel, D., Smith, E., Wilson, R., and Aguirre, G. 1978. Congenital stationary night blindness: An animal model. *Investigative Ophthalmology and Visual Science* 17:788–795.

220. Pickett, J., Lindley, D., Boosinger, T., and Toivio-Kinnucan, M. 1991. Stationary night blindness in a Collie. *Progress in Veterinary and Comparative Ophthalmology* 1:303–308.

221. Narfström, K., Wrigstad, A., Ekesten, B., and Nilsson, S.E. 1994. Hereditary retinal dystrophy in the Briard dog: Clinical and hereditary characteristics. *Veterinary and Comparative Ophthalmology* 4:85–92.

222. Aguirre, G., Baldwin, V., Pearce-Kelling, S., Narfström, K., Ray, K., and Acland, G. 1998. Congenital stationary night blindness in the dog: Common mutation in the RPE65 gene indicates founder effect. *Molecular Vision* 4:23–36.

223. Wrigstad, A., Nilsson, S.E., and Narfström, K. 1992. Ultrastructural changes of the retina and the retinal pigment epithelium in Briard dogs with hereditary congenital night blindness and partial day blindness. *Experimental Eye Research* 55:805–818.

224. Riis, R., and Siakotos, A. 1989. Inherited lipid retinopathy within a dog breed. *Investigative Ophthalmology and Visual Science* 30(Supplement):308.

225. Watson, P., Simpson, K., and Bedford, P. 1993. Hypercholesterolaemia in Briards in the United Kingdom. *Research in Veterinary Science* 54:80–85.

226. Parry, H. 1954. Degeneration of the dog retina. VI. Central progressive atrophy with pigment epithelial dystrophy. *British Journal of Ophthalmology* 38:653–668.

227. Aguirre, G., and Laties, A. 1976. Pigment epithelial dystrophy in the dog. *Experimental Eye Research* 23:247–256.

228. Curtis, R. 1988. Retinal diseases in the dog and cat: An overview and update. *Journal of Small Animal Practice* 29:397–415.

229. Bedford, P. 1984. Retinal pigment epithelial dystrophy (CPRA): A study of the disease in the Briard. *Journal of Small Animal Practice* 25:129–138.

230. Barnett, K. 1969. Genetic anomalies of the posterior segment of the canine eye. *Transactions of the Ophthalmology Society* 89:301–313.

231. Barnett, K. 1969. Primary retinal dystrophies in the dog. *Journal of the American Veterinary Medical Association* 154:804–808.

232. McLellan, G.J., Elks, R., Lybaert, P., Watte, C., Moore, D.L., and Bedford, P.G. 2002. Vitamin E deficiency in dogs with retinal pigment epithelial dystrophy. *The Veterinary Record* 151(22):663–667.

233. McLellan, G.J., and Bedford, P.G. 2012. Oral vitamin E absorption in English Cocker Spaniels with familial vitamin E deficiency and retinal pigment epithelial dystrophy. *Veterinary Ophthalmology* 15(Suppl 2):48–56.

234. Grahn, B.H., Philibert, H., Cullen, C.L., Houston, D.M., Semple, H.A., and Schmutz, S.M. 1998. Multifocal retinopathy of Great Pyrenees dogs. *Veterinary Ophthalmology* 1:211–221.

235. Gornik, K.R., Pirie, C.G., Duker, J.S., and Boudrieau, R.J. 2014. Canine multifocal retinopathy caused by a BEST1 mutation in a Boerboel. *Veterinary Ophthalmology* 17(5):368–372.

236. Grahn, B.H., Sandmeyer, L.L., and Breaux, C. 2008. Retinopathy of Coton de Tulear dogs: Clinical manifestations, electroretinographic, ultrasonographic, fluorescein and indocyanine green angiographic, and optical coherence tomographic findings. *Veterinary Ophthalmology* 11(4):242–249.

237. Rah, H., Maggs, D.J., Blankenship, T.N., Narfstrom, K., and Lyons, L.A. 2005. Early-onset, autosomal recessive, progressive retinal atrophy in Persian cats. *Investigative Ophthalmology and Visual Science* 46(5):1742–1747.

238. Carlile, J., Carrington, S., and Bedford, P. 1984. Six cases of progressive retinal atrophy in Abyssinian cats. *Journal of Small Animal Practice* 25:415–420.

239. Narfström, K. 1985. Progressive retinal atrophy in the Abyssinian cat. *Investigative Ophthalmology and Visual Science* 26:193–200.

240. Narfström, K., and Nilsson, S. 1986. Progressive retinal atrophy in the Abyssinian cat. *Investigative Ophthalmology and Visual Science* 27:1569–1576.

241. Narfström, K. 1983. Hereditary progressive retinal atrophy in the Abyssinian cat. *Journal of Heredity* 74:273–276.

242. Barnett, K. 1982. Progressive retinal atrophy in the Abyssinian cat. *Journal of Small Animal Practice* 23:763–766.

243. Rubin, L., and Lipton, D. 1973. Retinal degeneration in kittens. *Journal of the American Veterinary Medical Association* 62:467–469.

244. West-Hyde, L., and Buyukmihci, N. 1982. Photoreceptor degeneration in a family of cats. *Journal of the American Veterinary Medical Association* 181:243–247.

245. Kelly, D., and Lewis, D. 1985. Rapidly progressive diffuse retinal degeneration in a kitten. *Journal of Small Animal Practice* 26:317–322.

246. Valle, D., Boison, A., Jezyk, P., and Aguirre, G. 1981. Gyrate atrophy of the choroids and retina in a cat. *Investigative Ophthalmology and Visual Science* 20:251–254.

247. Kohyama, M., Yabuki, A., Ochiai, K. et al. 2016. In situ detection of GM1 and GM2 gangliosides using immunohistochemical and immunofluorescent techniques for auxiliary diagnosis of canine and feline gangliosidoses. *BMC Veterinary Research* 2016 Mar 31;12:67.

248. Murray, J., Blakemore, W., and Barnett, K. 1977. Ocular lesions in cats with GM1-gangliosidosis with visceral involvement. *Journal of Small Animal Practice* 18:1–10.

249. Wang, C.Y., and Smith, B.F. 2007. Development of quantitative polymerase chain reaction assays for allelic discrimination of gangliosidoses in cats. *American Journal of Veterinary Research* 68(3):231–235.

250. Cowell, K., Jezyk, P., Haskins, M., and Patterson, D. 1976. Mucopolysaccharidosis in a cat. *Journal of the American Veterinary Medical Association* 169:334–339.

251. Langweiler, M., Haskins, M., and Jezyk, P. 1978. Mucopolysaccharidosis in a litter of cats. *Journal of the American Animal Hospital Association* 14:748–751.

252. Haskins, M., Jezyk, P., Desnick, R., McDonough, S., and Patterson, D. 1979. Mucopolysaccharidosis in a domestic shorthaired cat, a disease distinct from that seen in the Siamese cat. *Journal of the American Veterinary Medical Association* 175:384–387.

253. Breton, L., Guerin, P., and Morin, M. 1983. A case of mucopolysaccharidosis VI in a cat. *Journal of the American Animal Hospital Association* 19:891–896.

254. Newkirk, K.M., Atkins, R.M., Dickson, P.I., Rohrbach, B.W., and McEntee, M.F. 2011. Ocular lesions in canine mucopolysaccharidosis I and response to enzyme replacement therapy. *Investigative Ophthalmology and Visual Science* 52(8):5130–5135.

255. Cummings, J.F., Wood, P.A., de Lahunta, A., Walkley, S.U., and Le Boeuf, L. 1988. The clinical and pathologic heterogeneity of feline α-mannosidosis. *Journal of Veterinary Internal Medicine* 2(4):163–70.

256. Siakotos, A., Armstrong, D., Koppang, N., and Connole, E. 1978. Studies on the retina and the pigment epithelium in hereditary canine ceroid lipofuscinosis. II. The subcellular distribution of lysosomal hydrolases and other enzymes. *Investigative Ophthalmology and Visual Science* 17:618–633.

257. Berson, E., and Watson, G. 1980. Electroretinograms in English Setters with neuronal ceroid lipofuscinosis. *Investigative Ophthalmology and Visual Science* 19:87–90.

258. Sisk, D., Levesque, D., Wood, P., and Styer, E. 1990. Clinical and pathologic features of ceroid lipofuscinosis in two Australian Cattle Dogs. *Journal of the American Veterinary Medical Association* 197:361–364.

259. Smith, R.E., Sutton, R.H., Jolly, R.D., and Smith, K.R. 1996. A retinal degeneration associated with ceroid

lipofuscinosis in adult Miniature Schnauzers. *Veterinary and Comparative Ophthalmology* 6:187–191.

260. Minatel, L., Underwood, S.C., and Carfagnini, J.C. 2000. Ceroid lipofuscinosis in a Cocker Spaniel dog. *Veterinary Pathology* 37:488–490.

261. Narfstrom, K., Wrigstad, A., Ekesten, B., and Berg, A.L. 2007. Neuronal ceroid lipofuscinosis: Clinical and morphologic findings in nine affected Polish Owczarek Nizinny (PON) dogs. *Veterinary Ophthalmology* 10(2):111–120.

262. Rabin, A., Hayes, K., and Berson, E. 1973. Cone and rod responses in nutritionally-induced retinal degeneration in the cat. *Investigative Ophthalmology* 12:694–704.

263. Hayes, K., Carey, R., and Schmidt, S. 1975. Retinal degeneration associated with taurine deficiency in the cat. *Science* 188:949–951.

264. Anderson, P., Baker, D., Corbin, J., and Helper, L. 1979. Biochemical lesions associated with taurine deficiency in the cat. *Journal of Animal Science* 49:1227–1234.

265. Wen, G., Sturman, J., Wisniewski, H., Lidsky, A., Cornwell, A., and Hayes, K. 1979. Tapetum disorganization in taurine-depleted cats. *Investigative Ophthalmology and Visual Science* 18:1200–1206.

266. Pion, P., Kittleson, M., Rogers, Q., and Morris, J. 1987. Myocardial failure in cats associated with low plasma taurine: A reversible cardiomyopathy. *Science* 237:764–768.

267. Williams-Retz, L., and O'Brien, S. 1990. The role of taurine in the feline well being. *Iowa State University Veterinarian* 52:23–26.

268. Morris, M. 1965. Feline degenerative retinopathy. *Cornell Veterinarian* 60:295–308.

269. Brucker, R. 1949. Uber den ophthalmoskopischen nachweis von fovea und arei bei tieren. *Ophthalmologica* 118:969–980.

270. Bellhorn, R., and Fischer, C. 1970. Feline central retinal degeneration. *Journal of the American Veterinary Medical Association* 157:842–849.

271. Soure, E. 1972. Observations of feline retinal degenerations. *Veterinary Medicine/Small Animal Clinician* 67:983–986.

272. Bellhorn, R., Aguirre, G., and Bellhorn, M. 1974. Feline central retinal degeneration. *Investigative Ophthalmology* 13:608–616.

273. Berson, E., Hayes, K., Rabin, A., and Watson, G. 1976. Retinal degeneration in cats fed casein. II. Supplementation with methionine, cysteine, or taurine. *Investigative Ophthalmology* 15:52–58.

274. Schmidt, S., Berson, E., and Hayes, K. 1976. Retinal degeneration in cats fed casein. I. Taurine deficiency. *Investigative Ophthalmology* 15:47–52.

275. Barnett, K., and Burger, I. 1980. Taurine deficiency retinopathy in the cat. *Journal of Small Animal Practice* 21:521–534.

276. Ricketts, J. 1983. Feline central retinal degeneration in the domestic cat. *Journal of Small Animal Practice* 24:221–227.

277. Brewer, N. 1982. Nutrition of the cat. *Journal of the American Veterinary Medical Association* 180:1179–1182.

278. Erbersdobler, V.H. 1983. Durch taurinmangel bedingte augenkrankheiten bei katzen sowie zur taurinversorgung von katzen. *Tierarztliche Umschau* 38:340–344.

279. Hickman, M.A. 2000. Bioavailability of taurine for cats. *Compendium on Continuing Education for the Practicing Veterinarian* 22:33–35.

280. Aguirre, G. 1978. Retinal degeneration associated with the feeding of dog foods to cats. *Journal of the American Veterinary Medicial Association* 172:791–796.

281. da Costa, P., and Hoskin, J. 1990. The role of taurine in cats: Current concepts. *Compendium on Continuing Education for the Practicing Veterinarian* 12:1235–1240.

282. Loew, F., Martin, C., Dunlap, R., Mapletoft, R., and Smith, S. 1970. Naturally occurring and experimental thiamine deficiency in cats receiving commercial cat food. *Canadian Veterinary Journal* 11:109–113.

283. Rubin, L. 1974. *Atlas of Veterinary Ophthalmology*. Lea and Febiger: Philadelphia, pp. 1–470.

284. Hayes, K., Rousseau, J., and Hegsted, D. 1970. Plasma tocopherol concentrations and vitamin E deficiency in dogs. *Journal of the American Veterinary Medical Association* 157:64–71.

285. Riis, R., Sheffy, B., Loew, E., Kern, T., and Smith, J. 1981. Vitamin E deficiency retinopathy in dogs. *American Journal of Veterinary Research* 42:74–86.

286. Davidson, M.G., Geoly, E.J., Gilger, B.C., McLellan, G.J., and Whitley, W. 1998. Retinal degeneration associated with vitamin E deficiency in hunting dogs. *Journal of the American Veterinary Medical Association* 213:645–651.

287. Nell, B., and Walde, I. 2010. Posterior segment diseases. *Equine Veterinary Journal* Suppl(37):69–79.

288. Tvedten, H., and Whitehair, C. 1977. *Torulopsis glabrata* and vitamin A deficiency in dogs. *American Journal of Veterinary Research* 38:1941–1948.

289. Paulsen ,M., Johnson, L., and Young, S. 1989. Blindness and sexual dimorphism associated with vitamin A deficiency in feedlot cattle. *Journal of the American Veterinary Medical Association* 194:933–937.

290. Moore, L., Huffman, C., and Duncan, C. 1935. Blindness in cattle associated with a constriction of the optic nerve and probably of nutritional origin. *Journal of Nutrition* 9:533–551.

291. Wetzel, J., and Moore, L. 1940. Blindness in cattle due to papilledema. *American Journal of Ophthalmology* 23:499–513.

292. Blakemore, F., Ottaway, C., Sellers, K., Eden, E., and Moore, T. 1957. The effects of a diet deficient in vitamin A on the development of the skull, optic nerves, and brain of cattle. *Journal of Comparative Pathology* 67:277–288.

293. Hayes, K., Nielsen, S., and Eaton, H. 1968. Pathogenesis of the optic nerve lesion in vitamin A-deficient calves. *Archives of Ophthalmology* 80:777–787.

294. Spratling, F., Bridge, P., Barnett, K., Abrams, J., and Palmer, A. 1965. Experimental hypovitaminosis-A in calves. *Veterinary Record* 77:1532–1542.

295. Barnett, K., Palmer, A., Abrams, J., Bridge, P.L., Spratling, F., and Sharman, I. 1970. Ocular changes associated with hypovitaminosis A in cattle. *British Veterinary Journal* 126:561–573.

296. Moore, I. 1941. Some ocular changes and deficiency manifestations in mature cows fed a ration deficient in vitamin A. *Journal of Dairy Science* 24:893–902.

297. Divers, T., Blackmon, D., Martin, C., and Worrell, D. 1986. Blindness and convulsions associated with vitamin A deficiency in feedlot steers. *Journal of the American Veterinary Medical Association* 189:1579–1582.

298. Van Donkersgoed, J., and Clark, E. 1988. Blindness caused by hypovitaminosis A in feedlot cattle. *Canadian Veterinary Journal* 29:925–927.

299. Schaller, J., Wyman, M., Weisbrode, S., and Olsen, R. 1981. Induction of retinal degeneration in cats by methylnitrosurea and ketamine hydrochloride. *Veterinary Pathology* 18:239–247.

300. Gelatt, K.N., van der Woerdt, A., Ketring, K.L., Andrew, S.E., Brooks, D.E., Biros, D.J., Denis, H.M., and Cutler, T.J. 2001. Enrofloxacin-associated retinal degeneration in cats. *Veterinary Ophthalmology* 4(2):99–106.

301. Ford, M.M., Dubielzig, R.R., Giuliano, E.A., Moore, C.P., and Narfstrom, K.L. 2007. Ocular and systemic manifestations after oral administration of a high dose of enrofloxacin in cats. *American Journal of Veterinary Research* 68(2):190–202.

302. Wiebe, V., and Hamilton, P. 2002. Fluoroquinolone-induced retinal degeneration in cats. *Journal of the American Veterinary Medical Association* 221(11):1568–1571.

303. Ramirez, C.J., Minch, J.D., Gay, J.M., Lahmers, S.M., Guerra, D.J., Haldorson, G.J., Schneider, T., and Mealey, K.L. 2011. Molecular genetic basis for fluoroquinolone induced retinal degeneration in cats. *Pharmacogenet Genomics* 21(2):66–75.

304. Barclay, S., and Riis, R. 1979. Retinal detachment and reattachment associated with ethylene glycol intoxication in a cat. *Journal of the American Animal Hospital Association* 15:719–124.

305. Hopkins, K., Marcella, K., and Strecker, A. 1990. Ivermectin toxicosis in a dog. *Journal of the American Veterinary Medical Association* 197:93–94.

306. Meekins, J.M., Guess, S.C., and Rankin, A.J. 2015. Retinopathy associated with ivermectin toxicosis in five cats. *Journal of the American Veterinary Medical Association* 246(11):1238–1241.

307. Kenny, P.J., Vernau, K.M., Puschner, B., and Maggs, D.J. 2008. Retinopathy associated with ivermectin toxicosis in two dogs. *Journal of the American Veterinary Medical Association* 233(2):279–284.

308. Ketring, K. 1990. Presumed ocular toxicity of ivermectin. *Proceedings of the Kal Kan Symposium*, Colombus, OH 13, pp. 109–110.

309. Epstein, S.E., and Hollingsworth, S.R. 2013. Ivermectin-induced blindness treated with intravenous lipid therapy in a dog. *Journal of Veterinary Emergency and Critical Care (San Antonio)* 23(1):58–62.

310. Kidwell, J.H., Buckley, G.J., Allen, A.E., and Bandt, C. 2014. Use of IV lipid emulsion for treatment of ivermectin toxicosis in a cat. *Journal of the American Animal Hospital Association* 50(1):59–61.

311. Van Kampen, K., and James, L. 1971. Ophthalmic lesions in locoweed poisoning of cattle, sheep, and horses. *American Journal of Veterinary Research* 32:1293–1295.

312. Watson, W., Barnett, K., and Terlecki, S. 1972. Progressive retinal degeneration (bright blindness) in sheep: A review. *Veterinary Record* 91:665–670.

313. Rosen, E., Edgar, J., and Smith, J. 1970. Male fern retrobullar neuropathy in cattle. *Journal of Small Animal Practice* 10:619–625.

314. Quigley, H., and Addicks, E. 1980. Chronic experimental glaucoma in primates. II. Effect of extended intraocular pressure elevation on optic nerve head and axonal transport. *Investigative Ophthalmology and Visual Science* 19:137–152.

315. Williams, L., Gelatt, K., Gum, G., Samuelson, S., and Merideth, R. 1980. Orthograde rapid axoplasmic transport and ultrastructural changes of the optic nerve of normotensive, acute ocular hypertensive, and glaucomatous Beagles. *Proceedings of the Scientific Meeting of the American College of Veterinary Ophthalmologists* 11, pp. 172–206.

316. Minckler, D., and Spaeth, G. 1981. Optic nerve damage in glaucoma. *Survey of Ophthalmology* 26:128–148.

317. Whiteman, A., Klaus, G., Miller, P.E., and Dubielzig, R. 2002. Morphologic features of degeneration and cell death in the neurosensory retina in dogs with primary angle-closure glaucoma. *American Journal of Veterinary Research*. 63(2):257–61.

318. Heywood, R., Hepworth, P., and van Abbe, N. 1976. Age changes in the eyes of the Beagle dog. *Journal of Small Animal Practice* 17:171–177.

319. Bellhorn, R., and Haring, B. 1974. Peripheral retinal cysts. *Veterinary Medicine/Small Animal Clinician* 69:1528–1530.

320. Okun, E., Rubin, L., and Collins, E. 1961. Retinal breaks in the senile dog eye. *Archives of Ophthalmology* 66:702–707.

321. van der Woerdt, A., Nasisse, M., and Davidson, M. 1991. Sudden acquired retinal degeneration in the dog: Clinical and laboratory findings in 36 cases. *Progress in Veterinary and Comparative Ophthalmology* 1:11–18.

322. Komaromy, A.M., Abrams, K.L., Heckenlively, J.R., Lundy, S.K., Maggs, D.J., Leeth, C.M., MohanKumar, P.S., Petersen-Jones, S.M., Serreze, D.V., and van der Woerdt, A. 2016. Sudden acquired retinal degeneration syndrome (SARDS)—A review and proposed strategies toward a better understanding of pathogenesis, early diagnosis, and therapy. *Veterinary Ophthalmology* 19(4):319–31.

323. Holt, E., Feldman, E., and Buyukmihci, N. 1999. The prevalence of hyperadrenocorticism (Cushing's syndrome) in dogs with sudden acquired retinal degeneration (SARD). *Proceedings of the Scientific Meeting of the American College of Veterinary Ophthalmologists* 30, p. 35.

324. Abrams, K., Gareen, I., and Marchand, K. 2001. Factors associated with canine sudden acquired retinal detachment syndrome (SARDS): 350 cases. *Proceedings of the Scientific Meeting of the American College of Ophthalmologists* 32, p. 17.

325. Carter, R.T., Oliver, J.W., Stepien, R.L., and Bentley, E. 2009. Elevations in sex hormones in dogs with sudden acquired retinal degeneration syndrome (SARDS). *Journal of the American Animal Hospital Association* 45(5):207–214.

326. Bellhorn, R., Murphy, C., and Thirkill, C. 1988. Antiretinal immunoglobulins in canine ocular diseases. *Seminars in Veterinary Medicine and Surgery* 3:28–32.

327. Keller, R.L., Kania, S.A., Hendrix, D.V., Ward, D.A., and Abrams, K. 2006. Evaluation of canine serum for the presence of antiretinal autoantibodies in sudden acquired retinal degeneration syndrome. *Veterinary Ophthalmology* 9(3):195–200.

328. Gilmour, M.A., Cardenas, M.R., Blaik, M.A., Bahr, R.J., and McGinnis, J.F. 2006. Evaluation of a comparative pathogenesis between cancer-associated retinopathy in humans and sudden acquired retinal degeneration syndrome in dogs via diagnostic imaging and Western blot analysis. *American Journal of Veterinary Research* 67(5):877–881.

329. Miller, P.E., Glbreath, E.J., Kehren, J.C., Steinberg, H., and Dubielzig, R. 1998. Photoreceptor cell death by apoptosis in dogs with sudden acquired retinal degeneration syndrome. *American Journal of Veterinary Research* 59:149–152.

330. Gooley, J.J., Lu, J., Fischer, D., and Saper, C.B. 2003. A broad role for melanopsin in nonvisual photoreception. *Journal of Neuroscience* 23(18):7093–7106.

331. Gooley, J.J., Lu, J., Chou, T.C., Scammell, T.E., and Saper, C.B. 2001. Melanopsin in cells of origin of the retinohypothalamic tract. *Nature Neuroscience* 4(12):1165.

332. Grozdanic, S.D., Matic, M., Sakaguchi, D.S., and Kardon, R.H. 2007. Evaluation of retinal status using chromatic

pupil light reflex activity in healthy and diseased canine eyes. *Investigative Ophthalmology & Visual Science* 48(11):5178–5183.

333. Spatola, R.A., Nadelstein, B., Leber, A.C., and Berdoulay, A. 2015. Preoperative findings and visual outcome associated with retinal reattachment surgery in dogs: 217 cases (275 eyes). *Veterinary Ophthalmology* 18(6): 485–496.

334. van der Woerdt, A., Wilkie, D., and Myer, C. 1993. Ultrasonographic abnormalities in the eyes of dogs with cataracts: 147 cases (1986–1992). *Journal of the American Veterinary Medical Association* 203:838–841.

335. Hendrix, D.V., Nasisse, M., Cowen, P., and Davidson, M. 1993. Clinical signs, concurrent diseases, and risk factors associated with retinal detachment in dogs. *Progress in Veterinary and Comparative Ophthalmology* 3:87–91.

336. Peiffer, R., Wilcock, B., and Yin, H. 1990. The pathogenesis and significance of preiridal fibrovascular membrane in domestic animals. *Veterinary Pathology* 27:41–45.

337. Nelms, S.R., Nasisse, M.P., Davidson, M.G., and Kirschner, S.E. 1993. Hyphema associated with retinal disease in dogs: 17 cases (1986–1991). *Journal of the American Veterinary Medical Association* 202:1289–1292.

338. Netland, P.A., Mukai, S., and Covington, H. 1994. Elevated intraocular pressure secondary to rhegmatogenous retinal detachment. *Survey of Ophthalmology* 39:234–240.

339. Johnstone, N., and Ward, D.A. 2005. The incidence of posterior capsule disruption during phacoemulsification and associated postoperative complication rates in dogs: 244 eyes (1995–2002). *Veterinary Ophthalmology* 8(1):47–50.

340. Strobel, B.W., Wilkie, D.A., and Gilger, B.C. 2007. Retinal detachment in horses: 40 cases (1998–2005). *Veterinary Ophthalmology* 10(6):380–385.

341. Smith, P.J., Mames, R.N., Samuelson, D.A., Lewis, P.A., and Brooks, D.E. 1997. Photoreceptor outer segments in aqueous humor from dogs with rhegmatogenous retinal detachments. *Journal of the American Veterinary Medical Association* 211:1254–1256.

342. Dietrich, U.M. 2013. Ophthalmic examination and diagnostic: Part 3: Diagnostic ultrasonography. In: Gelatt, K.N., Gilger, B.C., and Kern, T.J., editors. *Veterinary Ophthalmology* 5th edition. Wiley-Blackwell: Ames, IA, pp. 669–683.

343. Scotty, N.C. 2005. Ocular ultrasonography in horses. *Clinical Techniques in Equine Practice* 4:106–113.

344. Penninck, D., Daniel, G.B., Brawer, R., and Tidwell, A.S. 2001. Cross-sectional imaging techniques in veterinary ophthalmology. *Clinical Techniques in Small Animal Practice* 16:22–39.

345. Vainisi, S.J., and Wolfer, J.C. 2004. Canine retinal surgery. *Veterinary Ophthalmology*, 7(5):291–306.

346. Schmidt, G.M., and Vainisi, S.J. 2004. Retrospective study of prophylactic random transscleral retinopexy in the Bichon Frise with cataract. *Veterinary Ophthalmology*, 7(5):307–310.

347. Parry, H. 1954. Degenerations of the dog retina. IV. Retinopathies associated with distemper-complex virus infections. *British Journal of Ophthalmology* 38:295–309.

348. Jubb, K., Saunders, L., and Coates, H. 1957. The intraocular lesions of canine distemper. *Journal of Comparative Pathology* 67:21–29.

349. Fischer, C. 1971. Retinal and retinochoroidal lesions in early neuropathic canine distemper. *Journal of the American Veterinary Medical Association* 158:740–752.

350. MacMillian, A. 1974. Retinal dysplasia and degeneration in the young cat: Feline panleukopenia virus as an etiologic agent. *Davis, PhD dissertation*, University of California.

351. Percy, D., Scott, F., and Albert, D. 1975. Retinal dysplasia due to feline panleukopenia virus infection. *Journal of the American Veterinary Medical Association* 167:935–937.

352. Severin, G. 1995. *Severin's Veterinary Ophthalmology Notes.* Design Pointe Communications: Fort Collins, CO, pp. 1–546.

353. Albert, D., Lahav, M., and Carmichael, L. 1976. Canine herpes-induced retinal dysplasia and associated ocular anomalies. *Investigative Ophthalmology* 15:267–278.

354. Townsend, W.M., Jacobi, S., Tai, S.H., Kiupel, M., Wise, A.G., and Maes, R.K. 2013. Ocular and neural distribution of feline herpesvirus-1 during active and latent experimental infection in cats. *BMC Veterinary Research* 9:185.

355. Doherty, M. 1971. Ocular manifestations of feline infectious peritonitis. *Journal of the American Veterinary Medical Association* 159:417–424.

356. Albert, D.M., Lahav, M., Colby, E.D., Shadduck, J.A., and Sang, D.N. 1977. Retinal neoplasia and dysplasia. I. Induction by feline leukemia virus. *Investigative Ophthalmology & Visual Science* 16(4):325–337.

357. Bistner, S., Rubin, L., and Saunders, L. 1970. The ocular lesions of bovine viral diarrhea mucosal disease. *Veterinary Pathology* 7:275–286.

358. Martin, C. 1981. Retinopathies of food animals. In: Howard, J., editor, *Current Therapy of Food Animals.* WB Saunders: Philadelphia, PA, pp. 1067–1072.

359. Brown, T.T., Bistner, S.I., de Lahunta, A., Scott, F.W., and McEntee, K. 1975. Pathogenetic studies of infection of the bovine fetus with bovine viral diarrhea virus. II. Ocular lesions. *Veterinary Pathology* 12(56):394–404.

360. Jubb, K., Saunders, L., and Stenius, P. 1960. Die histologischen augenveranderungen beim bosartigen kartarrhalfieber des rindes. *Schweizer Archiv fur Tierheilkunde* 102:392–400.

361. Whiteley, H., Young, S., Liggitt, H., and Demartini, J. 1985. Ocular lesions of bovine malignant catarrhal fever. *Veterinary Pathology* 22:219–225.

362. Meyers, S., Wagnild, J., Wallow, I. et al. 1978. Septic choroiditis with serous detachment of the retina in dogs. *Investigative Ophthalmology and Visual Science* 17:1104–1109.

363. Hatfield, C., Rebhun, W., Dietze, A., and Carlisle, M. 1987. Endocarditis and optic neuritis in a Quarter horse mare. *Compendium on Continuing Education for the Practicing Veterinarian* 9:451–454.

364. Formston, C. 1994. Retinal detachment and bovine tuberculosis in cats. *Journal of Small Animal Practice* 35:5–8.

365. Michau, T.M., Breitschwerdt, E.B., Gilger, B.C., and Davidson, M.G. 2003. *Bartonella vinsonii* subspecies berkhoffi as a possible cause of anterior uveitis and choroiditis in a dog. *Veterinary Ophthalmology* 6(4):299–304.

366. MacDonald, D., Christian, R., and Chalmers, G. 1973. Infectious thromboembolic meningoencephalitis: Literature review and occurrence in Alberta. *Canadian Veterinary Journal* 14:57–61.

367. Deeg, C.A., Ehrenhofer, M., Thurau, S.R., Reese, S., Wildner, G., and Kaspers, B. 2002. Immunopathology of recurrent uveitis in spontaneously diseased horses. *Experimental Eye Research* 75(2):127–1.

368. Roberts, S. 1962. Fundus lesions in equine periodic ophthalmia. *Journal of the American Veterinary Medical Association* 141:229–239.

369. Townsend, W.M., Stiles, J., and Krohne, S.G. 2006. Leptospirosis and panuveitis in a dog. *Veterinary Ophthalmology* 9(3):169–173.

370. Walde, V., and Burtscher, H. 1980. Ablatio retinae infolge kryptokokkose beim hund. *Kleintier Praxis* 25:251–264.

371. Finn, M.J., Stiles, J., and Krohne, S.G. 2007. Visual outcome in a group of dogs with ocular blastomycosis treated with systemic antifungals and systemic corticosteroids. *Veterinary Ophthalmology* 10(5):299–303.

372. Bloom, J.D., Hamor, R.E., and Gerding, P.A. 1996. Ocular blastomycosis in dogs: 73 cases, 108 eyes (1985–1993). *Journal of the American Veterinary Medical Association* 209:1271–1274.

373. Brooks, D.E., Legendre, A.M., Gum, G.G. et al. 1991. The treatment of canine ocular blastomycosis with systemically administered itraconazole. *Progress in Veterinary and Comparative Ophthalmology* 1:263–268.

374. Bromel, C., and Sykes, J.E. 2005. Histoplasmosis in dogs and cats. *Clinical Techniques in Small Animal Practice* 20(4):227–232.

375. Gelatt, K., Chrisman, C., Samuelson, D., Shell, L., and Buergelt, C. 1991. Ocular and systemic aspergillosis in a dog. *Journal of the American Animal Hospital Association* 27:427–431.

376. Migaki, G., Font, R., and Sauer, R. 1982. Canine protothecosis: A review of the literature and report of an additional case. *Journal of the American Veterinary Medical Association* 181:794–797.

377. Schultze, A.E., Ring, R.D., Morgan, R.V., and Patton, C.S. 1998. Clinical, cytologic, and histopathologic manifestations of protothecosis in two dogs. *Veterinary Ophthalmology* 1:239–243.

378. Stenner, V.J., Mackay, B., King, T., Barrs, V.R., Irwin, P., Abraham, L., Swift, N. et al. 2007. Protothecosis in 17 Australian dogs and a review of the canine literature. *Medical Mycology* 45(3):249–266.

379. Glaze, M., and Gaunt, S. 1986. Uveitis associated with *Ehrlichia platys* infection in a dog. *Journal of the American Veterinary Medical Association* 188:916–918.

380. Swanson, J., and Dubielzig, R. 1986. Clinical and histopathological characteristics of acute canine ocular ehrlichiosis. *Proceedings of the Scientific Meeting of the American College of Veterinary Ophthalmologists* 117, pp. 219–232.

381. Leiva, M., Naranjo, C., and Pena, MT. 2005. Ocular signs of canine monocytic ehrlichiosis: A retrospective study in dogs from Barcelona, Spain. *Veterinary Ophthalmology* 8(6):387–393.

382. Komnenou, A.A., Mylonakis, M.E., Kouti, V., Tendoma, L., Leontides, L., Skountzou, E., Dessiris, A., Koutinas, A.F., and Ofri, R. 2007. Ocular manifestations of natural canine monocytic ehrlichiosis (Ehrlichia canis): A retrospective study of 90 cases. *Veterinary Ophthalmology* 10(3):137–142.

383. Martin, C. 1982. Ocular signs of systemic diseases. *Modern Veterinary Practice* 63:799–804.

384. Ellett, E., Playter, R., and Pierce, K. 1973. Retinal lesions associated with induced canine ehrlichiosis: A preliminary report. *Journal of the American Animal Hospital Association* 9:214–218.

385. Davidson, M.G., Breitschwerdt, E.B., Walker, D.H., Levy, M.G., Carlson, C.S., Hardie, E.M., Grindem, C.A., and Nasisse, M.P. 1990. Vascular permeability and coagulation during Rickettsia rickettsii infection in dogs. *American Journal of Veterinary Research* 51(1):165–170.

386. Davidson, M.G., Breitschwerdt, E.B., Nasisse, M.P., and Roberts, S.M. 1989. Ocular manifestations of Rocky Mountain spotted fever in dogs. *Journal of the American Veterinary Medical Association* 194(6):777–781.

387. Vainisi, S., and Campbell, H. 1969. Ocular toxoplasmosis in cats. *Journal of the American Veterinary Medical Association* 154:141–152.

388. Powell, C.C., and Lappin, M.R. 2001. Clinical ocular toxoplasmosis in neonatal kittens. *Veterinary Ophthalmology* 4(2):87–92.

389. Pennisi, M.G. 2015. Leishmaniosis of companion animals in Europe: An update. *Veterinary Parasitology* 208(1–2):35–47.

390. Pena, M.T., Naranjo, C., Klauss, G., Fondevila, D., Leiva, M., Roura, X., Davidson, M.G., and Dubielzig, R.R. 2008. Histopathological features of ocular leishmaniosis in the dog. *The Journal of Comparative Neurology* 138(1):32–39.

391. Macintire, D.K., Vincent-Johnson, N., Dillon, A.R. et al. 1997. Hepatozoonosis in dogs: 22 cases (1989–1994). *Journal of the American Veterinary Medical Association* 210:916–922.

392. Rubin, L., and Saunders, L. 1965. Intraocular larva migrans in dogs. *Veterinary Pathology* 2:566–573.

393. Hughes, P., Dubielzig, R., and Kazacos, K. 1987. Multifocal retinitis in New Zealand Sheepdogs. *Veterinary Pathology* 24:22–27.

394. Perry, A.W., Hertling, R., and Kennedy, M.J. 1991. Angiostrongylosis with disseminated larval infection associated with signs of ocular and nervous disease in an imported dog. *The Canadian Veterinary Journal* 32(7):430–431.

395. King, M.C.A., Grose, R.M.R., and Startup, G. 1994. Angiostrongylus vasorum in the anterior chamber of a dog's eye. *Journal of Small Animal Practice* 35(6):326–328.

396. Brooks, D., Wolf, E., and Merideth, R. 1984. Ophthalmoyiasis interna in two cats. *Journal of the American Animal Hospital Association* 20:157–160.

397. Cello, R. 1971. Ocular onchocerciasis in the horse. *Equine Veterinary Journal* 3:148–153.

398. Weisse, I., Seitz, R., and Stegmann, H. 1981. Eine multifokale serose chorioretinitis beim Beagle. *Veterinary Pathology* 18:1–12.

399. Giger, U., Werner, L., Millichamp, N., and Gorman, N. 1985. Sulfadiazine-induced allergy in six Doberman Pinschers. *Journal of the American Veterinary Medical Association* 186:479–484.

400. Gwin, R., Wyman, M., Ketring, K., and Winston, S. 1980. Idiopathic uveitis and exudative retinal detachment in the dog. *Journal of the American Animal Hospital Association* 16:163–170.

401. Andrew, S.E., Abrams, K.L., Brooks, D.E., and Kubilis, P.S. 1997. Clinical features of steroid-responsive retinal detachments in twenty-two dogs. *Veterinary and Comparative Ophthalmology* 7:82–87.

402. Wilcock, B., and Peiffer, R. 1987. The pathology of len-induced uveitis in dogs. *Veterinary Pathology* 24:549–553.

403. Fischer, C., and Jones, G. 1972. Optic neuritis in dogs. *Journal of the American Veterinary Medical Association* 160:68–79.

404. Walde, V., and Swoboda, R. 1980. Die, plotzliche Erblindung des hundes, diagnostik-therapie-prognose. *Kleintier Praxis* 25:61–78.

405. Nell, B. 2008. Optic neuritis in dogs and cats. *The Veterinary Clinics of North America Small Animal Practice* 38(2):403–415, viii.

406. Richards, T.R., Whelan, N.C., Pinard, C.L., Alcala, F.C., and Wolfe, K.C. 2011. Optic neuritis caused by canine distemper virus in a Jack Russell terrier. *The Canadian Veterinary Journal* 52(4):398–402.

407. Stadtbaumer, K., Leschnik, M.W., and Nell, B. 2004. Tick-borne encephalitis virus as a possible cause of optic neuritis in a dog. *Veterinary Ophthalmology* 7(4):271–277.

408. Fischer, C., and Si-Kwang, L. 1971. Neuro-ophthalmologic manifestations of primary reticulosis of the central nervous system in a dog. *Journal of the American Veterinary Medical Association* 158:1240–1248.

409. Russo, M. 1979. Primary reticulosis of the central nervous system in dogs. *Journal of the American Veterinary Medical Association* 174:492–500.

410. Garmer, N., Naeser, P., and Bergman, A. 1981. Reticulosis of the eyes and the central nervous system in a dog. *Journal of Small Animal Practice* 22:39–45.

411. Bailey, C., and Higgins, R. 1986. Characteristics of cerebrospinal fluid associated with canine granulomatous meningoencephalomyelitis: A retrospective study. *Journal of the American Veterinary Medical Association* 188:418–421.

412. Palmer, A., Malinowski ,W., and Barnett, K. 1974. Clinical signs including papilloedema associated with brain tumors in twenty-one dogs. *Journal of Small Animal Practice* 15:359–386.

413. Crook, K.I., Early, P.J., Messenger, K.M., Munana, K.R., Gallagher, R., and Papich, M.G. 2013. The pharmacokinetics of cytarabine in dogs when administered via subcutaneous and continuous intravenous infusion routes. *Journal of Veterinary Pharmacology and Therapeutics* 36(4):408–411.

414. Adamo, F.P., and O'Brien, R.T. 2004. Use of cyclosporine to treat granulomatous meningoencephalitis in three dogs. *Journal of the American Veterinary Medical Association* 225(8):1211–1216. 1196.

415. Hayreh, S. 1978. Fluids in the anterior part of the optic nerve in health and disease. *Survey of Ophthalmology* 23:1–24.

416. Saunders, L., Bistner, S., and Rubin, L. 1972. Proliferative optic neuropathy in the horse. *Veterinary Pathology* 9:368–378.

417. Chandler, K.J., Billson, F.M., and Mellor, D.J. 2003. Ophthalmic lesions in 83 geriatric horses and ponies. *The Veterinary Record* 153(11):319–322.

418. Vestre, W., Turner, T., and Carlton, W. 1982. Proliferative optic neuropathy in a horse. *Journal of the American Veterinary Medical Association* 181:490–491.

419. Platt, H., Barnett, K., Barry, D., and Bell, A. 1983. Degenerative lesions of the optic nerve in Equidae. *Equine Veterinary Journal Supplement* 2:91–97.

420. Hardy, J., Robertson, J., and Wilkie, D. 1990. Ischemic optic neuropathy and blindness after arterial occlusion for treatment of guttural pouch mycosis in two horses. *Journal of the American Veterinary Medical Association* 196:1631–1634.

421. Martin, C., Leipold, H., and Radostits, O. 1972. Polycythemia in a calf: Ocular findings. *Veterinary Medicine/Small Animal Clinician* 67:885–889.

422. Lombard, C., and Twitchell, M. 1978. Tetralogy of fallot, persistent left cranial vena cava, and retinal detachment in a cat. *Journal of the American Animal Hospital Association* 14:624–630.

423. Shull, R., Osborne, C., Barrett, R. et al. 1978. Serum hyperviscosity syndrome associated with IgA multiple myeloma in two dogs. *Journal of the American Animal Hospital Association* 14:58–70.

424. Center, S., and Smith, J. 1982. Ocular lesions in a dog with serum hyperviscosity secondary to an IgA myeloma.

425. Bublot, M., Thiriart, C., Grauwels, M. et al. 1985. Myelome multiple a IgG complilque du syndrome d'hyperviscosite chez un chien. *Annales de Medicine Veterinaire* 129:555–564.

426. Hendrix, D.V., Gelatt, K., Smith, P.J., Brooks, D.E., and Whittaker, C. 1998. Ophthalmic disease as the presenting complaint in five dogs with multiple myeloma. *Journal of the American Animal Hospital Association* 34:121–128.

427. Fischer, C.A. 1970. Retinopathy in anemic cats. *Journal of the American Veterinary Medical Association* 156(10):1415–1427.

428. Gelatt, K. 1979. Neuroretinopathy in the horse. *Equine Medicine and Surgery* 3:91–96.

429. Seider, M.I., and Damato, B.E. 2015. Leukemic retinopathy. *Journal of the American Medical Association Ophthalmology* 133(4):e144534–5.

430. Kern, T., and Riis, R. 1980. Ocular manifestations of secondary hyperlipidemia associated with hypothyroidism and uveitis in a dog. *Journal of the American Animal Hospital Association* 16:907–914.

431. Wyman, M., and McKissick, G. 1973. Lipemia retinalis in a dog and cat: Case reports. *Journal of the American Animal Hospital Association* 9:288–291.

432. Rogers, W., Donovan, D., and Kociba, G. 1975. Idiopathic hyperlipoproteinemia in dogs. *Journal of the American Veterinary Medical Association* 166:1087–1091.

433. Halenda, R.M., and Moore, C.P. 1998. Presumed lipid retinopathy in a diabetic dog. *Veterinary Ophthalmology* 1:171–174.

434. Gwin, R., Gelatt, K., Terrell, T., and Hood, C. 1978. Hypertensive retinopathy associated with hypothyroidism, hypercholesterolemia, and renal failure in a dog. *Journal of the American Animal Hospital Association* 14:200–209.

435. Maggio, F., DeFrancesco, T.C., Atkins, C.E., Pizzirani, A., Gilger, B.C., and Davidson, M.G. 2000. Ocular lesions associated with systemic hypertension in cats: 69 cases (1985–1998). *Journal of the American Veterinary Medical Association* 217:695–702.

436. Manning, P. 1979. Thyroid gland and arterial lesions of Beagles with familial hypothyroidism and hyperlipoproteinemia. *American Journal of Veterinary Research* 40:820–828.

437. Brown, S., Atkins, C., Bagley, R., Carr, A., Cowgill, L., Davidson, M., Egner, B. et al. 2007. Guidelines for the identification, evaluation, and management of systemic hypertension in dogs and cats. *Journal of Veterinary Internal Medicine* 21(3):542–558. 360.

438. Kobayashi, D., Peterson, M., Graves, T., Lesser, M., and Nichols, C. 1990. Hypertension in cats with chronic renal failure or hyperthryoidism. *Journal of Veterinary Internal Medicine* 4:58–62.

439. Maher, E.R.Jr., and McNiel, E.A. 1997. Pheochromocytoma in dogs and cats. *The Veterinary Clinics of North America. Small Animal Practice* 27:359–380.

440. Stiles, J., Polzin, D.J., and Bistner, S.I. 1994. The prevalence of retinopathy in cats with systemic hypertension and chronic renal failure or hyperthyroidism. *Journal of the American Animal Hospital Association* 30:564–572.

441. Van der Woerdt, A., and Peterson, M.E. 1998. Prevalence of ocular abnormalities in cats with hyperthyroidism. *Proceedings of the Scientific Meeting of the American College of Veterinary Ophthalmologists* 29, p. 26.

442. Sansom, J., Barnett, K.C., Dunn, K.A., Smith, K.C., and Dennis, R. 1994. Ocular disease associated with

hypertension in 16 cats. *Journal of Small Animal Practice* 35:604–611.

443. Turner, L., Brogdon, J., Lees, G., and Greco, D. 1990. Idiopathic hypertension in a cat with secondary hypertensive retinopathy associated with a high-salt diet. *Journal of the American Animal Hospital Association* 26:647–651.

444. Dukes, J. 1992. Hypertension: A review of the mechanisms, manifestations, and management. *Journal of Small Animal Practice* 33:119–129.

445. Javadi, S., Djajadiningrat-Laanen, S.C., Kooistra, H.S. et al. 2005. Primary hyperaldosteronism, a mediator of progressive renal disease in cats. *Domestic Animal Endocrinology* 28:85–104.

446. Ash, R.A., Harvey, A.M., and Tasker, S. 2005. Primary hyperaldosteronism in the cat: A series of 13 cases. *Journal of Feline Medicine and Surgery* 7:173–182.

447. Bovee, K., Littman, M., Crabtree, B., and Aguirre, G. 1989. Essential hypertension in a dog. *Journal of the American Veterinary Medical Association* 195:81–86.

448. Paulsen, M., Allen, T., Jaenke, R., Ching, S., Severin, G., and Hammond, T. 1989a. Arterial hypertension in two canine siblings: Ocular and systemic manifestations. *Journal of the American Animal Hospital Association* 25:287–295.

449. Ortega, T., Feldman, D., Nelson, R., Willits, N., and Cowgill, L. 1996. Systemic arterial blood pressure and urine protein/creatinine ratio in dogs with hperadrenocorticism. *Journal of the American Veterinary Medical Association* 209:1724–1729.

450. Elliott, J., Barber, P., Syme, H., Rawlings, J., and Markwell, P. 2001. Feline hypertension: Clinical findings and response to antihypertensive treatment in 30 cases. *Journal of Small Animal Practice* 42:122–129.

451. Keyes, J., and Goldblatt, H. 1938. Experimental hypertension. VIII. Vascular changes in the eyes. *Archives of Ophthalmology* 20:812–825.

452. Hayreh, S., Servais, G., and Virdi, P. 1985. Fundus lesions in malignant hypertension. III. Arterial blood pressure, biochemical, and fundus changes. *Ophthalmology* 92:45–59.

453. Hayreh, S., Servais, G., and Virdi, P. 1985. Fundus lesions in malignant hypertension. IV. Focal intraretinal periarteriolar transudates. *Ophthalmology* 92:60–73.

454. Crispin, S.M., and Mould, J.R. 2001. Systemic hypertensive disease and the feline fundus. *Veterinary Ophthalmology* 4(2):131–40.

455. Wolfer, J., Grahn, B.H., and Arrington, K. 1997. Diagnostic ophthalmology. Hypertensive retinopathy. *The Canadian Veterinary Journal* 38(8):519–520.

456. Ross, L. 1990. Hypertensive disease. In: Kirk, R., editor. *Current Veterinary Therapy*, 10th edition. WB Saunders: Philadelphia, PA, pp. 2047–2056.

457. Herring, I.P., Panciera, D.L., and Werre, R. 2014. Longitudinal prevalence of hypertension, proteinuria, and retinopathy in dogs with spontaneous diabetes mellitus. *Journal of Veterinary Internal Medicine* 28(2):488–489.

458. Engerman, R., and Bloodworth, J. 1965. Experimental diabetic retinopathy in dogs. *Archives of Ophthalmology* 73:205–210.

459. Patz, A., Berkow, J., Maumenee, A., and Cox, J. 1965. Studies on diabetic retinopathy. II. Retinopathy and nephropathy in spontaneous canine diabetes. *Diabetes* 14:700–708.

460. Gepts, W., and Toussaint, D. 1967. Spontaneous diabetes in dogs and cats: A pathologic study. *Diabetologia* 3:249–265.

461. Sibay, T., and Hausler, H. 1967. Eye findings in two spontaneously diabetic related dogs. *American Journal of Ophthalmology* 63:289–294.

462. Toole, D., Miller, G., and Hazel, S. 1984. Bilateral retinal microangiopathy in a dog with diabetes mellitus and hypoadrenocorticism. *Veterinary Pathology* 21:120–121.

463. Barnett, K. 1981. Diabetic retinopathy in the dog. *British Journal of Ophthalmology* 65:312–314.

464. Monti, F., Bellan, B., Berardi, S., and Peruccio, C. 1976. The clinical picture of diabetic retinopathy in the dog. *Folia Veteriniaria Latina* 6:249–274.

465. Herrtage, M., Barnett, K., and MacDougall, D. 1985. Diabetic retinopathy in a cat with megestrol acetate-induced diabetes. *Journal of Small Animal Practice* 26:595–601.

466. Takahashi, Y., Wyman, M., Ferris, F., and Kador, P. 1992. Diabetes-like preproliferative retinal changes in galactose-fed dogs. *Archives of Ophthalmology* 110:1295–1302.

467. Kador, P.F., Akagi, Y., Terubayashi, H., Wyman, M., and Kinoshita, J.H. 1988. Prevention of pericyte ghost formation in retinal capillaries of galactose-fed dogs by aldose reductase inhibitors. *Archives of Ophthalmology* 106:1099–1102.

468. Kador, P.F., Akagi, Y., Takahashi, Y., Ikebe, H., Wyman, W., and Kinoshita, J.H. 1990. Prevention of retinal vessel changes associated with diabetic retinopathy in galactose-fed dogs by aldose reductase inhibitors. *Archives of Ophthalmology* 108:1301–1309.

469. Mansour, S.Z., Hatchell, D.L., Chandler, D., Saloupis, P., and Hatchell, M.C. 1990. Reduction of basement membrane thickening in diabetic cat retina by sulindac. *Investigative Ophthalmology and Visual Science* 31:457–563.

470. Schiavo, D., and Field, W. 1975. Retinal arteriolar macroaneurysms in a Beagle dog. *Veterinary Medicine/Small Animal Clinician* 70:733–736.

471. Patz, A. 1965. The effect of oxygen on immature retinal vessles. *Investigative Ophthalmology* 4:988–999.

472. McLeod, D.S., D'Anna, S.A., and Lutty, G.A. 1998. Clinical and histopathologic features of canine oxygen-induced proliferative retinopathy. *Investigative Ophthalmology and Visual Science* 39:1918–1932.

473. Chan-Ling, T., Tout, S., Hollander, H., and Stone, J. 1992. Vascular changes and their mechanisms in the feline model of retinopathy of prematurity. *Invest Ophthalmol Vis Sci* 33(7):2128–2147.

474. Kremer, I., Levitt, A., Goldberg, G., Wilunsky, E., Merlob, P., and Nissenkorn, I. 1992. The effect of light on oxygen-induced vasoproliferative retinopathy in newborn kittens. *Invest Ophthalmol Vis Sci* 33(5):1595–1598.

475. Martin, C., Kaswan, R., and Chapman, W. 1986. Four cases of traumatic optic nerve blindness in the horse. *Equine Veterinary Journal* 18:133–137.

476. Byrne, S.F., and Green, R.L. 2010. Trauma and postsurgical findings. In: Byrne, S.D., and Green, R.L., editors, *Ultrasound of the Eye and Orbit* 2nd edition: Jaypee Brothers Medical Publishers (P) Ltd.: New Dheli, pp. 87–114.

477. Ossoining, K.C., Bigar, F., Kaefring, S.L. et al. 1975. Echographic detection and localization of BB shots in the eye and orbit. *Bibliotheca Ophthalmologica* 83:109–18.

478. Sawada, A., Frazier, S.L., and Ossoining, K.C. 1977. The role of ultrasound in the management of ocular foreign bodies. In: White, D., and Brown, R.E, editors. *Ultraosund in Medicine*. Plenum Press: New York, p. 3A:1003.

479. Davidson, M., Nasisse, M., Jamieson, V., English, R., and Olivero, D. 1991. Traumatic anterior lens

capsule disruption. *Journal of the American Animal Hospital Association* 27:410–414.

480. Braughler, J.M., Hall, E.D., Means, E.D., Waters, T.R., and Anderson, D.K. 1987. Evaluation of an intensive methylprednisolone sodium succinate dosing regimen in experimental spinal-cord injury. *Journal of Neurosurgery* 67:102–105. [PubMed: 3598657].

481. Hall, E.D., and Braughler, J.M. 1984. Corticosteroid-therapy in experimental cord injury. *Journal of Neurosurgery* 61:805–806. [PubMed: 6470796].

482. Bains, M., and Hall, E.D. 2012. Antioxidant therapies in traumatic brain and spinal cord injury. *Biochimica et Biophysica Acta (BBA)-Molecular Basis of Disease* 1822:675–684. [PubMed: 22080976].

483. Collinson, P.N., and Peiffer, R.L. 1993. Clinical presentation, morphology, and behavior of primary choroidal melanomas in eight dogs. *Progress in Veterinary and Comparative Ophthalmology* 3:158–164.

484. Schoster, J.V., Dubielzig, R.R., and Sullivan, L. 1993. Choroidal melanoma in a dog. *Journal of the American Veterinary Medical Association* 203:89–91.

485. Harris, B.P., and Dubielzig, R.R. 1999. Atypical primary ocular melanoma in cats. *Veterinary Ophthalmology* 2:121–124.

486. Bourguet, A., Piccicuto, V., Donzel, E., Carlus, M., and Chahory, S. 2014. A case of primary choroidal malignant melanoma in a cat. *Veterinary Ophthalmology* 18(4), pp. 345–349. doi: 10.1111/vop.12233.

487. Semin, M.O., Serra, F., Mahe, V., Deviers, A. et al. 2011 Choroidal melanocytoma in a cat. *Veterinary Ophthalmology* 14:205–208.

488. Hyman, J.A., Koch, S.A., and Wilcock, B.P. 2002. Canine choroidal melanoma with metastases. *Veterinary Ophthalmology* 5(2):113–117. E Lim, C.C., Cullen, C.L., Grahn, B.H. 2006. Choroidal melanoma in the right eye with focal retinal detachment. *The Canadian Veterinary Journal* 47(1):85–86.

489. Miwa, Y., Matsunaga, S., Kato, K., Ogawa, H., Nakayama, H., Tsujimoto, S., and Sasaki, N. 2005. Choroidal melanoma in a dog. *Journal of Veterinary Medical Science* 67(8):821–823.

490. Steinmetz, A., Ellenberger, K., Marz, I., Ludewig, E., and Oechtering, G. 2012. Oculocardiac reflex in a dog caused by a choroidal melanoma with orbital extension. *Journal of the American Animal Hospital Association* 48(1):66–70.

491. Weisse, V., and Stotzer, H. 1971. Intraokulares melanom bei einem jungen Beagle kasuistische mitteilung. *Berliner und Munchener Tierarztliche Wochenschrift* 84(17):328–330.

492. O'Toole, D., and Murphy, J. 1983. Spindle B cell melanoma in the choroid of a dog. *Journal of Small Animal Practice* 24:561–567.

493. Aguirre, G., Brown, G., Shields, J., and Dubielzig, R. 1984. Melanoma of the choroid in a dog. *Journal of the American Animal Hospital Association* 20:471–476.

494. Dubielzig, R., Aguirre, G., Gross, S., and Diters, R. 1985. Choroidal melanomas in dogs. *Veterinary Pathology* 22:582–585.

495. Hogan, R.N., and Albert, D.M. 1991. Does retinoblastoma occur in animals? *Progress in Veterinary and Comparative Ophthalmology* 1:73–82.

496. Regan, D.P., Dubielzig, R.R., Zeiss, C.J., Charles, B., Hoy, S.S., and Ehrhart, E.J. 2013. Primary primitive neuroectodermal tumors of the retina and ciliary body in dogs. *Veterinary Ophthalmology* 16(Suppl 1:87–93.

497. Jensen, O.A., Kaarsholm, S., Prause, J.U., and Heegaard, S. 2003. Neuroepithelial tumor of the retina in a dog. *Veterinary Ophthalmology* 6(1):57–60.

498. Syed, N.A., Nork, M., Poulsen, G.L., Riis, R.C., George, C., and Albert, D.M. 1997. Retinoblastoma in a dog. *Archives of Ophthalmology* 115:758–763.

499. Mowat, F.M., Langohr, I.M., Bilyk, O., Koterbay, A., Pierce, K.E., and Petersen-Jones, S.M. 2012. Bilateral uveal metastasis of a subcutaneous fibrosarcoma in a cat. *Veterinary Ophthalmology* 15(6):391–397.

500. Szymanski, C.M. 1972. Bilateral metastatic intraocular hemangiosarcoma in a dog. *Journal of the American Animal Hospital Association* 161(7):803–805.

501. Labelle, A.L., and Labelle, P. 2013. Canine ocular neoplasia: A review. *Veterinary Ophthalmology* 16(Suppl 1):3–14.

502. Labelle, P., and Holmberg, B.J. 2010. Ocular myxoid leiomyosarcoma in a cat. *Veterinary Ophthalmology* 13(1):58–62.

503. Nerschbach, V., Eule, J.C., Eberle, N., Hoinghaus, R., and Betz, D. 2016. Ocular manifestation of lymphoma in newly diagnosed cats. *Veterinary and Comparative Oncololgy* 14(1):58–66.

504. Krohne, S.G., Henderson, N.M., Richardson, R.C. et al. 1992. Prevalence of ocular involvement in dogs with multicentric lymphoma: Prospective evaluation of 94 cases. *Veterina and Comparative Ophthalmology* 4:127–135.

505. Cassotis, N.J., Dubielzig, R.R., Gilger, B.C., and Davidson, M.G. 1999. Angioinvasive pulmonary carcinoma with posterior segment metastasis in four cats. *Veterinary Ophthalmology* 2:125–131.

PRESUMED INHERITED OCULAR DISEASES

SHANNON D. BOVELAND

INTRODUCTION

Diagnosis and clinical assessment of visual changes in the dog are important aspects of small animal practice. Pet owners often assume that an eye problem affects an animal to the same extent as it would a person. Thus, the owner can become extremely apprehensive about the disorder.

Knowing or suspecting that the underlying cause of a disorder is heritable has considerable influence on the advice a veterinarian gives an owner or a breeder.[1,2] To provide an accurate diagnosis and prognosis, and to offer genetic counseling, veterinarians should be aware of breed predispositions and inheritability of ocular diseases. Signalment, history, and ophthalmic examination findings form the diagnostic database.

The Canine Eye Registry Foundation (CERF), which was established in 1974, served as a data collection agency for purebred dogs. The CERF also functioned as a registry for "clear-eyed dogs" (dogs free of major heritable eye diseases such as cataracts, PRA, and corneal dystrophies). In 2012, the American College of Veterinary Ophthalmologists (ACVO) announced the use of a new Eye Certification Registry (ECR). The new ECR is a joint effort between the Orthopedic Foundation for Animals (OFA) and the ACVO to better centralize the eye exam info/data with other screening testing (cardiology, orthopedics) and accessibility of data for tracking and research worldwide. This combined toolset will allow responsible breeders to make informed breeding decisions to reduce the incidence and prevalence of inheritable diseases in animals.[3]

Currently, to register a dog with the OFA-ERC, an owner must have the dog examined by a member of the ACVO before applying for an OFA-ECR registry number. The examination is performed after the pupils are dilated, utilizing slit lamp biomicroscopy and indirect ophthalmoscopy. The registration is valid for 1 year from the date of examination. An OFA-ECR number is evidence that the dog was examined and determined to be phenotypically free of major hereditary eye disease as of the date examined.

The CERF and the veterinary medical database at Purdue University started an equine eye registry mainly for certification of Rocky Mountain horses in 1999.[4] Now, the Equine Eye Registry Foundation works with the ACVO to maintain a registry of horses. Horse owners too receive a registration number and certificate, providing horse buyers and breeders certification of the ophthalmic examination and maintaining the integrity of high-quality bloodlines.

The European College of Veterinary Ophthalmologists (ECVO; www.ecvo.org) has developed a process to certify animals free of inherited eye disease. A common certificate is used throughout Europe (Spiess B.M., personal communication, 2000; Stades F., personal communication, 2000). Examinations are performed by ECVO diplomates, ACVO diplomates, or non-ECVO diplomates who are trained and tested by the ECVO to become eye scheme examiners (ESEs), under the umbrella of the ECVO (Stades F., personal communication, 2000; Bedford P., personal communication, 2000). The eye examination is performed, following pharmacological mydriasis, using slit lamp biomicroscopy and indirect ophthalmoscopy. In some breeds in which iridocorneal angle anomalies occur, gonioscopy is also used. Currently, each country is collating data independently, but efforts are underway to exchange data between countries (Spiess B.M., personal communication, 2000).

Other countries are also making efforts to formalize certification schemes for inherited ocular diseases (Spiess B.M., personal communication, 2000; Ofri R., personal communication, 2000).

The utilization of molecular genetic techniques has revolutionized the diagnosis of hereditary ocular disease. Many of the first veterinary diagnostic DNA tests were developed in the field of veterinary ophthalmology, specifically in the diagnosis of inherited retinal degeneration. Genetic diagnostic techniques are now developed for other systemic hereditary diseases such as von Willebrand's disease, pyruvate kinase deficiency of Basenjis, and copper toxicosis of Bedlington terriers.[5]

If the specific mutation responsible for a given disease is known, then a mutation-based test can be developed that can very precisely identify the presence or absence of that mutation in a given dog's test sample. In autosomal recessive diseases, two copies of the mutant allele are necessary for expression of the given disease. Dogs that are "carriers" do not have the disease but carry one copy of the mutant gene that they can pass to offspring. Most canine hereditary retinal degenerations are caused by autosomal recessive disorders. Mutation-based tests can identify with 100% accuracy dogs that are genetically normal with respect to a particular gene, dogs that are carriers, or dogs that are affected. These tests can be performed at a very early age, even before the onset of clinical signs of the disease (Petersen-Jones S., personal communication, 2000).

Commercially available mutation-based tests currently exist for three specific forms of retinal degeneration in the dog. In Irish setters, rod–cone dysplasia 1 (rcd-1) is characterized by abnormal development of rod and cone photoreceptors due to a mutation in the cGMP phosphodiesterase β-subunit,[6,7] an essential component of phototransduction in the retina. Through the technique of mismatch polymerase chain reaction (PCR), the test is able to determine whether a dog is genetically "clear," is a carrier that will never develop rcd-1, or is affected due to the presence of two copies of the mutant allele.

Rod–cone dysplasia type 3 (rcd-3) is a disease of Cardigan Welsh Corgis that is caused by a mutation in the α-subunit of cGMP phosphodiesterase (PDE6A), leading to nonfunctional, prematurely truncated protein product.[8] The rod photoreceptors are abnormally formed, whereas the cones initially develop normally but are quick to degenerate.[6] The technique of allele-specific PCR is employed in the commercially available tests offered by multiple genetic testing companies (Table 15.1). Allele-specific PCR utilizes two sets of primers, one to amplify only the normal gene and one to amplify only the mutant gene.[9] It is therefore possible to determine whether a given sample contains only normal copies of the genes (genetically "clear" or normal), one normal copy and one mutant copy (carrier), or only mutant copies (affected).

Congenital stationary night blindness is an autosomal recessive disease of Briard dogs caused by a mutation in RPE65, a highly conserved gene that is expressed in the RPE of the retina.[10] Affected Briards are congenitally night blind and have varying degrees of visual impairment in bright light conditions. The disease is a progressive disorder that does not cause ophthalmoscopic abnormalities until later in life.[11] The test amplifies a 135-base pair segment of DNA across the mutation site using PCR. The mutant gene copy will be four-base pairs shorter than a normal DNA segment. This four-base pair difference can be visualized on a high-resolution agarose gel, allowing accurate identification of the presence of normal as well as mutant copies of the gene (Petersen-Jones S., personal communication, 2000).

Progressive rod–cone degeneration (prcd), a widespread form of retinal degeneration that affects many breeds of dogs, displays significant genetic heterogeneity within as well as between breeds.[12] Prcd is an autosomal recessive disorder that generally causes night blindness by 2–5 years of age and complete blindness by 5–12 years of age. Since it affects many breeds of dogs, the phenotypic expression of the disease can vary according to the breed. Various forms of progressive retinal atrophy (PRA) have been documented in more than 100 dog breeds.[12] At least 21 disease-causing mutations in 18 genes have been identified to be associated with prcd.[13] Currently, there are numerous breeds where genetic testing for prcd are available.[14]

Primary lens luxation (PLL) is another inherited condition that is common in several breeds of terriers that a mutation-based test is used to identify affected carriers. In 2007, the Veterinary Medical Database and the CERF found the diagnosis of PLL recorded in 85 breeds for 10 years (1996–2005).[15] A mutation associated with PLL in the miniature bull terrier and the Lancashire heeler dog has been identified.[15–17] A mutation on the same chromosome causes the disease in other breeds including the Parson and Jack Russell terriers as well as the Tibetan terrier.[18,19] PLL is considered to be recessively inherited in the Tibetan terrier and in other breeds as well.[18,19] The ADAMTS17 mutation has been associated with primary lens luxation widespread among terrier breeds.[17,20]

The implications of genetic testing for breeding are tremendous. By selectively breeding normals to carriers, phenotypic expression of disease can be avoided. The argument may also be made that even affected dogs can be used for breeding to genetically normal dogs, since the resultant puppies will be carriers, but may not be affected by disease. Affected dogs with other exceptional traits may, therefore, still be able to pass these valuable traits on to future generations. Significant narrowing of the gene pool has previously occurred in some breeds when breeders were trying to eliminate hereditary defects by eliminating known carriers from the breeding population. In some cases, this narrowing of the gene pool has resulted in the promotion of other genetically based diseases.

This chapter provides a list of breed predispositions for ocular disease in various domestic species and genetic testing laboratories (**Tables 15.1–15.5**). The information is derived from current veterinary ophthalmic texts, journal articles, newsletters, personal communication with colleagues, and personal experience. Although the authors suspect these disorders are inherited, inheritance has not been proved in all instances.

Table 15.1 Genetic testing laboratories for canine ocular disorders.

List compiled from data from the ACVO Genetics Committee (as of July 25, 2016)

OptiGen, LLC

Cornell Business & Technology Park

767 Warren Road, Suite 300

Ithaca, NY 14850

Tel: 607-257-0301

Fax: 607-257-0353

Email: genetest@optigen.com

www.optigen.com

Animal Health Trust

Lanwades Park

Kentford

Newmarket

Suffolk

United Kingdom

CB8 7UU

Tel: 01638 55 56 21 (UK)

Fax: 01638 55 56 66 (UK)

www.aht.org.uk

Animal Genetics Inc.

1336 Timberlane Road

Tallahassee, FL 32312-1766

Tel: 1-866-922-6436

Email: contact@animalgenetics.us

www.animalgenetics.us/

DOGenes Inc.

161 Sherin Ave.

Peterborough, ON K9J 7V5

Canada

Tel: 705-748-0089

www.dogenes.com

Genetic Testing at Gluck

1400 Nicholasville Road

Lexington, KY 40546-0099

Tel: 859-218-1165

www.getgluck.ca.uky.edu

GenSol Diagnostics

125 North Main Street Unit 1846

Table 15.1 (*Continued*) Genetic testing laboratories for canine ocular disorders.

Clayton, GA 30525

Tel: 844-369-3686

Email: info@gensoldx.com

www.gensoldx.com

Goldstein Molecular and Genetics Laboratory

Cornell University

Richard E. Goldstein

Tel: 607-253-4480

Fax: 607-253-3534

Email: phpt@cornell.edu

HealthGene Corp.

9131 Keele Street, Unit A2

Concord, ON L4 K 0G7

Canada

Tel: 1-877-371-1551 (toll free)

Fax: 289-553-5232

Email: info@healthgene.com

www.healthgene.com

MSU - Laboratory of Comparative Medical Genetics

Michigan State University

2209 Biomedical Physical Sciences

East Lansing, MI, 48824

Tel: 517-844-5348

Email: fyfe@cvm.msu.edu

MU - Animal Molecular Genetics Lab

University of Missouri College of Veterinary Medicine

321 Connaway Hall

Columbia, MO 65211

Tel: 573-884-3712

Fax: 573-884-5414

Email: hansenl@missouri.edu

www.caninegeneticdiseases.net/

Orthopedic Foundation for Animals

2300 E Nifong Boulevard

Columbia, MO 65201-3806

Tel: 573-442-0418

Fax: 573-875-5073

Email: ofa@offa.org

www.offa.org

(Continued)

Table 15.1 (*Continued*) **Genetic testing laboratories for canine ocular disorders.**

Paw Print Genetics

220 E. Rowan Ave.

Suite 220

Spokane, WA 99207

Tel: 509-483-5950

Email: askus@pawprintgenetics.com

www.pawprintgenetics.com

PennGen

School of Veterinary Medicine

University of Pennsylvania

3900 Delancey St

Philadelphia, PA 19104

Tel: 215-898-3375

Fax: 215-573-2162

PennGen@vet.upenn.edu

UC-Davis, Veterinary Genetics Lab

Veterinary Genetics Laboratory

PO Box 1102

Davis, CA 95617-1102

Tel: 530-752-2211

Fax: 530-752-3556

www.vgl.ucdavis.edu

VetGen

3728 Plaza Drive, Suite 1

Ann Arbor, MI 48108

Tel: 1-800-483-8436 (toll free)

Fax: 734-669-8441

www.vetgen.com

Table 15.2 **Breed predisposition to eye disease in dogs.**

Affenpinscher

Cataracts (rare)

Distichiasis[21]

Persistent pupillary membranes[22]

Afghan Hound

Cataracts: Recessive trait[23,24]

Congenital retinal detachment (complete retinal dysplasia)[23]

Corneal dystrophy[23,25–27]

Distichiasis[21]

Eversion of the third eyelid

Medial canthal pocket syndrome[23]

Mesodermal dysgenesis (goniodysgenesis) (some affected dogs may develop glaucoma)[28]

Oversized palpebral fissure (euryblepharon)[25,29]

Persistent pupillary membranes[23,25]

Progressive retinal atrophy

Airedale Terrier

Cataracts

Chronic superficial keratitis (pannus)[23,26,27]

Congenital retinal detachment (complete retinal dysplasia)[23,30]

Corneal dystrophy[30]

Distichiasis[23,25,27,29]

Entropion[23]

Persistent pupillary membranes

Progressive retinal atrophy

Vitreous degeneration[31]

Akbash Dog

Cataracts[26]

Akita

Cataracts[26]

Corneal dystrophy[23,32]

Distichiasis[33]

Entropion[23,26,34]

Eversion of the cartilage of the third eyelid[2]

Glaucoma[23]

Multiple ocular anomalies: Microphthalmia, congenital cataracts, posterior lenticonus, retinal dysplasia[26,35]

Persistent pupillary membranes[26,36]

Progressive retinal atrophy (most commonly diagnosed in 2- to 3-year-old males)[26,37]

Retinal dysplasia: Retinal folds[23,26]

Strabismus[38]

Uveodermatologic syndrome (vitiligo and uveitis syndrome)[26,39–45]

Alaskan Klee Kai

Corneal dystrophy[14]

Distichiasis[46]

(*Continued*)

Table 15.2 (Continued) Breed predisposition to eye disease in dogs.

Persistent pupillary membranes[21,33,47]

Vitreous degeneration[14]

Alaskan Malamute

Cataracts[23,26]

Coloboma of the optic nerve[23,26]

Corneal dystrophy[48]

Distichiasis[26]

Glaucoma[26,36]

Hemeralopia (cone dysplasia): Autosomal recessive trait[23,26,49–54]

Persistent pupillary membranes[26,48]

Progressive retinal atrophy (diagnosed at 2–4 years of age)

Refractory superficial corneal ulcer[2,23]

Retinal dysplasia[26]

American Bulldog

Ceroid lipofuscinosis[55–57]

Distichiasis[58]

Glaucoma[59]

Multifocal retinopathy (autosomal recessive cmr1 gene; DNA test available)[60]

American Cocker Spaniel

Cataracts: Recessive trait[26,61–65]

Corneal dystrophy: Posterior polymorphous, epithelial/stromal[25,26]

Distichiasis: Dominant trait suspected[26,63,66,67]

Ectopic cilium

Ectropion[26]

Ectropion/entropion

Encircling third eyelid

Entropion[26]

Euryblepharon/macroblepharon[26]

Exposure keratopathy syndrome[26]

Glaucoma[26,68,69]

Imperforate lacrimal punctum

Keratoconjunctivitis sicca/dry eye[26,63]

Keratitis: Secondary[21,26]

Lens subluxation (secondary glaucoma)[25,70]

Mesodermal dysgenesis glaucoma

Microphakia, nuclear and perinuclear cataracts, and persistent pupillary membranes

Optic nerve coloboma[2]

Optic nerve hypoplasia

Oversized palpebral fissure (macroblepharon)

Persistent pupillary membranes[26,33]

Posterior polymorphous dystrophy[23]

Progressive retinal atrophy: Autosomal recessive prcd; DNA test available[26,71–73]

Table 15.2 (Continued) Breed predisposition to eye disease in dogs.

Prolapse of the gland of the third eyelid[26,74]

Proliferative episcleritis (fibrous histiocytoma)

Redundant forehead skin[29]

Retinal dysplasia: Geographic/detachment, retinal folds; autosomal recessive trait[26,27,75]

Trichomegaly: Inherited trait

American Eskimo Dog

Cataracts[26]

Lens luxation (DNA test available)[20]

Retinal atrophy (autosomal recessive prcd; DNA test available)[26,73]

American Hairless Terrier

Cataracts[48]

Distichiasis[48]

Lens luxation (DNA test available)[17,20]

Persistent pupillary membranes[48]

American Lamalese

Corneal dystrophy

American Pit Bull Terrier

Persistent pupillary membranes[58]

Progressive retinal atrophy (autosomal recessive crd2; DNA test available)[13,76,77]

Retinal dysplasia[58]

American Staffordshire Terrier

Cataracts[26,78,79]

Ceroid lipofuscinosis[80]

Distichiasis[36]

Entropion[26,27]

Persistent hyperplastic primary vitreous[26,27,81,82]

Persistent pupillary membranes[36,83]

Progressive retinal atrophy (autosomal recessive rcd1b; DNA test available)[13,23,76,77]

Retinal dysplasia[36]

American Water Spaniel

Cataracts[23,26]

Distichiasis[26]

Entropion[26]

Microphthalmia[26]

Persistent pupillary membranes[36]

Retinal dysplasia: Retinal folds[23,26,27]

Argentine Dogo

Persistent pupillary membranes[36]

Australian Cattle Dog (Queensland Heeler, Blue Heeler)

Cataracts[26,27]

Ceroid lipofuscinosis[26,84]

Corneal dystrophy[47]

Table 15.2 (*Continued*) **Breed predisposition to eye disease in dogs.**

Glaucoma[68]

Lens luxation (DNA test available)[17,20,26]

Persistent pupillary membranes[23,48]

Progressive retinal atrophy (autosomal recessive prcd/rcd4; DNA tests available)[26,73,85,86]

Retinal dysplasia[36]

Australian Kelpie

Cataracts[36]

Progressive retinal atrophy[27,48]

Australian Shepherd Dog

Cataracts: Anterior cortical, nuclear (5–8 years of age),[23] posterior polar subcapsular, triangular (18 months–3 years of age):[1,23] Autosomal codominant (toy breed); DNA test available[26,87,88]

Ceroid lipofuscinosis[89,90]

Choroidal hypoplasia (Collie eye anomaly): Autosomal recessive; DNA test available[21,23,26,91–94]

    Staphyloma/coloboma

    Retinal detachment

    Retinal hemorrhage

    Optic nerve coloboma

Corectopia/dyscoria/coloboma/equatorial staphyloma (homozygous merle): Autosomal recessive trait[95]

Corneal dystrophy[36,96]

Distichiasis[21,26,95,97–100]

Iris coloboma: Toy breed[26]

Iris hypoplasia: Toy breed[46]

Microcornea[101]

Microphthalmia/heterochromia (with multiple ocular defects; presumed autosomal recessive with incomplete penetrance: Toy breed)[26,95,97–100]

Micropapilla[47]

Multifocal retinopathy: Autosomal recessive cmr1; DNA test available[102]

Ocular coloboma/staphyloma without microphthalmia[26,27]

Persistent hyaloid artery[36]

Persistent pupillary membranes[26,36]

Progressive retinal atrophy (prcd, generalized)/cone degeneration (2–7 years of age):[54] Autosomal recessive; DNA tests available[26,46,58,73]

Retinal detachment

Retinal dysplasia: Retinal folds[36]

Uveodermatologic syndrome (vitiligo and uveitis syndrome)[39]

Australian Stumpy Tail Cattle Dog

Progressive retinal atrophy (prcd, generalized); DNA test available[73]

Australian Terrier

Cataracts[36]

Persistent pupillary membranes[47]

Progressive retinal atrophy

Retinal dysplasia: Retinal folds[23]

Table 15.2 (*Continued*) **Breed predisposition to eye disease in dogs.**

Basenji

Cataracts[26]

Corneal dystrophy: Endothelial, epithelial/stromal[26]

Optic nerve coloboma[26,103]

Persistent pupillary membranes: Inherited trait[21,23,26,48,103–106]

Posterior segment coloboma[26]

Progressive retinal atrophy (autosomal recessive Bas_PRA1; DNA test available)[23,26,107,108]

Retinal detachment[23,26,104]

Basset Hound

Cataracts[26]

Distichiasis[48]

Ectropion[26,33,109]

Entropion[26]

Eversion of the cartilage of the third eyelid[2,110]

Iris cysts[111]

Macroblepharon[33,109]

Mesodermal dysgenesis glaucoma[28,112]

Oversized palpebral fissure[29]

Persistent hyaloid artery[33]

Persistent pupillary membranes[21,26,36,47]

Primary glaucoma (narrow- or closed-angle); DNA test available for POAG[26,113–119]

Progressive retinal atrophy

Redundant forehead skin[29]

Retinal dysplasia[33]

Secondary glaucoma (subluxation of the lens)[25]

Beagle

Cataracts: Incomplete dominant trait[33,120,121]

Corneal dystrophy: Epithelial/stromal[122–127]

Congenital stationary night blindness (autosomal recessive)[128]

Distichiasis[23,26]

Ectropion[32]

Encircling third eyelid

Iris cyst[111]

Micropapilla

Microphthalmia/multiple ocular anomalies[26,129]

Optic nerve hypoplasia

Oval corneal opacity (corneal dystrophy)

Palpebral neoplasia[130]

Persistent pupillary membranes[33]

Primary glaucoma (open- or narrow-angle): Autosomal recessive trait (DNA test available)[26,117,131–141]

Progressive retinal atrophy[26]

Prolapse of the gland of the third eyelid[26]

Retinal dysplasia[26]

Tapetal cell degeneration: Autosomal recessive trait[142–145]

(Continued)

Table 15.2 (*Continued*) **Breed predisposition to eye disease in dogs.**

Bearded Collie

Cataracts (2- to 5-year-old males)[23,26]

Congenital retinal detachment (complete retinal dysplasia)[146]

Corneal dystrophy[26]

Choroidal hypoplasia (Collie eye anomaly: Autosomal recessive; DNA test available)[36,48,92,93]

   Optic nerve coloboma

   Staphyloma/coloboma

   Retinal detachment

   Retinal hemorrhage

Persistent pupillary membranes[23,26,36]

Progressive retinal atrophy

Retinal dysplasia: Retinal folds[26,27]

Bedlington Terrier

Cataracts[26]

Distichiasis[26]

Entropion[147]

Imperforate lacrimal punctum[26,148]

Micropalpebral fissure

Microphthalmia[26]

Nasolacrimal duct stenosis[23]

Persistent pupillary membranes[36,48]

Progressive retinal atrophy

Retinal dysplasia and detachment: Autosomal recessive[23,26,149,150]

Retinal dysplasia: Retinal folds[26]

Belgian Laekenois

Distichiasis[47]

Belgian Malinois

Cataracts[83]

Chronic superficial keratitis/pannus[48]

Persistent pupillary membranes[36]

Progressive retinal atrophy[27,36,48]

Retinal dysplasia: Retinal folds[83]

Vitreous degeneration[110]

Belgian Sheepdog (Belgian Shepherd Dog – Groenendael)

Achiasmic optic nerves with nystagmus: Autosomal recessive[151]

Cataracts[23,26]

Chronic superficial keratitis (pannus)[2,26,152]

Corneal dystrophy (Epithelial/stromal)[26]

Micropapilla[26]

Persistent pupillary membranes[26,36]

Progressive retinal atrophy[26,153]

Retinal dysplasia: Retinal folds[36]

Retinopathy (congenital blindness): Recessive trait?

Table 15.2 (*Continued*) **Breed predisposition to eye disease in dogs.**

Belgian Tervuren

Cataracts[23]

Chronic superficial keratitis (pannus)[26,154]

Distichiasis[36]

Micropapilla[26,27]

Persistent pupillary membranes[26,36]

Progressive retinal atrophy[26]

Retinal dysplasia[36,83]

Berger Picard (Picardy Shepherd-Picardie)

Cataracts[110]

Corneal dystrophy: Epithelial/stroma[58]

Distichiasis[110]

Nictitans cartilage anomaly/eversion[58]

Persistent pupillary membranes[110]

Retinal atrophy[58]

Retinal dysplasia[46]

Retinopathy[58]

Bernese Mountain Dog

Cataracts[36,48]

Cataracts/retinal detachment[111]

Distichiasis[48]

Entropion[26]

Ectropion[36,83]

Persistent pupillary membranes[36]

Progressive retinal atrophy[26,155]

Systemic histiocytosis[156–160]

Bichon Frise

Cataracts[26,161,162]

Corneal dystrophy: Epithelial/stromal[23,26]

Distichiasis[26]

Entropion[23]

Persistent pupillary membranes[26,36]

Strabismus (exotropia)[23,32]

Retinal dysplasia: Retinal folds[26]

Vitreous degeneration[21,26]

Black and Tan Coonhound

Cataracts[26]

Retinal dysplasia: Retinal folds[36]

Black Russian Terrier

Cataracts[21,47]

Persistent pupillary membranes[58]

Bloodhound

Cataracts[48]

Ectropion[25,26,65]

Ectropion/entropion

(*Continued*)

Table 15.2 (*Continued*) **Breed predisposition to eye disease in dogs.**

Entropion[26,65,163]
Eversion of the cartilage of the third eyelid
Persistent pupillary membranes[23,36,48]
Prolapse of the gland of third eyelid[26,27,65]
Keratoconjunctivitis sicca[1]
Macroblepharon[26,65]
Redundant forehead skin[25,70]
Retinal dysplasia: Retinal folds[36,48]
Boerboel
Multifocal retinopathy (autosomal recessive cmr1; DNA test available)[164]
Bolognese
Cataracts[58]
Corneal dystrophy: Epithelial/stroma[58]
Distichiasis[36]
Persistent pupillary membranes[36]
Border Collie
Cataracts (4–6 years of age)[23,26]
Central progressive retinal atrophy (1–3 years of age)
Ceroid lipofuscinosis; DNA test available[165,166]
Collie eye anomaly (choroidal hypoplasia) autosomal recessive; DNA test available[23,92,93,167]
Optic nerve coloboma
Retinal detachment
Retinal hemorrhage
Corneal dystrophy: Epithelial/stroma[47]
Distichiasis[47]
Fibrous histiocytoma
Lens luxation[168]
Persistent pupillary membranes[26,36]
Progressive retinal atrophy (2–5 years of age), suggested X-linked[26,71,169]
Proliferative keratoconjunctivitis[25,29]
Retinal dysplasia: Retinal folds[26]
Vitreous degeneration[14]
Border Terrier
Cataracts: DNA test available[23,26,27,48,87]
Distichiasis[47]
Persistent pupillary membranes[36,83]
Progressive retinal atrophy
Retinal dysplasia: Retinal folds[23]
Vitreous degeneration[48]
Borzoi
Cataracts (posterior pole; 1–4 years of age)[23,36]
Chronic superficial keratitis[2] (pannus)
Corneal dystrophy: Epithelial/stroma[83]

Table 15.2 (*Continued*) **Breed predisposition to eye disease in dogs.**

Micropapilla[83]
Microphthalmia (multiple ocular anomalies)
Optic nerve hypoplasia[83]
Persistent pupillary membranes[23,83]
Progressive retinal atrophy
Retinal degeneration[26]
Retinal dysplasia
Retinopathy[170]
Boston Terrier
Cataracts, congenital: Juvenile; late-onset (autosomal recessive; DNA test available)[26,32,78,79,87,152,171,172]
Corneal endothelial dystrophy (average age 7.5 years)[26,173]
Corneal dystrophy: Epithelial/stromal[26]
Distichiasis[26]
Entropion (medial)[25]
Glaucoma[26,29,68,117]
Hypertrophy (prolapse) of the gland of the third eyelid
Imperforate lacrimal puncta[58]
Iris cyst[2,111]
Keratoconjunctivitis sicca
Persistent pupillary membranes[26,36]
Progressive retinal atrophy
Refractory superficial corneal ulcer[23,174]
Strabismus (exotropia)[23,29]
Vitreous degeneration[36,46]
Bouvier des Flandres
Cataracts (congenital)[26,175]
Corneal dystrophy: Epithelial/stroma[47]
Distichiasis[48]
Entropion[23,26,36]
Glaucoma[26,176–178]
Mesodermal dysgenesis glaucoma
Persistent hyperplastic tunica vasculosa lentis[26,179]
Persistent hyperplastic primary vitreous[26,179]
Persistent pupillary membranes[26,36]
Retinal dysplasia[48]
Vitreous degeneration[47]
Boxer
Cataracts[23,26]
Central progressive retinal atrophy[2,23]
Corneal dystrophy: Epithelial/stromal[26]
Corneal dystrophy: Epithelial erosion[26,180–182]
Distichiasis[26]
Ectopic cilia[33]
Ectropion[26]

Table 15.2 (*Continued*) **Breed predisposition to eye disease in dogs.**

Entropion

Euryblepharon/macroblepharon[36,48]

Nonpigmented third eyelid

Persistent pupillary membrane[33]

Progressive retinal atrophy

Prolapse of the gland of the third eyelid

Refractory superficial corneal ulcer (basement membrane dystrophy)

Vitreous degeneration[58]

Boykin Spaniel

Cataracts[26,27]

Choroidal hypoplasia (Collie eye anomaly): Autosomal recessive; DNA test available[21,47,93]

   Staphyloma/coloboma

   Retinal detachment

   Retinal hemorrhage

Corneal dystrophy: Epithelial/stromal[26]

Distichiasis[26]

Persistent hyaloid artery[36]

Persistent pupillary membrane[36]

Progressive retinal atrophy (retinal atrophy; generalized)[26]

Retinal dysplasia: Retinal folds[26]

Bracco Italiano

Cataracts[110]

Distichiasis[58]

Retinal dysplasia: Retinal folds[33]

Briard

Cataracts

Congenital stationary night blindness (hereditary retinal dystrophy in Briards): Autosomal recessive CSNB: DNA test available)[10,26,183–187]

Corneal dystrophy: Epithelial/stromal[26]

Central progressive retinal atrophy (inherited vitamin E deficiency) (McLellan G., personal communication, 2002)[188,189]

Persistent pupillary membranes[33,36]

Progressive retinal atrophy[26]

Brittany

Cataracts[26]

Distichiasis[23,83]

Glaucoma[28]

Iris cyst[25]

Lens luxation[26,27]

Persistent pupillary membranes[36]

Progressive retinal atrophy

Retinal dysplasia: Retinal folds/geographic[21,33]

Vitreous degeneration[33]

Table 15.2 (*Continued*) **Breed predisposition to eye disease in dogs.**

Brussels Griffon

Cataracts[26]

Distichiasis[25,29,36,48]

Ectopic cilium[27]

Exposure keratopathy syndrome/macroblepharon[26]

Lens luxation[36,48]

Optic nerve coloboma[26]

Persistent hyaloid artery[36]

Persistent pupillary membranes[26,36]

Progressive retinal atrophy[23,36,48]

Retinal dysplasia: Geographic[21]

Vitreous degeneration[21,26,47]

British Bulldog

Cataracts[23,26]

Distichiasis[26]

Ectopic cilia[26]

Ectropion[26]

Ectropion/entropion

Entropion[26,163]

Euryblepharon/macroblepharon[26]

Iris cysts[111]

Keratoconjunctivitis sicca/dry eye[26,190,191]

Nasal fold trichiasis

Persistent pupillary membranes[25]

Prolapse of the gland of the third eyelid[26,65,74,192]

Redundant forehead skin[29]

Retinal dysplasia: Retinal folds[26]

Bullmastiff

Cataracts[26,27]

Distichiasis[26]

Ectropion[48]

Entropion[26]

Euryblepharon/macroblepharon[48]

Eversion of the cartilage of the third eyelid

Glaucoma[23,26]

Micropapilla[48]

Multifocal retinopathy (autosomal recessive cmr1; DNA test available)[60]

Optic nerve hypoplasia[48]

Persistent pupillary membranes[26,36]

Progressive retinal atrophy (autosomal dominant; DNA test available)[193]

Retinal dysplasia: Retinal folds[26]

Bull Terrier

Cataracts[48]

Ectropion[26]

(*Continued*)

Table 15.2 (*Continued*) **Breed predisposition to eye disease in dogs.**

Entropion

Keratoconjunctivitis sicca[194]

Lens luxation[33]

Micropalpebral fissure (blepharophimosis)

Persistent pupillary membranes[36,48]

Progressive retinal atrophy

Prolapse (hypertrophy) of the gland of the third eyelid[27]

Bull Terrier (Miniature)

Cataracts[48]

Entropion[26]

Persistent pupillary membranes[36,48]

Lens luxation[16,33]

Cairn Terrier

Cataracts[23,26]

Ectopic cilium[25]

Lens luxation with secondary glaucoma

Persistent hyaloid artery[36]

Persistent pupillary membranes[36,83]

Pigmentary glaucoma (ocular melanosis with/without secondary glaucoma): Presumed autosomal dominant[26,48,195]

Progressive retinal atrophy: Recessive trait[196]

Retinal dysplasia[23]

Canaan Dog

Cataracts[36,48]

Distichiasis[33]

Persistent pupillary membranes[36]

Cardigan Welsh Corgi

Cataracts[26]

Central progressive retinal atrophy

Distichiasis[26]

Entropion[23]

Lens luxation with secondary glaucoma

Persistent corneal epithelial erosion[1,23]

Persistent pupillary membranes[36,48,83]

Progressive retinal atrophy (rod–cone dysplasia type 3): Recessive trait rcd3; DNA test available[8,9,26,196,197]

Refractory superficial corneal ulcer

Retinal dysplasia: Focal or multifocal[9,23,27]

Cavalier King Charles Spaniel

Cataracts[23,26,79]

Congenital KCS and ichthyosiform dermatosis: Autosomal recessive[198,199]

Corneal dystrophy: Epithelial/stromal[26,200]

Distichiasis[26,29]

Entropion[33]

Exposure pigmentary keratitis/macroblepharon[26]

Table 15.2 (*Continued*) **Breed predisposition to eye disease in dogs.**

Keratoconjunctivitis sicca/dry eye[201]

Microphthalmia with multiple ocular anomalies[26,202]

Persistent pupillary membrane[36]

Posterior lenticonus, cataracts, and microphthalmia (reported in Sweden)[202]

Progressive retinal atrophy (1–5 years of age)[23,26]

Retinal dysplasia: Geographic/detachment, retinal folds[23,26]

Vitreous degeneration[33]

Cesky Terrier

Corneal dystrophy: Epithelial/stromal[21,47]

Distichiasis[83]

Chesapeake Bay Retriever

Cataracts: Dominant trait with incomplete penetrance[26,203]

Central progressive retinal atrophy[29]

Distichiasis[26]

Entropion: Lateral canthus, lower eyelid[26]

Eversion of the cartilage of the third eyelid

Persistent pupillary membranes[26,27,36,83]

Progressive retinal atrophy: Recessive prcd[26,73]

Retinal dysplasia: Geographic/detachment, retinal folds[23,26]

Chihuahua

Cataracts[26]

Ceroid lipofuscinosis[204]

Corneal endothelial dystrophy (average age of onset 9.5 years)[26,173]

Distichiasis[46]

Entropion

Glaucoma[23]

Iridal atrophy[25]

Keratoconjunctivitis sicca

Lens luxation and secondary glaucoma

Persistent pupillary membranes[26,36]

Progressive retinal atrophy

Trichiasis[2]

Vitreous degeneration[26]

Chinese Crested Dog

Cataracts[26]

Ceroid lipofuscinosis[205]

Lens luxation: DNA test is available[17,20]

Persistent pupillary membranes[36,48]

Retinal atrophy: Autosomal recessive prcd; DNA test available[12,36,73]

Vitreous degeneration[17,20,27,36,73]

Chinese Foo Dog

Lens luxation: DNA test is available[20]

Chinook

Cataracts[36]

Persistent pupillary membranes[36]

(*Continued*)

Table 15.2 (Continued) Breed predisposition to eye disease in dogs.

Retinal dysplasia[36]

Vitreous degeneration[33,110]

Chow Chow

Anterior chamber cleavage syndrome[2]

Cataracts[26,206]

Chronic superficial keratitis (pannus) (Hamor R., personal communication, 1990)

Corneal dystrophy, endothelial[26,27]

Displaced lacrimal punctum[25]

Ectropion[21,23]

Entropion[26]

Entropion (lateral canthus)

Glaucoma[2,26,68,207]

Keratitis: Secondary, chronic[21,47]

Micropalpebral fissure (blepharophimosis)

Oversized palpebral fissure[29]

Persistent pupillary membranes: Inherited trait[26,36,110,208]

Progressive retinal atrophy

Redundant forehead skin

Clumber Spaniel

Amaurosis[23]

Cataracts[26]

Ectropion[26]

Entropion[26,209]

Distichiasis[26]

Keratitis: Secondary, chronic[26]

Keratoconjunctivitis sicca[21,26]

Macroblepharon[26]

Microphthalmia[26,27]

Persistent pupillary membranes[26,36]

Retinal dysplasia: Retinal folds[26,27]

Collie (Rough or Scotch, and Smooth)

Cataracts[23,26]

Central progressive retinal atrophy[23,29]

Collie eye anomaly: Autosomal recessive trait (choroidal hypoplasia, staphyloma/coloboma, retinal detachment, retinal hemorrhage, optic nerve coloboma)[26,92,93,210–233]

Corneal dystrophy: Epithelial/stromal[36]

Distichiasis[26]

Entropion secondary to enlarged orbit/enophthalmos

Fibrous histiocytoma

Microcornea[29]

Micropalpebral fissure (blepharophimosis)[234]

Microphthalmia[26,235]

Optic nerve hypoplasia[2]

Persistent hyaloid artery[33]

Table 15.2 (Continued) Breed predisposition to eye disease in dogs.

Persistent pupillary membranes[26,36,110]

Progressive retinal atrophy: Generalized[26]

Progressive retinal atrophy (rod–cone dysplasia type 2): Autosomal recessive trait; DNA test is available[236–240]

Proliferative keratoconjunctivitis[25,26,241,242]

Retinal dysplasia: Retinal folds[26]

Stationary night blindness: Presumed autosomal recessive[243]

Coonhound

Cataracts[23,26]

Central progressive retinal atrophy

Ectropion

Entropion[27]

Progressive retinal atrophy

Retinal dysplasia: Retinal folds[36]

Coonhound (Redbone Hound)

Central progressive retinal atrophy[2,25,29]

Ectropion

Entropion: inherited trait[26]

Coton de Tulear

Cataracts (Clerc B., personal communication, 2000)[36]

Corneal dystrophy: Epithelial, stromal[36]

Distichiasis[47]

Multifocal retinopathy: Autosomal recessive cmr2; DNA test is available[60,244]

Persistent pupillary membranes[36]

Retinal dysplasia: Retinal folds/bullae[26]

Retinal atrophy (generalized)[26]

Vitreous degeneration[36]

Curly Coated Retriever

Cataracts[2,26,65]

Choroidal hypolasia[83]

Corneal dystrophy: Epithelial/stromal[26]

Distichiasis[26]

Ectropion[23]

Entropion[25]

Optic nerve coloboma[83]

Persistent pupillary membranes[36]

Progressive retinal atrophy[2]

Retinal dysplasia: Retinal folds[83]

Vitreous degeneration[33,110]

Dachshund

Cataracts[23,26]

Ceroid lipofuscinosis[56,245]

Chronic superficial keratitis (pannus): Presumed autosomal recessive[26,29,152,246]

Coloboma/staphyloma (smooth standard only)[21]

(Continued)

Table 15.2 (*Continued*) **Breed predisposition to eye disease in dogs.**

Corneal dystrophy: Epithelial/stromal; endothelial[26,173,247]
Dermoid: Inherited trait[2,23,26,248]
Distichiasis[26]
Ectopic cilium
Entropion[23]
Glaucoma[23]
Iris coloboma[48]
Keratoconjunctivitis sicca[29]
Micropapilla[26,27,36]
Microphthalmia/multiple ocular defects[26,246,249]
Multiple ocular defects (homozygous merle)[27]
Optic nerve coloboma[26]
Optic nerve hypoplasia[2,36,210]
Persistent hyaloid artery[36,83]
Persistent pupillary membranes[36,48,110]
Progressive retinal atrophy: Recessive trait suspected; DNA test is available[25,26,107,250–259]
Punctate keratitis[26]
Recurrent epithelial erosion
Retinal dysplasia: Retinal fold[36,48]
Retinopathy: Associated with ceroid lipo fuscinosis[251]; DNA test is available[55,260]
Uveodermatologic syndrome[261]
Dachshund (Miniature)
Chronic superficial keratitis (pannus)
Progressive retinal atrophy (degeneration): Autosomal recessive[25,29,250]
Dalmatian
Cataracts[26,209]
Ceroid lipofuscinosis: Presumed autosomal recessive[117,165,262–264]
Corneal dystrophy: Epithelial/stromal[36]
Chronic superficial keratitis (pannus)[23]
Dermoid[26,29,209]
Distichiasis[23,36]
Entropion[2,26,209]
Glaucoma[26,70,117,209,263]
Iris coloboma[33]
Iris sphincter dysplasia: Folds[48]
Microphthalmia[111]
Persistent pupillary membranes[33]
Progressive retinal atrophy
Retinal dysplasia[33]
Dandie Dinmont Terrier
Cataracts
Entropion[23]
Glaucoma[265]

Table 15.2 (*Continued*) **Breed predisposition to eye disease in dogs.**

Mesodermal dysgenesis glaucoma[207]
Persistent pupillary membranes[36,48]
Refractory superficial corneal ulcer
Doberman Pinscher
Anterior chamber cleavage syndrome/microphthalmia/retinal dysplasia[2,266]
Cataracts[26]
Coloboma
Distichiasis[26]
Enophthalmos[23,30]
Entropion: Lower eyelid, secondary to enlarged orbit/enophthalmos/large zygoma
Eversion of the cartilage of the third eyelid[25,27]
Ligneous conjunctivitis[267]
Microphakia, nuclear cataracts (7 months of age)
Microphthalmia with multiple ocular anomalies[26,266,268–270]
Persistent hyperplastic primary vitreous: Presumed dominant/incomplete penetrance[26,271–278]
Persistent hyperplastic tunica vasculosa lentis: Presumed dominant/incomplete penetrance[26,175,271–278]
Persistent pupillary membranes[26,36,101]
Progressive retinal atrophy
Retinal dysplasia: Retinal folds[23,26]
Dogue de Bordeaux
Cataracts[48]
Distichiasis[48]
Ectropion[1,83]
Entropion
Persistent pupillary membranes[33]
Multifocal retinopathy: Autosomal recessive cmr1; DNA test available[164]
English Cocker Spaniel
Cataracts: Recessive trait suspected[26,61,79,279,280]
Central progressive retinal atrophy (inherited vitamin E deficiency)[23,188,189,281,282]
Corneal dystrophy: Epithelial/stromal[36]
Distichiasis: Dominant trait suspected[26]
Ectropion[26]
Ectropion/entropion
Entropion (lower eyelid)
Glaucoma (narrow-angle)[26,116,283]
Imperforate lacrimal punctum[26]
Keratoconjunctivitis sicca/dry eye[201]
Lens luxation[23]
Optic nerve coloboma (pits)
Persistent pupillary membranes[26,36,110,279]
Progressive retinal atrophy (progressive rod–cone degeneration, autosomal recessive); DNA test available[26,72,73,284,285]

(*Continued*)

Table 15.2 (*Continued*) **Breed predisposition to eye disease in dogs.**

Retinal dysplasia: Retinal folds[26,33]

English Setter

Cataracts[26,29]

Ceroid lipofuscinosis[27,165,286–290]

Chalazion

Corneal dystrophy: Epithelial/stromal[26]

Distichiasis[26]

Ectropion

Ectropion/entropion[2]

Entropion

Eversion of the cartilage of the third eyelid

Keratoconjunctivitis sicca[2]

Macroblepharon[23]

Palpebral neoplasia[130]

Persistent pupillary membranes[26,36]

Progressive retinal atrophy: Generalized[26,291]

Progressive retinal atrophy (rod–cone dysplasia type 4 rcd4): Autosomal recessive; DNA test available[86]

Retinal dysplasia: Retinal folds[26,110]

English Shepherd

Choroidal hypoplasia (Collie eye anomaly): Autosomal recessive; DNA test is available[26,93,292]

   Optic nerve coloboma

   Retinal detachment

   Retinal hemorrhage

   Staphyloma/coloboma

Persistent pupillary membranes[26]

Progressive retinal atrophy (prcd): Autosomal recessive; DNA test is available[73]

English Springer Spaniel

Cataracts[23,26]

Cataracts/lenticonus[2]

Central progressive retinal atrophy

Chronic superficial keratitis (pannus)[23]

Coloboma of the optic nerve[23]

Corneal dystrophy: Epithelial/stromal[26]

Distichiasis[29,83]

Ectropion[2]

Entropion[25,26]

Glaucoma[26,293]

Optic nerve hypoplasia[294]

Persistent hyaloid artery[33,47]

Persistent pupillary membranes[26,29,36]

Progressive retinal atrophy: Generalized[26,295]

Progressive retinal atrophy: Autosomal recessive cord-1; DNA test available[296]

Table 15.2 (*Continued*) **Breed predisposition to eye disease in dogs.**

Refractive error[297,298]

Retinal dysplasia: Retinal folds; autosomal recessive trait[26,299–301]

   Geographic detachment: Autosomal recessive trait[26,299–301]

Vitreous degeneration[295]

English Toy Spaniel (King Charles, Prince Charles, Ruby, Blenheim)

Cataracts[26,27]

Corneal dystrophy: Epithelial/stromal[26]

Distichiasis[26]

Entropion[26]

Euryblepharon/macroblepharon[21]

Persistent hyaloid artery[26]

Persistent hyperplastic primary vitreous/persistent hyperplastic tunica vasculosa lentis: Presumed dominant/incomplete penetrance[26]

Persistent pupillary membranes[58]

Pigmentary keratitis[47]

Retinal dysplasia: Retinal folds; presumed autosomal recessive[26,27]

Vitreous degeneration[110]

Entlebucher Mountain Dog

Cataracts: Presumed autosomal recessive[26,302,303]

Corneal dystrophy: Epithelial/stromal[304]

Glaucoma[302]

Persistent pupillary membrane[33,305]

Progressive retinal atrophy: Autosomal recessive (prcd); DNA test available[73,83,302,303]

Retinal dysplasia: Retinal folds[21]

Eurasier

Distichiasis[33]

Glaucoma[306,307]

Field Spaniel

Cataracts[23,26]

Corneal dystrophy: Epithelial/stroma[14]

Distichiasis[26]

Entropion[47]

Ectropion[47]

Euryblepharon/macroblepharon[33]

Persistent pupillary membranes[36,83]

Progressive retinal atrophy[27]

Retinal dysplasia: Retinal folds, geographic[26,27]

Fila Brasileiro

Ectropion[2]

Entropion

Finnish Lapphund

Cataracts[22]

Persistent pupillary membranes[33]

Retinal atrophy: Autosomal recessive (prcd); DNA test available[33,73]

(Continued)

Table 15.2 (*Continued*) **Breed predisposition to eye disease in dogs.**

Finnish Spitz

Cataracts[26]

Flat Coated Retriever

Cataracts[23,26]

Corneal dystrophy: Epithelial/stroma[83]

Distichiasis[26]

Ectropion[23]

Entropion[26]

Glaucoma[26,308,309]

Persistent pupillary membranes[83]

Progressive retinal atrophy[27]

Retinopathy[310]

Fox Terrier (Smooth)

Cataracts[26,311]

Corneal epithelial dystrophy[29]

Glaucoma[26]

Lens luxation with secondary glaucoma: DNA test available

Persistent pupillary membranes

Progressive retinal atrophy[23]

Trichiasis

Fox Terrier (Toy)

Lens luxation with secondary glaucoma: DNA test available[20]

Persistent pupillary membranes[110]

Trichiasis[29]

Fox Terrier (Wire)

Cataracts (juvenile)[26]

Corneal endothelial dystrophy

Corneal epithelial dystrophy[29]

Distichiasis[29]

Entropion[23]

Glaucoma[2,26,312]

Lens luxation with secondary glaucoma (3–7 years of age): DNA test available[2,20]

Persistent pupillary membranes[36,48]

Progressive retinal atrophy

Refractory corneal ulcer[2]

French Bulldog

Cataracts[26,87]

Corneal dystrophy: Epithelial/ stromal[31]

Distichiasis[26,27]

Entropion[96]

Pigmentary keratitis[14]

Persistent pupillary membranes[48,96,110]

Prolapsed of the gland of the third eyelid[192]

Retinal dysplasia: Retinal folds[26]

German Pinscher

Cataracts[26,48,313,314]

Corneal dystrophy, epithelial/stromal[26]

Micropapilla[36,83]

Optic nerve hypoplasia[36,83]

Persistent pupillary membranes[33]

Persistent hyperplastic tunica vasculosa lentis (PHTVL)[313,314]

Vitreous degeneration[48]

German Shepherd Dog

Cataracts: Congenital (presumed autosomal dominant),[26,79,315] cortical (presumed autosomal recessive)[26,315]

Central progressive retinal atrophy (reported in Europe)

Chronic superficial keratitis (pannus)[26,152,316–319]

Coloboma

Cone degeneration: Hemeralopia/achromatopsia autosomal recessive[320]

Corneal dystrophy: Epithelial/stromal[23,26,200]

Dermoid, conjunctiva, cornea, eyelid

Distichiasis[48]

Ectropion[23]

Eversion of the cartilage of the third eyelid

Lens luxation[23]

Limbal melanoma[47,321]

Micropapilla[110]

Optic nerve hypoplasia[2,23,26]

Oversized palpebral fissure (euryblepharon), juvenile, transient[29]

Persistent pupillary membranes[36,83]

Plasmoma/atypical pannus[58]

Progressive retinal atrophy[26,71,107,209]

Retinal dysplasia: Retinal folds, geographic[26,27,322]

Third eyelid conjunctivitis (plasma cell infiltration)[25]

German Shorthaired Pointer

Cataracts[23,26]

Cone degeneration/ achromatopsia: Autosomal recessive; DNA test available[54]

Corneal dystrophy

Distichiasis[26]

Entropion (lower eyelid)

Eversion of the cartilage of the third eyelid[323]

Hemeralopia[26]

Nictitans cartilage anomaly/eversion[26,323]

Persistent hyperplastic primary vitreous/persistent hyperplastic tunica vasculosa lentis[26]

Persistent pupillary membranes[26,36]

Progressive retinal atrophy[26,107]

Strabismus[25]

Retinal dysplasia: Retinal folds[26]

(*Continued*)

Table 15.2 (*Continued*) Breed predisposition to eye disease in dogs.

German Wirehaired Pointer

Cataracts[23,26]

Entropion

Retinal dysplasia: Retinal folds[83]

Glen of Imaal Terrier

Cataracts[96]

Cone rod dystrophy: Autosomal recessive crd3; DNA test available[324,325]

Distichiasis[83]

Retinal atrophy[77,83,96]

Golden Retriever

Cataracts[26,78,79,326–330]

Central progressive retinal atrophy

Ceroid lipofuscinosis[331]

Coloboma of the optic nerve[23]

Corneal dystrophy: Epithelial/stromal[23,26,174]

Distichiasis[2,26]

Ectropion

Enophthalmos

Entropion[26]

Glaucoma[26]

Iris cyst

Limbal melanoma[332]

Optic nerve hypoplasia[23]

Persistent pupillary membranes[26,96,208]

Progressive retinal atrophy: Autosomal recessive; three DNA tests available[26,333,334]

Pigmentary keratitis[26]

Pigmentary uveitis[26,83,335–338]

Retinal dysplasia: Retinal folds, geographic/detachment[26,322,339]

Uveal cysts[26,335–337]

Uveodermatologic syndrome (vitiligo and uveitis syndrome)[39]

Gordon Setter

Cataracts[23,26]

Cone degeneration/achromatopsia[340]

Distichiasis[48]

Ectropion[26]

Entropion (lower eyelid)/macroblepharon[26]

Keratoconjunctivitis sicca[2]

Persistent hyaloid artery[48]

Persistent pupillary membranes[26,36,48]

Progressive retinal atrophy[341–343]

Retinal atrophy: Autosomal recessive rod–cone dysplasia type 4 (rcd4); DNA test available[86]

Retinal dysplasia: Retinal folds[2,26]

Uveal cysts[48]

Table 15.2 (*Continued*) Breed predisposition to eye disease in dogs.

Great Dane

Cataracts[26]

Ciliary body cyst[26]

Distichiasis[26]

Ectropion[26]

Ectropion/entropion

Enophthalmos

Entropion secondary to enlarged orbit/enophthalmos[26]

Euryblepharon/macroblepharon[36]

Eversion of the cartilage of the third eyelid[2]

Glaucoma[2,26,28,36,344]

Hemeralopia[23]

Mesodermal dysgenesis

Microphthalmia[26,235]

Multiple ocular anomalies (homozygous merle): Presumed autosomal dominant[26,235,328]

Nictitans cartilage anomaly/eversion[26]

Persistent hyperplastic primary vitreous/persistent hyperplastic tunica vasculosa lentis[14]

Persistent pupillary membranes[36]

Progressive retinal atrophy[26]

Prolapse of the gland of the third eyelid[192]

Retinal dysplasia (harlequin)

Uveal cysts[36,345]

Great Pyrenees (Pyrenean Mountain Dog)

Cataracts[26,48]

Corneal dystrophy: Epithelial/stromal[21]

Distichiasis[96]

Ectropion (lateral aspect of the eyelid)/entropion (medial aspect of the eyelid)

Entropion[48]

Micropapilla[21]

Multifocal retinopathy: Autosomal recessive cmr1; DNA test available[110,346,347]

Persistent pupillary membranes[26,48,96,110]

Progressive retinal atrophy: Presumed autosomal recessive[27,48]

Retinal dysplasia: Retinal folds, presumed autosomal recessive[48]

Retinal dysplasia: Geographic/detached [96]

Greater Swiss Mountain Dog

Cataracts[26]

Distichiasis[26]

Entropion[58]

Persistent pupillary membranes[48,83,96]

Retinal dysplasia[96]

Greyhound

Cataracts[96]

(*Continued*)

Table 15.2 (*Continued*) **Breed predisposition to eye disease in dogs.**

Chronic superficial keratitis (pannus)[26,348,349]
Corneal dystrophy
Distichiasis
Lens luxation[26,33]
Optic nerve hypoplasia[26]
Persistent hyperplastic primary vitreous[350]
Progressive retinal atrophy[26,351]
Vitreous degeneration[83]
Griffon
See Brussels Griffon
Harrier
Cataracts[21]
Persistent pupillary membranes[36,48]
Havana Silk Dog
Cataracts[26,352]
Distichiasis[26]
Persistent pupillary membranes[26,36]
Progressive retinal atrophy[26]
Retinal dysplasia[21]
Vitreous degeneration[26,110]
Havanese (Toy)
Cataracts[26,352]
Distichiasis[26]
Persistent pupillary membranes[23,26,36]
Progressive retinal atrophy[26]
Retinal detachment[27]
Retinal dysplasia[21]
Vitreous degeneration[26,110]
Ibizan Hound
Cataracts[23,26,27]
Persistent pupillary membranes[22,36,83]
Retinal dysplasia: Presumed autosomal recessive[2,26,46]
Icelandic Sheepdog
Cataracts[110]
Persistent pupillary membranes[36]
Retinal dysplasia[33]
Irish Setter (also Red and White)
Amblyopia with quadriplegia: Autosomal recessive[353,354]
Anterior chamber cleavage[2] syndrome
Cataracts[26]
Central progressive retinal atrophy
Corneal dystrophy[29]
Distichiasis[26,48]
Enophthalmos
Entropion[26]

Table 15.2 (*Continued*) **Breed predisposition to eye disease in dogs.**

Entropion secondary to enlarged orbit/enophthalmos/large zygoma
Eversion of the cartilage of the third eyelid[23,26]
Lens luxation[2,23]
Optic nerve hypoplasia[2]
Persistent hyaloid artery[26]
Persistent hyperplastic primary vitreous[23]
Persistent pupillary membranes[26,110]
Progressive retinal atrophy (rod–cone dysplasia type 1 and type 4; rcd1; rcd4): Autosomal recessive trait; DNA test available[6,7,23,26,86,353–373]
Retinal dysplasia: Retinal folds[48]
Uveodermatologic syndrome (vitiligo and uveitis syndrome)[39]
Irish Terrier
Cataracts[26]
Progressive retinal atrophy[27]
Irish Water Spaniel
Cataracts[23,26]
Distichiasis[26]
Entropion[26]
Persistent pupillary membranes[36,83]
Progressive retinal atrophy[23,27]
Irish Wolfhound
Cataracts[23,26]
Corneal dystrophy: Epithelial/stromal[26]
Distichiasis[26]
Entropion[27]
Eversion of the cartilage of the third eyelid[23,26]
Micropapilla[26]
Optic nerve hypoplasia[31]
Persistent pupillary membranes[83]
Progressive retinal atrophy: Presumed autosomal recessive[31]
Retinal dysplasia: Retinal folds/geographic[36,47,83]
Uveal cysts[26]
Italian Greyhound
Cataracts[2,26]
Corneal dystrophy[23]
Glaucoma[27]
Iris cyst
Lens luxation[48]
Micropapilla
Optic nerve hypoplasia[23]
Persistent hyaloid artery[36]
Persistent pupillary membranes[33,47]
Progressive retinal atrophy: IG-PRA1; DNA test available[26]
Retinal degeneration (generalized)
Vitreous degeneration[26,27,48]

(*Continued*)

Table 15.2 (*Continued*) **Breed predisposition to eye disease in dogs.**

Jack Russell Terrier

Cataracts[26,110]

Corneal dystrophy: Epithelial/stromal[33]

Distichiasis[26]

Persistent pupillary membranes[36,48]

Lens luxation with secondary glaucoma: DNA test available[17,20,26,374–377]

Vitreous degeneration[36,110]

Jagdterrier

Lens luxation: DNA test avaialable[20]

Japanese Chin (Japanese Spaniel)

Cataracts[26]

Distichiasis[26,36,83]

Entropion[26]

Persistent hyaloid artery[26]

Persistent hyperplastic primary vitreous/persistent hyperplastic tunica vasculosa lentis[21]

Persistent pupillary membranes[21,36,83,110]

Pigmentary keratitis[26]

Progressive retinal atrophy[23,31]

Vitreous degeneration[36]

Karelian Bear Dog

Progressive retinal atrophy: autosomal recessive: DNA test available[31,73,378]

Keeshond

Cataracts[23,26]

Central progressive retinal atrophy

Distichiasis[26]

Ectopic cilium[25]

Entropion[36]

Glaucoma

Optic nerve hypoplasia[23]

Persistent pupillary membranes[21]

Progressive retinal atrophy

Kerry Blue Terrier

Cataracts[23,26]

Corneal dystrophy: Epithelial/stromal[33]

Distichiasis[33]

Entropion (lower eyelid)

Keratoconjunctivitis sicca[29,194]

Micropalpebral fissure (blepharophimosis)

Persistent pupillary membrane[33]

Progressive retinal atrophy

Trichiasis (upper lateral)[29]

Vitreous degeneration[36]

Table 15.2 (*Continued*) **Breed predisposition to eye disease in dogs.**

Komondor

Cataracts[23,26]

Entropion[33]

Persistent pupillary membranes[33]

Kuvasz

Cataracts[23,26]

Corneal dystrophy: Epithelial/stromal; endothelial[31,33]

Entropion[26]

Distichiasis[2,26]

Persistent pupillary membranes[26,36]

Progressive retinal atrophy: Autosomal recessive prcd; DNA test available[26,73]

Vitreous degeneration[33]

Labradoodle (Australian)

Achromatopsia type 1: Autosomal recessive; DNA test available[379]

Cataracts: Presumed dominant with incomplete penetrance; autosomal recessive[26,78,79,327,380,381]

Corneal dystrophy: Epithelial/stromal[26,382]

Distichiasis[26]

Ectropion[26]

Entropion[26,209,380]

Glaucoma[306]

Limbal melanoma[332]

Persistent hyaloid artery[26]

Persistent hyperplastic primary vitreous/persistent hyperplastic tunica vasculosa lentis[26]

Persistent pupillary membranes[26,36,47]

Progressive retinal atrophy: Autosomal recessive (prcd); DNA test available[26,72,73,383–385]

Retinal dysplasia: Presumed autosomal recessive (retinal folds); DNA test is available[26,208,386–393]

Retinal dysplasia: Presumed autosomal recessive (fold/geographic/without skeletal defects; DNA test available[26,208,386–393]

Retinal dysplasia: Presumed autosomal recessive with incomplete dominance for the eye (retinal fold/geographic/with skeletal defects; DNA test available[26,208,386–394]

Uveal cysts[36]

Vitreous degeneration[83,110]

Labrador Retriever

Achromatopsia type 1(ACHM-type 1): Autosomal recessive; DNA test available[379]

Cataracts: Autosomal recessive, dominant or incomplete dominant trait[26,78,79,209,327,380,381]

Central progressive retinal atrophy: Incomplete dominant trait suspected

Corneal dystrophy: Epithelial/stromal[26,382]

Corneal opacity[25,29]

Distichiasis[26,29]

(Continued)

Table 15.2 (*Continued*) **Breed predisposition to eye disease in dogs.**

Ectropion[23,26]

Enophthalmos

Entropion (lateral canthus)[26,209,380]

Entropion (lower eyelid)[2,26,209,380]

Glaucoma[306]

Iris melanoma

Limbal melanoma[332]

Nystagmus[29]

Persistent hyaloid artery[26]

Persistent hyperplastic primary vitreous/persistent hyperplastic tunica vasculosa lentis[26]

Persistent pupillary membranes[26,36,47]

Progressive retinal atrophy (progressive rod–cone degeneration): Autosomal recessive; DNA test available[26,72,73,383–385]

Retinal detachment (retinal dysplasia): Autosomal recessive; DNA test available[23]

Retinal dysplasia: Autosomal recessive trait; DNA test available

    Focal or geographic detachment, without skeletal dysplasia: Presumed autosomal recessive[26,208,386,388–393]

    Folds, geographic/detachment with skeletal defects: Presumed incomplete dominant trait[26,208,386–394]

Uveal cysts[36]

Vitreous degeneration[83,110]

Lagotto Romagnolo

Cataracts[26]

Distichiasis[26]

Persistent pupillary membranes[26,36]

Lakeland Terrier

Cataracts[23]

Distichiasis[29]

Lens luxation: DNA test available[20,375]

Persistent pupillary membranes[26,36,294]

Lancashire Heeler

Choroidal hypoplasia (Collie eye anomaly): Autosomal recessive; DNA test available[92,93,395]

    Staphyloma/coloboma

    Retinal detachment

    Retinal hemorrhage

    Optic nerve coloboma

Lens luxation: DNA test available[15,17,20]

Persistent pupillary membrane[33]

Lapponian Herder

Multifocal retinopathy (cmr3): Autosomal recessive; DNA test available[164]

Progressive retinal atrophy: Autosomal recessive; DNA test available[73]

Large Munsterlander

Cataracts

Table 15.2 (*Continued*) **Breed predisposition to eye disease in dogs.**

Leonberger

Cataracts[26,396]

Ciliary body cysts[21]

Distichiasis[36,83]

Ectropion[36]

Entropion[36,83,396]

Euryblepharon/macroblepharon[83,396]

Nictitans cartilage anomaly/eversion[33]

Persistent pupillary membranes[26,36,396]

Lhasa Apso

Aberrant dermis

Cataracts[2,23,26,64]

Ciliated caruncle[26]

Corneal dystrophy[23]

Distichiasis[26]

Ectopic cilium[2,26,29]

Entropion

Entropion (medial lower eyelid)[2]

Exposure keratopathy syndrome/macroblepharon[26]

Imperforate lacrimal puncta[26]

Keratoconjunctivitis sicca[26,194]

Lagophthalmos/exophthalmos

Macroblepharon

Persistent pupillary membranes[26,36]

Progressive retinal atrophy[27]

Prolapse of the gland of the third eyelid[26,74]

Traumatic proptosis

Louisiana Catahoula Leopard Dog

Iris coloboma[31]

Persistent pupillary membranes[36]

Retinal dysplasia: Retinal folds[31]

Lowchen

Cataracts[26]

Distichiasis[26,48]

Exposure/pigmentary keratitis[48]

Progressive retinal atrophy[27]

Persistent pupillary membranes[26,36]

Retinal atrophy (generalized)[26]

Vitreous degeneration[26,46]

Lucas Terrier

Lens luxation: DNA test available[20]

Maltese

Caruncular trichiasis[2]

Cataracts[26,64]

Distichiasis[31]

(*Continued*)

Table 15.2 (*Continued*) **Breed predisposition to eye disease in dogs.**

Entropion[26]

Epiphora

Glaucoma[23]

Persistent hyaloid remnant[26]

Persistent pupillary membranes[33]

Progressive retinal atrophy[26]

Retinal dysplasia: Retinal folds[2,23]

Manchester Terrier (Toy and Standard)

Cataracts[26,147]

Lens luxation with secondary glaucoma[23,311]

Progressive retinal atrophy

Mastiff[13]

Cataracts[26]

Corneal dystrophy[23,33]

Distichiasis[48]

Ectropion[26,29]

Entropion[26,163]

Macroblepharon/exposure keratopathy syndrome[26]

Multifocal retinopathy (cmr1): Autosomal recessive; DNA test available[60]

Persistent pupillary membranes[26,47,48]

Progressive retinal atrophy: Autosomal recessive; DNA test available[26,27,397]

Retinal dysplasia: Retinal folds[26]

Uveal cysts[47]

MI-KI

Cataracts[83]

Corneal dystrophy: Epithelial/stromal[21]

Distichiasis[33]

Entropion[21]

Persistent pupillary membrane[83]

Retinal dysplasia

Vitreous degeneration[36,83]

Miniature (Toy) American/Australian Shepherd

Cataracts: Autosomal codominant; DNA test available[26,87,88]

Choroidal hypoplasia (Collie eye anomaly): Autosomal recessive; DNA test available[21,26,91–93]

  Staphyloma/coloboma

  Retinal detachment

  Retinal hemorrhage

  Optic nerve coloboma

Coloboma/staphyloma without micophthalmia[26]

Cone degeneration: Autosomal recessive; DNA test available[54]

Corneal dystrophy[36]

Distichiasis[21,26]

Iris coloboma[26]

Table 15.2 (*Continued*) **Breed predisposition to eye disease in dogs.**

Iris hypoplasia[46]

Persistent hyaloid artery[36]

Persistent pupillary membranes[26,36]

Progressive retinal atrophy (prcd): Autosomal recessive; DNA test available[26,46,58,73]

Microphthalmia with multiple ocular defects: Presumed autosomal recessive with incomplete penetrance[26,95,97–100]

Micropapilla[47]

Multifocal retinopathy (cmr1): Autosomal recessive; DNA test available[102]

Retinal dysplasia[36]

Miniature Bull Terrier

Cataracts[36]

Corneal dystrophy: Endothelial[83]

Lens luxation: DNA test available[15–17,26]

Persistent pupillary membrane[26,36,110]

Progressive retinal atrophy[110]

Vitreous degeneration[36,83,110]

Miniature Pinscher

Cataracts[26]

Chronic superficial keratitis (pannus)[23]

Corneal dystrophy: Epithelial/stromal[26,27]

Entropion (medial canthus)[29]

Keratoconjunctivitis sicca

Micropapilla[48]

Optic nerve hypoplasia[48]

Persistent pupillary membranes[36,48]

Progressive retinal atrophy[25,48]

Vitreous degeneration[110]

Neapolitan Mastiff

Cataracts[27,48]

Dermoid

Distichiasis[48]

Ectropion/macroblepharon[27,48]

Entropion[48]

Eversion of the cartilage of the third eyelid[2]

Persistent pupillary membranes[48]

Progressive retinal atrophy

Prolapse of the gland of the third eyelid[2,398]

Newfoundland

Anterior chamber cleavage syndrome[23]

Cataracts[26,27]

Distichiasis[31]

Ectropion[26]

Ectropion (lateral aspect of the eyelid)/entropion (medial aspect of the eyelid)

(*Continued*)

Table 15.2 (*Continued*) **Breed predisposition to eye disease in dogs.**

Entropion (lateral canthus)[26]

Eversion of the cartilage of the third eyelid

Glaucoma[36,306]

Macroblepharon[26,27,234]

Persistent pupillary membranes[36]

Progressive retinal atrophy[399]

Prolapse of the gland of the third eyelid[26]

Retinal dysplasia: Retinal folds[26,36,48]

Uveal cysts[26]

Norrbottenspets

Cataracts[26]

Norfolk Terrier

Cataracts[23]

Coloboma of the optic disc[23]

Lens luxation: DNA test available[20,375]

Northern Inuit Dog

Oculoskeletal dysplasia[400]

Norwegian Buhund

Cataracts: Pulverulent; presumed autosomal dominant[26,401]

Retinal dysplasia[31]

Norwegian Elkhound

Cataracts[26]

Distichiasis[26,29]

Ectropion[46]

Entropion (lateral canthus)[2,402]

Glaucoma[2,26,68,117,312,403–406]

Lens luxation

Persistent pupillary membranes[26,36]

Progressive retinal atrophy(prcd): Autosomal recessive; DNA test available[31,73]

  Rod dysplasia: Autosomal recessive trait[26,407–410]

  Early rod degeneration: Autosomal recessive trait[26,411–415]

Retinal dysplasia: Retinal folds[26]

Uveal cysts[31]

Norwegian Lundehund

Persistent pupillary membranes[21]

Norwich Terrier

Cataracts[36]

Corneal dystrophy[23,36]

Distichiasis[36]

Lens luxation: DNA test available[17,20,375]

Persistent pupillary membranes[36]

Vitreous degeneration[36]

Nova Scotia Duck Tolling Retriever

Cataracts[26,27,416]

Table 15.2 (*Continued*) **Breed predisposition to eye disease in dogs.**

Choroidal hypoplasia (Collie eye anomaly): Autosomal recessive; DNA test available[47,92,93]

  Staphyloma/coloboma

  Retinal detachment

  Retinal hemorrhage

  Optic nerve coloboma

Corneal dystrophy: Epithelial/stromal[26]

Corneal dystrophy: Endothelial[48]

Distichiasis[26]

Micropapilla[48,96]

Persistent pupillary membranes[26,36]

Progressive retinal atrophy (prcd): Autosomal recessive; DNA test available[26,73,416]

Retinal dysplasia[48]

Uveal cysts[48]

Old English Sheepdog

Cataracts (congenital): Recessive trait suspected[304,417]

Coloboma/stapyloma[48]

Corneal dystrophy[36]

Distichiasis[25,83]

Entropion

Micropapilla[48]

Microphthalmia/cataracts: Multiple ocular anomalies[26,417]

Persistent hyperplastic primary vitreous/persistent hyperplastic tunica vasculosa lentis[48]

Persistent pupillary membranes[26,36]

Progressive retinal atrophy[23,26,29]

Retinal detachment/cataracts[27,36]

Retinal dysplasia: Retinal folds[23,26]

Uveodermatologic syndrome[26]

Vitreous degeneration

Papillon

Cataracts[23,26]

Corneal dystrophy[21,27]

Distichiasis[36,83]

Entropion

Micropapilla[48]

Persistent pupillary membranes[26,36]

Progressive retinal atrophy: Autosomal recessive; DNA test available[26,418–422]

Retinal dysplasia[58]

Vitreous degeneration[26]

Parson Russell Terrier

Cataracts[36,377]

Distichiasis[36]

Lens luxation: DNA test available[17,20]

(*Continued*)

Table 15.2 (*Continued*) **Breed predisposition to eye disease in dogs.**

Persistent pupillary membranes[36]

Progressive retinal atrophy[58]

Vitreous degeneration[47]

Patterdale Terrier

Lens luxation: DNA test available[20]

Pekingese

Aberrant dermis (medial canthus)

Caruncular trichiasis (ciliated caruncle)[23,27]

Cataracts[26]

Distichiasis: Dominant trait suspected[26,65,423]

Ectopic cilium[26,29]

Entropion (lower medial eyelid)[26]

Exposure keratopathy syndrome/macroblepharon[1,2,26]

Keratoconjunctivitis sicca[26]

Lacrimal punctum atresia

Lagophthalmos/exophthalmos

Lens luxation[23]

Macroblepharon

Nasal fold trichiasis

Pigmentary keratitis

Progressive retinal atrophy[26,107]

Traumatic proptosis

Trichiasis (lateral upper eyelid)

Ulcerative keratitis

Pembroke Welsh Corgi

Cataracts[23,26]

Corneal dystrophy (vascularization)[23]

Distichiasis[26]

Lens luxation

Persistent pupillary membranes[26,36,110]

Progressive retinal atrophy[27]

Retinal dysplasia: Retinal folds, geographic/detachment[23,26]

Vitreous degeneration[31]

Petit Basset Griffon Vendeen

Cataracts[21]

Corneal dystrophy: Epithelial/stromal/endothelial[26,36]

Glaucoma: Autosomal recessive; DNA test available[26,48,119]

Persistent hyaloid artery[14]

Persistent pupillary membranes[21,26,36,46,47]

Pigment deposition on posterior corneal surface; possible persistent pupillary membranes

Retinal dysplasia: Retinal folds[23,26]

Vitreous degeneration[36]

Pharaoh Hound

Cataracts[26]

Distichiasis[47]

Table 15.2 (*Continued*) **Breed predisposition to eye disease in dogs.**

Optic nerve hypoplasia[23]

Persistent pupillary membranes[21,47]

Retinal dysplasia[48]

Pointer

Cataracts: Dominant trait[26]

Chronic superficial keratitis (pannus)

Corneal dystrophy[23,48]

Entropion[23,29]

Persistent pupillary membranes[48]

Progressive retinal atrophy

Retinal dysplasia: Retinal folds[26]

Polski Owczarek Nizinny (Polish Owczarek Nizinny, Polish Lowland Sheepdog)

Cataracts[48]

Central progressive retinal atrophy[26]

Ceroid lipofuscinosis[424]

Corneal dystrophy[36,48,83]

Distichiasis[36,83]

Persistent pupillary membranes[26,36]

Progressive retinal atrophy (rod–cone dysplasia type 1): Autosomal recessive; DNA test available[86]

Pomeranian

Blepharophimosis[23]

Cataracts (2–4 years of age)[23,48]

Distichiasis[26,32,83]

Entropion[26]

Epiphora

Lacrimal punctum atresia

Persistent pupillary membranes[33]

Progressive retinal atrophy[27,110]

Trichiasis[32]

Vitreous degeneration[36]

Poodle (Miniature and Toy)

Caruncular trichiasis[23]

Cataracts (juvenile): Autosomal recessive[26,64]

Chronic superficial keratitis (pannus)

Corneal dystrophy: Endothelial, epithelial[25,32,48]

Distichiasis: Dominant trait suspected[26]

Entropion (medial lower eyelid)

Epiphora

Glaucoma (open- or narrow-angle)[26,68,117,425]

Hemeralopia (Miniature Poodle)

Imperforate lacrimal punctum[26]

Iridal atrophy[25,29]

Lens luxation[70]

Microphthalmia[26]

(*Continued*)

Table 15.2 (*Continued*) **Breed predisposition to eye disease in dogs.**

Optic nerve hypoplasia[26,210,426,427]

Optic nerve micropapilla[26]

Persistent pupillary membranes[26,36]

Progressive retinal atrophy (progressive rod–cone degeneration): Autosomal recessive; DNA test available[26,71–73,110,383,413,428–438]

Recurrent epithelial erosion (basement membrane dystrophy)[32]

Retinal detachment[23]

Trichomegaly[25,29]

Vitreous degeneration[26,110]

Poodle (Standard)

Cataracts: Recessive trait suspected[26,64,439,440]

Congenital night blindness[23]

Corneal dystrophy: Epithelial/stromal[48]

Distichiasis[26]

Entropion

Glaucoma[26,68,117,425]

Imperforate lacrimal punctum[26]

Microphthalmia[26,27]

Microphthalmia/cataracts/persistent pupillary membranes/keratopathy[2]

Optic nerve hypoplasia[2,26,426,427]

Optic nerve micropapilla[26]

Persistent pupillary membranes[26,36]

Progressive retinal atrophy: Autosomal recessive; DNA test available[26,71–73,110,383,413,429,431–438]

Vitreous degeneration[26,110]

Portuguese Podengo Pequeno

Distichiasis[14]

Persistent pupillary membranes[58]

Vitreous degeneration[14]

Portuguese Water Dog

Cataracts[26,27]

Distichiasis[26]

Corneal dystrophy[58]

Microphthalmia and multiple congenital anomalies[23,26,27,441]

Persistent pupillary membranes[26,36]

Progressive retinal atrophy (progressive rod–cone degeneration): Autosomal recessive; DNA test available[26,36,73,442]

Retinal dysplasia[36]

Pug

Aberrant dermis (medial)[1,23]

Caruncular trichiasis[23]

Cataracts[64,83]

Corneal dystrophy[29]

Distichiasis[2,26]

Entropion (medial lower eyelid)[26]

Table 15.2 (*Continued*) **Breed predisposition to eye disease in dogs.**

Exposure keratopathy syndrome/macroblepharon[26,443]

Lagophthalmos/exophthalmos/macroblepharon

Micropapilla[48]

Nasal fold trichiasis

Persistent pupillary membranes[83]

Pigmentary keratitis

Progressive retinal atrophy[27]

Retinal dysplasia: Presumes autosomal recessive[46,110]

Traumatic proptosis

Vitreous degeneration[83]

Trichiasis[2]

Ulcerative keratitis

Puli

Cataracts[23,48]

Corneal dystrophy[36,83]

Persistent hyaloid artery[48]

Persistent pupillary membranes[36]

Progressive retinal atrophy[23]

Retinal dysplasia: Retinal folds[26]

Pyrenean Shepherd

Cataracts[48]

Choroidal hypoplasia[31,48]

Lens luxation[48]

Persistent pupillary membranes[48]

Retinal dysplasia[31]

Rat Terrier

Cataracts[48]

Distichiasis[48]

Lens luxation: DNA test available[17,20]

Persistent pupillary membranes[48]

Rhodesian Ridgeback

Cataracts[23,26]

Distichiasis[26]

Entropion[444]

Eversion of the cartilage of the third eyelid

Persistent pupillary membranes[36,48,83]

Progressive retinal atrophy[27]

Rottweiler

Amaurosis[26]

Cataracts: Congenital, inherited[2,26,445,446]

Corneal dystrophy: Epithelial/stromal[26]

Distichiasis

Entropion, lateral canthus and lower eyelid,[2,26,29,32,163] secondary to enlarged orbit/enophthalmos/large zygoma

Iris coloboma (inherited)[27]

(*Continued*)

Table 15.2 (Continued) Breed predisposition to eye disease in dogs.

Iris/uvealcyst[23,26,146,446]

Microphthalmia

Oversized palpebral fissure (macroblepharon)

Persistent pupillary membranes[33]

Progressive retinal atrophy[26,146]

Refractory superficial corneal ulcer[23]

Retinal degeneration

Retinal detachment[23]

Retinal dysplasia: Retinal folds[26,27,146]

Russell Terrier

Lens luxation: DNA test available[20]

Saint Bernard

Cataracts[26]

Dermoid[26,109,447,448]

Distichiasis

Ectropion[26]

Ectropion (lateral aspect of the lower eyelid)/entropion (medial aspect of the lower eyelid)

Entropion (lateral canthus)[26,32,109,163]

Eversion of the cartilage of the third eyelid

Microphthalmia

Multiple ocular anomalies[26,27,449]

Oversized palpebral fissure (macroblepharon)[29,48]

Persistent pupillary membranes[47]

Prolapse of the gland of the third eyelid

Redundant facial skin[25,29]

Uveodermatologic syndrome (vitiligo and uveitis syndrome)[39]

Saluki

Cataracts[27,83]

Corneal dystrophy (Lavach J., personal communication, 1985)

Entropion[26]

Glaucoma (iridocorneal angle abnormality)[33]

Persistent pupillary membranes[36,83]

Posterior suture line imperfection[2]

Progressive retinal atrophy

Retinal detachment[25]

Retinal dysplasia[29]

Samoyed

Cataracts[26]

Coloboma of the optic nerve

Corneal dystrophy: Stromal, epithelial[2,26,101,200]

Distichiasis[23,26]

Entropion

Glaucoma[26,28,68,450–454]

Mesodermal dysgenesis (goniodysgenesis)[28]

Microphthalmos

Table 15.2 (Continued) Breed predisposition to eye disease in dogs.

Persistent pupillary membranes[26,29,36]

Primary glaucoma

Progressive retinal atrophy (3 years of age at onset): X-linked recessive; DNA test available[26,455,456]

Refractory superficial corneal ulcer[2,23]

Retinal detachment and cataracts with skeletal dwarfism[23]

Retinal dysplasia: Retinal folds/detachment with skeletal dwarfism autosomal recessive with incomplete dominance for the eye; DNA test available[26,394,457]

    Geographic/detachment, presumed autosomal recessive[25,26,32,457]

Uveodermatologic syndrome[26,40,458]

Schapendoes

Progressive retinal atrophy (CCDC66): Autosomal recessive; DNA test available[459,460]

Schipperke

Cataracts[23,26]

Distichiasis[36,83]

Entropion

Narrow palpebral fissure[29]

Persistent pupillary membranes[21,26,36]

Progressive retinal atrophy[26]

Retinal dysplasia[33]

Vitreous degeneration[21,47]

Schnauzer (Giant)

Cataracts[23,26]

Glaucoma[23]

Nictitans cartilage anomaly/eversion[26]

Persistent pupillary membranes[36]

Progressive retinal atrophy: Autosomal recessive prcd; DNA test available

Retinal dysplasia: Retinal folds[36]

Schnauzer (Miniature)

Cataracts: congenital (microphthalmia, posterior lenticonus): Simple autosomal recessive trait[26,305,461,462]

    Juvenile: Autosomal recessive trait[26,27,147,463–465]

Ceroid lipofuscinosis: Presumed autosomal recessive[26,165,466]

Corneal dystrophy[25,58]

Distichiasis[305]

Entropion (medial lower eyelid)[32]

Keratoconjunctivitis sicca[83]

Lacrimal punctum atresia

Microcornea

Optic nerve hypoplasia[23]

Persistent hyperplastic primary vitreous[32]

Persistent pupillary membranes[29,83]

Progressive retinal atrophy (rod–cone dysplasia)[26,256,467,468]

Retinal atrophy: Low-amplitude electroretinogram[26]

(Continued)

Table 15.2 (*Continued*) **Breed predisposition to eye disease in dogs.**

Retinal dysplasia: Retinal folds[23,469]

Vitreous degeneration[58]

Schnauzer (Standard)

Cataracts[26]

Congenital cataracts and microcornea[23]

Corneal dystrophy: Epithelial/stromal[26]

Distichiasis[26]

Persistent hyperplastic primary vitreous[25]

Persistent pupillary membranes[110]

Retinal atrophy (generalized): Presumed autosomal recessive[26]

Retinal dysplasia: Retinal folds[26]

Vitreous degeneration[31]

Scottish Deerhound

Cataracts[23]

Scottish Terrier

Cataracts[26]

Lens luxation

Ligneous conjunctivitis[267,470]

Persistent pupillary membranes[26,29,36,83]

Progressive retinal atrophy[27]

Vitreous degeneration[33]

Sealyham Terrier

Cataracts: Recessive trait suspected[36]

Distichiasis[83]

Glaucoma[2,28]

Imperforate lacrimal punctum

Lens luxation with secondary glaucoma: DNA test available[20,26,209,375,471]

Persistent pupillary membrane[36,48,83]

Progressive retinal atrophy

Retinal dysplasia: Retinal folds; presumed autosomal recessive[26,472]

   Geographic/detachment: Presumed autosomal recessive[23,26,472]

Chinese Shar Pei

Blepharitis

Cataracts[26]

Corneal dystrophy: Epithelial/stromal[26,473,474]

Ectropion/entropion

Entropion[26,473–476]

Glaucoma[26]

Keratitis (secondary, chronic)[36]

Lens luxation: Autosomal recessive[26,477]

Mesodermal dysgenesis glaucoma

Persistent pupillary membranes[36]

Progressive retinal atrophy[26,27]

Prolapse of the gland of the third eyelid[26]

Table 15.2 (*Continued*) **Breed predisposition to eye disease in dogs.**

Redundant facial skin

Retinal dysplasia (cataracts)[23]

Strabismus (esotropia)

Shetland Sheepdog

Amaurosis[23]

Cataracts[27]

Central progressive retinal atrophy[111]

Choroidal hypoplasia (Collie eye anomaly): Autosomal recessive; DNA test available[26,93,292]

   Staphyloma/coloboma

   Retinal detachment

   Retinal hemorrhage

   Optic nerve coloboma

Corneal dystrophy (bilateral, central, circular) (6 months–4 years at diagnosis)[2,23,26,200]

Distichiasis[2,26]

Ectopic cilium[25]

Micropalpebral fissure (blepharophimosis)[25]

Optic nerve coloboma[26]

Optic nerve hypoplasia[23]

Persistent pupillary membranes[26,36,110]

Progressive retinal atrophy (CNGA1-PRA): Autosomal recessive; DNA test available[478]

Retinal dysplasia: Retinal folds[2,23]

Slowly progressive retinopathy[479]

Uveodermatologic syndrome[26,40,42]

Shiba Inu

Cataracts[26]

Corneal dystrophy[36,83]

Distichiasis[26]

Exposure pigmentary keratitis[33]

Glaucoma[58,480,481]

Persistent pupillary membranes[26,36]

Vitreous degeneration[83]

Shih Tzu

Aberrant dermis

Caruncular trichiasis (ciliated caruncle)[23,26]

Cataracts[23,26]

Corneal dystrophy[36]

Distichiasis[26]

Ectopic cilium[26]

Entropion (medial lower eyelid)[26]

Exophthalmos/lagophthalmos

Exposure keratopathy syndrome/macroblepharon[14,26]

Glaucoma[480]

Keratoconjunctivitis sicca[26,201]

(*Continued*)

Table 15.2 (*Continued*) **Breed predisposition to eye disease in dogs.**

Micropapilla[48]

Optic nerve hypoplasia[48,482]

Oversized palpebral fissure (macroblepharon)

Persistent hyaloid artery[58]

Persistent pupillary membranes[110]

Progressive retinal atrophy[26,483]

Retinal detachment[23,483,484]

Traumatic proptosis

Ulcerative keratitis

Vitreous degeneration[23,110,484]

Shiloh Shepherd

Corneal dystrophy[48]

Chronic superficial keratitis (pannus)[46]

Siberian Husky

Cataracts[26,485]

Chronic superficial keratitis (pannus)[29]

Corneal dystrophy: Endothelial[32]

    Epithelial/stromal: Presumed autosomal recessive[26,127,247,486,487]

Distichiasis[26]

Entropion[26]

Glaucoma (goniodysgenesis)[2,26,68,117,207,403,404,485]

Lens luxation[26]

Palpebral neoplasia

Persistent hyperplastic primary vitreous[26,488]

Persistent pupillary membranes[2,29,36,48,58]

Progressive retinal atrophy: Presumed X-linked; DNA test available[26,27,456,489]

Retinal dysplasia: Retinal folds geographic/detached presumed autosomal recessive[23,26,58]

Uveitis[26]

Uveodermatologic syndrome[26,39,40,458]

Vitreous degeneration[58]

Silken Windhound

Choroidal hypoplasia (Collie eye anomaly): Autosomal recessive; DNA test available[14,93]

    Staphyloma/coloboma

    Retinal detachment

    Retinal hemorrhage

    Optic nerve coloboma

Silky Terrier

Cataracts[33,64,83,305]

Corneal dystrophy[33,83]

Persistent pupillary membranes[23,33,83]

Progressive retinal atrophy: Autosomal recessive prcd; DNA test available[73]

Vitreous degeneration[33,304,305]

Table 15.2 (*Continued*) **Breed predisposition to eye disease in dogs.**

Skye Terrier

Distichiasis

Lens luxation[23]

Sloughi

Progressive retinal atrophy (rcd1a): Autosomal recessive; DNA test available[490]

Smooth Fox Terrier

Cataracts[26]

Glaucoma[26,312]

Lens luxation: DNA test available[26,209,374,375,471]

Persistent pupillary membrane[36]

Soft-Coated Wheaten Terrier

Cataracts[23,26,491]

Choroidal hypoplasia[110]

Corneal dystrophy[36]

Distichiasis[26]

Microphthalmia with multiple ocular anomalies[26,491]

Optic nerve hypoplasia[23]

Persistent hyaloid artery[26,491]

Persistent pupillary membranes[26,36,491]

Progressive retinal atrophy[27]

Retinal dysplasia: Retinal folds[26]

Spanish Water Dog

Persistent pupillary membranes[14]

Progressive retinal atrophy: Autosomal recessive prcd; DNA test available[58,73]

Spinone Italiano

Cataracts[26]

Distichia[21,47]

Ectropion[27]

Persistent pupillary membranes[36,48]

Spitz

Progressive retinal atrophy

Staffordshire Bull Terrier (English)

Cataracts (juvenile): Recessive trait suspected[26,78,79,83,88]

Distichiasis[48]

Entropion[27]

Lens luxation

Persistent hyaloid artery[48]

Persistent hyperplastic primary vitreous and lenticonus[26,81,82]

Persistent pupillary membranes[36,83]

Progressive retinal atrophy

Vitreous degeneration[14]

Sussex Spaniel

Cataracts

Distichiasis[83]

(*Continued*)

Table 15.2 (*Continued*) **Breed predisposition to eye disease in dogs.**

Ectropion[48]

Entropion[27]

Macroblepharon[83]

Iris coloboma[83]

Persistent hyaloid artery[48]

Retinal dysplasia: Retinal folds[23,27,48]

Swedish Lapphund

Progressive retinal atrophy: Autosomal recessive prcd; DNA test available[73]

Swedish Vallhund

Cataracts[33]

Corneal dystrophy[21]

Distichiasis[21,47]

Persistent pupillary membranes[36,48]

Retinal dysplasia[21]

Retinopathy: Presumed autosomal recessive; DNA test available[14,46,492,493]

Vitreous degeneration[33,110]

Swiss Hound

Progressive retinal atrophy (rare)[26]

Teddy Roosevelt Terrier

Lens luxation: DNA test available[20]

Tenterfield Terrier

Lens luxation: DNA test available[20]

Tibetan Mastiff

Persistent pupillary membranes[23]

Tibetan Spaniel

Cataracts[26]

Ceroid lipofuscinosis[494]

Distichiasis[26]

Entropion[26]

Exposure/pigmentary keratitis[31]

Micropapilla

Microphthalmia[23]

Persistent pupillary membranes[23,36,48]

Progressive retinal atrophy: Autosomal recessive; DNA test available[23,26,27,446,495]

Tibetan Terrier

Cataracts[26]

Central progressive retinal atrophy (rare)[23]

Ceroid lipofuscinosis[494,496]

Corneal dystrophy[36]

Distichiasis[26]

Lens luxation: Autosomal recessive trait suspected; DNA test available[15,18–20,26,375]

Persistent pupillary membranes[26,29,36]

Progressive retinal atrophy: DNA test available[26,85,495,497,498]

Nyctalopia: Autosomal recessive rcd4; DNA test available[497]

Progressive retinal atrophy (rod–cone dysplasia rcd4): Autosomal recessive; DNA test is available[86]

Retinal dysplasia: Geographic[27]

Vitreous degeneration[58]

Vizsla (Wirehaired)

Cataracts[26,27,306]

Corneal dystrophy: Epithelial/stromal[26]

Distichiasis[33]

Entropion[23,26]

Persistent pupillary membranes[26,36,83]

Prolapse of the gland of the third eyelid[31]

Progressive retinal atrophy

Vitreous degeneration[31]

Volpino Italiano

Lens luxation: DNA test availabale[20]

Weimaraner

Cataracts and retinal dysplasia[23,26]

Corneal dystrophy (1–8 years of age)[23,36,48]

Distichiasis[2,26]

Enlarged orbit

Entropion: Lower eyelid,[32] secondary to enlarged orbit/enophthalmos[26]

Eversion of the cartilage of the third eyelid[26]

Medial canthal pocket syndrome[23]

Persistent pupillary membranes[36]

Progressive retinal atrophy[23,26]

Refractory superficial corneal ulcer[23,174]

Welsh Springer Spaniel

Cataracts: Autosomal recessive trait[26,79,499]

Corneal dystrophy[36,83]

Distichiasis[26,27]

Entropion[36,83]

Glaucoma: Autosomal dominant trait[26,68,293,500]

Persistent pupillary membranes[23,26,36]

Progressive retinal atrophy (5–7 years of age)[26,107]

Retinal dysplasia[36]

Vitreous degeneration[33]

Welsh Terrier

Cataracts[23,26]

Distichiasis[26]

Glaucoma[26,293]

Keratoconjunctivitis sicca[26]

Lens luxation (secondary glaucoma): DNA test available[20,25,26,70,79,375]

Persistent pupillary membranes[26,36,48]

(*Continued*)

Table 15.2 (*Continued*) **Breed predisposition to eye disease in dogs.**

West Highland White Terrier

Cataracts: Autosomal recessive trait[26,501]

Keratoconjunctivitis sicca[26,190,191,502]

Lens luxation

Microphthalmia[23,26]

Persistent pupillary membranes[23,26,36]

Retinal atrophy (generalized)[26]

Retinal dysplasia: Retinal folds[26]

Vitreous degeneration[31]

Whippet

Cataracts[23,26,27]

Choroidal hypoplasia (Collie eye anomaly): Autosomal recessive; DNA test available[92,93]

    Staphyloma/coloboma

    Retinal detachment

    Retinal hemorrhage

    Optic nerve coloboma

Corneal stromal lipid dystrophy

Lens luxation (8–10 years of age)[1]

Micropapilla[23]

Persistent pupillary membrane[36,48]

Progressive retinal atrophy[503]

Vitreous degeneration[21,26,27,36]

Wirehaired Pointing Griffon

Corneal dystrophy[88]

Yorkshire Terrier

Cataracts (3–6 years of age)[26]

Corneal dystrophy: Epithelial/stromal[23,26,504]

Distichiasis[25,36]

Entropion

Keratoconjunctivitis sicca[26,505]

Lens luxation: DNA test available[17,20]

Ligneous conjunctivitis[506]

Persistent pupillary membranes[26,36]

Progressive retinal atrophy (5–11 years of age): DNA test available[2,23,26,27]

Retinal dysplasia: Geographic/detachment[23,504,507] (reported in Europe); hereditary/recessive trait suspected

Subepithelial geographic corneal dystrophy (in puppies)[2,23]

Table 15.3 **Breed predisposition to eye disease in cats.**

Abyssinian

Retinal degeneration[508,509]

Birman

Cataracts[510]

Corneal sequestrum[511]

Dermoid[512]

Burmese

Corneal sequestrum[511]

Dermoid[512]

Eyelid coloboma[513]

Glaucoma[514,515]

Third eyelid gland prolapse[513]

Uveal cysts[516]

Himalayan

Cataracts[517]

Corneal sequestration[511]

Manx

Corneal dystrophy[518]

Persian

Cataracts[519]

Corneal sequestration[511]

Eyelid coloboma[520]

Glaucoma[521]

Progressive retinal atrophy: Autosomal recessive[522,523]

Proliferative vitreoretinopathy[524]

Siamese

Corneal sequestration[511]

Lens luxation (primary)[525]

Open angle glaucoma[526]

Retinal dystrophy[527]

Somali

Multifocal retinal dysplasia[510]

Table 15.4 **Breed predisposition to eye disease in horses.**

American Saddlebred

Cataracts[528]

Appaloosa

Cataracts[529,530]

Congenital hypertropia[531]

Congenital stationary night blindness[532]

Equine recurrent uveitis[530]

Glaucoma optic disc coloboma

Iris hypoplasia[4]

Microphthalmos[4]

Scleral ectasia[4]

Arabian

Cataracts

Belgian Draft Horse

Aniridia (iris hypoplasia)[533,534]

Cataracts[70]

Limbal dermoid[4]

Comtois

Cataracts[535]

Cornea globosa[535]

Iridociliary cysts[535]

Iris stromal hypoplasia[535]

Retinal detachment[535]

Friesian

Corneal dystrophy (pellucid marginal degeneration)[536]

Icelandic Horses

Cataracts[537]

Iridociliary cysts[537]

Iris stromal hypoplasia[537]

Megaloglobus[537]

Pectinate ligament dysplasia[537]

Retinal dysplasia[537]

Kentucky Mountain Saddle Horse

Cataracts: Presumed semidominant

Choroidal hypoplasia

Ciliary body cyst[538]

Dyscoria: Presumed semidominant

Goniosynechiae /absence of iridocorneal angle/primary pectinate ligament dysplasia[4,539]

Iris coloboma

Iris hypoplasia: Presumed semidominant[538]

Hypertelorism

Macroblepharon

Macrocornea (cornea globosa): Presumed semidominant[538]

Microphthalmos with multiple ocular anomalies

Table 15.4 (*Continued*) **Breed predisposition to eye disease in horses.**

Miosis

Optic nerve hypoplasia

Persistent pupillary membranes

Lens subluxation

Retinal cyst

Retinal dysplasia: Presumed semidominant

Retinal detachment[538]

Retinal pigment epithelial proliferation ("high-water marker") of previous retinal detachment[539]

Vitreous degeneration

Miniature Horse

Cataracts: Presumed semidominant[540]

Choroidal hypoplasia

Ciliary body cyst[540]

Dyscoria: Presumed semidominant[539,540]

Goniosynechia/absence of iridocorneal angle/primary pectinate ligament dysplasia[4,539,540]

Hypertelorism

Iris coloboma

Iris cyst[540]

Iris hypoplasia: Presumed semidominant[540]

Lens subluxation

Macroblepharon

Macrocornea (cornea globosa): Presumed semidominant[539,540]

Macrophthalmos with multiple ocular anomalies

Miosis[540]

Optic nerve hypoplasia

Persistent pupillary membranes

Retinal cyst[540]

Retinal detachment

Retinal dysplasia: Presumed semidominant[540]

Retinal pigment epithelial proliferation ("high-water marker") of previous retinal detachment[539,540]

Vitreous degeneration

Morgan Horse

Cataracts, nuclear[541]

Glaucoma

Retinal dysplasia and detachment

Mountain Pleasure Horse

Cataracts: Presumed semidominant

Choroidal hypoplasia[539]

Ciliary body cyst

Dyscoria: Presumed semidominant

Goniosynechiae/absence of iridocorneal angle/primary pectinate ligament dysplasia[4,539]

Hypertelorism

(*Continued*)

Table 15.4 (*Continued*) **Breed predisposition to eye disease in horses.**
Iris coloboma
Iris hypoplasia: Presumed semidominant
Lens subluxation
Macroblepharon
Macrocornea (cornea globosa): Presumed semidominant[539]
Macrophthalmos with multiple ocular anomalies
Miosis
Optic nerve hypoplasia[4]
Persistent pupillary membranes
Retinal cyst
Retinal detachment
Retinal dysplasia: Presumed semidominant[4,539]
Retinal pigment epithelial proliferation ("high-water marker") of previous retinal detachment[539]
Vitreous degeneration
Paso Fino
Congenital stationary night blindness[542]
Glaucoma[528]
Quarter Horse
Cataracts[529,543]
Coloboma
Entropion
Iris hypoplasia (aniridia)[530]
Limbal dermoid[4]
Rocky Mountain Horse
Anterior segment dysgenesis[539]
Cataracts: Presumed semidominant[4,535,539]
Choroidal hypoplasia
Ciliary body cyst[535,538,539]
Dyscoria: Presumed semidominant
Goniosynechiae/absence of iridocorneal angle/primary pectinate ligament dysplasia[4,539]
Hypertelorism
Iris coloboma
Iris hypoplasia: Presumed semidominant[535,538,539]
Lens subluxation[539]
Macroblepharon[539]
Macrocornea (cornea globosa): Presumed semidominant[535,538,539]
Macrophthalmos with multiple ocular anomalies[539]
Miosis[539]
Optic nerve hypoplasia
Persistent pupillary membranes
Retinal cyst[539]
Retinal detachment[535,538,539]
Retinal dysplasia: Presumed semidominant[539]

Table 15.4 (*Continued*) **Breed predisposition to eye disease in horses.**
Retinal pigment epithelial proliferation ("high-water marker") of previous retinal detachment[4,539]
Vitreous degeneration
Shetland Pony
Cataracts: Presumed semidominant[4]
Choroidal hypoplasia
Ciliary body cyst
Dyscoria: Presumed semidominant
Goniosynechiae/absence of iridocorneal angle/primary pectinate ligament dysplasia[4,539]
Hypertelorism
Iris coloboma
Iris hypoplasia: Presumed semidominant
Lens subluxation
Macroblepharon
Macrocornea (cornea globosa): Presumed semidominant[539]
Macrophthalmos with multiple ocular anomalies
Miosis
Optic nerve hypoplasia
Persistent pupillary membranes
Retinal cyst
Retinal detachment
Retinal dysplasia: Presumed semidominant
Retinal pigment epithelial proliferation ("high-water marker") of previous retinal detachment[539]
Vitreous degeneration
Standardbred
Congenital stationary night blindness
Retinal detachments[528]
Thoroughbred
Cataracts: Presumed dominant trait[529,543]
Nuclear: Presumed dominant trait[4]
Entropion
Microphthalmia associated with multiple ocular anomalies
Progressive retinal atrophy[532,544]
Retinal dysplasia and detachment[544]
Warmbloods
Glaucoma[528]
Pigment retinopathy[545]

Table 15.5 Breed disposition to eye disease in cattle.
Aberdeen Angus
Heterochromia iridis
Retinitis pigmentosa-1 (RP1)[546]
Abondance
Retinitis pigmentosa-1 (RP1)[546]
Austrian Murboden
Heterochromia iridis[547]
Ayrshire
Esotropia[548–550]
Heterochromia iridis[547]
Beef Booster Composite
Retinitis pigmentosa-1 (RP1)[546]
Belgian Blue
Retinitis pigmentosa-1 (RP1)[546]
Brown Swiss (Braunvieh)
Esotropia[549,550]
Heterochromia iridis[547]
Supernumerary openings of the nasolacrimal system[551]
Charolais
Coloboma[552,553]
Retinitis pigmentosa-1 (RP1)[546]
Gelbvieh
Retinitis pigmentosa-1 (RP1)[546]
Guernsey
Heterochromia iridis[547]
Hereford
Coloboma with albinism[554]
Congenital cataracts[555]
Dermoid[556]
Retinal dysplasia

Table 15.5 (*Continued*) Breed disposition to eye disease in cattle.
Holstein
Esotropia[548–550]
Heterochromia iridis[547]
Lenticular coloboma[557]
Nuclear cataracts[557]
Persistent pupillary membranes[557]
Iris to lens
Posterior lenticonus[557]
Retinitis pigmentosa-1 (RP1)[546]
Holstein–Friesian
Congenital cataracts[555]
Jersey
Aniridia
Congenital cataracts: Autosomal recessive[555]
Convergent strabismus with exophthalmia: Recessive[548,550,558]
Microphthalmia
Multiple ocular anomalies[559]
Maine Anjou
Retinitis pigmentosa-1 (RP1)[546]
Montbeliarde
Retinitis pigmentosa-1 (RP1)[546]
Normande
Retinitis pigmentosa-1 (RP1)[546]
Red Angus
Retinitis pigmentosa-1 (RP1)[546]
Shorthorn
Convergent strabismus with exophthalmia[548,550,558]
Multiple ocular anomalies[560–562]
Retinal dysplasia with multiple ocular anomalies[560,561]
Vosgienne
Retinitis pigmentosa-1 (RP1)[546]

ACKNOWLEDGMENTS

This chapter was made possible in part by the previous contributions of R. David Whitley and Kristina R. Vyganta, as well as, Raymond and Margaret Hammond, Ponte Vedra Beach, FL; the K-9 Obedience Club of Jacksonville, Jacksonville, FL; Seminole Dog Fanciers Association, Longwood, FL; Greater Orange Park Dog Club, Orange Park, FL; Greater Daytona Dog Fanciers Association, Daytona Beach, FL; Brevard Kennel Club, Coca, FL; Treasure Coast Kennel Club of Florida, Fort Pierce, FL; and Okaloosa Kennel Club, Fort Walton Beach, FL. Current additions to this book have been made possible by the continuous contributions and additions of ocular diseases proven or suspected to be inherited in purebred dogs by the Genetics Committee of the ACVO and the Orthopedic Foundation for Animals (OFA), Canine Eye Registration Foundation (CERF).

REFERENCES

1. Whitley, R.D. 1988. Focusing on eye disorders among purebred dogs. *Veterinary Medicine* 83:50–63.
2. Whitley, R.D., McLaughlin, S., and Gilger, B. 1995. Update on eye disorders among purebred dogs. *Veterinary Medicine*.
3. American College of Veterinary Ophthalmologists. Orthopedic Foundation for Animals (OFA)—Eye Certification Registry Information ACVO Website2017. Available from: acvo.org.

4. ACVO Genetics Committee, editor. 1999. *Ocular Disorders Presumed to Be Inherited in Purebred Horses.* Equine Eye Registration Foundation: Baton Rouge, LA.

5. Mostoskey, U.V., Padgett, G.A., Stinson, A.W., Brewer, G.J., and Duffendack, J.C. 2000. Canine molecular genetic diseases. *Compendium on Continuing Education for the Practising Veterinarian.* 22(5):480-+.

6. Aguirre, G., and Rubin, L. 1975. Rod-cone dysplasia (progressive retinal atrophy) in Irish Setters. *Journal of the American Veterinary Medical Association.* 166(2):157.

7. Aguirre, G., Farber, D., Lolley, R., O'Brien, P., Alligood, J., Fletcher, R.T. et al. 1982. Retinal degenerations in the dog III. abnormal cyclic nucleotide metabolism in rod-cone dysplasia. *Experimental Eye Research.* 35(6):625–642.

8. Petersen-Jones, S.M., Entz, D.D., and Sargan, D.R. 1999. cGMP phosphodiesterase-α mutation causes progressive retinal atrophy in the Cardigan Welsh Corgi dog. *Investigative Ophthalmology & Visual Science.* 40(8):1637–1644.

9. Petersen-Jones, S.M., and Zhu, F.X. 2000. Development and use of a polymerase chain reaction-based diagnostic test for the causal mutation of progressive retinal atrophy in Cardigan Welsh Corgis. *American Journal of Veterinary Research.* 61(7):844–846.

10. Aguirre, G.D., Baldwin, V., Pearce-Kelling, S., Narfström, K., Ray, K., and Acland, GM. 1998. Congenital stationary night blindness in the dog: common mutation in the RPE65 gene indicates founder effect. *Molecular Vision.* 4:23.

11. Narfstrom, K., Wrigstad, A., Ekesten, B., and Nilsson, S. 1994. Hereditary retinal dystrophy in the Briard dog: Clinical and hereditary characteristics. *Progress in Veterinary & Comparative Ophthalmology.*

12. Downs, L.M., Hitti, R., Pregnolato, S., and Mellersh, C.S. 2014. Genetic screening for PRA-associated mutations in multiple dog breeds shows that PRA is heterogeneous within and between breeds. *Veterinary Ophthalmology.* 17(2):126–130.

13. Miyadera, K., Acland, G.M., and Aguirre, G.D. 2012. Genetic and phenotypic variations of inherited retinal diseases in dogs: the power of within-and across-breed studies. *Mammalian Genome.* 23(1–2):40–61.

14. ACVO Genetics Committee, editor 2015 and/or Data from OFA All-Breeds Report, 2014–2015. The Blue Book: Ocular Disorders Presumed to be Inherited in Purebred Dogs. 2015. 8th edition. *ACVO Annual Conference*; 2015; Coeur d'Alene, ID.

15. Sargan, D.R., Withers, D., Pettitt, L., Squire, M., Gould, D.J., and Mellersh, C.S. 2007. Mapping the mutation causing lens luxation in several terrier breeds. *Journal of Heredity.* 98(5):534–538.

16. Curtis, R., Barnett, K., and Startup, F. 1983. Primary lens luxation in the Miniature Bull Terrier. *The Veterinary Record.* 112(14):328–330.

17. Farias, F.H., Johnson, G.S., Taylor, J.F., Giuliano, E., Katz, M.L., Sanders, D.N. et al. 2010. An ADAMTS17 splice donor site mutation in dogs with primary lens luxation. *Investigative Ophthalmology & Visual Science.* 51(9):4716–4721.

18. Willis, M., Curtis, R., Barnett, K., and Tempest, W. 1979. Genetic aspects of lens luxation in the Tibetan Terrier. *The Veterinary Record.* 104(18):409–412.

19. Curtis, R. 1983. Aetiopathological aspects of inherited lens dislocation in the Tibetan Terrier. *Journal of Comparative Pathology.* 93(1):151–163.

20. Gould, D., Pettitt, L., McLaughlin, B., Holmes, N., Forman, O., Thomas, A. et al. 2011. ADAMTS17 mutation associated with primary lens luxation is widespread among breeds. *Veterinary Ophthalmology.* 14(6):378–384.

21. ACVO Genetics Committee, editor 2008 and/or Data from CERF All-Breeds Report, 2003–2007. The Blue Book: Ocular Disorders Presumed to Be Inherited in Purebred Dogs. 2015, 8th edition. *ACVO Annual Conference*; 2008; Boston, MA.

22. ACVO Genetics Committee, editor, 2011 and/or Data from CERF All-Breeds Report, 2009. The Blue Book: Ocular Disorders Presumed to Be Inherited in Purebred Dogs. 2011 *ACVO Annual Conference*; 2011, 2015; Hilton Head, SC.

23. Rubin, L.F. 1989. *Inherited Eye Diseases in Purebred Dogs.* Williams and Wilkins, Baltimore, MD.

24. Roberts, S., and Helper, L. 1972. Cataracts in Afghan hounds. *Journal of the American Veterinary Medical Association.* 160(4):427–432.

25. Blogg, J.R. 1980. *The Eye in Veterinary Practice. Volume I. Extraocular Disease Appendix A.* WB Saunders: London.

26. ACVO Genetics Committee, editor 1999 and/or Data from CERF All-Breeds Report, 1991–1998. The Blue Book: Ocular Disorders Presumed to be Inherited in Purebred Dogs. 2015, 8th edition. *ACVO Annual Conference*; 1999; Chicago, IL.

27. ACVO Genetics Committee, editor Ocular Disorders Proven or suspected to be Hereditary in Dogs. The Blue Book: Ocular Disorders Presumed to be Inherited in Purebred Dogs. 2015, 8th edition. *ACVO Annual Conference*; 1992; Baton Rouge, LA.

28. Brooks, D. 1986. Canine and feline glaucomas. In: Kirk, R.W. editor. *Current Veterinary Therapy IX (Small Animal Practice).* IX edition. WB Saunders: Philadelphia, PA, pp. 656–659.

29. Slatter, D. 2001. *Appendix 1. Fundamentals of Veterinary Ophthalmology.* 3rd edition. WB Saunders: Philadelphia, PA, pp. 609–616.

30. Gelatt, K. 1991. *Textbook of Veterinary Ophthalmology.* 2nd edition. Lea & Febiger: Philadelphia, PA.

31. ACVO Genetics Committee, editor 2014 and/or Data from OFA/CERF All-Breeds Report, 2013–2014. The Blue Book: Ocular Disorders Presumed to be Inherited in Purebred Dogs. 2015, 8th edition. *ACVO Annual Conference*; 2014; Fort Worth, TX.

32. Bistner, S.I., Aguirre, G., and Batik, G. 1977. *Appendix 1: Atlas of Veterinary Ophthalmic Surgery.* WB Saunders, Philadelphia, PA, pp. 279–290.

33. ACVO Genetics Committee, editor 2006 and/or Data from CERF All-Breeds 2001–2005. The Blue Book: Ocular Disorders Presumed to be Inherited in Purebred Dogs. 2015, 8th edition. *ACVO Annual Conference*; 2006; San Antonio, TX.

34. Startup, F. 1986. Hereditary eye problems in the Japanese Akita. *The Veterinary Record.* 118(9):251.

35. Laratta, L., Riis, R., Kern, T., and Koch, S. 1985. Multiple congenital ocular defects in the Akita dog. *The Cornell Veterinarian.* 75(3):381.

36. ACVO Genetics Committee, editor 2005 and/or Data from CERF All-Breeds Report 2003–2004. The Blue Book: Ocular Disorders Presumed to be Inherited in Purebred Dogs. 2015, 8th edition. *ACVO Annual Conference*; 2005; Nashville, TN.

37. Toole, D., and Roberts, S. 1984. Generalized progressive retinal atrophy in two Akita dogs. *Veterinary Pathology.* 21(5):457–462.

38. Allgoewer, I., Blair, M., Basher, T., Davidson, M., Hamilton, H., Jandeck, C. et al. 2000. Extraocular muscle

myositis and restrictive strabismus in 10 dogs. *Veterinary Ophthalmology.* 3(1):21–26.

39. Kern, T., Walton, D., Riis, R., Manning, T., Laratta, L., and Dziezyc, J. 1985. Uveitis associated with poliosis and vitiligo in six dogs. *Journal of the American Veterinary Medical Association.* 187(4):408–414.

40. Bussanich, M., Rootman, J., and Dolman, C. 1982. Granulomatous pan uveitis and dermal depigmentation in dogs. *Journal of the American Animal Hospital Association.* 22:121–124.

41. Romatowski, J. 1985. A uveodermatological syndrome in an Akita dog. *Journal of the American Animal Hospital Association.* 21:777–780.

42. Campbell, K., McLaughlin, S., and Reynolds, H. 1986. Generalized leukoderma and poliosis following uveitis in a dog. *Journal of the American Animal Hospital Association.* 22(1):121–124.

43. Bellhorn, R.W., Murphy, C.J., and Thirkill, C.E., editors. 1988. Anti-retinal immunoglobulins in canine ocular diseases. *Seminars in Veterinary Medicine and Surgery (Small Animal),* 3:28–32.

44. Murphy, C.J., Bellhorn, R., and Thirkill, C. 1991. Anti-retinal antibodies associated with Vogt-Koyanagi-Harada-like syndrome in a dog. *Journal of the American Animal Hospital Association.* 27(4):399–402.

45. Morgan, R. 1989. Vogt-Koyanagi-Harada syndrome in humans and dogs. *Compendium on Continuing Education for the Practising Veterinarian.*

46. ACVO Genetics Committee, editor 2011 and/or Data from CERF All-Breeds Report, 2010. The Blue Book: Ocular Disorders Presumed to be Inherited in Purebred Dogs. 2015, 8th edition. *ACVO Annual Conference*; 2011; Hilton Head, SC.

47. ACVO Genetics Committee, editor 2007 and/or Data from CERF All-Breeds Report 2002–2006. The Blue Book: Ocular Disorders Presumed to be Inherited in Purebred Dogs. 2015, 8th edition. *ACVO Annual Conference*; 2007; Kona, HI.

48. ACVO Genetics Committee, editor 2000–2002 and/or Data from CERF All-Breeds Report, 2000–2002. The Blue Book: Ocular Disorders Presumed to be Inherited in Purebred Dogs. 2015, 8th edition. *ACVO Annual Conference*; 2002; Denver, CO.

49. Rubin, L. 1971. Hemeralopia in Alaskan Malamute pups. *Journal of the American Veterinary Medical Association.*

50. Rubin, L. 1971. Clinical features of hemeralopia in the adult Alaskan Malamute. *Journal of the American Veterinary Medical Association.* 158(10):1696–1698.

51. Aguirre, G., and Rubin, L. 1974. Pathology of hemeralopia in the Alaskan Malamute dog. *Investigative Ophthalmology & Visual Science.* 13(3):231–235.

52. Aguirre, G., and Rubin, L. 1975. The electroretinogram in dogs with inherited cone degeneration. *Investigative Ophthalmology & Visual Science.* 14(11):840–847.

53. Seddon, J., Hampson, E., Smith, R., and Hughes, I. 2006. Genetic heterogeneity of day blindness in Alaskan Malamutes. *Animal Genetics.* 37(4):407–410.

54. Sidjanin, D.J., Lowe, J.K., McElwee, J.L., Milne, B.S., Phippen, T.M., Sargan, D.R. et al. 2002. Canine CNGB3 mutations establish cone degeneration as orthologous to the human achromatopsia locus ACHM3. *Human Molecular Genetics.* 11(16):1823–1833.

55. Awano, T., Katz, M.L., O'Brien, D.P., Sohar, I., Lobel, P., Coates, J.R. et al. 2006. A frame shift mutation in canine TPP1 (the ortholog of human CLN2) in a juvenile Dachshund with neuronal ceroid lipofuscinosis. *Molecular Genetics and Metabolism.* 89(3):254–260.

56. Awano, T., Katz, M.L., O'Brien, D.P., Taylor, J.F., Evans, J., Khan, S. et al. 2006. A mutation in the cathepsin D gene (CTSD) in American Bulldogs with neuronal ceroid lipofuscinosis. *Molecular Genetics and Metabolism.* 87(4):341–348.

57. Evans, J., Katz, M.L., Levesque, D., Shelton, G.D., Lahunta, A., and O'Brien, D. 2005. A variant form of neuronal ceroid lipofuscinosis in American Bulldogs. *Journal of Veterinary Internal Medicine.* 19(1):44–51.

58. ACVO Genetics Committee, editor 2013–2014 and Data from OFA All-Breeds Report, 2013–2014. The Blue Book: Ocular Disorders Presumed to be Inherited in Purebred Dogs. 2015, 8th edition. *ACVO Annual Conference*; 2013; Rio Mar Beach, Puerto Rico.

59. Pumphrey, S.A., Pizzirani, S., Pirie, C.G., and Needle, D.B. 2013. Glaucoma associated with uveal cysts and goniodysgenesis in American Bulldogs: A case series. *Veterinary Ophthalmology.* 16(5):377–385.

60. Guziewicz, K.E., Zangerl, B., Lindauer, S.J., Mullins, R.F., Sandmeyer, L.S., Grahn, B.H. et al. 2007. Bestrophin gene mutations cause canine multifocal retinopathy: a novel animal model for best disease. *Investigative Ophthalmology & Visual Science.* 48(5):1959–1967.

61. Olesen, H., Jensen, O., and Norn, M. 1974. Congenital hereditary cataract in Cocker Spaniels. *Journal of Small Animal Practice.* 15(12):741–750.

62. Yakely, W. 1978. A study of heritability of cataracts in the American Cocker Spaniel [Dogs]. *Journal of the American Veterinary Medical Association.*

63. Williams, L., Peiffer Jr., R., Gelatt, K., and Gum, G. 1979. A survey of ocular findings in the American Cocker Spaniel [Dogs]. *Journal of the American Animal Hospital Association.*

64. Gelatt, K.N., and MacKay, E.O. 2005. Prevalence of primary breed-related cataracts in the dog in North America. *Veterinary Ophthalmology.* 8(2):101–111.

65. Barnett, K.C. 1976. Comparative aspects of canine hereditary eye disease. *Advances in Veterinary Science and Comparative Medicine.*

66. Bedford, P. 1979. The treatment of canine distichiasis by the method of partial tarsal plate excision. *Journal of the American Animal Hospital Association.*

67. Lavach, J., and Gelatt, K. 1979. Diseases of the eyelids (Part II). *Compendium on Continuing Education for the Practising Veterinarian.* 1:485–492.

68. Gelatt, K.N., and MacKay, E.O. 2004. Prevalence of the breed-related glaucomas in pure-bred dogs in North America. *Veterinary Ophthalmology.* 7(2):97–111.

69. Lovekin, L.G., and Belhorn R. 1968. Clinicopathologic changes in primary glaucoma in Cocker Spaniel. *American Journal of Veterinary Research.* 29(2):379–&.

70. Slatter, D. 2001. *Lens. Fundamentals of Veterinary Ophthalmology.* 3rd edition. WB Saunders: Philadelphia, PA, pp. 393–410.

71. Barnett, K. 1965. Canine retinopathies III. The other breeds. *Journal of Small Animal Practice.* **6**(3):185–196.

72. Aguirre, G.D., and Acland, G.M. 1988. Variation in retinal degeneration phenotype inherited at the prcd locus. *Experimental Eye Research.* 46(5):663–687.

73. Zangerl, B., Goldstein, O., Philp, A.R., Lindauer, S.J., Pearce-Kelling, S.E., Mullins, R.F. et al. 2006. Identical mutation in a novel retinal gene causes progressive rod–cone degeneration in dogs and retinitis pigmentosa in humans. *BMC Genomics.* 88(5):551–563.

74. Morgan, R., Duddy, J., and McClurg, K. 1993. Prolapse of the gland of the third eyelid in dogs: a retrospective study of 89 cases (1980 to 1990). *Journal of the American Animal Hospital Association.*

75. MacMillan, A., and Lipton, D. 1978. Heritability of multifocal retinal dysplasia in American Cocker Spaniels. *Journal of the American Veterinary Medical Association.* 172(5):568–572.

76. Goldstein, O., Mezey, J.G., Schweitzer, P.A., Boyko, A.R., Gao, C., Bustamante, C.D. et al. 2013. IQCB1 and PDE6B mutations cause similar early onset retinal degenerations in two closely related Terrier dog breeds retinal degenerations and terrier dog breeds. *Investigative Ophthalmology & Visual Science.* 54(10):7005–7019.

77. Kijas, J.K., Zangerl, B., Miller, B., Nelson, J., Kirkness, E.F., Aguirre, G.D. et al. 2004. Cloning of the canine ABCA4 gene and evaluation in canine cone-rod dystrophies and progressive retinal atrophies. *Molecular Vision.* 10:223.

78. Barnett, K. 1978. Hereditary cataract in the dog. *Journal of Small Animal Practice.* 19(1–12):109–120.

79. Barnett, K. 1985. The diagnosis and differential diagnosis of cataract in the dog. *Journal of Small Animal Practice.* 26(6):305–316.

80. Siso, S., Navarro, C., Hanzlíček, D., and Vandevelde, M. 2004. Adult onset thalamocerebellar degeneration in dogs associated to neuronal storage of ceroid lipopigment. *Acta Neuropathologica.* 108(5):386–392.

81. Leon, A., Curtis, R., and Barnett, K. 1986. Hereditary persistent hyperplastic primary vitreous in the Staffordshire Bull Terrier. *Journal of the American Animal Hospital Association.* 22(6):765–774.

82. Curtis, R., Barnett, K., and Leon, A. 1984. Persistent hyperplastic primary vitreous in the Staffordshire Bull Terrier. *The Veterinary Record.* 115(15):385.

83. ACVO Genetics Committee, editor 2002–2003 and/or Data from CERF All-Breeds Report, 2002–2003. The Blue Book: Ocular Disorders Presumed to be Inherited in Purebred Dogs. 2015, 8th edition. *ACVO Annual Conference*; 2003 Coeur d'Alene, ID.

84. Wood, P.A., Sisk, D.B., Styer, E., Baker, H.J., and Prieur, D.J. 1987. Animal model: Ceroidosis (ceroid-lipofuscinosis) in Australian Cattle dogs. *American Journal of Medical Genetics. Part A.* 26(4):891–898.

85. Dekomien, G., and Epplen, J. 2000. Exclusion of the PDE6A gene for generalised progressive retinal atrophy in 11 breeds of dog. *Animal Genetics.* 31(2):135–139.

86. Downs, L., Bell, J., Freeman, J., Hartley, C., Hayward, L., and Mellersh C. 2013. Late-onset progressive retinal atrophy in the Gordon and Irish Setter breeds is associated with a frameshift mutation in C2orf71. *Animal Genetics.* 44(2):169–177.

87. Mellersh, C.S., Pettitt, L., Forman, O.P., Vaudin, M., and Barnett, K.C. 2006. Identification of mutations in HSF4 in dogs of three different breeds with hereditary cataracts. *Veterinary Ophthalmology.* 9(5):369–378.

88. Mellersh, C.S., McLaughlin, B., Ahonen, S., Pettitt, L., Lohi, H., and Barnett, K.C. 2009. Mutation in HSF4 is associated with hereditary cataract in the Australian Shepherd. *Veterinary Ophthalmology.* 12(6):372–378.

89. Katz, M.L., Farias, F.H., Sanders, D.N., Zeng, R., Khan, S., Johnson, G.S. et al. 2010. A missense mutation in canine CLN6 in an Australian Shepherd with neuronal ceroid lipofuscinosis. *BioMed Research International.* 2011:1–6.

90. O'Brien, D., and Katz, M. 2008. Neuronal ceroid lipofuscinosis in 3 Australian shepherd littermates. *Journal of Veterinary Internal Medicine.* 22(2):472–475.

91. Rubin, L., Nelson, B., and Sharp, C. 1991. Collie eye anomaly in Australian Shepherd dogs. *Progress in Veterinary & Comparative Ophthalmology.* 1:105–108.

92. Lowe, J.K., Kukekova, A.V., Kirkness, E.F., Langlois, M.C., Aguirre, G.D., Acland, G.M. et al. 2003. Linkage mapping of the primary disease locus for Collie eye anomaly. *BMC Genomics.* 82(1):86–95.

93. Parker, H.G., Kukekova, A.V., Akey, D.T., Goldstein, O., Kirkness, E.F., Baysac, K.C. et al. 2007. Breed relationships facilitate fine-mapping studies: a 7.8-kb deletion cosegregates with Collie eye anomaly across multiple dog breeds. *Genome Research.* 17(11):1562–1571.

94. Munyard, K.A., Sherry, C.R., and Sherry, L. 2007. A retrospective evaluation of congenital ocular defects in Australian Shepherd dogs in Australia. *Veterinary Ophthalmology.* 10(1):19–22.

95. Gelatt, K., Powell, N., and Huston, K. 1981. Inheritance of microphthalmia with coloboma in the Australian Shepherd dog. *American Journal of Veterinary Research.* 42(10):1686–1690.

96. ACVO Genetics Committee, editor 2003–2004 and/or Data from CERF All-Breeds Report, 2005. The Blue Book: Ocular Disorders Presumed to be Inherited in Purebred Dogs. 2015, 8th edition. *ACVO Annual Conference*; 2004; Washington, DC.

97. Gelatt, K., and Veith, L. 1970. Hereditary multiple ocular anomalies in Australian Shepherd dogs. *Veterinary Medicine, Small Animal Clinician.* 65:39–42.

98. Gelatt, K., and McGill, L. 1973. Clinical characteristics of microphthalmia with colobomas of the Australian Shepherd Dog. *Journal of the American Veterinary Medical Association.* 162(5):393–396.

99. Bertram, T., Coignoul, F., and Cheville, N. 1984. Ocular dysgenesis in Australian Shepherd dogs. *Journal of the American Animal Hospital Association.* 20(1):177–182.

100. Cook, C., Burling, K., and Nelson, E. 1991. Embryogenesis of posterior segment colobomas in the Australian Shepherd dog. *Progress in Veterinary & Comparative Ophthalmology.* 1:163–170.

101. Nelson, D., and MacMillan, A. 1986. Diseases of the cornea. In: R.W. Kirk (editor), *Current Veterinary Therapy IX: Small Animal Practice.* WB Saunders: Philadelphia, PA, pp. 642–649.

102. Hoffmann, I., Guziewicz, K.E., Zangerl, B., Aguirre, G.D., and Mardin, C.Y. 2012. Canine multifocal retinopathy in the Australian Shepherd: A case report. *Veterinary Ophthalmology.* 15(S2):134–138.

103. Barnett, K., and Knight, G. 1969. Persistent pupillary membrane and associated defects in the Basenji. *The Veterinary Record.* 85(9):242–248.

104. Bistner, S., Rubin, L., and Roberts, S. 1971. A review of persistent pupillary membranes in the Basenji dog. *Animal Hospital.*

105. Roberts, S.R., and Bistner, S. 1968. Persistent pupillary membrane in Basenji dogs. *Journal of the American Veterinary Medical Association.* 153(5):533–542.

106. Mason, T. 1976. Persistent pupillary membrane in the Basenji. *Australian Veterinary Journal.* 52(8):343–344.

107. Priester, W. 1974. Canine progressive retinal atrophy: occurrence by age, breed, and sex. *American Journal of Veterinary Research.*

108. Goldstein, O., Jordan, J.A., Aguirre, G.D., and Acland, G.M. 2013. A non-stop S-antigen gene mutation is associated with late onset hereditary retinal degeneration in dogs. *Molecular Vision*. 18:1871.

109. Priester, W. 1972. Congenital ocular defects in cattle, horses, cats, and dogs. *Journal of the American Veterinary Medical Association*. 160(11):1504–1511.

110. ACVO Genetics Committee, editor 2009 and/or Data from CERF All-Breeds Report, 2008. The Blue Book: Ocular Disorders Presumed to be Inherited in Purebred Dogs. 2015, 8th edition. *ACVO Annual Conference*; 2009; Chicago, IL.

111. Wyman, M. 1986. *Manual of Small Animal Ophthalmology*. Churchill Livingstone, New York.

112. Wyman, M., and Ketring, K. 1976. Congenital glaucoma in the Basset Hound: a biologic model. *American Academy of Ophthalmology and Otolaryngology*. 81(4 Pt 1):OP645.

113. Ahram, D.F., Cook, A.C., Kecova, H., Grozdanic, S.D., and Kuehn, M.H. 2014. Identification of genetic loci associated with primary angle-closure glaucoma in the Basset Hound. *Molecular Vision*. (20):497–510.

114. Ahram, D.F., Grozdanic, S.D., Kecova, H., Henkes, A., Collin, R.W., and Kuehn, M.H. 2015. Variants in nebulin (NEB) are linked to the development of familial primary angle closure glaucoma in basset hounds. *PloS One*. 10(5):e0126660.

115. Bedford, P. 1980. The aetiology of canine glaucoma. *The Veterinary Record*. 107(4):76–82.

116. Bedford, P. 1977. A gonioscopic study of the iridocorneal angle in the English and American breeds of Cocker Spaniel and the Basset Hound. *Journal of Small Animal Practice*. 18(10):631–642.

117. Slater, M., and Erb, H. 1986. Effects of risk factors and prophylactic treatment on primary glaucoma in the dog. *Journal of the American Veterinary Medical Association*. 188(9):1028–1030.

118. Martin, C., and Wyman, M. 1968. Glaucoma in the Basset Hound. *Journal of the American Veterinary Medical Association*. 153(10):1320.

119. Oliver, J.A., Forman, O.P., Pettitt, L., and Mellersh, C.S. 2015. Two independent mutations in ADAMTS17 are associated with primary open angle glaucoma in the Basset Hound and Basset Fauve de Bretagne breeds of dog. *PloS One*. 10(10):e0140436.

120. Heywood, R. 1971. Juvenile cataracts in the Beagle dog. *Journal of Small Animal Practice*. 12(3):171–177.

121. Hirth, R., Greenstein, E., and Peer, R. 1974. Anterior capsular opacities (spurious cataracts) in Beagle dogs. *Veterinary Pathology*. 11(2):181–194.

122. American Kennel Club. 1989. *American Kennel Club Genetic Disease Registry*. University of Pennsylvania, Pennsylvania.

123. Roth, A.M., Ekins, M.B., Waring, G., Gupta, L.M., and Rosenblatt, L. 1981. Oval corneal opacities in Beagles. III. Histochemical demonstration of stromal lipids without hyperlipidemia. *Investigative Ophthalmology & Visual Science*. 21(1):95–106.

124. Ekins, M.B., Sgoutas, D.S., Waring, G.O., and Kanes, G.J. 1983. Oval lipid corneal opacities in Beagles: VI. Quantitation of excess stromal cholesterol and phospholipid. *Experimental Eye Research*. 36(2):279–286.

125. Morrin, L., Waring III, G., and Spangler, W. 1982. Oval lipid corneal opacities in Beagles: ultrastructure of normal Beagle cornea. *American Journal of Veterinary Research*. 43(3):443–453.

126. Spangler, W., Waring, G., and Morrin, L. 1982. Oval lipid corneal opacities in Beagles: V. Ultrastructure. *Veterinary Pathology*. 19(2):150–159.

127. Waring, G., Ekins, M., Spangler, W., Roth, A., and MacMillan, A. 1979. Oval lipid corneal opacities in Beagles and crystalline lipid corneal opacities in Siberian Huskies. *Metabolic and Pediatric Ophthalmology*. 3(2-4):203–&.

128. Kondo, M., Das, G., Imai, R., Santana, E., Nakashita, T., Imawaka, M. et al. 2015. A naturally occurring canine model of autosomal recessive congenital stationary night blindness. *PloS One*. 10(9):e0137072.

129. Andersen, A., and Shultz, F.T. 1958. Inherited (congenital) cataract in the dog. *American Journal of Pathology*. 34(5):965.

130. Roberts, S., Severin, G., and Lavach, J. 1986. Prevalence and treatment of palpebral neoplasms in the dog: 200 cases (1975–1983). *Journal of the American Veterinary Medical Association*. 189(10):1355–1359.

131. Gelatt, K., and Gum, G. 1981. Inheritance of primary glaucoma in the Beagle. *American Journal of Veterinary Research*. 42(10):1691–1693.

132. Gelatt, K. 1972. Familial glaucoma in the Beagle dog. *Animal Hospital*.

133. Gelatt, K.N., Peiffer, R., Gwin, R.M., Gum, G.G., and Williams, L.W. 1977. Clinical manifestations of inherited glaucoma in the Beagle. *Investigative Ophthalmology & Visual Science*. 16(12):1135–1142.

134. Peiffer Jr., R., Gum, G., Grimson, R., and Gelatt, K. 1980. Aqueous humor outflow in Beagles with inherited glaucoma: Constant pressure perfusion. *American Journal of Veterinary Research*. 41(11):1808–1813.

135. Brooks, D., Samuelson, D., and Gelatt, K. 1989. Ultrastructural changes in laminar optic nerve capillaries of Beagles with primary open-angle glaucoma. *American Journal of Veterinary Research*. 50(6):929–935.

136. Brooks, D., Samuelson, D., Gelatt, K., and Smith, P. 1989. Morphologic changes in the lamina cribrosa of Beagles with primary open-angle glaucoma. *American Journal of Veterinary Research*. 50(6):936–941.

137. Samuelson, D.A., Gum, G.G., and Gelatt, K. 1989. Ultrastructural changes in the aqueous outflow apparatus of Beagles with inherited glaucoma. *Investigative Ophthalmology & Visual Science*. 30(3):550–561.

138. Brooks, D.E., Strubbe, D.T., Kubilis, P.S., MacKay, E.O., Samuelson, D.A., and Gelatt, K.N. 1995. Histomorphometry of the optic nerves of normal dogs and dogs with hereditary glaucoma. *Experimental Eye Research*. 60(1):71–89.

139. Gum, G., Gelatt, K., and Knepper, P. 1993. Histochemical localization of glycosaminoglycans in the aqueous outflow pathways in normal Beagles and Beagles with inherited glaucoma. *Progress in Veterinary & Comparative Ophthalmology*. 3(2):52–57.

140. Gelatt, K., Gum, G., Mackay, E., and Gelatt, K. 1996. Estimations of aqueous humor outflow facility by pneumatonography in normal, genetic carrier and glaucomatous Beagles. *Progress in Veterinary & Comparative Ophthalmology*.

141. Kuchtey, J., Olson, L.M., Rinkoski, T., MacKay, E.O., Iverson, T., Gelatt, K.N. et al. 2011. Mapping of the disease locus and identification of ADAMTS10 as a candidate gene in a canine model of primary open angle glaucoma. *PLoS Genetics*. 7(2):e1001306.

142. Bellhorn, R.W., Bellhorn, M.B., Swarm, R.L., and Impellizzeri, C.W. 1975. Hereditary tapetal abnormality in the Beagle. *Ophthalmic Research*. 7(4):250–260.

143. Wen, G.Y., Sturman, J.A., Wisniewski, H.M., MacDonald, A., and Niemann, W.H. 1982. Chemical and ultrastructural changes in tapetum of Beagles with a hereditary abnormality. *Investigative Ophthalmology & Visual Science.* 23(6):733–742.

144. Burns, M.S., Tyler, N.K., and Bellhorn, R.W. 1988. Melanosome abnormalities of ocular pigmented epithelial cells in Beagle dogs with hereditary tapetal degeneration. *Current Eye Research.* 7(2):115–123.

145. Burns, M.S., Bellhorn, R.W., Impellizzeri, C.W., Aguirre, G.D., and Laties, A.M. 1988. Development of hereditary tapetal degeneration in the Beagle dog. *Current Eye Research.* 7(2):103–114.

146. Bedford, P. 1982. Multifocal retinal dysplasia in the Rottweiler. *The Veterinary Record.* 111(13):304–305.

147. Rubin, L.F., Koch, S.A., and Huber, R. 1969. Hereditary cataracts in Miniature Schnauzers. *Journal of the American Veterinary Medical Association.*

148. Barnett, K. 1979. Imperforate and micro-lachrymal puncta in the dog. *Journal of Small Animal Practice.* 20(8):481–490.

149. Rubin, L. 1968. Heredity of retinal dysplasia in Bedlington Terriers. *Journal of the American Veterinary Medical Association.* 152(3):260–&.

150. Rubin, L. 1963. Hereditary retinal detachment in Bedlington Terriers. *A Preliminary Report Small Animal Clinician.* 3:387–389.

151. Hogan, D., and Williams, R.W. 1995. Analysis of the retinas and optic nerves of achiasmatic Belgian Sheepdogs. *Journal of Comparative Neurology.* 352(3):367–380.

152. Slatter, D.H., and Lavach, J. 1977. Überreiter's syndrome (chronic superficial keratitis) in dogs in the Rocky Mountain area—A study of 463 cases. *Journal of Small Animal Practice.* 18(12):757–772.

153. Miller, T., Samuelson, D., and Turner, L. 1986. Generalized retinopathy in the Belgian Sheepdog. *Investigative Ophthalmology & Visual Science.* 27:310.

154. Chavkin, M., Roberts, S., Salman, M., Severin, G., and Scholten, N. 1994. Risk factors for development of chronic superficial keratitis in dogs. *Journal of the American Veterinary Medical Association.* 204(10):1630–1634.

155. Chaudieu, G., and Molon-Noblot, S. 2004. Early retinopathy in the Bernese Mountain dog in France: Preliminary observations. *Veterinary Ophthalmology.* 7(3):175–184.

156. Scherlie Jr., P., Smedes, S., Feltz, T., Dougherty, S., and Riis, R. 1992. Ocular manifestation of systemic histiocytosis in a dog. *Journal of the American Veterinary Medical Association.* 201(8):1229–1232.

157. Moore, P., and Rosin, A. 1986. Malignant histiocytosis of Bernese Mountain dogs. *Veterinary Pathology.* 23(1):1–10.

158. Padgett, G., Madewell, B., Keller, E., Jodar, L., and Packard, M. 1995. Inheritance of histiocytosis in Bernese Mountain dogs. *Journal of Small Animal Practice.* 36(3):93–98.

159. Paterson, S., Boydell, P., and Pike, R. 1995. Systemic histiocytosis in the Bernese Mountain dog. *Journal of Small Animal Practice.* 36(5):233–236.

160. Rosin, A., Moore, P., and Dubielzig, R. 1986. Malignant histiocytosis in Bernese Mountain dogs. *Journal of the American Veterinary Medical Association.* 188(9):1041–1045.

161. Gelatt, K.N., Wallace, M.R., Andrew, S.E., MacKay, E.O., and Samuelson, D.A. 2003. Cataracts in the Bichon Frise. *Veterinary Ophthalmology.* 6(1):3–9.

162. Schmidt, G.M., and Vainisi, S.J. 2004. Retrospective study of prophylactic random transscleral retinopexy in the Bichon Frise with cataract. *Veterinary Ophthalmology.* 7(5):307–310.

163. ACVO Genetics Committee, editor 2001 and/or Data from CERF All-Breeds Report, 2001. The Blue Book: Ocular Disorders Presumed to be Inherited in Purebred Dogs. 2015, 8th edition. *ACVO Annual Conference;* 2001; Sarasota, FL.

164. Zangerl, B., Wickström, K., Slavik, J., Lindauer, S.J., Ahonen, S., Schelling, C. et al. 2010. Assessment of canine BEST1 variations identifies new mutations and establishes an independent bestrophinopathy model (cmr3). *Molecular Vision.* 16:2791.

165. Jolly, R., Palmer, D., Studdert, V., Sutton, R., Kelly, W., Koppang, N. et al. 1994. Canine ceroid lipofuscinoses: A review and classification. *Journal of Small Animal Practice.* 35(6):299–306.

166. Melville, S.A., Wilson, C.L., Chiang, C.S., Studdert, V.P., Lingaas, F., and Wilton, A.N. 2005. A mutation in canine CLN5 causes neuronal ceroid lipofuscinosis in Border collie dogs. *BMC Genomics.* 86(3):287–294.

167. Bedford, P. 1982. Collie eye anomaly in the Border Collie. *The Veterinary Record.* 111(2):34–35.

168. Foster, S., Curtis, R., and Barnett, K. 1986. Primary lens luxation in the Border Collie. *Journal of Small Animal Practice.* 27(1):1–6.

169. Vilboux, T., Chaudieu, G., Jeannin, P., Delattre, D., Hedan, B., Bourgain, C. et al. 2008. Progressive retinal atrophy in the Border Collie: A new XLPRA. *BMC Veterinary Research.* 4(1):10.

170. Storey, E.S., Grahn, B.H., and Alcorn, J. 2005. Multifocal chorioretinal lesions in Borzoi dogs. *Veterinary Ophthalmology.* 8(5):337–347.

171. Curtis, R. 1984. Late-onset cataract in the Boston terrier. *The Veterinary Record.* 115(22):577–578.

172. Mellersh, C.S., Graves, K.T., McLaughlin, B., Ennis, R.B., Pettitt, L., Vaudin, M. et al. 2007. Mutation in HSF4 associated with early but not late-onset hereditary cataract in the Boston Terrier. *Journal of Heredity.* 98(5):531–533.

173. Martin, C., and Dice, P. 1982. Corneal endothelial dystrophy in the dog. *Journal of the American Animal Hospital Association.*

174. Whitley, R., and Gilger, B. 1999. Diseases of the canine cornea and sclera. *Veterinary Ophthalmology.* 3:635–673.

175. Stades, F. 1986. Diseases of the lens and vitreous. In: *Current Veterinary Therapy IX.* WB Saunders: Philadelphia, PA, pp. 660–669.

176. Boeve, M., and Stades, F. 1985. Glaucoom bij hond en kat: Overzicht en retrospectieve evaluatie van 421 patienten. I. Pathobiologische achtergronden, indeling en raspredisposities. *Tijdschrift voor Diergeneeskunde.*

177. Van der Linde-Sipman, J. 1987. Dysplasia of the pectinate ligament and primary glaucoma in the Bouvier des Flandres dog. *Veterinary Pathology.* 24(3):201–206.

178. Dubin, A., Bentley, E., Buhr, K., and Miller, P. 2014. Evaluation and identification of risk factors for primary angle-closure glaucoma (PACG) in Bouvier des Flandres dogs. *Veterinary Ophthalmology.* 17(6):E33.

179. Van Rensburg, I., Petrick, S., Van Der Lugt, J., and Smit, M. 1992. Multiple inherited eye anomalies including persistent hyperplastic tunica vasculosa lentis in Bouvier des Flandres. *Progress in Veterinary & Comparative Ophthalmology.* 2:133–139.

180. Roberts, S.R. 1965. Superficial indolent ulcer of the cornea in Boxer dogs. *Journal of Small Animal Practice.* 6(2):111–115.

181. Gelatt, K., and Samuelson, D. 1982. Recurrent corneal erosions and epithelial dystrophy in the Boxer dog. *Journal of the American Animal Hospital Association*.

182. Kirschner, S., Niyo, Y., and Betts, D. 1989. Idiopathic persistent corneal erosions: Clinical and pathological findings in 18 dogs. *Journal of the American Animal Hospital Association*.

183. Narfström, K. 1998. Retinal dystrophy or "congenital stationary night blindness" in the Briard dog. *Veterinary Ophthalmology*. 2(1):75–76.

184. Narfström, K., Wrigstad, A., and Nilsson, S. 1989. The Briard dog: A new animal model of congenital stationary night blindness. *British Journal of Ophthalmology*. 73(9):750–756.

185. Veske, A., Nilsson, S.E.G., Narfström, K., and Gal, A. 1999. Retinal dystrophy of Swedish Briard/Briard–Beagle dogs is due to a 4-bp deletion in RPE65. *BMC Genomics*. 57(1):57–61.

186. Wrigstad, A., Narfström, K., and Nilsson, S.E.G. 1994. Slowly progressive changes of the retina and retinal pigment epithelium in Briard dogs with hereditary retinal dystrophy. *Documenta Ophthalmologica*. 87(4):337–354.

187. Lightfoot, R., Cabral, L., Gooch, L., Bedford, P., and Boulton, M. 1996. Retinal pigment epithelial dystrophy in Briard dogs. *Research in Veterinary Science*. 60(1):17–23.

188. Bedford, P. 1984. Retinal pigment epithelial dystrophy (CPRA): A study of the disease in the Briard. *Journal of Small Animal Practice*. 25(3):129–138.

189. McLellan, G., Richelle, M., Elks, R., Lybaert, P., and Bedford, P., editors. 1997. Vitamin E deficiency in canine retinal epithelial dystrophy (RPED)- Results of the oral vitamin E tolerance test in clinically normal dogs and in RPED affected cocker spaniels. *Proceedings: World Small Animal Veterinary Association Congress*; Birmingham, UK.

190. Kaswan, R., Martin, C., and Chapman Jr., W. 1984. Keratoconjunctivitis sicca: histopathologic study of nictitating membrane and lacrimal glands from 28 dogs. *American Journal of Veterinary Research*. 45(1):112–118.

191. Sansom, J., Barnett, K., Neumann, W., Schulte-Neumann, A., Clerc, B., Jegou, J. et al. 1995. Treatment of keratoconjunctivitis sicca in dogs with cyclosporine ophthalmic ointment: A European clinical field trial. *The Veterinary Record*. 137(20):504–507.

192. Mazzucchelli, S., Vaillant, M., Wéverberg, F., Arnold-Tavernier, H., Honegger, N., Payen, G. et al. 2012. Retrospective study of 155 cases of prolapse of the nictitating membrane gland in dogs. *The Veterinary Record*. 170(17):443.

193. Kijas, J.W., Cideciyan, A.V., Aleman, T.S., Pianta, M.J., Pearce-Kelling, S.E., Miller, B.J. et al. 2002. Naturally occurring rhodopsin mutation in the dog causes retinal dysfunction and degeneration mimicking human dominant retinitis pigmentosa. *Proceedings of the National Academy of Sciences*. 99(9):6328–6333.

194. Kern, T. 1986. Disorders of the lacrimal system. In: R.W. Kirk (editor), *Current Veterinary Therapy IX*. WB Saunders: Philadelphia, PA, pp. 634–641.

195. Petersen-Jones, S.M., Forcier, J., and Mentzer, A. 2007. Ocular melanosis in the Cairn Terrier: clinical description and investigation of mode of inheritance. *Veterinary Ophthalmology*. 10(S1):63–69.

196. Keep, J. 1972. Clinical aspects of progressive retinal atrophy in the Cardigan Welsh Corgi. *Australian Veterinary Journal*. 48(4):197–199.

197. Petersen-Jones, S.M., and Entz, D.D. 2002. An improved DNA-based test for detection of the codon 616 mutation in the alpha cyclic GMP phosphodiesterase gene that causes progressive retinal atrophy in the Cardigan Welsh Corgi. *Veterinary Ophthalmology*. 5(2):103–106.

198. Hartley, C., Donaldson, D., Smith, K.C., Henley, W., Lewis, T.W., Blott, S. et al. 2012. Congenital keratoconjunctivitis sicca and ichthyosiform dermatosis in 25 Cavalier King Charles Spaniel dogs. Part I: Clinical signs, histopathology, and inheritance. *Veterinary Ophthalmology*. 15(5):315–326.

199. Barnett, K. 2006. Congenital keratoconjunctivitis sicca and ichthyosiform dermatosis in the Cavalier King Charles spaniel. *Journal of Small Animal Practice*. 47(9):524–528.

200. Crispin, S., and Barnett, K. 1983. Dystrophy, degeneration and infiltration of the canine cornea. *Journal of Small Animal Practice*. 24(2):63–83.

201. Sanchez, R., Innocent, G., Mould, J., and Billson, F. 2007. Canine keratoconjunctivitis sicca: disease trends in a review of 229 cases. *Journal of Small Animal Practice*. 48(4):211–217.

202. Narfstrom, K., and Dubielzig, R. 1984. Posterior lenticonus, cataracts and microphthalmia; congenital ocular defects in the Cavalier King Charles Spaniel. *Journal of Small Animal Practice*. 25(11):669–677.

203. Gelatt, K., Whitley, R., Lavach, J., Barrie, K., and Williams, L. 1979. Cataracts in Chesapeake Bay Retrievers. *Journal of the American Veterinary Medical Association*. 175(11):1176.

204. Ashwini, A., D'Angelo, A., Yamato, O., Giordano, C., Cagnotti, G., Harcourt-Brown, T. et al. 2016. Neuronal ceroid lipofuscinosis associated with an MFSD8 mutation in Chihuahuas. *Molecular Genetics and Metabolism*. 118(4):326–332.

205. Guo, J., O'Brien, D.P., Mhlanga-Mutangadura, T., Olby, N.J., Taylor, J.F., Schnabel, R.D. et al. 2015. A rare homozygous MFSD8 single-base-pair deletion and frameshift in the whole genome sequence of a Chinese crested dog with neuronal ceroid lipofuscinosis. *BMC Veterinary Research*. 10(1):960.

206. Collins, B., Collier, L., Johnson, G., Shibuya, H., Moore, C., and da Silva, C.J. 1992. Familial cataracts and concurrent ocular anomalies in Chow Chows. *Journal of the American Veterinary Medical Association*. 200(10):1485–1491.

207. Corcoran, K., Koch, S., and Peiffer, R. 1995. Primary glaucoma in the Chow Chow. *Ophthalmic Literature*. 1(48):62.

208. Nelson, D., and MacMillan, A. 1983. Multifocal retinal dysplasia in field trial Labrador Retrievers. *Journal of the American Animal Hospital Association*.

209. Hodgman, S. 1963. Abnormalities and defects in pedigree dogs–I. An investigation into the existence of abnormalities in pedigree dogs in the British Isles. *Journal of Small Animal Practice*. 4(6):447–456.

210. Moore, C., and Whitley, R. 1984. Visual disturbance in the dog. II. Diseases of the retina and optic papilla. *Compendium on Continuing Education for the Practising Veterinarian*.

211. Magrane, W. 1953. Congenital anomaly of the optic nerve in Collies. *North American Veterinarian*. 34:646.

212. Roberts, S.R. 1960. Congenital posterior ectasia of the sclera in Collie dogs. *American Journal of Ophthalmology*. 50(3):451–465.

213. Donovan, E., and Wyman, M. 1965. Ocular fundus anomaly in the Collie. *Journal of the American Veterinary Medical Association*. 147(12):1465.

214. Roberts, S.R., and Dellaporta, A. 1965. Congenital posterior ectasia of the sclera in Collie dogs. Part I. Clinical features. *American Journal of Ophthalmology*. 59(2):180185–3186.

215. Freeman, H.M., Donovan, R.H., and Schepenss, CL. 1966. Retinal detachment, chorioretinal changes, and staphyloma in the Collie: I. Ophthalmoscopic findings. *Archives of Ophthalmology*. 76(3):412–421.

216. Roberts, S.R., Dellaporta, A., and Winter, F.C. 1966. The Collie ectasia syndrome: Pathology of eyes of young and adult dogs. *American Journal of Ophthalmology*. 62(4):728–752.

217. Roberts, S.R., Dellaporta, A., and Winter, F.C. 1966. The Collie ectasia syndrome: Pathologic alterations in the eyes of puppies one to fourteen days of age. *American Journal of Ophthalmology*. 61(6):1458–1466.

218. Roberts, S.R. 1967. Color dilution and hereditary defects in Collie dogs. *American Journal of Ophthalmology*. 63(6):1762–1775.

219. Yakely, W., Wyman, M., Donovan, E., and Fechheimer, N. 1968. Genetic transmission of an ocular fundus anomaly in Collies. *Journal of the American Veterinary Medical Association*. 152(5):457.

220. Donovan, R., Freeman, H.M., and Schepens, C.L. 1969. Anomaly of the Collie eye. *Journal of the American Veterinary Medical Association*. 155(6):872–877.

221. Freeman, H., Donovan, R., and Schepens, C. 1968. Chorioretinal changes, juxtapapillary staphyloma, and retinal detachment in the Collie. *Bibliotheca Ophthalmologica: Supplementa ad Ophthalmologica*. 79:111–117.

222. Latshaw, W., Wyman, M., and Venzke, W. 1969. Embryologic development of an anomaly of ocular fundus in the Collie dog. *American Journal of Veterinary Research*. 30(2):211.

223. Roberts, S. 1969. The collie eye anomaly. *Journal of the American Veterinary Medical Association*. 155(6):859.

224. Wyman, M., and Donovan, E. 1969. Eye anomaly of the Collie. *Journal of the American Veterinary Medical Association*. 155(6):866–870.

225. Blogg, J. 1970. Collie eye anomaly. *Australian Veterinary Journal*. 46(11):530–532.

226. Bjerkås, E. 1991. Collie eye anomaly in the Rough Collie in Norway. *Journal of Small Animal Practice*. 32(2):89–92.

227. Yakely, W. 1972. Collie eye anomaly: decreased prevalence through selective breeding. *Journal of the American Veterinary Medical Association*. 161(10):1103–1107.

228. Barnett, K. 1979. Collie eye anomaly (CEA). *Journal of Small Animal Practice*. 20(9):537–542.

229. Brown, G.C., Shields, J.A., Patty, B.E., and Goldberg, R.E. 1979. Congenital pits of the optic nerve head: I. Experimental studies in Collie dogs. *Archives of Ophthalmology*. 97(7):1341–1344.

230. Bedford, P. 1982. Collie eye anomaly in the United Kingdom. *The Veterinary Record*. 111(12):263–270.

231. Stades, F., and Barnett, K. 1981. Collie eye anomaly in Collies in the Netherlands. *Veterinary Quarterly*. 3(2):66–73.

232. Vainisi, S., Peyman, G., Wolf, E., and West, C. 1989. Treatment of serous retinal detachments associated with optic disk pits in dogs. *Journal of the American Veterinary Medical Association*. 195(9):1233–1236.

233. Wallin-Håkanson, B., Wallin-Hakanson, N., and Hedhammar, Å. 2000. Influence of selective breeding on the prevalence of chorioretinal dysplasia and coloboma in the Rough Collie in Sweden. *Journal of Small Animal Practice*. 41(2):56–59.

234. Munger, R. 1983. Disease of the eyelid. In: Kirk, R.W., editor. *Current Therapy VIII (Small Animal Practice)*. WB Saunders: Philadelphia, PA, pp. 537–543.

235. Gwin, R., Wyman, M., Lim, D., Ketring Jr., K., and Werling, K. 1981. Multiple ocular defects associated with partial albinism and deafness in the dog. *Journal of the American Animal Hospital Association*.

236. Kukekova, A.V., Goldstein, O., Johnson, J.L., Richardson, M.A., Pearce-Kelling, S.E., Swaroop, A. et al. 2009. Canine RD3 mutation establishes rod-cone dysplasia type 2 (rcd2) as ortholog of human and murine rd3. *Mammalian Genome*. 20(2):109–123.

237. Acland, G.M., Ray, K., Mellersh, C.S., Gu, W., Langston, A.A., Rine, J. et al. 1998. Linkage analysis and comparative mapping of canine progressive rod–cone degeneration (prcd) establishes potential locus homology with retinitis pigmentosa (RP17) in humans. *Proceedings of the National Academy of Sciences*. 95(6):3048–3053.

238. Santos-Anderson, R.M., Tso, M., and Wolf, E.D. 1980. An inherited retinopathy in Collies. A light and electron microscopic study. *Investigative Ophthalmology & Visual Science*. 19(11):1281–1294.

239. Wolf, E., Vainisi, S., and Santos-Anderson, R. 1978. Rod-cone dysplasia in the Collie. *Journal of the American Veterinary Medical Association*. 173(10):1331.

240. Woodford, B., Liu, Y., Fletcher, R., Chader, G., Farber, D., Santos-Anderson, R. et al. 1982. Cyclic nucleotide metabolism in inherited retinopathy in Collies: A biochemical and histochemical study. *Experimental Eye Research*. 34(5):703–714.

241. Smith, J., Bistner, S., and Riis, R. 1976. Infiltrative corneal lesions resembling fibrous histiocytoma: Clinical and pathologic findings in six dogs and one cat. *Journal of the American Veterinary Medical Association*. 169(7):722.

242. Paulsen, M., Lavach, J., Snyder, S., Severin, G., and Eichenbaum, J. 1987. Nodular granulomatous episclerokeratitis in dogs: 19 cases (1973–1985). *Journal of the American Veterinary Medical Association*. 190(12):1581–1587.

243. Pickett, J., Lindley, D., and Boosinger, T. 1991. Stationary night blindness in a Collie. *Progress in Veterinary & Comparative Ophthalmology*. 1:303–308.

244. Grahn, B.H., Sandmeyer, L.L., and Breaux, C. 2008. Retinopathy of Coton de Tulear dogs: Clinical manifestations, electroretinographic, ultrasonographic, fluorescein and indocyanine green angiographic, and optical coherence tomographic findings. *Veterinary Ophthalmology*. 11(4):242–249.

245. Sanders, D.N., Farias, F.H., Johnson, G.S., Chiang, V., Cook, J.R., O'Brien, D.P. et al. 2010. A mutation in canine PPT1 causes early onset neuronal ceroid lipofuscinosis in a Dachshund. *Molecular Genetics and Metabolism*. 100(4):349–356.

246. Dausch, D., Wegner, W., Michaelis, M., and Reetz, I. 1977. Ophthalmological findings in merle Dachshunds. *DTW Deutsche tierarztliche Wochenschrift*. 84(12):468–475.

247. Cooley, P.L., and Dice, P.F. 1990. Corneal dystrophy in the dog and cat. *The Veterinary Clinics of North America. Small Animal Practice*. 20(3):681–692.

248. Brandsch, H., and Schmidt, V. 1982. Analysis of heredity of dermoid in dog eye. *Monatsh Veterinarmed*. 37(8):305–306.

249. Sorsby, A., and Davey, J. 1954. Ocular associations of dappling (or merling) in the coat colour of dogs. *Brazilian Journal of Genetics*. 52(2):425.

250. Curtis, R., and Barnett, K. 1993. Progressive retinal atrophy in Miniature Longhaired Dachshund dogs. *The British Veterinary Journal*. 149(1):71–85.

251. Mellersh, C., Boursnell, M., Pettitt, L., Ryder, E., Holmes, N., Grafham, D. et al. 2006. Canine RPGRIP1 mutation establishes cone–rod dystrophy in Miniature Longhaired Dachshunds as a homologue of human Leber congenital amaurosis. *BMC Genomics*. 88(3):293–301.

252. Ropstad, E.O., Narfstrom, K., Lingaas, F., Wiik, C., Bruun, A., and Bjerkas, E. 2008. Functional and structural changes in the retina of wire-haired Dachshunds with early-onset cone–rod dystrophy. *Investigative Ophthalmology & Visual Science*. 49(3):1106–1115.

253. Miyadera, K., Kato, K., Boursnell, M., Mellersh, C.S., and Sargan, D.R. 2012. Genome-wide association study in RPGRIP1–/– dogs identifies a modifier locus that determines the onset of retinal degeneration. *Mammalian Genome*. 23(1–2):212–223.

254. Wiik, A.C., Wade, C., Biagi, T., Ropstad, E.-O., Bjerkås, E., Lindblad-Toh, K. et al. 2008. A deletion in nephronophthisis 4 (NPHP4) is associated with recessive cone-rod dystrophy in standard wire-haired Dachshund. *Genome Research*. 18(9):1415–1421.

255. Wiik, A., Thoresen, S., Wade, C., Lindblad-Toh, K., and Lingaas, F. 2009. A population study of a mutation allele associated with cone–rod dystrophy in the standard wire-haired Dachshund. *Animal Genetics*. 40(4):572–574.

256. Zhang, Q., Acland, G.M., Parshall, C.J., Haskell, J., Ray, K., and Aguirre, G.D. 1998. Characterization of canine photoreceptor phosducin cDNA and identification of a sequence variant in dogs with photoreceptor dysplasia. *Oncogene*. 215(2):231–239.

257. Turney, C., Chong, N.V., Alexander, R.A., Hogg, C.R., Fleming, L., Flack, D. et al. 2007. Pathological and electrophysiological features of a canine cone–rod dystrophy in the Miniature Longhaired Dachshund. *Investigative Ophthalmology & Visual Science*. 48(9):4240–4249.

258. Miyader,a K., Kato, K., Aguirre-Hernández, J., Tokuriki, T., Morimoto, K., Busse, C. et al. 2009. Phenotypic variation and genotype-phenotype discordance in canine cone–rod dystrophy with an RPGRIP1 mutation. *Molecular Vision*. 15:2287–2305.

259. Kuznetsova, T., Iwabe, S., Boesze-Battaglia, K., Pearce-Kelling, S., Chang-Min, Y., McDaid, K. et al. 2012. Exclusion of RPGRIP1 ins44 from primary causal association with early-onset cone–rod dystrophy in dogs. *Investigative Ophthalmology & Visual Science*. 53(9):5486–5501.

260. Pearce, J., Whiting, R.E., Castaner, L., Narfström, K., Johnson, G., and Katz, M. 2013. Multifocal retinopathy in a colony of Miniature Longhaired Dachshunds with late infantile neuronal ceroid lipofuscinosis. *Veterinary Ophthalmology*. 16(1):E16.

261. Herrera, H.D., and Duchene, AG. 1998. Uveodermatological syndrome (Vogt–Koyanagi–Harada -like syndrome) with generalized depigmentation in a Dachshund. *Veterinary Ophthalmology*. 1(S1):47–51.

262. Goebel, H.H., Bilzer, T., Dahme, E., Malkusch, F., Opitz, J.M., Reynolds, J.F. et al. 1988. Morphological studies in canine (Dalmatian) neuronal ceroid-lipofuscinosis. *American Journal of Medical Genetics. Part A*. 31(5):127–139.

263. Goebel, H.H., and Dahme, E. 1986. Ultrastructure of retinal pigment epithelial and neural cells in the neuronal ceroid-lipofuscinosis affected Dalmatian dog. *Retina*. 6(3):179–188.

264. Goebel, H., and Dahme, E. 1985. Retinal ultrastructure of neuronal ceroid-lipofuscinosis in the Dalmatian dog. *Acta Neuropathologica*. 68(3):224–229.

265. Ahonen, S.J., Pietilä, E., Mellersh, C.S., Tiira, K., Hansen, L., Johnson, G.S. et al. 2013. Genome-wide association study identifies a novel canine glaucoma locus. *PloS One*. 8(8):e70903.

266. Peiffer Jr., R., and Fischer C. 1983. Microphthalmia, retinal dysplasia, and anterior segment dysgenesis in a litter of Doberman Pinschers. *Journal of the American Veterinary Medical Association*. 183(8):875.

267. Ramsey, D.T., Ketring, K.L., Glaze, M.B., Knight, B., and Render, J.A. 1996. Ligneous conjunctivitis in four Doberman Pinschers. *Journal of the American Animal Hospital Association*. 32(5):439–447.

268. Arnbjerg, J., and Jensen, O. 1982. Spontaneous microphthalmia in two Doberman puppies with anterior chamber cleavage syndrome. *Journal of the American Animal Hospital Association*.

269. Bergsjø, T., Arnesen, K., Heim, P and., Nes, N. 1984. Congenital blindness with ocular developmental anomalies, including retinal dysplasia, in Doberman Pinscher dogs. *Journal of the American Veterinary Medical Association*. 184(11):1383.

270. Lewis, D., Kelly, D., and Sansom, J. 1986. Congenital microphthalmia and other developmental ocular anomalies in the Dobermann. *Journal of Small Animal Practice*. 27(9):559–566.

271. Van der Linde-Sipman, J., Stades, F., and de Wolff-Rouendaal, D. 1983. Persistent hyperplastic tunica vasculosa lentis and persistent hyperplastic primary vitreous in the Doberman Pinscher: pathological aspects. *Journal of the American Animal Hospital Association*. 2:163–172.

272. Stades, F. 1980. Persistent hyperplastic tunica vasculosa lentis and persistent hyperplastic primary vitreous (PHTVL/PHPV) in 90 closely related Doberman Pinschers: Clinical aspects. *Journal of the American Animal Hospital Association*. 16(5):739–751.

273. Stades, F. 1983. Persistent hyperplastic tunica vasculosa lentis and persistent hyperplastic primary vitreous in Doberman Pinschers: techniques and results of surgery. *Journal of the American Animal Hospital Association*. 16(5):739–751.

274. Stades, F. 1983. Persistent hyperplastic tunica vasculosa lentis and persistent hyperplastic primary vitreous in Doberman Pinschers-genetic-aspects. *Journal of the American Animal Hospital Association*. 19(6):957–964.

275. Boeve, M., Van der Linde-Sipman, J., Stades, F., and Vrensen, G. 1990. Early morphogenesis of persistent hyperplastic tunica vasculosa lentis and primary vitreous. A transmission electron microscopic study. *Investigative Ophthalmology & Visual Science*. 31(9):1886–1894.

276. Boeve, M.H., Van der Linde-Sipman, T., and Stades, F. 1988. Early morphogenesis of persistent hyperplastic tunica vasculosa lentis and primary vitreous. The dog as an ontogenetic model. *Investigative Ophthalmology & Visual Science*. 29(7):1076–1086.

277. Stades, F., Boeve, M., Van Den Brom, W., and van der Linde-Sipman, J. 1991. The incidence of PHTVL/PHPV in Doberman and the results of breeding rules. *Veterinary Quarterly*. 13(1):24–29.

278. Boeve, M., Stades, F., Van Der Linde-Sipman, J., and Vrensen, G. 1992. Persistent hyperplastic tunica vasculosa lentis and primary vitreous (PHTVL/PHPV) in the dog: A comparative review. *Progress in Veterinary & Comparative Ophthalmology*. 2:163–172.

279. Strande, A., Nicolaissen, B., and Bjerkas, I. 1988. Persistent pupillary membrane and congenital cataract in a litter of

English Cocker Spaniels. *Journal of Small Animal Practice.* 29(4):257–260.

280. Engelhardt, A., Stock, K.F., Hamann, H., Brahm, R., Grußendorf, H., Rosenhagen, C.U. et al. 2008. A retrospective study on the prevalence of primary cataracts in two pedigrees from the German population of English Cocker Spaniels. *Veterinary Ophthalmology.* 11(4):215–221.

281. McLellan, G.J., and Bedford, P.G. 2012. Oral vitamin E absorption in English Cocker Spaniels with familial vitamin E deficiency and retinal pigment epithelial dystrophy. *Veterinary Ophthalmology.* 15(S2):48–56.

282. McLellan, G., Cappello, R., Mayhew, I., Elks, R., Lybaert, P., Watte, C. et al. 2003. Clinical and pathological observations in English Cocker Spaniels with primary metabolic vitamin E deficiency and retinal pigment epithelial dystrophy. *The Veterinary Record.* 153(10):287–292.

283. Bedford, P. 1975. The aetiology of primary glaucoma in the dog. *Journal of Small Animal Practice.* 16(1–12):217–239.

284. Aguirre, G., and Acland, G., editors. 1983. Progressive retinal atrophy in the English cocker spaniel. *Proceedings of the American College of Veterinary Ophthalmologists.* 158(2):208–218.

285. Gould, D., Petersen-Jones, S., Lin, C., and Sargan, D. 1997. Cloning of canine rom-1 and its investigation as a candidate gene for generalized progressive retinal atrophies in dogs. *Animal Genetics.* 28(6):391–396.

286. Narfström, K., and Wrigstad, A. 1995. Clinical, electrophysiological, and morphological findings in a case of neuronal ceroid lipofuscinosis in the Polish Owczarek Nizinny (PON) dog. *Veterinary Quarterly.* 17(Suppl):46–41.

287. Nilsson, S.E.G., and Wrigstad, A. 1997. Electrophysiology in some animal and human hereditary diseases involving the retinal pigment epithelium. *Contact Lens & Anterior Eye.* 11(5):698–706.

288. Koppang, N. 1969. Neuronal ceroid-lipofuscinosis in English Setters juvenile amaurotic familiar idiocy (AFI) in English Setters. *Journal of Small Animal Practice.* 10(11):639–644.

289. Koppang, N., Opitz, J.M., and Pullarkat, R.K. 1988. The English Setter with ceroid-lipofuscinosis: A suitable model for the juvenile type of ceroid-lipofuscinosis in humans. *American Journal of Medical Genetics.* 31(S5):117–125.

290. Armstrong, D., Koppang, N., and Nilsson, S.E. 1982. Canine hereditary ceroid lipofuscinosis. *European Neurology.* 21(3):147–156.

291. Bjerkas, E. 1990. Generalised progressive retinal atrophy in the English Setter in Norway. *The Veterinary Record.* 126(9):217.

292. Barnett, K., and Stades, F. 1979. Collie eye anomaly in the Shetland Sheepdog in the Netherlands. *Journal of Small Animal Practice.* 20(6):321–329.

293. Cottrell, B.D., and Barnett, K. 1988. Primary glaucoma in the Welsh Springer Spaniel. *Journal of Small Animal Practice.* 29(3):185–199.

294. OptiGen®. OptiGen for the genetic advantage 2000 Available from http://www.optigen.com/.

295. Lhériteau, E., Petit, L., Weber, M., Le Meur, G., Deschamps, J.-Y., Libeau, L. et al. 2014. Successful gene therapy in the RPGRIP1-deficient dog: A large model of cone–rod dystrophy. *Cytokines Cellular & Molecular Therapy.* 22(2):265–277.

296. Narfström, K., Jeong, M., Hyman, J., Madsen, R.W., and Bergström, T.F. 2012. Assessment of hereditary retinal degeneration in the English Springer Spaniel dog and disease relationship to an RPGRIP1 mutation. *Stem Cells International.*

297. Kubai, M.A., Bentley, E., Miller, P.E., Mutti, D.O., and Murphy, C.J. 2008. Refractive states of eyes and association between ametropia and breed in dogs. *American Journal of Veterinary Research.* 69(7):946–951.

298. Kubai, M.A., Labelle, A.L., Hamor, R.E., Mutti, D.O., Famula, T.R., and Murphy, C.J. 2013. Heritability of lenticular myopia in English Springer Spaniels lenticular myopia in English Springer Spaniels. *Investigative Ophthalmology & Visual Science.* 54(12):7324–7328.

299. Schmidt, G., Ellersieck, M., Wheeler, C., Blanchard, G., and Keller, W. 1979. Inheritance of retinal dysplasia in the English Spring Spaniel. *Journal of the American Veterinary Medical Association.* 174(10):1089.

300. Lavach, J., Murphy, J., and Severin, G. 1978. Retinal dysplasia in English Springer Spaniel. *Journal of the American Animal Hospital Association.* 14(2):192 199.

301. Toole, D., Young, S., Severin, G., and Neumann, S. 1983. Retinal dysplasia of English Springer Spaniel dogs: light microscopy of the postnatal lesions. *Veterinary Pathology.* 20(3):298–311.

302. Spiess, B. 1993. Inherited eye diseases in the Entlebucher Mountain dog. *Schweizer Archiv fuer Tierheilkunde.* 136(3):105–110.

303. Heitmann, M., Hamann, H., Brahm, R., Grussendorf, H., Rosenhagen, C., and Distl, O. 2005. Analysis of prevalence of presumed inherited eye diseases in Entlebucher Mountain Dogs. *Veterinary Ophthalmology.* 8(3):145–151.

304. Koch, S. 1972. Cataracts in interrelated old English Sheepdogs. *Journal of the American Veterinary Medical Association.* 160(3):299.

305. Gelatt, K., Samuelson, D., Barrie, K., Das, N., Wolf, E., Bauer, J. et al. 1983. Biometry and clinical characteristics of congenital cataracts and microphthalmia in the Miniature Schnauzer. *Journal of the American Veterinary Medical Association.* 183(1):99–102.

306. Strom, A.R., Hässig, M., Iburg, T.M., and Spiess, B.M. 2011. Epidemiology of canine glaucoma presented to University of Zurich from 1995 to 2009. Part 1: Congenital and primary glaucoma (4 and 123 cases). *Veterinary Ophthalmology.* 14(2):121–126.

307. Rosolen, S., Boillot, T., Dulaurent, T., Goulle, F., Neveux, N., Lafarge-beurlet, S. et al. 2014. Morphological, biometrical and biochemical susceptibilities for glaucoma in healthy Eurasier dogs. *Veterinary Ophthalmology.* 17(6):E23.

308. Read, R., Wood, J., and Lakhani, K. 1998. Pectinate ligament dysplasia (PLD) and glaucoma in Flat Coated Retrievers. I. Objectives, technique and results of a PLD survey. *Veterinary Ophthalmology.* 1(2–3):85–90.

309. Wood, J., Lakhani, K., and Read, R. 1998. Pectinate ligament dysplasia and glaucoma in Flat Coated Retrievers. II. Assessment of prevalence and heritability. *Veterinary Ophthalmology.* 1(2–3):91–99.

310. ACVO Genetics Committee, editor 2014–2015 and/or Data from OFA All-Breeds Report 2014–2015. The Blue Book: Ocular Disorders Presumed to be Inherited in Purebred Dogs. 2015, 8th edition. *ACVO Annual Conference;* 2015; Coeur d'Alene, ID.

311. Helper, L. 1989. *Appendix 1. Magrane's Canine Ophthalmology.* 4th edition. Lea & Febiger: Philadelphia, PA, pp. 275–277.

312. Martin, C.L., and Wyman, M. 1978. Primary glaucoma in the dog. *The Veterinary Clinics of North America. Small Animal Practice.* 8(2):257–286.

313. Leppänen, M., Mårtenson, J., and Mäki, K. 2001. Results of ophthalmologic screening examinations of German Pinschers in Finland–A retrospective study. *Veterinary Ophthalmology*. 4(3):165–169.

314. Pfahler, S., Menzel, J., Brahm, R., Rosenhagen, C.U., Hafemeister, B., Schmidt, U. et al. 2015. Prevalence and formation of primary cataracts and persistent hyperplastic tunica vasculosa lentis in the German Pinscher population in Germany. *Veterinary Ophthalmology*. 18(2):135–140.

315. Barnett, K. 1986. Hereditary cataract in the German Shepherd dog. *Journal of Small Animal Practice*. 27(6): 387–395.

316. Campbell, L., Okuda, H., Lipton, D., and Reed, C. 1975. Chronic superficial keratitis in dogs: Detection of cellular hypersensitivity. *American Journal of Veterinary Research*. 36(5):669.

317. Bedford, P., and Longstaffe, J. 1979. Corneal pannus (chronic superficial keratitis) in the German Shepherd dog. *Journal of Small Animal Practice*. 20(1):41–56.

318. Eichenbaum, J., Lavach, J., Gould, D., Severin, G., Paulsen, M., and Jones, R. 1986. Immunohistochemical staining patterns of canine eyes affected with chronic superficial keratitis. *American Journal of Veterinary Research*. 47(9):1952–1955.

319. Jokinen, P., Rusanen, E.M., Kennedy, L.J., and Lohi, H. 2011. MHC Class II risk haplotype associated with canine chronic superficial keratitis in German Shepherd dogs. *Veterinary Immunology and Immunopathology*. 140(1):37–41.

320. Tanaka, N., Dutrow, E.V., Miyadera, K., Delemotte, L., MacDermaid, C.M., Reinstein, S.L. et al. 2015. Canine CNGA3 gene mutations provide novel insights into human achromatopsia-associated channelopathies and treatment. *PloS One*. 10(9):e0138943.

321. Martin, C. 1981. Canine epibulbar melanomas and their management. *Journal of the American Animal Hospital Association*.

322. Aguirre, G. 1999. The geographic form of retinal dysplasia in dogs is not always a congenital abnormality. *Veterinary Ophthalmology*. 2:61–66.

323. Martin, C., and Leach, R. 1970. Everted membrana nictitans in German Shorthaired Pointers. *Journal of the American Veterinary Medical Association*. 157:1229–1232.

324. Goldstein, O., Mezey, J.G., Boyko, A.R., Gao, C., Wang, W., Bustamante, C.D. et al. 2010. An ADAM-9 mutation in canine cone-rod dystrophy 3 establishes homology with human cone-rod dystrophy 9. *Molecular Vision*. 1(16):1549–1569.

325. Kropatsch, R., Petrasch-Parwez, E., Seelow, D., Schlichting, A., Gerding, W.M., Akkad, D.A. et al. 2010. Generalized progressive retinal atrophy in the Irish Glen of Imaal Terrier is associated with a deletion in the ADAM-9 gene. *Molecular and Cellular Probes*. 24(6):357–363.

326. Barnett, K. 1980. Cataract in the Golden Retriever. *The Veterinary Record*. 106:315.

327. Curtis, R., and Barnett, K. 1989. A survey of cataracts in Golden and Labrador Retrievers. *Journal of Small Animal Practice*. 30(5):277–286.

328. Rubin, L.F. 1974. Cataract in Golden Retrievers [dogs]. *Journal of the American Veterinary Medical Association*.

329. Bona S. 1995. *A population genetic study in the breeding situation and on hereditary determined diseases, especially eye and joint diseases, in the Golden and Labrador Retriever.* International Information System for the Agricultural Science and Technology: Agris.

330. Gelatt, K. 1972. Cataracts in the Golden Retriever dog. *Veterinary Medicine, Small Animal Clinician*. 67(10):1113.

331. Gilliam, D., Kolicheski, A., Johnson, G., Mhlanga-Mutangadura, T., Taylor, J., Schnabel, R. et al. 2015. Golden Retriever dogs with neuronal ceroid lipofuscinosis have a two-base-pair deletion and frameshift in CLN5. *Molecular Genetics and Metabolism*. 115(2):101–109.

332. Donaldson, D., Sansom, J., Scase, T., Adams, V., and Mellersh, C. 2006. Canine limbal melanoma: 30 cases (1992–2004). Part 1. Signalment, clinical and histological features and pedigree analysis. *Veterinary Ophthalmology*. 9(2):115–119.

333. Downs, L.M., Wallin-Håkansson, B., Boursnell, M., Marklund, S., Hedhammar, Å., Truvé, K. et al. 2011. A frameshift mutation in Golden Retriever dogs with progressive retinal atrophy endorses SLC4A3 as a candidate gene for human retinal degenerations. *PloS One*. 6(6):e21452.

334. Downs, L.M., Wallin-Håkansson, B., Bergström, T., and Mellersh, C.S. 2014. A novel mutation in TTC8 is associated with progressive retinal atrophy in the Golden Retriever. *Canine Genetics and Epidemiology*. 1(1):4.

335. Townsend, W.M., and Gornik, K.R. 2013. Prevalence of uveal cysts and pigmentary uveitis in Golden Retrievers in three Midwestern states. *Journal of the American Veterinary Medical Association*. 243(9):1298–1301.

336. Deehr, A.J., and Dubielzig, R.R. 1998. A histopathological study of iridociliary cysts and glaucoma in Golden Retrievers. *Veterinary Ophthalmology*. 1(2–3):153–158.

337. Holly, V.L., Sandmeyer, L.S., Bauer, B.S., Verges, L., and Grahn, B.H. 2015. Golden Retriever cystic uveal disease: A longitudinal study of iridociliary cysts, pigmentary uveitis, and pigmentary/cystic glaucoma over a decade in western Canada. *Veterinary Ophthalmology*. 19(3):237–244.

338. Sapienza, J., Simo, F., and Prades-Sapienza, A. 2000. Golden Retriever uveitis: 75 cases (1994–1999). *Veterinary Ophthalmology*. 3(4):241–246.

339. Long, S., and Crispin, S. 1999. Inheritance of multifocal retinal dysplasia in the Golden Retriever in the UK. *The Veterinary Record*. 145(24):702–704.

340. Good, K.L., Komáromy, A.M., Kass, P.H., and Ofri, R. 2015. Novel retinopathy in related Gordon Setters: A clinical, behavioral, electrophysiological, and genetic investigation. *Veterinary Ophthalmology*. 19(5):398–408.

341. Magnusson, H. 1909. On night blindness in the dog following inbreeding. *Svensk Veterinärtidning*. 14:462–466.

342. Magnusson, H. 1911. Uber retinitis pigmentosa und konsanquinitat beinm hunde. *Archiv Fur Vergleichende Ophtalmologie*. 2:147–163.

343. Magnusson, H. 1917. Noch ein fall von nachtblindheit beim hunde. *Graefe's Archive for Clinical and Experimental Ophthalmology*. 93(4):404–411.

344. Wood, J.L., Lakhani, K.H., Mason, I.K., and Barnett, K.C. 2001. Relationship of the degree of goniodysgenesis and other ocular measurements to glaucoma in Great Danes. *American Journal of Veterinary Research*. 62(9):1493–1499.

345. Spiess, B., Bolliger, J., Guscetti, F., Haessig, M., Lackner, P., and Ruehli, M. 1998. Multiple ciliary body cysts and secondary glaucoma in the Great Dane: A report of nine cases. *Veterinary Ophthalmology*. 1(1):41–45.

346. Grahn, B., Philibert, H., Cullen, C., Houston, D., Semple, H., and Schmutz, S. 1998. Multifocal retinopathy of Great Pyrenees dogs. *Veterinary Ophthalmology*. 1(4):211–221.

347. Grahn, B.H., and Cullen, C.L. 2001. Retinopathy of Great Pyrenees dogs: Fluorescein angiography, light microscopy

and transmitting and scanning electron microscopy. *Veterinary Ophthalmology.* 4(3):191–199.

348. Peiffer, R., Gelatt, K., and Gwin, R. 1977. Chronic superficial keratitis (pannus) in related Greyhounds. *Veterinary Medicine, Small Animal Clinician.* 72(1):35–37.

349. Peiffer, R., Gelatt, K., and Gwin, R. 1977. Chronic superficial keratitis. *Veterinary Medicine, Small Animal Clinician: VM, SAC.* 72(1):35.

350. Grimes, T., and Mullaney, J. 1969. Persistent hyperplastic primary vitreous in a Greyhound. *The Veterinary Record.* 85(22):607–610.

351. Slatter, D., Blogg, J., and Constable, I. 1980. Retinal degeneration in Greyhounds. *Australian Veterinary Journal.* 56(3):106–115.

352. Starr, A.N., Famula, T.R., Markward, N.J., Baldwin, J.V., Fowler, K.D., Klumb, D.E. et al. 2007. Hereditary evaluation of multiple developmental abnormalities in the Havanese dog breed. *Journal of Heredity.* 98(5):510–517.

353. Palmer, A., Payne, J., and Wallace, M.E. 1973. Hereditary quadriplegia and amblyopia in the Irish Setter. *Journal of Small Animal Practice.* 14(6):343–352.

354. Sakai, T., Harashima, T., Yamamura, H., Nitaya, R., and Ikeda, T. 1994. Two cases of hereditary quadriplegia and amblyopia in a litter of Irish Setters. *Journal of Small Animal Practice.* 35(4):221–223.

355. Aguirre, G. 1976. Inherited retinal degenerations in the dog. *Proceedings of the American Academy of Ophthalmology and Otolaryngology.* 81(4 Pt 1):667–676.

356. Hodgman, S. 1949. Progressive retinal atrophy in dogs. 1. The disease of Iris Setters (red). *The Veterinary Record.* 61:185–189.

357. Parry, H. 1953. Degenerations of the dog retina: II. Generalized progressive atrophy of hereditary origin. *British Journal of Ophthalmology.* 37(8):487.

358. Lewis, D. 1977. Reappearance of PRA in the Irish Setter. *The Veterinary Record.* 101(6):122–123.

359. Acland, G.M. 1979. Involvement of cyclic GMP phosphodiesterase activator in an hereditary retinal degeneration. *Bionature.* 280:62.

360. Lee, R., Lieberman, B., Hurwitz, R., and Lolley, R. 1985. Phosphodiesterase-probes show distinct defects in rd mice and Irish Setter dog disorders. *Investigative Ophthalmology & Visual Science.* 26(11):1569–1579.

361. Lolley, R.N., Lee, R.H., and Hurwitz, R.L. 1985. Biochemical and immunological characteristics of photoreceptor phosphodiesterase in inherited retinal degeneration of rd mice and affected Irish setter dogs. In: *Retinal Degeneration: Experimental and Clinical Studies.* Alan R. Liss: New York, pp. 133–146.

362. Schmidt, S., and Aguirre, G. 1985. Reductions in taurine secondary to photoreceptor loss in Irish Setters with rod-cone dysplasia. *Investigative Ophthalmology & Visual Science.* 26(5):679–683.

363. Schmidt, S.Y., Andley, U.P., Heth, C.A., and Miller, J. 1986. Deficiency in light-dependent opsin phosphorylation in Irish Setters with rod-cone dysplasia. *Investigative Ophthalmology & Visual Science.* 27:1551–1559.

364. Fletcher, R.T., Sanyal, S., Krishna, G., Aguirre, G., and Chader, G.J. 1986. Genetic expression of cyclic GMP phosphodiesterase activity defines abnormal photoreceptor differentiation in neurological mutants of inherited retinal degeneration. *Journal of Neurochemistry.* 46(4):1240–1245.

365. Barbehenn, E., Gagnon, C., Noelker, D., Aguirre, G., and Chader G. 1988. Inherited rod-cone dysplasia: Abnormal distribution of cyclic GMP in visual cells of affected Irish Setters. *Experimental Eye Research.* 46(2):149–159.

366. Cunnick, J., Rider, M., Takemoto, L., and Takemoto, D. 1988. Rod/cone dysplasia in Irish Setters. Presence of an altered rhodopsin. *Biochemical Journal.* 250(2):335–341.

367. Farber, D.B., Danciger, J.S., and Aguirre, G. 1992. The β subunit of cyclic GMP phosphodiesterase mRNA is deficient in canine rod-cone dysplasia 1. *Neuron.* 9(2):349–356.

368. Clements, P.J., Gregory, C.Y., Peterson-Jones, S.M., Sargan, D.R., and Bhattacharya, S.S. 1993. Confirmation of the rod cGMP phosphodiesterase β subunit (PDEβ) nonsense mutation in affected rcd-1 Irish Setters in the UK and development of a diagnostic test. *Current Eye Research.* 12(9):861–866.

369. Suber, M.L., Pittler, S.J., Qin, N., Wright, G.C., Holcombe, V., Lee, R.H. et al. 1993. Irish Setter dogs affected with rod/cone dysplasia contain a nonsense mutation in the rod cGMP phosphodiesterase beta-subunit gene. *Proceedings of the National Academy of Sciences.* 90(9):3968–3972.

370. Ray, K., Baldwin, V.J., Acland, G.M., and Aguirre, G.D. 1995. Molecular diagnostic tests for ascertainment of genotype at the rod cone dysplasia 1 (rcd1) locus in Irish Setters. *Current Eye Research.* 14(3):243–247.

371. Ray, K., Baldwin, V.J., Acland, G.M., Blanton, S.H., and Aguirre, G.D. 1994. Cosegregation of codon 807 mutation of the canine rod cGMP phosphodiesterase beta gene and rcd1. *Investigative Ophthalmology & Visual Science.* 35(13):4291–4299.

372. Petersen-Jones, S., Clements, P., Barnett, K., and Sargan, D. 1995. Incidence of the gene mutation causal for rod-cone dysplasia type 1 in Irish Setters in the UK. *Journal of Small Animal Practice.* 36(7):310–314.

373. Djajadiningrat-Laanen, S., Boevé, M., Stades, F., and van Oost, B. 2003. Familial non-rcd 1 generalised retinal degeneration in Irish Setters. *Journal of Small Animal Practice.* 44(3):113–116.

374. Lawson, D. 1969. Luxation of the crystalline lens in the dog. *Journal of Small Animal Practice.* 10(8):461–463.

375. Curtis, R., and Barnett, K. 1980. Primary lens luxation in the dog. *Journal of Small Animal Practice.* 21(12):657–668.

376. Curtis, R., Barnett, K., and Lewis, S. 1983. Clinical and pathological observations concerning the aetiology of primary lens luxation in the dog. *The Veterinary Record.* 112(11):238–246.

377. Oberbauer, A.M., Hollingsworth, S.R., Belanger, J.M., Regan, K.R., and Famula, T.R. 2008. Inheritance of cataracts and primary lens luxation in Jack Russell Terriers. *American Journal of Veterinary Research.* 69(2):222–227.

378. Ahonen, S.J., and Lohi, H. 2014. Progressive retinal atrophy in the Karelian Bear Dog: A large animal model for retinitis pigmentosa. *Investigative Ophthalmology & Visual Science* 55(13):3270.

379. Dixon, C.J. 2016. Achromatopsia in three sibling Labrador Retrievers in the UK. *Veterinary Ophthalmology.* 19(1):68–72.

380. Johnston, D., and Cox, B. 1970. The incidence in purebred dogs in Australia of abnormalities that may be inherited. *Australian Veterinary Journal.* 46(10):465–474.

381. Kraijer-Huver, I.M., Gubbels, E.J., Scholten, J., Djajadiningrat-Laanen, S.C., Boevé, M.H., and Stades F.C. 2008. Characterization and prevalence of cataracts in Labrador Retrievers in The Netherlands. *American Journal of Veterinary Research.* 69(10):1336–1340.

382. Tetas, R., Pettitt, L., Downs, L., Busse, C., Kafarnik, C., Dulaurent, T. et al. 2014. Mutation in the carbohydrate sulfotransferase-6 (chst6) gene causing macular corneal dystrophy in the dog. *Veterinary Ophthalmology*. 17(6):E16.

383. Barnett, K. 1965. Two forms of hereditary and progressive retinal atrophy in the dog. I. The Miniature Poodle. II. The Labrador Retriever. *Journal of the American Animal Hospital Association*. 1:234–245.

384. Kommonen, B., and Karhunen, U. 1990. A late receptor dystrophy in the Labrador Retriever. *Vision Research*. 30(2):207–213.

385. Kommonen, B., Kylmä, T., Karhunen, U., Dawson, W.W., and Penn, J.S. 1997. Impaired retinal function in young Labrador Retriever dogs heterozygous for late onset rod-cone degeneration. *Vision Research*. 37(3):365–370.

386. Barnett, K., Bjorck, G., and Kock, E. 1969. Hereditary retinal dysplasia in the Labrador Retriever in England and Sweden. *Journal of Small Animal Practice*. 10(12):755–759.

387. Kock, E. 1974. *Retinal dysplasia: A comparative study in human beings and dogs*. Stockholm.

388. Carrig, C., MacMillan, A., Brundage, S., Pool, R., and Morgan, J. 1977. Retinal dysplasia associated with skeletal abnormalities in Labrador Retrievers. *Journal of the American Veterinary Medical Association*. 170(1):49–57.

389. Carrig, C., Sponenberg, D., Schmidt, G., and Tvedten, H. 1988. Inheritance of associated ocular and skeletal dysplasia in Labrador Retrievers. *Journal of the American Veterinary Medical Association*. 193(10):1269–1272.

390. Carrig, C.B., Schmidt, G.M., and Tvedten, H.W. 1990. Growth of the radius and ulna in Labrador Retriever dogs with ocular and skeletal dysplasia. *Veterinary Radiology & Ultrasound*. 31(3):165–168.

391. Blair, N.P., Dodge, J.T., and Schmidt, G.M. 1985. Rhegmatogenous retinal detachment in Labrador retrievers: I. Development of retinal tears and detachment. *Archives of Ophthalmology*. 103(6):842–847.

392. Blair, N.P., Dodge, J.T., and Schmidt, G.M. 1985. Rhegmatogenous retinal detachment in Labrador retrievers: II. Proliferative vitreoretinopathy. *Archives of Ophthalmology*. 103(6):848–854.

393. Gionfriddo, J., Betts, D., and Niyo, Y. 1992. Retinal and skeletal dysplasia in a field trial Labrador Retriever puppy. *Canine Practice*.

394. Goldstein, O., Guyon, R., Kukekova, A., Kuznetsova, T.N., Pearce-Kelling, S.E., Johnson, J. et al. 2010. COL9A2 and COL9A3 mutations in canine autosomal recessive oculoskeletal dysplasia. *Mammalian Genome*. 21(7–8):398–408.

395. Bedford, P. 1998. Collie eye anomaly in the Lancashire Heeler. *The Veterinary Record*. 143(13):354–356.

396. Heinrich, C.L., Lakhani, K.H., Featherstone, H.J., and Barnett, K.C. 2006. Cataract in the UK Leonberger population. *Veterinary Ophthalmology*. 9(5):350–356.

397. Kijas, J., Miller, B., Pearce-Kelling, S., Aguirre, G., and Acland, G. 2003. Canine models of ocular disease: outcross breedings define a dominant disorder present in the English Mastiff and Bull Mastiff dog breeds. *Journal of Heredity*. 94(1):27–30.

398. ACVO Genetics Committee, editor Consensus agreed/supportive vote. The Blue Book: Ocular Disorders Presumed to be Inherited in Purebred Dogs. 2015, 8th edition.

399. Dekomien, G., and Epplen, J.T. 2003. Evaluation of the canine RPE65 gene in affected dogs with generalized progressive retinal atrophy. *Molecular Vision*. 9:601–605.

400. Stavinohova, R., Ricketts, S., Hartley, C., Pettitt, L., Tetas, R., Burmeister, L. et al., editors. 2017. Genetic investigation of oculoskeletal dysplasia in the Northern Inuit Dog. *European College of Veterinary Ophthalmologists Annual Scientific Meeting*; Estoril, Portugal, May 18–21, 2017.

401. Bjerkas, E., and Haaland, M. 1995. Pulverulent nuclear cataract in the Norwegian Buhund. *Journal of Small Animal Practice*. 36(11):471–474.

402. Schmidt, G. 1977. Diseases of the eyelids. In: Kirk, R.W., editor. *Current Veterinary Therapy VI (Small Animal Practice)*. WB Saunders: Philadelphia, PA, pp. 603–604.

403. Brooks, D.E. 1990. Glaucoma in the dog and cat. *The Veterinary Clinics of North America. Small Animal Practice*. 20(3):775–797.

404. Whitley, R., editor. 1987. Recent advances in glaucoma therapy. *World Small Animal Veterinary Association Congress*; Montreal, Canada.

405. Ekesten, B., Bjerkas, E., Kongsengen, K., and Narfstrom, K. 1997. Primary glaucoma in the Norwegian Elkhound. *Progress in Veterinary & Comparative Ophthalmology*.

406. Ahonen, S.J., Kaukonen, M., Nussdorfer, F.D., Harman, C.D., Komáromy, A.M., and Lohi, H. 2014. A novel missense mutation in ADAMTS10 in Norwegian Elkhound primary glaucoma. *PloS One*. 9(11):e111941.

407. Cogan, D.G., and Kuwabara, T. 1965. Photoreceptive abiotrophy of the retina in the Elkhound. *Pathologia Veterinaria*. 2(2):101–128.

408. Aguirre, G., and Rubin, L. 1971. Progressive retinal atrophy (rod dysplasia in the Norwegian Elkhound). *Journal of the American Veterinary Medical Association*. 158(2):208–218.

409. Aguirre, G.D., and Rubin, L.F. 1971. An electrophysiologic approach for early diagnosis of progressive retinal atrophy in the Norwegian Elkhound. *Journal of the American Animal Hospital Association*. 7:136.

410. Aguirre, G.D., and Rubin, L. 1971. The early diagnosis of rod dysplasia in the Norwegian Elkhound. *Journal of the American Veterinary Medical Association*. 159(4):429–433.

411. Acland, G., and Aguirre, G. 1987. Retinal degenerations in the dog: IV. Early retinal degeneration (erd) in Norwegian Elkhounds. *Experimental Eye Research*. 44(4):491–521.

412. Moghrabi, W.N., Kedzierski, W., and Travis, G.H. 1995. Canine homolog and exclusion of retinal degeneration slow (rds) as the gene for early retinal degeneration (erd) in the dog. *Experimental Eye Research*. 61(5):641–643.

413. Ray, K., Acland, G.M., and Aguirre, G.D. 1996. Nonallelism of erd and prcd and exclusion of the canine RDS/peripherin gene as a candidate for both retinal degeneration loci. *Investigative Ophthalmology & Visual Science*. 37(5):783–794.

414. Kukekova, A.V., Aguirre, G.D., and Acland, G.M. 2003. Cloning and characterization of canine SHARP1 and its evaluation as a positional candidate for canine early retinal degeneration (erd). *Oncogene*. 312:335–343.

415. Goldstein, O., Kukekova, A.V., Aguirre, G.D., and Acland, G.M. 2010. Exonic SINE insertion in STK38L causes canine early retinal degeneration (erd). *BMC Genomics*. 96(6):362–368.

416. Nova Scotia Duck Tolling Retriever Club of Canada. 1990. The Blue Book 8th edition: Ocular Disorders Presumed to be Inherited in Purebred Dogs 2015. In: Committee AG, editor.: ACVO.

417. Barrie, K., Peiffer, R., Gelatt, K., and Williams, L. 1979. Posterior lenticonus, microphthalmia, congenital cataracts, and retinal folds in an Old English Sheepdog. *Journal of the American Animal Hospital Association*.

418. Hakanson, N., and Narfstrom, K. 1995. Progressive retinal atrophy in Papillon dogs in Sweden: A clinical survey. *Progress in Veterinary & Comparative Ophthalmology.*

419. Narfström, K., and Ekesten, B. 1998. Electroretinographic evaluation of Papillons with and without hereditary retinal degeneration. *American Journal of Veterinary Research.* 59(2):221–226.

420. Petersen-Jones, S., Bartoe, J., and Winkler, P. 2011. Characterization of retinal dystrophies in papillons. *Veterinary Ophthalmology.* 14(4):280–281.

421. Ahonen, S.J., Arumilli, M., and Lohi, H. 2013. A CNGB1 frameshift mutation in Papillon and Phalene dogs with progressive retinal atrophy. *PloS One.* 8(8):e72122.

422. Winkler, P.A., Ekenstedt, K.J., Occelli, L.M., Frattaroli, A.V., Bartoe, J.T., Venta, P.J. et al. 2013. A large animal model for CNGB1 autosomal recessive retinitis pigmentosa. *PloS One.* 8(8):e72229.

423. Gelatt, K.N. 1973. Pediatric ophthalmology in small animal practice. *The Veterinary Clinics of North America.* 3(3):321.

424. Narfström, K., Wrigstad, A., Ekesten, B., and Berg, A.L. 2007. Neuronal ceroid lipofuscinosis: clinical and morphologic findings in nine affected Polish Owczarek Nizinny (PON) dogs. *Veterinary Ophthalmology.* 10(2):111–120.

425. Gelatt, K.N., and MacKay, E.O. 2004. Secondary glaucomas in the dog in North America. *Veterinary Ophthalmology.* 7(4):245–259.

426. Kern, T., and Riis, R. 1981. Optic nerve hypoplasia in three Miniature Poodles. *Journal of the American Veterinary Medical Association.* 178(1):49.

427. Vestre, W., and Brightman, A. 1980. Congenital blindness due to optic nerve hypoplasia [dogs]. *Canine Practice.*

428. Acland, G., Boughman, J., and Aguirre, G., editors. 1981. Inheritance of progressive rod-cone degeneration: A case of genetic selection. *Scientific Meeting of the American College of Veterinary Ophthalmology.*

429. Barnett, K. 1962. Hereditary retinal atrophy in the Poodle. *The Veterinary Record.* 74:672–675.

430. Aguirre, G., Alligood, J., O'Brien, P., and Buyukmihci, N. 1982. Pathogenesis of progressive rod-cone degeneration in Miniature Poodles. *Investigative Ophthalmology & Visual Science.* 23(5):610–630.

431. Aguirre, G., Acland, G., and Chader, G. 1981. Hereditary retinal degenerations in the dog: Specificity of abnormal cyclic nucleotide metabolism to diseases of arrested photoreceptor development. *Birth Defects Original Article Series.* 18(6):119–133.

432. Parkes, J., Aguirre, G., Rockey, J., and Liebman, P. 1982. Progressive rod-cone degeneration in the dog: Characterization of the visual pigment. *Investigative Ophthalmology & Visual Science.* 23(5):674–678.

433. Sandberg, M., Pawlyk, B., and Berson, E. 1986. Full-field electroretinograms in Miniature Poodles with progressive rod-cone degeneration. *Investigative Ophthalmology & Visual Science.* 27(7):1179–1184.

434. Aguirre, G., and O'Brien, P. 1986. Morphological and biochemical studies of canine progressive rod-cone degeneration. 3H-fucose autoradiography. *Investigative Ophthalmology & Visual Science.* 27(5):635–655.

435. Alvarez, R.A., Aguirre, G.D., Acland, G.M., and Anderson, R.E. 1994. Docosapentaenoic acid is converted to docosahexaenoic acid in the retinas of normal and prcd-affected miniature poodle dogs. *Investigative Ophthalmology & Visual Science.* 35(2):402–408.

436. Kemp, C., and Jacobson, S. 1992. Rhodopsin levels in the central retinas of normal Miniature Poodles and those with progressive rod-cone degeneration. *Experimental Eye Research.* 54(6):947–956.

437. Wetzel, M., Fahlman, C., Maude, M., Alvarez, R., O'Brien, P., Acland, G. et al. 1988. Fatty acid metabolism in normal Miniature Poodles and those affected with progressive rod-cone degeneration (prcd). *Progress in Clinical and Biological Research.* 314:427–439.

438. Gaiddon, J., Lallement, P., and Peiffer, R. 1995. Positive correlation between coat color and electroretinographically diagnosed progressive retinal atrophy in Miniature Poodles in southern France. *Progress in Veterinary & Comparative Ophthalmology.*

439. Rubin, L., and Flowers, R. 1972. Inherited cataract in a family of Standard Poodles. *Journal of the American Veterinary Medical Association.* 161(2):207.

440. Barnett, K., and Startup, F. 1985. Hereditary cataract in the Standard Poodle. *The Veterinary Record.* 117(1):15–16.

441. Pennsylvania SoVMUo. 2014. A new form of early-onset pra in Portuguese water dogs: ABSTRACT NO.: 65 *Veterinary Ophthalmology.* 17(6):E26.

442. Miyadera, K., and Aguirre, G. 2014. A new form of early-onset pra in Portuguese Water dogs. *Veterinary Ophthalmology.* 17(6):E26.

443. Labelle, A.L., Dresser, C.B., Hamor, R.E., Allender, M.C., and Disney, J.L. 2013. Characteristics of, prevalence of, and risk factors for corneal pigmentation (pigmentary keratopathy) in Pugs. *Journal of the American Veterinary Medical Association.* 243(5):667–674.

444. Rhodesian Ridgeback Breed Club. Breed Club Request to ACVO Genetics Committee, 2008. In: Committee AG, editor. The Blue Book 8th edition: Ocular Disorders Presumed to be Inherited in Purebred Dogs 20152008. p. 811–812.

445. Bjerkas, E., and Bergsjo, T. 1991. Hereditary cataract in the Rottweiler dog. *Progress in Veterinary & Comparative Ophthalmology.* 1:7–10.

446. Bjerkas, E. 1991. Progressive retinal atrophy in dogs in Norway. *Norsk Veterinaertidsskrift.* 103:601–610.

447. Gelatt, K. 1971. Bilateral corneal dermoids and distichiasis in a dog. *Veterinary Medicine, Small Animal Clinician.* 66(7):658–659.

448. Szczulowska, M. 1967. Dermoid cyst in the eye in relation to heredity and overfeeding. *Medical Veterinarian.* 23:567.

449. Martin, C., and Leipold, H. 1974. Aphakia and multiple ocular defects in Saint Bernard puppies. *Veterinary Medicine, Small Animal Clinician.* 69(4):448–453.

450. Ekesten, B., and Narfström, K. 1991. Correlation of morphologic features of the iridocorneal angle to intraocular pressure in Samoyeds. *American Journal of Veterinary Research.* 52(11):1875–1878.

451. Ekesten, B., and Narfstrom, K. 1992. Age-related changes in intraocular pressure and iridocorneal angle in Samoyeds. *Progress in Veterinary & Comparative Ophthalmology.* 2:37–40.

452. Ekesten, B. 1993. Correlations of intraocular distances to the iridocorneal angle in Samoyeds with special reference to angle-closure glaucoma. *Progress in Veterinary & Comparative Ophthalmology.* 3:67–73.

453. Ekesten, B., and Torrång, I. 1995. Heritability of the depth of the opening of the ciliary cleft in Samoyeds. *American Journal of Veterinary Research.* 56(9):1138–1143.

454. Ekesten, B. 1993. Biological variability and measurement error variability in ocular biometry in Samoyed dogs. *Acta Veterinaria Scandinavica.* 35(4):427–433.

455. Dice, P. 1980. Progressive retinal atrophy in the Samoyed. *Modern Veterinary Practice.* 61(1):59–60.

456. Zhang, Q., Acland, G.M., Wu, W.X., Johnson, J.L., Pearce-Kelling, S., Tulloch, B. et al. 2002. Different RPGR exon ORF15 mutations in Canids provide insights into photoreceptor cell degeneration. *Human Molecular Genetics.* 11(9):993–1003.

457. Meyers, V., Aguirre, G., and Patterson, D. 1983. Short-limbed dwarfism and ocular defects in the Samoyed dog. *Journal of the American Veterinary Medical Association.* 183(9):975–979.

458. Halliwell, R. 1982. Autoimmune diseases in domestic animals. *Journal of the American Veterinary Medical Association.* 181(10):1088.

459. Dekomien, G., Vollrath, C., Petrasch-Parwez, E., Boevé, M.H., Akkad, D.A., Gerding, W.M. et al. 2010. Progressive retinal atrophy in Schapendoes dogs: Mutation of the newly identified CCDC66 gene. *Journal of Neurogenetics.* 11(2):163–174.

460. Lippmann, T., Jonkisz, A., Dobosz, T., Petrasch-Parwez, E., Epplen, J.T., and Dekomien, G. 2007. Haplotype-defined linkage region for gPRA in Schapendoes dogs. *Molecular Vision.* 13:174–180.

461. Gelatt, K., Samuelson, D., Bauer, J., Das, N., Wolf, E., Barrie, K. et al. 1983. Inheritance of congenital cataracts and microphthalmia in the Miniature Schnauzer. *American Journal of Veterinary Research.* 44(6):1130–1132.

462. Shastry, B.S., and Reddy, V. 1994. Studies on congenital hereditary cataract and microphthalmia of the Miniature Schnauzer dog. *Biochemical and Biophysical Research Communications.* 203(3):1663–1667.

463. Samuelson, D., Noveen, D., Bauer, J., Joyce, J., and Gelatt, K. 1987. Prenatal morphogenesis of the congenital cataracts in the Miniature Schnauzer. *Lens Resolution.* 4(4):231–250.

464. Barnett, K. 1985. Hereditary cataract in the Miniature Schnauzer. *Journal of Small Animal Practice.* 26(11):635–644.

465. Monaco, M., Samuelson, D., and Gelatt, K. 1984. Morphology and postnatal development of the normal lens in the dog and congenital cataract in the Miniature Schnauzer. *Lens Resolution.* 2(4):393–433.

466. Smith, R., Sutton, R., Jolly, R., and Smith, K. 1996. A retinal degeneration associated with ceroid-lipofuscinosis in adult Miniature Schnauzers. *Progress in Veterinary & Comparative Ophthalmology.*

467. Aguirre, G., Parshall, C., Acland, G., Notarfrancesco, K., Nitroy, S., and Chader, G., editors. 1985. Progressive retinal atrophy in the Miniature Schnauzer. *Proceedings of the American College of Veterinary Ophthalmologists.*

468. Parshall, C.J., Wyman, M., Nitroy, S., Acland, G.M., and Aguirre, G.D. 1991. Photoreceptor dysplasia: an inherited progressive retinal atrophy of Miniature Schnauzer dogs. *Progress in Veterinary & Comparative Ophthalmology.* 1(3):187.

469. Grahn, B.H., Storey, E.S., and McMillan, C. 2004. Inherited retinal dysplasia and persistent hyperplastic primary vitreous in Miniature Schnauzer dogs. *Veterinary Ophthalmology.* 7(3):151–158.

470. Mason, S.L., McElroy, P., and Nuttall, T. 2012. Ligneous membranitis in Scottish Terriers. *The Veterinary Record.* 171(6):160.

471. Formston, C. 1945. Observations on subluxation and luxation of the crystalline lens in the dog. *Journal of Comparative Pathology and Therapeutics.* 55:168IN7–84IN8.

472. Ashton, N., Barnett, K., and Sachs, D. 1968. Retinal dysplasia in the Sealyham Terrier. *American Journal of Pathology.* 96(2):269–272.

473. Lenarduzzi, R. 1983. Management of eyelid problems in Chinese Shar-Pei puppies. *Veterinary Medicine.* 78(4):548–550.

474. Bedford, P. 1984. Entropion in Shar Peis. *The Veterinary Record.* 115(25–26) p. 666.

475. Startup, F. 1985. Entropion in the Shar Pei. *The Veterinary Record.* p. 57.

476. Barnett, K. 1988. Inherited eye disease in the dog and cat. *Journal of Small Animal Practice.* 29(7):462–475.

477. Lazarus, J., Pickett, J., and Champagne, E. 1998. Primary lens luxation in the Chinese Shar Pei: Clinical and hereditary characteristics. *Veterinary Ophthalmology.* 1(2–3):101–107.

478. Wiik, A., Ropstad, E., Ekesten, B., Karlstam, L., Wade, C., and Lingaas, F. 2015. Progressive retinal atrophy in Shetland Sheepdog is associated with a mutation in the CNGA1 gene. *Animal Genetics.* 46(5):515–521.

479. Karlstam, L., Hertil, E., Zeiss, C., Ropstad, E.O., Bjerkås, E., Dubielzig, R.R. et al. 2011. A slowly progressive retinopathy in the Shetland Sheepdog. *Veterinary Ophthalmology.* 14(4):227–238.

480. Kanemaki, N., Tchedre, K.T., Imayasu, M., Kawarai, S., Sakaguchi, M., Yoshino, A. et al. 2013. Dogs and humans share a common susceptibility gene SRBD1 for glaucoma risk. *PloS One.* 8(9):e74372.

481. Kato, K., Sasaki, N., Matsunaga, S., Mochizuki, M., Nishimura, R., and Ogawa, H. 2006. Possible association of glaucoma with pectinate ligament dysplasia and narrowing of the iridocorneal angle in Shiba Inu dogs in Japan. *Veterinary Ophthalmology.* 9(2):71–75.

482. Garcia da Silva, E., Dubielzig, R., Zarfoss, M.K., and Anibal, A. 2008. Distinctive histopathologic features of canine optic nerve hypoplasia and aplasia: A retrospective review of 13 cases. *Veterinary Ophthalmology.* 11(1):23–29.

483. Itoh, Y., Maehara, S., Yamasaki, A., Tsuzuki, K., and Izumisawa, Y. 2010. Investigation of fellow eye of unilateral retinal detachment in Shih-Tzu. *Veterinary Ophthalmology.* 13(5):289–293.

484. Hendrix, D., Nasisse, M., Cowen, P., and Davidson, M. 1993. Clinical signs, concurrent diseases, and risk factors associated with retinal detachment in dogs. *Progress in Veterinary & Comparative Ophthalmology.* 3(3):87–91.

485. Stanley, R., and Blogg, J. 1991. Eye diseases in Siberian Husky dogs. *Australian Veterinary Journal.* 68(5):161–162.

486. Waring III, G., MacMillan, A., and Reveles, P. 1986. Inheritance of crystalline corneal dystrophy in Siberian Huskies. *Journal of the American Animal Hospital Association.*

487. MacMillan, A., Waring III, G., Spangler, W., and Roth, A. 1979. Crystalline corneal opacities in the Siberian Husky. *Journal of the American Veterinary Medical Association.* 175(8):829–832.

488. Ori, J.-I., Yoshikai, T., Yoshimura, S., and Takenaka, S. 1998. Persistent hyperplastic primary vitreous (PHPV) in two Siberian Husky dogs. *Journal of Veterinary Medical Science.* 60(2):263–265.

489. Acland, G.M., Blanton, S.H., Hershfield, B., and Aguirre, G.D. 1994. XLPRA: A canine retinal degeneration inherited as an X-linked trait. *American Journal of Medical Genetics.* 52(1):27–33.

490. Dekomien, G., Runte, M., Goedde, R., and Epplen, J.T. 2000. Generalized progressive retinal atrophy of Sloughi

dogs is due to an 8-bp insertion in exon 21 of the PDE6B gene. *Cytogenetic and Genome Research.* 90(3–4):261–267.

491. Van der Woerdt, A., Stades, F., Van der Linde-Sipman, J., and Boeve, M. 1995. Multiple ocular anomalies in two related litters of Soft Coated Wheaten Terriers. *Progress in Veterinary & Comparative Ophthalmology.*

492. Cooper, A.E., Ahonen, S., Rowlan, J.S., Duncan, A., Seppälä, E.H., Vanhapelto, P. et al. 2014. A novel form of progressive retinal atrophy in Swedish Vallhund dogs. *PloS One.* 9(9):e106610.

493. Ahonen, S.J., Arumilli, M., Seppälä, E., Hakosalo, O., Kaukonen, M.K., Komáromy, A.M. et al. 2014. Increased expression of MERTK is associated with a unique form of canine retinopathy. *PloS One.* 9(12):e114552.

494. Katz, M.L., Narfström, K., Johnson, G.S., and O'Brien, D.P. 2005. Assessment of retinal function and characterization of lysosomal storage body accumulation in the retinas and brains of Tibetan Terriers with ceroid-lipofuscinosis. *American Journal of Veterinary Research.* 66(1):67–76.

495. Downs, L.M., and Mellersh, C.S. 2014. An Intronic SINE insertion in FAM161A that causes exon-skipping is associated with progressive retinal atrophy in Tibetan Spaniels and Tibetan Terriers. *PloS One.* 9(4):e93990.

496. Drögemüller, C., Wöhlke, A., and Distl, O. 2005. Characterization of candidate genes for neuronal ceroid lipofuscinosis in dog. *Journal of Heredity.* 96(7):735–738.

497. Loew, E., and Riis, R. 1983. Congenital nyctalopia in the Tibetan Terrier. *Transactions of the 14th Annual Scientific Program of the American College of Veterinary Ophthalmologists,* Chicago, pp. 83–97.

498. Millichamp, N.J., Curtis, R., and Barnett, K.C. 1988. Progressive retinal atrophy in Tibetan Terriers. *Journal of the American Veterinary Medical Association.* 192(6):769–776.

499. Barnett, K. 1980. Hereditary cataract in the Welsh Springer Spaniel. *Journal of Small Animal Practice.* **21**(11):621–625.

500. Oliver, J., Pettitt, L., and Mellersh, C. 2014. Goniodysgenesis and glaucoma in the Welsh Springer Spaniel: a candidate gene study. *Veterinary Ophthalmology.* 17(6):E31–E2.

501. Narfström, K. 1981. Cataract in the West Highland white Terrier. *Journal of Small Animal Practice.* 22(7):467–471.

502. Baker, G.J., and Formston, C. 1968. An evaluation of transplantation of the parotid duct in the treatment of kerato-conjunctivitis sicca in the dog. *Journal of Small Animal Practice.* 9(6):261–268.

503. Somma, A.T., Moreno, J.C.D., Sato, M.T., Rodrigues, B.D., Bacellar-Galdino, M., Occelli, L.M. et al. 2016. Characterization of a novel form of progressive retinal atrophy in Whippet dogs: a clinical, electroretinographic, and breeding study. *Veterinary Ophthalmology.* 20(5):450–459.

504. Walde, I. 1997. Retinal and corneal dysplasias in the Yorkshire Terrier and other dog breeds in Austria. *Tierarztliche Praxis.* 25(1):62–67.

505. Herrera, H.D., Weichsler, N., Gómez, J.R., Jalón, D., and García, J.A. 2007. Severe, unilateral, unresponsive keratoconjunctivitis sicca in 16 juvenile Yorkshire Terriers. *Veterinary Ophthalmology.* 10(5):285–288.

506. Torres, M.D., Leiva, M., Tabar, M.D., Naranjo, C., Pastor, J., and Peña, T. 2009. Ligneous conjunctivitis in a plasminogen-deficient dog: Clinical management and 2-year follow-up. *Veterinary Ophthalmology.* 12(4):248–253.

507. Stades, F. 1978. Hereditary retinal dysplasia (RD) in a family of Yorkshire Terriers. *Tijdschrift voor Diergeneeskunde.* 103(20):1087.

508. Narfström, K. 1985. Progressive retinal atrophy in the Abyssinian cat. Clinical characteristics. *Investigative Ophthalmology & Visual Science.* 26(2):193–200.

509. Seeliger, M.W., and Narfström, K. 2000. Functional assessment of the regional distribution of disease in a cat model of hereditary retinal degeneration. *Investigative Ophthalmology & Visual Science.* 41(7):1998–2005.

510. Narfström, K. 1999. Hereditary and congenital ocular disease in the cat. *Journal of Feline Medicine and Surgery.* 1(3):135–141.

511. Startup, F. 1988. Corneal necrosis and sequestration in the cat: A review and record of 100 cases. *Journal of Small Animal Practice.* 29(7):476–486.

512. Hendy-Ibbs, P. 1985. Familial feline epibulbar dermoids. *The Veterinary Record.* 116(1):13–14.

513. Koch, S. 1979. Congenital ophthalmic abnormalities in the Burmese cat. *Journal of the American Veterinary Medical Association.* 174(1):90–91.

514. Jacobi, S., and Dubielzig, R.R. 2008. Feline primary open angle glaucoma. *Veterinary Ophthalmology.* 11(3):162–165.

515. Hampson, E., Smith, R., and Bernays, M. 2002. Primary glaucoma in Burmese cats. *Australian Veterinary Journal.* 80(11):672–680.

516. Blacklock, B.T., Grundon, R.A., Meehan, M., Tetas Pont, R., and Hartley, C. 2016. Uveal cysts in domestic cats: A retrospective evaluation of thirty-six cases. *Veterinary Ophthalmology.*

517. Rubin, L. 1986. Hereditary cataract in Himalayan cats. *Feline Practice.* 16(1):14–15.

518. Bistner, S.I., Aguirre, G., and Shively, J.N. 1976. Hereditary corneal dystrophy in the Manx cat: A preliminary report. *Investigative Ophthalmology & Visual Science.* 15(1):15–26.

519. Collier, L., Bryan, G., and Prieur, D. 1979. Ocular manifestations of the Chediak–Higashi syndrome in four species of animals. *Journal of the American Veterinary Medical Association.* 175(6):587–590.

520. Bellhorn, R., Barnett, K., and Henkind, P. 1971. Ocular colobomas in domestic cats. *Journal of the American Veterinary Medical Association.*

521. Walde, I., and Rapp, E. 1993. Feline glaucoma. Clinical and morphological aspects (a retrospective study of 38 cases). *European Journal of Companion Animal Practice.* 4:87–105.

522. Lyons, L.A., Creighton, E.K., Alhaddad, H., Beale, H.C., Grahn, R.A., Rah, H. et al. 2016. Whole genome sequencing in cats, identifies new models for blindness in AIPL1 and somite segmentation in HES7. *BMC Genomics.* 17(1):265.

523. Rah, H., Maggs, D.J., Blankenship, T.N., Narfstrom, K., and Lyons, L.A. 2005. Early-onset, autosomal recessive, progressive retinal atrophy in Persian cats. *Investigative Ophthalmology & Visual Science.* 46(5):1742–1747.

524. Dubielzig, R.R., Hoffman, A., Ehrhart, E., and Zarfoss, M. 2011. A spontaneous neovascular proliferative vitreoretinopathy in cats with features similar to retinopathy of prematurity. *Investigative Ophthalmology & Visual Science.* 52(14):3154.

525. Olivero, D., Riis, R., Dutton, A., Murphy, C., Nasisse, M., and Davidson, M. 1991. Feline lens displacement: A retrospective analysis of 345 cases. *Progress in Veterinary & Comparative Ophthalmology.* 1(4):239–244.

526. McLellan, G., Betts, D., Sigle, K., and Grozdanic, S. 2005. Congenital glaucoma in the Siamese Cat–A novel spontaneous animal model for glaucoma research. *Investigative Ophthalmology & Visual Science.* 46(13):134.

527. Narfström, K., Menotti Raymond, M., and Seeliger, M. 2011. Characterization of feline hereditary retinal dystrophies using clinical, functional, structural and molecular genetic studies. *Veterinary Ophthalmology.* 14(S1):30–36.

528. Brooks, D. 1999. Equine ophthalmology. In: Gelatt, K.N., editor. *Veterinary Ophthalmology.* 3rd edition. Lippincott Williams & Wilkins: Philadelphia, PA, pp. 1053–116.

529. Whitley, R., Meek, L.A., Millichamp, N., McRae, E.E., and Priehs, D. 1990. Cataract surgery in the horse: A review of six cases. *Equine Veterinary Journal.* 22(S10):85–90.

530. McLaughlin, S., Whitley, R., and Gilger, B. 1992. Diagnosis and treatment of lens diseases. *The Veterinary Clinics of North America. Equine Practice.* 8(3):575–585.

531. Gelatt, K., and McClure, J. 1979. Congenital strabismus and its correction in 2 Appaloosa horses. *Journal of Equine Veterinary Science.* 3(5):240–244.

532. Rebhun, W., Loew, E., Riis, R., and Laratta, L. 1984. Clinical manifestations of night blindness in the Appaloosa horse. *Compendium on Continuing Education for the Practising Veterinarian.*

533. Eriksson, K. 1955. Hereditary aniridia with secondary cataract in horses. *Nordisk Veterinaermedicin.* 7:773–779.

534. Joyce, J. 1983. Aniridia in Quarter horses. *Equine Veterinary Journal.* (Supplement 2:21–22.

535. Ségard, E.M., Depecker, M.C., Lang, J., Gemperli, A., and Cadoré, J.L. 2013. Ultrasonographic features of PMEL17 (Silver) mutant gene–associated multiple congenital ocular anomalies (MCOA) in Comtois and Rocky Mountain horses. *Veterinary Ophthalmology.* 16(6):429–435.

536. Lassaline-Utter, M., Gemensky-Metzler, A.J., Scherrer, N.M., Stoppini, R., Latimer, C.A., MacLaren, N.E. et al. 2014. Corneal dystrophy in Friesian horses may represent a variant of pellucid marginal degeneration. *Veterinary Ophthalmology.* 17(S1):186–194.

537. Andersson, L.S., Axelsson, J., Dubielzig, R.R., Lindgren, G., and Ekesten, B. 2011. Multiple congenital ocular anomalies in Icelandic horses. *BMC Veterinary Research.* 7(1):21.

538. Grahn, B.H., Pinard, C., Archer, S., Bellone, R., Forsyth, G., and Sandmeyer, L.S. 2008. Congenital ocular anomalies in purebred and crossbred Rocky and Kentucky Mountain horses in Canada. *The Canadian Veterinary Journal.* 49(7):675.

539. Ramsey, D.T., Ewart, S.L., Render, J.A., Cook, C.S., and Latimer, C.A. 1999. Congenital ocular abnormalities of Rocky Mountain horses. *Veterinary Ophthalmology.* 2(1):47–59.

540. Plummer, C.E., and Ramsey, D.T. 2011. A survey of ocular abnormalities in miniature horses. *Veterinary Ophthalmology.* 14(4):239–243.

541. Beech, J., Aguirre, G., and Gross, S. 1984. Congenital nuclear cataracts in the Morgan horse. *Journal of the American Veterinary Medical Association.* 184(11):1363–1365.

542. Rebhun, W. 1992. Retinal and optic nerve diseases. *The Veterinary Clinics of North America. Equine Practice.* 8(3):587–608.

543. Barnett, K. 1975. The eye of the newborn foal. *Journal of Reproduction and Fertility Supplement.* (23):701–703.

544. Rubin, L.F. 1974. *Atlas of Veterinary Ophthalmoscopy.* Lea & Febiger, Philadelphia.

545. Finno, C.J., Kaese, H.J., Miller, A.D., Gianino, G., Divers, T., and Valberg, S.J. 2016. Pigment retinopathy in warmblood horses with equine degenerative myeloencephalopathy and equine motor neuron disease. *Veterinary Ophthalmology.* 20(4):304–309.

546. Michot, P., Chahory, S., Marete, A., Grohs, C., Dagios, D., Donzel, E. et al. 2016. A reverse genetic approach identifies an ancestral frameshift mutation in RP1 causing recessive progressive retinal degeneration in European cattle breeds. *Genetics, Selection, Evolution.* 48(1):56.

547. Huston, K., Leipold, H., and Freeman, A. 1968. Heterochromia irides in dairy cattle. *Finnish Journal of Dairy Science.* 51(7):1101–1102.

548. Regan, W., Gregory, P., and Mead, S. 1944. Hereditary strabismus in Jersey cattle. *Journal of Heredity.* 35(8):233–234.

549. Willoughby, R., and Gibbons, W.E. 1970. The eye and its adnexa. *Bovine Medicine and Surgery.*

550. Rebhun, W. 1979. Diseases of the bovine orbit and globe. *Journal of the American Veterinary Medical Association.* 175(2):171.

551. Heider, L., Wyman, M., Burt, J., Root, C., and Gardner, H. 1975. Nasolacrimal duct anomaly in calves. *Journal of the American Veterinary Medical Association.* 167(2):145.

552. Barnett, K., and Ogien, A. 1972. Ocular colobomata in Charolais cattle. *The Veterinary Record.* 91(24):592.

553. McCormack, J., Powers, R., and Albert, R. 1975. Typical colobomas in Charolais cattle [congenital defects]. *Veterinary Medicine, Small Animal Clinician.*

554. Gelatt, K., Huston, K., and Leipold, H. 1969. Ocular anomalies of incomplete albino cattle: Ophthalmoscopic examination. *American Journal of Veterinary Research.* 30(8):1313.

555. Gelatt, K.N. 1971. Cataracts in cattle. *Journal of the American Veterinary Medical Association.* 159(2):195–200.

556. Barkyoumb, S.D., and Leipold, H. 1984. Nature and cause of bilateral ocular dermoids in Hereford cattle. *Veterinary Pathology.* 21(3):316–324.

557. Grahn, B., Leis, M., Bauer, B., Sandmeyer, L., Buchanan, F., Schumann, F., and Petrie, L., editors. 2016. Congenital lenticular anomalies in a purebred Holstein dairy herd. *Annual Scientific Meeting of the European College of Veterinary Ophthalmologists*; 2016. Veterinary Ophthalmology: Budapest, Hungary.

558. Willoughby, R.A. 1968. Congenital eye defects in cattle. *Modern Veterinary Practice.* (49):36–40.

559. Saunders, L., and Fincher, M. 1951. Hereditary multiple eye defects in grade Jersey calves. *The Cornell Veterinarian.* 41(4):351.

560. Leipold, H. 1971. Multiple ocular anomalies and hydrocephalus in grade beef short-horn cattle. *American Journal of Veterinary Research.* 32:1019–1026.

561. Greene, H., and Leipold, H. 1974. Hereditary internal hydrocephalus and retinal dysplasia in Shorthorn calves. *The Cornell Veterinarian.* 64(3):367.

562. Miller, T., and Gelatt, K. 1991. Food animal ophthalmology. In: Gelatt, K.N., editor. *Veterinary Ophthalmology,* pp. 642–643.

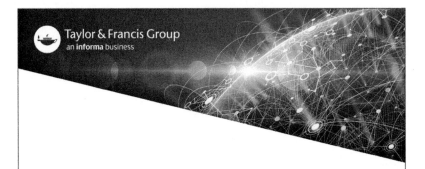